T0296666

GRAINGER & ALLISON'S DIAGNOSTIC RADIOLOGY

SIXTH EDITION

The Chest and Cardiovascular System

GRAINGER & ALLISON'S DIAGNOSTIC RADIOLOGY

SIXTH EDITION

The Chest and Cardiovascular System

EDITED BY

Cornelia M. Schaefer-Prokop, MD, PhD

Adrian K. Dixon, MD, MD(Hon caus), FRCP, FRCR, FRCS, FFRRCSI(Hon), FRANZCR(Hon), FACR(Hon), FMedSci

ELSEVIER

London New York Oxford Philadelphia St Louis Sydney Toronto

ELSEVIER

ISBN: 978-0-7020-6940-6

Executive Content Strategist: Michael Houston
Content Development Specialist: Louise Cook
Project Manager: Andrew Riley
Design: Christian Bilbow
Marketing Manager: Rachael Pignotti

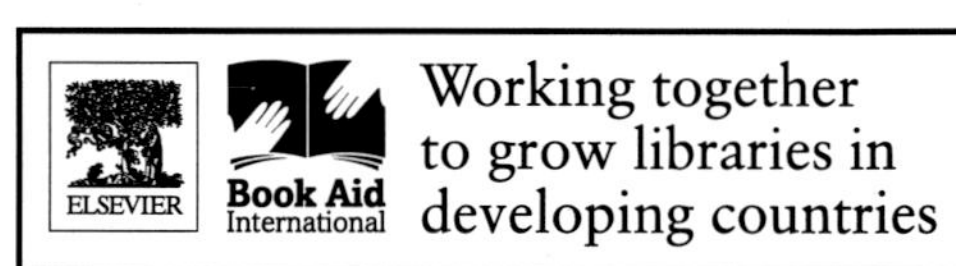

Contents

Preface

The 17 chapters in this book have been selected from the contents of the Chest and Cardiovascular System section in *Grainger & Allison's Diagnostic Radiology, Sixth Edition*. These chapters provide a succinct up-to-date overview of current imaging techniques and their clinical applications in daily practice and it is hoped that with this concise format the user will quickly grasp the fundamentals they need to know. Throughout these chapters, the relative merits of different imaging investigations are described, variations are discussed and recent imaging advances are detailed.

Grainger & Allison's Diagnostic Radiology has long been recognized as the standard general reference work in the field, and it is hoped that this book, utilizing the content from the latest sixth edition of this classic reference work, will provide radiology trainees and practitioners with ready access to the most current information, written by internationally recognized experts, on what is new and important in the radiological diagnosis of chest and cardiovascular disorders.

List of Contributors

Zelena A. Aziz, MRCP, FRCR, MD
Consultant Chest Radiologist, London Chest Hospital, Barts Health NHS Trust, London, UK

Catherine Beigelman-Aubry, MD
Priva Docent-Maitre d'enseignement et recherche, Radiodiagnostic and Interventional Radiology, Centre Hospitalier Universitaire Vaudois, Lausanne, Switzerland

Sanjeev Bhalla, MD
Chief, Cardiothoracic Radiology, Mallinckrodt Institute of Radiology, Washington University in St Louis, St Louis, MO, USA

Jan Bogaert, MD, PhD
Professor of Medicine, Department of Radiology, University Hospital Gasthuisberg, University of Leuven, Leuven, Belgium

Susan J. Copley, MBBS, MD, FRCR, FRCP
Consultant Radiologist and Reader in Thoracic Imaging, Hammersmith Hospital, Imperial College NHS Trust, London, UK

Albert de Roos, MD
Professor of Radiology, Department of Radiology, Leiden University Medical Center, Leiden, The Netherlands

Sujal R. Desai, MD, MRCP, FRCR
Consultant Radiologist, King's College Hospital, London, UK

Christoph Engelke, MD
Geschäftsführender Oberarzt, Abteilung Diagnostische Radiologie, Universitätsmedizin Göttingen, Germany

Rossella Fattori, MD
Professor of Radiology; Director, Invasive Cardiology, Emergency Department, San Salvatore Hospital, Pesaro, Italy

Tomás Franquet, MD
Chief Section of Thoracic Imaging, Department of Radiology, Hospital de Sant Pau; Associate Professor of Radiology, Universitat Autonoma de Barcelona, Barcelona, Spain

Fergus Gleeson, MD
Radiologist, Department of Radiology, Churchill Hospital, Oxford, UK

Philippe A. Grenier, MD
Professor, Radiology, Hôpital Pitié-Salpêtrière, Paris, France

David M. Hansell, MD, FRCP, FRCR, FRSM
Professor of Thoracic Imaging, Radiology, Royal Brompton Hospital, London, UK

Ieneke J.C. Hartmann, MD, PhD
Radiologist, Radiology, Maasstad Hospital, Rotterdam, The Netherlands

Cylen Javidan-Nejad, MD
Associate Professor of Cardiothoracic Radiology, Mallinckrodt Institute of Radiology, Washington University in St Louis, St Louis, MO, USA

Hefin Jones, MRCP, FRCR
Radiologist, Department of Clinical Radiology, University Hospital Birmingham, New Queen Elizabeth Hospital, Birmingham, UK

Lucia J.M. Kroft, MD, PhD
Radiologist, Department of Radiology, Leiden University Medical Center, Leiden, The Netherlands

Olga Lazoura, MD, PhD
Consultant Radiologist, Royal Free Hospital, London, UK

Luigi Lovato, MD
Radiologist, Cardiovascular Radiology Unit, Cardiothoracic Radiology, Cardiovascular-Thoracic Department, S. Orsola Hospital, Bologna, Italy

Katharina Marten-Engelke, MD
Professor of Radiology, Diagnostic Breast Centre, Göttingen, Germany

Agostino Meduri, MD
Adjunct Professor, Bioimaging and Radiological Sciences, Catholic University of the Sacred Heart, Rome, Italy

Arjun Nair, MB ChB, MRCP, FRCR
Fellow in Thoracic Imaging, Department of Radiology, Royal Brompton Hospital, London, UK

Luigi Natale, MD
Researcher and Aggregate Professor of Radiology, Radiological Sciences Department, Catholic University of Sacred Heart, Rome, Italy

Simon P.G. Padley, MBBS, BSc, MRCP, FRCR
Consultant Radiologist, Chelsea and Westminster Hospital and Royal Brompton Hospital; Reader in Radiology, Imperial College School of Medicine, London, UK

Nadeem Parkar, MD
Fellow in Cardiothoracic Imaging, Mallinckrodt Institute of Radiology, Washington University in St Louis, St Louis, MO, USA

Michael A. Quail, MSc, MB ChB(Hons), MRCPCH
British Heart Foundation Clinical Research Training Fellow, Centre for Cardiovascular Imaging, UCL Institute of Cardiovascular Science; Paediatric Cardiology Academic Clinical Fellow, Department of Cardiology, Great Ormond Street Hospital, London, UK

John H. Reynolds, MMedSci, FRCR, DMRD
Consultant Radiologist, Department of Radiology, Birmingham Heartlands Hospital, Birmingham, UK

Cornelia M. Schaefer-Prokop, MD, PhD
Professor of Radiology, Meander Medical Centre, Amersfoort, The Netherlands

Hans-Marc J. Siebelink, MD, PhD
Non-Invasive Imaging, Department of Cardiology, Leiden University Medical Center, Leiden, The Netherlands

Nicola Sverzellati, PhD
Researcher, Department of Surgical Sciences, Radiology Section, University of Parma, Parma, Italy

Andrew M. Taylor, BA(Hons), BM BCh, MRCP, FRCR
Professor of Cardiovascular Imaging, Centre for Cardiovascular Imaging, UCL Institute of Cardiovascular Science and Great Ormond Street Hospital for Children, London, UK

Johny A. Verschakelen, MD, PhD
Director, Chest Radiology, Department of Radiology, University Hospitals Leuven, Leuven, Belgium

Jos J.M. Westenberg, PhD
Assistant Professor, Department of Radiology, Leiden University Medical Center, Leiden, The Netherlands

CHAPTER 1

Techniques in Thoracic Imaging

Arjun Nair • Zelena A. Aziz • David M. Hansell

CHAPTER OUTLINE

Chest radiography and computed tomography (CT) remain the imaging tests of choice for the evaluation of respiratory disease. The basic technique of chest radiography has changed little over the past century, but continuing developments in image receptor technology have resulted in the more efficient acquisition of chest radiographs with the benefit of a lower radiation dose. Radiographs are now mainly produced in digital format, thus facilitating their incorporation into picture archiving and communications systems (PACS). Evolving CT technology has meant that multidetector row CT (MDCT) systems have largely replaced single-detector CT. Newer dual-energy CT (DECT) systems may provide new applications, although these have not yet been fully validated. These developments have resulted in larger volume CT data sets increasingly becoming the norm. Protocols for MDCT continue to be developed and refined to ensure the correct balance is struck between the imperatives of obtaining adequate information and dose minimisation. Ultrasound and magnetic resonance imaging (MRI) may have specific but limited roles in the investigation of thoracic disease. Positron emission tomography (PET) fused with CT (PET-CT) now has an established role in the investigation of neoplastic disease, enabling the simultaneous assessment of metabolic function, anatomical location and unsuspected extrathoracic metastatic disease.

CHEST RADIOGRAPHY

Equipment Considerations

Chest radiography remains the commonest diagnostic radiographic procedure. Chest radiographs were traditionally acquired with conventional film-screen radiography systems that provide, at low cost, good image quality and high spatial resolution.[1,2] However, film-screen radiography is limited by a relatively narrow exposure range and consequent high retake rate, as well as inflexibility in image display and manipulation.[1] The exponential advances in computational power, storage capacity and detector technology have led to the replacement of film-screen radiography by PACS and digital imaging systems in most modern imaging departments.

Early digital imaging systems introduced over 30 years ago (generally termed 'computed radiography' (CR)) used a photostimulable phosphor image receptor plate,[3] and continue to be used in some departments because of their compatibility with conventional radiography equipment. However, CR systems have largely been superseded by direct radiography (DR) systems (Table 1-1). DR systems employ either direct or indirect methods for converting X-ray photons into electrical charges, thereby generating an electrical signal that can be read directly.[4] Direct conversion may be achieved by photoconductors within flat-panel detectors (most commonly amorphous selenium), or using a selenium drum. Indirect conversion involves the use of a scintillator associated with either a charge-couple device (CCD) or flat-panel detector (FPD). Scintillators most commonly use thallium-doped caesium iodide-based, or more recently gadolinium-based compounds.

Both CR and DR systems offer many advantages over conventional film-screen radiography. Chief among these is the wide dynamic range or latitude of the image plate; consequently, exposure errors are reduced and the need for repeat examinations is lessened. Also, both CR and DR systems employ reusable detectors, manual optimisation of the display features desired for the anatomical part selected can be performed immediately and there is more efficient image archiving, retrieval and transmission when integrated into PACS. While there are conflicting reports with respect to dose and image quality for CR imaging of the thorax as compared with conventional radiography,[1,5,6] DR systems undoubtedly offer superior image quality compared with both CR and film-screen combinations, with the added advantages of rapid image display and generally higher detector quantum efficiency. The latter efficiency allows a significant reduction in exposure, and consequently in effective dose.[7] Among DR systems, indirect conversion FPDs provide the highest image quality.

TABLE 1-1 **Methods of Computed Radiography and Direct Radiography**

	Computed Radiography (CR)	Direct Radiography (DR)	
X-Ray Conversion Method	Indirect conversion	Indirect conversion	Direct conversion
Devices	Removable image plates using storage phosphors (analogous to conventional film cassettes)	Scintillator-thin-film transistor array	Selenium drum
		Scintillator-charge-coupled device	Photoconductor flat-panel detector
Image Readout	Separate readout process: detector layer must be analysed by laser (point scan or line-scan); resulting output is converted into electrical signal	Direct readout process: X-rays are converted immediately into electrical signal and read	

Additional Radiographic Views

Frontal and lateral projections of the chest are adequate for most purposes. Other radiographic views are increasingly less frequently performed because of the ready availability of cross-sectional imaging. One projection that is still occasionally used is the lateral decubitus view, taken as a frontal projection with a horizontal beam and the patient lying on his/her side. It may be used to identify an effusion that is not visible on an erect chest radiograph, to demonstrate the movement of fluid in the pleural space or to localise or confirm an equivocal opacity seen on a frontal projection, especially when CT is unavailable.

Portable supine lateral shoot-through radiographs can be valuable in identifying suspected pneumothorax in critically ill patients unsafe for CT.[8] Less commonly, expiratory radiographs may be performed to enhance visualisation of pneumothoraces, but the real value of this practice has been questioned.[9]

Radiographs exposed in expiration may be valuable in the investigation of air trapping, particularly in paediatric practice in the context of a suspected inhaled foreign body.[10]

Portable Chest Radiography

The imaging problems associated with portable chest radiography are (A) scattered radiation; (B) the inability of the radiograph to capture all relevant information; and (C) the lack of control over the overall optical density of the resulting image when there is slight over- or under-exposure. Additionally, the shorter focus–detector distance results in undesirable, and sometimes misleading, magnification of structures. High kilovoltage techniques cannot be used because portable machines are unable to deliver a sufficiently high kilovoltage, and as the maximum current is limited, long exposure times are needed, increasing movement artefact. CR systems provide solutions to some of the limitations of portable chest radiography by controlling optical density and contrast, but are unable to overcome the problem of scatter. CR systems remain the most widely used portable radiography system.

Portable DR detectors using FDPs with gadolinium-based scintillators have been available since 2001.[11] Despite this, FDP detectors have not yet been widely adopted because of (A) prohibitive costs, and (B) the hitherto restricted positioning of DR detectors in a portable bedside setting. However, an increasing array of portable DR detectors is now being made available, including those that can be integrated into existing CR cassettes for flexible positioning, and those with wireless transmission capabilities to allow immediate transfer to PACS,[4,12] which may substantially improve technologists' workflow.[12] Such developments are likely to encourage the uptake of portable DR systems in the near future.

Novel Radiographic Techniques

The new techniques of digital tomosynthesis, dual-energy subtraction radiography and temporal subtraction radiography have potential clinical application, chiefly for nodule detection to varying degrees, but at present are confined mainly to research studies.

Digital tomosynthesis of the chest involves the capture of a series of radiographic acquisitions with a digital detector system and computer-controlled apparatus, from which an unlimited number of section images at arbitrary depths and focus can be reconstructed.[13] In this way, an object such as a pulmonary nodule may be rendered more conspicuous, with an exposure equivalent to that of a single film-screen lateral chest radiograph,[14] and therefore with a dose substantially lower than that of CT. Preliminary data suggest improved sensitivity as compared with standard chest radiography for the detection of pulmonary nodules.[14,15]

Dual-energy subtraction radiography is essentially a bone suppression technique that takes advantage of the differential attenuation of X-ray photons of high atomic number materials (such as calcium and iodine) at different photon energies.[13] Such differential attenuation causes the contrast from calcium and bone in a high kVp image to be reduced. As such, subtraction of the low-energy from the high-energy image allows subtraction of obscuring bony structures, potentially increasing pulmonary nodule conspicuity (Fig. 1-1). Low- and high-kVp images can be generated in two ways. First, a single shot exposure, using a two-panel storage phosphor detection system with a copper filter, can be used to generate low- (usually 60) and high- (usually 120) kVp exposures, which can then be subtracted from each other. Alternatively, digital detectors are used to capture a sequential exposure, first at low and then high tube voltages, in a short interval.[16]

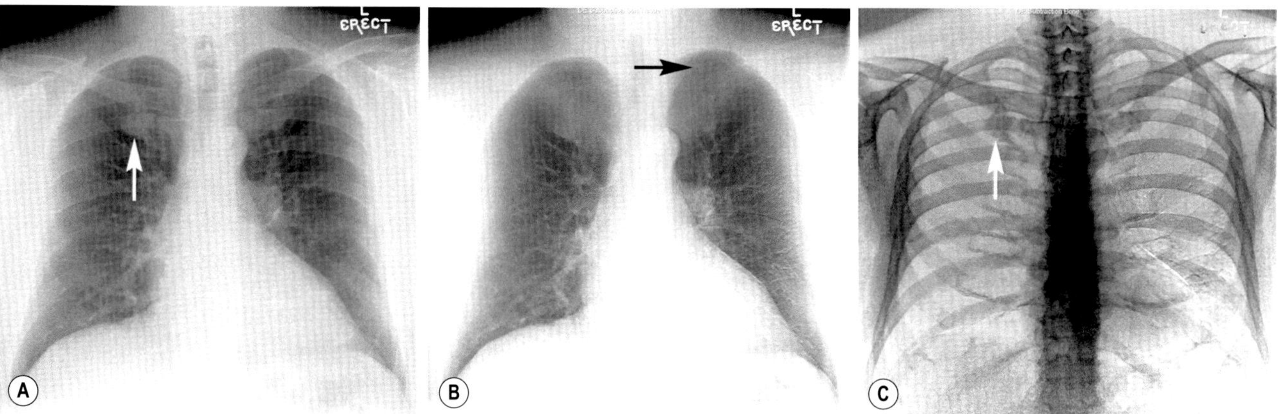

FIGURE 1-1 ■ **Series of dual-energy subtraction chest radiographs in a healthy man.** A right apical opacity is seen on a conventional posteroanterior radiograph (A), but a soft-tissue nodule in the left apex only becomes conspicuous on a bone-subtracted image (B). Additionally, a soft-tissue subtracted image (C) reveals that the right apical opacity is actually calcification of the first costochondral junction. (With permission from McAdams HP, Samei E, Dobbins J III, et al 2006 Recent advances in chest radiography. Radiology 241(3): 663–683.)

Temporal subtraction radiography involves the subtraction of a current and a previous radiograph to generate a difference image, so that any temporal change (such as a new lesion) is made more conspicuous. This technique relies heavily on co-registration of the two images using computer-generated techniques.[16]

COMPUTED TOMOGRAPHY OF THE THORAX

The introduction of spiral (helical) CT in the early 1990s constituted a fundamental evolutionary step in the ongoing refinement of CT imaging, replacing the discontinuous acquisition of data in conventional CT with volumetric data acquisition. In 1998 several CT manufacturers introduced MDCT systems, which provided considerable improvement in acquisition speed, coverage and temporal and spatial resolution.[17–19] These systems typically offered simultaneous acquisition of four sections with a gantry rotation time of as low as 0.5 s. Since then, there has been further rapid improvement in CT performance with increased numbers of detector rows and faster tube rotation; currently, systems with up to 320 active detector rows are available.[20] Rotation times of the X-ray tubes have decreased from 0.5 to 0.33 s per rotation. Recent developments in CT technology have not decreased this rotation time further, but instead use novel methods for increasing temporal and spatial resolution, with either dual-source technology (with two X-ray sources mounted at 90° to each other), a 'flying focal spot' (converting a 128-detector row array into a virtual 256-detector row array), or wide-area detectors, effectively providing 320-detector row coverage.[21] The faster data acquisition enables not only better coverage in a single breath-hold but also results in a significant reduction in patient movement artefacts. In paediatric practice this has meant less frequent need for sedation.[22]

The introduction of MDCT has expanded the clinical indications for CT; these are summarised in Table 1-2.

TABLE 1-2 **Indications for CT of the Chest**

In the Acute Setting

- Chest trauma
- Evaluation of acute aortic syndromes (dissection, transection)
- Demonstration of pulmonary embolism
- Identification of complications after thoracic surgery (mediastinal haematomas, complex pleural collections)

In the Non-Acute Setting

- Evaluation of nodules, hilar or mediastinal masses identified on a chest radiograph
- Lung cancer diagnosis and staging
- Detection of pulmonary metastases from known extrathoracic malignancy
- Characterization of interstitial lung disease
- Identification of bronchiectasis/small airways disease
- Emphysema quantification and preoperative evaluation for lung volume reduction surgery
- Preoperative evaluation of thoracic cage deformities
- Assessment of congenital anomalies of the thoracic great vessels
- Coronary calcium scoring and CT coronary angiography

MDCT systems permit reconstructions of varying slice thickness by collimating and adding together the signals of neighbouring detector rows, with overlap between these rows if necessary. Hence, from the same data set, both narrow sections (0.6–1.25 mm thickness) for high spatial resolution detail or three-dimensional (3D) post-processing and wide sections (2.5–5 mm) for better contrast resolution or quick review can be produced. The convenience of a single protocol is particularly useful for patients with suspected focal and interstitial lung disease. Thin section reconstructions are recommended for volumetric assessment[23] and characterisation[24] of pulmonary nodules, the evaluation of interstitial lung disease and the evaluation of pulmonary embolism,[25] whereas 3- to 5-mm reconstructions are usually adequate for the initial assessment of mediastinal masses and for lung cancer staging

TABLE 1-3 **Post-Processing Techniques and Examples of Clinical Application**

Technique	Technical Considerations	Examples of Use
Multiplanar and curved multiplanar reconstructions (MPR and CMPR)	2D techniques that provide alternate viewing perspectives, usually with conventional window settings. Images are obtained by a reordering of the voxels into 1-voxel-thick tomographic sections, excluding those voxels outside the imaging plane	Evaluation of the large airways and pulmonary emboli, particularly for interpretative difficulties on axial sections due to either partial volume averaging or the inability to differentiate periarterial from endoluminal abnormalities
Maximum intensity projection (MIP)	A ray is cast through the CT data and only data above an assigned value are displayed, thus reducing all data in the line of the ray to a single plane. Sliding slabs of 5–10 mm are commonly used	Mainly used in vascular imaging and in the evaluation of micronodular disease (more accurate identification of nodules versus vessels, and more precise characterization of nodule distribution) (Fig. 1-2)
Mininum intensity projection (MinIP)	Similar to MIP, but only data below an assigned value are displayed and thus it is best suited for showing areas of low density	May improve conspicuity of subtle density differences of lung parenchyma and therefore highlight regions of emphysema or air trapping
Shaded surface display (SSD)	Data reformatted around a threshold that defines the interface of tissues. SSD does not reveal any internal detail	Evaluation of airway abnormalities
Volume rendering	Histogram-based classification is applied to attenuation values in the entire CT data set. CT attenuation can be mapped to brightness, opacity and colour to display a structure of interest. Voxels partially filled with a density of interest are also included. The resultant images contain depth information whilst maintaining 3D spatial relationships	Used in angiographic examinations and also to evaluate large airway abnormalities
Virtual bronchoscopy	Surface rendering and volume rendering are used to produce endoscopic simulations of the airway	Virtual endoscopic or perspective volume rendering images are not widely applied as they seldom give information that cannot be obtained by MPR. However, virtual CT bronchoscopy can provide a view 'through' an obstructing lesion to visualise the airway distal to it, which may not be possible with conventional bronchoscopy
Computer-aided detection	Computerised complex pattern recognition employing a combination of image processing, segmentation and pattern classifiers to identify lesions of interest	Detection and volumetric assessment of pulmonary nodules and pulmonary emboli
Quantitative lung parenchymal assessment	Quantification of parenchymal lung density using techniques such as density masks and histogram analysis to allow objective parenchymal assessment	Emphysema quantification
Dual-energy CT pulmonary blood volume assessment	Generation of iodine maps that act as a surrogate of lung perfusion and therefore of pulmonary blood volume on dual-energy CT	Assessment of perfusion defects in acute and chronic pulmonary thromboembolism
Dual-energy CT virtual unenhanced imaging	Removal of iodine from post-contrast dual-energy acquisitions to generate virtual unenhanced images	Evaluation of apparent enhancement in pulmonary nodules without need for two separate pre- and post-contrast CT acquisitions

studies. In younger patients, however, a more critical approach should be adopted with the CT examination being tailored to the specific clinical question being asked (e.g. interspaced sections when possible), to avoid unnecessary radiation dose.

The introduction of 16- and 64-detector MDCT systems allowed the goal of truly isotropic imaging to be realised: each image data element (voxel) is of equal dimension in all three axes, and forms the basis for allowing image display in any arbitrarily chosen imaging plane. The acquisition of volumetric high-resolution data has permitted new methods of 2D and 3D reconstruction that can complement conventional axial image review, particularly in the display of airways and vascular structures. Furthermore, isotropic imaging has facilitated the development of computer-aided detection and diagnosis systems for the detection and evaluation of pulmonary nodules[26,27] and pulmonary emboli,[28] as well as automated quantification of disease processes, most notably emphysema.[29]

Table 1-3 summarises the various post-processing techniques used in evaluating thoracic disease.

Dual-Energy CT

The concept of DECT was first explored in the 1970s although initial efforts were hampered by limitations in the CT hardware and computational power available at the time. New CT technology has permitted the development of DECT systems over the past seven years. The principles underpinning DECT are the same as for

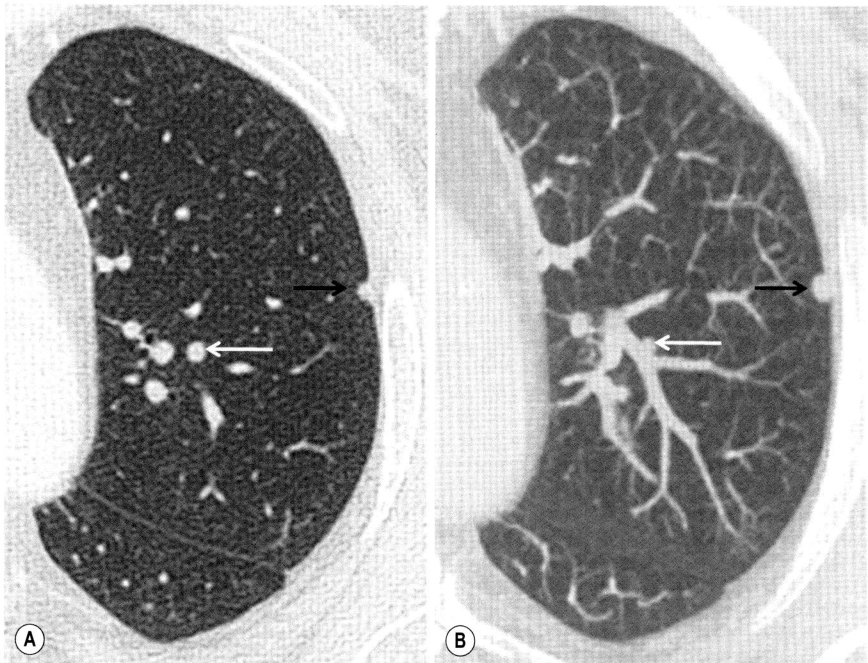

FIGURE 1-2 ■ **Suspected pulmonary metastases in a man with poorly differentiated adenoid cystic carcinoma.** On a 1-mm-thin section image (A), a subpleural nodule (black arrow) is easily seen, but a central nodule (white arrow) can be mistaken for a pulmonary vessel. Scrolling through 10-mm-thick maximum intensity projection (MIP) images (B) can show the central nodule as distinct from the adjacent vessel (white arrow), and make the subpleural nodule more conspicuous (black arrow).

dual-energy subtraction radiography (discussed earlier). DECT allows materials to be differentiated by analysing their attenuation properties at different photon energies, using the material decomposition theory.[30] This theory is particularly applicable to high atomic number materials such as iodine or calcium owing to the photoelectric effect, as they exhibit different degrees of attenuation at different energies.

Different methods for achieving DECT acquisitions are currently used. A dual-source CT system with two X-ray tubes mounted at 90° to each other can provide a dual-energy acquisition by operating the tubes at different kilovoltages (typically 80 or 100 kVp and 140 kVp, respectively)[31] (Fig. 1-3). DECT imaging with single-source CT currently uses either rapid switching between two kilovoltages[32] or a dual-layer ('sandwich') detector, with different detector layers absorbing the different energy spectra.[33]

Regardless of the acquisition technology employed, these DECT systems are all able to generate material-specific image data sets or subtraction images, from a single CT acquisition. In doing so, the need for pre- and post-contrast imaging can be obviated, thus reducing dose while simultaneously avoiding problems arising from misregistration between acquisitions before and after intravenous contrast agents. For example, material differentiation of iodine makes it possible to create a virtual unenhanced image data set. This may have potential clinical application in pulmonary nodule characterisation,[34] for example. Alternatively, by creating an 'iodine only' image data set, a map of pulmonary blood volume can be generated from a contrast-enhanced thoracic DECT acquisition. The latter may demonstrate perfusion defects in acute and chronic pulmonary thromboembolism[35–37] analogous to, and potentially comparable with, that depicted by perfusion scintigraphy.[35,37] While promising, these potential clinical applications of DECT in thoracic imaging have yet to undergo extensive validation.

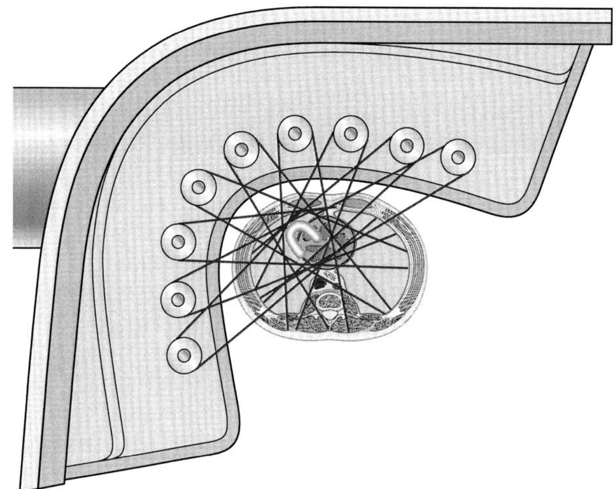

FIGURE 1-3 ■ **Geometry of a dual-source CT system.** The two tubes are positioned at 90° to each other, diametrically opposite their detector arrays.

Dose Considerations

It is important to appreciate some fundamental principles of CT acquisition and factors affecting radiation dose, before considering strategies for dose reduction.

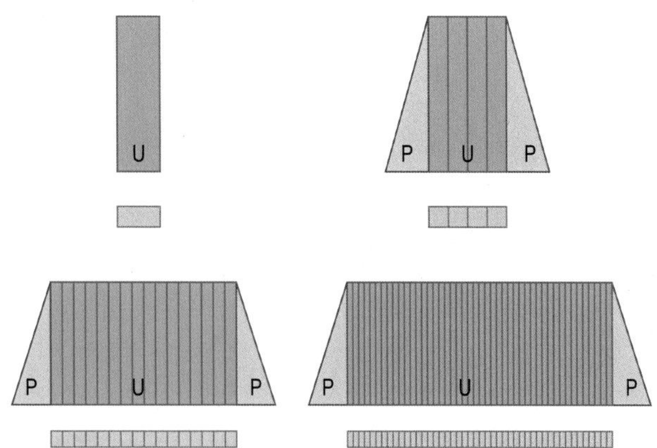

FIGURE 1-4 ■ Geometry and dose profile for spiral, 4-, 16- and 64-slice CT. In spiral CT, the whole dose within the umbral region (U) contributes to image reconstruction with no wastage. In 4-slice CT, wastage occurs within the penumbral regions (P). The relative contribution of the penumbral region decreases with an increasing number of simultaneously acquired sections. The effect of this wastage is minimised in 64-slice CT.

In a CT X-ray tube, a small area on the anode plate emits X-rays that penetrate the patient and are registered by the detector. A collimator between the X-ray tube and the patient, the pre-patient collimator, is used to shape the beam and establish the dose profile. In general, the collimated dose profile is a trapezoid in the longitudinal direction, resulting in umbral and penumbral regions within the area of coverage. In the umbral region, X-rays emitted from the entire area of the focal spot fall on the detector; however, in the penumbral regions at the edge of the beam, only a part of the focal spot illuminates the detector—the pre-patient collimator blocking off other parts.

Despite its undoubted clinical benefit, MDCT carries an increased radiation exposure burden compared with conventional single-slice CT. The increase in radiation arises primarily as a result of wasted radiation dose, due to decreased geometric efficiency of MDCT. Geometric efficiency indicates the proportion of the X-ray beam used in image formation. Lower efficiency thus means that increased doses will be required to maintain similar image quality.[38] With MDCT, only the plateau (umbral) region of the dose profile is used to ensure an equal signal level for all detector elements—the penumbral region is discarded, either by a post-patient collimator or by the intrinsic self-collimation of the MDCT, and represents 'wasted' dose[39] (Fig. 1-4). The relative contribution of the penumbral region decreases with increasing section width (due to a decrease in the incident beam width) and with an increasing number of simultaneously acquired images, in 4- to 16-section MDCT systems.[40] However, with 64-channel MDCT, the incident beam width remains constant over both narrow and wide collimation acquisitions; therefore, geometric efficiency of 64-MDCT is high, with consequently little penalty by way of increased dose.[40]

Another factor that decreases geometric efficiency in MDCT arises from gaps between detector elements in the multidetector array. Photons incident on these regions do not contribute to image signal, and are another form of wasted dose. In general, the number of gaps increases with increasing numbers of sections, thus decreasing the efficiency.[39]

TABLE 1-4 Dose Reduction Strategies in Thoracic CT

Tube current modulation using:
Automatic exposure control
Weight-based modulation
Size-based modulation
Automatic exposure control (AEC)
Gated modulation, e.g. prospective ECG-gating in CT coronary angiography
Tube current reduction in low-dose examinations
Tube potential reduction
Beam-shaping filters (e.g. bowtie filters)
Restricting length of coverage to area of interest
Higher pitch (by increasing table speed), wider collimation where possible
Faster gantry rotation time
New detectors with higher radiation sensitivity, to decrease exposure time
Patient shielding
Statistical iterative reconstruction techniques (e.g. adaptive statistical iterative reconstruction)

Dose reduction strategies are summarised in Table 1-4. The CT parameters that directly affect radiation dose include gantry geometry, rotation time, tube current and voltage, acquisition modes, *z*-axis coverage, pitch, section collimation and section overlap or interval. Factors that indirectly affect dose include reconstruction methods and image filters.

Reduction in tube current is the most practical means of decreasing CT radiation dose, provided this does not compromise image quality due to increased noise. A 50% reduction in tube current can halve effective radiation dose.[41] Authors of several studies using MDCT have suggested that it is possible to reduce tube current markedly (to tube current-time products of between 40 and 70 milliampere seconds, or mAs) in chest examinations without significantly affecting image quality.[42–44] In the paediatric population, some institutions favour the use of a tube current manually tailored to body weight,[45] for instance 1 mAs kg^{-1} for imaging the thorax, an approach that significantly reduces radiation dose.

Tube potential (peak voltage) determines the incident X-ray mean energy, and variation in tube potential causes a substantial change in CT radiation dose. The effect of tube voltage on image quality is complex, since it affects both image noise and tissue contrast. Thus, the image quality ramifications of a decrease in tube voltage to reduce radiation exposure must be carefully examined before being implemented. For chest examinations, 120 kVp is commonly used. In thin patients (<50 kg) and in the paediatric population, 100 kVp is recommended; the use of 80 kVp has been found to be associated with unacceptable beam hardening even in the smallest of patients.[46]

The feasibility of low-dose CT for lung cancer screening has been the subject of renewed interest in recent

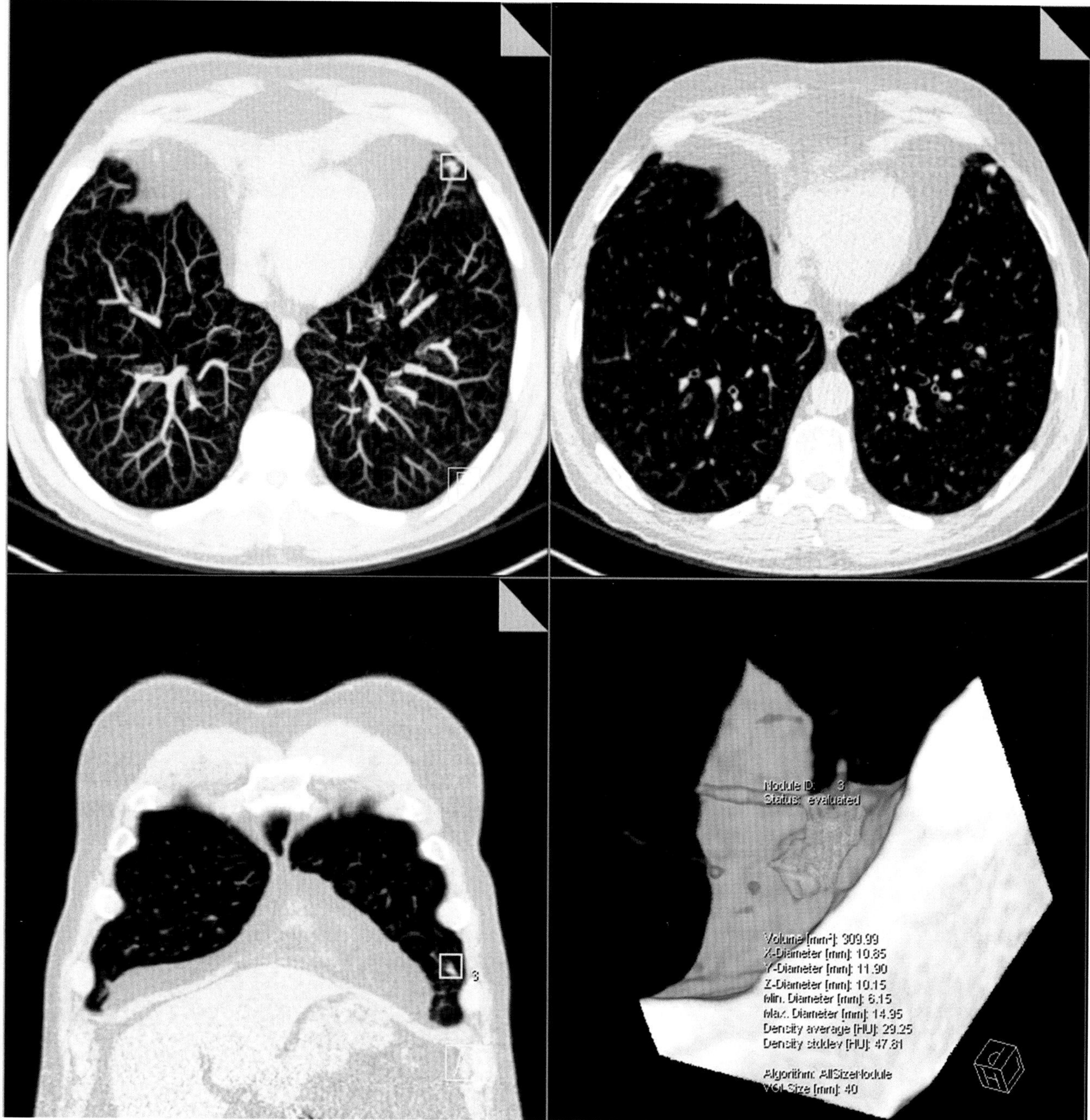

FIGURE 1-5 ■ **Screenshot from volumetric analysis of a low-dose CT study in a lung cancer screening trial.** The CT parameters were based on the patient's body weight, with the effective mAs kept at 22 mAs and a tube potential of 120 kVp.

years. Many authors[47–49] have already proven the efficacy of low-dose CT for pulmonary nodule detection, with tube current–time products as low as 20 mAs still providing acceptable diagnostic images for pulmonary nodule detection. This is due to the inherent high contrast between air and lesions within the lung parenchyma, limiting the obscuring effects of quantum noise. Current low-dose CT screening studies using MDCT use low-dose protocols that adapt tube potential to body weight, and modify tube currents to achieve predetermined effective doses.[50,51] For example, the current UK lung screening pilot study stratifies patients into three groups: <50 kg, 50–80 kg and >80 kg body weight. Tube potentials of 90, 120 and 140 kVp, respectively, are used, and tube current is modified such that effective doses delivered are less than 0.4, 0.8 and 1.6 mSv, respectively[51] (Fig. 1-5).

With helical CT systems, beam collimation, table speed and pitch are interlinked parameters that affect diagnostic image quality. Faster table speed for a given collimation, resulting in a higher pitch, is associated with a reduced radiation dose (if other data acquisition parameters, including tube current, are held constant) because of a shorter exposure time. However, this is not true for some multidetector systems that use an effective mAs setting (defined as mAs divided by pitch). Here, the effective mAs level is held constant (by automatic tube current adjustment) irrespective of pitch value, so that radiation dose does not vary as pitch is changed.[52] Caution should be exercised when extrapolating dose reduction strategies from single- to multidetector CT systems.

Automatic tube current modulation, by means of automatic exposure control (AEC), is a technical innovation that can substantially reduce patient dose. There are three basic methods used currently with MDCT systems: patient-size AEC, *z*-axis AEC and angular (*x*- and *y*-axes) AEC.[53] In patient-size AEC, the appropriate tube current is selected for a given patient size. In *z*-axis AEC, tube current is adjusted to maintain a user-selected noise level in the image data, independent of patient size and anatomy. In angular AEC, the tube current is adjusted to minimise X-rays in projections (angles) that have less importance for the reduction of overall image noise content. With angular AEC, a mean reduction of 36% in dose without loss of image quality in CT imaging studies in children has been reported.[54] MDCT imaging usually has two or more combinations of AEC methods available.

Reconstruction techniques that diminish noise can indirectly contribute to dose reduction, since they help achieve sufficiently diagnostic images from low-dose examinations. These techniques include noise reduction filters utilised within the traditional filtered back projection (FBP) reconstruction techniques, and more recently, statistical iterative reconstruction techniques. Iterative reconstruction, while more computationally intensive, has shown promise in aiding dose reduction in coronary[55] and thoracic[56,57] CT. For example, Pontana et al. recently showed that a mean dose reduction of 35% was possible using iterative reconstruction as compared with FBP with no loss in image quality.[57]

Ultimately, the complexity of the interrelationships between the different CT parameters and dose requires a close collaboration between radiologists and medical physicists to ensure that the radiation burden to patients is as low as possible without diagnostic accuracy being compromised.

Intravenous Contrast Medium Enhancement and Timing of CT Data Acquisition

Intravenous enhancement is used routinely for thoracic CT examinations, most frequently for lung cancer staging, CT pulmonary angiography (CTPA), CT coronary angiography (CTCA) and aortic evaluation. Intravenous enhancement in general is influenced by several factors. These include

- Patient factors, such as body size (as measured by body mass index and body surface area),[58] and cardiac output;
- Contrast medium factors, including the iodine delivery rate[59] (itself a product of iodine concentration, injected contrast volume and the rate of injection);
- Timing of acquisition, depending on whether automated bolus triggering, test bolus or a set delay is used to initiate the CT data acquisition;[60] and
- Changes in respiration, e.g. suboptimal pulmonary artery opacification in CTPA on deep inspiration, due to a variety of suggested mechanisms.[61]

With single-detector CT, a volume of 100 mL of 150 mg mL^{-1} of iodine injected at a rate of 2.5 mL s^{-1} after a 25-s delay was recommended for general thoracic work,[62] while 120–140 mL of 240–300 mg mL^{-1} of iodine injected at a rate of 3–4 mL s^{-1},[63] with either a fixed delay or the use of automated triggering mechanisms, was recommended for CTPA. However, it has been necessary to redesign contrast administration protocols and the timing of acquisition, caused by: (A) the reduced acquisition time brought about by MDCT; (B) newer technology, such as dual-energy CT; (C) the need to reduce contrast dose to minimise potential nephrotoxicity; and (D) the increasing feasibility of 'triple-rule-out' CT to provide simultaneous evaluation of the coronary arteries, pulmonary arteries and aorta, as well as other intrathoracic pathological features in patients presenting with acute chest pain.[64]

In general, the faster acquisition times of MDCT require a higher iodine delivery rate to achieve speedier peak arterial contrast enhancement. If contrast volume is to be reduced, a higher rate can be achieved by a faster injection rate and a higher concentration of contrast medium. In addition, biphasic injection protocols are now preferred. Single-bolus (i.e. monophasic) contrast administration can cause thoracic MDCT acquisitions to suffer from streak and beam-hardening artefacts, due to the dense contrast medium within the brachiocephalic veins during CT data acquisition. To overcome this, biphasic injection protocols are now the norm, using dual-headed power injectors to deliver both contrast medium and a saline chaser to dilute the contrast density in the peripheral veins, thus overcoming the artefacts, as well as providing a more homogeneous enhancement profile.[65] For 64-slice thoracic MDCT acquisitions, typical injection parameters are 60–120 mL of 320–400 mg mL^{-1} of iodine injected at 3.5–5 mL s^{-1}, followed by 20–40 mL of normal saline injected at the same rate.

For triple-rule-out studies, variations in the number of phases, timing, volume and composition of the chaser (e.g. using a mixture of 50:50 contrast material and saline) are employed. For example, a triphasic protocol comprising an initial injection of undiluted contrast medium, followed by a second phase with a mixture of contrast media and saline and, finally, a third pure saline flush may be used.[66]

Window Settings

The density within each voxel is represented by a Hounsfield unit (HU) value. In the thorax these units encompass a wide range, from aerated lung (approximately −800 HU) to ribs (+700 HU). No single-window setting can depict this wide range of densities on a single image. For this reason, a thoracic CT examination requires viewing in at least two settings in order to demonstrate the lung parenchyma and the soft tissues of the mediastinum. Furthermore, it may be necessary to adjust the window settings to improve the demonstration of a particular structure or abnormality. Preferred window settings for thoracic CT vary between institutions, but some generalisations can be made. For the soft tissues of the mediastinum and chest wall a window width of 300–500 HU and a centre of +40 HU are appropriate. For the lungs a wide window of approximately 1500 HU or more at a centre of approximately −600 HU is usually satisfactory. The window settings have a profound influence on the visibility and apparent size of normal and abnormal structures. The most accurate representation of an object appears to be achieved if the value of the window level is halfway between the density of the structure to be measured and the density of the surrounding tissue. For example, the diameter of a pulmonary nodule, measured on soft-tissue settings appropriate for the mediastinum, will be grossly underestimated.[67] It is also important to remember that when inappropriate window settings are used, smaller structures (e.g. peripheral pulmonary vessels) are proportionately much more affected than larger structures.

HIGH-RESOLUTION COMPUTED TOMOGRAPHY

The fundamental components of a high-resolution CT (HRCT) technique are thin collimation, usually 1–2 mm, and a high spatial frequency algorithm reconstruction. A third component concerns the interval between slices. For the majority of patients being investigated exclusively for suspected interstitial lung disease, interspaced (as opposed to volumetric) HRCT remains an adequate examination and should be used for younger patients. This is because the dose of interspaced HRCT is considerably lower than a volumetric high-resolution acquisition.[68,69] Even when techniques are optimised for dose, volumetric HRCT of the chest incurs a dose that is four to ten times higher than interspaced HRCT.[69–71] For example, a study comparing volumetric and axial 1.25-mm interspaced HRCT images in children reported an effective dose of 7.6 mSv for the volumetric acquisition compared with 0.57 mSv for the interspaced technique, despite adapting tube voltage and current to body weight.[71] Thin collimation improves spatial resolution and consequently enhances the detection of key morphological features in HRCT interpretation: thickened interlobular septa, ground-glass opacification, small nodules and abnormally thickened or dilated airways. Reducing the section thickness below 1 mm will not yield any significant further improvement in spatial resolution and at the same time will reduce the signal-to-noise ratio of the image. A sharp reconstruction algorithm reduces image smoothing and makes structures visibly sharper, although image noise becomes more obvious.[72] Intravenous contrast medium should be avoided unless there is another clinical indication necessitating its use (such as pulmonary embolism) since it can spuriously increase parenchymal opacification and interfere with interpretation, especially in comparison examinations (Fig. 1-6).

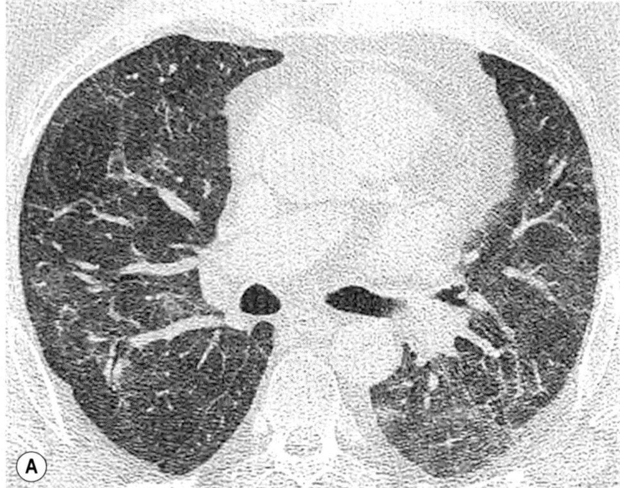

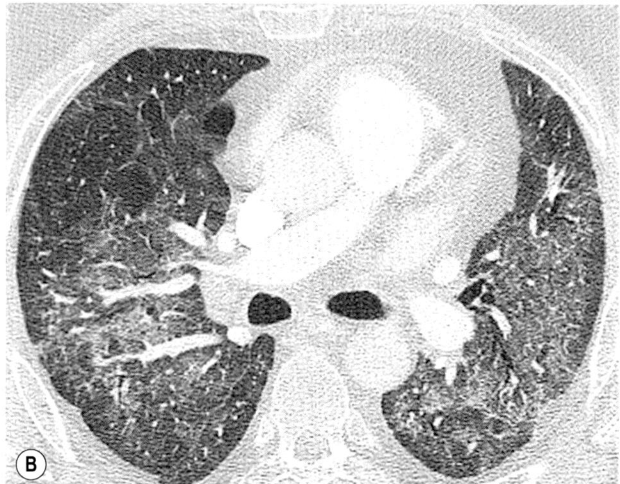

FIGURE 1-6 (A) Unenhanced and (B) intravenously enhanced volumetric 1-mm section HRCT images in a patient with biopsy-proven non-specific interstitial pneumonia, taken one week apart. Generally, increased ground-glass opacity is seen in both lungs, but it is difficult to determine whether this represents new parenchymal opacification, or whether it is purely the consequence of contrast enhancement.

Images are usually obtained in the supine position from the apices to the lung bases at full inspiration and at 10- or 20-mm intervals. When early interstitial fibrosis is suspected, HRCT is often performed in the prone position to prevent confusion with the increased opacification often seen in the dependent posterobasal segments in the usual supine position (Fig. 1-7). However, there is no advantage in prone CT if there is obvious diffuse lung disease on a contemporary chest radiograph.[73]

The necessity of expiratory CT sections is somewhat controversial. Although images at end-expiration can reveal small or subtle areas of air trapping (Fig. 1-8), the mosaic attenuation pattern attributable to small airways disease is usually apparent, albeit less conspicuous, on inspiratory images in most patients with clinically significant small airways disease.

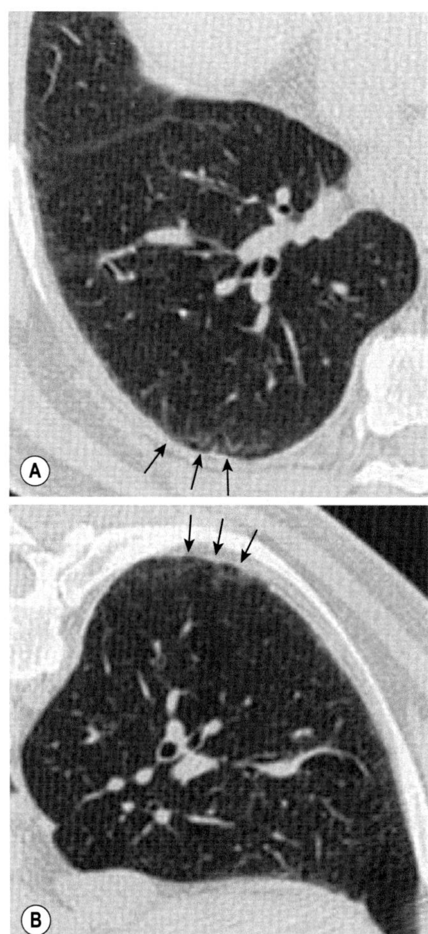

FIGURE 1-7 ■ HRCT for suspected asbestosis. (A) HRCT image in the supine position demonstrates fine reticulation and increased subpleural density (arrows). (B) These changes (arrows) persist on the prone image and may represent early asbestosis in this patient who had an appropriate asbestos exposure.

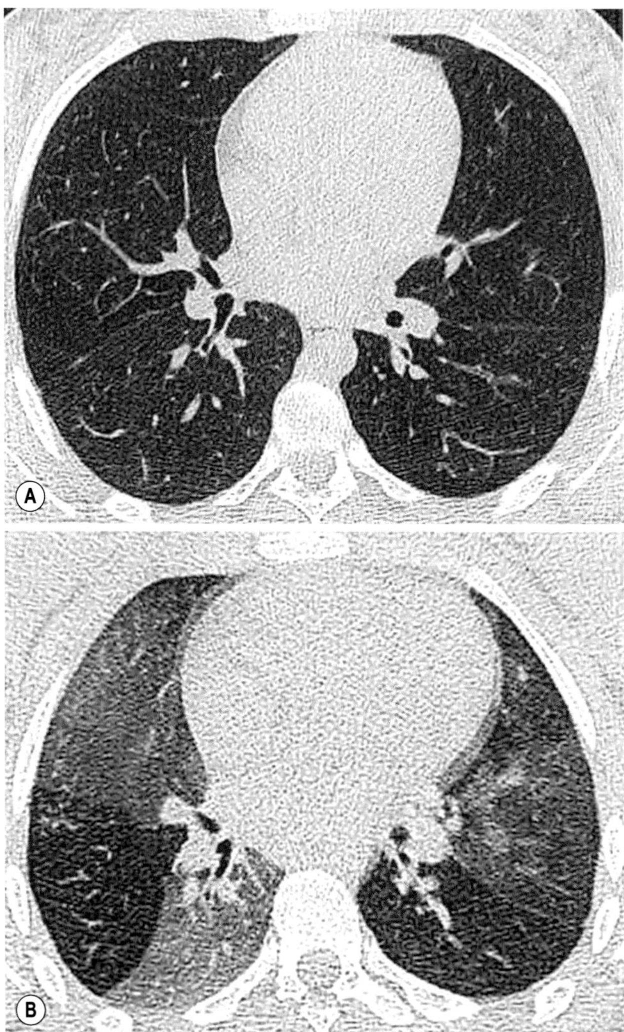

FIGURE 1-8 ■ Mosaic attenuation in a patient with bronchiectasis in the lower lobes (not shown). HRCT image taken in inspiration (A) shows subtle mosaicism, emphasised in the section acquired at end-expiration (B), indicating small airways disease.

ULTRASOUND

The main advantages of chest ultrasound are its bedside availability, absence of radiation and the ease of guided aspiration of pleural fluid and some solid tumours. Visualisation of the chest wall requires a high-frequency linear probe (5–7.5 MHz), whereas pleural and pulmonary disease is better detected with a sector or phased-array probe with a lower frequency (3.5 MHz). Most pleural fluid collections of clinical significance are readily identified on standard chest radiographs, but in the intensive care setting even small effusions may cause respiratory compromise and ultrasound (US) is an effective way of detecting and subsequently guiding aspiration. US is also valuable in identifying loculated collections which may require drainage by multiple catheters. The identification of septations and increased echogenicity within pleural effusions frequently suggest an exudate[74] (Fig. 1-9) but does not correlate with purulence or the need for surgical intervention.[75] With real-time US, the movement of the diaphragm may be observed and the reduced motion of paralysis may be of diagnostic value. US is also a quick

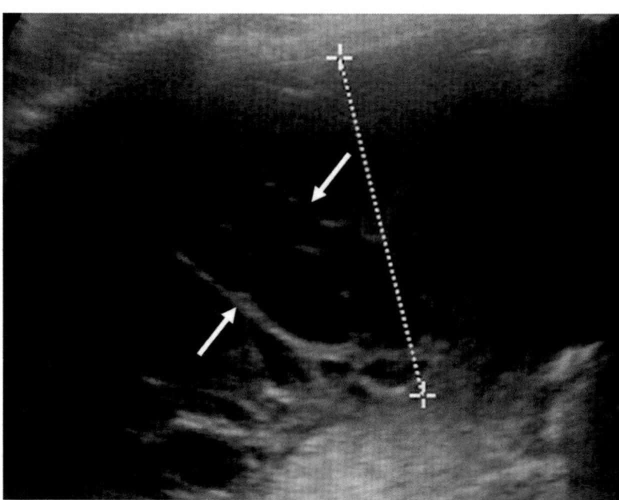

FIGURE 1-9 ■ Ultrasound evaluation of empyema. Multiple septations (arrows) are present within the anechoic pleural collection.

and effective way of guiding percutaneous needle biopsy of peripheral lung, pleural or chest wall lesions, but cannot be used if there is any aerated lung between the ultrasound probe and the lesion.

Endoscopic and Endobronchial Ultrasound

For endoscopic ultrasound (EUS), a high-frequency US transducer is incorporated into the tip of an endoscope to provide high-resolution images of the gastrointestinal wall and structures in close proximity to the gastrointestinal tract. Linear echoendoscopes that can image parallel to the long axis of the instrument allow visualisation of a projecting needle, relative to adjacent tissue, making EUS-guided aspiration or intervention possible. Transoesophageal EUS-guided real-time fine-needle aspiration (FNA) of mediastinal lymph nodes (particularly subaortic, subcarinal, paraoesophageal and pulmonary ligament nodes) has become a useful, minimally invasive and safe method for staging the mediastinum,[76,77] to confirm or refute N2 or N3 disease in patients with non-small cell lung cancer. EUS-FNA has a pooled sensitivity and specificity of 84 and 99.5%, respectively, for the detection of malignant mediastinal lymph nodes in lung cancer.[78]

Endobronchial ultrasound (EBUS) is another relatively new technique that allows ultrasound-guided sampling of mediastinal lymph nodes. EBUS-transbronchial needle aspiration (EBUS-TBNA) can be performed with real-time guidance using a bronchoscope with a convex ultrasound probe[79] (Fig. 1-10). EBUS-TBNA is particularly useful for sampling high mediastinal, paratracheal, subcarinal, hilar and interlobar nodes, with a pooled sensitivity of 90% for mediastinal lymph node staging. Recently, Herth et al. evaluated a combined mediastinal staging approach using both EUS-FNA and EBUS-TBNA performed by a single operator in a single sitting, and found a combined sensitivity of 96%, higher than that for either technique alone.[80] Such combined minimally invasive approaches may find wider clinical applicability in appropriately selected lung cancer patients in the future.

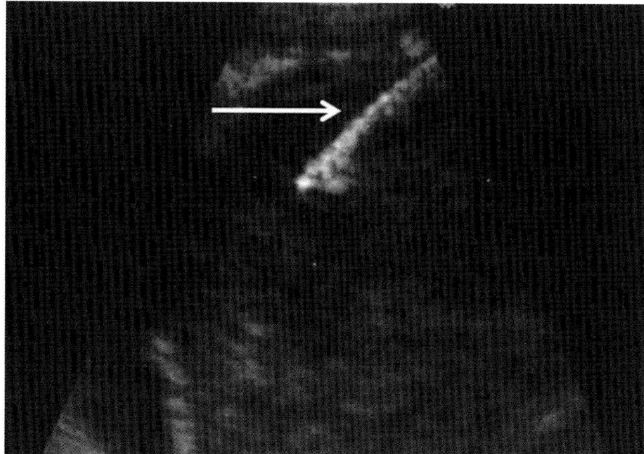

FIGURE 1-10 ■ Endobronchial ultrasound-transbronchial aspiration (EBUS-TBNA) of a subcarinal node in a patient with mediastinal lymphadenopathy. The needle is visualised as a linear focus of high echoreflectivity (arrow). (Courtesy of Dr Pallav Shah, Royal Brompton Hospital.)

MAGNETIC RESONANCE IMAGING

General technical considerations of magnetic resonance imaging are outlined elsewhere and its specific applications in the chest are described where appropriate in the following chapters. This section will summarise the spectrum of MRI techniques used in thoracic imaging.

The general advantages of MRI are its excellent soft-tissue contrast and lack of ionising radiation. However, in the lungs these advantages are greatly outweighed by significant limiting factors, not least of which are the relatively poor spatial resolution of MRI, the extremely low proton density of normal lung, the further decrease of signal by strong susceptibility artefacts induced by the multiple air–soft tissue interfaces within the lung and the consequences of cardiac and respiratory movement. As such, it is now accepted that MRI is no substitute for CT in the investigation of most thoracic conditions that require cross-sectional imaging. The high-resolution multiplanar reconstructions facilitated by isotropic MDCT acquisitions have widened the scope for MDCT to be used in most aspects of thoracic imaging, including areas previously thought to be the domain of 'problem-solving' MRI. The main indications for MRI in the chest include the evaluation of the heart, aorta and pulmonary arteries (particularly in the setting of pulmonary hypertension); demonstrating pulmonary embolism if radiation and intravenous contrast medium need to be avoided; characterisation of mediastinal lesions that are equivocal on CT; and evaluation of superior sulcus tumours, particularly if brachial plexus involvement is suspected.

No generic protocol can be prescribed for MR of the thorax; individualised protocols should always be tailored to the clinical question being asked. Traditional imaging sequences have included T1-weighted spin echo (SE) with or without contrast enhancement with gadolinium chelates (for the initial detection of abnormalities or the demonstration of anatomy) and T2-weighted fast spin echo (FSE) (for further characterisation of abnormalities). Occasionally, a fat-saturation MRI technique (phase-shift gradient-echo imaging or proton-selective fat-saturation imaging) can be useful for detecting fat and distinguishing it from haemorrhage in the evaluation of mediastinal masses. MRI is useful in confirming the cystic nature of mediastinal lesions that appear solid on CT (cysts containing non-serous fluid can have high attenuation on CT) as these cysts will have characteristically high signal intensity when imaged with T2-weighted sequences regardless of the nature of the cyst contents[81] (Fig. 1-11).

To overcome the problem of respiratory motion, other sequences (fast low-angle shot (FLASH) and half Fourier turbo-spin echo (HASTE)) that can be acquired in one breath-hold with acquisition times well below 30 s have been developed. Additional techniques to compensate for

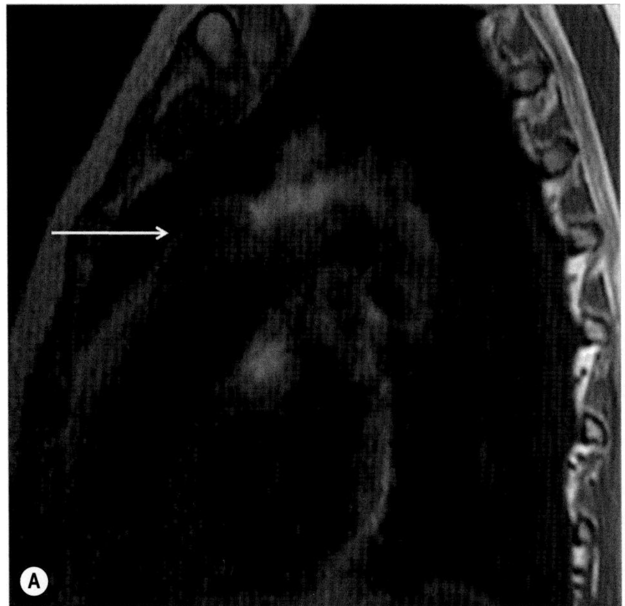

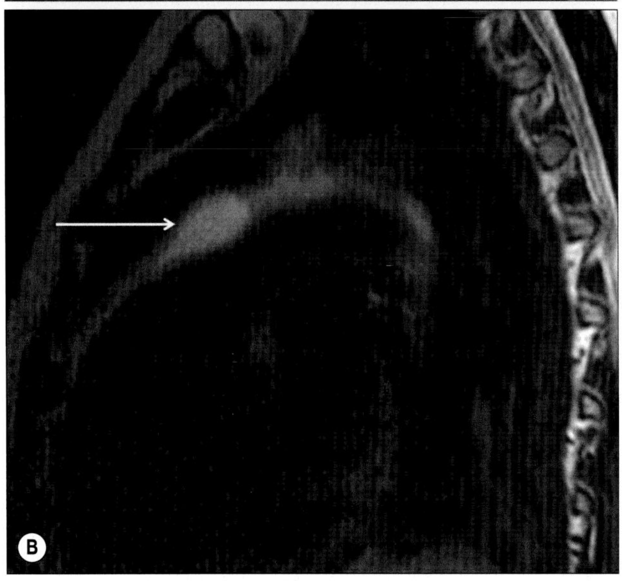

FIGURE 1-11 ■ Anterior mediastinal mass in a 54-year-old woman incidentally discovered during MRI of the thoracolumbar spine. A well-circumscribed ovoid anterior mediastinal lesion is present (arrows) that is hypointense on T1-weighted (A) and markedly hyperintense on T2-weighted (B) sagittal MR images relative to muscle. The appearances are consistent with a thymic cyst.

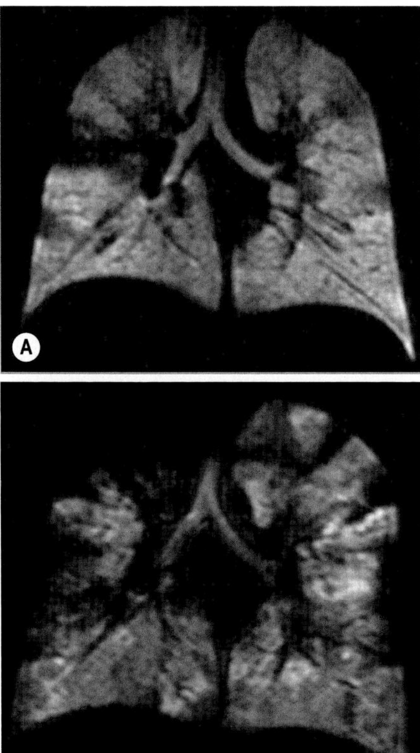

FIGURE 1-12 ■ Coronal hyperpolarised ^{3}He MR images of 24-year-old (A) and 17-year-old (B) patients with cystic fibrosis, with FEV1 of 109 and 52%, respectively. Both patients demonstrate multiple ventilation defects, but the patient in (B) with the poorer FEV1 shows defects which are both larger and more widespread. (With permission from Ohno Y, Koyama H, Yoshikawa T, et al 2011 Pulmonary magnetic resonance imaging for airway diseases. J Thorac Imaging 26(4): 301–316.)

respiratory motion in non-breath-hold MRI have also been evaluated. Three-dimensional gradient-recalled echo (GRE) and volume-interpolated breath-hold examination (VIBE) sequences[82,83] can be used to potentially evaluate lung morphology with high spatial resolution and fewer artefacts.

A few sophisticated MR imaging techniques demonstrate promise but are still largely research tools without wide clinical availability. Hyperpolarised noble gas imaging with either ^{3}He or ^{129}Xe has been used to increase proton density (and so signal-to-noise ratio) in the lung. This can be used to demonstrate parts of the lung that participate in ventilation, and so enable the evaluation of structure–function relationships in lung disease such as cystic fibrosis[84] (Fig. 1-12). Diffusion-sensitive MRI techniques allow mapping of the 'apparent diffusion coefficient' (ADC) of ^{3}He within lung spaces, where ADC is physically related to local bronchoalveolar dimensions. ADC values are increased in fibrosis and emphysema, and show good agreement with predicted lung function. In the evaluation of solitary pulmonary nodules, dynamic contrast-enhanced MR imaging demonstrates good correlation with lesion angiogenesis, and so can help in nodule characterisation.[85]

MRI is thus still clinically most applicable to the imaging of the heart and pulmonary vasculature, and the specific techniques required for this are dealt with elsewhere.

VENTILATION–PERFUSION SCINTIGRAPHY

Ventilation–perfusion (V/Q) scintigraphy is a non-invasive technique for the assessment of the distribution of pulmonary blood flow and alveolar ventilation and has primarily been used for the diagnosis of pulmonary embolism. Lung scintigraphy remains part of the diagnostic algorithm in the investigation of patients with pulmonary embolism, and guidelines suggest that it may be considered, subject to its availability, as the initial imaging investigation provided the chest radiograph is normal and there is no significant symptomatic concurrent cardiopulmonary disease.[86]

Perfusion scintigraphy is performed following the intravenous injection of ^{99m}Tc-labelled protein microparticles which, because of their size, undergo microembolisation in the pulmonary vascular bed. Agents for ventilation scintigraphy include krypton-81m, ^{99m}Tc-diethylenetriaminepentaacetic acid, ^{99m}Tc-labelled carbon microparicles (Technegas) and ^{133}xenon. Krypton-81m is in many ways the ideal agent of choice for ventilation imaging but it has a very short half-life, is expensive to produce and accumulates progressively in regions of lung with a low ventilatory turnover. The lung can be imaged in multiple projections and in each projection, perfusion and ventilation images can be acquired sequentially, or, with the newer digital cameras, simultaneously. Technegas is an ultrafine and scintigraphically more efficient aerosol that is considered to behave truly like a gas because the mean aerodynamic diameter of the particles are between 30 and 90 nm.

Ventilation–perfusion lung scintigraphy performed using single photon emission CT (SPECT) technique (as opposed to merely using planar acquisitions) has shown that diagnostic accuracy for pulmonary embolism is at least comparable with,[87] and may exceed,[88] that of CT pulmonary angiography with MDCT (4- to 16-detector MDCT). However, the lack of availability of this technique means it is unlikely to be frequently used for patients with suspected pulmonary embolism.

REFERENCES

1. Rong XJ, Shaw CC, Liu X, et al. Comparison of an amorphous silicon/cesium iodide flat-panel digital chest radiography system with screen/film and computed radiography systems—a contrast-detail phantom study. Med Phys 2001;28(11):2328–35.
2. Garmer M, Hennigs SP, Jager HJ, et al. Digital radiography versus conventional radiography in chest imaging: diagnostic performance of a large-area silicon flat-panel detector in a clinical CT-controlled study. AJR Am J Roentgenol 2000;174(1):75–80.
3. Rowlands JA. The physics of computed radiography. Phys Med Biol 2002;47(23):R123–R66.
4. Cowen AR, Kengyelics SM, Davies AG. Solid-state, flat-panel, digital radiography detectors and their physical imaging characteristics. Clin Radiol 2008;63(5):487–98.
5. Kroft LJ, Veldkamp WJ, Mertens BJ, et al. Comparison of eight different digital chest radiography systems: variation in detection of simulated chest disease. AJR Am J Roentgenol 2005;185(2):339–46.
6. Bernhardt TM, Otto D, Reichel G, et al. Detection of simulated interstitial lung disease and catheters with selenium, storage phosphor, and film-based radiography. Radiology 1999;213(2):445–54.
7. Bacher K, Smeets P, Bonnarens K, et al. Dose reduction in patients undergoing chest imaging: digital amorphous silicon flat-panel detector radiography versus conventional film-screen radiography and phosphor-based computed radiography. AJR Am J Roentgenol 2003;181(4):923–9.
8. Morgan RA, Owens CM, Collins CD, et al. Detection of pneumothorax with lateral shoot-through digital radiography. Clin Radiol 1993;48(4):249–52.
9. Seow A, Kazerooni EA, Pernicano PG, Neary M. Comparison of upright inspiratory and expiratory chest radiographs for detecting pneumothoraces. AJR Am J Roentgenol 1996;166(2):313–16.
10. Hilliard T, Sim R, Saunders M, et al. Delayed diagnosis of foreign body aspiration in children. Emerg Med J 2003;20(1):100–1.
11. Puig S. [Digital radiography of the chest in pediatric patients]. Radiologe 2003;43(12):1045–50.
12. Lehnert T, Naguib NN, Ackermann H, et al. Novel, portable, cassette-sized, and wireless flat-panel digital radiography system: initial workflow results versus computed radiography. AJR Am J Roentgenol 2011;196(6):1368–71.
13. McAdams HP, Samei E, Dobbins J III, et al. Recent advances in chest radiography. Radiology 2006;241(3):663–83.
14. James TD, McAdams HP, Song JW, et al. Digital tomosynthesis of the chest for lung nodule detection: interim sensitivity results from an ongoing NIH-sponsored trial. Med Phys 2008;35(6):2554–7.
15. Vikgren J, Zachrisson S, Svalkvist A, et al. Comparison of chest tomosynthesis and chest radiography for detection of pulmonary nodules: human observer study of clinical cases. Radiology 2008;249(3):1034–41.
16. MacMahon H, Li F, Engelmann R, et al. Dual energy subtraction and temporal subtraction chest radiography. J Thorac Imaging 2008;23(2):77–85.
17. Hu H, He HD, Foley WD, Fox SH. Four multidetector-row helical CT: image quality and volume coverage speed. Radiology 2000;215(1):55–62.
18. Flohr TG, Schaller S, Stierstorfer K, et al. Multi-detector row CT systems and image-reconstruction techniques. Radiology 2005;235(3):756–73.
19. McCollough CH, Zink FE. Performance evaluation of a multi-slice CT system. Med Phys 1999;26(11):2223–30.
20. Hsiao EM, Rybicki FJ, Steigner M. CT coronary angiography: 256-slice and 320-detector row scanners. Curr Cardiol Rep 2010;12(1):68–75.
21. Gupta R, Grasruck M, Suess C, et al. Ultra-high resolution flat-panel volume CT: fundamental principles, design architecture, and system characterization. Eur Radiol 2006;16(6):1191–205.
22. Pappas JN, Donnelly LF, Frush DP. Reduced frequency of sedation of young children with multisection helical CT. Radiology 2000;215(3):897–9.
23. Wormanns D, Kohl G, Klotz E, et al. Volumetric measurements of pulmonary nodules at multi-row detector CT: in vivo reproducibility. Eur Radiol 2004;14(1):86–92.
24. Brandman S, Ko JP. Pulmonary nodule detection, characterization, and management with multidetector computed tomography. J Thorac Imaging 2011;26(2):90–105.
25. Remy-Jardin M, Pistolesi M, Goodman LR, et al. Management of suspected acute pulmonary embolism in the era of CT angiography: a statement from the Fleischner Society. Radiology 2007;245(2):315–29.
26. Rubin GD, Lyo JK, Paik DS, et al. Pulmonary nodules on multi-detector row CT scans: performance comparison of radiologists and computer-aided detection. Radiology 2005;234(1):274–83.
27. Roos JE, Paik D, Olsen D, et al. Computer-aided detection (CAD) of lung nodules in CT scans: radiologist performance and reading time with incremental CAD assistance. Eur Radiol 2010;20(3):549–57.
28. Walsham AC, Roberts HC, Kashani HM, et al. The use of computer-aided detection for the assessment of pulmonary arterial filling defects at computed tomographic angiography. J Comput Assist Tomogr 2008;32(6):913–18.
29. Madani A, Zanen J, de MV, Gevenois PA. Pulmonary emphysema: objective quantification at multi-detector row CT—comparison with macroscopic and microscopic morphometry. Radiology 2006;238(3):1036–43.
30. Zatz LM. The effect of the kVp level on EMI values. Selective imaging of various materials with different kVp settings. Radiology 1976;119(3):683–8.
31. Flohr TG, McCollough CH, Bruder H, et al. First performance evaluation of a dual-source CT (DSCT) system. Eur Radiol 2006;16(2):256–68.
32. Geyer LL, Scherr M, Korner M, et al. Imaging of acute pulmonary embolism using a dual energy CT system with rapid kVp switching: initial results. Eur J Radiol 2011;81(12):3711–18.
33. Eliahou R, Hidas G, Duvdevani M, Sosna J. Determination of renal stone composition with dual-energy computed tomography: an emerging application. Semin Ultrasound CT MR 2010;31(4):315–20.

34. Chae EJ, Song JW, Seo JB, et al. Clinical utility of dual-energy CT in the evaluation of solitary pulmonary nodules: initial experience. Radiology 2008;249(2):671–81.
35. Nakazawa T, Watanabe Y, Hori Y, et al. Lung perfused blood volume images with dual-energy computed tomography for chronic thromboembolic pulmonary hypertension: correlation to scintigraphy with single-photon emission computed tomography. J Comput Assist Tomogr 2011;35(5):590–5.
36. Hoey ET, Gopalan D, Ganesh V, et al. Dual-energy CT pulmonary angiography: a novel technique for assessing acute and chronic pulmonary thromboembolism. Clin Radiol 2009;64(4):414–19.
37. Thieme SF, Graute V, Nikolaou K, et al. Dual energy CT lung perfusion imaging-correlation with SPECT/CT. Eur J Radiol 2010;81(2):360–5.
38. Lewis M. Radiation dose issues in multi-slice CT scanning. ImPACT technology update no. 3. 2005. Available at: <http://www.impactscan.org/download/msctdose.pdf>. Accessed 1 December 2011.
39. Mayo JR, Aldrich J. Radiation exposure in thoracic CT. In: Schoepf UJ, editor. Multidetector-Row CT of the Thorax. 1st ed. Heidelberg: Springer; 2006. pp. 25–34.
40. Dalrymple NC, Prasad SR, El-Merhi FM, Chintapalli KN. Price of isotropy in multidetector CT. Radiographics 2007;27(1): 49–62.
41. Kalra MK, Maher MM, Toth TL, et al. Strategies for CT radiation dose optimization. Radiology 2004;230(3):619–28.
42. Jung KJ, Lee KS, Kim SY, et al. Low-dose, volumetric helical CT: image quality, radiation dose, and usefulness for evaluation of bronchiectasis. Invest Radiol 2000;35(9):557–63.
43. Yi CA, Lee KS, Kim TS, et al. Multidetector CT of bronchiectasis: effect of radiation dose on image quality. AJR Am J Roentgenol 2003;181(2):501–5.
44. Takahashi M, Maguire WM, Ashtari M, et al. Low-dose spiral computed tomography of the thorax: comparison with the standard-dose technique. Invest Radiol 1998;33(2):68–73.
45. Yu L, Bruesewitz MR, Thomas KB, et al. Optimal tube potential for radiation dose reduction in pediatric CT: principles, clinical implementations, and pitfalls. Radiographics 2011;31(3):835–48.
46. Cody DD, Moxley DM, Krugh KT, et al. Strategies for formulating appropriate MDCT techniques when imaging the chest, abdomen, and pelvis in pediatric patients. AJR Am J Roentgenol 2004; 182(4):849–59.
47. Diederich S, Lenzen H, Windmann R, et al. Pulmonary nodules: experimental and clinical studies at low-dose CT. Radiology 1999;213(1):289–98.
48. Itoh S, Ikeda M, Arahata S, et al. Lung cancer screening: minimum tube current required for helical CT. Radiology 2000;215(1): 175–83.
49. Gartenschlager M, Schweden F, Gast K, et al. Pulmonary nodules: detection with low-dose vs conventional-dose spiral CT. Eur Radiol 1998;8(4):609–14.
50. Xu DM, Gietema H, de Koning H, et al. Nodule management protocol of the NELSON randomised lung cancer screening trial. Lung Cancer 2006;54(2):177–84.
51. Baldwin DR, Duffy SW, Wald NJ, et al. UK Lung Screen (UKLS) nodule management protocol: modelling of a single screen randomised controlled trial of low-dose CT screening for lung cancer. Thorax 2011;66(4):308–13.
52. Mahesh M, Scatarige JC, Cooper J, Fishman EK. Dose and pitch relationship for a particular multislice CT scanner. AJR Am J Roentgenol 2001;177(6):1273–5.
53. Lee CH, Goo JM, Ye HJ, et al. Radiation dose modulation techniques in the multidetector CT era: from basics to practice. Radiographics 2008;28(5):1451–9.
54. Greess H, Lutze J, Nomayr A, et al. Dose reduction in subsecond multislice spiral CT examination of children by online tube current modulation. Eur Radiol 2004;14(6):995–9.
55. Leipsic J, Labounty TM, Heilbron B, et al. Estimated radiation dose reduction using adaptive statistical iterative reconstruction in coronary CT angiography: the ERASIR study. AJR Am J Roentgenol 2010;195(3):655–60.
56. Singh S, Kalra MK, Gilman MD, et al. Adaptive statistical iterative reconstruction technique for radiation dose reduction in chest CT: a pilot study. Radiology 2011;259(2):565–73.
57. Pontana F, Duhamel A, Pagniez J, et al. Chest computed tomography using iterative reconstruction vs filtered back projection (Part 2): image quality of low-dose CT examinations in 80 patients. Eur Radiol 2011;21(3):636–43.
58. Bae KT, Seeck BA, Hildebolt CF, et al. Contrast enhancement in cardiovascular MDCT: effect of body weight, height, body surface area, body mass index, and obesity. AJR Am J Roentgenol 2008;190(3):777–84.
59. Keil S, Plumhans C, Behrendt FF, et al. MDCT angiography of the pulmonary arteries: intravascular contrast enhancement does not depend on iodine concentration when injecting equal amounts of iodine at standardized iodine delivery rates. Eur Radiol 2008;18(8):1690–5.
60. Ramos-Duran LR, Kalafut JF, Hanley M, Schoepf UJ. Current contrast media delivery strategies for cardiac and pulmonary multidetector-row computed tomography angiography. J Thorac Imaging 2010;25(4):270–7.
61. Mortimer AM, Singh RK, Hughes J, et al. Use of expiratory CT pulmonary angiography to reduce inspiration and breath-hold associated artefact: contrast dynamics and implications for scan protocol. Clin Radiol 2011;66(12):1159–66.
62. Leung AN. Spiral CT of the thorax in daily practice: optimization of technique. J Thorac Imaging 1997;12(1):2–10.
63. Remy-Jardin M, Remy J, Artaud D, et al. Peripheral pulmonary arteries: optimization of the spiral CT acquisition protocol. Radiology 1997;204(1):157–63.
64. Halpern EJ. Triple-rule-out CT angiography for evaluation of acute chest pain and possible acute coronary syndrome. Radiology 2009;252(2):332–45.
65. Cademartiri F, Mollet N, van der Lugt A, et al. Non-invasive 16-row multislice CT coronary angiography: usefulness of saline chaser. Eur Radiol 2004;14(2):178–83.
66. Litmanovich D, Zamboni GA, Hauser TH, et al. ECG-gated chest CT angiography with 64-MDCT and tri-phasic IV contrast administration regimen in patients with acute non-specific chest pain. Eur Radiol 2008;18(2):308–17.
67. Harris KM, Adams H, Lloyd DC, Harvey DJ. The effect on apparent size of simulated pulmonary nodules of using three standard CT window settings. Clin Radiol 1993;47(4):241–4.
68. Kelly DM, Hasegawa I, Borders R, et al. High-resolution CT using MDCT: comparison of degree of motion artifact between volumetric and axial methods. AJR Am J Roentgenol 2004;182(3):757–9.
69. Studler U, Gluecker T, Bongartz G, et al. Image quality from high-resolution CT of the lung: comparison of axial scans and of sections reconstructed from volumetric data acquired using MDCT. AJR Am J Roentgenol 2005;185(3):602–7.
70. Mayo JR, Aldrich J, Muller NL. Radiation exposure at chest CT: a statement of the Fleischner Society. Radiology 2003;228(1): 15–21.
71. Bastos M, Lee EY, Strauss KJ, et al. Motion artifact on high-resolution CT images of pediatric patients: comparison of volumetric and axial CT methods. AJR Am J Roentgenol 2009;193(5): 1414–18.
72. Murata K, Khan A, Rojas KA, Herman PG. Optimization of computed tomography technique to demonstrate the fine structure of the lung. Invest Radiol 1988;23(3):170–5.
73. Volpe J, Storto ML, Lee K, Webb WR. High-resolution CT of the lung: determination of the usefulness of CT scans obtained with the patient prone based on plain radiographic findings. AJR Am J Roentgenol 1997;169(2):369–74.
74. Yang PC, Luh KT, Chang DB, et al. Value of sonography in determining the nature of pleural effusion: analysis of 320 cases. AJR Am J Roentgenol 1992;159(1):29–33.
75. Kearney SE, Davies CW, Davies RJ, Gleeson FV. Computed tomography and ultrasound in parapneumonic effusions and empyema. Clin Radiol 2000;55(7):542–7.
76. Gress FG, Savides TJ, Sandler A, et al. Endoscopic ultrasonography, fine-needle aspiration biopsy guided by endoscopic ultrasonography, and computed tomography in the preoperative staging of non-small-cell lung cancer: a comparison study. Ann Intern Med 1997;127(8 Pt 1):604–12.
77. Micames CG, McCrory DC, Pavey DA, et al. Endoscopic ultrasound-guided fine-needle aspiration for non-small cell lung cancer staging: a systematic review and metaanalysis. Chest 2007;131(2):539–48.
78. Detterbeck FC, Jantz MA, Wallace M, et al. Invasive mediastinal staging of lung cancer: ACCP evidence-based clinical practice guidelines (2nd edn). Chest 2007;132(3 Suppl):202S–20S.

79. Herth F, Becker HD, Ernst A. Conventional vs endobronchial ultrasound-guided transbronchial needle aspiration: a randomized trial. Chest 2004;125(1):322–5.
80. Herth FJ, Krasnik M, Kahn N, et al. Combined endoscopic-endobronchial ultrasound-guided fine-needle aspiration of mediastinal lymph nodes through a single bronchoscope in 150 patients with suspected lung cancer. Chest 2010;138(4):790–4.
81. Murayama S, Murakami J, Watanabe H, et al. Signal intensity characteristics of mediastinal cystic masses on T1-weighted MRI. J Comput Assist Tomogr 1995;19(2):188–91.
82. Bader TR, Semelka RC, Pedro MS, et al. Magnetic resonance imaging of pulmonary parenchymal disease using a modified breath-hold 3D gradient-echo technique: initial observations. J Magn Reson Imaging 2002;15(1):31–8.
83. Karabulut N, Martin DR, Yang M, Tallaksen RJ. MR imaging of the chest using a contrast-enhanced breath-hold modified three-dimensional gradient-echo technique: comparison with two-dimensional gradient-echo technique and multidetector CT. AJR Am J Roentgenol 2002;179(5):1225–33.
84. Eichinger M, Heussel CP, Kauczor HU, et al. Computed tomography and magnetic resonance imaging in cystic fibrosis lung disease. J Magn Reson Imaging 2010;32(6):1370–8.
85. Schaefer JF, Schneider V, Vollmar J, et al. Solitary pulmonary nodules: association between signal characteristics in dynamic contrast enhanced MRI and tumor angiogenesis. Lung Cancer 2006;53(1):39–49.
86. British Thoracic Society. British Thoracic Society guidelines for the management of suspected acute pulmonary embolism. Thorax 2003;58(6):470–83.
87. Reinartz P, Wildberger JE, Schaefer W, et al. Tomographic imaging in the diagnosis of pulmonary embolism: a comparison between V/Q lung scintigraphy in SPECT technique and multislice spiral CT. J Nucl Med 2004;45(9):1501–8.
88. Gutte H, Mortensen J, Jensen CV, et al. Detection of pulmonary embolism with combined ventilation-perfusion SPECT and low-dose CT: head-to-head comparison with multidetector CT angiography. J Nucl Med 2009;50(12):1987–92.

CHAPTER 2

The Normal Chest

Simon P.G. Padley • Katharina Marten-Engelke • Christoph Engelke

CHAPTER OUTLINE

THE LUNGS

Each lung is divided into lobes surrounded by pleura. There are two lobes on the left: the upper and lower, separated by the major (oblique) fissure; and three on the right: the upper, middle and lower lobes, separated by the major (oblique) and minor (horizontal) fissures. The fissures are frequently incomplete, particularly medially, containing localised defects which form an alveolar pathway for collateral air drift and the spread of disease.

For a fissure to be visualised on conventional radiographs, the X-ray beam must be tangential to the fissure. In most people, some of the minor fissure is seen in the frontal projection, but neither major fissure can be identified. In the lateral view, both the major and minor fissures are often identified, but usually only part of any fissure is seen; in fact, it is very unusual to see both left and right major fissures in their entirety.

The major fissures have similar anatomy on the two sides. They run obliquely anteriorly and inferiorly from approximately the fifth thoracic vertebra to pass through the hilum and contact the diaphragm 0–3 cm behind the anterior costophrenic angle. Each major fissure follows a gently curving plane somewhat similar to a propeller blade (Fig. 2-1), with the upper portion facing anterolaterally, and the lower portion facing anteromedially. Owing to the undulating course of the major fissure, either fissure may be seen as two lines on the lateral view. Consequently, it may appear to the unwary that a fissure is displaced when it is, in fact, in its normal position, or both fissures may appear to be in their normal positions when in reality one of them is so displaced that it is no longer visible.

The inferior portion of either or both major fissures may be widened due to fat or pleural thickening between the leaves of the pleura. In these circumstances the contact with the diaphragm will often be broadened and lead to a localised loss of silhouette, an appearance referred to as the juxtaphrenic peak.

With modern multidetector computed tomography (CT), the normal major fissures are frequently visible, but if not clearly defined the position can be inferred from the presence of a relatively avascular zone that forms the outer cortex of the lobe. With high-resolution CT (HRCT), a normal major fissure is seen as a thin line traversing the avascular zone,[1] although it may be represented as two parallel lines on at least one level in approximately one-third of the population because of an artefact related to cardiac and respiratory motion.[2]

The minor fissure fans out anteriorly and laterally from the right hilum in a horizontal direction to reach the chest wall. On a standard chest radiograph, the minor fissure contacts the chest wall at the axillary portion of the right sixth rib. The fissure curves gently, with its anterior and lateral portion usually curving downwards. Because of the curvature of the major fissure described above, part of the minor fissure may be projected posterior to the right major fissure on the lateral view.

On CT the minor fissure position is represented by an oval area of reduced vascularity at the level of the bronchus intermedius (Figs. 2-1 and 2-2). The normal minor fissure is not seen as a line on axial CT imaging but is apparent on multiplanar reformats.

In 1% of the population an accessory fissure,[3] called the 'azygos lobe fissure' (Fig. 2-3), is seen. This fissure contains the azygos vein at its lower end and results from failure of normal migration of the azygos vein from the chest wall to its usual position in the tracheobronchial angle and persistence of the invaginated visceral and parietal pleurae. There is no corresponding alteration in the segmental architecture of the lung, so the term 'lobe' is a misnomer. The azygos lobe may, however, be smaller and therefore less transradiant than corresponding normal lung.[4] On CT the altered course of the azygos vein can be seen traversing the lung (Figs. 2-3A–D). Other accessory fissures are occasionally identified (Fig. 2-2).[3] A minor fissure may separate the lingular segments from the remainder of the upper lobe, similar to the right minor fissure. A horizontally orientated fissure, a superior accessory fissure, may separate the apical segment from the basal segments of either lower lobe. An inferior accessory fissure is sometimes seen in one or other lower

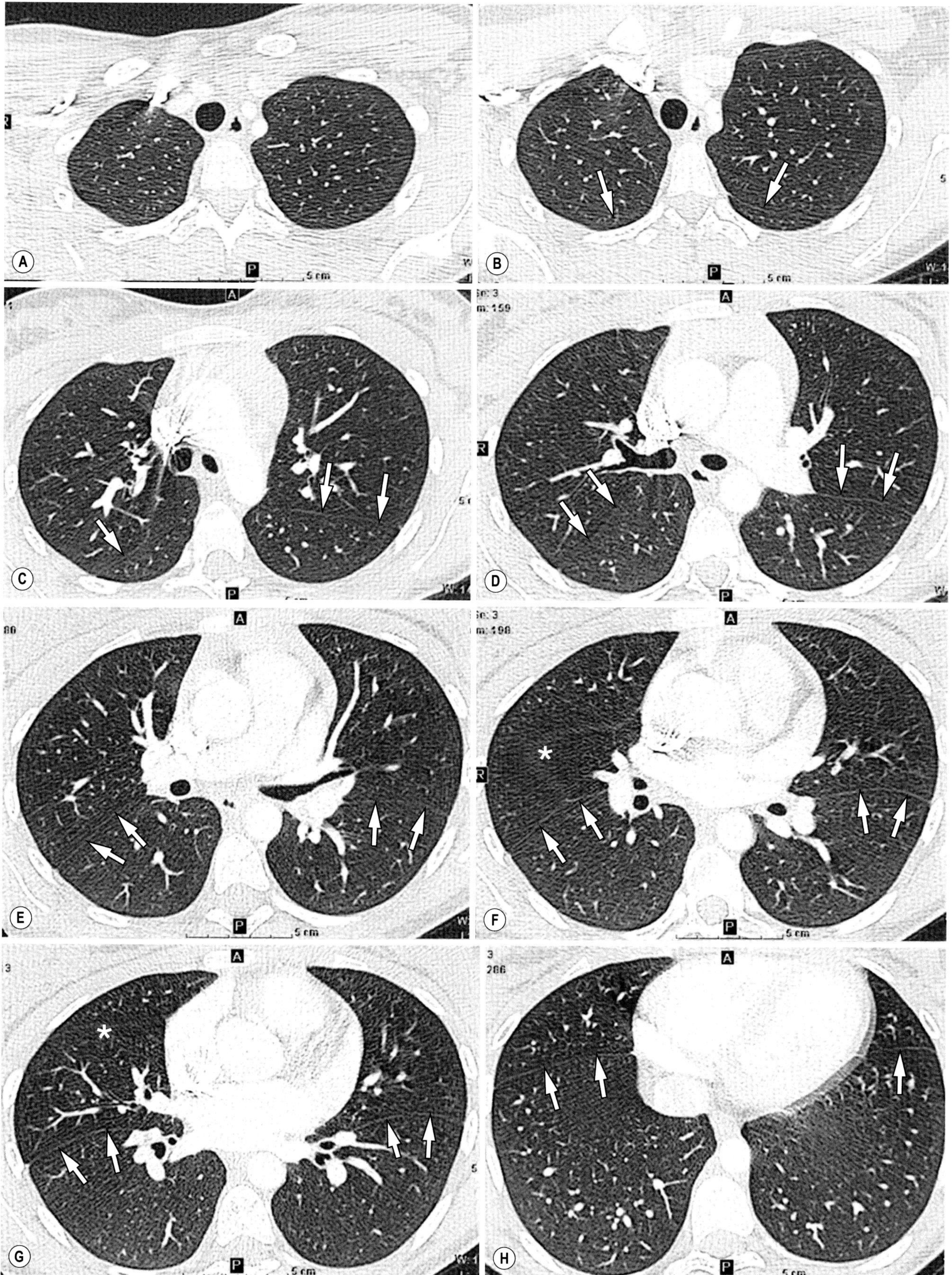

FIGURE 2-1 ■ **The position and shape of the major fissures (arrows) in the lower and the upper zones is best shown by CT.** Note that above the hila, the major fissures bow backwards (B, C), whereas below the hila, the major fissures bow forwards (D to H). The minor fissure (F, G) is apparent as an area of avascularity anterior to the major fissure. In this example the slightly bowed horizontal fissure undulates through the plane of the slice (asterisks). The images are high-resolution 0.625-mm-thin CT sections from a 64-row multislice CT study.

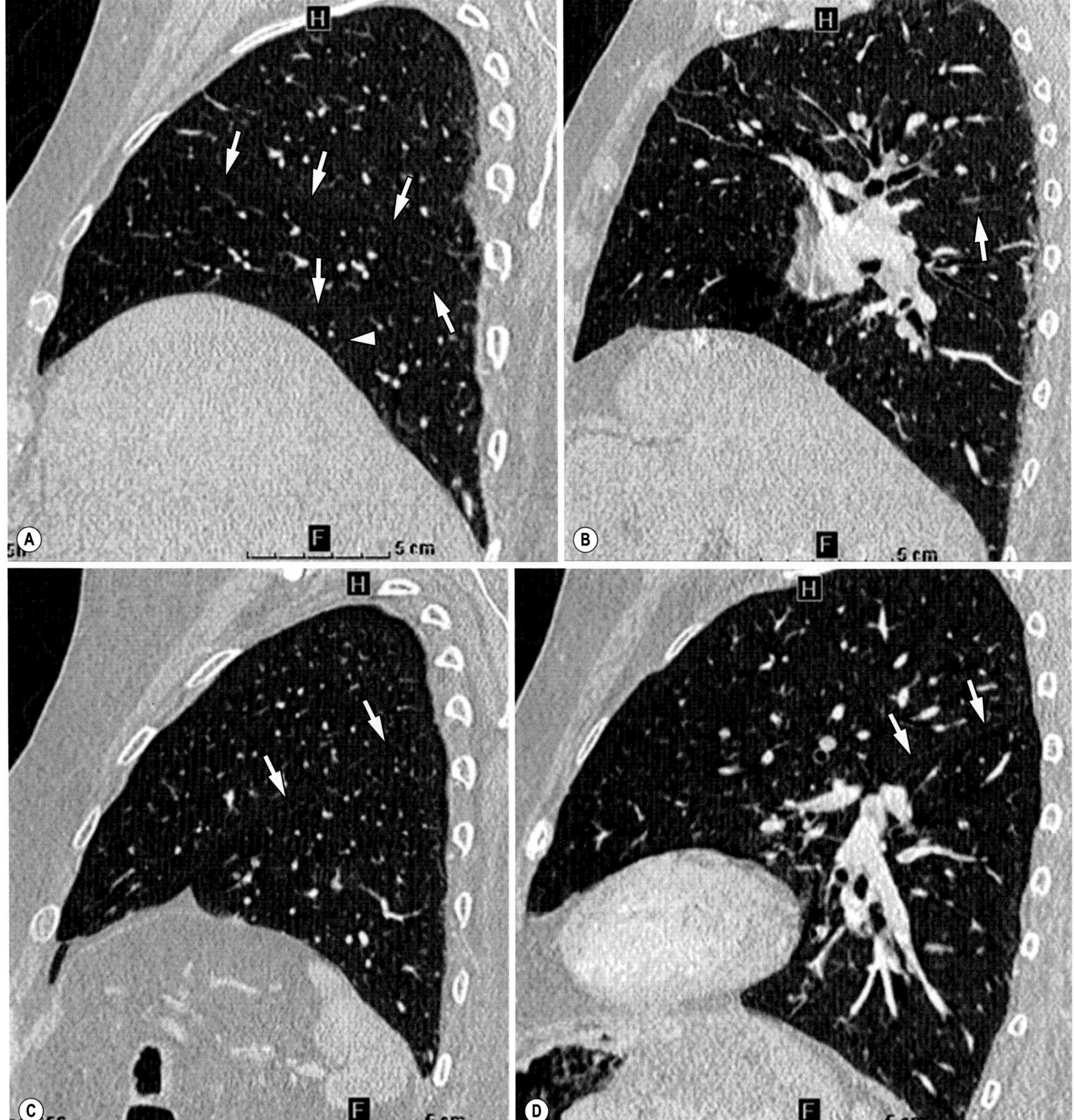

FIGURE 2-2 The position of fissures is often best shown in additional sagittal reformats (arrows) taken of the right lung (A, B) and the left lung (C, D). Note the course of the major and minor fissures together with an accessory cardiac fissure on the right (arrowhead), and the major fissure on the left (arrows).

lobe, usually the right, separating the medial and anterior basal segments. This fissure runs obliquely upward and medially towards the hilum from the diaphragm.

The inferior pulmonary ligaments[5] are pleural reflections from the mediastinum which hang down from the hila and are analogous in shape to many peritoneal reflections. These two layers of pleura may extend down to the diaphragm or may have a free inferior edge. The intersegmental septum of the lower lobe, a septum within the lung immediately beneath the inferior pulmonary ligament, is often visible on CT (Fig. 2-4).[6] When the inferior pulmonary ligament reaches the diaphragm it may contain a small amount of fat. This may efface the diaphragm, resulting in a juxtaphrenic peak. Otherwise, neither the intersegmental septum nor the inferior pulmonary ligament is visible on plain radiographs.

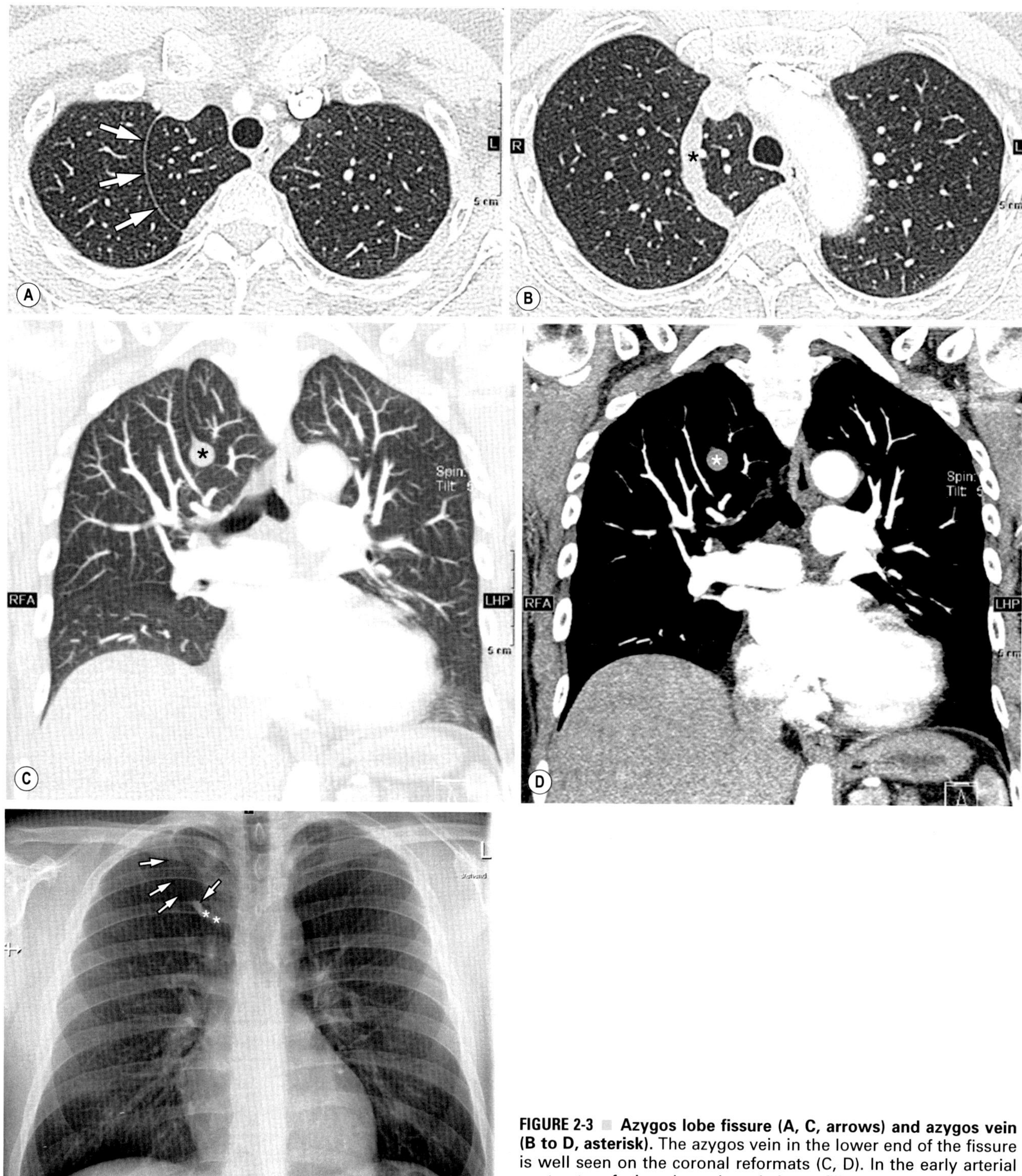

FIGURE 2-3 ■ Azygos lobe fissure (A, C, arrows) and azygos vein (B to D, asterisk). The azygos vein in the lower end of the fissure is well seen on the coronal reformats (C, D). In the early arterial contrast perfusion phase the vein is not filled with contrast media (D) displaying a soft-tissue-like attenuation. Occasionally on conventional plain film radiography (E) the course of the azygos vein from the mediastinum to the lower end of the fissure (arrowhead) can be appreciated as a vascular band (asterisk).

THE CENTRAL AIRWAYS

The trachea is a straight tube that, in children and young adults, passes inferiorly and posteriorly in the midline. In subjects with unfolding and ectasia of the aorta the trachea may deviate to the right and may also bow forward. In cross-section the trachea is usually round, oval or oval with a flattened posterior margin. Maximum coronal and sagittal diameters in adults on plain chest radiography are 21 and 23 mm, respectively, for women,

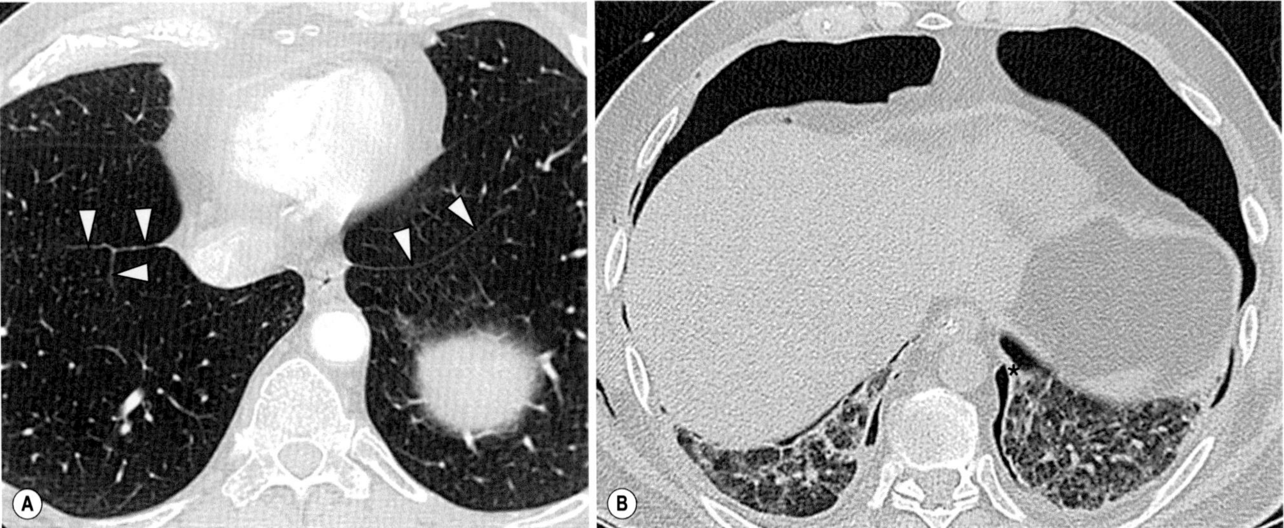

FIGURE 2-4 ■ Intersegmental bilateral septa deep to the inferior pulmonary ligament (A). Note the bifurcated T-shape of the septum on the right indicating the boundaries of the segments 9 and 10 (arrowheads). The function of the inferior pulmonary ligament fixating the lower lobe to the paraoesophageal mediastinum (asterisk) is well appreciated in another patient with pneumothorax (B).

and 25 and 27 mm for men.[7] On CT, which allows precise assessment of diameters and cross-sectional areas without magnification, the mean transverse diameter is 15.2 mm (SD 1.4) for women and 18.2 mm (SD 1.2) for men, the lower limit of normal being 12.3 mm for women, and 15.9 mm for men.[8] The diameters in growing children and young adults have been documented.[9] Calcification of the cartilage rings of the trachea is a common normal finding after the age of 40 years, increasing in frequency with age. The trachea divides into the two mainstem bronchi at the carina. In children the angles are symmetrical, but in adults the right mainstem bronchus has a steeper course than the left. The range of angles is wide, and alterations in angle can be diagnosed only by right–left comparisons, not by absolute measurement. The left main bronchus extends up to twice as far as the right main bronchus before giving off its upper lobe division.

The lobar and segmental branching pattern is shown in Fig. 2-5. There are many variations of the segmental and subsegmental branches.[10,11] Airways to subsegmental level can be routinely identified on volumetric thin-collimation CT.

THE LUNGS BEYOND THE HILA

The usual method of deciding normal lung density in the frontal view is by comparison with equivalent areas on the opposite side. Since this is not possible on the lateral chest radiograph, the detection of subtle densities is more difficult, but the density over the spine should decrease gradually as the eye travels down the spine until the diaphragm is reached. Certain other comparisons can be made, but are less reliable: the density of the high retrosternal areas is approximately equal to that of the area immediately posterior to the left ventricle; the density over the heart is usually similar to that over the shoulders; and, apart from the cardiac fat pads and overlying ribs, there should be no abrupt change in density over the heart shadow.

The segmental bronchi divide into smaller and smaller divisions until after 6–20 divisions they become bronchioles and no longer contain cartilage in their walls. The bronchioles divide and the last of the purely conducting airways are known as the terminal bronchioles, beyond which lie the alveoli. The walls of the segmental bronchi are invisible on the chest radiograph unless seen end-on, when they may cause ring shadows (Fig. 2-6).

The acinus, which is 5–6 mm in diameter, comprises respiratory bronchioles, alveolar ducts and alveoli. The acini are grouped together in lobules of three to five acini, which, in the lung periphery, are separated by septa and together compose the secondary pulmonary lobule. These peripheral interlobular septa, when thickened by disease, are the so-called septal or Kerley B lines.

The bronchopulmonary segments are based on the divisions of the bronchi. The boundaries between segments are complex in shape and have been likened to the pieces of a three-dimensional (3D) jigsaw puzzle; there is no septation between them (except in the rare instance of a patient with accessory fissures). Atelectasis or pneumonia may predominate in one or other segment, but rarely conforms precisely to the whole of just one segment, since collateral air drift occurs across the segmental boundary. The position of the segments as seen on standard radiographs is illustrated in Fig. 2-7.

The pulmonary blood vessels (Fig. 2-8) are responsible for branching linear markings within the lungs on both conventional radiographs and CT. It is not possible to distinguish arteries from veins in the outer two-thirds of the lungs on plain radiographs. Centrally, the orientations of the arteries and veins differ: the lower lobe veins run more horizontally and the lower lobe arteries more vertically. In the upper lobes, the arteries and veins show a similar gently curving vertical orientation, but the upper lobe veins lie lateral to the arteries and can

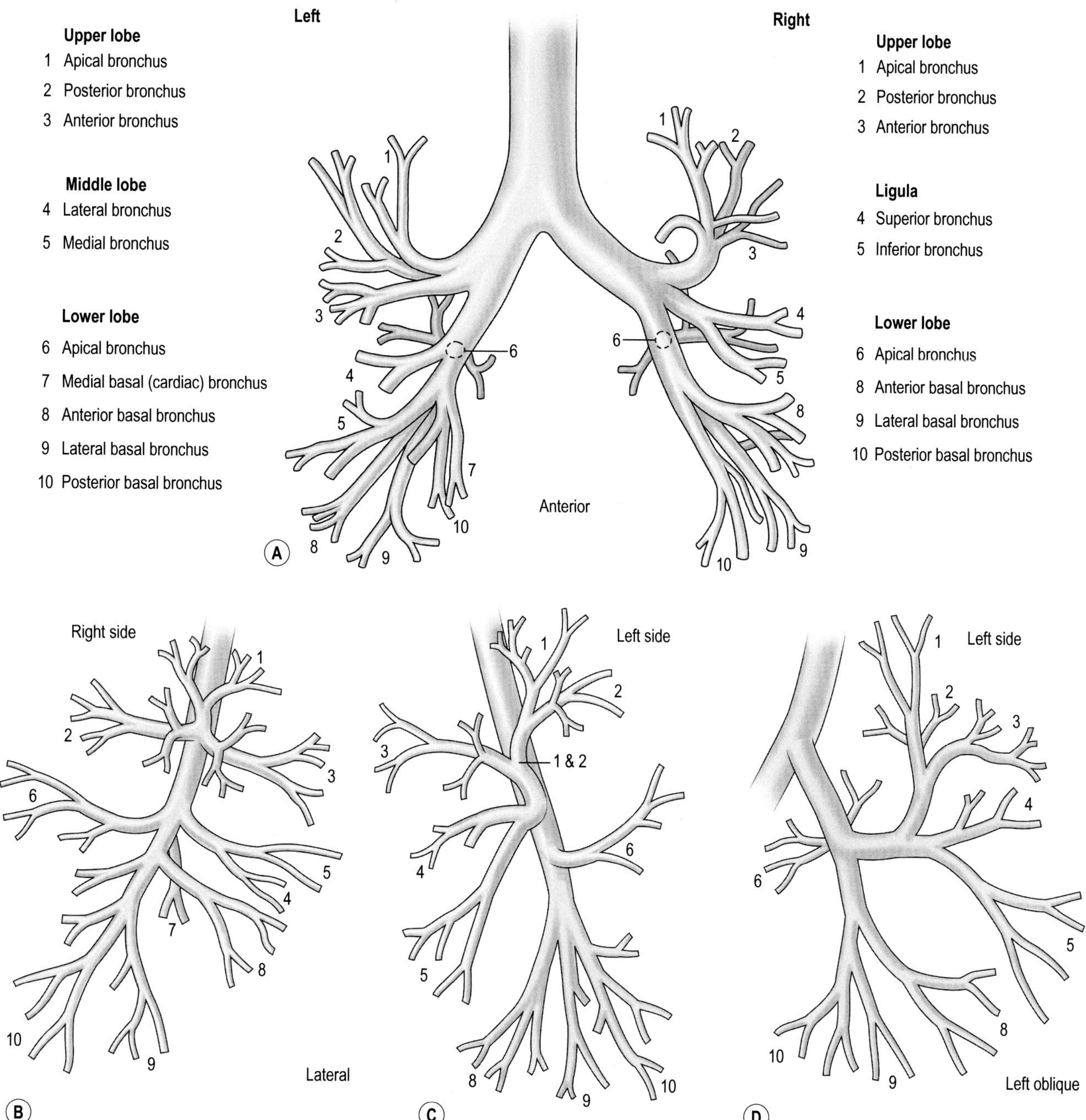

FIGURE 2-5 ■ **Diagram illustrating the anatomy of the main bronchi and segmental divisions.** The nomenclature is that approved by the British Thoracic Society. (Courtesy of the Editors of *Thorax*.)

sometimes be traced to the main venous trunk, the superior pulmonary vein.

The diameter of the blood vessels beyond the hilum varies with the position of the patient and with various haemodynamic factors. On plain chest radiographs taken in the upright position, there is a gradual increase in the relative diameter of vessels equivalent in distance from the hilum as the eye travels from apex to base. The differences are abolished when the patient lies supine. These observations correlate with physiological studies of perfusion which show that in the erect position there is a gradation of blood flow (the lower zones showing greater blood flow than the upper zones) from apex to base, a difference that is less obvious in the supine patient.

While a general statement regarding these differences in zonal blood vessel size can be made, it is difficult to draw conclusions from the size of any particular peripheral pulmonary vessel. Certain measurements have, however, been suggested for upright chest radiographs:

1. The artery and bronchus of the anterior segment of either or both upper lobes are frequently seen end-on. The diameter of the artery is usually much the same as the diameter of the bronchus (4–5 mm). In the authors' experience, an end-on vessel with a

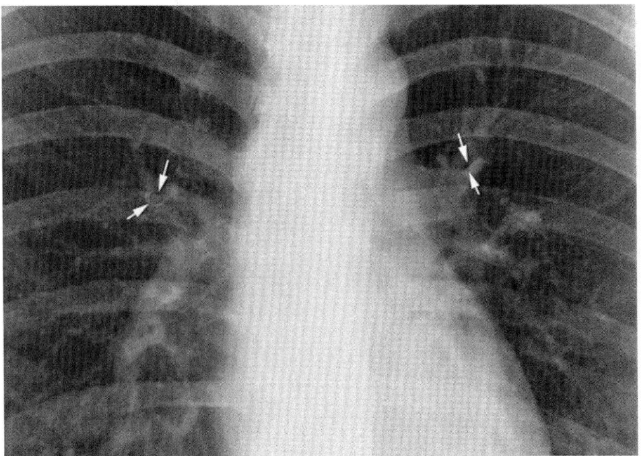

FIGURE 2-6 ■ Ring shadows (arrowheads) due to end-on bronchial projection as a normal finding on chest radiography. Note the delicate appearance in a patient without interstitial oedema.

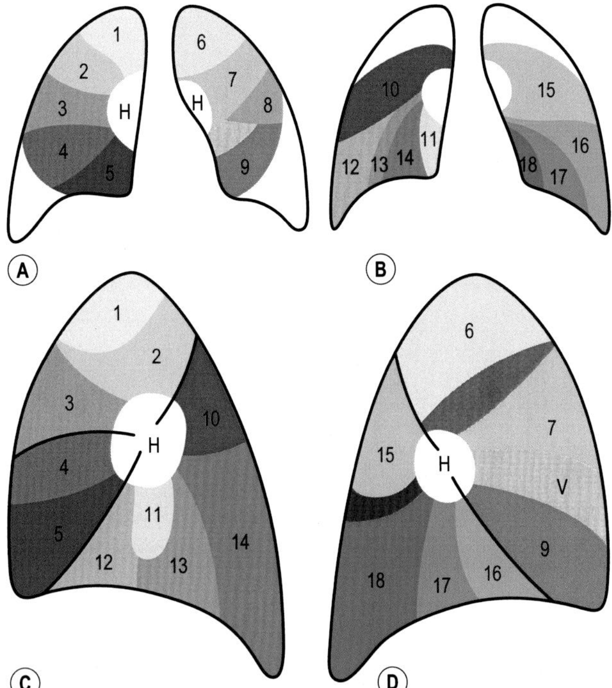

FIGURE 2-7 ■ Diagrams of position of segments seen on plain frontal and lateral chest radiographs. There is substantial overlap of the projected images of the segments in both views; this overlap is worse in the frontal than the lateral projection. (A) shows only the segments in the upper lobes and the middle lobe; (B) shows only the segments in the lower lobes; (C, D) show all the segments in the right and left lung, respectively, in the lateral view. H = hila, 1 = apical segment of right upper lobe (RUL), 2 = posterior segment of RUL, 3 = anterior segment of RUL, 4 = lateral segment of right middle lobe (RML), 5 = medial segment of RML, 6 = apical posterior segment of left upper lobe (LUL), 7 = anterior segment of LUL, 8 = superior segment of lingula, 9 = inferior segment of lingula, 10 = apical (superior) segment of right lower lobe (RLL), 11 = medial basal segment of RLL, 12 = anterior basal segment of RLL, 13 = lateral basal segment of RLL, 14 = posterior basal segment of RLL, 15 = apical (superior) segment of left lower lobe (LLL), 16 = anterior basal segment of LLL, 17 = lateral basal segment of LLL, 18 = posterior basal segment of LLL.

diameter of over 1.5 times the diameter of the adjacent bronchus indicates that the vessel is increased in size.

2. Vessels in the first anterior interspace should not exceed 3 mm in diameter.

A rich network of lymphatic vessels drains the lung and pleura to the hilar lymph nodes. The subpleural lymphatics are found beneath the pleura at the junction of the interlobular septa with the pleura. These vessels connect with each other and with the lymphatic vessels accompanying the veins in the interlobular septa. Lymph then flows to the hilum via deep lymphatic channels that run peribronchially and in the deep septa of the lungs. In normal circumstances the lymphatic network is invisible radiographically but when thickened the septa are seen as line shadows known as septal or Kerley lines. Thickened interlobular septa correspond to Kerley B lines and thickened deep septa correspond to Kerley A lines.

There are a few intrapulmonary lymph nodes, but they are small and cannot be identified on a chest radiograph but may be seen as small, peripherally located ellipsoid nodules on CT.[12,13]

THE HILA

Understanding the normal hilum on plain radiography, CT and magnetic resonance imaging (MRI) requires an appreciation of the anatomy of the major blood vessels (Figs. 2-9 to 2-13).

On plain radiograph and CT the densities of the normal hilum are due mainly to blood vessels (Figs. 2-9D to 2-11 and 2-13). Normal lymph nodes cannot be recognised as discrete structures, and the bronchial walls contribute little to the bulk of the hila, being thin and easily recognised for what they are. On MRI (Fig. 2-14), the lack of signal from fast-flowing blood within the vessels or from air in the bronchi means that there is relatively little signal generated from normal hilar structures on standard spin-echo sequences. The only signal will be from slow-flowing blood in the vessels (Fig. 2-14E), from the bronchial walls and from the fat and hilar nodes. Normal lymph nodes of just a few millimetres in size are often evident as discrete structures on modern multidetector CT. The major points to remember when viewing the hila (Fig. 2-15) are the following:

1. The transverse diameter of the lower lobe arteries before their segmental divisions can be determined with reasonable accuracy: they measure 9–16 mm on the normal postero-anterior (PA) chest radiograph (Fig. 2-11).
2. The posterior walls of the right main bronchus and its division into the right upper lobe bronchus and bronchus intermedius are outlined by air and appear as a thin stripe on lateral plain radiographs (Fig. 2-13) and on CT (Fig. 2-12). The posterior walls of the equivalent bronchi on the left are rarely visible on the plain radiograph because the left lower lobe artery intervenes between the lung and the bronchial tree. The lung does, in fact, frequently invaginate between the left lower lobe artery and the descending aorta to contact the

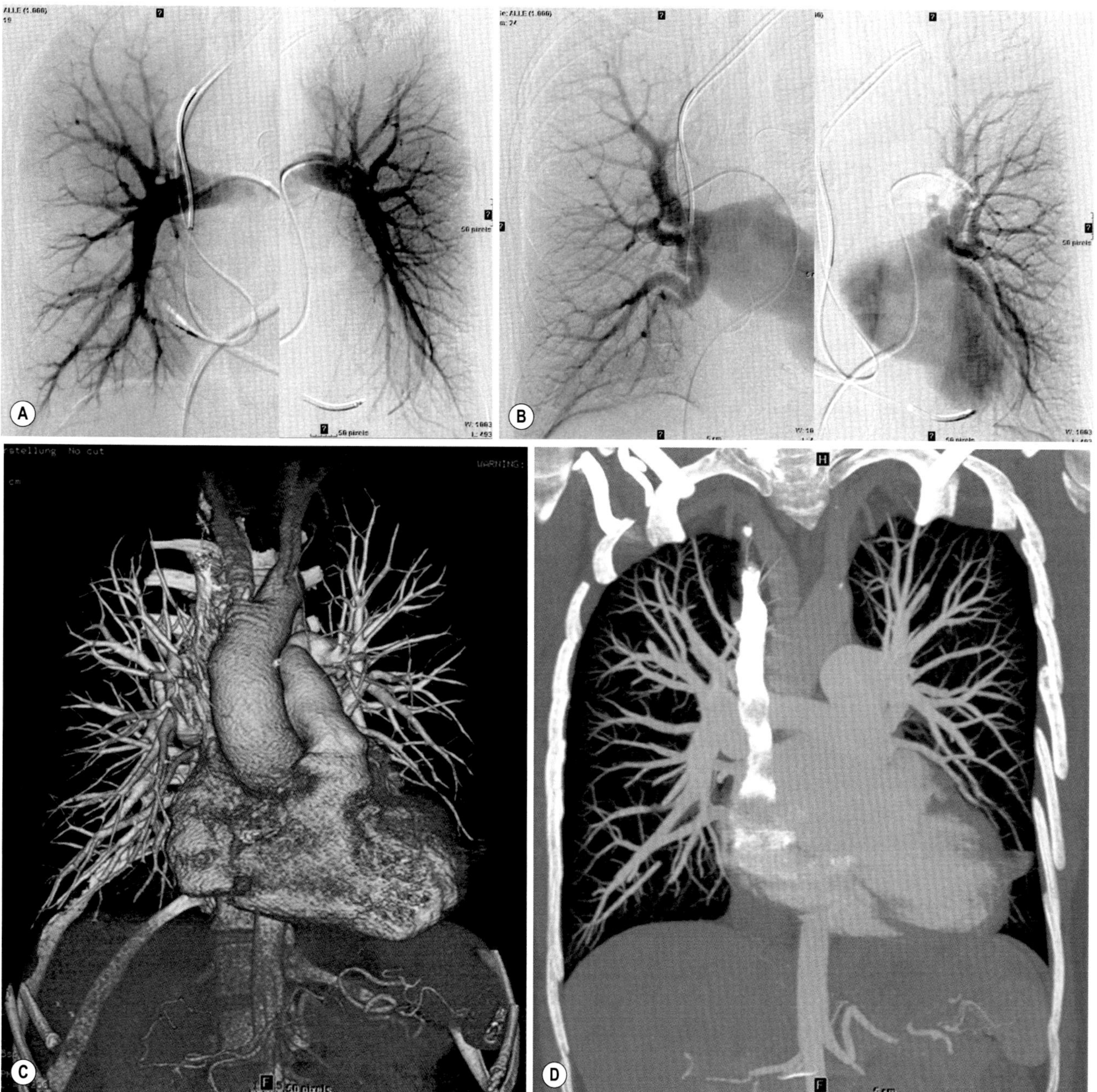

FIGURE 2-8 ■ **Pulmonary angiography.** Conventional digital subtraction angiography using selective right and left injections (A, B). Composed image obtained during (A) the arterial phase and (B) the venous phase. Note the difference in arrangement of the central arteries and veins, whereas anatomic differences are not perceptible in the lung periphery. Also note the biventricular ICD device overlying the projection in this patient with cardiac arrhythmia. On CT pulmonary angiography the anatomical relation of arterial and venous systems can be appreciated interactively on one image using volume rendering (C) or thick-slab maximum intensity imaging (D).

posterior wall of the left lower lobe bronchus, but this is usually only visible on CT or MRI.

3. The right pulmonary artery passes anterior to the major bronchi, whereas the left pulmonary artery arches superior to the left main bronchus (Figs. 2-8C, D and 2-9A). The central portion of the right hilum consists of a combination of the right pulmonary artery and the superior pulmonary vein. Since these two vessels are immediately adjacent to one another (on the left, the left main bronchus lies between them), they may be responsible for a density that is sufficiently great to be confused with a mass on lateral plain radiographs and even, on occasion, on CT.
4. On lateral chest radiographs the angles between the middle and right lower lobe bronchi on the right, and the upper and lower lobe bronchi on the left, do not contain any large end-on vessels; a rounded

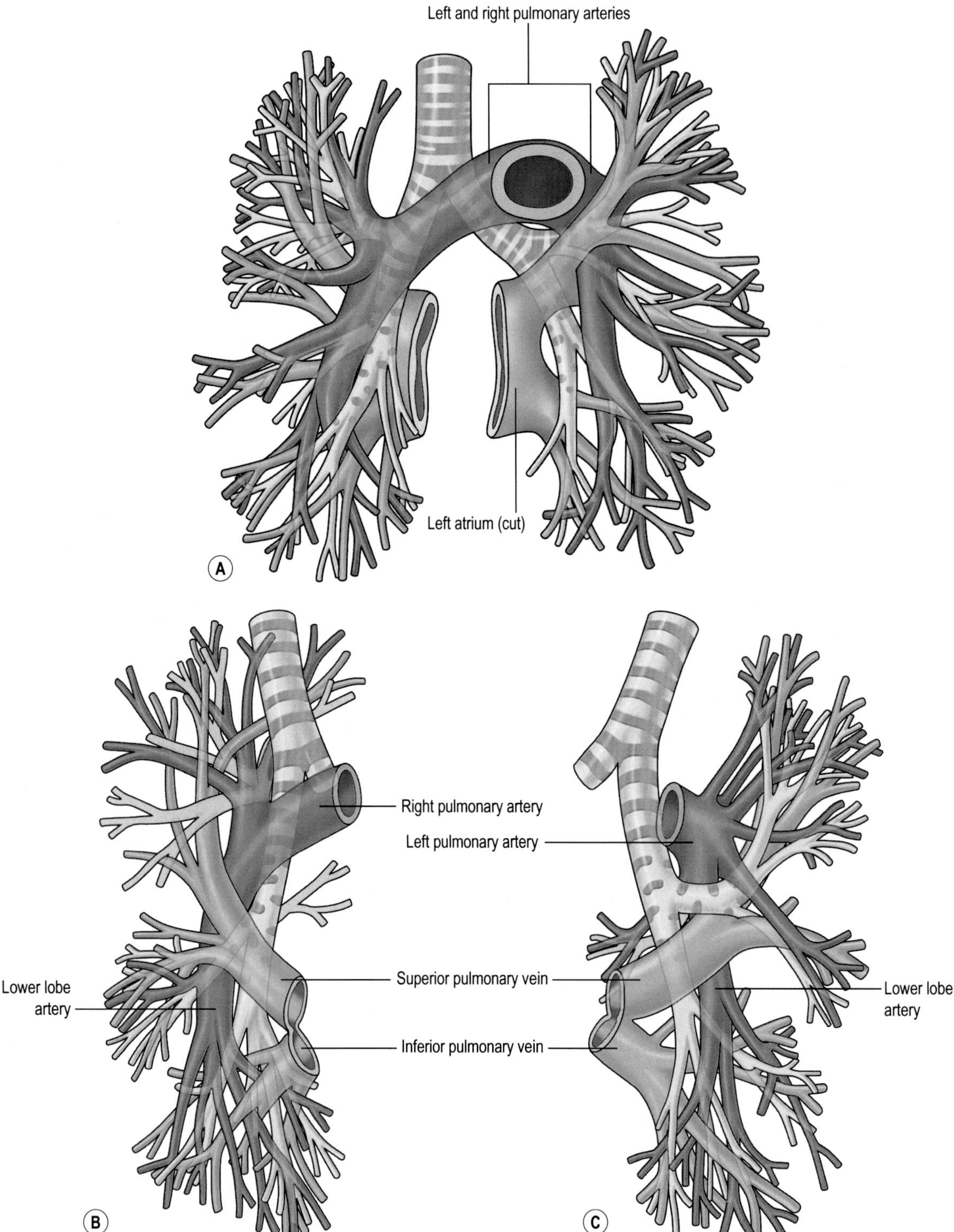

FIGURE 2-9 ■ **Diagrams of the relationships between the hilar blood vessels and bronchi.** (A) Frontal view. (B) Right posterior oblique view of right hilum. (C) Left posterior oblique view of left hilum.

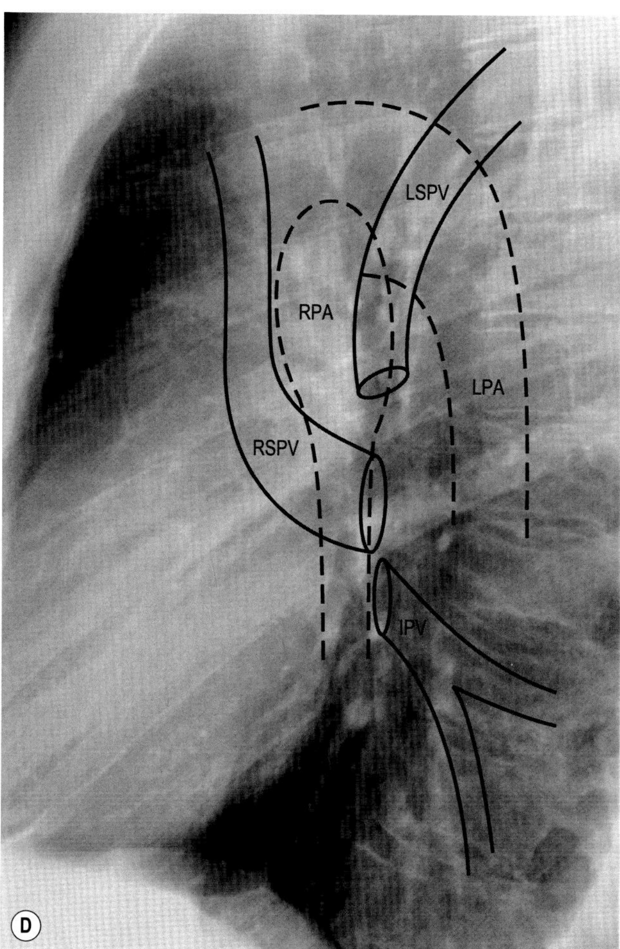

FIGURE 2-9, Continued ■ (D) Lateral chest radiograph with major blood vessels drawn in. IPV = inferior pulmonary vein—only one has been drawn in since they are superimposed, LPA = left pulmonary artery, LSPV = left superior pulmonary vein, RPA = right pulmonary artery, RSPV = right superior pulmonary vein. (Diagrams drawn by Ron Ervin and reproduced with permission from Armstrong P (ed) 1983 Critical problems in diagnostic radiology. Lippincott, Philadelphia.)

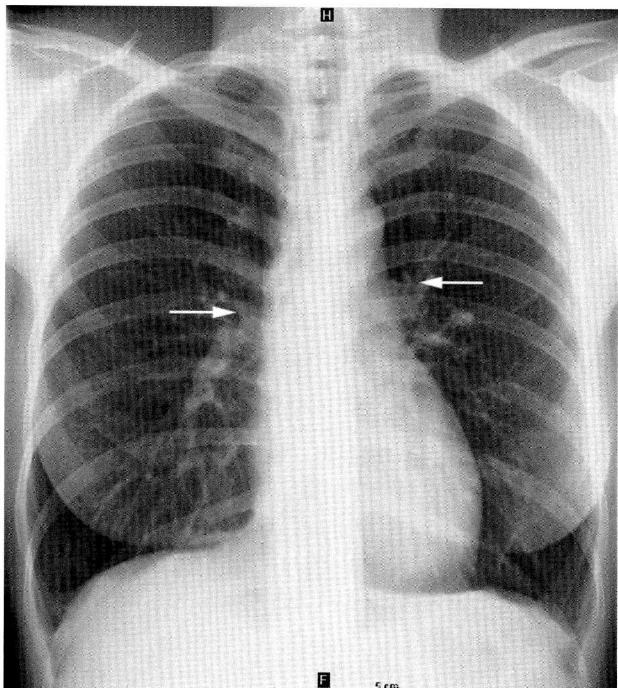

FIGURE 2-10 ■ Normal digital PA chest radiograph demonstrating position and density of the hilar structures. Arrows indicate the hilar points where the superior pulmonary vein crosses the descending lower lobe artery, the left normally being level with or slightly higher than the right.

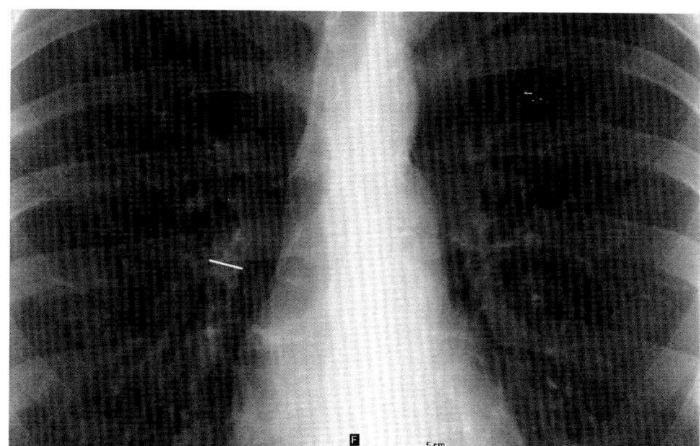

FIGURE 2-11 ■ Frontal view of the hila in a plain chest radiograph. The measurement points for the diameter of the right lower lobe artery are indicated.

shadow of greater than 1 cm in these angles is, therefore, unlikely to be a normal vessel.[14]

5. The pulmonary veins are similar on the two sides (Fig. 2-9). The superior pulmonary vein is the anterior structure in the upper and mid-hilum on both sides. Since, however, the central portions of the pulmonary arteries are so differently organised on the two sides, the relationships of the major veins to the arteries differ. On the right the superior pulmonary vein is separated from the central bronchi by the lower division of the right pulmonary artery, whereas on the left the superior pulmonary vein is separated from the pulmonary artery by the bronchial tree.

Both inferior pulmonary veins travel obliquely anteriorly and superiorly, inferior to the branches of the left lower lobe artery, to enter the left atrium. They are slightly posterior to the plane of the left lower lobe bronchi. They may be seen either end-on or in oblique cross-section in PA, lateral and oblique projections and may, therefore, simulate a mass.

THE MEDIASTINUM

The radiographic anatomy of the mediastinum can be described from many points of view, depending on the technique that is under discussion. In this chapter only plain radiographs, CT and MRI will be considered in any detail, CT and MRI being illustrated first because an appreciation of the cross-sectional anatomy of the

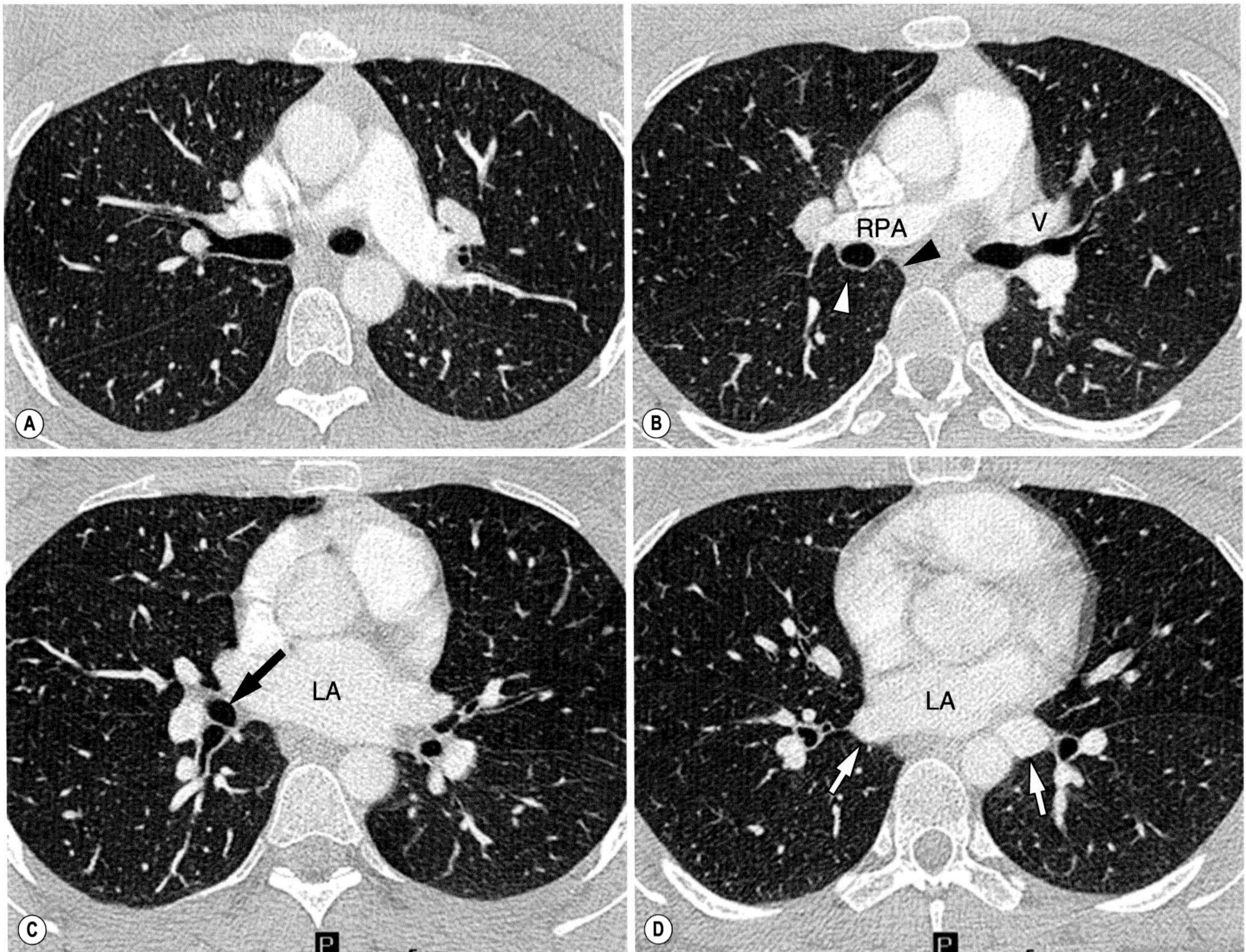

FIGURE 2-12 ■ **CT of normal hila.** High-resolution CT images (0.625 mm) have been obtained through the hilar structures during contrast medium injection and displayed on lung windows (L-500, W 1500). (A) Section just below the tracheal carina at the origin of the right upper lobe bronchus, immediately posterior to the upper lobe vein (v). (B) Section through level of right main pulmonary artery (RPA) and bronchus intermedius (arrowhead). Note the tongue of lung that contacts the left main bronchus between the aorta (B) and the left lower lobe artery (black arrowhead). Note also that the right lung contacts the posterior wall of the bronchus intermedius as it extends into the azygo-oesophageal recess. (C) Section through the level of the middle lobe bronchus (long arrow) at the point of origin of the bronchus to the superior segment of the right lower lobe. Note that the middle lobe bronchus separates the right lower lobe artery from the right superior pulmonary vein as it enters the left atrium (LA). The lung contacts the posterior wall of the right lower lobe bronchus as it extends into the azygo-oesophageal recess. (D) Section through the level of the inferior pulmonary veins (arrows). At this level the lower lobe arteries have bilaterally divided into basal segmental divisions; each are less than 10 mm in diameter.

mediastinum helps in understanding the appearances on plain chest radiographs.

The mediastinum is conventionally divided into superior, anterior, middle and posterior compartments. The exact anatomical boundaries of these divisions are unimportant to the radiologist (indeed, they vary according to different authors), since they do not provide a clear-cut guide to disease and their boundaries do not form any barriers to the spread of the disease.

Computed Tomography and Magnetic Resonance Imaging

The blood vessels, trachea and main bronchi make up the bulk of the mediastinum, and the CT/MRI anatomy of these structures is illustrated in Figs. 2-12 to 2-16.

The thymus is situated anterior to the aorta and right ventricular outflow tract or pulmonary artery; it is often best appreciated on a section through the aortic arch or great vessels (Figs. 2-12, 2-16 and 2-17). Before puberty[15] the thymus fills in most of the mediastinum in front of the great vessels. During this period of life the gland varies so greatly in size that measurement is of little value in deciding normality. Approximate symmetry is the rule. Also, the thymus fills in the spaces between the great vessels and the anterior chest wall as if moulded by these structures. In adults the thymus is bilobed or triangular in shape. The maximum width and thickness of each lobe decreases with advancing age. Between the ages of 20 and 50, the average thickness as measured by CT decreases from 8–9 mm to 5–6 mm, the maximum thickness of each lobe being up to 15 mm. These diameters are

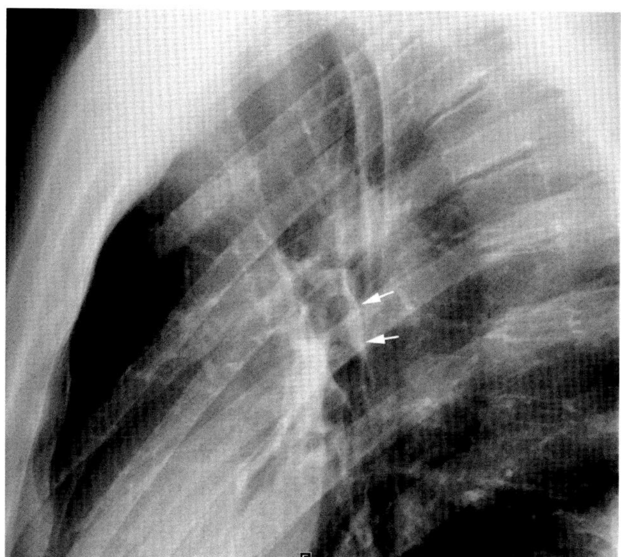

FIGURE 2-13 ■ **Lateral view of the hila showing normal thickness of the posterior wall of the bronchus intermedius (arrows).**

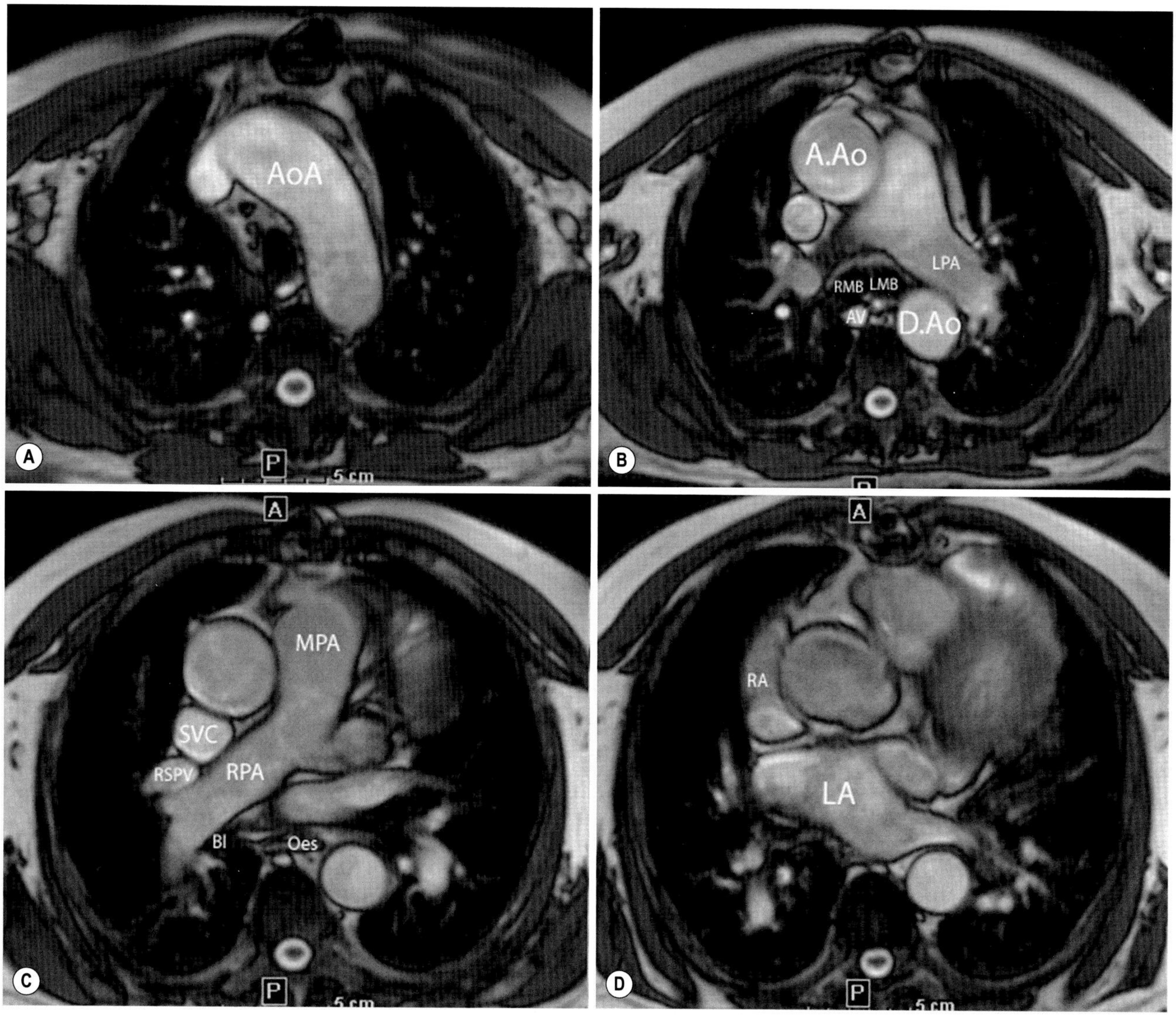

FIGURE 2-14 ■ **MRI of normal mediastinum and hila.** Four transverse and four coronal sections have been chosen to show the important anatomical features: (A–D, G, H) gradient echo post gadolinium iv; (E, F) T1-weighted gradient echo sequence). (A) is 1 cm above the tracheal carina; (B) is just below (A); (C) is at the level of the right main pulmonary artery; (D) is at the level of the mid left atrium. A.Ao = ascending aorta; AV = azygos vein; BI = bronchus intermedius; D.Ao = descending aorta; LA = left atrium; LCA = left carotid artery; LMB = left main bronchus; LPA = left pulmonary artery; LV = left ventricle; MPA = main pulmonary artery; Oes = oesophagus; RA = right atrium; RMB = right main bronchus; RSPV = right superior pulmonary vein; SVC = superior vena cava; T = trachea.

Continued on following page

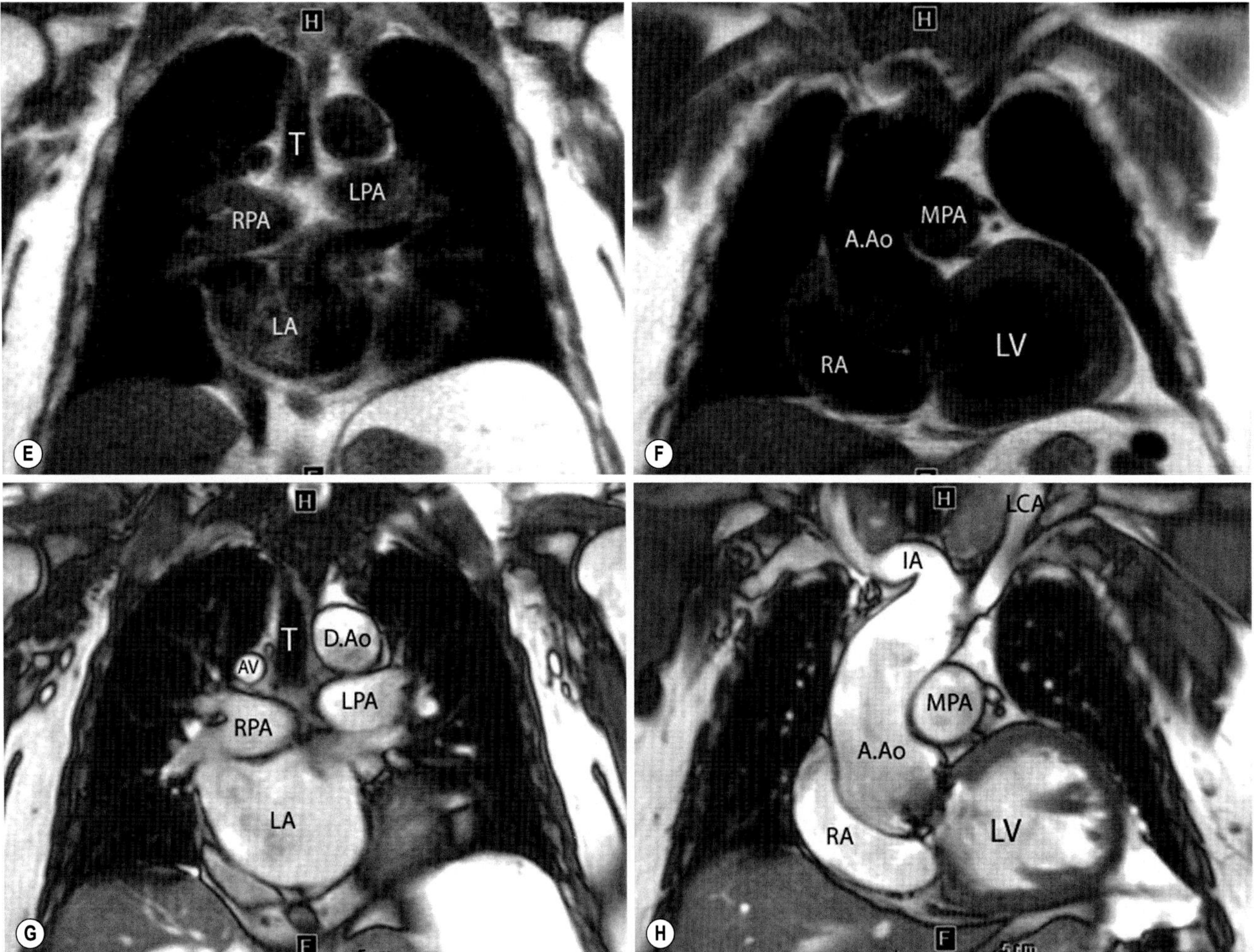

FIGURE 2-14, Continued

greater on MRI, presumably because MRI demonstrates the thymic tissue even when it is partially replaced by fat. On MRI, sagittal images demonstrate the gland to be 5–7 cm long in its craniocaudad dimension.

In younger patients, the CT density of the thymus is homogeneous and close to that of other soft tissues, but after puberty the density gradually decreases owing to fatty replacement, so that above 40 years of age the thymus usually has an attenuation value identical to that of fat and is often indistinguishable from the adjacent mediastinal fat, apart from some residual thymic parenchyma, which may be visible as streaky or nodular densities within the fat (Fig. 2-17).[16,17] On MRI the intensity of the thymus in T1-weighted images is similar to that of muscle and appreciably lower than that of mediastinal fat, although, as would be expected, this difference decreases with age. On T2-weighted images, the intensity differences are slight and do not vary with age.

Lymph nodes are widely distributed in the mediastinum. Ninety-five per cent of normal mediastinal lymph nodes are less than 10 mm in diameter, and the remainder, with few exceptions, are less than 15 mm in diameter.[18–22] Lymph nodes in the paraspinal areas, in the region of the brachiocephalic veins and in the space behind the diaphragmatic crura are generally smaller, 6 mm or less, whereas nodes in the aortopulmonary window, pretracheal and lower paratracheal spaces and subcarinal compartment are often 6–10 mm in diameter.

Lymph nodes encircle the trachea and main bronchi except where the aorta, pulmonary artery or oesophagus is in direct contact with the airway. There is no clear division between the various nodes, but they can be categorised according to site.

The nomenclature of mediastinal lymph nodes should accord with the international lymph node map in the seventh edition of the TNM classification for lung cancer proposed by the International Association for the Study of Lung Cancer (IASLC)[23,24] (Figs. 2-18, 2-19; Table 2-1). This classification groups nodal stations into seven anatomic zones: supraclavicular, upper, aortopulmonary, subcarinal, lower, hilar and peripheral. The supraclavicular zone extends from the lower margin of the cricoids cartilage to the clavicles and, in the midline, the upper border of the manubrium (station 1R, right-sided nodes; station 1L, left-sided nodes). The upper zone includes

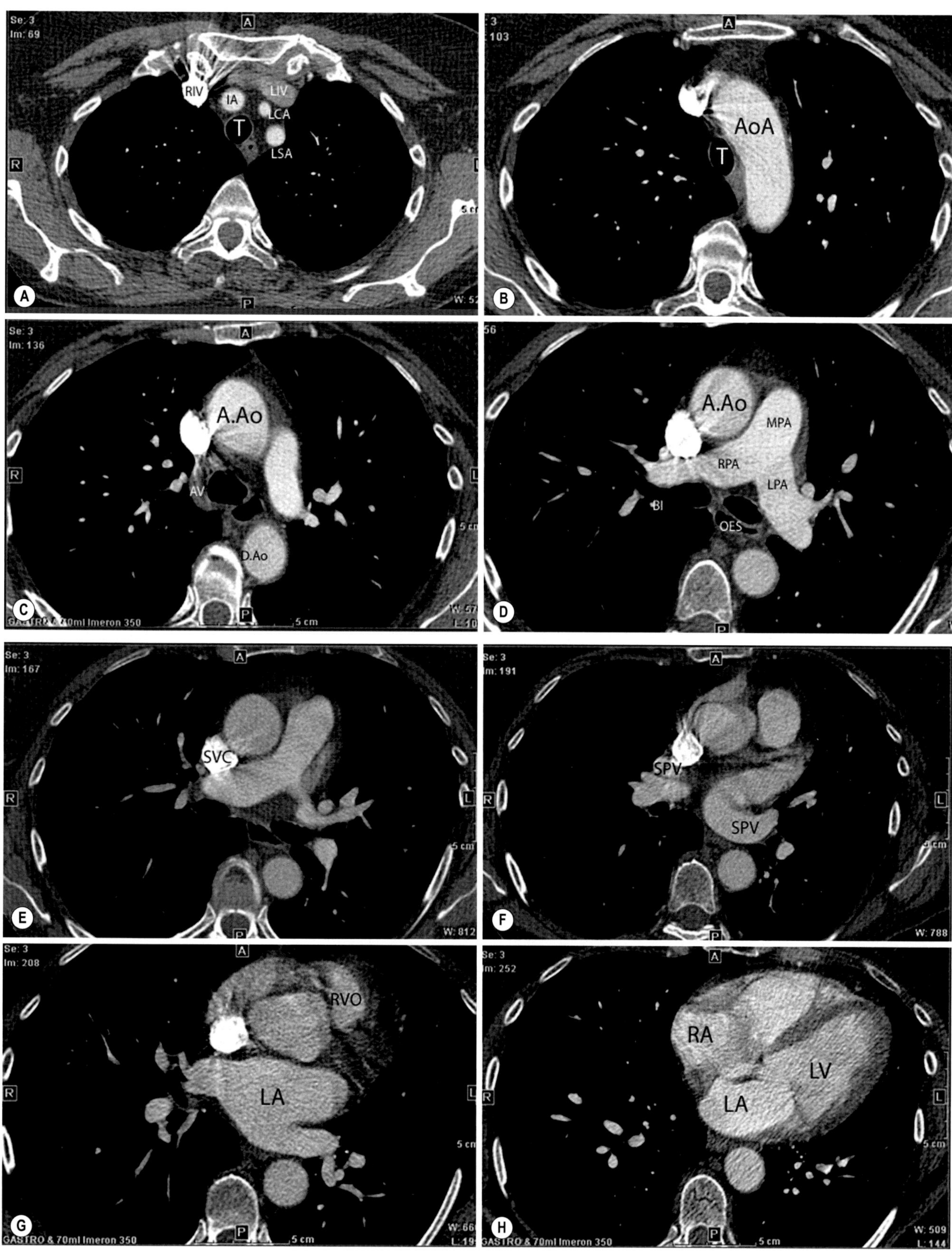

FIGURE 2-15 ■ **CT of normal mediastinum.** (A–I) Five 1-cm-thick sections have been selected to show the important anatomical features. The level of each section is illustrated in the diagram. A.Ao = ascending aorta; AoA = aortic arch; AV = azygos vein; D.Ao = descending aorta; IA = innominate artery; LA = left atrium; LCA = left carotid artery; LIV = left innominate vein; LPA = left pulmonary artery; LSA = left subclavian artery; MPA = main pulmonary artery; OES = oesophagus; RA = right atrium; RIV = right innominate vein; RPA = right pulmonary artery; RVO = right ventricular outflow tract; SPV = superior pulmonary vein; SVC = superior vena cava; T = trachea.

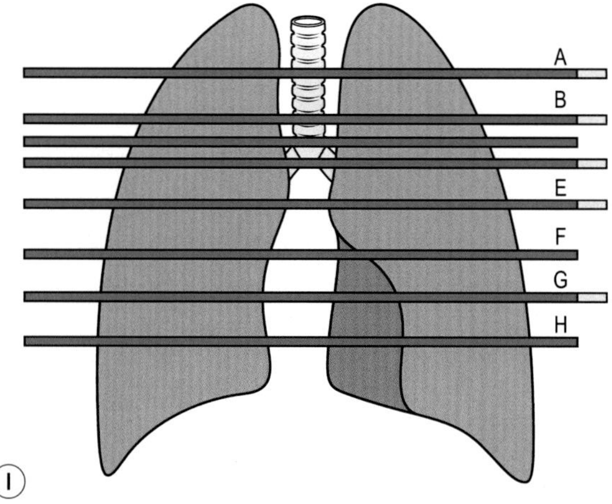

FIGURE 2-15, Continued

upper paratracheal (stations 2R and 2L, above the superior border of the aortic arch or the intersection of the innominate vein with the trachea, respectively), prevascular (station 3a), retrotracheal (station 3p) and lower paratracheal nodes (station 4R, station 4L, below the superior border of the aortic arch or the intersection of the innominate vein with the trachea, respectively). Aortopulmonary window nodes (stations 5, 6) lie subaortic or paraaortic; subcarinal nodes (station 7) lie beneath the main bronchi within the mediastinal pleura, but superior to the upper border of the lower lobe bronchus (left) or the bronchus intermedius (right). The lower zone extends downwards to the diaphragm and includes paraesophageal (station 8) and pulmonary ligament nodes (station 9). Nodes are also present in the hila (station 10), and in the lung periphery (stations 12–14).

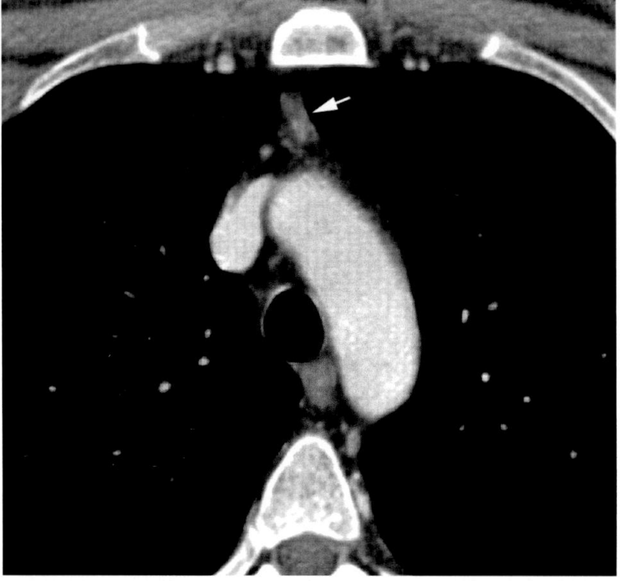

FIGURE 2-16 CT of normal thymus (arrow) in a young adult man.

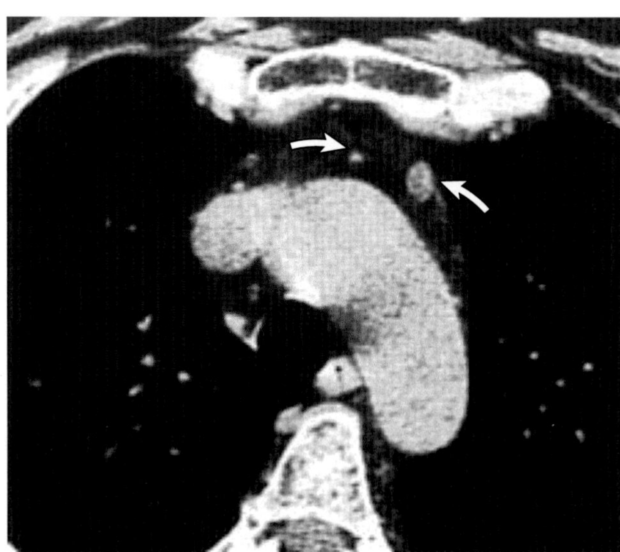

FIGURE 2-17 Thymic residues (curved arrows) shown by CT.

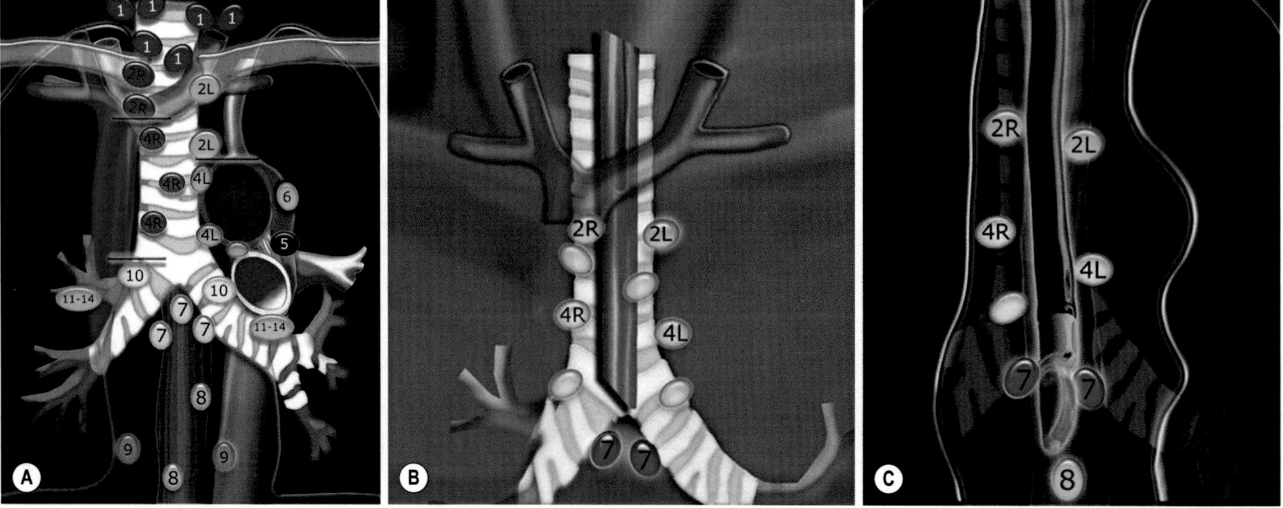

FIGURE 2-18 The International Association for the Study of Lung Cancer (IASLC) lymph node map grouping the lymph node stations into 'zones' for purpose of prognostic analysis (from: <http://www.radiologyassistant.nl/en/4646f1278c26f>). Please see explanations in Table 2-1.

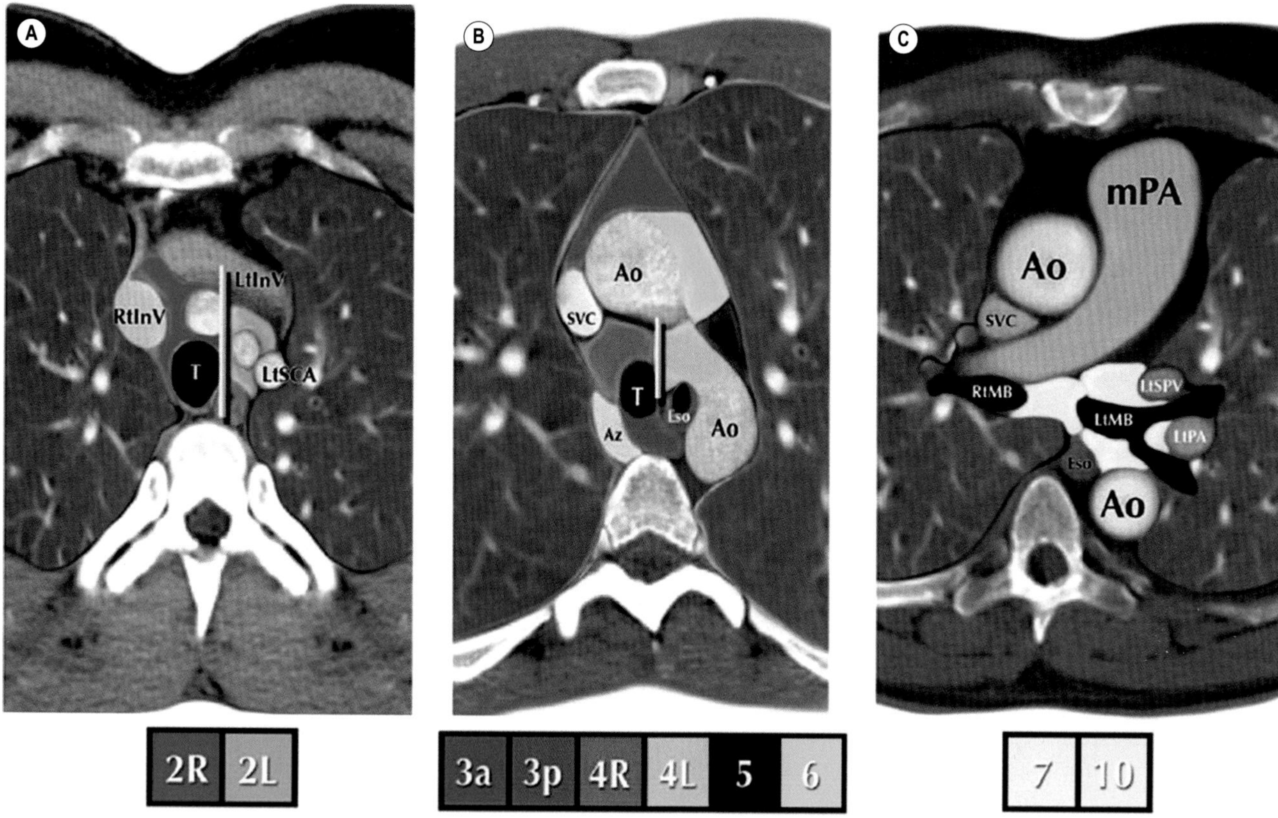

FIGURE 2-19 ■ The IASLC lymph node map can be applied to clinical staging by computed tomography in axial (A–C) views. The border between the right and left paratracheal region is shown in (A) and (B). Ao = aorta; Az = azygos vein; MB = main bronchus; Eso = oesophagus; IV = innominate vein; LtInV = left innominate vein; LtSCA = left subclavian artery; PA = pulmonary artery; SPV = superior pulmonary vein; RtInV = right innominate vein; SVC = superior vena cava; T = trachea. (With permission from Rusch VW, Asamura H, Watanabe H et al 2009 The IASLC lung cancer staging project. J Thorac Oncol 4: 568–577.)

TABLE 2-1 **IASLC Map for Regional Lymph Nodes***

Zone	Side	Border	Anatomical Structure
1		Upper	Lower margin of cricoid cartilage
1		Lower	Clavicles/manubrium
1		Left/right	Midline of trachea
2R	Right	Upper	Apex of right lung/upper border of manubrium
2R	Right	Lower	Intersection of caudal margin of innominate vein with trachea/nodes to left lateral border of trachea
2L	Left	Upper	Apex of left lung/upper border of manubrium
2L	Left	Lower	Superior border of aortic arch
3a	Anterior	Upper	Apex of chest
3a	Anterior	Lower	Level of carina
3a	Anterior	Anterior	Posterior aspect of sternum
3a	Anterior	Posterior	Anterior border of superior vena cava
3a	Anterior	Upper	Apex of chest
3a	Anterior	Lower	Level of carina
3a	Anterior	Anterior	Posterior aspect of sternum
3a	Anterior	Posterior	Left carotid artery
3p	Posterior	Upper	Apex of chest
3p	Posterior	Lower	Carina
4R	Right	Para-/pretracheal—upper	Intersection of caudal margin of innominate vein with trachea
4R	Right	Right para-/pretracheal—lower	Lower border of azygos vein
4L	Left	Left paratracheal to lig. art.—upper	Upper margin of aortic arch
4L	Left	Left paratracheal to lig. art.—lower	Upper rim of left main pulmonary artery
5		Subaortic lateral to lig. art.—upper	Lower border of aortic arch
5		Subaortic lateral to lig. art.—lower	Upper rim of left main pulmonary artery
6		Anterior and lateral to ascending aorta and aortic—upper	Line tangential to upper border of aortic arch
6		Anterior and lateral to ascending aorta and aortic—lower	Lower border of aortic arch

Continued on following page

TABLE 2-1 **IASLC Map for Regional Lymph Nodes (Continued)**

Zone	Side	Border	Anatomical Structure
7		Mediastinal subcarinal—upper	Carina of trachea
7	Right	Mediastinal subcarinal—lower	Lower border of bronchus intermedius
7	Left	Mediastinal subcarinal—lower	Upper border of lower lobe bronchus
8	Right	Paraoesophageal excluding subcarinal—upper	Lower border of bronchus intermedius
8	Left	Paraoesophageal excluding subcarinal—upper	Upper border of lower lobe bronchus
8		Paraoesophageal excluding subcarinal—lower	Diaphragm
9		Within pulmonary ligament incl. inf. pulm. vein—upper	Inferior pulmonary vein
9		Within pulmonary ligament incl. inf. pulm. vein—lower	Diaphragm
10	Right	Hilar—adjacent to mainstem bronchi and hilar vessels—upper	Lower rim of azygos vein
10	Left	Hilar—adjacent to mainstem bronchi and hilar vessels—lower	Upper rim of pulmonary artery
10		Hilar—adjacent to mainstem bronchi and hilar vessels	Interlobar region bilaterally
11	Right	Interlobar—superior subgroup	a#11s: between upper lobe bronchus and bronchus intermedius
11	Right	Interlobar—inferior subgroup	a#11i: between middle and lower lobe bronchi
11	Left	Interlobar	Between upper lobe bronchus and lower lobe bronchi
12		Lobar	Adjacent to lobar bronchi
13		Segmental	Adjacent to segmental bronchi
14		Subsegmental	Adjacent to subsegmental bronchi

*International lymph node map in the seventh edition of the TNM classification for lung cancer.

The oesophagus is visible on all axial CT and MRI sections from the root of the neck down to the diaphragm. It may contain a small amount of air in approximately 80% of normal people. If there is sufficient mediastinal fat, the entire circumference of the oesophagus can be identified, and if air is present in the lumen, the uniform thickness of the wall can be appreciated. Without air, the collapsed oesophagus appears circular or oval in shape and measures approximately 1 cm in its narrowest diameter. On MRI the signal intensity on T1-weighted images is similar to that on muscle but on T2-weighted images the oesophagus often shows much higher signal intensity than muscle.

Radiographic Appearances

Plain chest radiographs provide limited information regarding mediastinal anatomy, since only the interfaces between the lung and the mediastinum are visualised (Figs. 2-9, 2-10, 2-13, and 2-20).

Junction Lines[25,26]

When there is only a small amount of fat anterior to the ascending aorta and its major branches, the two lungs may be separated anteriorly by little more than the four intervening layers of pleura. In such patients an anterior junction line is visible on frontal chest radiographs (Fig. 2-20). The line diverges and fades out superiorly and cannot be identified above the level of the clavicles. It descends for a variable distance, usually deviating to the left, but never extending lower than the point where the two lungs separate to envelop the right ventricular outflow tract.

The lungs may also come close together behind the oesophagus, forming the posterior junction line (Figs. 2-20 and 2-21). This line, unlike the anterior junction line, separates to envelop the aortic arch. It may reform below the aortic arch where the two lungs occasionally abut behind the oesophagus. Superiorly, the posterior junction line extends to the level of the lung apices where it diverges and disappears, a level appreciably higher than the medial ends of the clavicles. The differences in the superior extent of the anterior and posterior junction lines are related to the sloping boundary between the root of the neck and the thorax.

The major value of being able to identify the anterior and posterior junction lines is that a mass, or other space-occupying process, in the junctional areas can be excluded if these lines are visible. Since both junction lines are inconsistently seen, however, the *lack* of visualisation of one or both is not a reliable sign of disease.

Right Mediastinum above the Azygos Vein

The right superior mediastinal border is formed by the right brachiocephalic (innominate) vein and the superior vena cava. With aortic or brachiocephalic (innominate) artery ectasia or unfolding, either of these veins may be pushed laterally or the mediastinal border may be formed by the aorta or the right brachiocephalic artery. The right paratracheal region can be seen through the right brachiocephalic vein and superior vena cava because the lung contacts the right tracheal wall from the level of the clavicles down to the azygos vein, producing a visible stripe of uniform thickness known as the right paratracheal stripe (Fig. 2-21), between the tracheal air column and the lung. This stripe, which should be no

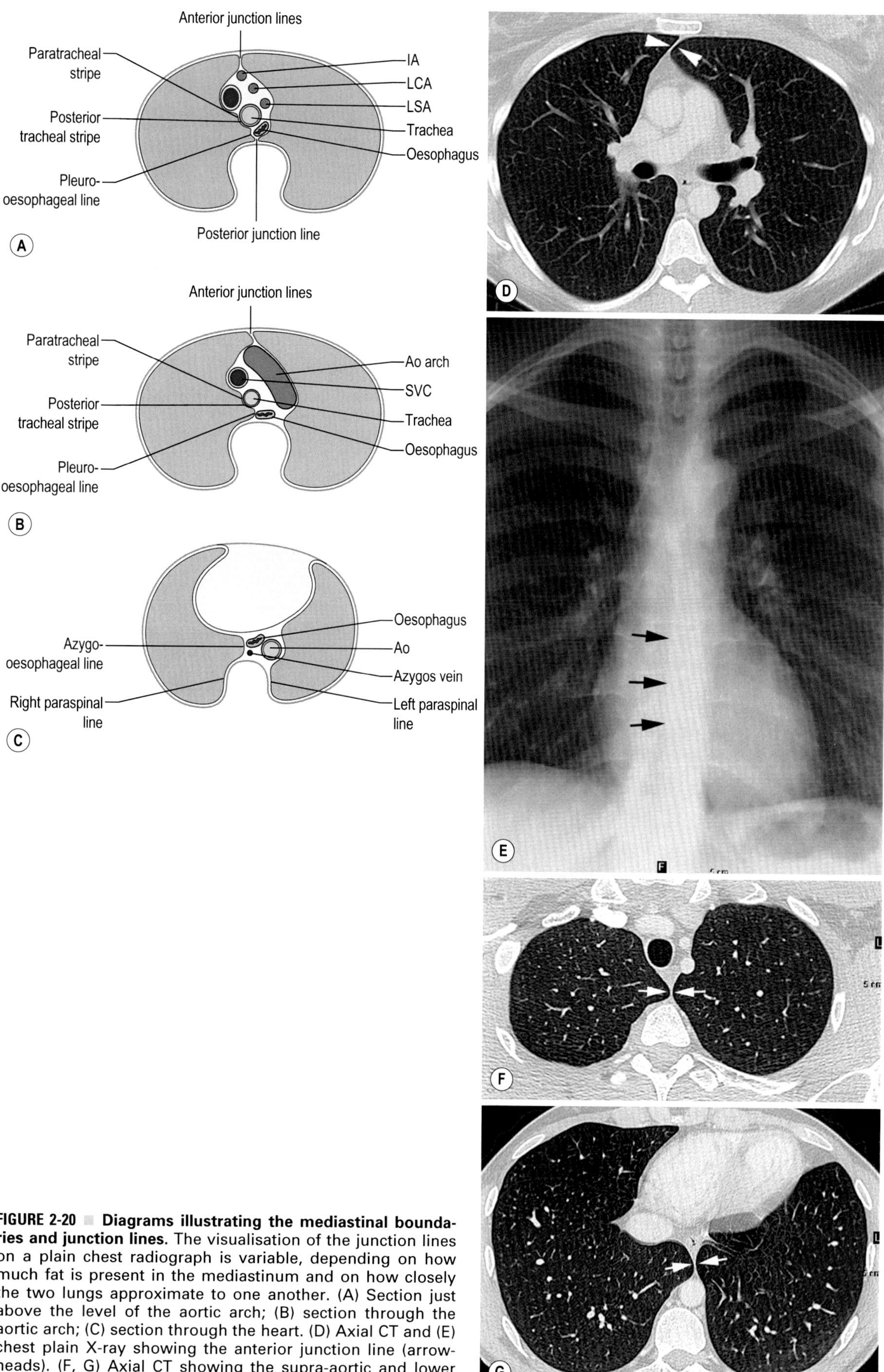

FIGURE 2-20 ■ **Diagrams illustrating the mediastinal boundaries and junction lines.** The visualisation of the junction lines on a plain chest radiograph is variable, depending on how much fat is present in the mediastinum and on how closely the two lungs approximate to one another. (A) Section just above the level of the aortic arch; (B) section through the aortic arch; (C) section through the heart. (D) Axial CT and (E) chest plain X-ray showing the anterior junction line (arrowheads). (F, G) Axial CT showing the supra-aortic and lower posterior junction line (arrows).

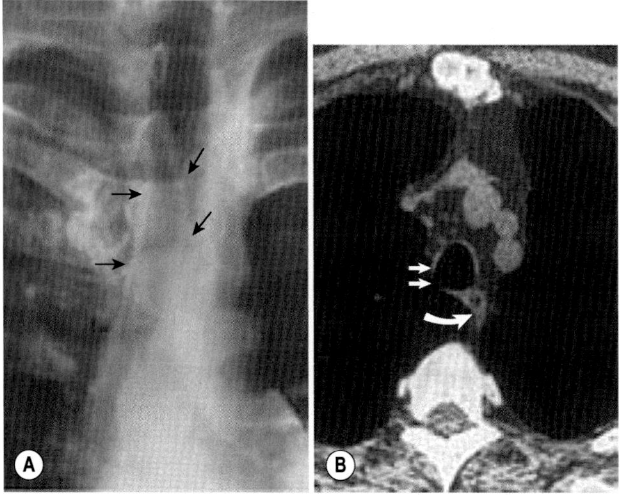

FIGURE 2-21 ■ Right tracheal stripe (straight arrows) and pleuro-oesophageal line (curved arrows) demonstrated on (A) plain radiograph and (B) unenhanced CT.

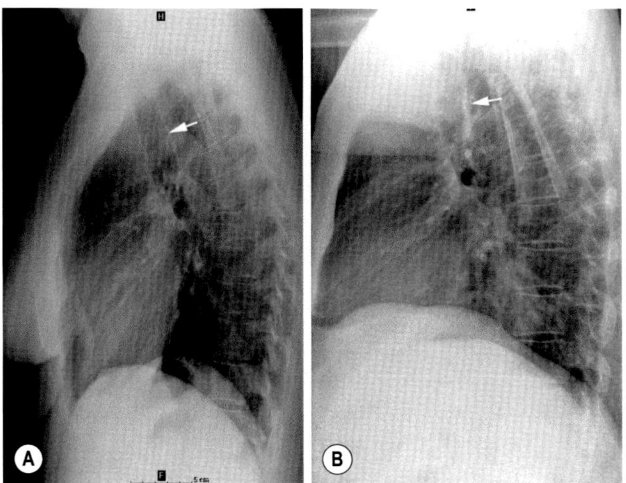

FIGURE 2-22 ■ **Lateral view of trachea and major bronchi.** (A) In this example, the posterior wall of the trachea is outlined by lung posterior to it (arrow). (B) In this example, the collapsed oesophagus is between the lung and the trachea (arrow).

more than 5 mm wide, is visible in approximately two-thirds of normal people. It consists of the wall of the trachea and the adjacent mediastinal fat, but no focal bulges because individual paratracheal lymph nodes can be seen. As with the junction lines, the diagnostic value of this stripe is that its presence excludes a space-occupying process in the area where the stripe is visible. The azygos vein is outlined by air in the lung at the lower end of the right paratracheal stripe. The diameter of the azygos vein in the tracheobronchial angle is variable: it may be considered normal when its diameter is 10 mm or less. The nodes immediately beneath the azygos vein are known as azygos nodes and are not recognisable on the normal chest radiograph.

The lung posterior to the trachea contacts the right wall of the oesophagus so that a recognisable border may be seen in the frontal projection. If the oesophagus at this level contains air, then the right wall of the oesophagus is seen as a stripe, the so-called oesophageal–pleural stripe,[27] curving superiorly and laterally behind the tracheal air column (Fig. 2-21).

In summary, on a frontal radiograph three interfaces are potentially recognisable in the right mediastinum above the azygos vein: the superior vena cava border, the right wall of the trachea and the right wall of the oesophagus.

Left Mediastinum above the Aortic Arch

The mediastinal shadow to the left of the trachea above the aortic arch is of low density and is caused by the left carotid and left subclavian arteries together with the left brachiocephalic (innominate) and jugular veins. The usual appearance on the frontal projection is a gently curving border formed by the left subclavian artery, which fades out where the artery enters the neck. A separate interface may occasionally be discernible for the left carotid artery or left brachiocephalic vein. The outer margin of the left tracheal wall is virtually never outlined, because the lung is separated from the trachea by the aorta and other vessels listed above.

Trachea and Retrotracheal Area in the Lateral View

The air column in the trachea can be seen throughout its length as it descends obliquely inferiorly and posteriorly. The course of the trachea on a normal lateral view is straight, or bowed anteriorly in patients with aortic unfolding, with no visible indentation from adjacent vessels. Small indentations into the air column of the trachea from tracheal cartilage rings may be apparent on the lateral view. The carina cannot be identified on the lateral view (though the right main bronchus is often mistaken for it). Its anterior wall is visible in a minority of patients, but the posterior wall is usually seen because lung often passes behind the trachea, thereby permitting visualisation of the posterior tracheal (stripe) band.[28] The thickness of this stripe is 2–3 mm, provided it is formed solely by the tracheal wall and pleura (Fig. 2-22). If a large amount of air is present in the oesophagus, the posterior tracheal band may be much thicker, since it then comprises the combined thicknesses of the posterior tracheal wall and the anterior oesophageal wall. Alternatively, the lung may be separated from the trachea by the full width of a collapsed oesophagus, leading to a band of density measuring 10 mm or more (Fig. 2-22).

Supra-aortic Mediastinum on the Lateral View

A variable proportion of the aortic arch and its major branches is visible on the lateral view, depending largely on the degree of aortic unfolding. The brachiocephalic (innominate) artery is the only branch vessel that is recognisable with any frequency. It arises anterior to the tracheal air column; usually the origin is unclear but, after a variable length, the posterior wall can be seen as a

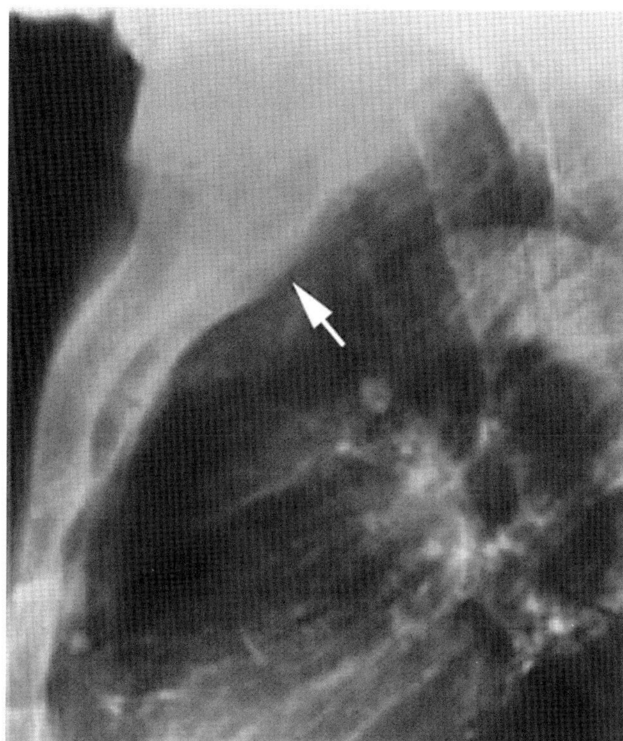

FIGURE 2-23 ■ **Bulge behind manubrium representing normal left innominate (brachiocephalic) vein (arrow).**

gently S-shaped interface as it crosses the tracheal air column. The left and right brachiocephalic (innominate) veins are also sometimes visible on the lateral view. The left brachiocephalic vein is seen as an extrapleural bulge behind the manubrium in a small proportion of normal people (Fig. 2-23).

Right Middle Mediastinal Border below the Azygos Arch

Below the azygos arch, the right lower lobe makes contact with the right wall of the oesophagus and the azygos vein as it ascends next to the oesophagus. This portion of the lung is known as the azygo-oesophageal recess, and the interface is known as the azygo-oesophageal line (Fig. 2-24). The shape of the azygos arch varies considerably in different subjects and therefore the shape of the upper portion of the azygo-oesophageal line varies accordingly. The upper few centimetres of the azygo-oesophageal line are, however, always straight or concave toward the lung, so that a convex shape suggests the presence of a subcarinal mass or left atrial enlargement. The azygo-oesophageal line can be traced down to the posterior costophrenic angle in normal subjects.

Left Cardiac Border below the Aortic Arch

This left cardiac border is formed by the main pulmonary artery and heart. The pleura smoothing the angle between the mid-portion of the aortic arch and the main and left pulmonary artery, the so-called aortic–pulmonary mediastinal stripe,[29] is the lateral extent of the aortopulmonary window. Because the aortopulmonary window is a

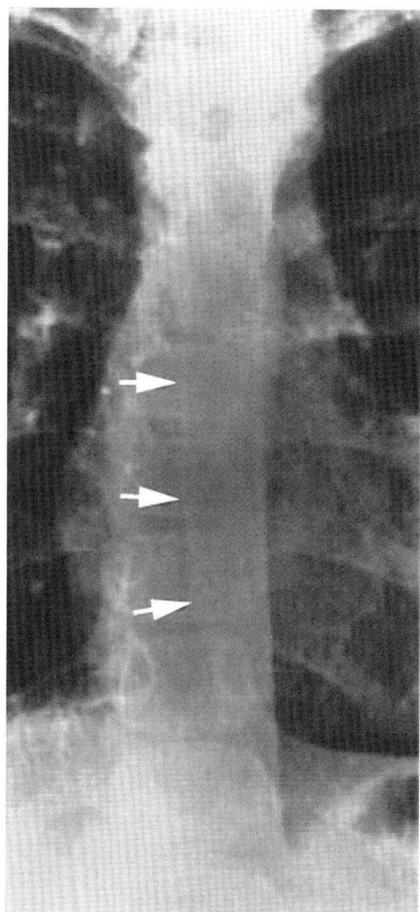

FIGURE 2-24 ■ **Azygo-oesophageal line (arrows).**

sensitive place to look for lymph node enlargement, Blank and Castellino[30] investigated the variable shape of this pleural reflection, as illustrated in Fig. 2-25.

A small 'nipple' may occasionally be seen projecting laterally from the aortic knuckle owing to the presence of the left superior intercostal vein.[31,32] The vein, which is formed by the junction of the left first to fourth intercostal veins, arches forward around the aorta just below the origin of the left subclavian artery to enter the left brachiocephalic vein. This normal nipple should not be misinterpreted as adenopathy projecting from the aortopulmonary window.

The interface between the lung and the left wall of the aorta can almost invariably be followed down to the level of the diaphragm, though contact with the proximal portion of the left pulmonary artery may silhouette a small portion of the interface. The shape varies with the degree of aortic unfolding. Though the lung invaginates between the heart and aorta to contact the left wall of the oesophagus, the interface with the oesophagus may be seen as a line if air is present within the lumen of the oesophagus.

Paraspinal Lines

Although lymph nodes and intercostal veins occupy the space between the spine and the lung, they cannot

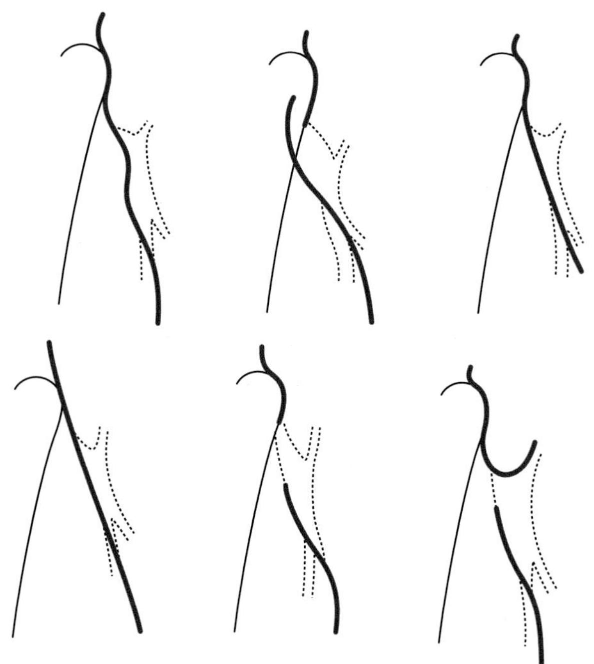

FIGURE 2-25 ■ Patterns of pleural reflection along the left border of the great vessels and heart. The heavy line indicates the visible pleural interface. (Adapted from Blank N, Castellino R A 1972 Patterns of pleural reflections of the left superior mediastinum: normal anatomy and distortions produced by adenopathy. Radiology 102: 585–589, with permission from the Radiological Society of North America.)

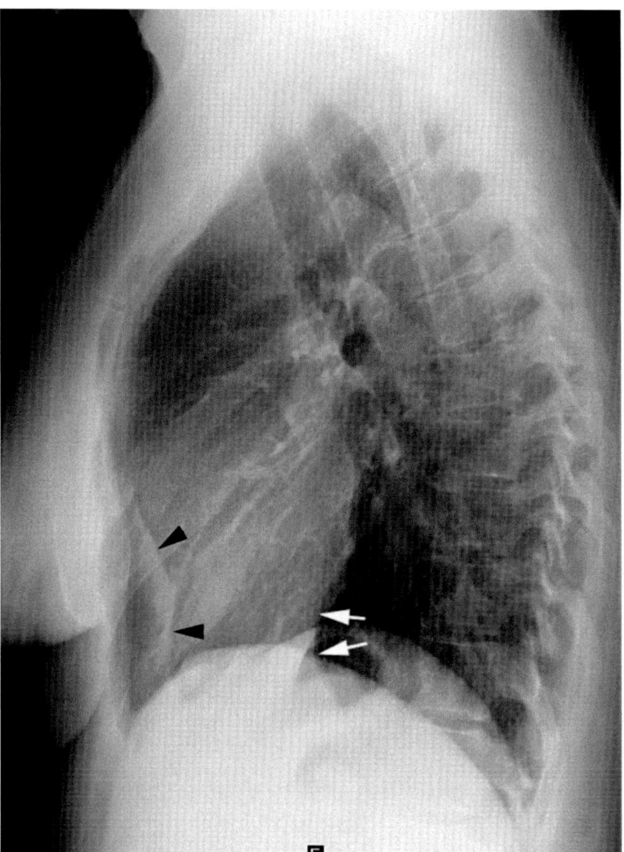

FIGURE 2-26 ■ Retrosternal stripe (arrowheads) and inferior vena cava in lateral projection (arrows).

normally be recognised individually. In individuals with little fat, the interfaces, known as the paraspinal lines, may closely reflect the undulations of the lateral spinal ligaments, but the more fat there is, the more these undulations are smoothed out. The thickness of the left paravertebral space is usually greater than that of the right and can be more than 10 mm in obese subjects. Aortic unfolding contributes to the thickness of the left paraspinal line; as the aorta moves posteriorly and laterally, it strips the pleura from its otherwise close contact with the profiled portions of the spine.

Retrosternal Line

The band-like opacity simulating pleural or extrapleural disease is often seen along the lower third of the anterior chest wall on a lateral chest radiograph (Fig. 2-26).[33] This density is due to mediastinal fat and to the differing anterior extent of the left and right lungs. The left lung does not contact the most anterior portion of the left thoracic cavity at these levels because the heart occupies the space. The band-like opacity is, therefore, accounted for by the normal heart and mediastinum, rather than by disease.

THE DIAPHRAGM

The diaphragm consists of a large dome-shaped central tendon surrounded by a sheet of striated muscle which is attached to ribs 7 to 12 and to the xiphisternum. The two diaphragmatic crura, which arise from the upper three lumbar vertebrae, arch superiorly and anteriorly to form the margins of the aortic and oesophageal hiatuses. The median arcuate ligament connecting the two crura forms the anterior margin of the aortic hiatus, and the crura themselves form its lateral boundary. The oesophageal hiatus lies anterior to the aortic hiatus, and anterior to that lies the hiatus for the inferior vena cava, which is situated within the central tendon immediately beneath the right atrium. In most individuals, the diaphragm has a smooth domed shape, but a scalloped outline is also common. The angle of contact with the chest wall is acute and sharp, but blunting of this angle can be normal in athletes, because they can depress their diaphragm to a remarkable degree on deep inspiration. The normal right hemidiaphragm is found at about the level of the anterior portion of the sixth rib, with a range of approximately one interspace above or below this level.[34] In most people, the right hemidiaphragm is 1.5–2.5 cm higher than the left, but the two hemidiaphragms are at the same level in some 9% of the population. In a few normal individuals the left hemidiaphragm is up to 1 cm higher than the right. The normal excursion of the diaphragm is usually between 1.5 and 2.5 cm, though greater degrees of movement are not uncommon

Transabdominal ultrasound, which is capable of providing accurate real-time measurement of movement,

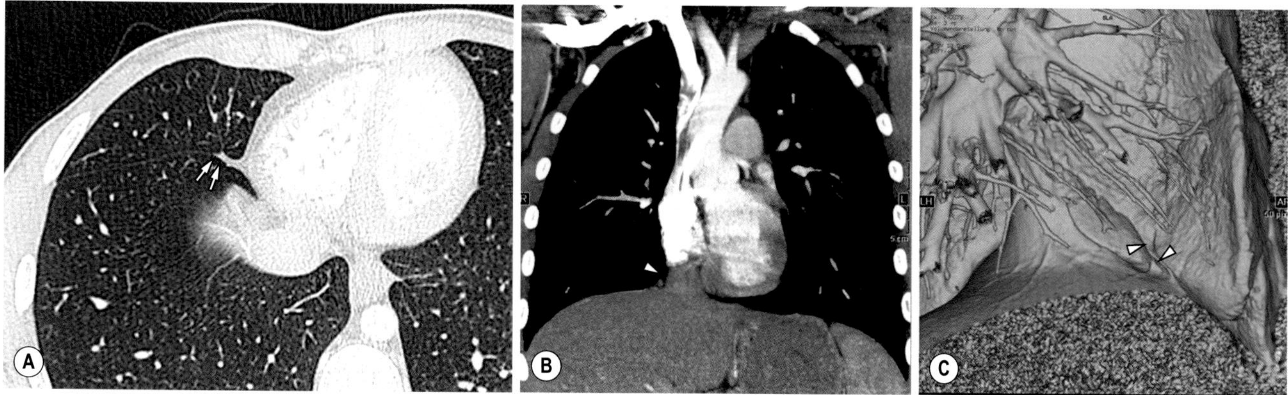

FIGURE 2-27 (A) Right phrenic nerve as it passes over the surface of the right hemidiaphragm (arrows). (B, C) Coronal secondary reformat and volume rendering showing the nerve as delicate structure crossing a lymph node in the mediastino-diaphragmatic angle (arrowheads).

shows a considerable normal range of between 2.0 and 8.6 cm, the mean excursion of the right hemidiaphragm on deep inspiration being 53 mm (SD 16.4) and that of the left being 46 mm (SD 12.4).[35]

Incomplete muscularisation, known as eventration, is also common. An eventration is composed of a thin membranous sheet replacing what should be muscle. Usually it is partial, involving one-half to one-third of the hemidiaphragm. The lack of muscle manifests itself radiographically as elevation of the affected portion of the diaphragm, and the usual appearance is one of a smooth hump on the contour of the diaphragm. Total eventration of a hemidiaphragm, which is much more common on the left than on the right, results in elevation of the whole hemidiaphragm; on fluoroscopy, hemidiaphragm movement is poor, absent or paradoxical, and severe cases of congenital eventration cannot be distinguished from acquired paralysis of the phrenic nerve.

A linear density arising from the lateral wall of the inferior vena cava (Fig. 2-27) is often seen coursing over the surface of the right hemidiaphragm. This line represents pleura and an envelope of fat investing the phrenic nerve, according to Berkman et al.,[36] or the inferior phrenic artery and vein, according to Ujita et al.[37]

REFERENCES

1. Glazer HS, Anderson DJ, DiCroce JJ, et al. Anatomy of the major fissure: evaluation with standard and thin-section CT. Radiology 1991;180:839–44.
2. Mayo JR, Muller NL, Henkelman RM. The double-fissure sign: a motion artifact on thin-section CT scans. Radiology 1987;165: 580–1.
3. Ariyurek OM, Gulsun M, Demirkazik FB. Accessory fissures of the lung: evaluation by high-resolution computed tomography. Eur Radiol 2001;11:2449–53.
4. Caceres J, Mata JH, Alegnet X. Increased density of the azygos lobe on frontal radiographs simulating disease: CT findings in seven patients. Am J Roentgenol 1993;160:245–8.
5. Rabinowitz JG, Cohen BA, Mendleson DS. The pulmonary ligament. Radiol Clin North Am 1984;22:659–72.
6. Berkman YM, Drossman SR, Marboe CC. Intersegmental (intersublobar) septum of the lower lobe in relation to the pulmonary ligament: anatomic, histologic, and CT correlations. Radiology 1993;185:389–93.
7. Breatnach E, Abbott GC, Fraser RE. Dimensions of the normal human trachea. Am J Roentgenol 1984;142:903–6.
8. Vock P, Spiegel T, Fram EK, et al. CT assessment of the adult intra-thoracic cross section of the trachea. J Comput Assist Tomogr 1984;8:1076–82.
9. Griscom NT, Wohl ME. Dimensions of the growing trachea related to age and gender. Am J Roentgenol 1986;146:233–7.
10. Jardin M, Remy J. Segmental bronchovascular anatomy of the lower lobes: CT analysis. Am J Roentgenol 1986;147:457–68.
11. Lee KS, Bae WK, Lee BH, et al. Bronchovascular anatomy of the upper lobes: evaluation with thin section CT. Radiology 1991;181: 765–72.
12. Oshiro Y, Kusumoto M, Moriyama N, et al. Intrapulmonary lymph nodes: thin-section CT features of 19 nodules. J Comput Assist Tomogr 2002;26:553–7.
13. Hyodo T, Kanazawa S, Dendo S, et al. Intrapulmonary lymph nodes: thin-section CT findings, pathological findings, and CT differential diagnosis from pulmonary metastatic nodules. Acta Med Okayama 2004;58:235–40.
14. Park C-K, Webb WR, Klein JS. Inferior hilar window. Radiology 1991;178:163–8.
15. Mendelson DS. Imaging of the thymus. Chest Surg Clin North Am 2001;11:269–93.
16. Dixon AK, Hilton CJ, Williams CT. Computed tomography and histological correlation of the thymic remnant. Clin Radiol 1981; 32:255–7.
17. Moore AV, Korobkin M, Olanow W, et al. Age-related changes in the thymus gland: CT-pathologic correlation. Am J Roentgenol 1983;141:241–6.
18. Genereux GP, Howie JL. Normal mediastinal lymph node size and number: CT and anatomic study. Am J Roentgenol 1984;142: 1095–100.
19. Glazer GM, Gross BH, Quint LE, et al. Normal mediastinal lymph nodes: number and size according to American Thoracic Society mapping. Am J Roentgenol 1985;144:261–5.
20. Schynder PA, Gamsu G. CT of the pretracheal retrocaval space. Am J Roentgenol 1982;136:303–8.
21. Ingram CE, Belli AM, Lewards MD, et al. Normal lymph node size in the mediastinum: a retrospective study in two patient groups. Clin Radiol 1989;40:35–39.
22. Murray JG, O'Driscoll M, Curtin JJ. Mediastinal lymph node size in an Asian population. Br J Radiol 1995;68:348–50.
23. Sobin LH, Gospodarowicz MK, Wittekind CH. TNM. Classification of Malignant Tumours. 7th ed. New York: Wiley; 2009.
24. Rusch VW, Asamura H, Watanabe H, et al. The IASLC lung cancer staging project. J Thorac Oncol 2009;4:568–77.
25. Proto AV, Simmons JD, Zylak CJ. The anterior junction anatomy. CRC Crit Rev Diagn Imaging 1983;19:111–73.
26. Proto AV, Simmons JD, Zylak CJ. The posterior junction anatomy. CRC Crit Rev Diagn Imaging 1983;20:121–73.
27. Cimmino CV. The oesophageal–pleural stripe: an update. Radiology 1981;140:607–13.
28. Bachman AL, Teixidor HS. The posterior tracheal band: a reflection of local mediastinal abnormality. Br J Radiol 1975;48:352–9.

29. Keats TE. The aortic–pulmonary mediastinal stripe. Am J Roentgenol 1975;116:107–9.
30. Blank N, Castellino RA. Patterns of pleural reflections of the left superior mediastinum: normal anatomy and distortions produced by adenopathy. Radiology 1972;102:585–9.
31. Lane EJ, Heitzman ER, Dinn WM. The radiology of the superior intercostal veins. Radiology 1976;120:263–7.
32. Abiru H, Ashizawa K, Hashmi R, et al. Normal radiographic anatomy of thoracic structures: analysis of 1000 chest radiographs in Japanese population. Br J Radiol 2005;78:398–404.
33. Whalen JP, Meyers MA, Oliphant M, et al. The retrosternal line. Am J Roentgenol 1973;117:861–72.
34. Lennon EA, Simon G. The height of the diaphragm in the chest radiograph of normal adults. Br J Radiol 1965;38:937–43.
35. Houston JG, Morris AD, Howie CA, et al. Quantitative assessment of diaphragmatic movement: a reproducible method using ultrasound. Clin Radiol 1992;46:405–7.
36. Berkman YM, Davis SD, Kazam E. Right phrenic nerve: anatomy, CT appearance, and differentiation from the pulmonary ligament. Radiology 1989;173:43–6.
37. Ujita M, Ojiri H, Arizumi M, et al. Appearance of the inferior phrenic artery and vein on CT scans of the chest: a CT and cadaveric study. Am J Roentgenol 1993;160:745–7.

CHAPTER 3

The Chest Wall, Pleura, Diaphragm and Intervention

Johny A. Verschakelen • Fergus Gleeson

CHAPTER OUTLINE

THE CHEST WALL

Although there are a wide variety of tissues and structures that make up the chest wall, based on their radiographic presentation, its components can be grouped into two major parts: the soft tissues and the bony structures.

SOFT TISSUES

On the chest radiograph the soft tissues present as areas of increased density that in part project next to the bony chest wall and in part overlay the different components of the chest. Abnormalities of the soft tissues will present as an abnormal increase or decrease in density often combined with the appearance of an abnormal contour or the disappearance of a normal contour.

Because of better density resolution and multiplanar reformatting, computed tomography (CT) can better demonstrate the different tissues of the chest wall. CT has the advantage over magnetic resonance imaging (MRI) of higher spatial resolution and the ability to better identify bony structures. MRI, however, yields greater soft-tissue contrast, which can be important.[1,2] Multiplanar imaging and three-dimensional (3D) reformation can be performed with both techniques.

Ultrasound may also be used to examine the chest wall. In general it provides less detailed and comprehensive information but it usually enables the lesion to be localised, allows a distinction to be made between cystic and solid lesions and enables guided aspiration/biopsy to be performed under imaging control.

Breasts

On the female chest radiograph it is mandatory to check that both breasts are present. Unilateral radical mastectomy is usually easy to detect because it generates a unilateral mid/lower zone transradiancy and an abnormally straight anterior axillary fold that passes upwards and inwards towards the mid clavicle (Fig. 3-1). Bilateral radical mastectomy is more difficult to identify, but an overall increase in basal transradiancy and axillary fold abnormalities should provide adequate clues. Surgical interventions short of radical mastectomy may be impossible to detect, but close attention to the relative transradiancy of the breast regions and to the breast contours may provide suggestive findings. In addition, the presence of vascular clips can be helpful.

Nipple shadows can mimic intrapulmonary nodules. A putative nipple should be checked for compatible size (5–15 mm), shape and location—its relation to the breast outline in a woman or the pectoralis opacity in a man.

Muscles

On the chest radiograph the pectoralis major produces a broad, band-like opacity extending downwards and medially from the axilla. Unilateral absence or hypoplasia of the pectoralis major results in a unilateral transradiancy and an abnormal anterior axillary fold as seen with mastectomy. In Poland's syndrome these changes are accompanied by ipsilateral hand and arm anomalies (particularly syndactyly) with or without absence of pectoralis minor, rib anomalies and hypoplasia of breast and nipple.

Soft-Tissue Calcification

Soft-tissue calcification may occur in the chest wall, and clues to its site and nature are provided by its morphology distribution and the clinical history. Possible causes to consider include granulomatous lymph nodes, parasites

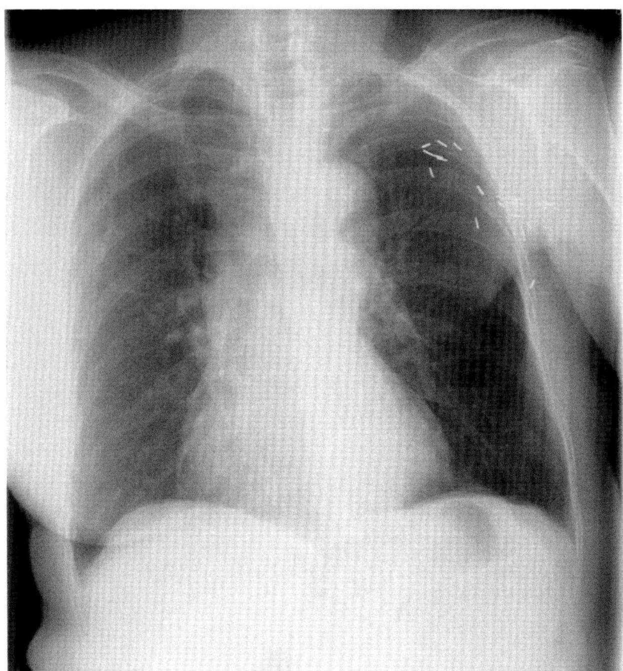

FIGURE 3-1 ■ **Left mastectomy.** The lower part of the left hemithorax is more transradiant than the right.

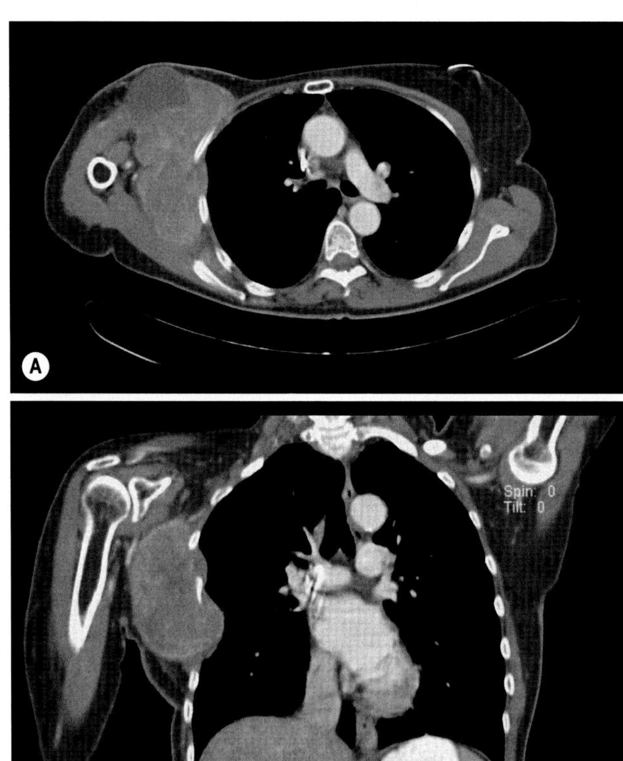

FIGURE 3-2 ■ **Chest wall fibrosarcoma.** (A, B) Axial and coronal CT of the chest show a large mass with heterogeneous density in the chest wall invading ribs, pleura and right lung. Patient underwent mastectomy and radiation therapy two years earlier.

(*Taenia solium* and *Dracunculus medinensis*), calcinosis universalis, childhood dermatomyositis, tuberculosis (spine, ribs or soft tissues) and bone neoplasms. Ossification is rare and most commonly seen in fibrodysplasia ossificans progressiva.

Subcutaneous Emphysema

Subcutaneous emphysema of the chest wall is not uncommon following surgery, pleural drain placement, trauma or in cases of spontaneous or acquired pneumomediastinum. Air dissects along tissue planes and between muscle bundles, giving an overall pattern of linear transradiancies which can significantly interfere with the interpretation of the underlying structures. In this way diagnosis of pneumothorax can become very difficult. In case of doubt, CT can be performed.

Soft-Tissue Tumours

A soft-tissue tumour of the chest wall gives rise to an opacity. Malignant and inflammatory lesions cause bony destruction and benign ones result in rib separation and notch-like remodelling from pressure erosion.

The most common benign chest wall tumour is a lipoma, but a variety of other mesenchymal tumours occur, including neurofibromas (focal or plexiform), neurilemmomas, haemangiomas and lymphangiomas (cystic hygromas). On CT, lipomas are well-demarcated homogeneous masses of low density (–90 to –150 HU). They contain few, if any, other soft-tissue components; the presence of the latter in a fatty tumour suggests a liposarcoma. MRI features are also characteristic, with high signal on T1-weighted images, intermediate signal on T2-weighted images and low signal with fat suppression.[1,2] Neurofibromas on CT characteristically have a lower density than muscle both before and after intravenous contrast medium. On MRI, neurofibromas give low-to-intermediate signal on T1-weighted images but high signal on T2-weighted images and marked contrast enhancement after gadolinium, which allows clear delineation of their extent. Haemangiomas are uncommon lesions that occasionally show phlebolithic calcification on plain radiography. Findings on CT include phleboliths, bone remodelling and an enhancing mass. MRI is the best investigation for delineating their extent. Lesions give an intermediate signal on T1-weighted images and a high signal on T2-weighted images, accompanied by artefacts generated by vessels, soft tissue and elements derived from haemorrhage.[1,2] Lymphangiomas on CT have the features of a fluid-filled cyst with or without septation. On MRI they have the features of a cyst with low protein content.

Malignant primary tumours arising in the soft tissues of the chest wall are unusual, the most common being lipo- or fibrosarcomas (Fig. 3-2).

Secondary tumours of the chest wall are common, particularly when due to local spread (carcinoma of the breast and lung, lymphoma); see bronchial carcinoma and Pancoast's tumour, below.

BONY STRUCTURES

Although depicting bone abnormalities is not the primary goal of a chest radiograph, the bony structures that are, as a result of the technique, often only partially visible should be carefully examined. CT, when indicated, is better at demonstrating congenital or acquired remodelling or complicated fractures; multidetector 2D or 3D reformations can be helpful.

Ribs

There are normally 12 pairs of ribs. Cervical ribs occur in 1–2% of the population and are commonly bilateral, though often asymmetrical.

Congenital abnormalities of modelling may be confined to one or two ribs or be generalised. One or a few upper ribs are commonly bifid, splayed, fused or hypoplastic. Usually occurring in isolation, these anomalies are occasionally part of a syndrome (e.g. basal cell naevus syndrome) or associated with other anomalies (e.g. Sprengel's deformity).

With acquired remodelling, abnormalities tend to be focal, affecting one or many ribs. Such acquired changes may follow fracture, surgery, osteomyelitis and empyema drainage, or result from external pressure (rib notching). The two main causes of rib notching are coarctation of the aorta and neurofibromatosis Type I.

Ribs may fracture and the callus formed can sometimes mimic an intrapulmonary opacity.

Destructive rib lesions occur most commonly in osteomyelitis or neoplastic disease. The former is uncommon and may be haematogenous (e.g. staphylococcal or tuberculous) or caused by direct spread from lung and pleural space (e.g. in actinomycosis). Bronchial carcinoma, including Pancoast's tumour, commonly spreads from lung to rib. In this latter condition MRI can be performed to study the extent of the disease, especially the relationship between the tumour and the plexus brachialis in case of a Pancoast's tumour[3] (Fig. 3-3). Multidetector CT (MDCT) can also play an important role, especially because it can better evaluate the invasion in the bony cortex of the ribs[4] (Fig. 3-3D). Also, 3D image reconstruction methods can be used in selected cases to clarify a complex relationship between the tumour invading the chest wall and vascular structures of the thoracic inlet.

Various primary and secondary tumours can affect ribs, causing localised lesions. Benign primary tumours are infrequent, and of these, the cartilaginous tumours (chondromas, osteochondromas) are the most common. They are predominantly anterior and may show characteristic cartilaginous calcification. Other lesions that broadly fall into this category include fibrous dysplasia, histiocytosis X, haemangioma and aneurysmal bone cyst[1] (Fig. 3-4).

The most common malignant rib tumours are metastatic deposits and myeloma. Primary malignant tumours are rare, chondrosarcomas being the least uncommon. Other malignancies that occur occasionally include lymphoma, osteosarcoma and round-cell tumours.

Sternum

This is well displayed in a lateral chest radiograph but is conspicuous in the frontal projection, in which only the manubrial margins are sometimes visible, giving rise to confusing shadows that may mimic mediastinal widening.

Various sternal deformities are described, and the most important radiologically is the depressed sternum

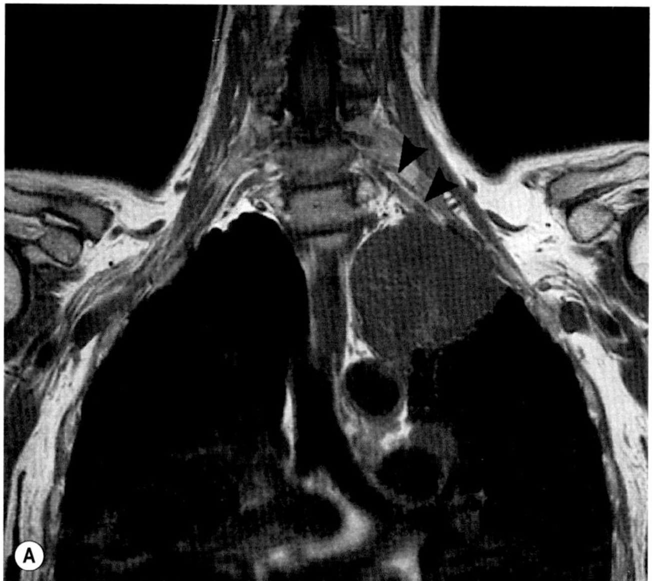

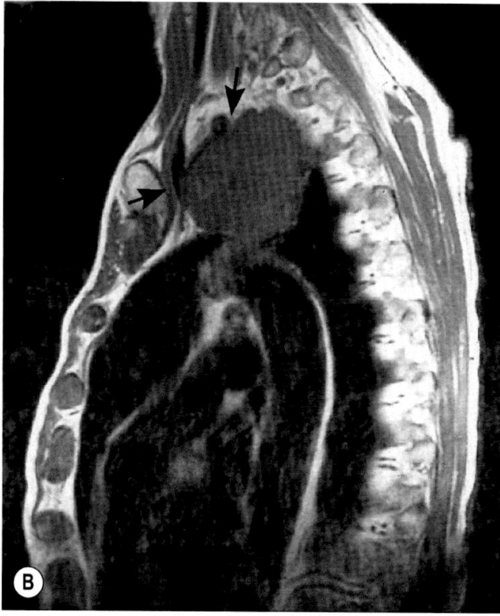

FIGURE 3-3 ■ **Pancoast's tumour.** (A, B) MRI. (A) Coronal and (B) sagittal image. Large tumour in the left upper lobe invading the soft tissues and displacing the vascular structures anteriorly (arrows). The brachial plexus has also been invaded (arrowheads).

Continued on following page

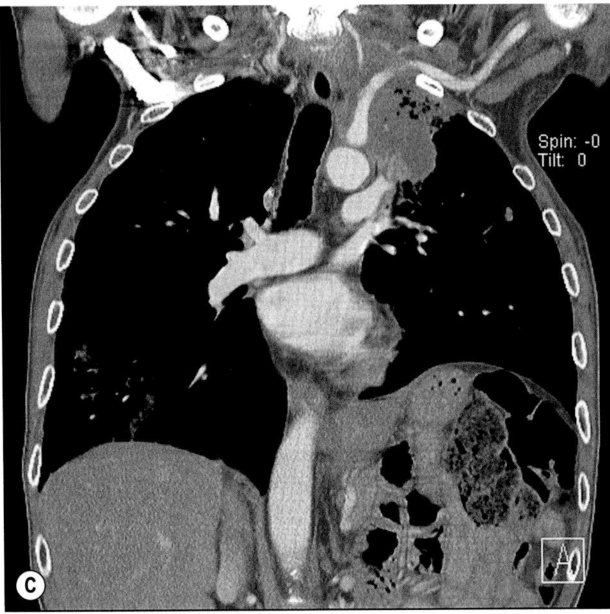

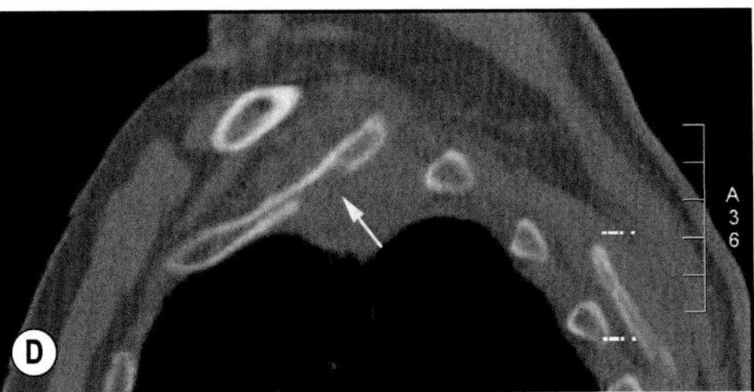

FIGURE 3-3, Continued (C, D) CT (different patient). (C) Coronal and (D) sagittal image bone window setting. Large tumour in the left upper lobe invading the soft tissues, displacing and invading the left subclavian artery and invading a rib (arrow).

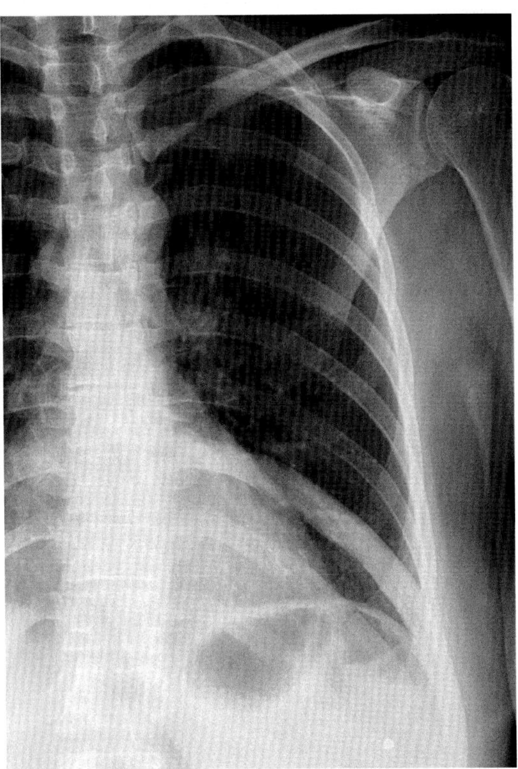

FIGURE 3-4 Fibrous dysplasia in a rib; chest radiograph detail of the left lung. Compared with the other ribs the ninth rib shows an increase in density and is slightly broadened.

(funnel chest, pectus excavatum) in which there is approximation of the lower half of the sternum and the spine (Fig. 3-5). This may be an isolated abnormality or it may be associated with other disorders such as Marfan's syndrome or congenital heart disease (particularly atrial septal defect (ASD)). The radiological signs on a postero-anterior (PA) chest radiograph consist of a shift of the heart to the left, straightening of the left heart border with prominence of the main pulmonary artery segment, loss of the descending aortic interface and an increased opacity in the right cardiophrenic angle, often accompanied by a loss of clarity of the right heart border which simulates right middle lobe disease. The diagnosis can be suspected on a PA radiograph from the steep inferior slope of the anterior ribs and undue clarity of the lower dorsal spine seen through the heart.

Pigeon chest (pectus carinatum) represents the reverse deformity and may be congenital or acquired.

Neoplasms of the sternum are usually malignant (myeloma, chondrosarcoma, lymphoma or metastatic carcinoma), the most common benign tumour being a chondroma. Non-neoplastic processes that may affect the sternum include osteomyelitis, histiocytosis X, Paget's disease, fibrous dysplasia, osteitis fibrosa cystica and intersternocostoclavicular hyperostosis.

CT is the best investigation for imaging the sternum because it eliminates overlapping structures, detects bony destruction, allows imaging of adjacent soft tissues (the parasternal–internal mammary zone) and has good contrast resolution superior to that of conventional radiography or tomography.

Clavicles

The medial clavicular ends are important landmarks used together with the spine in assessing rotation on a radiograph.

The joints at both ends are synovial but only the acromio-clavicular joint can be assessed with confidence on a chest radiograph. It may be eroded in any synovitis, particularly rheumatoid arthritis, and is also commonly fuzzy and ill-defined in hyperparathyroidism and rickets. Neoplasms of the clavicle are usually malignant (myeloma or metastatic). Other primary tumours and tumour-like

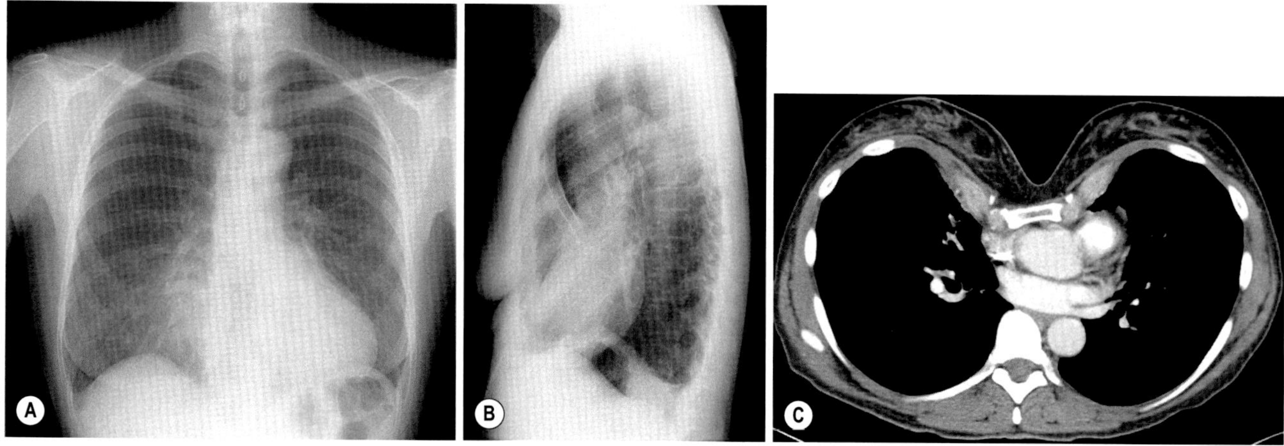

FIGURE 3-5 **Depressed sternum.** (A) PA chest radiograph. The depressed sternum displaces the heart to the left and rotates it so that the left heart border adopts a straight configuration. The right heart border becomes ill-defined and is bounded by a hazy opacity, simulating collapse of the right middle lobe. The ribs show their characteristic configuration—horizontal posteriorly and steeply oblique anteriorly. The posterior displacement of the sternum is better demonstrated on (B) the lateral chest radiograph and (C) the axial CT.

lesions include osteosarcoma, Ewing's sarcoma, post-radiation sarcoma, aneurysmal bone cyst, histiocytosis X and intersternocostoclavicular hyperostosis. Either CT or MRI is required to provide a full evaluation of the medial clavicular ends.

Spine

Kyphoscoliosis makes assessment of the chest radiograph difficult and CT is often necessary to evaluate possible thoracic disease.

THE PLEURA

The chest radiograph is still the most important and widely used means of demonstrating and following the progress of pleural disease, though ultrasound, CT and MRI can play a significant role in a number of specific situations. Pleural disease is manifest by the accumulation of fluid or air in the pleural space, by pleural thickening (with or without calcification), or by the presence of a pleural mass.

PLEURAL EFFUSION

A number of different types of fluid may accumulate in the pleural space, the most common being transudate, exudate (thin or thick), blood and chyle. Occasionally effusions are highly specific, not falling into any of the above categories and containing, for example, bile, cerebrospinal fluid or iatrogenic fluids. All types of pleural effusion are radiographically identical, though historical, clinical and other radiological features may help limit the diagnostic possibilities. Sometimes, also CT and MRI can help to specify the diagnosis.

Bilateral pleural effusions tend to be transudates because they develop secondary to generalised changes that affect both pleural cavities equally—a rise in capillary pressure or a fall in blood proteins, etc. Some bilateral effusions are exudates, however, and this is seen with metastatic disease, lymphoma, pulmonary embolism, rheumatoid disease, systemic lupus erythematosus (SLE), post-cardiac injury syndrome, myxoedema and some ascites-related effusions. Right-sided effusions are typically associated with ascites, heart failure and liver abscess, and left effusions with pancreatitis, pericarditis, oesophageal rupture and aortic dissection. Massive effusions are most commonly due to malignant disease, particularly metastases (lung or breast), but may also occur in heart failure, cirrhosis, tuberculosis, empyema and trauma.

Imaging Pleural Effusion[5]

Chest Radiograph

Free Pleural Fluid. A small amount of free fluid may be undetectable on an erect PA chest radiograph as it tends initially to collect under the lower lobes. Such small subpulmonary effusions can be demonstrated by ultrasound or CT.[6]

As the amount of effusion increases, the posterior and then the lateral costophrenic angles become blunted, by which time a 200- to 500-mL effusion is present. Following this the classical signs develop: homogeneous opacification of the lower chest with obliteration of the costophrenic angle and the hemidiaphragm. The superior margin of the opacity is concave to the lung and is higher laterally than medially. Above and medial to this meniscus there is a hazy increase in opacity owing to the presence of fluid posterior and anterior to the lungs (Fig. 3-6).

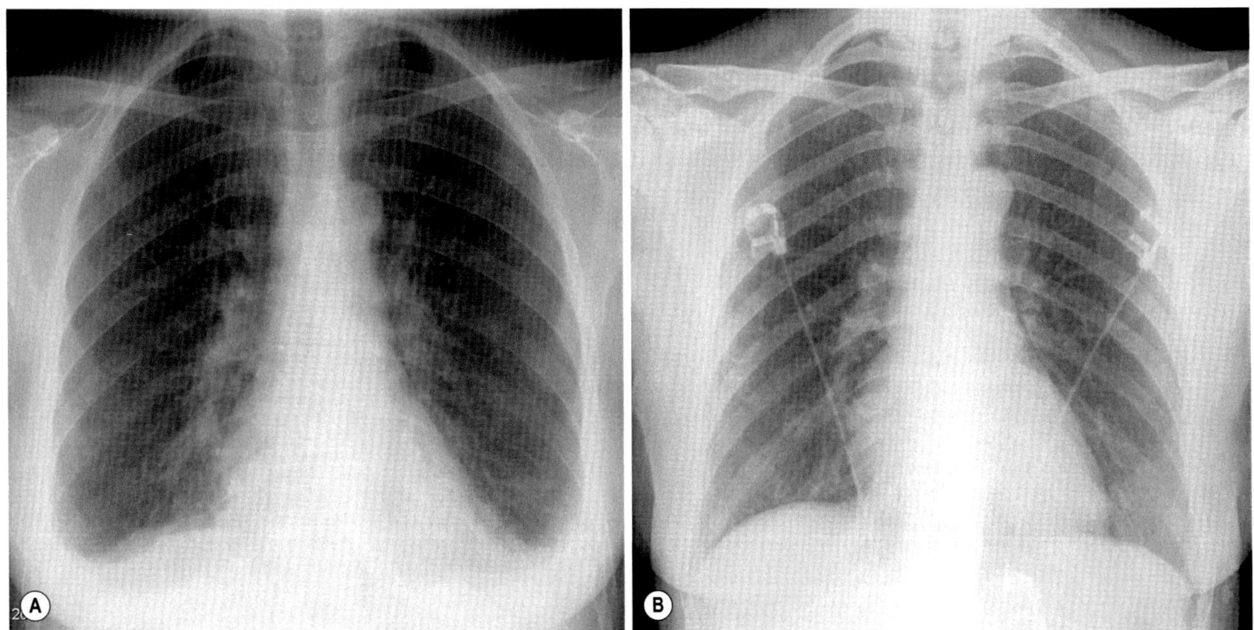

FIGURE 3-6 ■ Bilateral pleural effusion. (A) Erect and (B) supine chest radiograph. The pleural effusion obscures the diaphragm and both costophrenic angles. It has a curvilinear upper margin concave to lung and is higher laterally than medially. This is opposite to the findings on the supine chest radiograph where the pleural effusion is hardly visible as a hazy opacity affecting the lower part of the thorax. Note also that the costophrenic angles are not obscured and that the vascular opacities are preserved in the overlying lung.

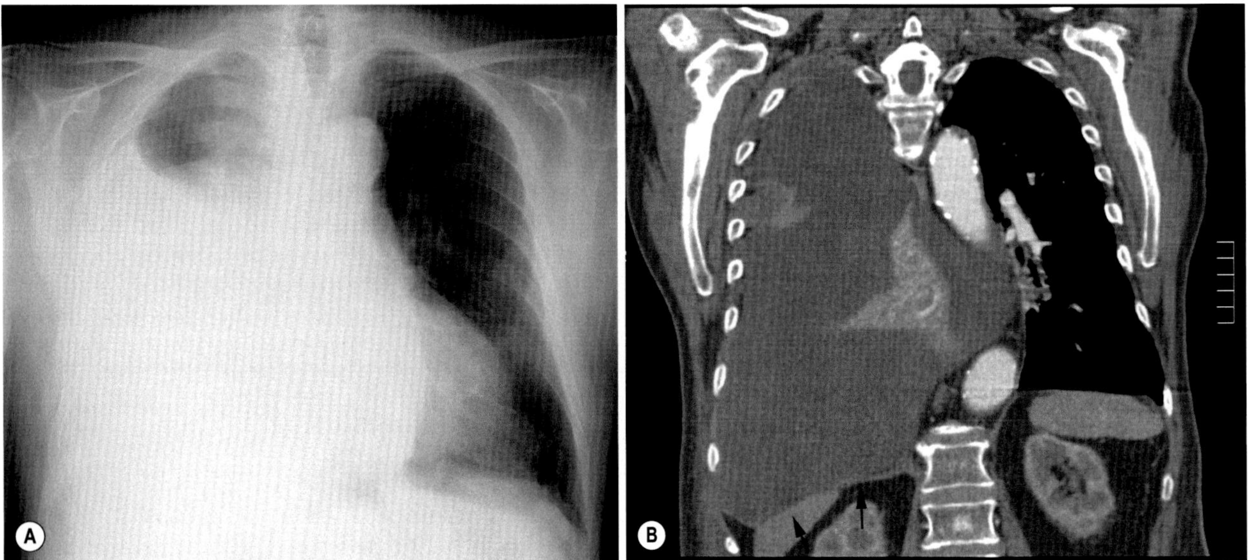

FIGURE 3-7 ■ Massive pleural effusion with mediastinal shift to the left. (A) Chest radiograph and (B) CT coronal reconstruction. A massive effusion displaces the mediastinum to the left. CT shows the important pleural effusion together with the enhanced atelectatic left lung. Note also the depression of the right hemidiaphragm (arrows).

Massive effusions cause dense opacification of the hemithorax with contralateral mediastinal shift (Fig. 3-7). Absence of mediastinal shift with a large effusion raises the strong possibility of obstructive collapse of the ipsilateral lung or extensive pleural malignancy, such as may be seen with mesothelioma or metastatic carcinoma (Table 3-1). Large effusions sometimes cause diaphragmatic inversion, particularly on the left where the diaphragm lacks the support of the liver.[7] Although pleural fluid collects initially under the lung, it is unusual for it to remain localised in this site once its volume exceeds 200–300 mL. This does happen occasionally, however, and may be suspected from an erect PA and lateral radiograph. On a PA radiograph this subpulmonary effusion[7] presents as a 'high hemidiaphragm' with an unusual contour that peaks more laterally than usual,

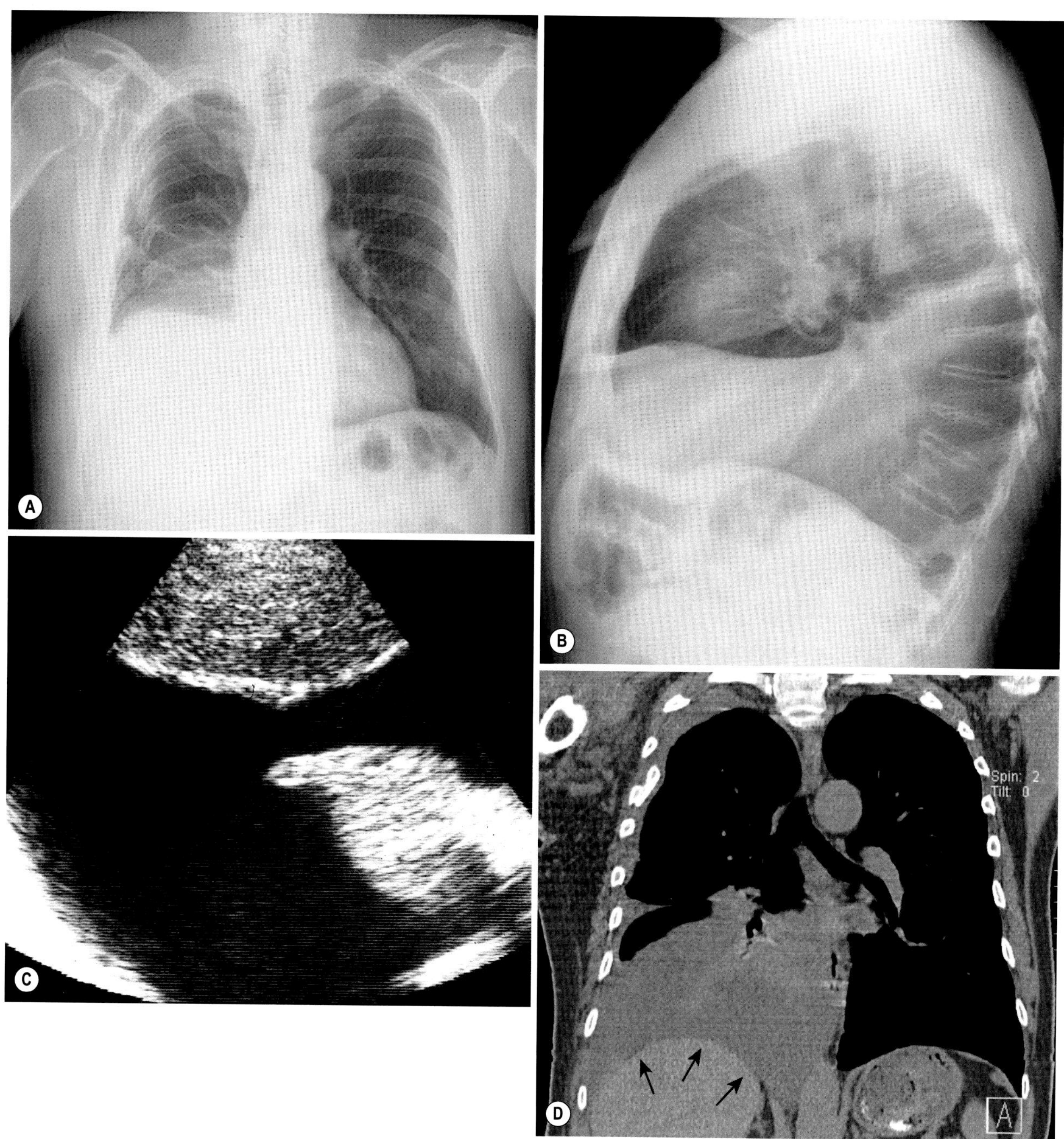

FIGURE 3-8 ■ **Subpulmonary pleural effusion.** On the (A) erect PA and (B) lateral radiograph the effusion simulates a high hemidiaphragm. (C) Ultrasound and (D) CT clearly show that the effusion is located above the diaphragm. Arrows = diaphragmatic area.

TABLE 3-1 **Causes of Opacification of a Hemithorax**
Pleural effusion
Consolidation
Collapse
Massive tumour
Fibrothorax
Combination of above lesions
Pneumonectomy
Lung agenesis

has a straight medial segment and falls away rapidly to the costophrenic angle laterally, which may or may not be blunted. Ultrasound or CT will confirm the diagnosis (see Fig. 3-8).

Loculated (Encysted, Encapsulated) Pleural Fluid. Fluid can loculate between visceral pleural layers in fissures or between visceral and parietal layers, usually against the chest wall. It is unusual for this to happen without some additional radiographic clue to the presence of pleural disease (Fig. 3-9). Both ultrasound and CT can be used to distinguish loculated fluid from solid lesions.

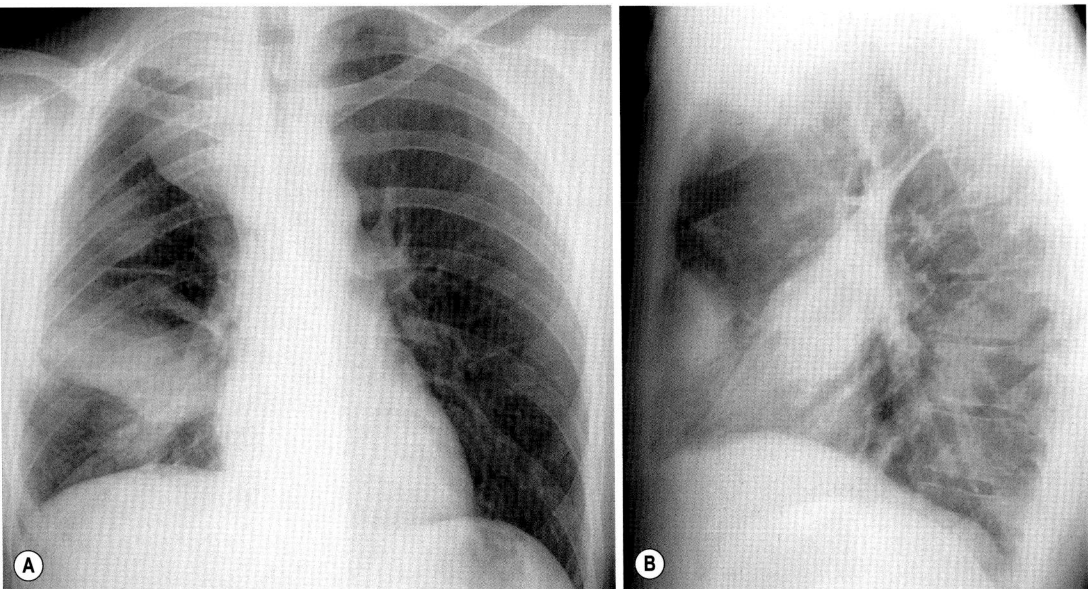

FIGURE 3-9 ■ Encapsulated fluid on (A) PA and (B) lateral chest radiographs. Pleural fluid is encapsulated in the major fissure and against the anterior chest wall. These encysted fluid collections can mimic a lung tumour.

Pleural Effusion in the Supine Patient. In the supine patient, pleural fluid layers out posteriorly and the meniscus effect, present from front to back, is not appreciated because of the projection. The main radiographic finding is a hazy opacity like a veil affecting the whole or the lower part of the hemithorax, with preserved vascular opacities in the overlying lung (see Fig. 3-6B). Additional signs include haziness of the diaphragmatic margin, blunting of the costophrenic angle, a pleural cap to the lung apex, thickening of the minor fissure and widening of the paraspinal interface.

Ultrasound[6,8]

Pleural fluid, especially when it is a transudate, is commonly echo-free and marginated on its deep aspect by a highly echogenic line at the fluid–lung interface. Exudative and haemorrhagic effusions may be echogenic and are often accompanied by pleural thickening. The pattern of echoes may be homogeneous, complex or septated. Features that help distinguish a fluid from a solid echogenic lesion include changes in shape with breathing, the presence of septa and fibrous strands and movement of components induced by breathing (Fig. 3-10). Occasionally, in the absence of such features, some echogenic fluid pleural effusions are indistinguishable from solid ones.[6]

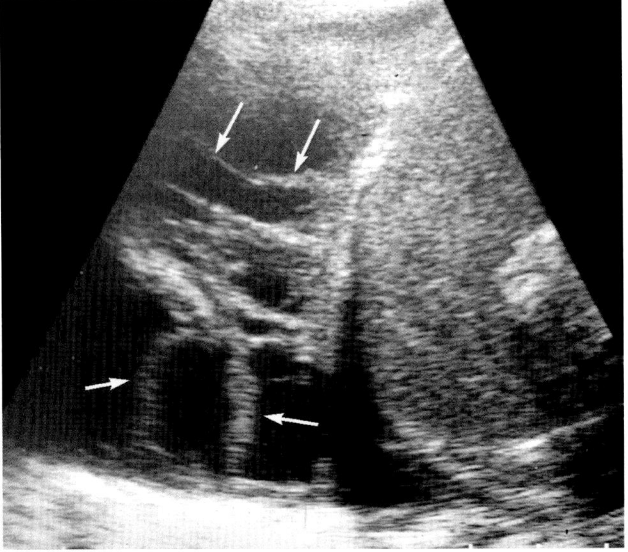

FIGURE 3-10 ■ Ultrasound of an empyema. The pleural fluid is separated by septa (arrows). Although the pleural fluid is echo-free in part, some areas return echoes owing to the turbid nature of the empyema fluid.

Ultrasound has a number of important roles in the evaluation and management of pleural fluid. It can be used to distinguish between pleural fluid, solid pleural (or extrapleural) lesions and peripheral lung lesions. In peripheral lung lesions, the presence of fluid bronchograms and vessels on Doppler examination will positively identify consolidation. In addition, pleural lesions characteristically make an *obtuse* angle with the chest wall, whereas with intrapulmonary lesions the angle is often *acute*. This ability of ultrasound to distinguish pulmonary lesions (collapse, consolidation, abscess) from pleural effusion is particularly useful when it comes to the evaluation of the opaque hemithorax. Ultrasound can also be used to identify small amounts of pleural fluid, or pleural fluid in unusual locations, as with a subpulmonary effusion (see Fig. 3-8C). Ultrasound is widely used to localise pleural fluid for aspiration and identify any solid components to allow guided biopsy. Furthermore, ultrasound may identify the cause of an effusion when it lies inside or even outside the chest (subphrenic abscess, metastasis, etc.).

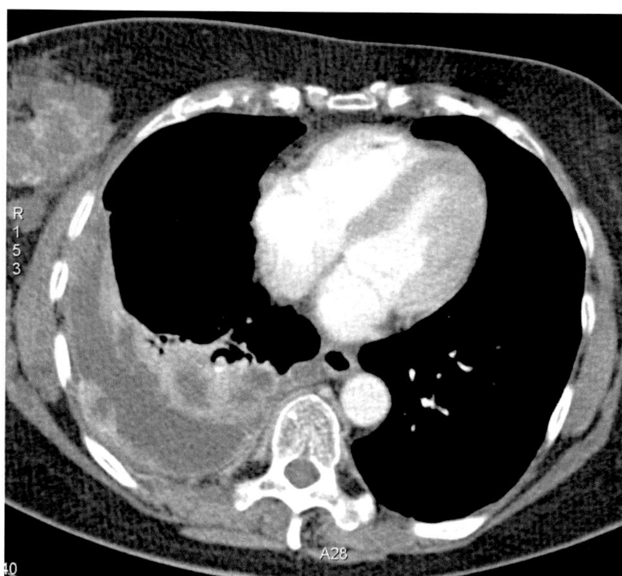

FIGURE 3-11 ■ **CT of malignant pleural disease.** In this right pleural effusion, CT identifies the extensive and irregular pleural thickening characteristic of a malignant process (pleural metastases). Note also the primary tumour in the right breast.

Computed Tomography[6,9]

CT is very sensitive in detecting pleural fluid and can distinguish between free and loculated fluid, identifying the extent and location of the latter. Accurate localisation of such loculated effusions is useful before drainage. CT distinguishes between parenchymal lung disease and pleural disease, a distinction often facilitated by administration of intravenous contrast medium. CT can characterise the morphology of pleural thickening that often accompanies a pleural effusion, distinguishing between malignant (nodular, with focal masses) and benign thickening, which is typically uniform. CT can also identify any underlying lung disease that might have provoked an effusion and it facilitates percutaneous aspiration and biopsy (Fig. 3-11).

A pleural effusion appears on CT as a dependent sickle-shaped opacity with a CT number lower than that of any adjacent pleural thickening or mass. CT numbers do not allow a distinction between transudate and exudate. However, parietal pleural thickening at contrast-enhanced CT almost always indicates the presence of pleural exudates. The higher density of clotted blood in a haemothorax is sometimes apparent. The fat-containing chylothorax does not have a CT number lower than normal, because of its protein content. Loculated effusions have a lenticular configuration with smooth margins and they displace the adjacent parenchyma.

Magnetic Resonance Imaging[6]

MRI has a limited role in the evaluation of pleural effusion. Pleural fluid has a low signal on T1-weighted sequences and a high signal on T2-weighted images, with a tendency for exudates to give a higher signal than transudates on T2-weighted sequences. In addition, complex exudates have greater signal intensity than simple exudates. It may also be possible to differentiate transudates from exudates using triple echo-pulse sequence, and benign from malignant changes using high-resolution MRI.[10] Chylous effusion can cause high signal intensity on T1-weighted images similar to subcutaneous fat. In the subacute and chronic stage, haematomas show bright signal intensity on T1-weighted images, surrounded by a dark rim caused by haemosiderin.

Some Specific Pleural Effusions

Exudates and Transudates

Pleural effusion is common in heart failure and tends to be more frequent and larger on the right.

All types of pericardial disease may be associated with pleural effusion, which is predominantly left-sided. Pleural effusion is a characteristic finding in the post-cardiac injury syndrome, seen in about 80% of patients. It may be bilateral or unilateral and is commonly accompanied by consolidation and pericardial effusion. Pulmonary embolism is commonly associated with pleural effusion, which is seen in 25–50% of cases.

A number of drugs have been described as causing pleural effusions. The most common agents are cytotoxics (methotrexate, procarbazine, mitomycin, busulfan, bleomycin and interleukin-2), nitrofurantoin, antimigraine drugs (ergotamine, methysergide), amiodarone, propylthiouracil, bromocriptine and gonadotrophins. With a number of these agents pleural thickening is more common than a pleural effusion.

Pleural effusion is also a recognised complication of hepatic cirrhosis. The principal mechanism of its production is the transdiaphragmatic passage of ascites, though other factors such as hypoalbuminaemia may contribute in a small number of cases.

Both acute and chronic pancreatitis are associated with pleural effusions which have high amylase levels. In acute pancreatitis, exudative and often blood-stained effusions form in 15% of patients, particularly on the left side where the diaphragm is closely related to the pancreatic tail. Associated elevation of the hemidiaphragm and basal lung consolidation are common. In chronic pancreatitis, effusions tend to be large and recurrent and patients present with dyspnoea, unlike effusions in acute pancreatitis in which abdominal symptoms predominate. The pathogenesis of pleural effusion in chronic pancreatitis is fistula formation following ductal rupture.

Pleural effusion is common with subphrenic abscess and occurs in about 80% of patients. The effusion is often accompanied by basal lung collapse and consolidation, an elevated hemidiaphragm and a subdiaphragmatic air–fluid level.

Pleural effusion may occur in a number of renal conditions. Exudative effusions may be seen in uraemia and are often accompanied by pericarditis. Effusions can be large or small and are often unilateral, behaving in a rather indolent fashion. In common with other hypoproteinaemic states, bilateral effusions develop in about 20% of patients with nephrotic syndrome. Peritoneal dialysis can produce pleural effusions by the direct

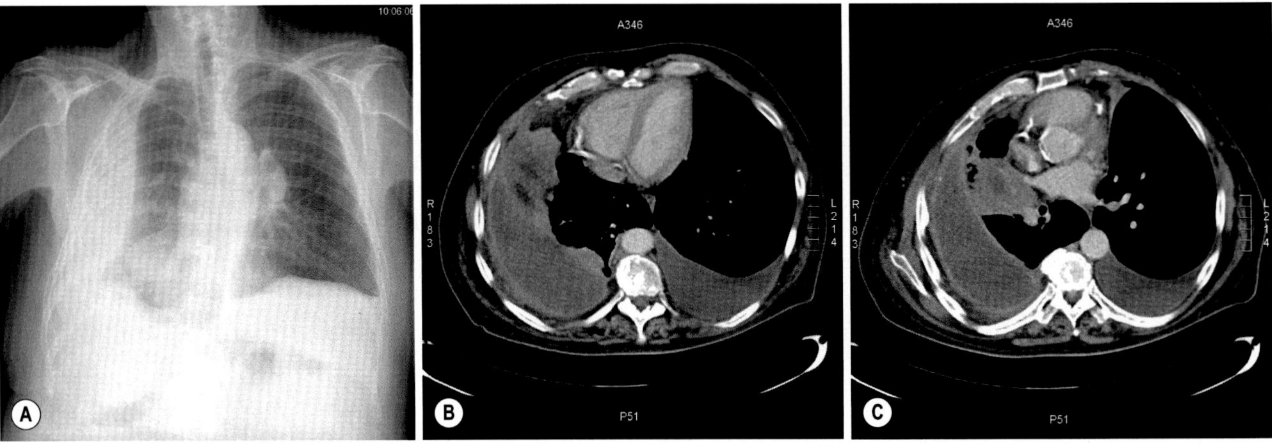

FIGURE 3-12 ■ **Empyema.** (A) Chest X-ray shows an encapsulated pleural effusion on the right and a free pleural effusion on the left. (B, C) An enhanced CT confirms this bilateral fluid collection. However, the pleura on the right is thickened but smooth and enhancing while subpleural fat is infiltrated and widened, which is the result of oedema. The empyema followed pneumonia, which can be seen in the middle lobe (C). Compare with non-complicated left pleural effusion.

transdiaphragmatic passage of fluid, as occurs with cirrhotic ascites. In common with other ascites-related effusions they are predominantly right-sided, but these effusions have a diagnostically high level of glucose.

Patients with acquired immune deficiency syndrome are at risk for a variety of pleural infections and neoplasms that can be associated with pleural effusion. These effusions are most frequently caused by pneumonic infections but can also be the result of non-Hodgkin's lymphoma. Empyema is a suppurative exudate usually parapneumonic. Less commonly it is caused by transdiaphragmatic extension of a liver abscess or by bronchopleural fistula (Fig. 3-12).

Bronchopleural Fistula

Bronchopleural fistula differs from a pneumothorax in that the communication with the pleural space is via airways rather than distal air spaces. It occurs in two main settings, following partial or complete lung resection and in association with necrotising infections.

Chylothorax

Chylous effusions are commonly milky because they contain triglycerides in the form of chylomicrons. Chylous and non-chylous pleural effusions are indistinguishable on the chest radiograph. In addition, despite its high fat content, the increased protein level of a chylothorax gives it an attenuation on CT similar to that of other pleural effusions. Chylous effusion can cause high signal intensity on T1-weighted images similar to subcutaneous fat. Chyle collects in the pleural space following rupture of the thoracic duct or seepage from collaterals. Rarely, it crosses the diaphragm from the abdomen in the presence of chylous ascites.

Haemothorax

On the plain chest radiograph an acute haemothorax is indistinguishable from other pleural fluid collections. Once the blood clots there is a tendency for loculation and occasionally a fibrin body will form. Pleural thickening and calcification are recognised sequelae. On CT a haemothorax may show areas of hyperdensity, and in the subacute or chronic stage it will appear on MRI as a high signal on T1- and T2-weighted images, possibly with a low signal rim caused by haemosiderin.

The most common cause of haemothorax is trauma, but it is seen in a number of other conditions, including ruptured aortic aneurysm, pneumothorax, extramedullary haematopoiesis and coagulopathies.

PNEUMOTHORAX

Air in the pleural space is a pneumothorax. When air and liquid are present the nomenclature depends on their relative volumes and the type of liquid. Small amounts of liquid are disregarded and the condition is still called a pneumothorax; otherwise, the prefix hydro-, haemo-, pyo- or chylo- is added, depending on the nature of the liquid.

Primary Spontaneous Pneumothorax

Iatrogenic causes apart, the most common type of pneumothorax in the adult is the so-called primary spontaneous pneumothorax (PSP). A pneumothorax occurring without an obvious precipitating event is spontaneous, and if the patient has essentially normal lungs it is in addition primary. PSP occurs predominantly in young adults (65% are between 20 and 40 years of age) and it is five times more common in men than women. Untreated, at least one-third of patients will have a recurrence, most commonly within a few years and on the ipsilateral side. PSP is nearly always caused by the rupture of an apical pleural bleb. Although not detectable on interval chest radiographs, one taken at the time of the pneumothorax will show one or more blebs projecting from the apical lung margin in 20% of patients; such

TABLE 3-2 **Causes of Adult Pneumothorax**

Spontaneous, Primary	
Spontaneous, Secondary	
Airflow obstruction	Asthma Chronic obstructive pulmonary disease Cystic fibrosis
Pulmonary infection	Cavitary pneumonia Tuberculosis Fungal disease AIDS Pneumatocele
Pulmonary infarction	
Neoplasm	Metastatic sarcoma
Diffuse lung disease	Histiocytosis X Lymphangioleiomyomatosis Fibrosing alveolitis Other diffuse fibroses
Hereditable disorders of fibrous connective tissue	Marfan's syndrome
Endometriosis (catamenial pneumothorax)	
Traumatic, Non-iatrogenic	
Ruptured oesophagus/trachea	
Closed chest trauma (± rib fracture)	
Penetrating chest trauma	
Traumatic, Iatrogenic	
Thoracotomy/thoracocentesis	
Percutaneous biopsy	
Tracheostomy	
Central venous catheterisation	

abnormal apical airspaces are much more commonly shown by interval CT.[11]

Secondary Spontaneous Pneumothorax

A large number of conditions predispose to pneumothorax (Table 3-2). In a number of these disorders pneumothorax occurs frequently.

Diagnosis

The diagnosis of pneumothorax is made with the chest radiograph, which also detects complications and predisposing conditions and helps in management[5] (Fig. 3-13).

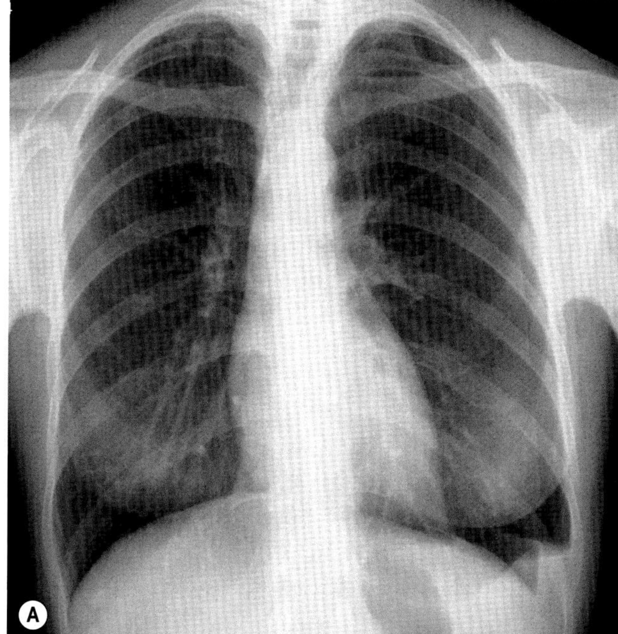

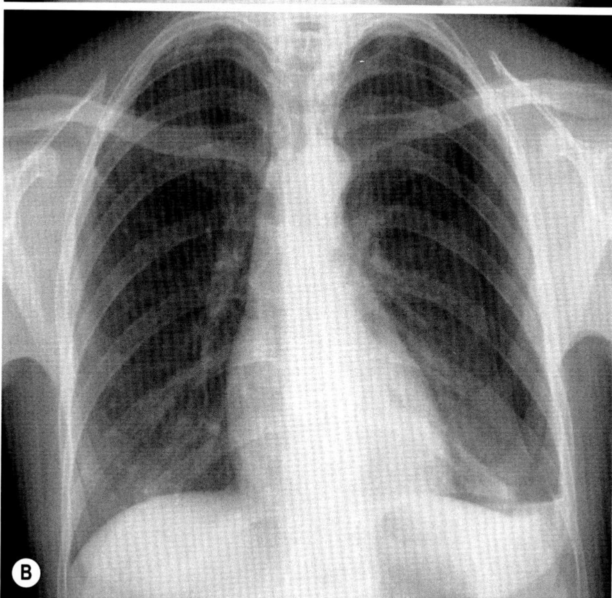

FIGURE 3-13 ■ **Left primary spontaneous pneumothorax.** Chest radiograph (A) at deep inspiration and (B) at deep expiration. The left lung has partially collapsed and an area of extreme low density without vascular markings becomes visible. The pneumothorax is accentuated on the chest radiograph at suspended deep expiration (B).

Typical Signs

These are seen on erect radiographs in which the pleural air rises to the lung apex. Under these conditions the visceral pleural line at the apex becomes separated from the chest wall by a transradiant zone devoid of vessels. Though this sounds a straightforward sign to assess, difficulties of interpretation can arise with avascular lung apices, as in bullous disease and when linear shadows are created by clothing or dressing artefacts, tubes and skin folds. Skin folds cause problems particularly in neonates and in old people radiographed slumped against a cassette in the AP projection (Fig. 3-14). Features that help identify artefacts and skin folds include extension of the 'pneumothorax' line beyond the margin of the chest cavity, laterally located vessels and an orientation of a line that is inconsistent with the edge of a slightly collapsed lung. In addition, the margin of skin folds tends to be much wider than the normally thin visceral pleural line. In indeterminate circumstances a repeat chest radiograph, an expiratory radiograph (see Fig. 3-13B) or one taken with the patient decubitus may clarify the situation. Should doubt still remain, then CT is particularly helpful in distinguishing between bullae and a pneumothorax.

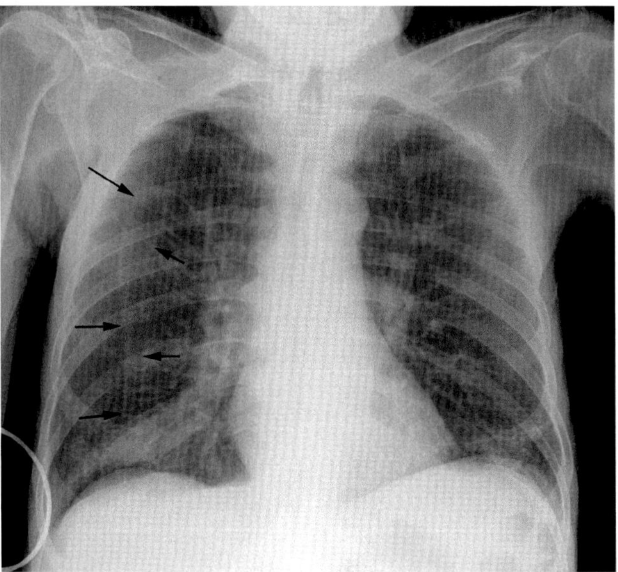

FIGURE 3-14 ■ **Skin folds mimicking a right pneumothorax (arrows).** The laterally located blood vessels, the wide margin of the lines, and the orientation of the lines that is inconsistent with the edge of a slightly collapsed lung help to differentiate them from a real pneumothorax.

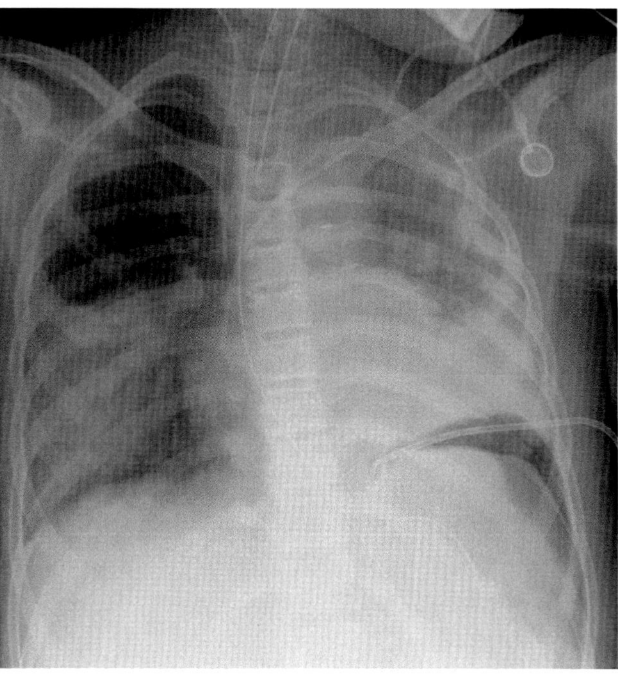

FIGURE 3-15 ■ **Supine pneumothorax.** Portable chest radiograph after development of a pneumothorax in a patient with a bilateral pneumonia. There is an increase of transradiancy at the left lung base and the costophrenic sulcus laterally is more pronounced ('deep sulcus sign').

Atypical Signs

These arise when the patient is supine or the pleural space partly obliterated. In the supine position, pleural air rises and collects anteriorly, particularly medially and basally, and may not extend far enough posteriorly to separate lung from the chest wall at the apex or laterally. Signs that suggest a pneumothorax under these conditions are[12,13] (Fig. 3-15):

- Ipsilateral transradiancy, either generalised or hypochondrial;
- A deep, finger-like costophrenic sulcus laterally;
- A visible anterior costophrenic recess seen as an oblique line or interface in the hypochondrium; when the recess is manifest as an interface it mimics the adjacent diaphragm ('double diaphragm sign');
- A transradiant band parallel to the diaphragm and/or mediastinum with undue clarity of the mediastinal border;
- Visualisation of the undersurface of the heart, and of the cardiac fat pads as rounded opacities suggesting masses; and
- Diaphragm depression.

In a patient who cannot stand, the presence of a pneumothorax can be confirmed with a lateral decubitus view or a supine decubitus projection with the cassette placed dorsolaterally at 45° and the X-ray tube angled perpendicular to the cassette. In experienced hands ultrasound may be able to detect small peripheral pneumothorax.[14]

When the pleural space is partly obliterated a pneumothorax may be loculated, and must be differentiated from other localised transradiancies. These include cysts, bullae, pneumatoceles, pneumomediastinum and local emphysema. These cannot always be differentiated by plain radiographs, but can be by CT.

Complications

Haemopneumothorax

This is a common complication of traumatic pneumothorax. Small amounts of serous or bloody fluid may also occur with a spontaneous pneumothorax, but only 2% of individuals develop a clinically significant haemothorax in these circumstances. Blood may clot in the pleural space, producing a mass which can mimic a pleural tumour.

Tension Pneumothorax

This life-threatening complication is present when intrapleural pressure becomes positive relative to atmospheric pressure for a significant part of the respiratory cycle. Tension has an adverse effect on gas exchange and cardiovascular performance, causing a rapid deterioration in the patient's clinical condition. The diagnosis is usually made clinically and treatment instituted without a radiograph. Should a chest radiograph be taken, it will show contralateral mediastinal shift and ipsilateral diaphragm depression. Mild degrees of contralateral mediastinal shift are not unusual with a non-tension pneumothorax because of the negative pressure in the normal pleural space. Moderate or gross mediastinal shift, however, should be taken as indicating tension, particularly if the ipsilateral hemidiaphragm is depressed. This latter sign is the more reliable and is almost invariably present with significant tension.

Pyopneumothorax

This unusual complication is seen most commonly following necrotising pneumonia or oesophageal perforation.

Adhesions

These generate straight band shadows extending from the lung margin to the chest wall. They limit collapse but at the same time may account for continued air leakage from the lung surface, and if they tear they may bleed. They can be identified with CT.

Re-expansion Oedema

This unusual complication is sometimes seen following the rapid therapeutic re-expansion of a lung that has been markedly collapsed for several days or more. Oedema comes on within hours of drainage, may progress for a day or two and clears within a week. It usually causes only mild morbidity.

PLEURAL THICKENING AND FIBROTHORAX[5]

Pleural thickening is common and usually represents the organised end stage of various active processes such as infective and non-infective inflammation (including asbestos exposure and pneumothorax) and haemothorax. When generalised and gross, it is termed a fibrothorax and may cause significant ventilatory impairment.

Radiologically, pleural thickening gives fixed shadowing of water density, most commonly located in the dependent parts of the pleural cavity. Viewed en profile, it appears as a band of soft-tissue density up to approximately 10 mm thick, more or less parallel to the chest wall and with a sharp lung interface. En face, it causes ill-defined, veil-like shadowing. Blunting of the costophrenic angle, often with tenting of the diaphragm, is a common finding. On ultrasound, benign pleural thickening produces an homogeneous echogenic layer just inside the chest wall. It is not reliably detected unless it is 1 cm or more thick. CT, on the other hand, is very sensitive at detecting pleural thickening, which is most easily assessed on the inside of the ribs, where there should normally be no soft-tissue opacity.

Fibrous pleural thickening is common in the apical pleural cupola. This may be secondary to tuberculosis or represent apical cap. Caps are age-related changes of unknown aetiology. Sometimes they have a scalloped contour or are associated with a tenting towards the lung. They are as commonly unilateral as bilateral. Caps should be distinguished from the companion shadows of the upper ribs, from extrapleural linear fat deposition and most importantly from a Pancoast's tumour. Companion shadows of the ribs are usually smoothly bordered towards the lung apex, while extrapleural fat is usually bilateral, symmetrical and also located along the lateral chest wall. Caps may be indistinguishable from Pancoast's tumour on the chest radiograph. In case of doubt, CT or MR should be performed.

Fibrous pleural thickening can be induced by asbestos exposure[15] (Fig. 3-16). This thickening can be diffuse or is more often multifocal. These pleural plaques can undergo hyaline transformation, calcify or ossify. They are most commonly found along the lower thorax and on the diaphragmatic pleura. In extensive disease also the anterior and ventral part of the thorax may be involved. Pleural plaques need to be large before they become visible on a chest X-ray (Fig. 3-16E). On CT they are visualised much earlier (Figs. 3-16A–D) and appear as circumscribed areas of pleural thickening separated from the underlying rib and extrapleural soft tissues by a thin layer of fat. Because of their higher density they can easily be differentiated from circumscribed increase of extrapleural fat, as sometimes seen in obese patients.

Diffuse pleural thickening is also a manifestation of asbestos exposure.

The radiographic definition of diffuse pleural thickening or fibrothorax is somewhat arbitrary. It has been suggested to consider as fibrothorax a smooth uninterrupted pleural density that extends over at least one-quarter of the chest wall. On CT, fibrothorax has been defined as a pleural thickening which extends more than 8 cm in the craniocaudal direction and 5 cm laterally and with a thickness of more than 3 mm. Common causes of fibrothorax are empyema, tuberculosis and haemorrhagic effusion. Asbestos exposure-related fibrothorax is less common than pleural plaques and is usually the sequel of a benign exudative effusion. CT may be helpful for finding the aetiology of the fibrothorax. Extensive calcification favours previous tuberculosis or empyema[5] (Fig. 3-17). Asbestos exposure-related fibrothorax is usually bilateral and rarely calcified. Generalised, postinflammatory pleural thickening must be distinguished from diffuse pleural malignancy caused by mesothelioma, metastatic disease (particularly adenocarcinoma), lymphoma and leukaemia. Mesothelioma and adenocarcinoma cause diffuse pleural thickening, which is often lobulated, and may surround the whole lung and extend into and along fissures. These features are frequently obscured by an effusion. The most useful signs on CT that indicate malignant as opposed to benign pleural thickening are circumferential thickening, nodularity, parietal thickening of more than 1 cm, and involvement of the mediastinal pleura[5] (see Figs. 3-18, 3-19). MRI signal intensity seems to be a valuable additional feature for differentiating benign from malignant disease, especially since MRI is often able to demonstrate the tumour extension into the chest wall. Signal hypointensity with long TR sequences is a reliable predictive sign of benign pleural disease.[16] Recent studies have shown that diffusion-weighted and dynamic contrast-enhanced MR imaging may be promising for differentiating malignant mesothelioma from benign pleural alterations.[17] FDG-PET CT combines metabolic and anatomic information and can be used to differentiate benign from malignant pleural thickening. However,[18] FDG-PET is not completely tumour-specific and uptake can be seen in benign inflammatory lesions as well.[19–21]

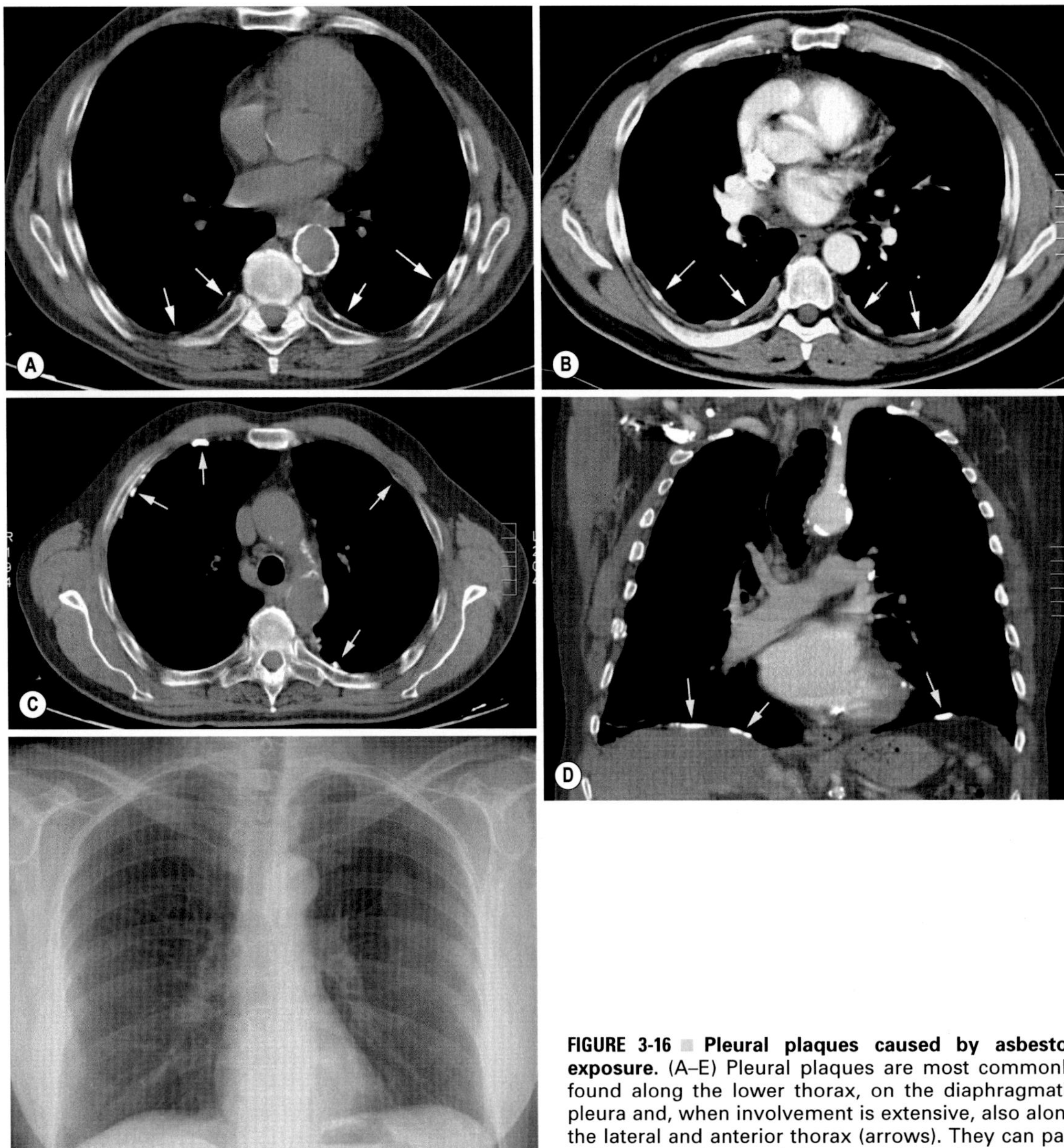

FIGURE 3-16 ■ Pleural plaques caused by asbestos exposure. (A–E) Pleural plaques are most commonly found along the lower thorax, on the diaphragmatic pleura and, when involvement is extensive, also along the lateral and anterior thorax (arrows). They can partially or completely calcify or ossify. In this situation, and when large, they can be seen on a chest radiograph (E).

FIGURE 3-17 ■ Pleural calcification. (A–C) On the chest radiograph (A) an extensive sheet-like calcification of the left pleura and a smaller localised calcification of the right pleura is seen together with focal calcifications of the diaphragmatic pleura (B, C). CT demonstrates the extent and thickness of the pleural calcification.

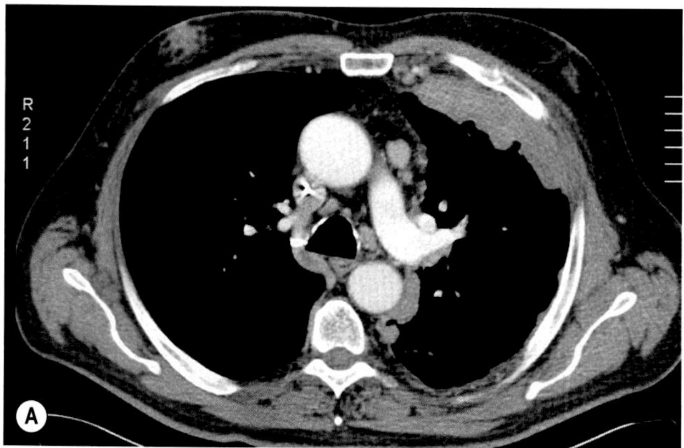

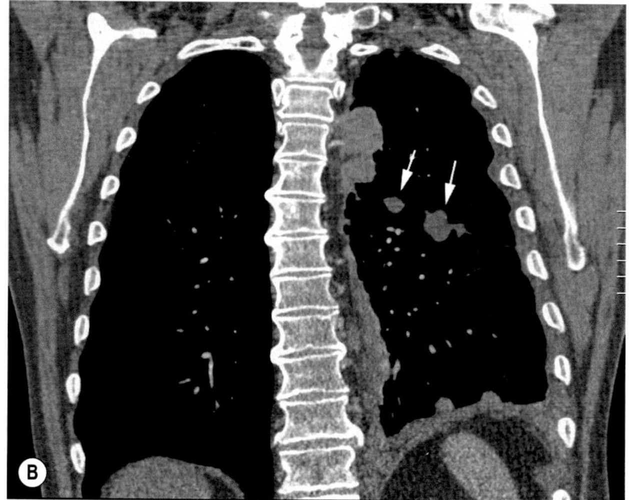

FIGURE 3-18 **Malignant mesothelioma.** (A) Axial and (B) coronal CT. Diffuse lobulated and nodular thickening of the pleura with tumour extension into the lobar fissure (arrows). Note the metastatic enlargement of some hilar and mediastinal lymph nodes.

PLEURAL CALCIFICATION

Pleural calcification is most commonly seen following asbestos exposure, empyema (usually tuberculous) and haemothorax (Fig. 3-17). In the last two conditions, calcification is irregular, resembles a plaque or sheet and is contained within thickened pleura. It may occur anywhere but is most common in the lower posterior half of the chest and is usually unilateral, unlike that found in silicosis, particularly of the asbestos-related type, where calcification occurs as more discrete collections within plaques and is usually bilateral.

PLEURAL TUMOURS

Localised Pleural Tumours[22]

These are relatively uncommon, the most common being a localised fibrous tumour (localised mesothelioma) (Fig. 3-20). These lesions most commonly present in middle age, about half the patients being asymptomatic. Hypertropic osteoarthropathy is a well-recognised

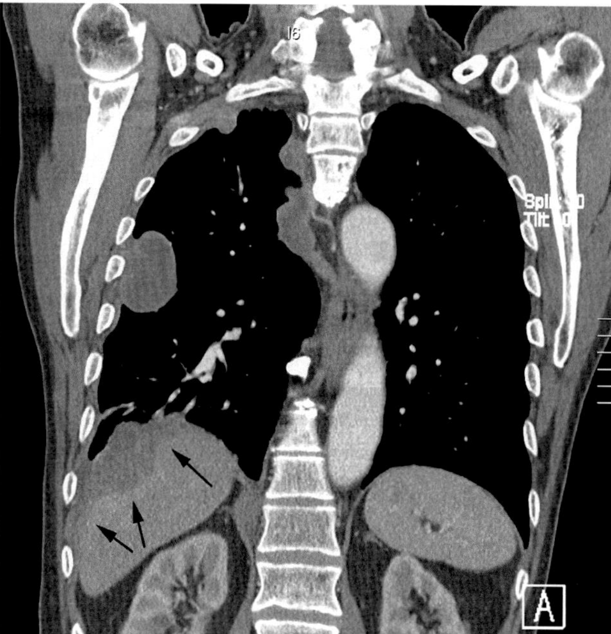

FIGURE 3-19 **Malignant pleural thickening caused by metastatic disease.** Malignant pleural thickening was caused by pleural metastases. Note the compression on the right hemidiaphragm and the extension of the tumour into the liver (arrows).

complication (10–30% of patients) and uncommonly the tumour produces hypoglycaemia. Microscopically, two-thirds are benign and one-third are malignant. The plain radiographic findings are of a pleurally based, well-demarcated, rounded and often slightly lobulated mass (2–20 cm diameter) which may, because of pedunculation, show marked positional variation with changes in posture and respiration. Pleural fibromas usually make an obtuse angle with the chest wall and may reach enormous sizes (Figs. 3-20A,B). Occasionally they may arise in a fissure. CT findings are similar to those observed on plain radiography: a mobile mass, often heterogeneous because of necrosis, haemorrhage, frequently enhancing after contrast medium administration, and rarely calcified. Malignant types are usually larger than 10 cm and may invade the chest wall. Typically, these tumours show low signal intensity on both T1- and T2-weighted images, although tumours with intermediate-to-high signal intensity have been described.[23]

Lipomas are asymptomatic benign tumours usually discovered incidentally on chest radiographs as sharply defined pleural masses. Diagnosis is easy with CT because this examination can delineate the pleural origin and the fatty composition. This fatty density is homogeneous. When heterogeneous and when also soft-tissue attenuation components are found, a liposarcoma or area of tumour infarction should be suspected. Pleural lipomas have high signal intensity on T1-weighted images. On T2-weighted images signal is moderately bright.

Diagnosis of pleural extension of bronchogenic carcinoma on a chest radiograph is very difficult. The only reliable indicator is rib destruction. With CT and MRI

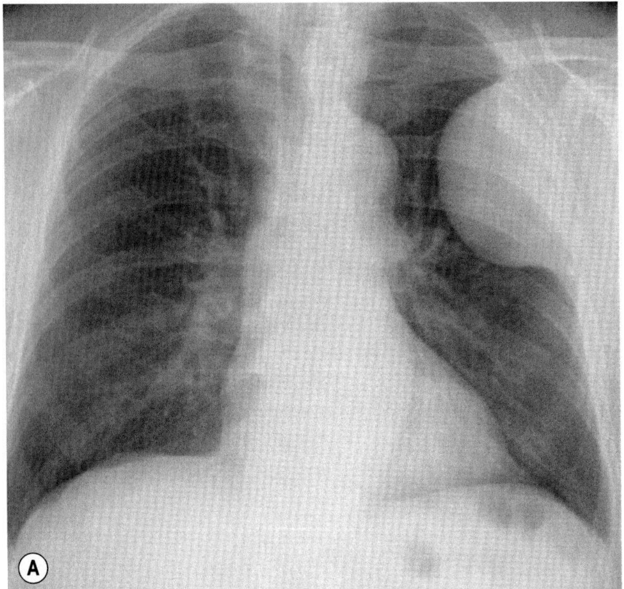

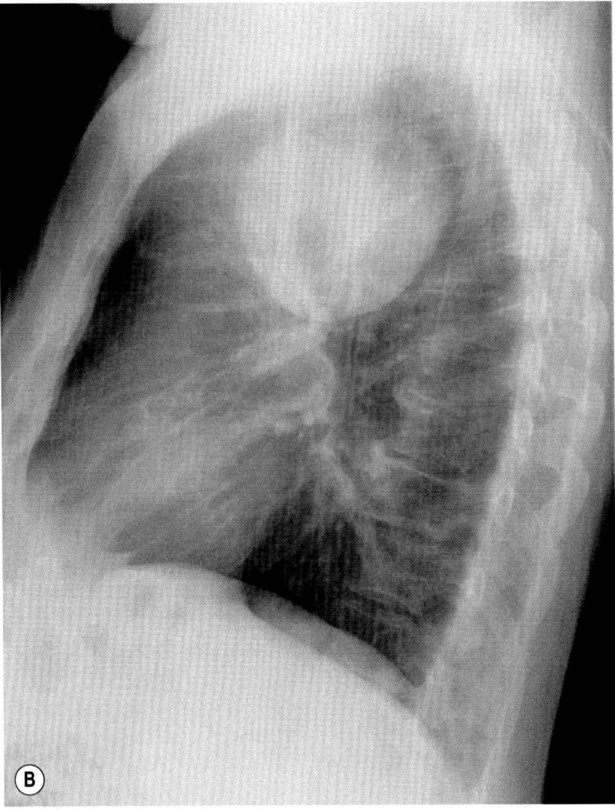

FIGURE 3-20 ■ **Large benign pleural fibroma.** (A) Frontal and (B) lateral radiographs show a large well-demarcated and homogeneous mass abutting the chest wall. Note the obtuse angle between the mass and the chest wall, suggesting the extrapulmonary origin of the mass.

also diagnosis can be difficult. Features such as a large contact (>3 cm) between the mass and the pleura, an obtuse angle between the tumour and the chest wall, an associated pleural thickening and the presence of pleural tags usually considered as signs of chest wall invasion also occur in benign lesions. The accuracy of CT can be increased by performing 2D and 3D reconstructions.

In cases where tumour invasion is obvious, 2D sagittal or coronal reconstructions can be helpful in ascertaining the extent of the mass. MRI has a slight advantage over CT in the evaluation of chest wall and pleura invasion. Before spiral CT, MRI was considered better for studying superior sulcus tumours and their extension to the chest wall (see Fig. 3-3). However, studies have shown that spiral CT and MRI showed comparable sensitivity but that spiral CT had higher specificity.

CT is superior in the detection of pleural calcifications and osseous destruction (see Fig. 3-3). MDCT can also be used in selected cases to clarify a complex relationship between tumour invading the chest wall and vascular structures of the thoracic inlet.

Pleural metastases are the most common pleural neoplasms. They are usually an adenocarcinoma with sites of origin including the ovary, stomach, breast and lung. Pleural metastatic disease can present as a solitary mass but more often multiple pleural locations are seen (Fig. 3-19). Pleural metastases are very often accompanied by pleural effusion, which can be the only finding on a chest radiograph. CT, MRI and ultrasound are more sensitive to demonstrate pleural metastasis as the cause of the pleural effusion.[9]

Diffuse Pleural Tumours

Diffuse tumoural thickening of the pleura can be caused by malignant mesothelioma or by pleural metastasis. Both entities are usually indistinguishable with imaging. Diffuse malignant mesothelioma is a rare primary neoplasm and its development is strongly related to asbestos exposure. It presents on a chest radiograph as an irregular and nodular pleural thickening with or without associated pleural effusion. Tumour extension into the interlobular fissures, accompanying pleural effusion, and invasion into the chest wall are better appreciated with CT (Fig. 3-19).

On CT, malignant mesothelioma presents as a nodular soft-tissue mass sometimes with hypodense areas corresponding with necrosis. Metastatic enlargement of hilar and mediastinal nodes is seen in up to 50% of patients. Malignant mesothelioma has a minimally increased signal on T1 and a moderately increased signal on T2. MRI may be superior to CT in determining extent of disease because it allows better evaluation of the relationship of the tumour to the structures of the chest wall, mediastinum and diaphragm. However, in most cases CT and MRI provide similar morphological information. Ultrasound may be a supplementary method for biopsy and surgery planning.[18,24] Finally, in many institutions, FDG-PET CT is used as a staging tool for malignant mesothelioma, although it should be emphasised again that FDG uptake is not entirely tumour-specific[19–21] (Fig. 3-21).

Intervention

Interventional procedures of the chest wall and pleura may be performed for both diagnostic and therapeutic

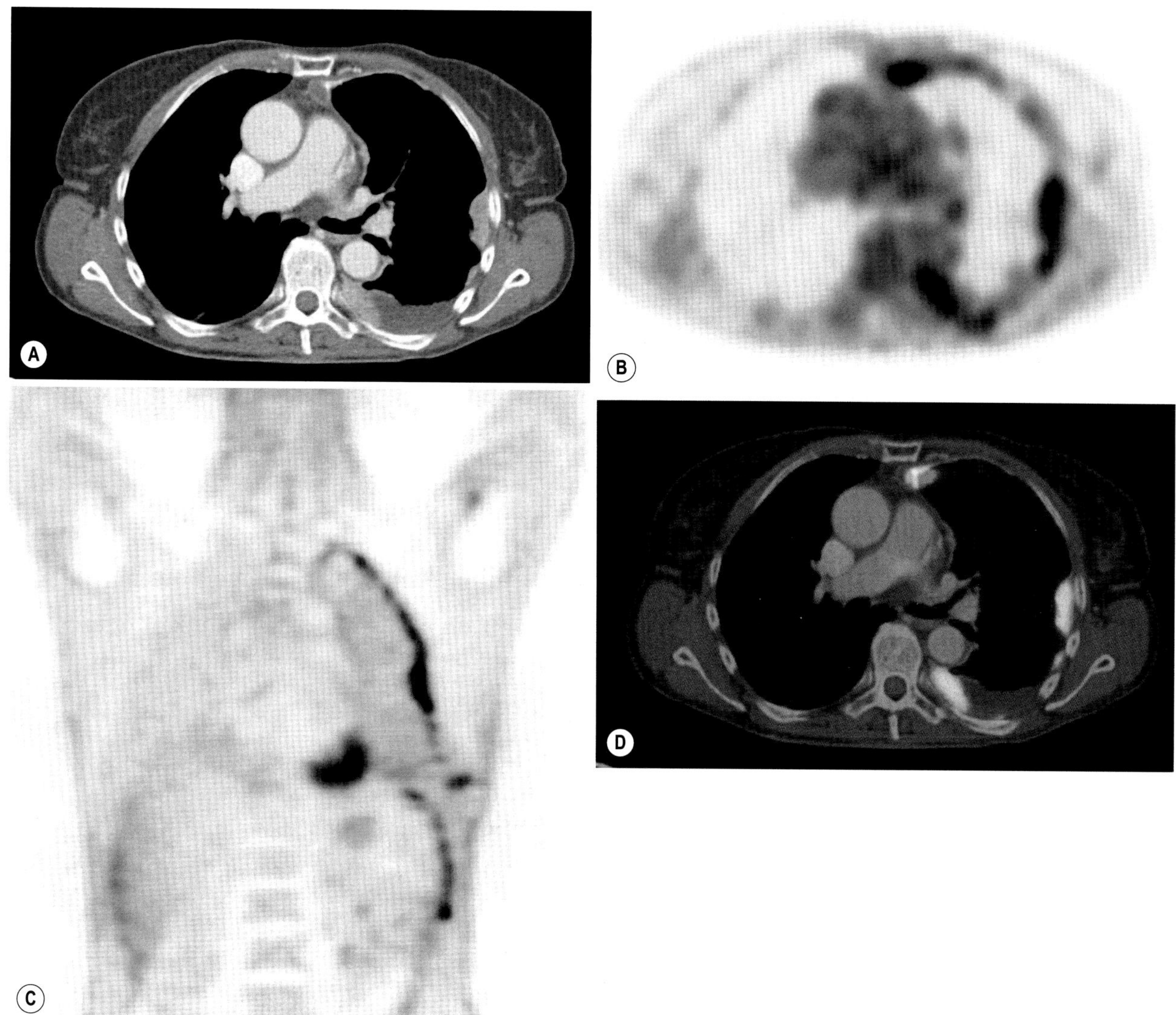

FIGURE 3-21 ■ **Malignant mesothelioma.** FDG-PET CT of a patient with malignant mesothelioma. CT (A), PET (B, C) and PET-CT fusion image (D) showing extent of the tumour.

reasons. Ultrasound or CT guidance is most commonly used, although fluoroscopy and, rarely, MRI have also been used. On occasion, PET-CT may be performed before biopsy to guide the procedure to a likely diagnostic site.

Chest Wall Intervention

It is usual to biopsy chest wall lesions, soft tissue and rib, using real-time ultrasound guidance. This has been shown to be safe and highly efficacious. Soft-tissue lesions are readily identified in most patients using ultrasound, with a prior diagnostic CT or MRI often used to help identify the site of abnormality if it is impalpable (Fig. 3-22). Rib lesions associated with a cortical break may be readily identified and biopsied, and this technique has been shown to be very useful in providing histological confirmation of primary and secondary malignancies when needed.[25]

Pleural Intervention

Pleural Aspiration. This is one of the commonest interventional procedures performed in hospital practice. It is usually performed to sample pleural fluid, but may also be performed for small pneumothoraces. Although regarded as a simple procedure, a number of studies have shown that it is associated with a complication rate of up to 10%, the commonest being pneumothorax, with less common complications being solid organ puncture and intercostal artery laceration.[26] The significance of the complications reported, including death from haemorrhage, and the frequency of the procedure have led to the recommendation that all pleural interventions are now guided by ultrasound.[27] This requirement has led to ultrasound now being part of the core curricula of chest physicians in training, and has been shown to reduce the incidence of complications.

Although it is a commonly held belief that the intercostal artery lies in the intercostal groove and is

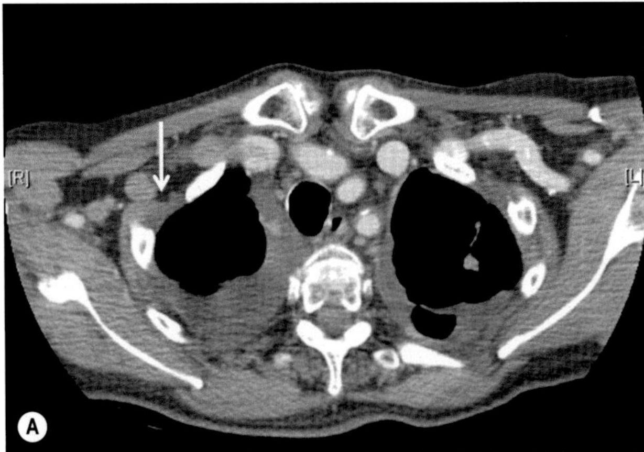

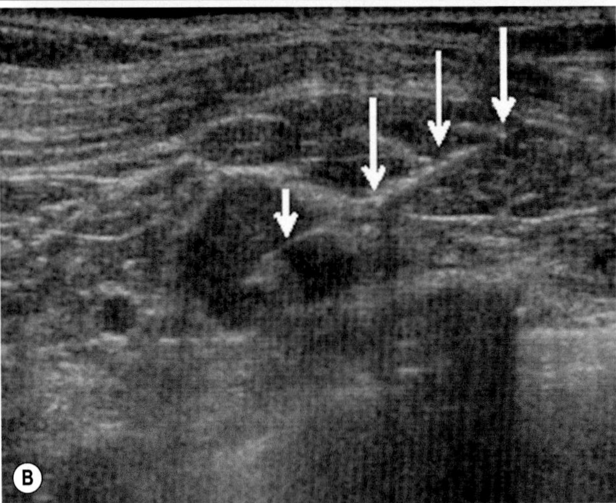

FIGURE 3-22 ■ (A) Contrast-enhanced CT, demonstrating a right subpectoral node, white arrow, in a patient with bilateral cytology negative pleural effusions and no histological diagnosis. (B) Ultrasound-guided biopsy of the same subpectoral node. The biopsy needle is arrowed passing through pectoralis, and its cutting needle bevel (short arrow) is clearly seen within the node.

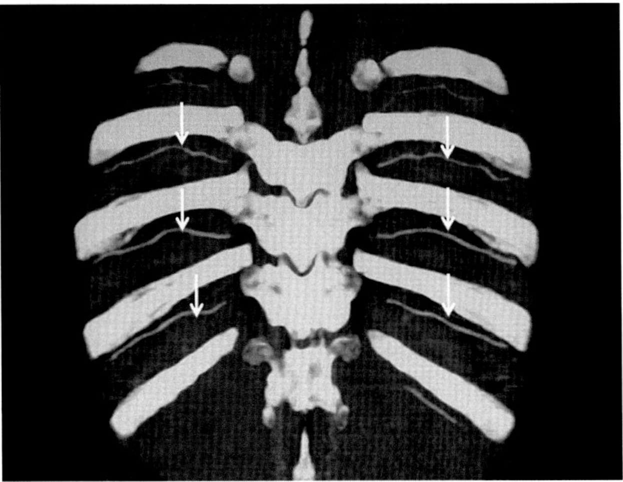

FIGURE 3-23 ■ 3D CT volumetric reformat of the posterior chest wall, demonstrating the intercostal arteries (Arrows), not protected by the flange of the rib medially. Note how tortuous the arteries are. This may become much more pronounced in the elderly.

protected by the flange of the rib, this is not absolutely correct. Gray described the intercostal artery arising from the aorta, and passing cranially and laterally until the angle of the rib, where it then lies in the intercostal groove.[28] This means that for a short distance posteriorly, the artery is exposed and may be lacerated when interventional procedures are performed. It has also been shown that intercostal arteries in the elderly may be tortuous and may be exposed for a greater distance before moving into the groove compared with that in the young[29] (Fig. 3-23). It is for these reasons that care should be taken when performing all pleural procedures, to ensure that the needle or cannula is as close as possible to the cranial surface of the rib and lateral to the angle of the rib.

Chest Drains. Patients with symptomatic pneumothoraces, large-volume pleural effusions, infected effusions and symptomatic malignant effusions require chest drain insertion.

For the most part, pneumothoraces are drained either as an emergency if under tension or because of trauma, on the ward or in Accident and Emergency departments. This is performed safely by clinicians using the safe triangle defined by anatomical landmarks. Occasionally, pneumothoraces may be small or loculated in patients with underlying lung disease such as cystic fibrosis or interstitial lung disease and drain insertion needs then to be performed under CT guidance to prevent underlying lung injury during insertion.

As with pleural aspiration, chest drains should be inserted under ultrasound guidance to avoid inadvertently puncturing lung or solid organs. For a substantial number of years there has been debate on whether large- or small-bore drains should be used in patients with infected pleural effusions. It would now appear that small-bore drains are at least as efficacious as large-bore drains.[30]

Both infected and malignant effusions may be uni- or multilocular and, or multiseptated. In these circumstances drain insertion alone may be insufficient to provide adequate drainage and the use of fibrinolytic therapy may be required.[31,32]

Pleural Biopsy. Although the aetiology of pleural thickening (or a combination of thickening and pleural effusion) will be determined in most patients by a combination of clinical history and imaging features making biopsy unnecessary, some patients require further investigation and histological confirmation (Fig. 3-24). This may either be by percutaneous biopsy or under direct visualisation at medical or video-assisted thoracoscopy. The use of closed needle pleural biopsy such as the Abram's biopsy has almost disappeared in all areas other than those endemic for tuberculosis, following evidence comparing its efficacy to image-guided cutting needle biopsy, particularly in patients with suspected pleural malignancy.[33] Whilst percutaneous biopsy has been shown to have a

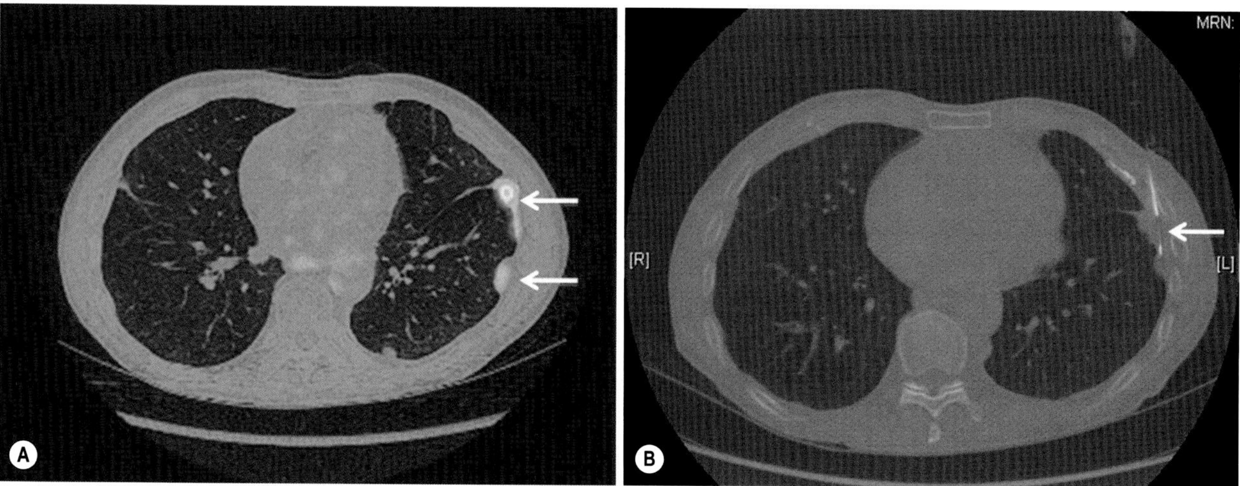

FIGURE 3-24 (A) PET-CT performed in a patient with suspected malignant pleural thickening, but the initial percutaneous biopsy was negative. Note how the two large left-sided pleural nodules, arrowed, have differing 18F-fluorodeoxyglucose avidity. (B) The more avid of the two nodules has been targeted for biopsy, arrowed.

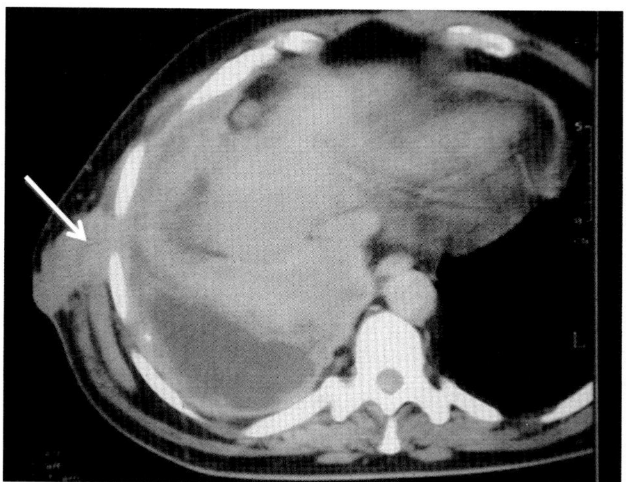

FIGURE 3-25 CT, demonstrating mesothelioma growing, arrowed, along the site of a prior pleural drain.

sensitivity of almost 90% for mesothelioma and for other pleural malignancies such as adenocarcinoma, it is unable to provide a tissue diagnosis and treat an associated pleural effusion in a single procedure. By comparison, medical thoracoscopy, which has become the technique of choice for patients with suspected malignant effusions, and percutaneous image-guided biopsy (mostly for patients unsuitable for thoracoscopy) allow combined diagnosis and therapy in a single procedure. In patients with suspected mesothelioma, a tissue diagnosis should be achieved using as few interventions as possible, because of the known incidence of biopsy and drain track tumour seeding[34] (Fig. 3-25).

THE DIAPHRAGM

The diaphragm is only seen because there is air-containing lung adjacent to it superiorly. It is 2–3 mm thick, but this will only be appreciated if there is air immediately beneath it, as with a pneumoperitoneum. Localised loss of clarity occurs when the diaphragm is not tangential to the X-ray beam, but usually indicates adjacent pulmonary or pleural disease; e.g. the costophrenic or costovertebral angles are obliterated by pleural fluid, and much of the diaphragmatic outline may be obliterated by basal pneumonia.

Each hemidiaphragm is normally represented on the PA radiograph by a smooth, curved line which is convex upwards. The lateral attachment of the diaphragm to the ribs is represented by the lateral costophrenic recess, a sharply defined acute angle. When the diaphragm is flat, as in emphysema, the most lateral muscle slips extend slightly upwards and may be seen as digitations. The costophrenic angle then becomes less acute, or even obtuse, and the appearance may simulate a small pleural effusion. Medially, the diaphragm meets the heart at the cardiophrenic angle. This is higher than the costophrenic angle and, unlike the latter, is often ill-defined owing to the presence of fat. On the right, this may simulate disease in the middle lobe, and on the left, disease in the lower lobe or lingula. Prominent fat pads at the cardiophrenic angles are an occasional cause of overestimation of the transverse cardiac diameter, particularly if the film is underexposed. On correctly exposed radiographs, the relatively low radio-opacity of the fat pad enables it to be distinguished from the cardiac apex.

On the lateral radiograph each dome makes an acute angle with the ribs posteriorly to form the posterior costophrenic recesses. The latter lie considerably lower than the highest part of each leaf—a point of great importance, as localised pulmonary or pleural disease adjacent to the posterior aspect of the diaphragm will often not be recognised on the PA radiograph, on which only the highest anterior portion of the diaphragmatic dome is represented. The right hemidiaphragm makes an upward curve as it extends anteriorly to the sternum. This part of its attachment is often poorly defined because of adjacent fat. Localisation of disease requires the correct identification of each leaf on the lateral radiographs. The left diaphragm is obscured anteriorly by the heart and usually has an air-distended gastric fundus beneath it; whichever leaf is nearer the film is related to the ribs least magnified by the diverging beam.

Level

In most people the diaphragm in the mid-lung field lies at the level of the fifth or sixth anterior rib interspace. It may lie at a lower level in normal young individuals, particularly those of an asthenic build and at a slightly higher level in the obese, the elderly and young infants. In over 90% of normal people the right hemidiaphragm is higher than the left. This difference in height on the PA film is usually about 15 mm, but may be as much as 30 mm.

Depression of the diaphragm occurs in emphysema and in acute severe asthma, but flattening only occurs in emphysema.

Inversion of the diaphragm is sometimes seen with a tension pneumothorax and with large basal bullae. It is also a common accompaniment of pleural effusions. Table 3-3 shows the most common causes of bilateral symmetrical elevation of the diaphragm.

Elevation of a single hemidiaphragm is usually secondary to adjacent pleural, pulmonary or subphrenic disease, or to phrenic nerve palsy (Table 3-4). A minor degree of diaphragmatic elevation is a common accompaniment of pleurisy, lower lobe pneumonia and pulmonary thromboembolism. In the latter there may be no visible change in the affected lung. Upper abdominal inflammatory processes and rib fractures may also cause a high diaphragm. A high hemidiaphragm may be mimicked by a subpulmonary pleural effusion (Fig. 3-8), a large well-defined tumour adjacent to the dome, or by combined middle and lower lobe collapse.

Eventration

In eventration a part of the normal diaphragmatic muscle is replaced by a thin layer of connective tissue and a few scattered muscle fibres.[35] The unbroken continuity differentiates it from diaphragmatic hernia. Some authors consider eventration to be a congenital anomaly resulting from failure of muscularisation of part or all of the diaphragmatic leaf. Most authors, however, also include within the definition elevation occurring as a result of acquired paralysis with atrophy of the diaphragmatic muscle, an inclusion justified by the fact that many adults with surgically proven eventration have previously had normal chest radiographs. Total eventration shows a marked left-sided predominance, for which there is no acceptable explanation.

Although eventration is a recognised cause of respiratory distress in the newborn, it is not usually associated with symptoms in the adult. Localised forms of the condition are relatively common, particularly in the elderly, and predominantly affect the right hemidiaphragm at its anteromedial aspect (Fig. 3-26). The distinction between a localised eventration and a small diaphragmatic hernia or a mass arising from the lung, pleura or diaphragm is best made using CT or MRI. The various causes of focal elevation or bulging of a diaphragm are given in Table 3-5.

TABLE 3-3 Causes of Bilateral Symmetrical Elevation of the Diaphragm

Supine position
Poor inspiration
Obesity
Pregnancy
Abdominal distension (ascites, intestinal obstruction, abdominal mass)
Diffuse pulmonary fibrosis
Lymphangitis carcinomatosa
Disseminated lupus erythematosus
Bilateral basal pulmonary emboli
Painful conditions (after abdominal surgery)
Bilateral diaphragmatic paralysis

TABLE 3-4 Causes of Unilateral Elevation of the Diaphragm

Posture—lateral decubitus position (dependent side)
Gaseous distension of stomach or colon
Dorsal scoliosis
Pulmonary hypoplasia
Pulmonary collapse
Phrenic nerve palsy
Eventration
Pneumonia or pleurisy
Pulmonary thromboembolism
Rib fracture and other painful conditions
Subphrenic infection
Subphrenic mass

TABLE 3-5 Causes of Focal Elevation (Bulge) of the Diaphragm

Partial eventration
Diaphragmatic hernia
Diaphragmatic tumour
Pleural tumour
Pulmonary tumour
Focal diaphragmatic dysfunction
Focal diaphragmatic adhesions

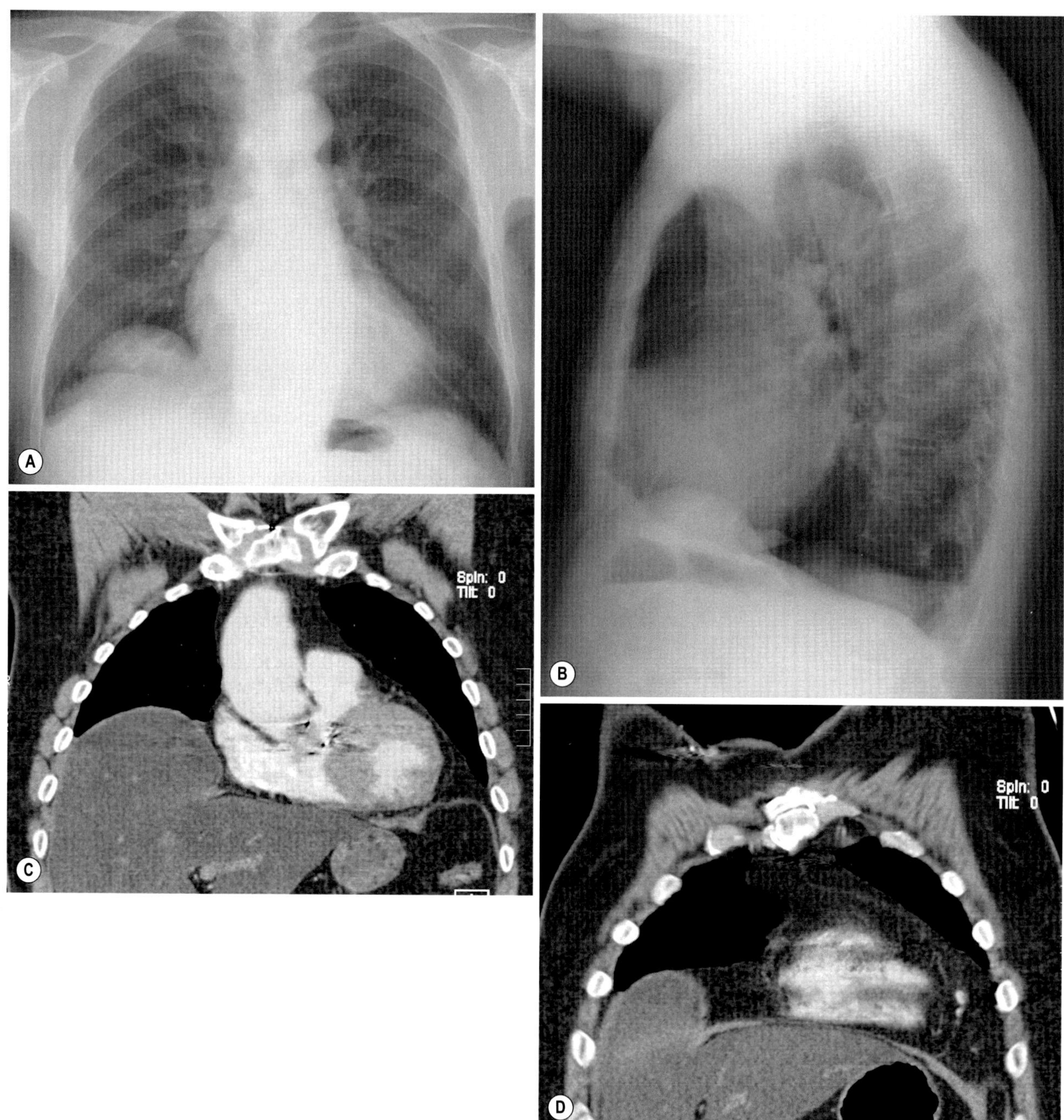

FIGURE 3-26 ■ **Focal eventration.** (A, B) PA and lateral chest radiograph reveal a soft-tissue opacity arising from the diaphragm. (C, D) CT shows the presence of liver under the elevated part of the diaphragm.

Movement and Paralysis

Unequal excursion of the two hemidiaphragms occurs in approximately 80% of normal people. However, this inequality of diaphragmatic excursion is less than 10 mm in most people. While normal young adults can move the diaphragm over at least 30 mm, this range is greatly reduced in the elderly.

As the chest radiograph is exposed at the end of a full inspiration, any severe unilateral limitation of diaphragmatic movement will be apparent on this static examination. Diaphragmatic movement is, however, better assessed by fluoroscopy, which should, ideally, be performed in both the AP and lateral projections with the patient erect and supine. The latter position is useful as the range of movement is usually greater than it is in the erect position. With the patient in the lateral position, any inequality of movement of the two leaves is readily assessed and localised restriction of movement identified better.[36] Restriction of diaphragmatic movement occurs secondary to disease of the phrenic nerve and secondary to inflammatory and painful conditions adjacent to the diaphragm, such as lower lobe pneumonia and subphrenic infection.

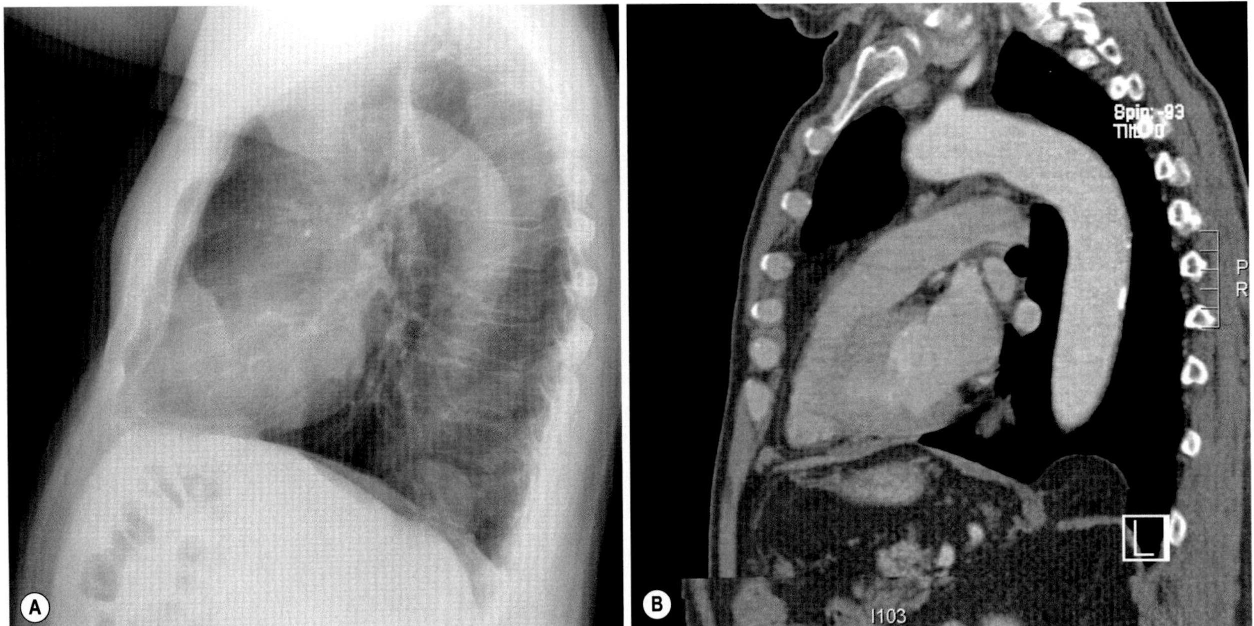

FIGURE 3-27 ■ **Bochdalek hernia.** (A) Lateral chest radiograph shows a focal bulge on the diaphragmatic contour just above the posterior costophrenic recess. (B) CT shows a fatty mass abutting the defect in the posteromedial aspect of the left hemidiaphragm.

Phrenic palsy is most commonly secondary to involvement of the phrenic nerve by tumour—usually a bronchial carcinoma. Phrenic nerve paresis may be caused by trauma (road accidents, birth injury, brachial plexus block and phrenic crush), irradiation and a variety of neurological conditions such as poliomyelitis, herpes zoster and cervical disc degeneration. The recognition of phrenic paresis depends upon finding a high hemidiaphragm which exhibits absent, restricted or paradoxical movement. The latter is particularly well demonstrated by sniffing. Diaphragmatic motion can also be examined with ultrasound.[36] Especially in patients who cannot come to the fluoroscopy room, bedside ultrasound is very useful. This technique has also a high accuracy to discover absent and paradoxical diaphragmatic motion. In addition, measurement of diaphragmatic thickness can be helpful to confirm diaphragmatic paralysis, since a paralysed diaphragm does not thicken during inspiration. An important mimic of phrenic paresis is eventration (usually left-sided, see above). In a significant small number of patients in whom there is little doubt that a phrenic paresis exists, no cause can be discovered. In this 'idiopathic' group the right leaf is more commonly affected than the left and it has been suggested that the palsy may be a legacy of previous viral neuritis.

Weakness or paralysis of both hemidiaphragms is most commonly seen in association with chronic neuromuscular disease and causes severe clinical disability. Bilateral paralysis may not be recognised by fluoroscopic examination, for passive descent of the diaphragm may occur with inspiration.

Diaphragmatic Hernias

Intrathoracic herniation of abdominal contents occurs through congenital defects in the muscle, through traumatic tears or, most commonly, through acquired areas of weakness at the central oesophageal hiatus. Congenital hernias presenting in childhood are discussed elsewhere. When the defect is small it may not come to attention until adulthood, when it usually presents as an incidental abnormality on the chest radiograph. Bochdalek defects through the pleuroperitoneal canal occur along the posterior aspect of the diaphragm and the hernia usually contains retroperitoneal fat or a portion of kidney or spleen[37] (Fig. 3-27). The majority occur on the left. A well-defined, dome-shaped, soft-tissue opacity is seen midway between the spine and lateral chest wall on the frontal view and above the posterior costophrenic recess on the lateral view. It may appear to 'come and go' on serial PA radiographs because of varying degrees of inspiration and differences in transdiaphragmatic pressure. It has been shown that asymptomatic small Bochdalek hernias are present in 6% of otherwise normal adults. These hernias appear on a lateral radiograph as a focal bulge centred approximately 4–5 cm anterior to the posterior diaphragmatic insertion. On CT and MRI the diagnosis can be made when a soft tissue or fatty mass is seen protruding through a small defect in the posteromedial aspect of either hemidiaphragm.

A Morgagni hernia presents in adulthood as an anterior opacity at the right cardiophrenic angle. It frequently contains omentum and may contain bowel. Its smooth, well-defined margin and soft-tissue radiodensity usually allow its differentiation from the much more common fat pad collection at this site. It is more difficult to differentiate from a low-lying pericardial cyst. Morgagni hernias containing gut can be diagnosed using barium, but the diagnosis is more simply established by means of CT or MRI. Hernias through the oesophageal hiatus are extremely common, particularly in the elderly in whom they may be an incidental finding on CT.

Diaphragmatic Trauma

Because diaphragmatic rupture is often associated with thoracic or abdominal injuries that require surgical treatment, many cases are diagnosed during surgery.[38] If surgery is not indicated, diaphragmatic tear can be missed, especially when it is small and when there is no herniation of abdominal structures to the chest. That is why suspicion is needed in all cases of trauma to the lower chest, but also in patients with severe pelvic trauma. The chest X-ray should be evaluated carefully. Special attention must be given to small changes in the diaphragm or to basal lung atelectasis or consolidation. If possible, the post-traumatic thorax should always be compared with previous chest X-rays.

The diagnostic tools are different in the acute and latent phase. In the acute phase surgical procedures are often necessary and if the patient has severe injuries bedside examinations, such as chest X-ray and ultrasound, should be relied upon. In the latent phase barium studies, spiral CT and MRI can give additional diagnostic information.

In the acute phase the chest X-ray is normal in about one-quarter of cases. In some cases gas and fluid shadows are seen in the thorax. Sometimes there is only a localised density in close relationship to the diaphragm (Fig. 3-29A), or an alteration in the diaphragmatic shape. The position of a nasogastric tube can help to localise the gastric fundus, but does not tell anything about the position of the diaphragm, which is essential in the diagnosis of a diaphragmatic tear. A follow-up X-ray of an acutely injured patient showing progressive opacification of one thorax side by a gas-filled structure is strongly suggestive for diaphragmatic rupture (Fig. 3-28).

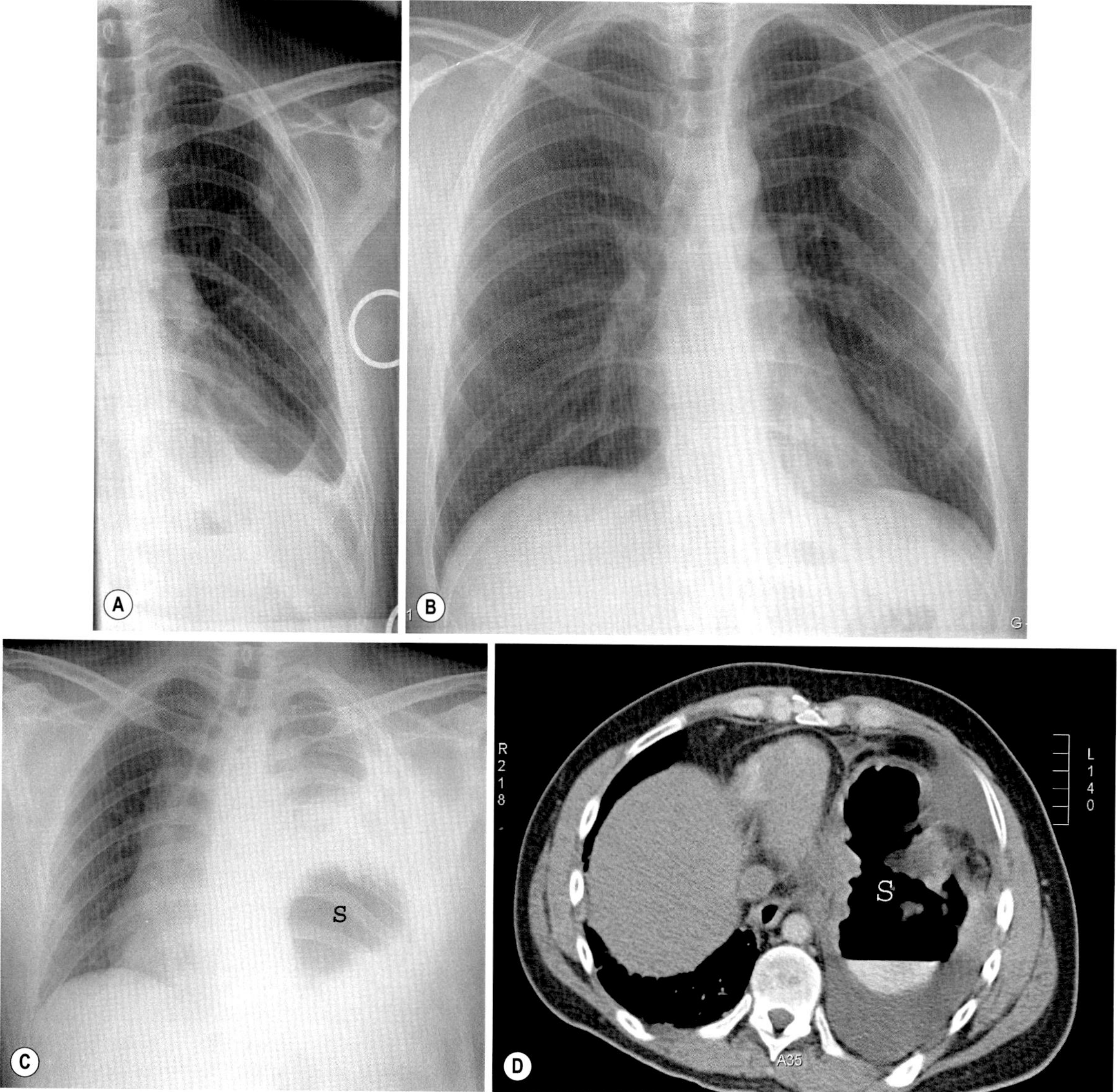

FIGURE 3-28 ■ Traumatic rupture of the diaphragm diagnosed 2 months after the trauma. (A) Detail of the left hemithorax. The supine chest radiograph immediately after the trauma shows multiple rib fractures, a pleural effusion and a poorly defined opacity at the left lung base. (B) One month after the trauma the chest radiograph is normal but (C) 2 months later a large gas-filled structure corresponding with the air-containing stomach (S) is seen in the left hemithorax, suggesting rupture and herniation. (D) CT confirmed the diagnosis of diaphragmatic rupture and shows the herniated stomach.

Barium studies can be very helpful in making the correct diagnosis, when an extrinsic narrowing occurs on the border of the stomach or bowel at the point where they pass the diaphragmatic tear. However, since barium studies cannot be used in emergency situations, they are predominantly indicated in the latent phase and eventually in the obstructive phase.

Pneumoperitoneum can be established by bringing a small amount of air into the abdominal cavity. If air shifts through the diaphragmatic tear and a pneumothorax occurs, the test is diagnostic for diaphragmatic rupture. However, no shift of air will occur when the tear is closed by adhesions or by the herniated organs themselves. In this case the exact position of the diaphragm can be visualised since it is delineated by the subdiaphragmatic air.

Ultrasound can be diagnostic if both the diaphragm and the herniated organs can be visualised. Examination of the right hemidiaphragm is facilitated by the presence of the liver, acting as an acoustic window. However, this technique is limited by the often minimal visualisation of the diaphragm itself, the tenderness over the upper abdomen and the presence of gas in herniated bowel.

The MDCT diagnosis of diaphragmatic rupture is largely based on the fact that abdominal organs are seen in the pleural space outside the diaphragm. However, the identification of the diaphragm on standard CT images can be very difficult; multiplanar CT reconstructions can help to show the defect directly. The more usual CT signs of diaphragmatic rupture include[39–43] discontinuity of the diaphragm with direct visualisation of the diaphragmatic injury ('absent diaphragm sign') possibly with inward curling of the torn hemidiaphragm ('dangling diaphragm sign'); herniation of abdominal organs with liver, bowel or stomach in contact with the posterior ribs ('dependent viscera sign'); thickening of the crus ('thick crus sign'); constriction of the stomach or bowel ('collar sign'); mushroom-like mass in the right hemithorax where the herniated liver is constricted by the tear ('hump sign') (Fig. 3-29C), linear lucency across the liver along the torn edges of the hemidiaphragm ('band sign') (Fig. 3-29B); active arterial extravasation of contrast material near the diaphragm; and in case of a penetrating diaphragmatic injury depiction of a missile or puncturing instrument trajectory.

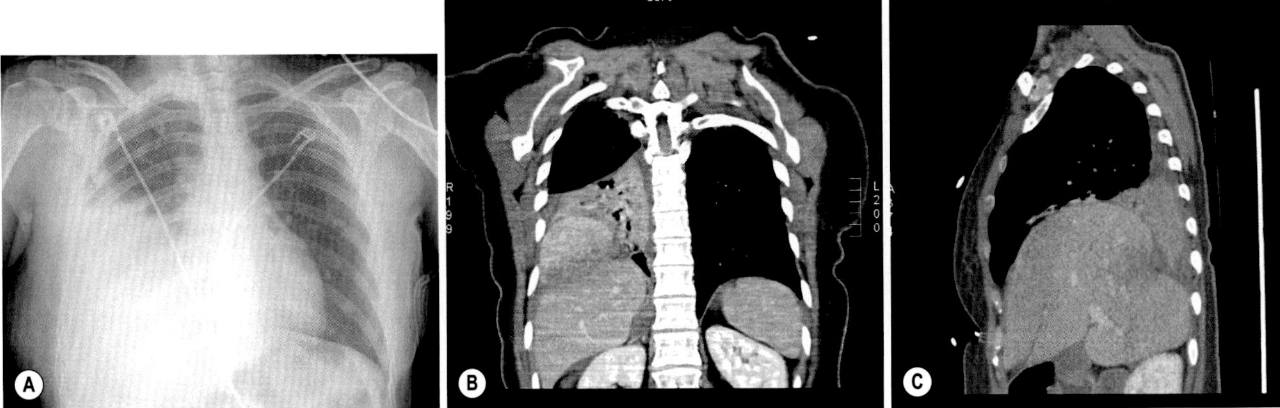

FIGURE 3-29 ■ **Traumatic diaphragmatic rupture.** (A) Chest radiograph shows an opacification of the lower part of the right hemithorax with disappearance of the diaphragmatic contour. CT (coronal (B) and sagittal (C) reconstructions) shows a consolidation of the right lower lobe and bulging of the liver into the chest. On the sagittal view (C) the posterior part of the herniated liver is somewhat constricted by the tear ('hump sign') while the coronal view (B) shows a linear lucency across the liver along the torn edges of the hemidiaphragm ('band sign').

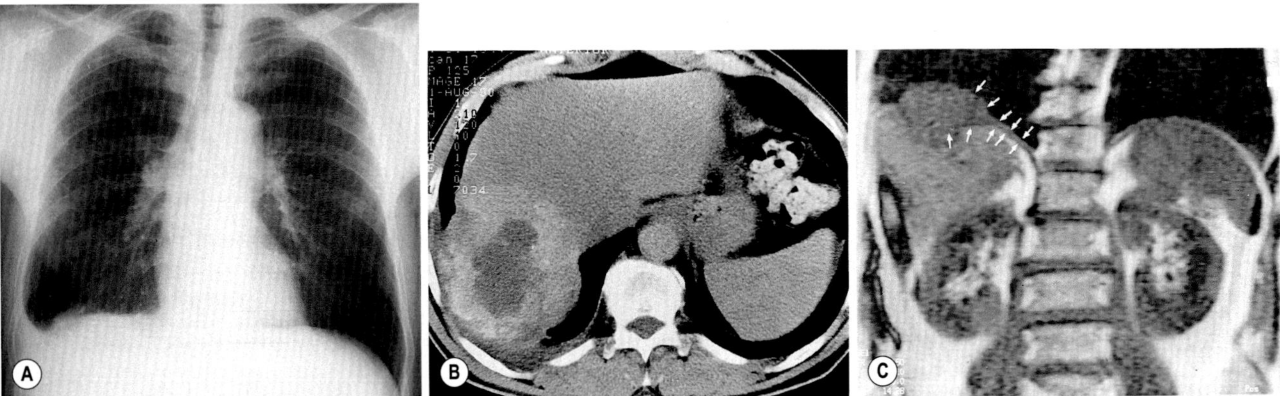

FIGURE 3-30 ■ **Primary malignant tumour of the diaphragm.** (A) PA chest radiograph shows a small focal bulge of the diaphragm in combination with a small pleural effusion. (B) CT and (C) MRI show an irregular mass with central necrosis in continuity with the right hemidiaphragm (arrows).

Because it is in most cases difficult to perform an MRI examination during the acute phase, this technique is more valuable in the latent phase. It allows both a static and a dynamic view of the diaphragm. However, as in CT, the parts of the diaphragm in contact with the liver and spleen are not visible.

Neoplasms of the Diaphragm

Primary tumours of the diaphragm are rare (Fig. 3-30). Both benign and malignant varieties are mostly derived from muscle, fibrous tissue, blood vessels, or fat. They are usually well defined and on the right may mimic an elevated diaphragm or local eventration. Calcification has been described in lipomas. Malignant tumours may present as a pleural effusion. Secondary invasion of the diaphragm by malignant tumours of the lung, pleura, stomach or pancreas may occur. Imaging with CT or MRI is particularly helpful in such patients.

REFERENCES

1. Kuhlman JE, Bouchardy L, Fishman EK, et al. CT and MR imaging evaluation of chest wall disorders. RadioGraphics 1994; 14:571–95.
2. Fortier M, Mayo JR, Swensen SJ, et al. MR imaging of the chest wall lesions. Radiographics 1994;14:597–606.
3. Takasugi JE, Rapoport S, Shaw C. Superior sulcus tumors: the role of imaging. J Thorac Imaging 1989;4:41–8.
4. Deschildre F, Petyt L, Remy-Jardin M, et al. Evaluation de la TDM par balayage spirale volumique (BSV) vs IRM dans le bilan d'extension pariétal des masses thoraciques. Rev Im Med 1994; 6(S):188.
5. Müller NL. Imaging the pleura. Radiology 1993;186:297.
6. McLoud TC, Flower CDR. Imaging the pleura: sonography CT, and MR imaging. Am J Roentgenol 1991;156:1145–53.
7. Fleischner FG. Atypical arrangement of free pleural effusion. Radiol Clin North Am 1963;1:347–62.
8. Lomas DJ, Padley SG, Flower CDR. The sonographic appearances of pleural fluid. Br J Radiol 1993;66:619–24.
9. McLoud TC. CT and MR in pleural disease. Clin Chest Med 1998;19:261–76.
10. Bittner RC, Schnoy N, Schonfeld N, et al. High-resolution magnetic resonance tomography (HR-MRT) of the pleura and thoracic wall: normal findings and pathological changes. Rofo Fortschr Geb Rontgenstr Neuen Bildgeb Verfahr 1995;162:296–303.
11. Lesur O, Delorme N, Fromaget JM, et al. Computed tomography in the etiologic assessment of idiopathic spontaneous pneumothorax. Chest 1990;98:341–7.
12. Gordon R. The deep sulcus sign. Radiology 1980;136:25–7.
13. Rhea JT, vanSonnenberg E, McLoud TC. Basilar pneumothorax in the supine adult. Radiology 1979;133:593–5.
14. Zanobetti M, Poggioni C, Pini R. Can chest ultrasonography replace standard chest radiography for evaluation of acute dyspnea in the ED? Chest 2011;139:1140–7.
15. Aberle DR, Gamsu G, Ray CS. High resolution CT of benign asbestos-related diseases: clinical and radiographic correlation. Am J Roentgenol 1988;151:883.
16. Falaschi F, Battolla L, Maschalchi M, et al. Usefulness of MR signal intensity in distinguishing benign from malignant pleural disease. Am J Roentgenol 1996;166:963–8.
17. Coolen J, De Keyzer F, Nafteux P, et al. Malignant pleural disease: diagnosis by using diffusion-weighted and dynamic contrast-enhanced MR imaging—initial experience. radiology 2012;263: 884–92.
18. Layer G, Schmitteckert H, Steudel A, et al. MRT, CT and sonography in the preoperative assessment of the primary tumor spread in malignant pleural mesothelioma. RoFo Fortschr Geb Rontgenstr Neuen Bildgeb Verfahr 1999;170:365–70.
19. Beyer T, Townsend DW, Brun T, et al. A combined PET/CT scanner for clinical oncology. J Nucl Med 2000;41:1369–79.
20. Erasmus JJ, Truong MT, Smythe WR, et al. Integrated computed tomography-positron emission tomography in patients with potentially resectable malignant pleural mesothelioma: Staging implications. J Thorac Cardiovasc Surg 2005;129:1364–70.
21. Jaruskova M, Belohlavek O. Role of FDG-PET and PET/CT in the diagnosis of prolonged febrile states. Eur J Nucl Med Mol Imaging 2006;33:913–18.
22. England DM, Hochholzer L, McCarthy MJ. Localized benign and malignant fibrous tumors of the pleura. A clinicopathologic review of 223 cases. Am J Surg Pathol 1989;13:640–58.
23. Kinoshita T, Ishii K, Miyasato S. Localized pleural mesothelioma: CT and MR findings. Magn Reson Imaging 1997;15:377–9.
24. Rusch VW, Godwin JD, Shuman WP. The role of computed tomography scanning in the initial assessment and the follow-up of malignant pleural mesothelioma. J Thorac Cardiovasc Surg 1988;96:171.
25. Targhetta R, Balmes P, Marty-Double C, et al. Ultrasonically guided aspiration biopsy in osteolytic bone lesions of the chest wall. Chest 1993;103:1403–8.
26. Diacon AH, Brutsche MH, Soler M. Accuracy of pleural puncture sites: a prospective comparison of clinical examination with ultrasound. Chest 2003;123:436–41.
27. Jones PW, Moyers JP, Rogers JT, et al. Ultrasound-guided thoracentesis: is it a safer method? Chest 2003;123:418–23.
28. Standring S, editor. Gray's Anatomy: The Anatomical Basis of Clinical Practise. 39th ed. Edinburgh: Elsevier: Churchill Livingstone; 2005.
29. Helm EJ, Rahman NM, Talakoub O, et al. Course and variation of the intercostal artery by CT scan. Chest 2012;143(3):634–9.
30. Rahman NM, Maskell NA, Hedley EL, et al. The relationship between chest tube size and clinical outcomes in pleural infection. Chest 2010;137:536–43.
31. Rahman NM, Maskell NA, West A, et al. Intrapleural use of tissue plasminogen activator and DNase in pleural infection. N Engl J Med 2011;365(6):518–26.
32. Davies CWH, Traill ZC, Gleeson FV, Davies RJO. Intrapleural streptokinase in the drainage of malignant multiloculated pleural effusions. Chest 1999;115:729–33.
33. Maskell NA, Gleeson FV, Davies RJO. Standard pleural biopsy versus CT-guided cutting needle biopsy for diagnosis of malignant disease in pleural effusions: a randomised controlled trial. Lancet 2003;361:1326–30.
34. Agarwal PP, Seeley JM, Matzinger FR, et al. Pleural mesothelioma: sensitivity and incidence of needle track seeding after image-guided biopsy versus surgical biopsy. Radiology 2006;241(2):589–94.
35. Deslauriers J. Eventration of the diaphragm. Chest Surg Clin North Am 1988;8:315–30.
36. Houston JG, Fleet M, Cowan MD, et al. Comparison of ultrasound with fluoroscopy in the assessment of suspected hemidiaphragmatic movement abnormality. Clin Radiol 1995;50:95–8.
37. Demartini WJ, House AJS. Partial Bochdalek herniation: computerized tomographic evaluation. Chest 1980;77:702–4.
38. Shah R, Sabanathan S, Mearns JA, et al. Traumatic rupture of diaphragm. Ann Thorac Surg 1995;60:1444–9.
39. Bergin D, Ennis R, Keogh C, et al. The 'dependent viscera' sign in CT diagnosis of blunt traumatic diaphragmatic rupture. Am J Roentgenol 2001;177:1137–40.
40. Leung JC, Nance ML, Schwab CW, et al. Thickening of the diaphragm: a new computed tomography sign of diaphragm injury. J Thorac Imaging 1999;14:126–9.
41. Mirvis SE, Shanmuganathan K. Imaging hemidiaphragmatic injury. Eur Radiol 2007;17:1411–21.
42. Desser TS, Edwards B, Hunt S, et al. The dangling diaphragm sign: sensitivity and comparison with existing CT signs of blunt traumatic diaphragmatic rupture. Emerg Radiol 2010;17:37–44.
43. Bodanapally UK, Shanmuganathan K, Mirvis SE, et al. MDCT diagnosis of penetrating diaphragm injury. Euro Radiol 2009;19: 1875–81.

CHAPTER 4

The Mediastinum, Including the Pericardium

Nadeem Parkar • Cylen Javidan-Nejad • Sanjeev Bhalla • Simon P.G. Padley

CHAPTER OUTLINE

The mediastinum is that anatomical region bounded laterally by the two lungs, anteriorly by the sternum, posteriorly by the vertebrae, superiorly by the thoracic inlet and inferiorly by the diaphragm.

MEDIASTINAL DISEASES

MEDIASTINAL MASSES

Incidence

The true prevalence of mediastinal masses is unknown as most surgical series are biased towards patients requiring surgery and do not include all aneurysms, intrathoracic goitres or lymph node masses in patients with established diagnoses such as lymphoma or sarcoidosis. In adult surgical series,[1–3] the most frequent tumours are of neurogenic (17–23%), thymic (20–25%) or lymph node (10–20%) origin (usually neoplastic). Developmental cysts, thyroid masses and germ-cell tumours constitute the next most frequent group (approximately 10% each). In children, neuroblastoma/ganglioneuroma, foregut cysts and germ-cell tumours account for over three-quarters of cases, whereas thymoma and thyroid masses are rare.

The mediastinum is divided into compartments to aid in developing a differential diagnosis. However, there are no physical boundaries between compartments. Anatomically the mediastinum is divided into superior and inferior compartments by an imaginary line traversing the manubriosternal joint and the lower margin of T4 vertebra. The inferior compartment is further divided into three parts: anterior, middle and posterior. The Felson method of division is based on lateral radiography. A line that extends from the thoracic inlet to the diaphragm along the posterior cardiac surface and anterior to the trachea separates the anterior from middle compartments. The middle and posterior compartments of the mediastinum are separated by a line that runs 1 cm behind the anterior margins of the vertebral bodies. A popular modification divides the entire mediastinum into anterior, middle and posterior compartments but does not have a separate superior compartment.[4] We find this latter approach helpful in our adult population.

Imaging Techniques

Mediastinal masses are often incidentally detected on chest radiograph. Despite diagnostic limitations, the chest X-ray (CXR) is important for detecting and localising mediastinal masses when suspected clinically.

Computed Tomography

CT is the most useful investigation for localising, characterising and demonstrating the extent of a mediastinal mass and its relationships. CT is also useful in delineating calcification, which can help generate a more refined differential diagnosis. Multidetector CT (MDCT) following intravenous contrast medium with multiplanar reformats provides an excellent assessment of mediastinal structures, including vessels in the coronal and sagittal planes (Fig. 4-1). CT may guide biopsy, plan resection and follow response to therapy.

Magnetic Resonance Imaging

Magnetic resonance (MR) remains useful for imaging suspected neurogenic tumours, demonstrating intraspinal extension of a mediastinal mass and further evaluating the relationship of a mass to the heart, pericardium and

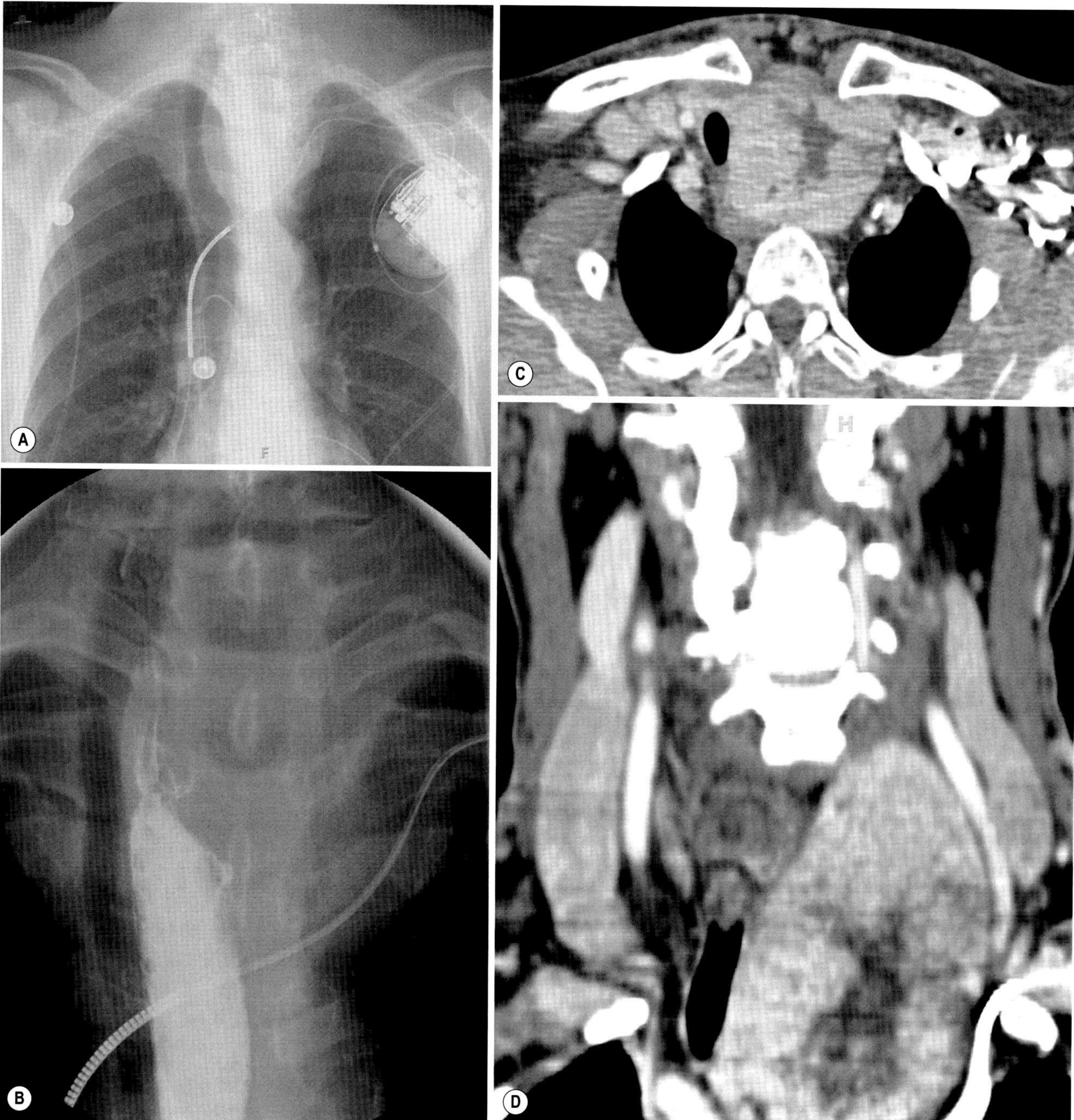

FIGURE 4-1 ■ **Value of multiplanar reformations.** A 45-year-old woman with dyspnoea: (A) frontal radiograph and (B) oesophogram demonstrate displacement of the trachea and oesophagus to the right, by a large mediastinal mass in the thoracic inlet. (C) Transaxial contrast medium-enhanced CT shows a large goitre arising from the left lobe of the thyroid. (D) Coronal reformat depicts the craniocaudal extent of the mass and its relationship with the adjacent structures.

larger intrathoracic vessels. MR may have advantages over contrast medium-enhanced CT for distinguishing between solid tissue and adjacent vessels (fast-flowing blood in vessels results in a signal void on spin-echo sequences) and may be useful for confirming that a mass is cystic. Unlike CT, MR is not as sensitive to the presence of calcification.

Ultrasound

Ultrasound of the mediastinum, including echocardiography and endoscopic ultrasound, may be of use in selected patients, in particular for distinguishing cystic from solid mediastinal masses and for distinguishing cardiac from paracardiac masses. Ultrasound is increasingly being used to guide mediastinal biopsy.

TABLE 4-1 **Approach to Mediastinal Masses by Location and Tissue Characterisation on CT or MR**

	Lesions	Fluid	Fat	Vascular
Anterior	Thymoma Lymphoma Germ-cell tumour Goitre	Thymic cyst Thymoma Pericardial cyst Germ-cell tumour Lymphoma	Germ-cell tumour Thymolipoma Fat pad Morgagni hernia	Thyroid Cardiac coronary aneurysm Ascending aortic aneurysm
Middle	Lymph nodes Duplication cyst Arch anomaly Oesophageal mass	Duplication cyst Necrotic nodes Pericardial recess	Lipoma Oesophageal fibrovascular polyp	Arch anomaly Azygos vein Vascular node
Posterior	Neurogenic Bone and marrow	Neuroenteric cyst Schwannoma Meningocele	Extramedullary hematopoiesis	Descending aorta
More than One Lesion	Infection Haemorrhage Lung Cancer	Lymphangioma Mediastinitis	Liposarcoma	Hemangioma

Radionuclide Examinations

Radionuclide examinations have a limited role in assessing mediastinal masses. Positron emission tomography (PET) and PET–CT using [F-18]2-deoxy-D-glucose (^{18}F-FDG) has proven useful in evaluating mediastinal lymph node involvement in lung cancer and lymphoma.[5,6] Radionuclide examinations may also be useful in imaging thyroid masses, neuroendocrine tumours and pheochromocytomas.

Approach to Mediastinal Masses

1. Localise to the mediastinum;
2. Localise within the mediastinum; and
3. Characterise on CT or MR.

Localise to the Mediastinum

The CXR is the first step in evaluating mediastinal diseases. Findings that help in localising the lesion to the mediastinum include:

1. No air bronchograms;
2. Obtuse margins with the lung;
3. Disruption of mediastinal lines; and
4. Abnormalities of spine, rib and sternum.

Localise within the Mediastinum

The information obtained from the relationship of the normal anatomical structures representing the 'mediastinal lines and stripes' on chest radiography aid in localising the lesion within the mediastinum to the anterior, middle or posterior mediastinum and generating a differential diagnosis before proceeding to a chest CT examination.[7]

Anterior mediastinal masses can be identified when both the hilum overlay sign and preservation of the posterior mediastinal lines are present. Widening of the right paratracheal stripe and convexity relative to the AP window reflection both indicate abnormality in the middle mediastinum. Disruption of the azygo-oesophageal recess can be caused by disease in either the middle or posterior mediastinum. Paravertebral masses disrupt the paraspinal lines, and the region of masses above the level clavicles can be inferred by their lateral margins: Posterior masses have sharp margins caused by their interface with lung, whereas anterior masses do not.[8]

Although there is no tissue plane separating the divisions of the mediastinum, attempting to localise an abnormality within the mediastinum helps in narrowing the differential diagnosis and determining appropriate further imaging.

Characterise on CT or MR

Mediastinal masses can be further characterised by CT or MR, depending on whether they contain fat, fluid or are vascular (Table 4-1).

Thyroid Masses

Most thyroid goitres are in the neck, yet between 3 and 17% of goitres extend into the thorax.[9,10]

Most thyroid masses in the mediastinum represent downward extensions of either a multinodular colloid goitre or, occasionally, an adenoma or carcinoma. Intrathoracic thyroid masses usually have a well-defined spherical or lobular outline (Fig. 4-1). Rounded or irregular, well-defined areas of calcification may be seen in benign areas, whereas amorphous cloud-like calcification is occasionally seen within carcinomas.

Almost all intrathoracic thyroid masses displace the trachea and may cause tracheal narrowing. The direction of displacement depends on the location of the mass. Thyroid masses are most commonly anterior and lateral to the trachea. Posteriorly, masses often separate the trachea and the oesophagus, and such separation by a localised mass rising into the neck is virtually diagnostic of a thyroid mass.

CT imaging features of mediastinal thyroid goitres are:

1. Continuity of the mass with the cervical thyroid gland;
2. Foci of heterogeneous attenuation (cystic areas and calcifications);
3. High attenuation on unenhanced CT (higher than muscle), reflecting high iodine content of thyroid tissue; and
4. Intense and prolonged enhancement.

The most important of these features is to demonstrate continuity of the mass with the cervical thyroid. It is usually possible to diagnose a thyroid origin by noting a well-defined mass in the paratracheal or retrotracheal region, almost invariably being continuous with the thyroid gland in the neck. It is not possible to distinguish between a benign and malignant mass on CT unless the tumour has clearly spread beyond the thyroid gland. It should, however, be noted that multiple masses are a feature of benign multinodular goitre, though carcinoma can develop in multinodular goitre. MRI of intrathoracic goitre, like CT, can identify cystic and solid components, and in addition can demonstrate haemorrhage. In most practices, evaluation of the questionable thyroid usually relies on ultrasound with biopsy.

Radionuclide imaging with ^{123}I or ^{131}I demonstrates the presence of thyroid tissue within the mediastinum in almost all intrathoracic goitres. Although radionuclide imaging is a sensitive and specific method of determining the thyroid nature of an intrathoracic mass, CT is more useful as the initial investigation because it provides more information should the mass prove to be something other than a thyroid lesion and is almost as specific as nuclear medicine in diagnosing a thyroid origin. CT optimally demonstrates the shape, size and position of the mass[11,12] (Fig. 4-2).

Parathyroid Masses

A parathyroid tumour is a rare cause of an anterior mediastinal mass. The parathyroid glands may migrate into the chest during fetal development. Mediastinal parathyroid tumours causing hyperparathyroidism are most commonly located in or around the thymus. In most patients with hyperparathyroidism, the aetiology lies within the parathyroid gland (either hyperplasia or a small adenoma) and escapes visualisation on CT. The role of CT or MR is for detection of ectopic adenoma, which is suspected when no lesion is detected by ultrasound or the hyperparathyroidism persists despite parathyroidectomy. The adenomas tend to be small and enhance homogeneously. Often, the CT is used in conjunction with ^{99m}Tc-sestamibi imaging[13,14] (Fig. 4-3).

Thymic Tumours

The thymus is a bilobed, triangular-shaped organ that occupies the retrosternal space and varies widely in size and shape depending on the age.[15] In subjects aged over 25, the thymus is no longer discretely recognised but seen as islands of soft-tissue attenuation within a background of fat. Although the thymus may still be seen as a discrete structure in adulthood, it usually involutes and is completely replaced by fat. Anterior mediastinal masses of thymic origin include thymomas, thymic carcinoma, thymolipoma, thymic lymphoma, thymic carcinoid and thymic hyperplasia. Thymic cysts may be simple cysts and occur in an otherwise normal gland, may lie within a thymoma or may follow thymic irradiation for Hodgkin's disease.[16]

Thymomas

Thymomas are the most common tumour of the thymus in adults, and the most common primary tumour of the anterior mediastinum in adults.[17] Thymomas are usually low-grade malignant tumours of thymic epithelium. Thymomas may be encapsulated (non-invasive thymomas) or may extend beyond the capsule (invasive type). The average age at diagnosis is approximately 50 years, earlier in those who present with myasthenia gravis. Thymomas are extremely unusual below the age of 15 and rare under 20. Up to 50% of patients with thymoma have myasthenia gravis, and approximately 10–20% of patients with myasthenia gravis have a thymoma. A variety of other syndromes are seen in patients with thymoma, including hypogammaglobulinaemia and pure red cell aplasia.[18,19]

Most thymomas (90%) arise in the upper anterior mediastinum. The mass is usually anterior to the ascending aorta, lying above the right ventricular outflow tract and pulmonary artery. A few are situated more inferiorly, projecting from the left or right heart border, or lying close to the cardiophrenic angles (Fig. 4-4). They are usually spherical or oval in shape and may show lobulated borders. Thymomas may contain one or more cysts and a few are predominantly cystic. Calcification, punctate or curvilinear, may be seen. All of these features are best demonstrated using CT,[20,21] which is the most sensitive technique for detecting thymoma in patients with myasthenia gravis.[22] Thymomas as small as 1.5–2.0 cm in diameter are readily identified in men and women over the age of 40, largely because the rest of the thymus is atropic. Diagnosing a small thymoma in those patients younger than age 40, and particularly younger than 30, can be difficult, because the normal gland is variable in size and in myasthenia gravis the associated hyperplasia may cause a bulky gland. Fortunately, thymoma is so infrequent in children that the potentially difficult problem of finding a thymoma in a child with myasthenia gravis rarely arises.

Thymomas usually show homogeneous density and uniform enhancement after contrast media injection and may occasionally be cystic. Invasion of the mediastinal fat and adjacent pleura may be identified with invasive thymomas, and while CT shows such invasion to advantage, it cannot reliably diagnose invasive thymoma if the tumour is still confined to the thymus.[23] Pleural metastases resulting from transpleural spread are a feature of invasive thymomas, and therefore the whole of the pleural cavity should be carefully examined.[23] On MR, the normal thymus in children and young adults characteristically demonstrates homogeneous and intermediate T1- and T2-weighted signal intensity, less intense than

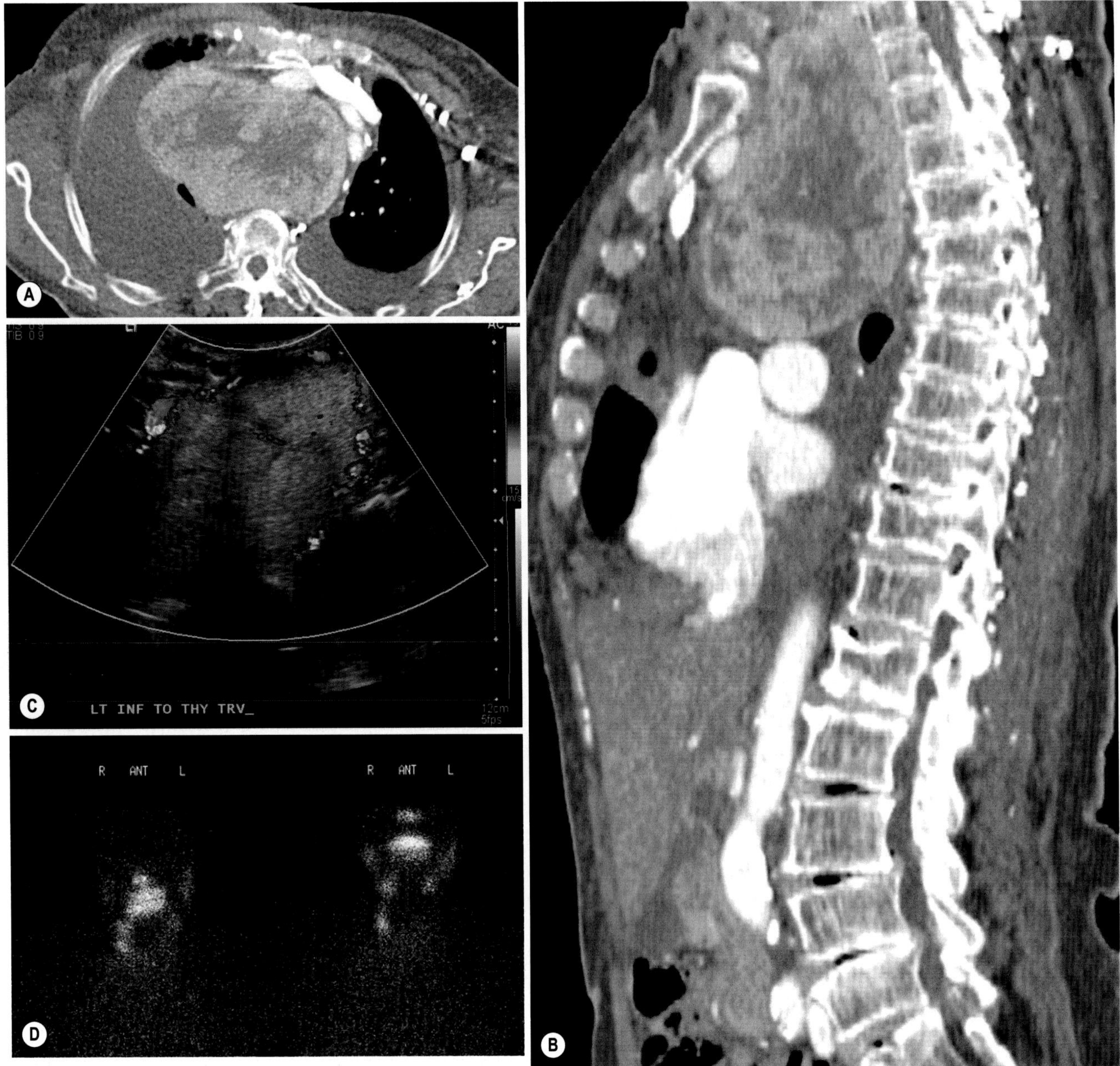

FIGURE 4-2 ■ Comparison of various techniques in assessment of goitre. A 90-year-old woman presents with swelling of her face and shortness of breath. (A) Transaxial and (B) sagittal reformatted images on contrast medium-enhanced CT imaging demonstrate a large intrathoracic goitre. Ultrasound evaluation of the neck using colour Doppler shows an enlarged left lobe of the thyroid with a mildly heterogeneous echogenicity. There are numerous tortuous venous collateral vessels surrounding the goitre, rendering safe fine-needle aspiration under ultrasound guidance impossible (C). ^{123}I radionuclide imaging of the face and neck demonstrates iodine uptake of the goitre (D).

mediastinal fat but greater than muscle. In older patients after puberty, the T1 and T2 signals increase with age because the thymus begins to involute and is replaced by fat.[24,25] Thymomas typically demonstrate low T1 signal intensity similar to muscle and relatively high T2 signal intensity. MR can be useful for showing mediastinal spread when there is doubt about the CT. T2-weighted images occasionally show lobulated internal architecture and scattered areas of high intensity that correspond to fibrous septa and cystic areas[26] (Fig. 4-4). Heterogeneity of signal intensity caused by septation, cystic change and haemorrhage is common.

Invasive thymomas invade beyond the capsule into the mediastinum and can involve the pleura and pericardium. Complete obliteration of the adjacent fat planes suggests mediastinal invasion (Fig. 4-5). On the contrary, complete preservation of the adjacent fat planes excludes extensive invasive disease but does not rule out minimal capsular invasion.[22] MR is superior to CT for defining the invasion of contiguous structures such as the pleura

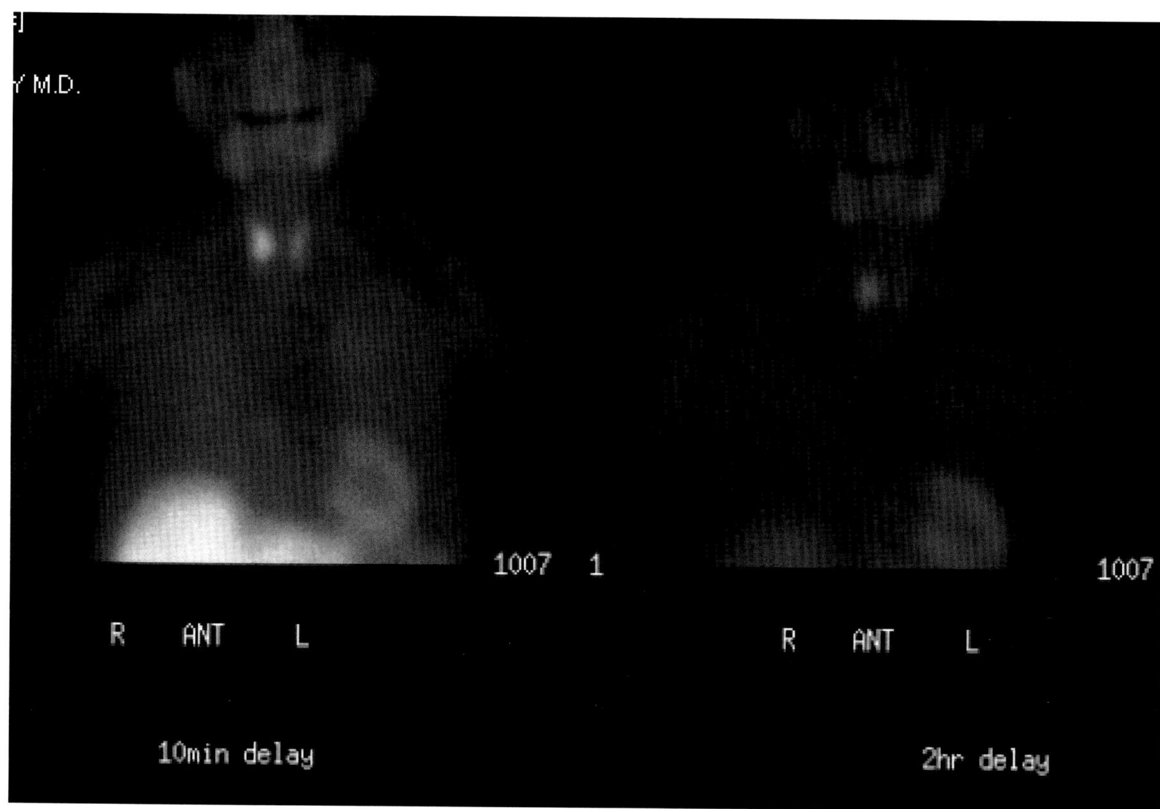

FIGURE 4-3 ■ **Role of scintigraphy in detecting parathyroid adenomas.** A 66-year-old woman with hypercalcaemia. CT (not shown) did not reveal a parathyroid adenoma. ^{99m}Tc-sestamibi radionuclide imaging demonstrates uptake in both thyroid and parathyroid parenchyma in the 10-minute delayed image (left); however, at 2-hour delay, imaging (right) demonstrates persistent uptake in the right lobe of the thyroid gland, representing the parathyroid adenoma.

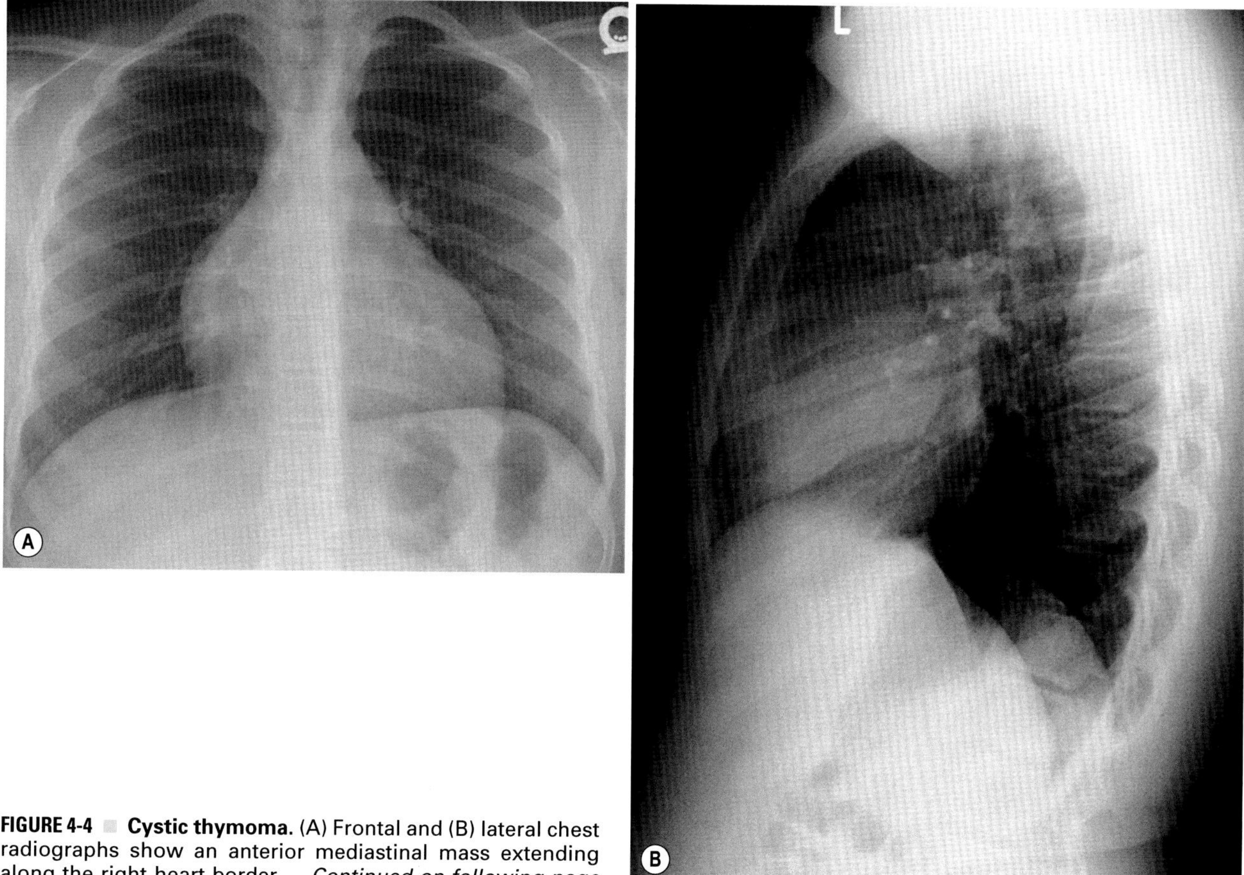

FIGURE 4-4 ■ **Cystic thymoma.** (A) Frontal and (B) lateral chest radiographs show an anterior mediastinal mass extending along the right heart border. *Continued on following page*

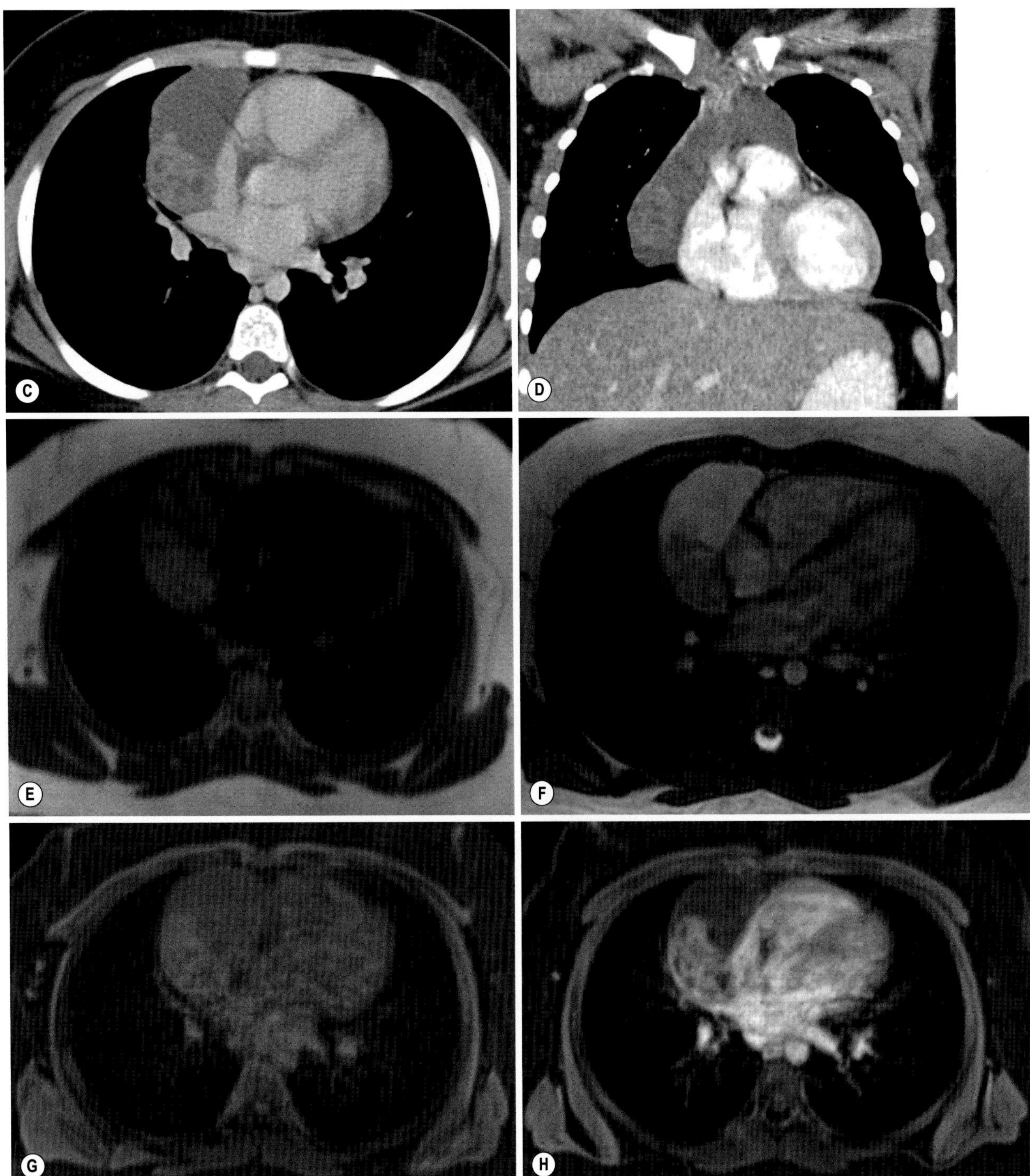

FIGURE 4-4, Continued ■ (C) Transaxial and (D) coronal reformatted CT images demonstrate the cystic and solid components of the mass. (E) T1- and (F) T2-weighted sequences reveal that the cystic portion has a low T1 and high T2 signal intensity and the solid portion is isointense to myocardium. T1-weighted, fat-saturated 3D acquisition (G) before and (H) after contrast media administration demonstrate heterogeneous enhancement of the solid component.

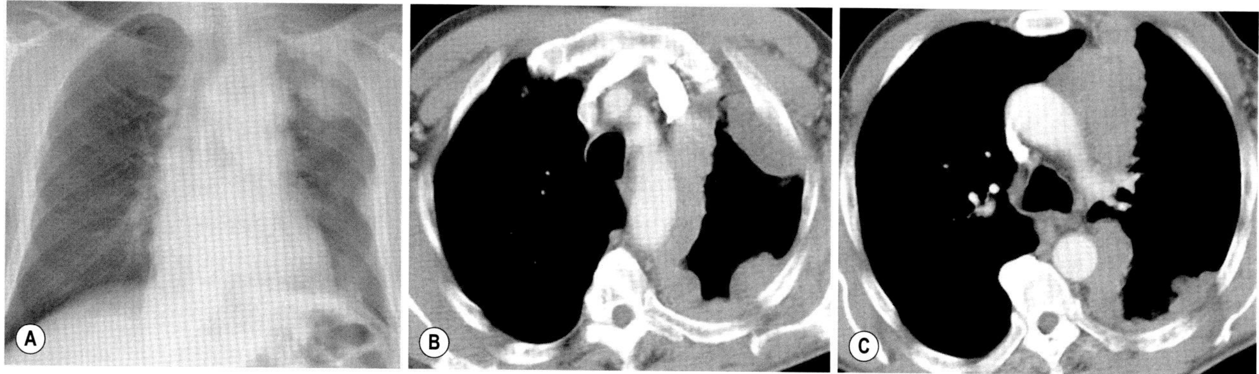

FIGURE 4-5 **Invasive thymoma.** A 74-year-old man with weight loss. (A) Chest radiograph displacement of the trachea and carina to the right and lobulation of the left pleura. CT demonstrates (B) multiple confluent pleural masses involving the medial and posterior pleura and (C) a mass arising from the thymus.

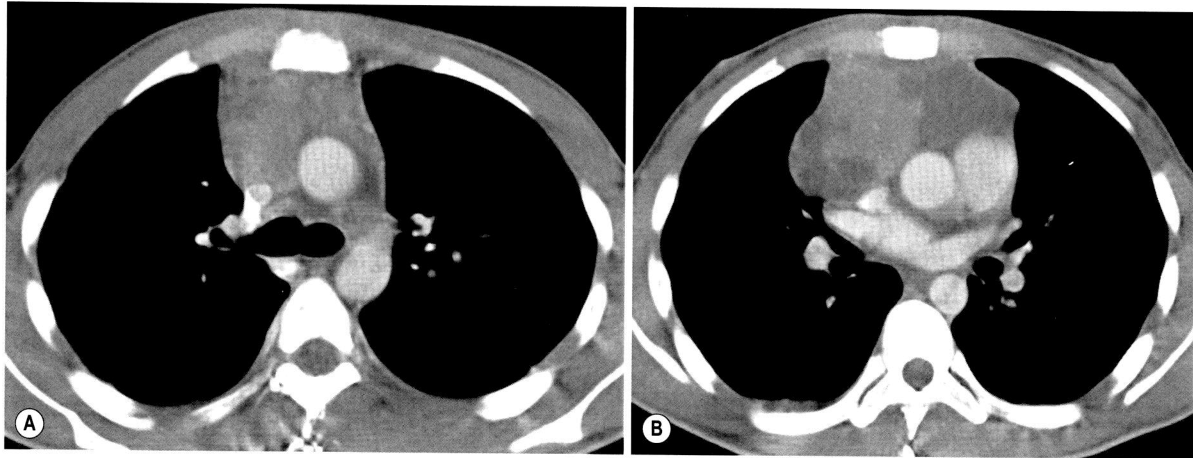

FIGURE 4-6 **Thymic carcinoma.** A 16-year-old man with history of weight loss and night sweats. Contrast medium-enhanced CT images show a heterogeneously enhancing anterior mediastinal mass arising from the right lobe of the thymus (A), with cystic (or necrotic) components. It extends inferiorly in the retrosternal space (B) and has no clear fat plane between it and the mediastinal structures (B). It was surgically excised and pathological examination revealed thymic carcinoma.

and pericardium in patients with invasive thymoma, but is not used in most cases.[27]

Thymic Carcinoma

Thymic carcinoma is a thymic epithelial tumour with a high degree of anaplasia, cell atypia and increased proliferation[28] and predominantly occurs in adults. Thymic carcinomas have a poor prognosis despite treatment with surgery and radiotherapy. Thymic carcinomas are aggressive, locally invasive malignancies that have frequently metastasised to regional lymph nodes and distant sites at presentation. They are typically large, heterogeneous masses, containing areas of necrosis and calcification, often demonstrating evidence of invasion of adjacent structures, in particular the mediastinum, pericardium and pleura[29,30] (Fig. 4-6). On MR, thymic carcinoma demonstrates intermediate signal intensity slightly higher than muscle on T1-weighted sequence and high signal intensity on T2-weighted sequence.[31] Thymic carcinomas are more commonly associated with mediastinal node and extrathoracic metastasis but less commonly associated with pleural implants compared with invasive thymomas.[30]

Thymic Neuroendocrine Tumour (Thymic Carcinoid)

Primary neuroendocrine tumours (carcinoids) of the thymus are rare and account for less than 5% of anterior mediastinal tumours. Unlike pulmonary carcinoids, these tumours are aggressive and at least 20% of patients have distant metastasis at presentation to the liver, lung, bone, pleura and pancreas.[32] Approximately 40% of patients have Cushing's syndrome because of adrenocorticotrophic hormone secretion by the tumour and up to 20% have multiple endocrine neoplasia (MEN) syndromes I and II.

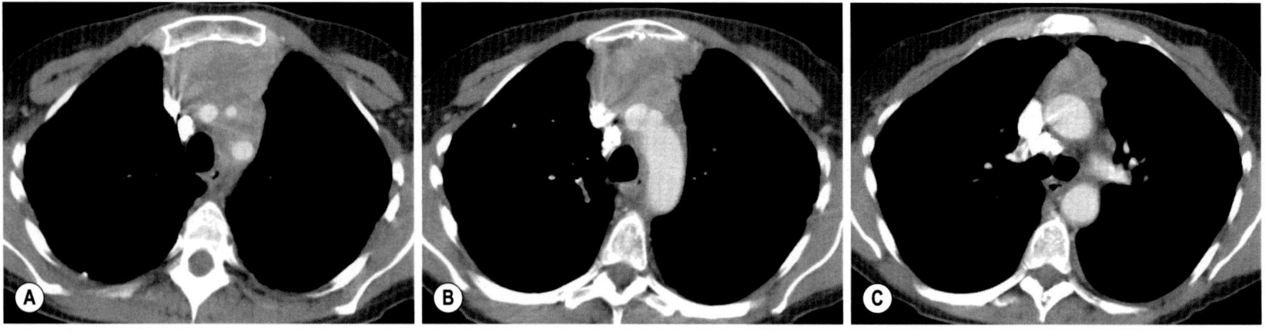

FIGURE 4-7 ■ **Thymic carcinoid.** A 58-year-old woman with palpitations. Contrast medium-enhanced CT images of the upper thorax (A–C) show an infiltrative soft-tissue mass arising from the anterior mediastinum, surrounding the mediastinal vasculature.

Thymic carcinoid is histologically distinct from thymoma, although their imaging features overlap. On CT or MR, the tumours appear as a lobulated thymic mass with heterogeneous enhancement (Fig. 4-7) and central areas of low attenuation secondary to necrosis or haemorrhage and may show local invasion. Bone metastasis is typically osteoblastic.

Thymolipomas

Thymolipomas are rare tumours composed of a mixture of mature fat and normal-looking or involuted thymic tissue. The reported age range is 3–60 years. The average age of the patient is 22–26 years and most patients are asymptomatic.[33] These tumours occur low in the anterior mediastinum, often in the cardiophrenic angle. Individual cases have been reported in association with a variety of conditions, including myasthenia gravis, aplastic anaemia, Graves' disease and hypogammaglobulinaemia. Thymolipomas can grow to a very large size before discovery and, being soft, mould themselves to the adjacent mediastinum and diaphragm, and may mimic cardiomegaly or lobar collapse.[34] CT shows the fatty nature of the mass, with islands of thymus and fibrous septa running through the lesion.[33,34] On MR, fat within the tumour appears as high signal intensity and soft tissue appears as low signal intensity bands coursing through the mass.[35]

Lymphofollicular Thymic Hyperplasia and Rebound Thymic Hyperplasia

The most common association of lymphofollicular thymic hyperplasia is myasthenia gravis (seen in 50% of patients with myasthenia gravis), but lymphofollicular thymic hyperplasia is also seen in other conditions, such as thyrotoxicosis, systemic lupus erythematosus, Hashimoto's thyroiditis and Addison's disease. Thymic hyperplasia is rarely severe enough to cause visible enlargement of the thymus. When it does enlarge the thymus, both lobes are enlarged, usually uniformly (Fig. 4-8). Only rarely, hyperplasia may mimic a thymic mass.

The thymus may atrophy because of stress or as a consequence of steroid or antineoplastic drug therapy.[36,37] The gland usually returns to its original size on recovery or cessation of treatment, but it may become larger than its original size (rebound thymic hyperplasia). Such rebound hyperplasia may be difficult to distinguish from neoplastic involvement. The diagnosis depends on a known reason for thymic rebound, the absence of clinical features to indicate tumour recurrence and the presence of an enlarged, normally shaped thymus.[37,38] In patients over 15 with an enlarged thymus, chemical shift MR and fat-suppressed T2-weighted or short tau inversion recovery (STIR) imaging can diagnose thymic hyperplasia by detecting fatty infiltration or fat in the thymus, helping to differentiate from a neoplastic process. In thymic hyperplasia there is a drop in signal intensity at opposed phase images, while in thymic tumours there is no such reduction in signal. Chemical shift MR can depict physiological fatty infiltration of the thymus in 50% of persons aged between 11 and 15, in 100% of those >15 but in none of those <15 years.[39,40]

Thymic Cyst

Thymic cysts are uncommon, representing 1% of all mediastinal masses. They can be congenital or acquired. Congenital thymic cysts are derived from a patent thymopharyngeal duct and are usually unilocular. Approximately 50% of thymic cysts are discovered in those < 20 years. Acquired thymic cysts are multilocular and occur in association with thymic tumours, Langerhans cell histiocytosis or radiation therapy for Hodgkin's disease. On chest radiographs, thymic cysts are indistinguishable from other thymic masses. On CT, simple congenital thymic cysts are seen as well-defined water attenuation masses with imperceptible walls. Multilocular thymic cysts appear as well-defined heterogeneous masses with imperceptible walls. On MR, thymic cysts demonstrate typical characteristics of fluid with low T1 and high T2 signal intensity (Fig. 4-9). If haemorrhage or infection occurs, then the cysts can demonstrate high signal on both T1- and T2-weighted images.

Germ-Cell Tumours of the Mediastinum

Germ-cell tumours account for 10–15% of anterior mediastinal masses in adults and approximately 25% in children. Germ-cell tumours of the mediastinum are believed to be derived from primitive germ-cell elements

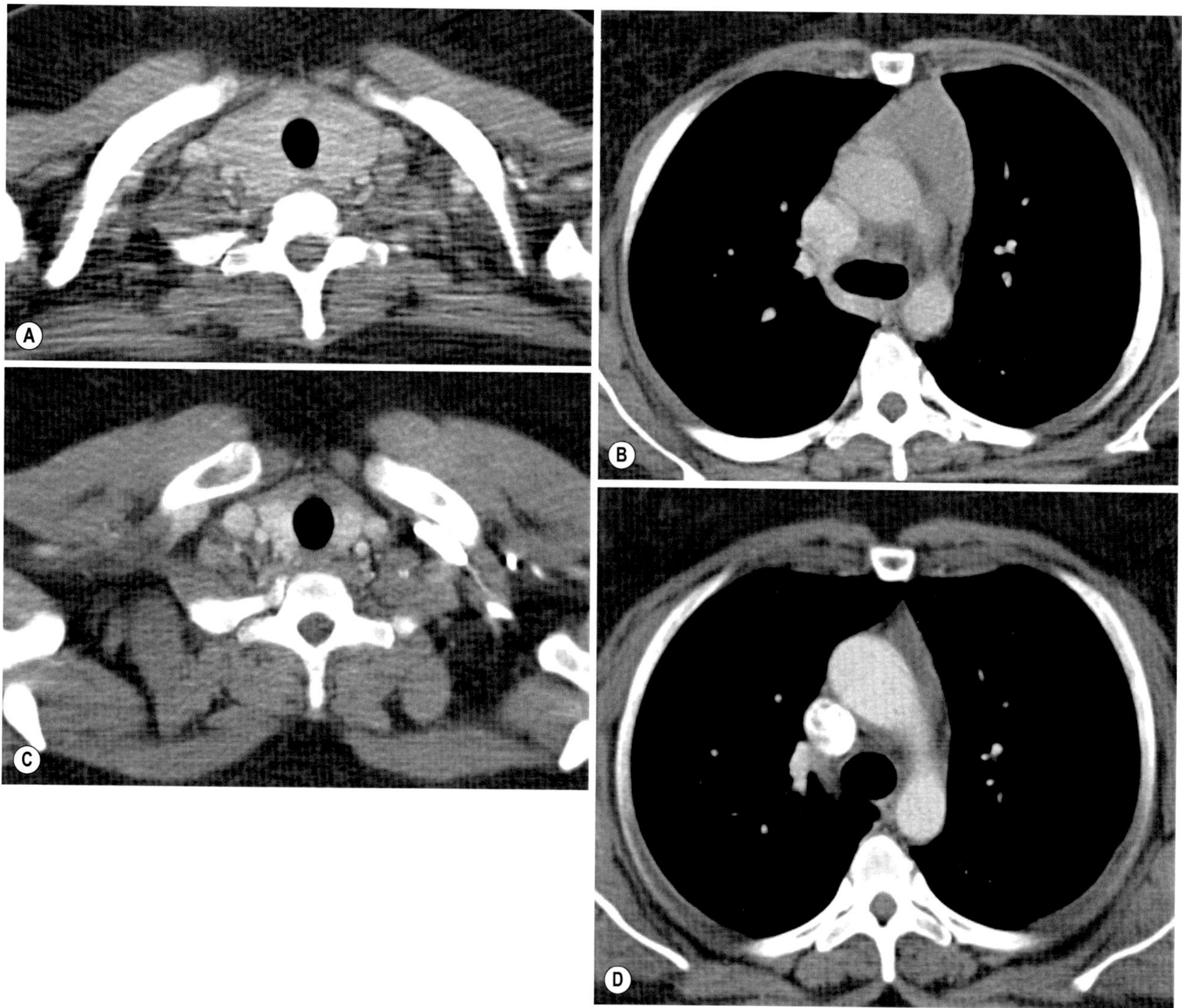

FIGURE 4-8 **Thymic hyperplasia with Graves' disease (thyrotoxicosis).** A 35-year-old woman with dysphagia, palpitations, tremors, exophthalmos and weight loss and elevated serum thyroid hormone. Contrast medium-enhanced CT demonstrates (A) enlarged thyroid and (B) thymus. Following treatment with I-131, (C) the thyroid gland and (D) thymus became much smaller.

left behind after embryonal cell migration. The mediastinum is the most common extragonadal site for these tumours, approximately 60% of which arise in the anterior mediastinum. Most germ-cell tumours present during the second to fourth decades of life. Mediastinal germ-cell tumours include teratoma and a number of malignant forms, chiefly seminoma and non-seminomatous germ-cell tumours such as embryonal carcinoma, choriocarcinoma, endodermal sinus tumour and tumours with mixtures of these cell types.[41] Malignant germ-cell tumours secrete human chorionic gonadotrophin and α-fetoprotein, which can be used as markers to diagnose and monitor the tumour. Malignant germ-cell tumours are almost always seen in male patients.

Teratomas

Teratomas contain elements of all three germinal layers: ectoderm (skin, teeth, hair), mesoderm (bone, cartilage, muscle) and endoderm (bronchial or GI epithelium). Teratomas usually have a benign course and surgical resection is the treatment of choice on the small chance that few malignant elements are present. Malignant teratomas have a poor prognosis. Teratomas are the most common mediastinal germ-cell tumour; most are cystic. Teratomas are found at all ages, particularly in adolescents and young adults, with women slightly outnumbering men.[42,43] They are usually asymptomatic and diagnosed incidentally on chest radiography or CT, but may give rise to cough, dyspnoea or chest pain if they compress the bronchial tree or superior vena cava (SVC), or if they rupture into the mediastinum or lung. Teratomas are usually stable, but haemorrhage or infection may lead to a rapid increase in size.

On chest radiograph or CT most teratomas present as a well-defined, rounded or lobulated mass, localised to the anterior mediastinum. Fat and calcification may rarely be identified on chest radiograph. CT appearances are variable. Combinations of fat, fluid, soft-tissue components and calcification may be seen[42] (Fig. 4-10).

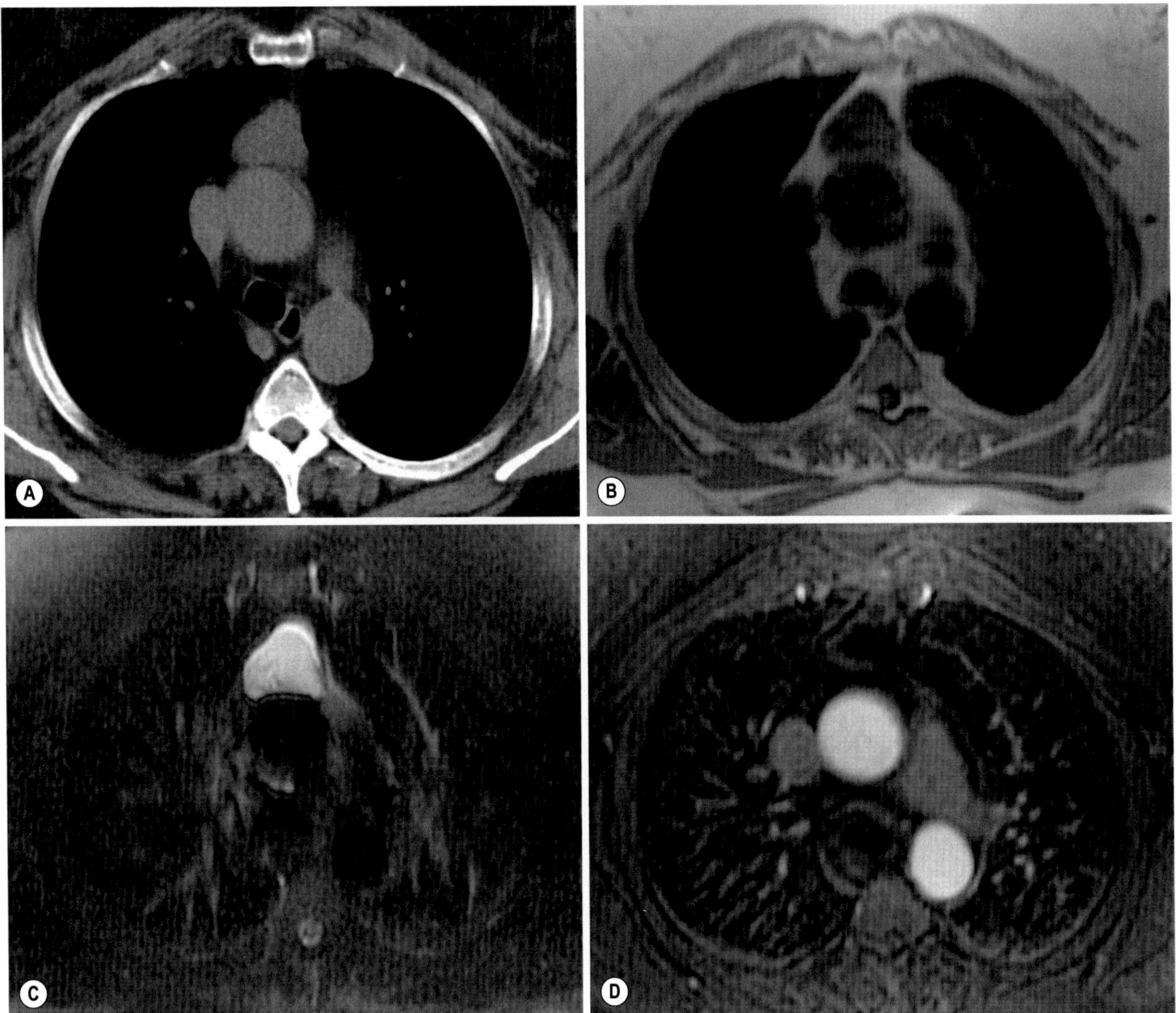

FIGURE 4-9 ■ **Thymic cyst.** Thoracic CT images (A) of a 64-year-old woman with diabetes and weight loss show an incidental finding of a well-circumscribed, low-attenuation anterior mediastinal mass. MR demonstrates low T1 signal intensity (B) and high T2 signal intensity (C) without evidence of enhancement following intravenous contrast medium administration (D).

MR is useful in differentiating teratoma from thymoma and lymphoma. Soft-tissue elements in the teratoma are isointense to muscle, cystic elements demonstrate low T1 intensity and high T2 intensity, and fat appears as high T1 intensity with signal loss on fat saturation sequence. Fat is virtually diagnostic of teratoma.[44]

Seminoma

Seminoma is the most common malignant mediastinal germ-cell tumour.[45] Seminomas occur almost exclusively in men during the second through fourth decades. They are usually well-defined solid masses with possible small foci of degenerative changes representing haemorrhage and necrosis[46] (Fig. 4-11). Symptoms are usually caused by mass effect on adjacent structures. On CT and MR seminomas have homogeneous attenuation and signal intensity and may have areas of haemorrhage and necrosis.

Non-Seminomatous Germ-Cell Tumours

Non-seminomatous germ-cell tumours include embryonal carcinoma, choriocarcinoma, endodermal sinus tumour and tumours with mixtures of these cell types. Malignant non-seminomatous germ-cell tumours are usually seen in young adults and are much more common in men (>90%) than in women. They are commonly more symptomatic than teratomas, from mass effect or invasion of adjacent structures.

The plain radiographic findings are similar, except that the malignant tumours are more often lobular in outline. Fat density and visible calcifications are rare. Because these are malignant tumours, they grow rapidly and metastasise readily to the lungs, bones or, less often, pleura (Fig. 4-12). CT often shows a lobular, asymmetric mass. The adjacent mediastinal fat planes may be obliterated, and the tumours either are of homogeneous soft-tissue density or show multiple areas of contrast media

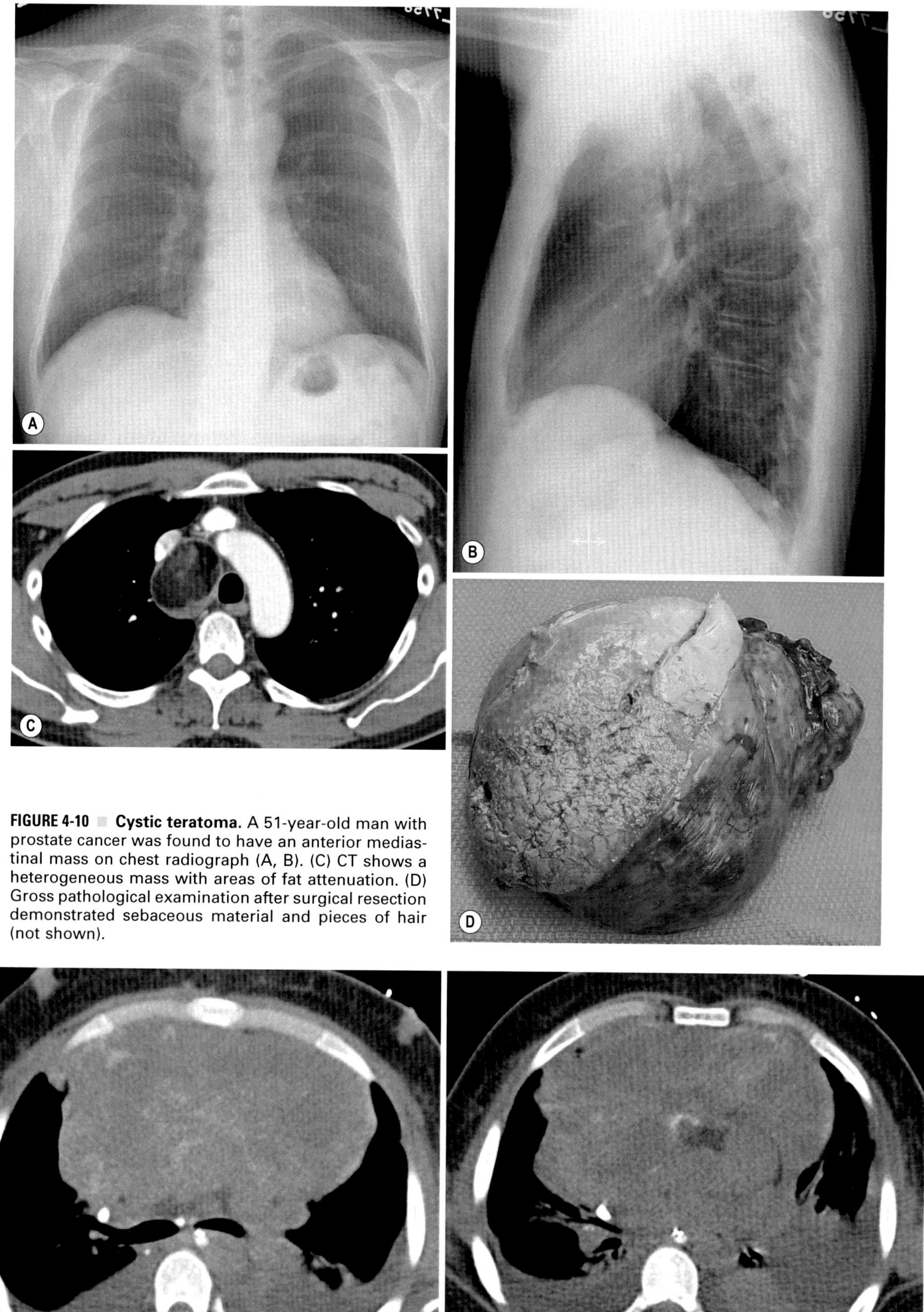

FIGURE 4-10 ■ **Cystic teratoma.** A 51-year-old man with prostate cancer was found to have an anterior mediastinal mass on chest radiograph (A, B). (C) CT shows a heterogeneous mass with areas of fat attenuation. (D) Gross pathological examination after surgical resection demonstrated sebaceous material and pieces of hair (not shown).

FIGURE 4-11 ■ **Seminoma.** A 19-year-old man with chest pain found to have a large anterior mediastinal mass on non-enhanced CT of the chest. The mass has a heterogeneous attenuation (A) and exerts mass effect upon the heart and airway (B).

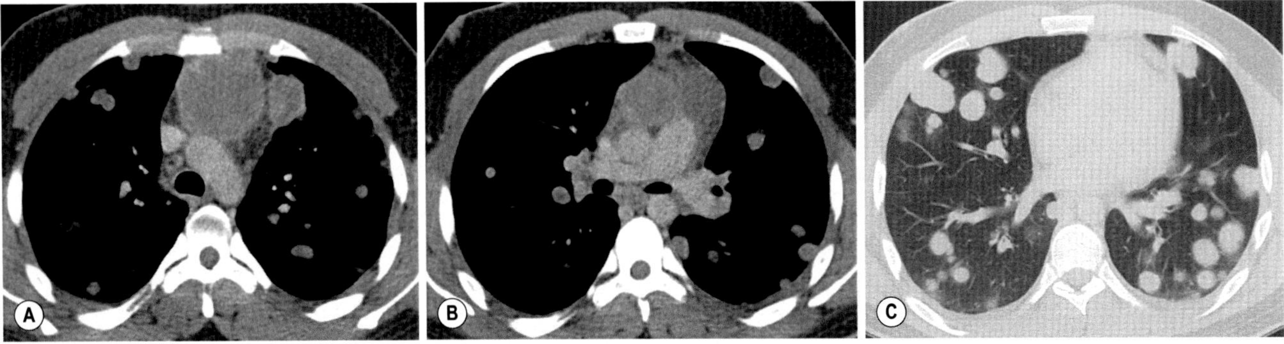

FIGURE 4-12 ■ **Metastatic choriocarcinoma.** A 23-year-old man presented with haemoptysis for 2 weeks. Chest CT demonstrates an anterior mediastinal mass of soft-tissue attenuation with slightly enhancing margins (A, B). (A) Mediastinal lymphadenopathy adjacent to the mass and (C) multiple pulmonary nodules dispersed throughout the lung are sites of metastases.

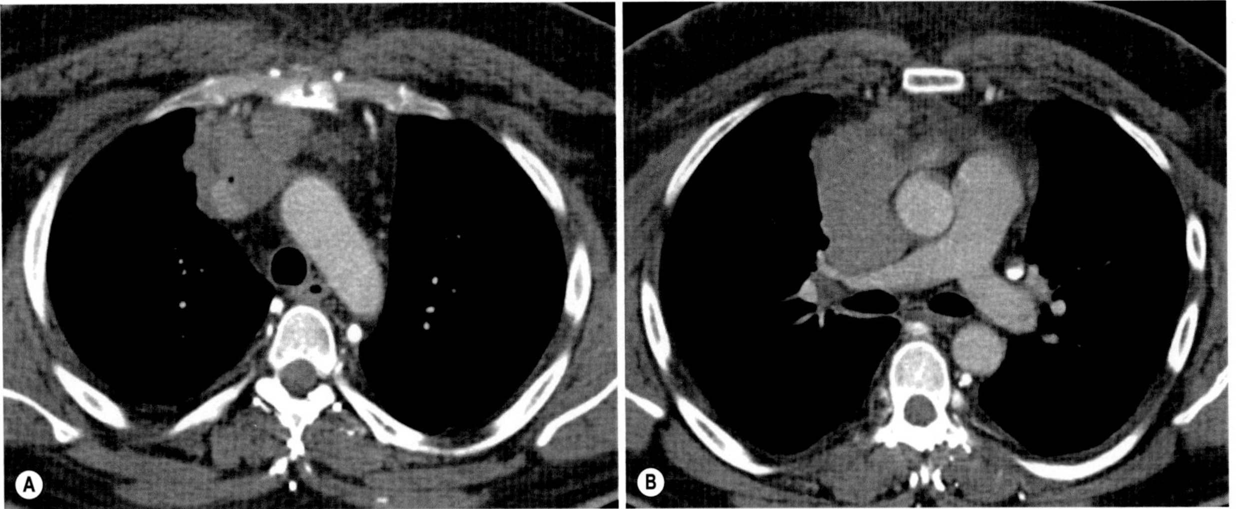

FIGURE 4-13 ■ **Large B-cell lymphoma.** A 33-year-old man found to have a lobular soft-tissue mass in the anterior mediastinum (A) extending to the right paratracheal and hilar regions (B).

enhancement interspersed with rounded areas of decreased attenuation caused by necrosis and haemorrhage.[47,48] On MR, these tumours may demonstrate heterogeneous intensities with areas of high T2 signal intensity corresponding to degenerative cystic changes.

Mediastinal Lymphadenopathy

Malignant Lymphoma and Leukaemia

Malignant lymphoma often involves mediastinal and hilar lymph nodes, multiple nodal groups usually being involved, particularly in Hodgkin's disease. Any intrathoracic nodal group may be enlarged and the following generalisations regarding plain radiograph, CT and MRI findings can be made:

1. The prevascular, para-aortic and paratracheal nodes are the groups most frequently involved (Fig. 4-13). The tracheobronchial and subcarinal nodes also may be enlarged in many cases. In most cases, the lymphadenopathy is bilateral but asymmetric. Hodgkin's disease, particularly the nodular sclerosing form, has a propensity to involve the prevascular, para-aortic and paratracheal nodes.
2. Hilar node enlargement is usually seen with mediastinal node enlargement. Hilar lymphadenopathy is rare without accompanying mediastinal node enlargement, particularly in Hodgkin's disease.
3. The posterior mediastinal nodes are infrequently involved—the enlarged nodes are often low in the mediastinum and contiguous retroperitoneal disease is likely.
4. The paracardiac nodes are rarely involved but become important as sites of recurrent disease because they may not be included in the initial radiation therapy fields.

Lymph node enlargement is also seen occasionally with leukaemia, the pattern being the same as with lymphoma. The lymph node enlargement in both lymphoma and leukaemia may resolve remarkably rapidly with therapy.

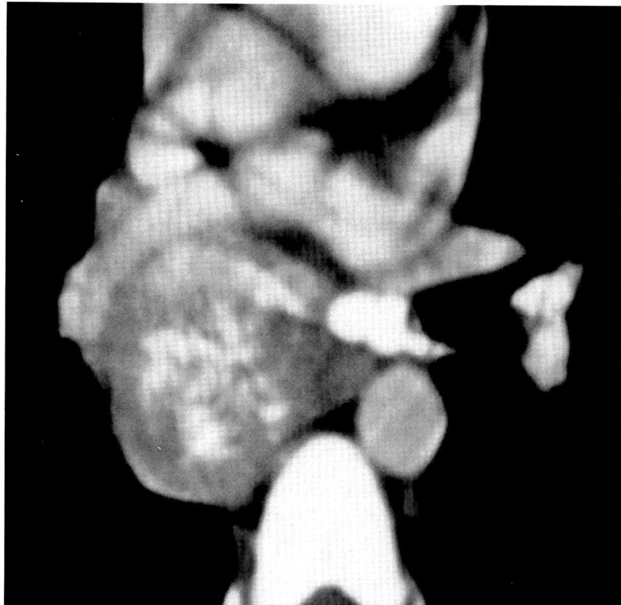

FIGURE 4-14 ■ **High-attenuation lymph nodes.** Transaxial image of chest CT shows a calcified mediastinal lymphadenopathy. Such dystrophic calcification is common as a sequela of *Histoplasma capsulatum* infection; however, it can also be seen with metastatic lymphadenopathy of mucinous adenocarcinomas.

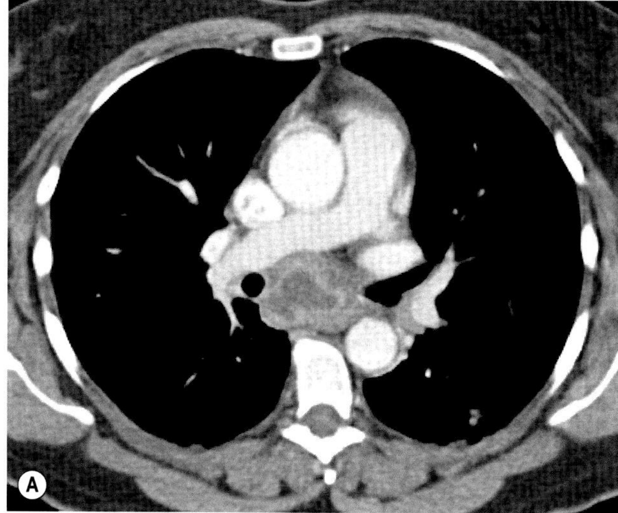

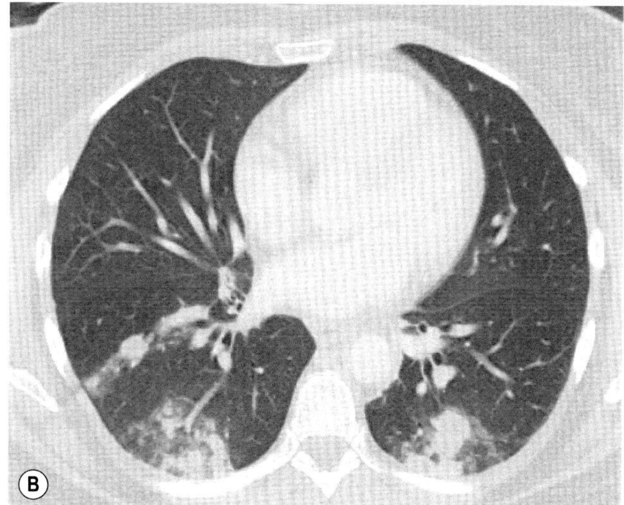

FIGURE 4-15 ■ **Low-attenuation lymph nodes.** Transaxial contrast medium-enhanced CT image of the chest in a 51-year-old woman with fever and chest pain shows subcarinal lymphadenopathy with central low attenuation caused by necrosis (A). Axial CT image in lung window setting lower in the chest reveals numerous confluent nodules in bilateral lower lobes caused by acute *Histoplasma capsulatum* (B).

Lymph Node Calcification

Extensive lymph node calcification is common following tuberculosis and fungal infection, and is occasionally seen with other infections (Fig. 4-14). It may also be encountered in a variety of other conditions, notably sarcoidosis, silicosis and amyloidosis. Although it may be seen in lymph node metastases from calcifying primary malignancies, such as osteosarcoma, chondrosarcoma and mucinous colorectal and ovarian tumours, lymph node calcification is rare in metastatic neoplasm. It is virtually unknown in untreated lymphoma though it is occasionally seen in nodes involved by Hodgkin's disease following therapy.

CT is the most sensitive technique for the detection of lymph node calcification. Two common patterns of calcification are coarse, irregularly distributed clumps within the node and homogeneous calcification of the whole node. A strikingly foamy appearance is rarely seen with *Pneumocystis jiroveci* (previously *Pneumocystis carinii*) infection in AIDS patients[49] and in some cases of metastatic mucinous neoplasms. Sometimes there is a ring of calcification at the periphery of the node—so-called 'eggshell calcification', which is a particular feature of sarcoidosis and of prolonged dust exposure (e.g. mining).

Low-Attenuation Nodes

On CT, areas of low attenuation within enlarged nodes, corresponding to necrosis, may be seen in a variety of conditions, particularly tuberculosis[50] and occasionally in fungal disease,[51] infections in immunocompromised patients, metastatic neoplasm (notably from testicular tumours[52]) and lymphoma[53] (Fig. 4-15). Necrotic lymph nodes are common in patients with active tuberculosis. They demonstrate central areas of low attenuation with peripheral enhancement when intravenous contrast medium has been administered. Attenuation values below that of water are seen in fatty replacement of inflammatory nodes and have been described in Whipple's disease.[54]

Enhancing Lymph Nodes

Castleman's disease is a rare cause of strikingly uniform enhancing lymph nodes. Castleman's disease (also referred to as angiofollicular lymph node hyperplasia) is a specific type of lymph node hyperplasia of uncertain aetiology which can cause substantial lymph node enlargement in many sites in the body. The lymph node mass is often localised to one area, can be huge and may be very vascular. The nodes may calcify and may show striking

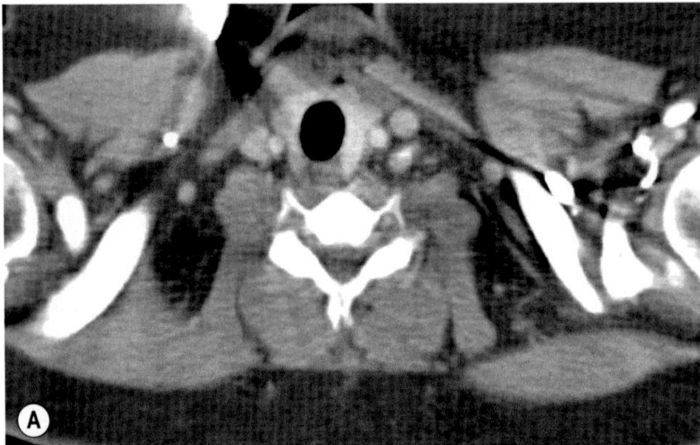

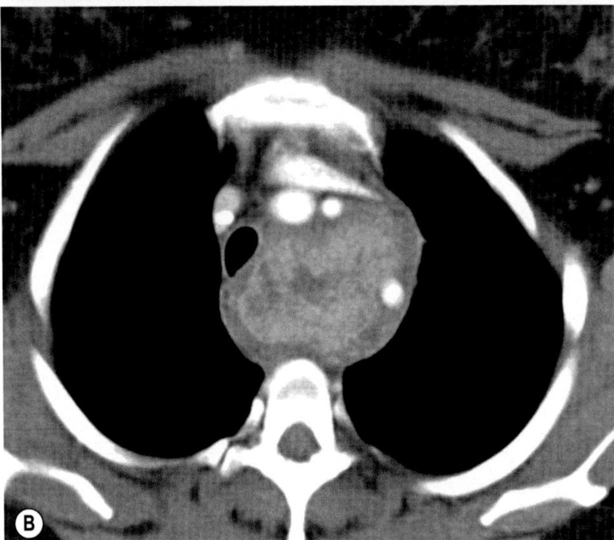

FIGURE 4-16 ■ **Castleman's disease.** A 33-year-old woman with shortness of breath was further evaluated by contrast medium-enhanced CT. Transaxial CT images show a normal thyroid (A), but narrowing and displacement of the trachea by a heterogeneously enhancing mediastinal mass located more inferiorly (B). The mass was surgically excised and pathological examination revealed hyaline vascular type of Castleman's disease.

contrast media enhancement on both CT and MRI[55,56] (Fig. 4-16). Histologically, there are two types: the hyaline vascular type and the plasma cell type.

In addition to Castleman's disease, marked lymph node enhancement may occur in hypervascular metastases from melanoma, renal cell carcinoma, carcinoid tumours, papillary thyroid cancer and Kaposi's sarcoma.[57]

Contrast media enhancement of enlarged nodes, when moderate in degree, is non-specific, being seen with inflammatory disorders, particularly tuberculosis, fungal disease, sarcoidosis and neoplasm. A low-density centre with rim enhancement of the enlarged node is a useful pointer towards the diagnosis of tuberculous or other granulomatous infections.

Lymph Node Enlargement

Normal-sized nodes are demonstrable at CT/MRI, but are not visible on CXR. The ease with which enlarged nodes can be recognised at CXR varies according to their location. Nodes in the right paratracheal group are readily identified: they show uniform or lobular widening of the right paratracheal stripe. Enlarged azygos nodes displace the azygos vein laterally and enlarge the shadow that normally represents the azygos vein to over 10 mm in its short-axis diameter. If the lymph nodes beneath the aortic arch become large enough to project beyond the aortopulmonary window they cause a local bulge in the angle between the aortic arch and the main pulmonary artery.

Hilar lymph node enlargement causes enlargement and/or lobulation of the outline of the hilar shadows. The diagnosis of lymph node enlargement on plain radiography depends on the recognition of the edge of a round or oval hilar mass, an analysis that requires a detailed understanding of the normal anatomy of the hilar blood vessels. Subcarinal lymph node enlargement widens the carinal angle and displaces the azygo-oesophageal line, so that the subcarinal portion of the azygo-oesophageal line, which is normally concave towards the lung, flattens or becomes convex towards the lung, an appearance that may be confused with left atrial enlargement. Subcarinal lymphadeonpathy can be appreciated on a lateral radiograph when it manifests with hilar lymphadenopathy. The combination of enlarged lymph nodes creates a rounded mass simulating a doughnut surrounding the mainstem bronchi.

Posterior mediastinal lymph node enlargement causes localised displacement of the paraspinal and para-oesophageal lines.

CT is an excellent method for detecting mediastinal lymph node enlargement. It is usually easy to distinguish between the normal vascular structures and enlarged lymph nodes using contrast medium-enhanced CT. The short-axis measurement provides the most representative guide to true size, because long-axis measurements vary to a significant degree according to the orientation of the lymph node within the CT section. In the assessment of lymph node enlargement, MRI provides essentially the same information as CT, although its use is limited to selected cases because of longer acquisition times and relatively limited spatial resolution (which may make measurement of individual nodes difficult). MR is not very helpful for detecting calcification. Although high T2 signal may be seen in lymphadenopathy, this finding is rarely specific.

Sarcoidosis. Sarcoidosis is a common cause of intrathoracic lymph node enlargement. Mediastinal lymph node enlargement occurs at some stage in most patients, with the hilar nodes being enlarged in almost all cases. Additionally, tracheobronchial, aortopulmonary and subcarinal nodes are enlarged in over half the patients. Anterior mediastinal nodes occasionally increase in size, but posterior mediastinal and internal mammary node enlargement is rare. One important diagnostic feature of lymphadenopathy in sarcoidosis is its symmetry. Lymph node calcification may have a stippled or egg-shell appearance.

Tuberculosis and Histoplasmosis. Lymph node enlargement caused by tuberculous or fungal infection may affect any of the nodal groups in the hila or mediastinum. One or more lymph nodes may be visibly enlarged and an associated area of pulmonary consolidation may be present. Lymph node enlargement is usually seen ipsilateral to the side of lung disease but involvement of the contralateral nodes may be present. Occasionally, widespread massive mediastinal and hilar node enlargement is seen. With healing, the nodes usually become smaller, often returning to normal size. Dense nodal calcification is frequent whether the nodes stay enlarged or shrink. The enlarged nodes, together with surrounding fibrosis, may compress the SVC or pulmonary veins and cause obstruction. Rim enhancement with a low-density centre may be seen with tuberculosis on contrast medium-enhanced CT.[50]

Metastatic Carcinoma. Mediastinal lymph node metastases can occur from primary bronchogenic carcinoma or from extrathoracic primary carcinomas. The extrathoracic tumours likely to metastasise to the mediastinum are head and neck cancer, breast cancer, genitourinary cancers and melanoma. In one large series, half the cases of mediastinal lymph node enlargement from extrathoracic primary carcinomas arose from tumours of the genitourinary tract, particularly the kidney and testis.[38] Most metastatic tumours cause lymph node enlargement without distinguishing characteristics. Calcified lymph node metastases are typical of mucinous adenocarcinoma or thyroid carcinoma.

Reactive Hyperplasia. Reactive hyperplasia in nodes draining infection/inflammation may cause mild enlargement, recognisable on CT but rarely on CXR.

Thoracic Lymphadenopathy in AIDS. Mediastinal lyphadenopathy is seen in 35–40% of HIV-infected patients and may raise concern for infection or malignancy.[58] Tuberculous and non-tuberculous mycobacterial disease and bacterial pneumonia are the primary infectious causes. Lymphoma and Kaposi's sarcoma are the major causes of malignancy. Lymphadenopathy without parenchymal lung disease may occur in patients with tuberculosis, *Mycobacterium avium-intracellulare* or cryptococcal infection.[59]

Foregut Duplication Cysts

'Foregut duplication cyst' is a term that covers various congenital cysts derived from the embryological foregut, including bronchogenic, and enteric cysts. Although attempts have been made to distinguish bronchogenic from oesophageal duplication cysts, prior infection or haemorrhage may denude the epithelium. The net effect is that even the pathologist may not be more specific than the diagnosis of *duplication cyst*.

Bronchogenic Cysts

Bronchogenic cysts are thought to result from abnormal budding of the developing tracheobronchia tree with separation of the buds from the normal airways.[60] Bronchogenic cysts are usually solitary asymptomatic mediastinal masses which may present at any age. Typically, they have a thin fibrous capsule, are lined with respiratory epithelium and contain cartilage, smooth muscle and glandular tissue. The cyst contents usually consist of thick mucoid material. Most are located adjacent to the trachea or main bronchi.[61] The subcarinal location is most frequent. The cysts can grow very large without causing symptoms, but they may compress surrounding structures, particularly the airways, and give rise to symptoms. In rare cases they become infected or haemorrhage occurs into the cyst; these complications may be life-threatening, particularly in infants and young children.

On CXR, duplication cysts present as spherical or oval masses with smooth outlines projecting from either side of the mediastinum (Fig. 4-17). Most are unilocular and do not have a lobulated outline. They usually contact the carina or main bronchi, but may be seen anywhere along the course of the trachea and larger airways, and frequently project into the middle mediastinum. Calcification of the wall is rare. Occasionally, duplication cysts can contain milk of calcium which creates a cyst–liquid calcium level within the cyst. Foregut duplication cysts frequently push the carina anteriorly and the oesophagus posteriorly—displacements that are almost never seen with other masses (the exceptions being thyroid masses and an aberrant left pulmonary artery).

CT is an excellent method of demonstrating the size, shape and position of a bronchogenic cyst and defining its extent and relation to key structures.[62] In some cases, it may demonstrate a thin-walled mass, with contents of uniform CT attenuation close to that of water (0 HU), thereby effectively making the diagnosis of a fluid-filled cyst[63] (Fig. 4-17). In other cases, the CT attenuation is similar to soft tissue and therefore to tumour, in which case the differential diagnosis becomes wider. Rarely, the cyst may show uniformly high density, probably caused by high protein content within the fluid.[64] In these cases, unenhanced CT images might be helpful.

T1-weighted MR images show that the intrinsic signal intensity varies from low to high, depending on the cyst contents. T2-weighted images demonstrate high signal intensity. The possibility of malignancy should be considered when a solid component is seen in the cyst. One advantage of MR is the ability to obtain fat-suppressed images before and after enhancement. The unenhanced images can be used as a mask and subtraction images can be created. Such subtraction images can be helpful to identify subtle areas of enhancement (making duplication cyst unlikely).

Oesophageal Duplication Cysts

Oesophageal duplication cysts are uncommon. They usually present first in childhood, but may not present until adulthood: initial presentation up to the age of 61 has been reported. They are distinguished from bronchogenic cysts pathologically by the presence of smooth

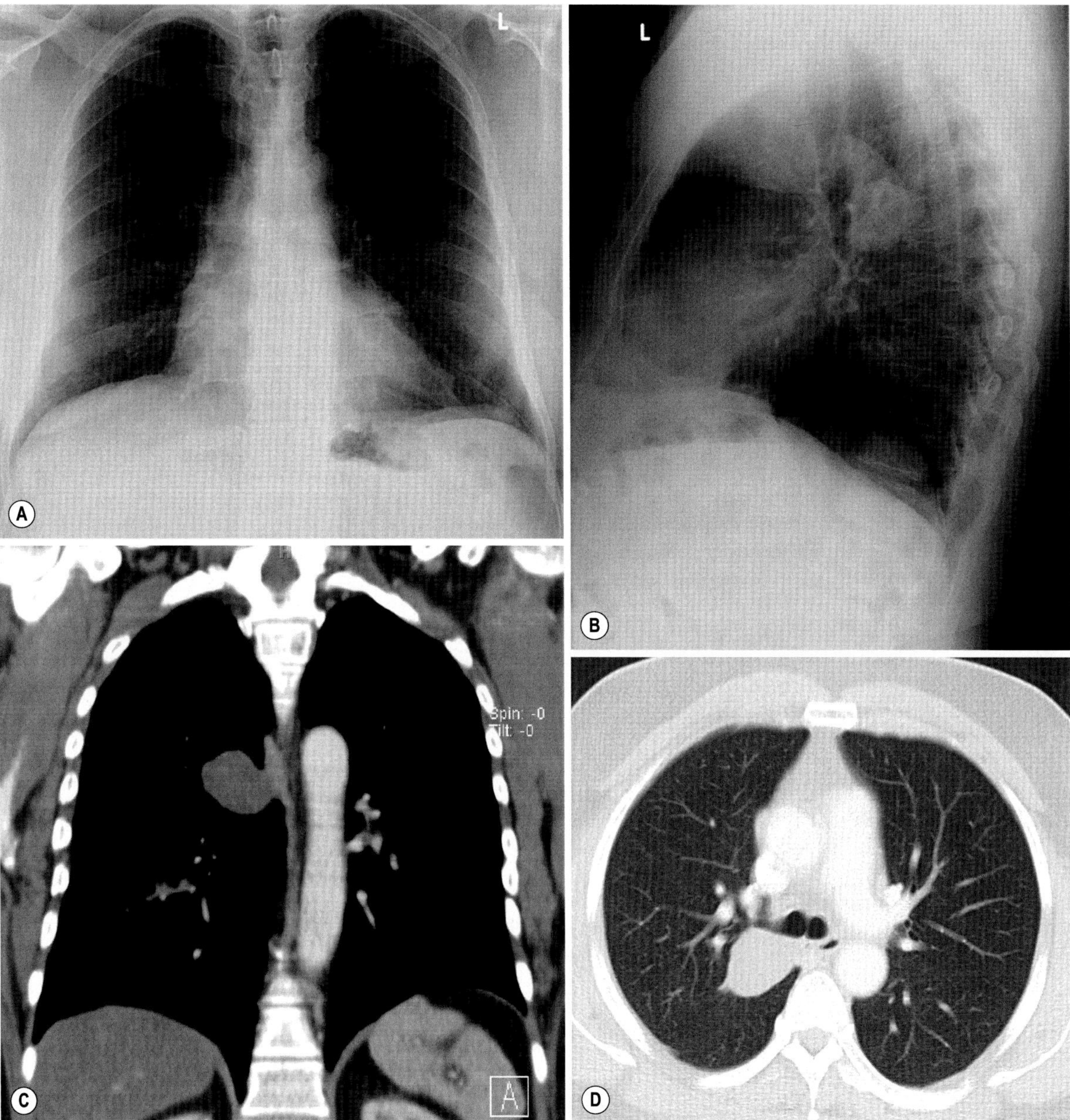

FIGURE 4-17 ■ **Bronchogenic cyst.** A 58-year-old man with hoarseness for several months. (A) Frontal and (B) lateral chest radiographs reveal a round middle mediastinal mass. (C) Coronal reformatted and (D) transaxial images of contrast medium-enhanced CT displayed in soft-tissue and lung-window settings, respectively, demonstrate a smooth-bordered, thin-walled mass of fluid attenuation located at the carina, closely associated with the right mainstem bronchus.

muscle in the walls, absence of cartilage and presence of mucosa resembling that of the oesophagus, stomach, or small intestine.[65] Many are clinically silent and are first discovered as an asymptomatic mass on thoracic imaging, but they may cause dysphagia, pain, or other symptoms caused by the compression of adjacent structures. A duplication cyst may become infected or ectopic gastric mucosa within the cyst may cause haemorrhage or perforation. The imaging features of oesophageal duplication cysts on CT and MRI are identical to those of bronchogenic cysts (Fig. 4-18) except that in the former, the wall of the lesion may be thicker, the cyst may assume a more tubular shape, and it may be in more intimate contact with the oesophagus.[61]

Neurenteric Cysts

Neurenteric cysts result from incomplete separation of the foregut from the notochord in early embryonic life and are far less common than oesophageal and bronchogenic cysts. The cyst wall contains both gastrointestinal and neural elements with an enteric epithelial

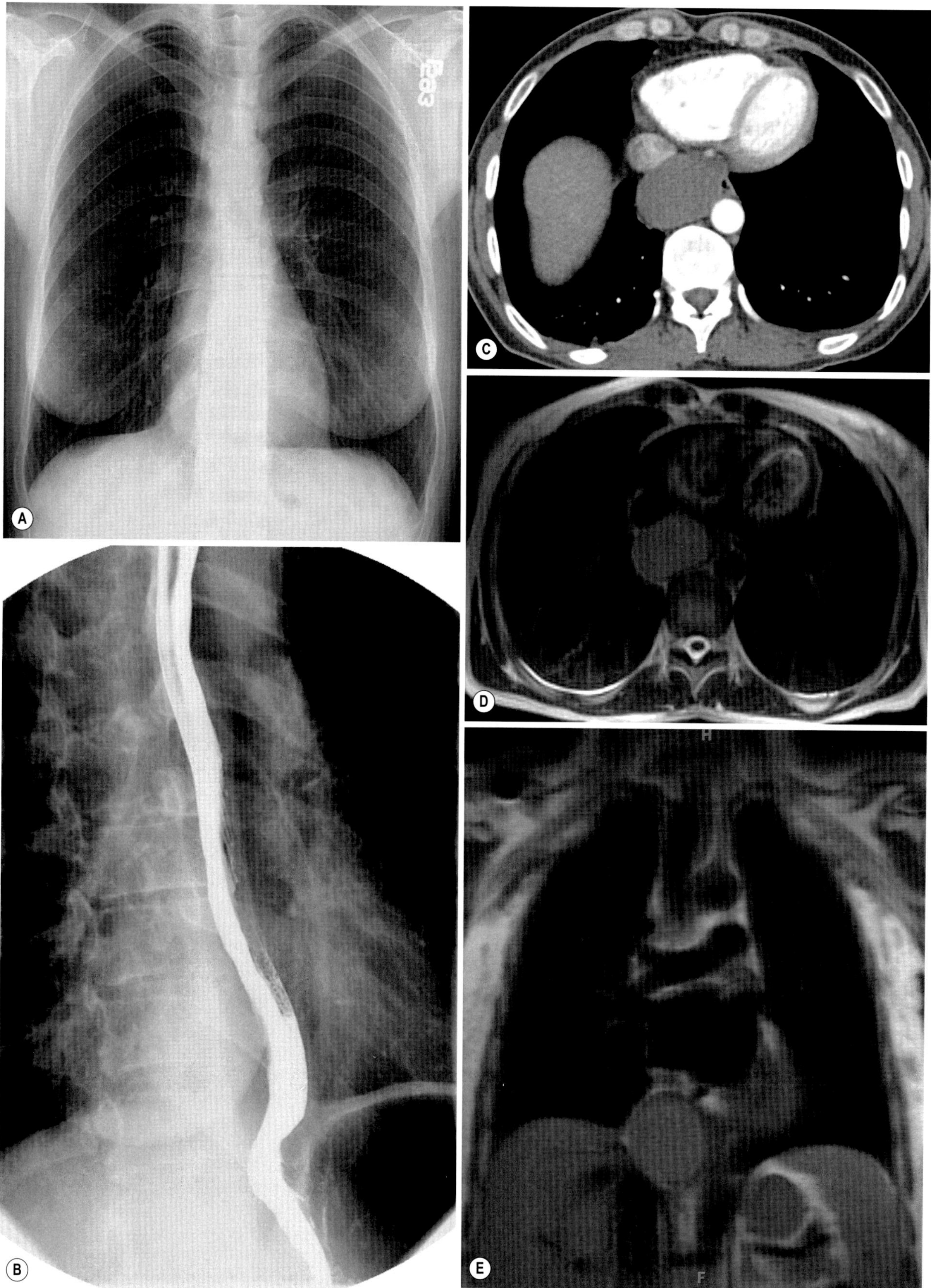

FIGURE 4-18 ■ **Oesophageal duplication cyst.** A 44-year-old woman presented with complaint of food stuck in her throat. (A) Chest radiograph shows an opacity causing rightward displacement of the azygo-oesophageal line. (B) Barium oesophogram demonstrates leftward deviation of distal oesophagus. (C) CT demonstrates a thin-walled cystic lesion abutting the oesophagus. (D) Axial and (E) coronal T2-weighted MR images demonstrate a homogeneous high T2 signal intensity of this mass and no enhancement on the T1-weighted contrast medium-enhanced sequence acquired after contrast agent administration (F).

Continued on following page

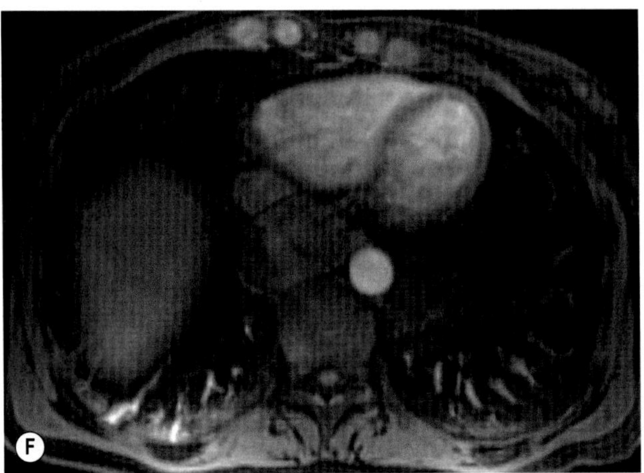

FIGURE 4-18, Continued

lining. There is usually a fibrous connection to the spine or an intraspinal component. Communication with the subarachnoid space or the gastrointestinal tract may be present, but communication with the oesophageal lumen is rare. There are typically associated vertebral body anomalies such as butterfly or hemivertebra. These cysts frequently produce pain and are often found early in life. Radiologically, a neurenteric cyst is a well-defined, round, oval or lobulated mass in the posterior mediastinum between the oesophagus (which is usually displaced) and the spine. Appearances on CT and MRI are similar to those of other foregut duplication cysts, with MRI being the investigation of choice for demonstrating the extent of intraspinal involvement.

Mediastinal Pancreatic Pseudocyst

On rare occasions, pancreatic pseudocysts extend into the mediastinum. Most patients are adults and have a history of pancreatitis; in children, the usual cause of the pseudocyst is trauma. Most patients also have left-sided or bilateral pleural effusions. The mediastinal component of the pseudocyst is usually in the middle or posterior mediastinum adjacent to the oesophagus, having gained access to the chest via the oesophageal or aortic hiatus. CT is the optimal method of demonstrating these thin-walled cysts, which may show continuity with the pancreas and any peripancreatic fluid collections. Isolated pancreatic mediastinal cysts are very rare. A history of pancreatitis will usually be present.

Neurogenic Tumours

Neurogenic tumours represent 20% of all adult and 35% of all paediatric mediastinal neoplasms. Neurogenic tumours are the most common tumours to arise in the posterior mediastinum, and most neurogenic tumours occur in this location.[61] Most neurogenic tumours in adults are benign and are discovered as asymptomatic masses on chest radiography, though some, particularly the malignant lesions, cause chest pain. They can be classified as tumours arising from peripheral nerves, including neurofibroma (Fig. 4-19), schwannoma and malignant tumours of nerve sheath origin (neurogenic sarcomas), or as tumours arising from sympathetic ganglia such as neuroblastomas and ganglioneuroblastomas. MRI is the best technique for imaging these tumours.[66] Neurofibromas or schwannomas are more common in adults, whereas neuroblastomas and ganglioneuroblastomas are more common in children. As a general guideline, peripheral nerve sheath tumours will have a craniocaudal dimension equal to their transverse dimension. Sympathetic ganglia tumours, however, tend to be longer in length than wide.

Peripheral Nerve Sheath Tumours

Peripheral nerve tumours are the most common mediastinal neurogenic tumours. They typically originate in an intercostal nerve in the paravertebral region. Most are benign. Radiologically, the benign tumours (neurofibromas and schwannomas) present as well-defined round or oval posterior mediastinal masses. Pressure deformity causing a smooth, scalloped indentation on the adjacent ribs, vertebral bodies, pedicles or transverse processes is common, particularly with larger lesions.[61,67] The scalloped cortex is usually preserved and is often thickened. These bone changes are diagnostic of a neurogenic lesion, the only differential diagnosis being that of a lateral thoracic meningocele. The rib spaces and the intervertebral foramina may be widened by the tumour.[61,67] On CT the tumours may be homogeneous or heterogeneous, usually enhancing heterogeneously. Punctate foci of calcification may be seen. Care must be taken on CT, however, as these lesions are often homogeneous and low in attenuation (from the myelin content). The net effect is a lesion that can mimic a duplication cyst. As a general rule, a posterior mediastinal lesion should not be called a cyst unless there is a clear vertebral anomaly or communication with the spinal canal.

On MR, neurofibromas and schwannomas have low-to-intermediate signal intensity on T1-weighted images and may have characteristic high signal intensity peripherally and low signal intensity centrally (target sign) on T2-weighted images;[68] and enhance after gadolinium. Ten percent of paravertebral neurofibroma extend into the spinal canal and appear as dumbbell-shaped masses with widening of the affected neural foramen.[69]

Malignant tumours of nerve sheath origin (Fig. 4-20) are rare spindle cell sarcomas, typically occurring in the third to fifth decades, although they may occur earlier in patients with neurofibromatosis type 1. Radiologically, the masses are usually larger than 5 cm in diameter.[61] Although MR cannot reliably differentiate benign from malignant neurogenic tumours, sudden change in size of a pre-existing mass, the development of heterogeneous signal intensity (caused by haemorrhage and necrosis) or infiltration of adjacent mediastinum or chest wall is cause for concern.[66] Haematogenous metastases to the lung have been reported but lymph node metastasis is rare.[61]

Sympathetic Ganglion Tumours

Sympathetic ganglion tumours are rare neoplasms representing a biological continuum ranging from benign ganglioneuroma to malignant neuroblastoma, with ganglioneuroblastoma being an intermediate form.[61] They originate from nerve cells rather than nerve sheaths and can occur in sympathetic ganglia and adrenal glands. Ganglioneuromas are benign neoplasms usually occurring in children and young adults. Ganglioneuroblastomas exhibit variable degrees of malignancy and usually occur in children.[70] Neuroblastomas are highly malignant tumours that typically occur in children younger than 5 years of age.[70] The posterior mediastinum is the most common extra-abdominal location of a neuroblastoma.

Ganglioneuromas and ganglioneuroblastomas usually arise from the sympathetic ganglia in the posterior mediastinum and therefore usually present radiologically as well-defined elliptical masses, with a vertical orientation, extending over the anterolateral aspect of three to five vertebral bodies.[61,71] Calcification occurs in approximately 25%. CT appearance is variable.[61] On MR, ganglioneuromas and ganglioneuroblastomas are usually of homogeneous intermediate signal intensity on T1- and T2-weighted images. Neuroblastomas are typically more heterogeneous, caused by areas of haemorrhage, necrosis,

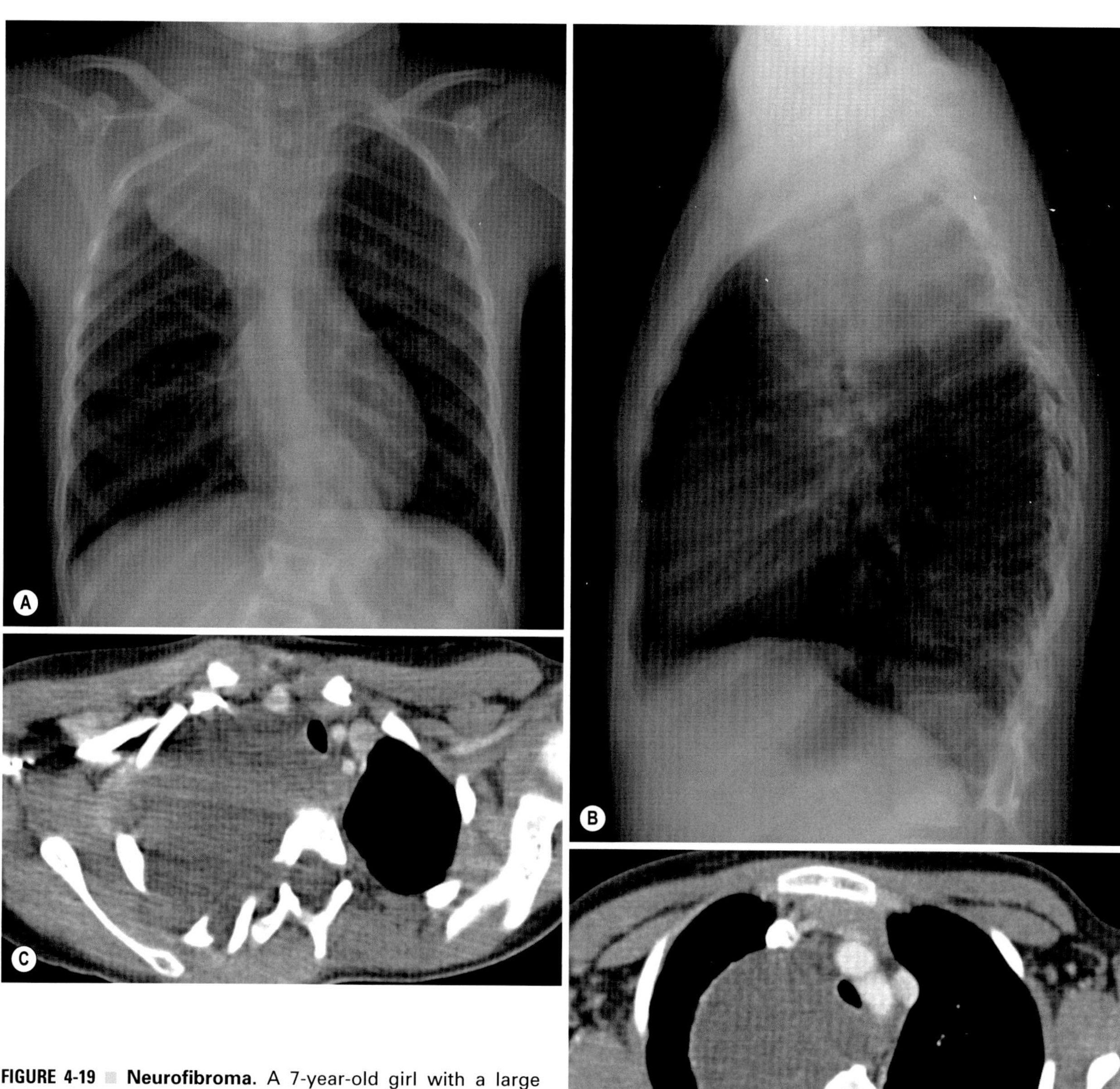

FIGURE 4-19 **Neurofibroma.** A 7-year-old girl with a large right apical mass associated with deformity of the adjacent ribs and scoliosis of the thoracic spine (A, B). CT demonstrates a homogeneous low-attenuation mass arising from the posterior mediastinum and extending to the right apex consistent with a plexiform neurofibroma causing mass effect on the trachea and vessels (C, D).

Continued on following page

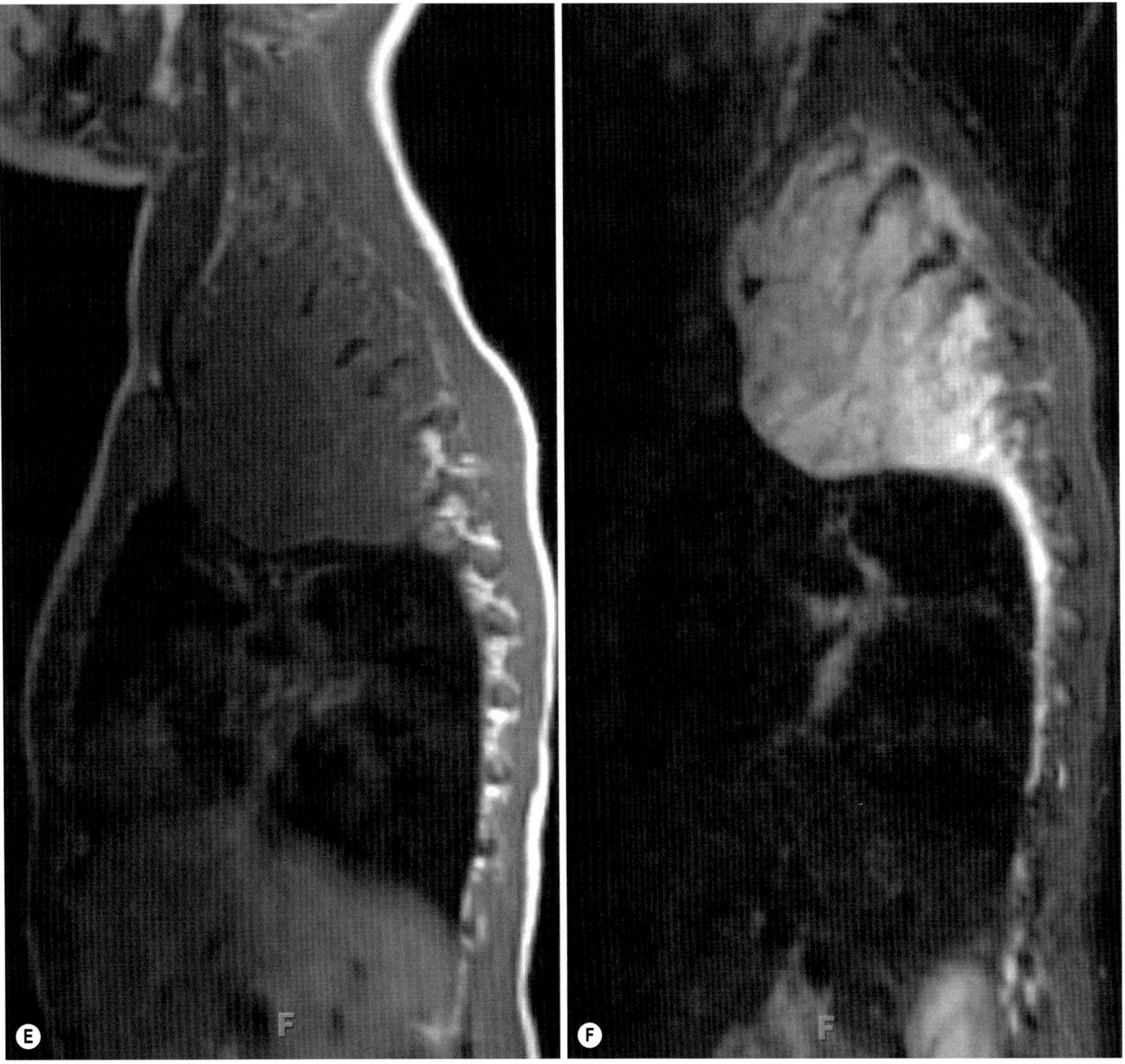

FIGURE 4-19, Continued ■ Sagittal images show that the mass has an isointense signal with chest wall musculature with T1-weighted sequence (E) and hyperintense signal with inversion-recovery sequence (F) imaging.

cystic degeneration and calcium. They may be locally invasive and have a tendency to cross the midline.

Mediastinal Paragangliomas

Intrathoracic paragangliomas are of two types: chemodectomas or phaeochromocytomas (functioning paragangliomas), either of which may be benign or malignant. Almost all intrathoracic chemodectomas are in a location close to the aortic arch and are classified as aortic body tumours. Other mediastinal chemodectomas are very rare.[72] They are usually single, but multicentric cases are reported.

Fewer than 2% of phaeochromocytomas occur in the chest. Most intrathoracic phaeochromocytomas are found in the posterior mediastinum or closely related to the heart, particularly in the wall of the left atrium or the interatrial septum. Approximately, one-third of mediastinal phaeochromocytomas are non-functioning and asymptomatic, the remainder presenting with the symptoms, signs and laboratory findings of overproduction of catecholamines.

The various paragangliomas have similar appearances on chest radiography, CT and MRI. They form rounded, soft-tissue masses, which are usually very vascular and therefore enhance intensely on CT.[73] On MR, phaeochromocytomas usually show a signal intensity similar to that of muscle on T1-weighted images and very high signal intensity on T2-weighted images.[74] MR is particularly useful for demonstrating intracardiac phaeochromocytomas. Radio-iodine MIBG (*meta*-iodobenzylguanidine) and somatostatin receptor scintigraphy both show

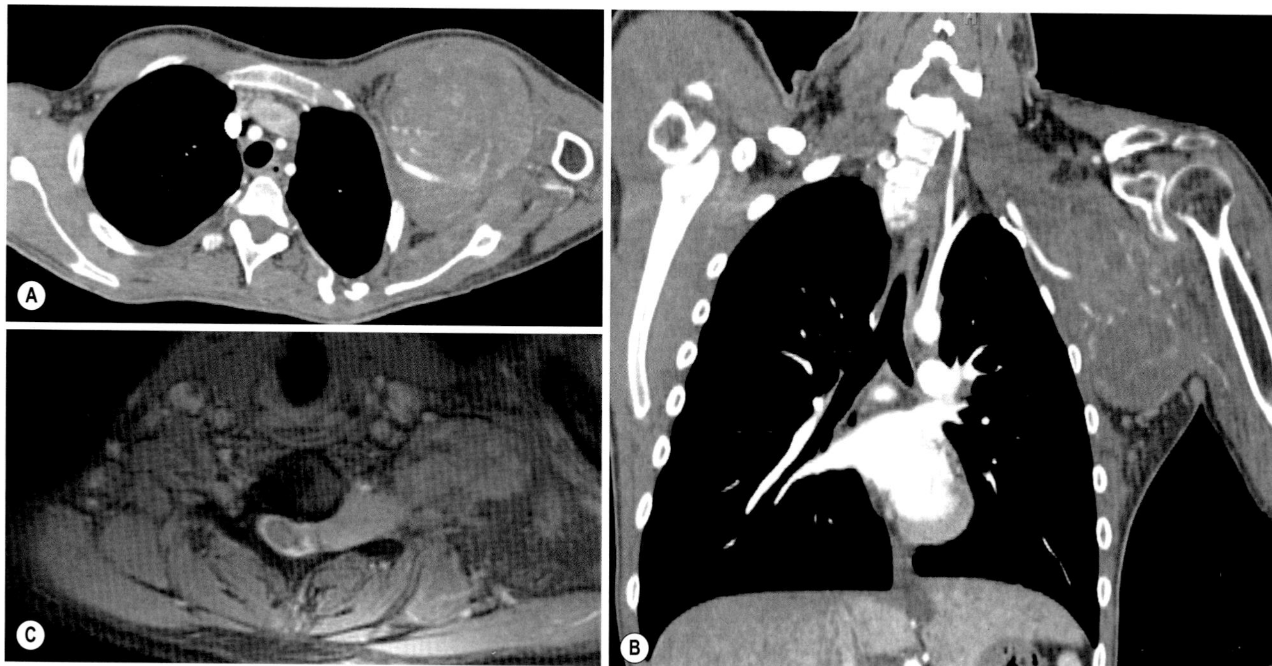

FIGURE 4-20 ■ **Malignant nerve sheath tumour.** A 23-year-old with left axillary mass and left shoulder pain. (A) Axial and (B) coronal contrast medium-enhanced CT images show a large heterogeneously enhancing mass in the left axilla, which encases the left subclavian artery. Axial contrast medium-enhanced MR image demonstrates that this enhancing mass expands the neural foramen of the spine, with no erosion of the vertebral body, suggesting that this is a neurogenic tumour (C).

increased activity in paragangliomas (Fig. 4-21) and are useful techniques for identifying extra-adrenal phaeochromocytomas.[74,75]

Lateral Thoracic Meningocele

Lateral thoracic meningoceles are rare posterior mediastinal cystic lesions characterised by redundant meninges (dura and arachnoid with small amounts of neural tissue within the wall) that protrude through the spinal foramen and are filled with cerebrospinal fluid. Like neurofibromas, they are commonly associated with neurofibromatosis.[76] They present as an asymptomatic mass, often with pressure deformity of the adjacent bone, indistinguishable on plain radiographs from neurofibromas. CT and MRI can both indicate the correct diagnosis by showing the mass to be fluid filled rather than solid[61] and demonstrating continuity between the CSF in the meningocele and that contained in the thecal sac. If necessary, the diagnosis can be established by CT with intrathecal contrast medium demonstrating flow into the lesion.

Extramedullary Haematopoiesis

Extramedullary haematopoiesis can result in paravertebral masses caused by compensatory expansion of bone marrow in patients with severe anaemia caused by inadequate production or excessive destruction of blood cells. The mechanism of marrow expansion is unknown. It can be seen in the presence of thalassaemia, hereditary spherocytosis, and sickle cell anaemia. The mass itself almost never causes symptoms. Radiographically,

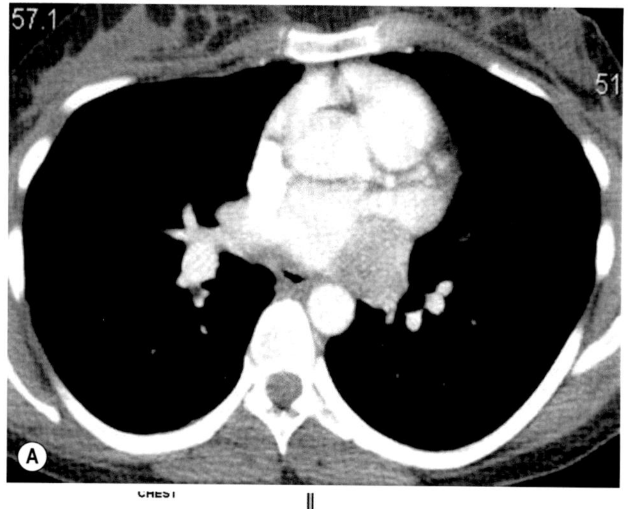

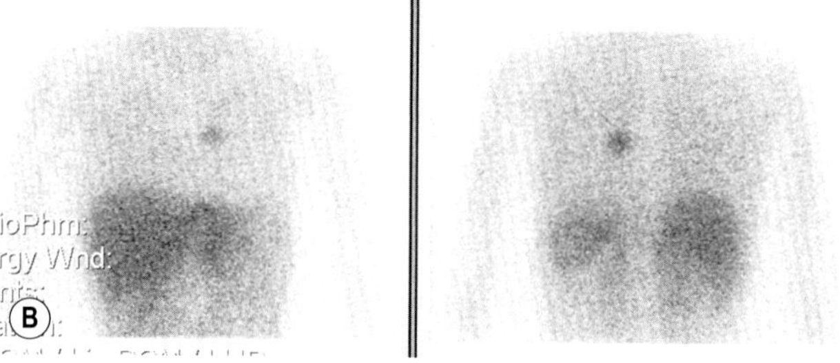

FIGURE 4-21 ■ **Paraganglioma.** CT of the chest demonstrates an enhancing mediastinal mass arising in the middle mediastinum adjacent to the left atrium, and protruding into it (A). I-131 *meta*-iodobenzylguanidine (MIBG) scintigraphy shows increased uptake, revealing that it is a paraganglioma (B).

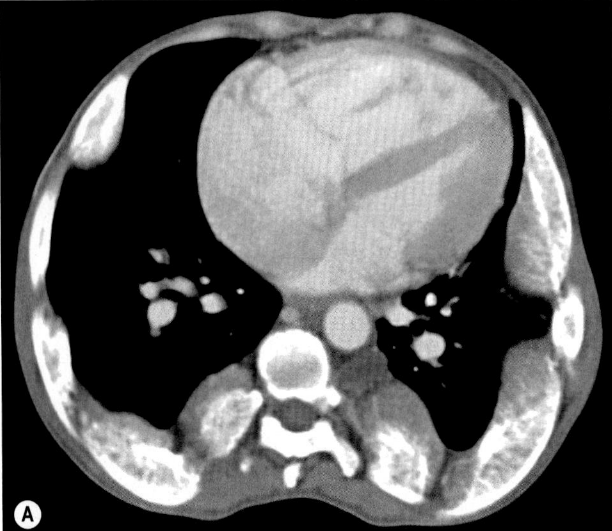

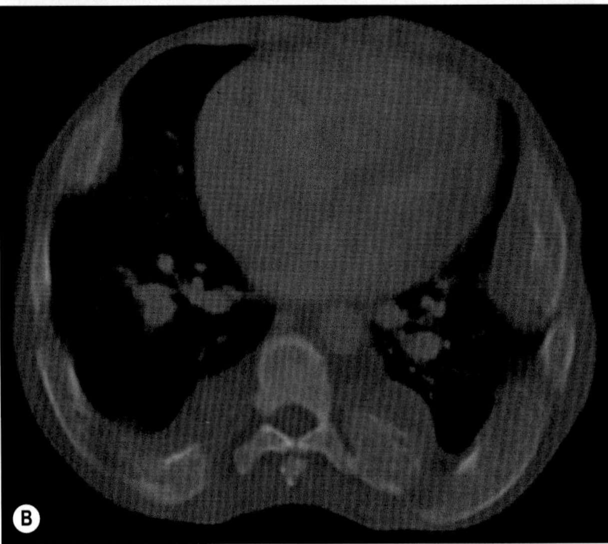

FIGURE 4-22 ■ **Extramedullary hematopoiesis.** Axial contrast medium-enhanced CT images optimised for (A) soft tissue and (B) bone of a 40-year-old woman with thalassaemia display bilateral soft-tissue masses closely associated with the ribs and the spine. The ribs are expanded by trabeculated bone.

lobulated paravertebral masses, usually multiple and bilateral and in the lower thoracic vertebra, are typically seen. They appear well marginated. The bones may be normal or may show an altered lace-like trabecular pattern caused by marrow expansion (Fig. 4-22). The masses are usually of homogeneous soft-tissue attenuation on CT, although occasionally, when the anaemia resolves, a fatty component may be visible.[77] Usually the masses are bilateral and reasonably symmetrical.

Mesenchymal Tumours and Tumour-Like Conditions

Lymphangiomas (Cystic Hygromas)

Lymphangiomas are rare, benign congenital malformations consisting of focal proliferations of well-differentiated lymphatic tissue comprising complex lymph channels or cystic spaces containing clear or straw-coloured fluid.[78] Most lymphangiomas are present at birth and detected in the first two years of life. Lymphangiomas are most common in the neck and axilla. Ten per cent of lymphangiomas in the neck extend into the mediastinum.[78,79] Lymphangiomas can occur in any part of the mediastinum, but are most common in the anterior or superior mediastinum. Mediastinal lymphangiomas may on occasion be wholly confined to the mediastinum but they are more frequently an extension from a lymphangioma in the neck Most cervicomediastinal lymphangiomas present in early life as a neck mass, whereas the purely mediastinal lymphangiomas usually present in older children and adults as an asymptomatic mediastinal mass. They are classified histologically as simple (capillary), cavernous or cystic (hygroma), depending on the size of the lymphatic channels they contain. Cystic lymphangiomas are most common. Lymphangiomas rarely produce symptoms caused by their soft consistency. However, compression of mediastinal structures can result in chest pain, cough and dyspnoea. Complications include airway compromise, infection, chylothorax and chylopericardium.[80] On CT, a lobulated smooth mass envelops the adjacent mediastinal structures rather than displaces them.[79] This feature can be useful in distinguishing lymphangiomas from other mediastinal cysts. Usually they have a homogeneous fluid attenuation (Fig. 4-23) but can have a combination of fluid and soft tissue.[81] Thin septations can sometimes be seen within the mass.[79,81] On MR the lesions may have heterogeneous T1 signal intensity but usually have high T2 signal intensity. Complete resection of lymphangiomas may be difficult because of their insinuating nature and follow-up may be needed to exclude recurrence.[82]

Haemangiomas

Haemangiomas are rare vascular tumours composed of interconnecting vascular channels with varying areas of thrombosis and fibrous stroma. Haemangiomas can be capillary, cavernous or venous with cavernous hemangiomas accounting for approximately 75% of the cases. Haemangiomas occur in young patients, with half of the patients being asymptomatic. Symptoms, when they occur, are caused by compression. On CT, enhancement following contrast media administration can be dense, focal or diffuse and peripheral or central. Phleboliths or punctate calcifications are seen in 10 to 20% of the cases.

Fatty Lesions in the Mediastinum

Fat is normally present in the mediastinum and its amount increases with age. Normal fat is equally distributed throughout the matrix of the mediastinum and is not encapsulated. Abnormalities of fat distribution in the mediastinum can be diffuse (mediastinal lipomatosis) or focal (fat-containing diaphragmatic hernia or mediastinal lipoma). Relatively large collections of fat are often present in the cardiophrenic angles, particularly in obese subjects. These cardiophrenic fat pads may resemble a mass.

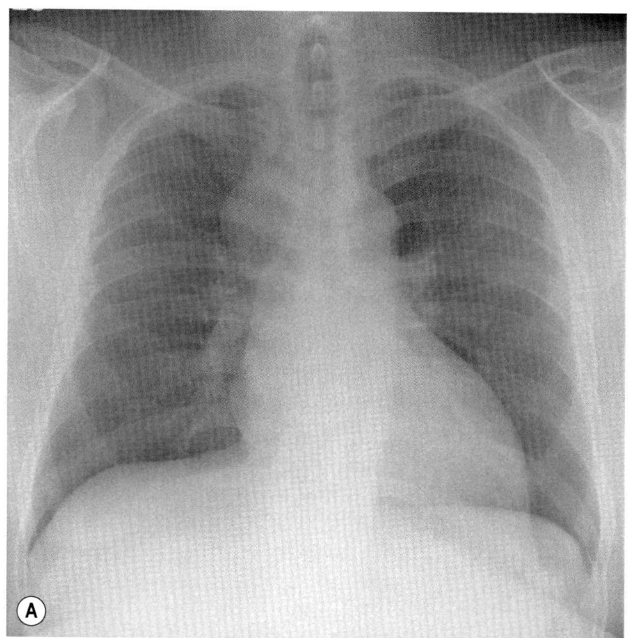

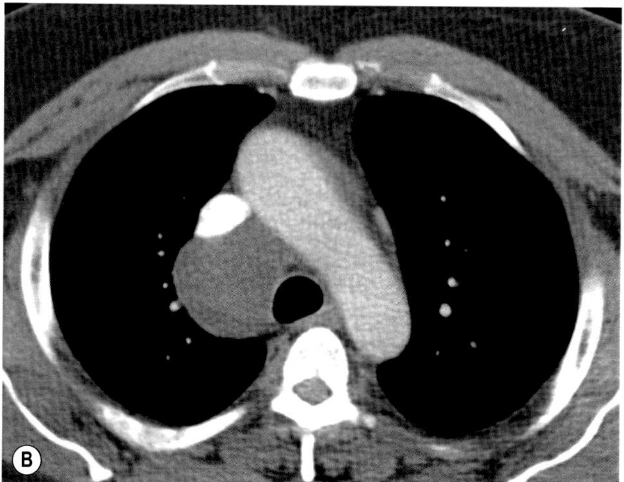

FIGURE 4-23 ■ **Lymphangioma.** A 56-year-old man found to have a right paratracheal opacity on chest radiograph (A). CT shows a smooth, well-defined right paratracheal lesion which has no perceptible wall and is of fluid attenuation (B). After surgical resection pathological examination revealed lymphagioma.

Mediastinal Lipomatosis

Mediastinal lipomatosis is a benign accumulation of excessive amount of unencapsulated histologically normal fat in the mediastinum. Mediastinal lipomatosis is a phenomenon seen particularly in Cushing's disease, in patients on steroid therapy and in obese subjects. When the fat deposits are extensive and symmetrical, the diagnosis is usually obvious. The excess fat deposition is most prominent in the upper mediastinum, resulting in a smooth symmetrical mediastinal widening on the chest radiograph. On CT, the fat should appear homogeneously low in attenuation, sharply outlining the mediastinal vessels and lymph nodes.

Fatty Tumours of the Mediastinum

Fatty tumours of the mediastinum are rare. On chest radiography, regardless of whether they are benign or malignant, fatty tumours are seen as well-defined round or oval mediastinal masses.

Mediastinal lipomas constitute 2% of all mediastinal tumours. They can occur in any part of the mediastinum but are most common in the prevascular space. Benign lipomas are soft and do not compress surrounding structures unless they are very large. On CT they show uniform fat attenuation.[83] Their boundaries are smooth and sharply demarcated from adjacent mediastinal structures.

Mediastinal liposarcomas are rare malignant fat-containing tumours. They may occur anywhere in the mediastinum. In contradistinction to benign lipomas, they usually contain large areas of soft-tissue density material. Histological differentiation between lipoma and liposarcoma depends on the presence of mitotic activity, cellular atypia, neovascularisation and tumour infiltration.

CT findings include heterogeneous attenuation with significant soft tissue within a mass with fat attenuation, poor definition of adjacent mediastinal structures and infiltration or invasion of mediastinal structures (Fig. 4-24).

Lipoblastoma, a benign tumour of childhood, contains fat and soft tissue.[84,85] Occasionally, the amount of fat attenuation is relatively small. CT findings are similar to liposarcomas.

Angiomyolipoma and myelolipoma are both benign tumours which may show a combination of soft-tissue and fat attenuation on CT and therefore can be indistinguishable from liposarcoma on imaging.[86,87] Angiomyolipomas and myelolipomas are rare in the mediastinum.

Fat-Containing Hernias

Herniation of omental fat is a common cause of a localised fatty mass in the mediastinum. Omental fat can herniate through the foramen of Morgagni and give the appearance of a cardiophrenic angle mass on the right. Fat herniation through the foramen of Bochdalek occurs most frequently on the left side posteriorly. The fat may herniate through the oesophageal hiatus as well. Such herniations are usually readily diagnosed because of their characteristic locations. On CT or MRI, appearances consistent with fat eliminate confusion with other mediastinal masses.[85]

OTHER MEDIASTINAL LESIONS

Acute Mediastinitis

Acute infection of the mediastinum is rare. The most common cause of acute mediastinitis is iatrogenic oesophageal perforation during diagnostic or therapeutic endoscopic procedures. Forceful vomiting may result in oesophageal perforation (Boerhaave's syndrome) and a

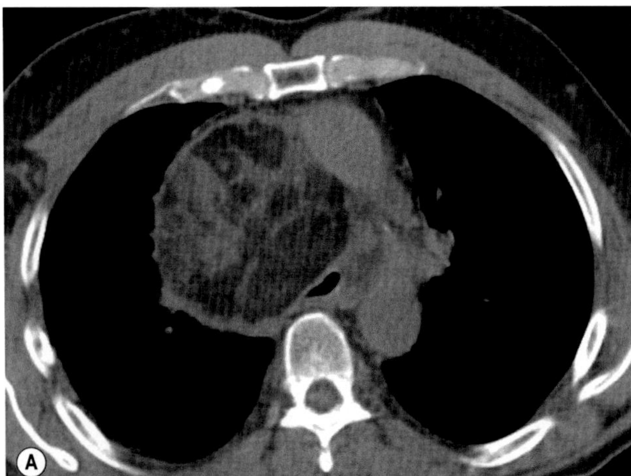

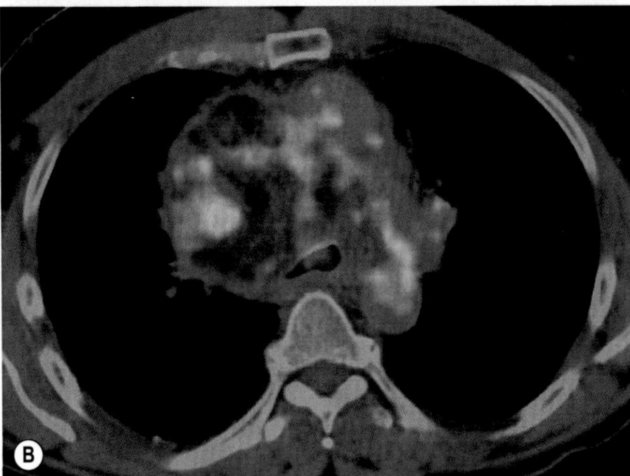

FIGURE 4-24 ■ **Liposarcoma.** A 58-year-old man with gradually worsening dyspnoea was found to have a large anterior mediastinal mass when evaluated by chest CT. This mass has a predominantly fat attenuation with internal thick septations and mural nodules and exerts significant mass effect upon the airway (A). PET-CT shows significant FDG uptake of the soft-tissue components of the mass (B).

leak into the mediastinum can result in acute mediastinitis. Such tears are almost invariably just above the gastro-oesophageal junction. Other causes of acute mediastinal infection are leakage from the oesophagus into the mediastinum through a necrotic neoplasm, and extension of infection from the neck, retroperitoneum or adjacent intrathoracic or chest wall structures into the mediastinum. Clinically, the patients are often very ill with an abrupt onset of high fever, tachycardia and chest pain. Diffuse mediastinitis has a very poor prognosis. The mortality associated with acute mediastinitis from oesophageal perforation is 5–30% even with appropriate treatment.[88]

The CXR may show widening and ill-defined mediastinal outline adjacent to the oesophagus. Streaks or collections of air may be seen within the mediastinum, and there may even be mediastinal air–fluid levels. Air may also be seen in the soft tissues of the neck. Pleural effusions are frequent and are usually on the left. Lower lobe pneumonia or atelectasis often complicates the radiographic picture. Radiologically, detection of oesophageal perforation relies on the presence of indirect signs, including pneumomediastinum, left pleural effusion and pneumothorax. An oesophagram using water-soluble contrast medium may show the site of perforation, with extravasation into the mediastinum.

CT is optimal in evaluating suspected mediastinitis and mediastinal abscess. CT shows obliteration of the normal mediastinal fat planes, oesophageal thickening and extraluminal gas bubbles within the mediastinum. In advanced cases there may be walled-off discrete fluid or air–fluid collections indicating abscess formation (Fig. 4-25). There may be an associated pleural effusion, empyema, subphrenic or pericardial collection. When acute mediastinitis is suspected following sternotomy, CT shows the extent of inflammation and any drainable mediastinal or pericardial fluid collections.[89] Distinguishing a retrosternal haematoma from reactive granulation tissue or cellulitis is difficult, as is distinguishing osteomyelitis from the direct effects of the surgical incision.[90] It should be remembered that substernal fluid collections and tiny pockets of air are normal in the first 20 days following sternotomy. Therefore, before gas-forming infections can be diagnosed, the air collections must appear de novo or must progressively increase in the absence of any other explanation.[91] In descending necrotising mediastinitis, CT shows solitary or multiple fluid collections, which may be contiguous with other fluid collections in the cervical region and diffuse obliteration of normal fat planes related to fasciitis.

Fibrosing Mediastinitis

Fibrosing mediastinitis (sclerosing mediastinitis or mediastinal fibrosis) is a disorder that results in proliferation of fibrous tissue and collagen within the mediastinum. It is usually caused by previous infection from histoplasmosis or tuberculosis.[92] Other causes include sarcoidosis, autoimmune diseases, retroperitoneal fibrosis, radiation and drugs such as methysergide. The most common clinical consequences are obstruction to the SVC and, occasionally, obstruction to the central pulmonary arteries or veins.

The CXR is non-specific and often underestimates the extent of mediastinitis. In fibrosing mediastinitis caused by previous tuberculous or fungal infection, the chest radiograph may show calcification of mediastinal or hilar lymph nodes. CT typically shows an infiltrative, often extensively calcified, hilar or mediastinal process, which may be relatively focal when disease is caused by previous histoplasmosis or tuberculosis (Fig. 4-26), and more diffuse in the idiopathic form.[93] Airway narrowing, vascular encasement and obstruction may also be seen. CT is excellent for the evaluation of the extent of mediastinal soft-tissue infiltration and to identify the degree of narrowing of the mediastinal structures (Fig. 4-26).

Two patterns of fibrosing mediastinits have been described: a focal pattern and a diffuse pattern.[93,94] The focal pattern caused by histoplasmosis, seen in 82% of

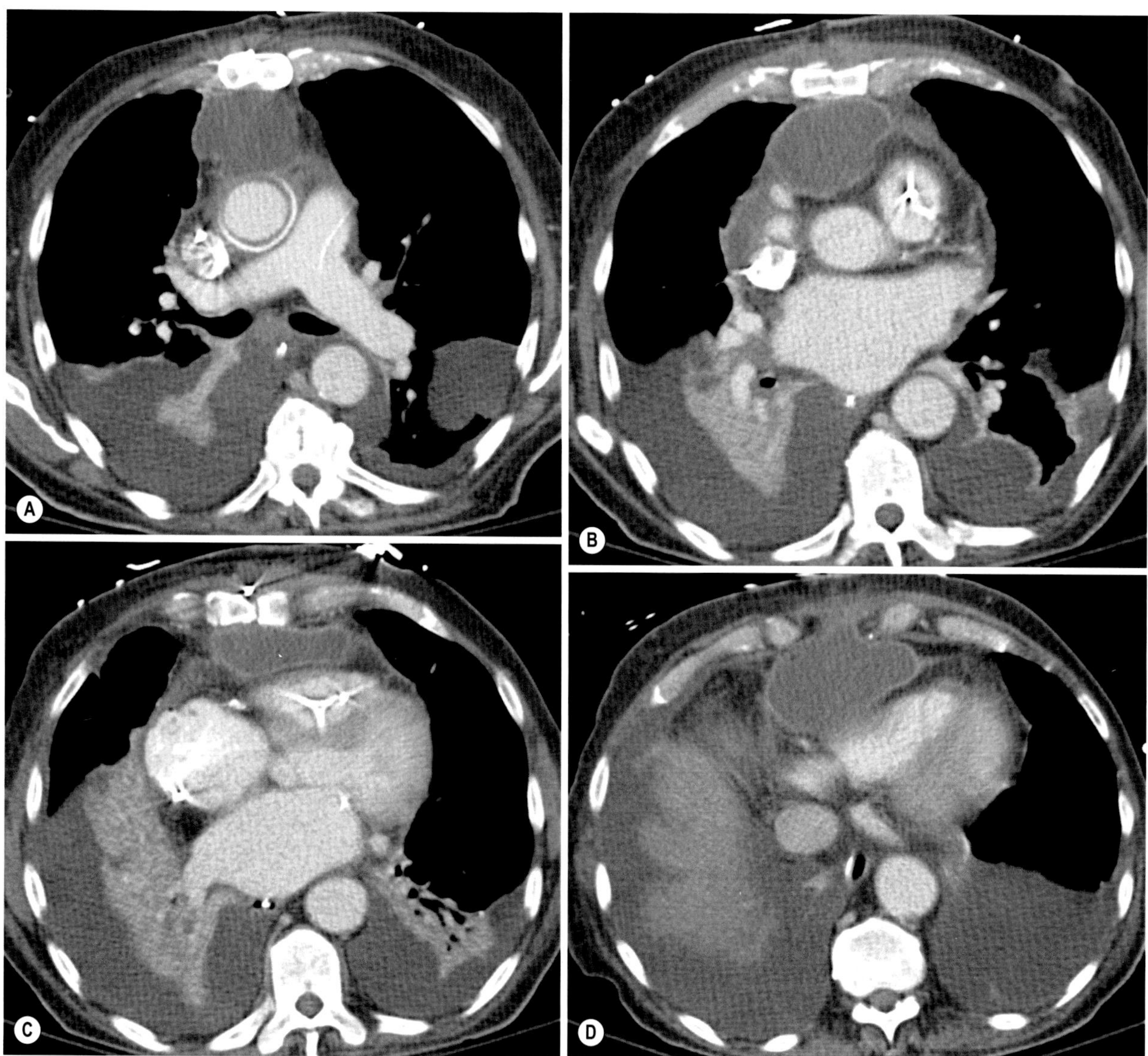

FIGURE 4-25 ■ **Mediastinal abscess.** An 83-year-old man had a contrast medium-enhanced CT of the chest (A–D) caused by persistent fever and chest pain following mitral valve replacement and ascending aortic graft repair. There is a large fluid collection with peripheral enhancement consistent with an abscess located posterior to the sternum and in close association with the aortic graft (A).

cases, manifests as a mass of soft-tissue attenuation that is frequently calcified (63% of cases) and is usually located in the right paratracheal, subcarinal or hilar regions. The diffuse pattern, not related to histoplasmosis, often occurs in the setting of retroperitoneal fibrosis seen in 18% of cases and manifests as a diffusely infiltrating, non-calcified mass that affects multiple mediastinal compartments.

Fibrosing mediastinitis typically demonstrates a heterogeneous, infiltrative mass of intermediate signal intensity on T1-weighted MR images. On T2-weighted MR images it is more variable, with areas of both increased and markedly decreased signal intensity seen in the same lesion.[95,96] Areas of decreased signal intensity represent calcification or fibrous tissue, and areas of increased signal intensity may indicate more active inflammation. Extensive regions of decreased signal intensity within the lesion, when present, help differentiate fibrosing mediastinitis from other infiltrative lesions of the mediastinum, such as metastatic carcinoma and lymphoma, that typically have increased T2 signal intensity. Heterogeneous enhancement of the mass may be seen after administration of a gadolinium-based contrast medium. MRI lacks sensitivity for detection of calcification, which is an important feature for differentiating fibrosing mediastinitis from other infiltrative disorders of the mediastinum, such as lymphoma and metastatic carcinoma.

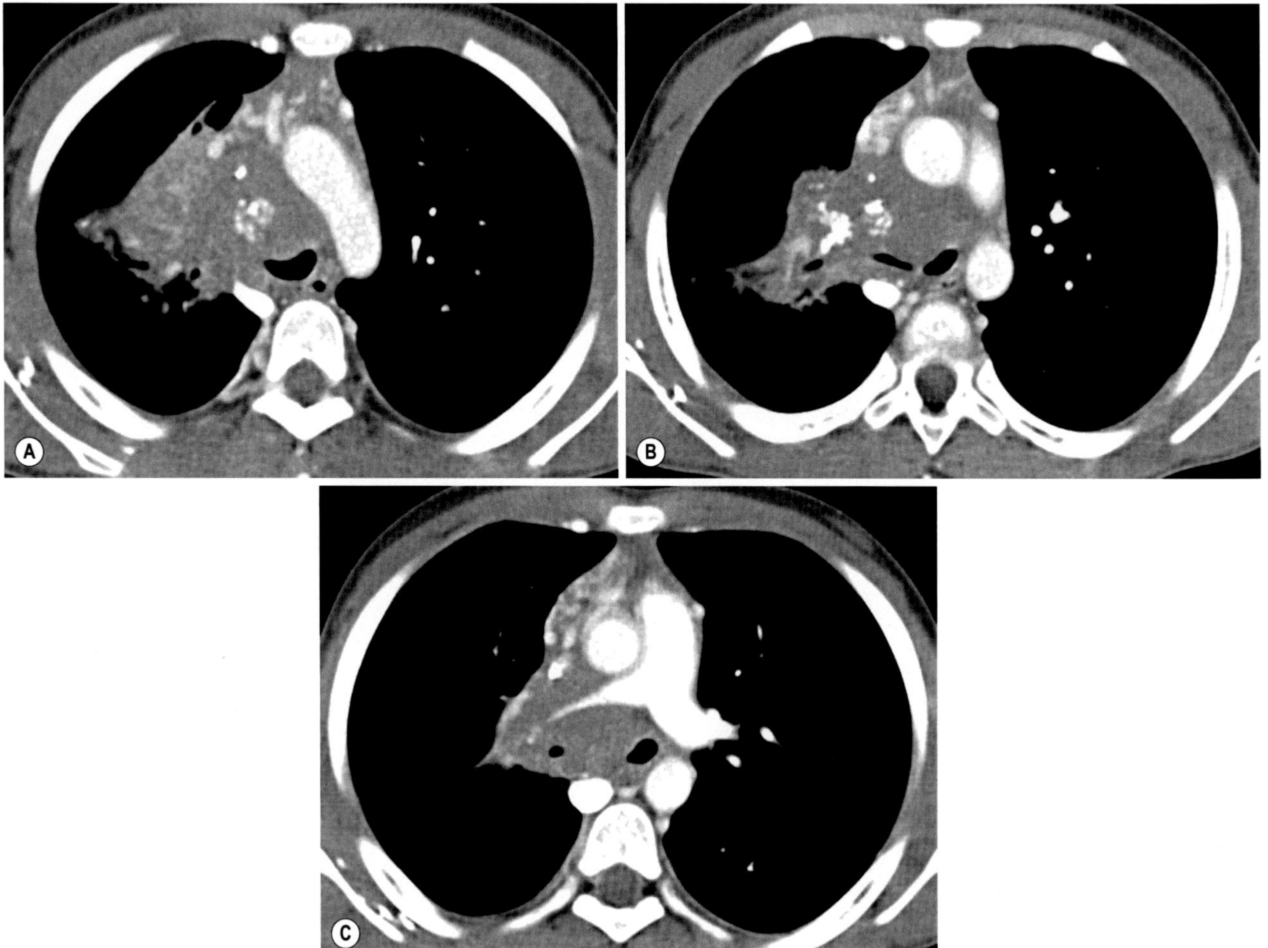

FIGURE 4-26 ■ **Fibrosing mediastinitis.** Contrast medium-enhanced CT shows a partially calcified mediastinal and hilar mass consistent with fibrosing mediastinitis secondary to histoplasmosis in a child with chronic cough and facial swelling. The mass causes stenosis of the superior vena cava (A), right upper lobe and mainstem bronchi (A, B) and right pulmonary artery (C). There are numerous mediastinal venous collaterals in the anterior mediastinum (A, B).

Mediastinal Haemorrhage

Mediastinal haemorrhage is most commonly caused by trauma to the arteries and veins within the mediastinum, with other causes including rupture of an aneurysm, aortic dissection and complications of central venous catheterisation.

Radiologically, haemorrhage produces an increase in the mediastinal diameter, which is maximal at the point of bleeding.[97] Blood may track through the mediastinum, frequently running over the apex of the left lung to produce a smooth and well-defined apical cap. When haemorrhage is severe, blood may rupture into the pleural cavity or dissect into lung along peribronchovascular sheaths, resulting in a radiographic pattern resembling interstitial oedema. On unenhanced CT, acute haemorrhage may appear of relative high attenuation. The appearance of mediastinal haematoma on MRI varies with the age of the haemorrhage.

Pneumomediastinum

Pneumomediastinum can be caused by intrathoracic and extrathoracic sources. Intrathoracic source of pneumomediastinum is seen in several clinical situations. In asthma, pneumomediastinum occurs from air trapping caused by mucus plugging or airway narrowing. Blunt trauma to the chest can cause pneumomediastinum secondary to rupture of the alveoli or a tear in the bronchus or trachea. Other situations include vomiting, weight lifting or straining against a closed glottis. Extrathoracic source can be dissection of air from the head and neck or the retroperitoneum. In many instances, however, a pneumomediastinum is the result of an air leak from a tear in a small intrapulmonary airway, the air dissecting through the lung via the hilum into the mediastinum. Asthma is the most common precipitating cause.

The presence of a pneumomediastinum is, in itself, of little significance (though it may be responsible for

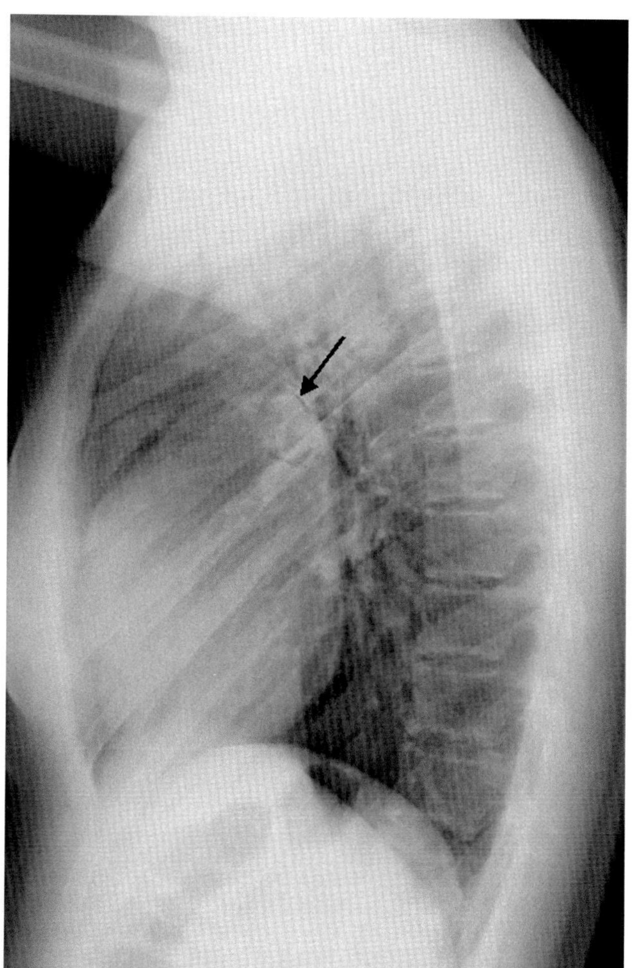

FIGURE 4-27 ■ Ring around the artery sign. A 13-year-old girl presented with chest pain and a burning sensation in the throat. Lateral projection of chest radiograph demonstrates a lucent line encircling the right pulmonary artery (black arrow), indicating that the mediastinal air is tracking into the right hilum.

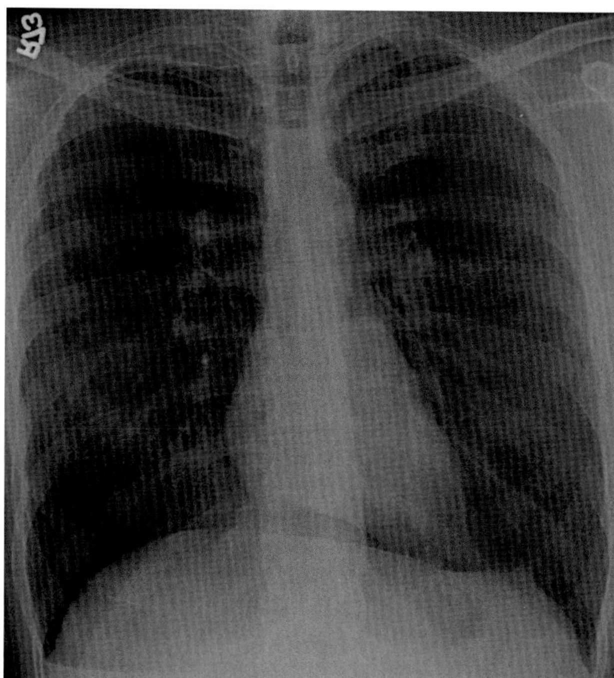

FIGURE 4-28 ■ Continuous diaphragm sign in pneumomediastinum. Frontal chest radiograph shows an uninterrupted outline of the diaphragm indicative of a pneumomediastinum.

substernal chest pain), but the condition causing the air leak (particularly bronchial, oesophageal, or pharyngeal perforation) may be of great significance to the patient.

The radiographic signs of pneumomediastinum depend on the anatomical structures outlined by the air. Air around the pulmonary artery (usually the right pulmonary artery) results in the 'ring around the artery sign'[98] (Fig. 4-27). Elevation of the thymus causes the 'sail sign'.[99] Air anterior to the pericardium is best seen on the lateral radiograph. The 'continuous diaphragm sign' is seen because of the air trapped posterior to the pericardium, giving the appearance of a continuous collection of air on the AP projection[100] (Fig. 4-28). Air from the mediastinum can extend laterally between the parietal pleura and the diaphragm to produce the 'extrapleural sign'.[101] Care must be taken not to confuse this sign for a pneumothorax. Usually the latter does not contain the webs and bands typical of pneumomediastinum. The 'tubular artery sign' occurs when there is air adjacent to the major branches of the aorta, the mediastinal air outlines the medial side and the aerated lung outlines the lateral side of the vessel. The 'double bronchial wall sign' is seen when the air adjacent to the bronchus allows clear depiction of the bronchial wall. Air can also dissect through the perivascular tissues and may track up into the neck, supraclavicular areas and axillae, as well as down into the retroperitoneum.

The differential diagnosis of a pneumomediastinum on chest radiograph includes a medially placed pneumothorax and a 'Mach effect' caused by the abrupt change in density between the lung and the adjacent heart and mediastinum. The Mach band effect is associated with convex surfaces, appearing as a region of lucency adjacent to structures with convex borders. The absence of an opaque line, which is typically seen in pneumomediastinum, can aid in differentiation. It is easy to appreciate why a medial pneumothorax can be mistaken for a pneumomediastinum, because in both instances there is a linear collection of air bounded on its lateral side by a thin line of pleura. Deciding whether the line is mediastinal parietal pleura or visceral pleura can be difficult; the distinction often depends on recognising the full extent of the air and looking carefully for a pneumothorax, or looking for evidence of air elsewhere in the mediastinum. Pneumomediastinum is easy to diagnose on CT as streaks or rounded collections of air surrounding vessels and other structures (Fig. 4-29).

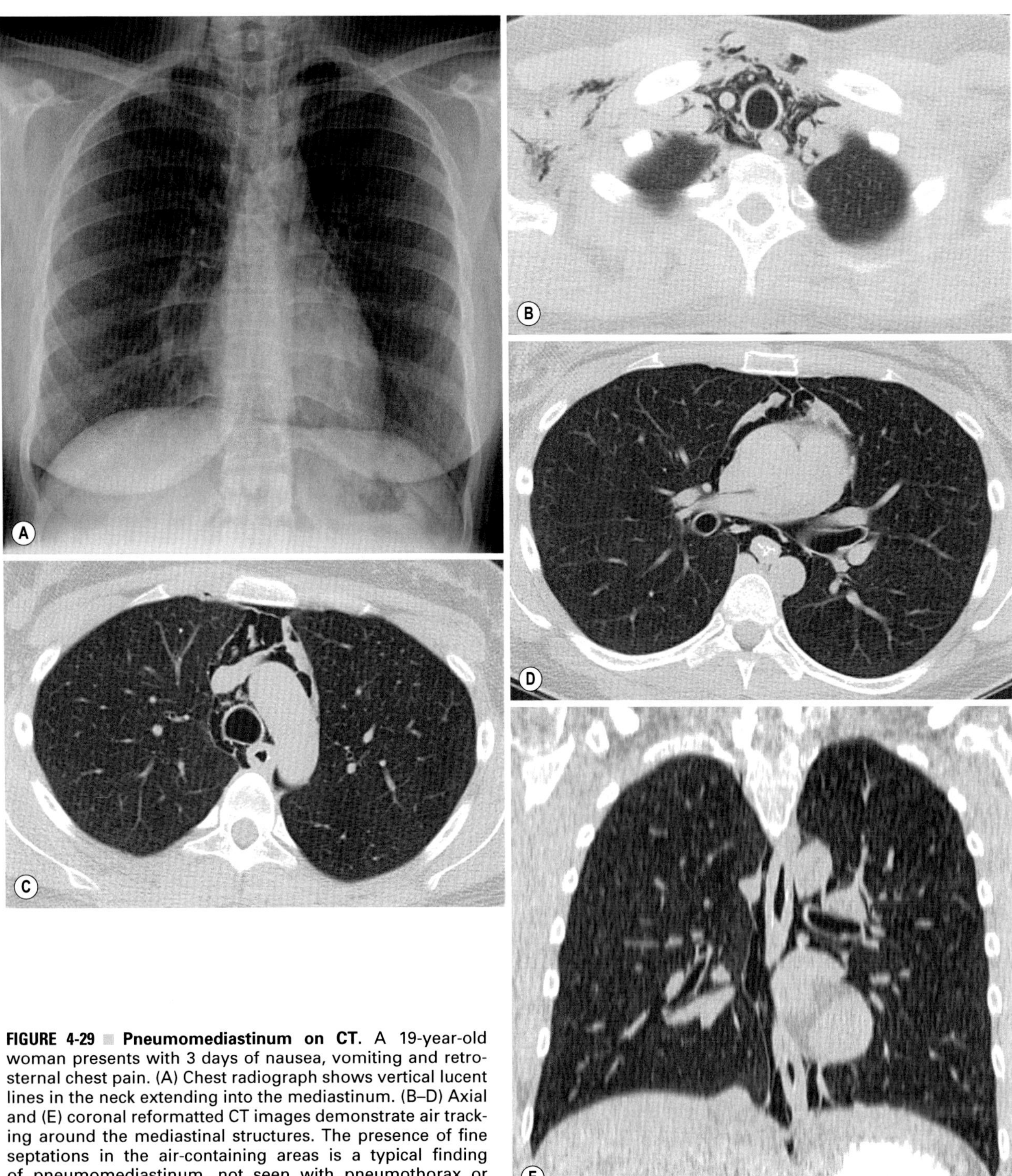

FIGURE 4-29 ■ **Pneumomediastinum on CT.** A 19-year-old woman presents with 3 days of nausea, vomiting and retrosternal chest pain. (A) Chest radiograph shows vertical lucent lines in the neck extending into the mediastinum. (B–D) Axial and (E) coronal reformatted CT images demonstrate air tracking around the mediastinal structures. The presence of fine septations in the air-containing areas is a typical finding of pneumomediastinum, not seen with pneumothorax or pneumopericardium.

PERICARDIUM

The pericardium is a compliant sac that consists of two layers, the parietal and visceral pericardium, separated by a small amount of fluid which is normally less than 50 mL.[102] The pericardium envelops the cardiac chambers and the origins of the great vessels. The left atrium is partially covered by the pericardium. The thickness of the normal pericardium as measured on CT and MR is less than 2 mm.[103,104] Pericardial sinuses may be seen on CT and MR containing small amounts of fluid in normal healthy individuals. The oblique pericardial sinus behind the left atrium may be misinterpreted (e.g. bronchogenic cyst).[105] The transverse pericardial sinus posterior to the ascending aorta may also be misinterpreted (aortic dissection, lymphadenopathy, etc.).[106,107] The superior pericardial recess lies posterior to the ascending aorta.

IMAGING PERICARDIAL DISEASE

Chest radiography is of limited use in the assessment of pericardial disease although pericardial effusions, calcification and secondary signs and complications of pericardial disease may be evident. Interval enlargement of the cardiac silhouette should raise the suspicion of pericardial effusion.

Transthoracic echocardiography (TTE) is usually the initial investigation of suspected pericardial disease. It is cheap and widely available and has high accuracy for detecting pericardial effusions and signs of tamponade. TTE is also helpful for guiding diagnostic or therapeutic pericardiocentesis. Restricted acoustic windows limit its evaluation of the entire pericardium; loculated collections, intrapericardial blood clot and pericardial thickening may be difficult to assess. It is not very accurate for depicting pericardial thickening, because echogenicity of the pericardium is similar to adjacent tissues. Transoesophageal echocardiography is limited by a narrow field of view. CT and MR have distinct advantages over echocardiography: larger field of view, higher contrast media resolution, excellent anatomical delineation and multiplanar reformats. MDCT with multiplanar reformats, particularly if ECG gated, provides excellent motion-free assessment of the pericardium; advantages include speed and wide availability and accessibility. CT can also detect pericardial calcifications which may be indicative of constrictive pericarditis. Disadvantages of CT include ionising radiation and the need for intravenous iodinated contrast agent. MRI can provide a comprehensive assessment of the pericardium. When T1- and T2-weighted sequences (some with ECG-gated breath-hold techniques) are combined with cine-based functional cardiac imaging, both pericardial disease and its impact on cardiac function can be assessed. MRI has some advantages over ultrasound and CT in detecting and characterising pericardial collections and masses. Limitations of MRI include its inability to reliably depict calcification and relatively long data acquisition times, especially with regard to breath-holding. Arrhythmias, which commonly occur in association with pericardial disease, may affect image acquisition and quality; nevertheless, CT or MR should be used when findings on echocardiography are difficult to interpret or non-diagnostic.

DEVELOPMENTAL ANOMALIES

Congenital Absence of the Pericardium

Compromise of the vascular supply to the pleuropericardial membrane during embryological development is associated with congenital defects in the pericardium. Pericardial defects are rare and usually asymptomatic. The defects vary in size from small communications between the pleural and pericardial cavities to complete (bilateral) absence of the pericardium. The most common form is complete absence of the left pericardium, with preservation of the pericardium on the right. Bilateral and isolated right-sided lesions are very rare. Absence of the pericardium is rarely associated with congenital anomalies of the heart and lungs, including atrial septal defect, tetralogy of Fallot, patent ductus arteriosus, bronchogenic cysts and pulmonary sequestration.[108] Pericardial defects are frequently associated with large defects in the parietal pleura, through which the left lung can herniate and surround the intrapericardial vascular structures.[78,79]

Complete absence of the pericardium is usually asymptomatic, whereas partial or localised absence of the pericardium may be complicated by herniation and entrapment of a cardiac chamber; in particular, the left atrial appendage in left-sided defects.

Chest radiograph findings are frequently subtle and non-specific.[109,110] In complete absence of the left pericardium they include displacement of the heart into the left chest and interposition of lung between the aorta and pulmonary artery (as well as between the left hemidiaphragm and cardiac silhouette). Both the medial and lateral borders of the main pulmonary artery may be visualised more clearly, caused by absence of the anterior pericardial reflection between the aorta and the pulmonary artery. Because of leftward displacement and rotation, the right cardiac border may not be seen. In partial pericardial defects, varying degrees of prominence of the pulmonary artery and/or left atrial appendage may be seen, while the heart retains its normal position in the thorax.[109] CT and MRI can depict herniation of cardiac structure through the defect. Discontinuation of the pericardial line can occasionally be detected in the partial form. The most reliable signs of complete absence of the left pericardium are interposition of lung between the aorta and main pulmonary artery, in the aortopulmonary window, and a rotation of the cardiac axis to the left side (rather like a right anterior oblique view).

Pericardial Cysts and Diverticula

Pericardial cysts are formed when a portion of the pericardium is pinched off during early development and are thought to be the result of persistence of blind-ending ventral parietal pericardial recesses. Those cysts that communicate with the pericardial space are termed pericardial diverticula. With increase or decrease in pericardial fluid, diverticula can change in size. They almost invariably appear as a well-defined, oval or occasionally lobulated mass attached to the pericardium.[111] More occur in the right cardiophrenic angle (approximately 70%) than on the left (approx. 20%); some are seen higher in the mediastinum. They contain clear fluid and can be recognised as fluid-filled cysts surrounded by normal pericardium on echocardiography, CT or MRI[104]

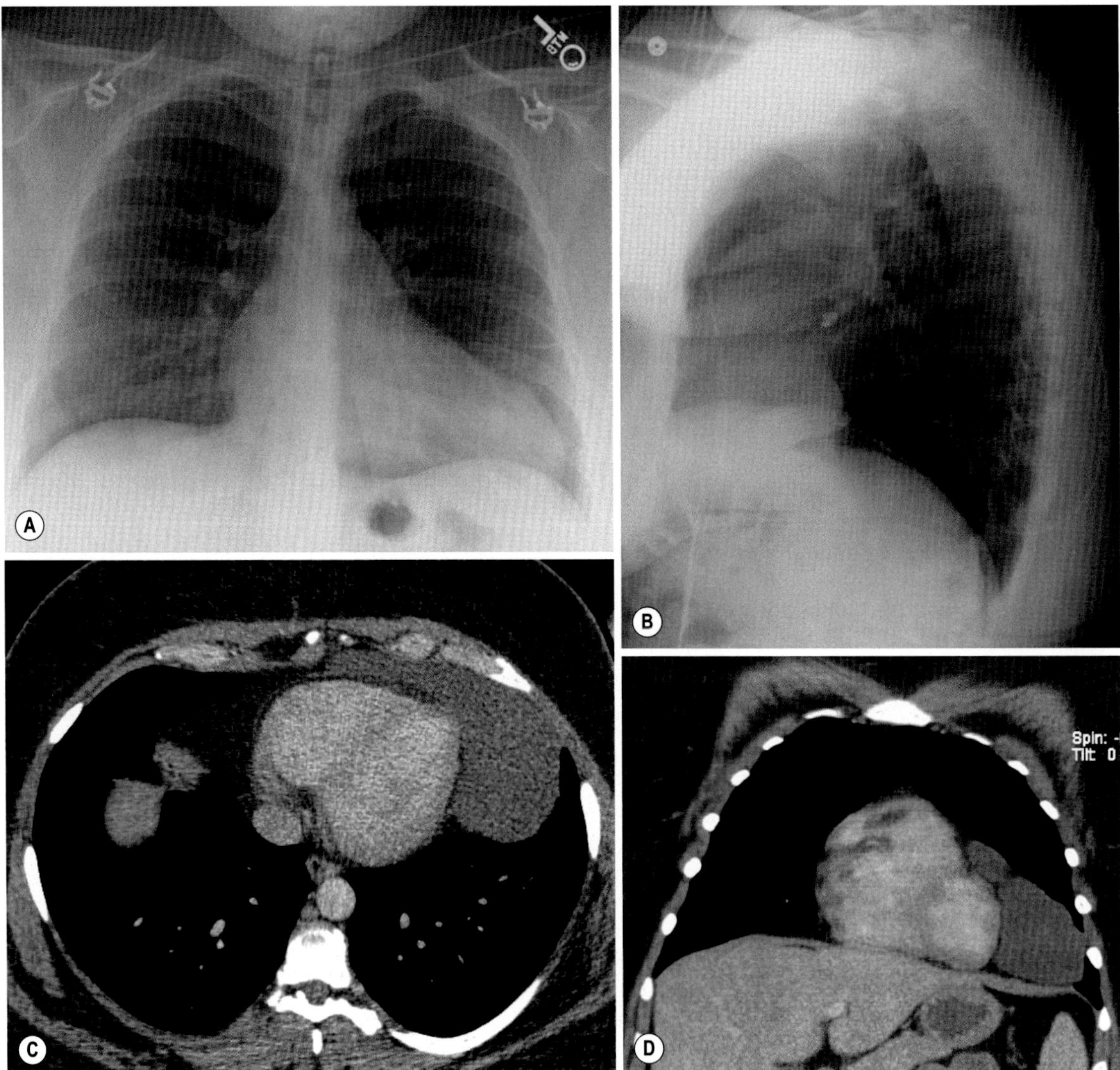

FIGURE 4-30 ■ **Pericardial cyst.** (A, B) Frontal and lateral chest radiographs of a 33-year-old woman show an abnormal mass-like contour of the left ventricle. (C) Axial and (D) coronal contrast medium-enhanced CT images demonstrate a mass of fluid attenuation without internal enhancement and no perceptible wall, located anterior and to the left of the heart.

(Fig. 4-30). On MRI, they have low-to-intermediate T1 signal intensity and homogeneous high T2 signal intensity. They do not enhance following intravenous gadolinium administration.

ACQUIRED PERICARDIAL DISEASE

Pericardial Effusion

Pericardial effusions are transudative or exudative accumulations of fluid in the pericardial space. Common causes of pericardial effusion include heart failure, renal insufficiency, infection (bacterial, viral or tuberculous), neoplasm (carcinoma of lung, breast or lymphoma) and injury (trauma and myocardial infarction). Transudative pericardial effusions may develop after cardiac surgery or in congestive heart failure, radiation, uraemia, post-pericardiectomy syndrome, myxoedema and collagen–vascular diseases. Haemopericardium may be caused by trauma, aortic dissection, aortic rupture or neoplasm. Interval enlargement of the cardiac silhouette on a radiograph over a short period of time should raise the suspicion of pericardial effusion. Filling in of the retrosternal space, effacement of the normal cardiac borders, development of a 'flask' or 'water bottle' cardiac configuration and bilateral hilar overlay are features of pericardial effusion. The epicardial fat pad sign may be seen on the lateral projection that demonstrates an anterior pericardial stripe (bordered by epicardial fat posteriorly and mediastinal fat anteriorly) thicker than 2 mm. This sign represents pericardial thickening or fluid[112,113] (Fig. 4-31). TTE is highly sensitive and specific for evaluating pericardial disease, although visualisation may be limited

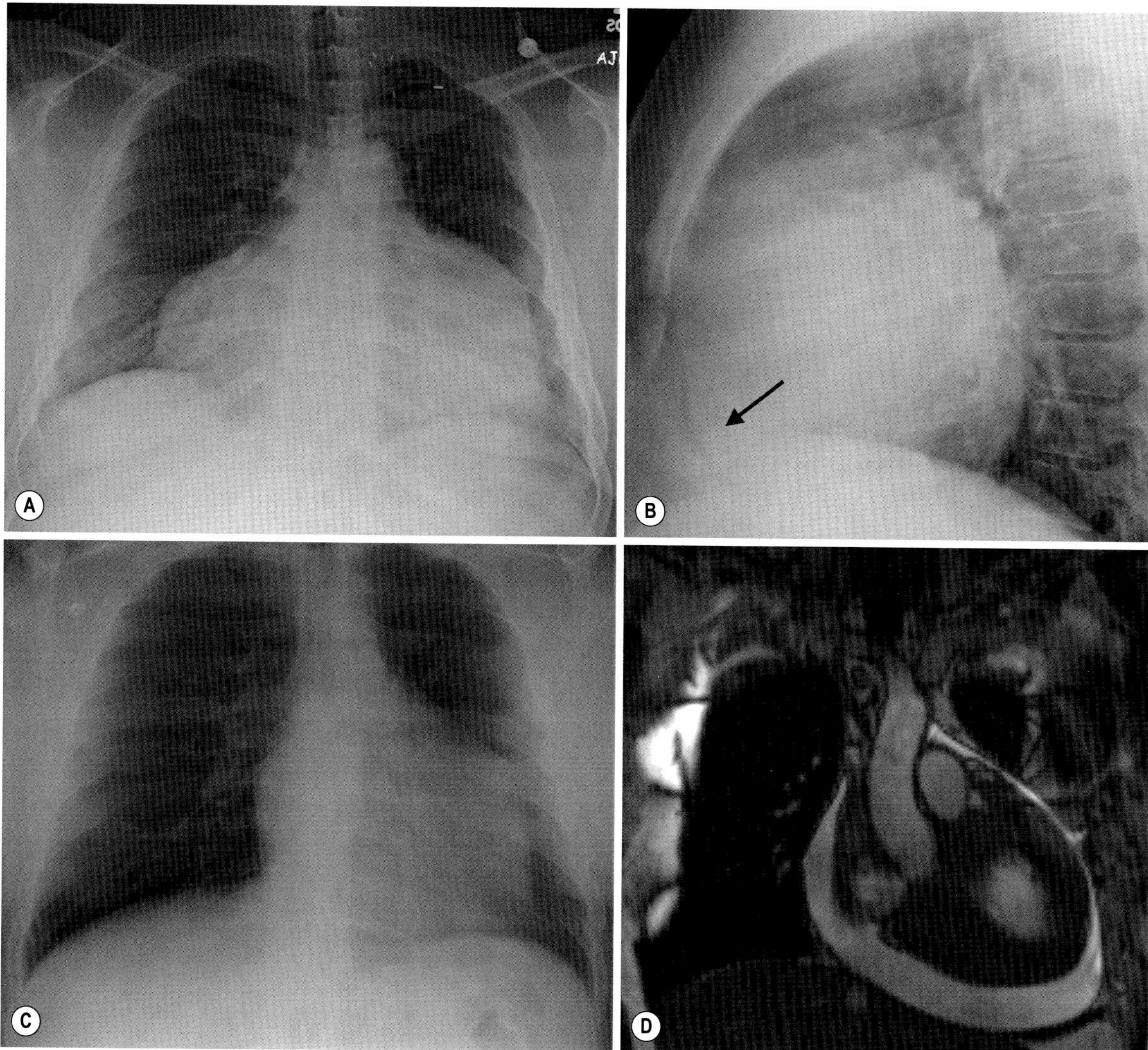

FIGURE 4-31 ■ **Pericardial effusion.** A 27-year-old man with chronic kidney disease presented with dyspnoea. Chest radiographs (A, B) of an enlarged cardiac silhouette since prior examination 6 months ago (C). The 'sandwich sign' (arrow) represents the pericardial effusion (B). (D) Steady-state free precession coronal MR image demonstrates uniformly hyperintense fluid in the pericardial sac, confirming the pericardial effusion.

in some obese or emphysematous patients; loculated collections and intrapericardial clot in postoperative patients may be difficult to detect.[114] CT and MR are indicated when TTE is inconclusive or when loculated or haemorrhagic effusion or pericardial thickening is suspected.[103,115] Increased attenuation in a pericardial effusion on CT suggests haemorrhage[116] (Fig. 4-32). When pericardial effusion is seen in patients with malignancy, the pericardium should be carefully evaluated for nodular (possibly metastatic) thickening of the pericardium. MRI is useful to differentiate small pericardial effusion from pericardial thickening. On spin-echo MRI, the signal characteristics of pericardial collections vary, depending on the composition of the fluid. In the absence of haemorrhage, effusions are typically of predominantly low T1 signal intensity, although intermediate signal intensity may be seen in inflammatory conditions such as uraemia, tuberculosis or trauma, possibly reflecting high protein content and when more focal, the presence of adhesions limiting normal flow of pericardial fluid in the pericardial space. In haemorrhagic effusions, signal intensity varies, depending on the age of blood products.

Cardiac Tamponade

Gradual accumulation of pericardial fluid may fail to produce clinical signs or symptoms for an extended period of time. However, *rapid* accumulation of as little as 100–200 mL of fluid can cause a haemodynamically significant compression of the heart, which severely impedes diastolic filling, resulting in pericardial tamponade. Despite the fact that the left ventricular contractility

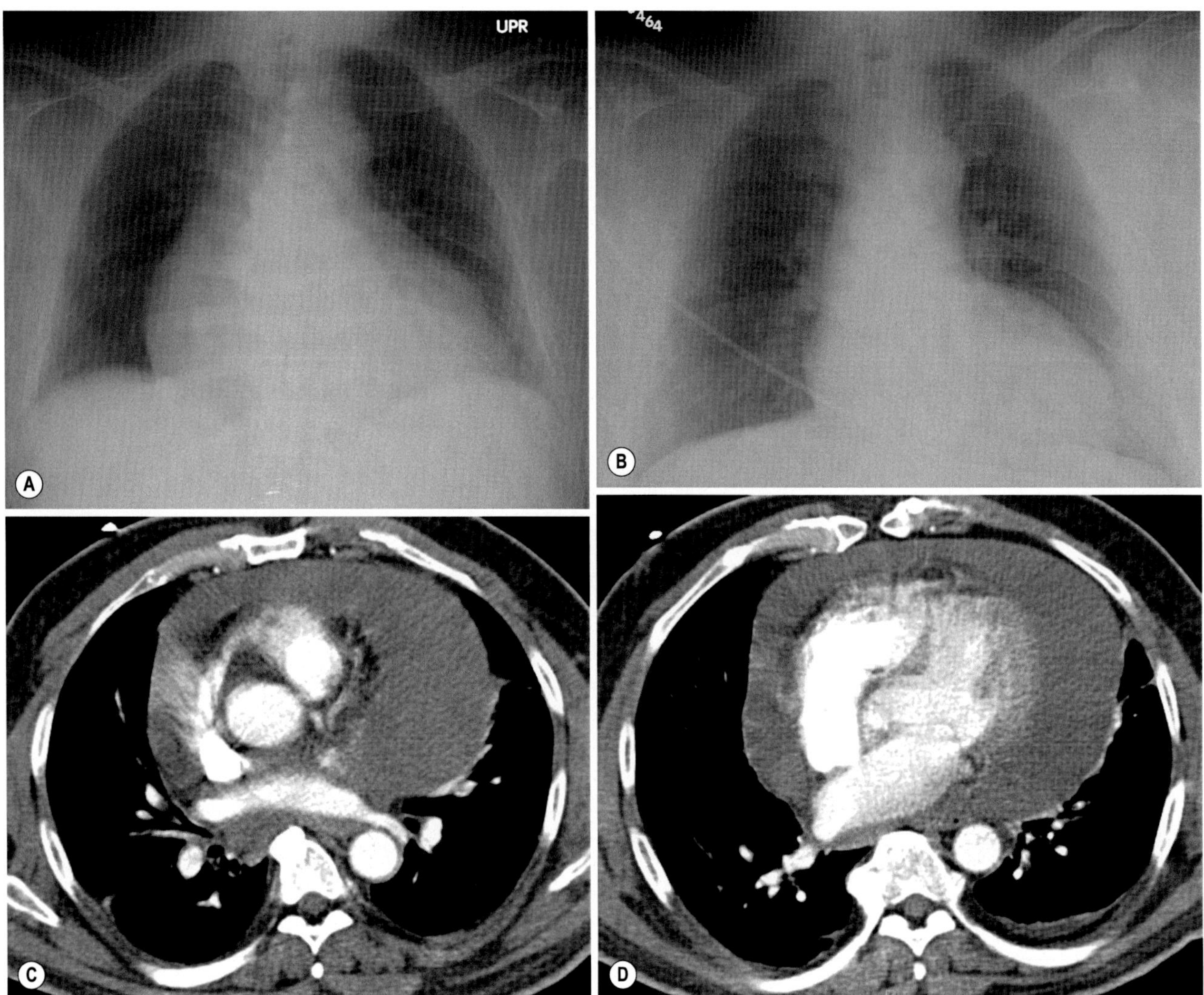

FIGURE 4-32 ■ **Pericardial haemorrhage.** A 63-year-old with diaphoresis and tachypnoea. Chest radiograph (A) shows enlargement of the cardiac silhouette since a previous radiograph obtained 10 months ago (B). Contrast medium-enhanced axial CT images (C, D) demonstrate a large high-attenuation fluid collection in the pericardium representing haemorrhage. The patient's symptoms suggest that there is tamponade physiology.

is normal, the stroke volume is decreased because of the diminished end diastolic volume, resulting in decreased cardiac output.

Because acute tamponade may occur with small effusions, clinically important pericardial enlargement may be difficult to detect on CXR. Subtle changes in cardiac contour may only be detectable by comparison with previous studies. If there is decreased pulmonary vascularity despite the cardiac enlargement or if the SVC and azygos veins are dilated, tamponade may be suspected.

Echocardiographic demonstration of pericardial effusion and the clinical findings are usually sufficient to make the diagnosis of tamponade. CT and MRI are frequently useful for determining the cause of the effusion, such as haemorrhage, neoplastic involvement, inflammation caused by tuberculosis, or other infectious processes.

Pericarditis

Inflammation of the pericardium (pericarditis) may occur in response to a variety of insults. Viral infection is the most common cause of pericarditis in the United States, the most common agents being Coxsackie group B and echoviruses. Pericarditis typically results in cellular proliferation, or the production of fluid (pericardial effusion) or fibrin, either alone or in combination. Thickening of the pericardium occurs because of fibrinous exudates and oedema. Causes include myocardial infarction (acute or post-myocardial infarction referred to as Dressler's syndrome), pericardiotomy, mediastinal irradiation, infection (viral or bacterial), connective tissue disease (rheumatoid arthritis, systemic lupus erythematosus), metabolic disorders (uraemia, hypothyroidism), neoplasia and AIDS.

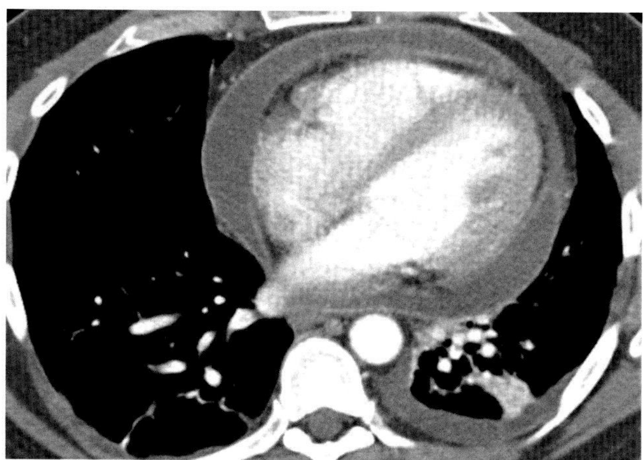

FIGURE 4-33 ■ **Pericarditis.** A 30-year-old man with new-onset of left-sided chest pain. Axial contrast medium-enhanced CT shows diffuse pericardial thickening and a moderate-sized pericardial effusion. This was caused by viral pericarditis.

The most common imaging manifestation of acute pericarditis is a pericardial effusion, the nature of the fluid varying with the underlying cause. Thickened inflamed pericardium can appear as moderate-to-high signal intensity on spin-echo MRI, and pericardial enhancement may be seen on either MRI or CT performed after intravenous contrast medium administration. Delayed images on contrast medium-enhanced CT are useful for demonstrating pericardial enhancement (Fig. 4-33).

Constrictive Pericarditis

Constrictive pericarditis presents with symptoms of heart failure such as dyspnoea, orthopnoea and fatigue. The most common causes of constrictive pericarditis are cardiac surgery and radiation therapy.[117] Other causes include infection (viral, tuberculous), connective tissue disease, uraemia, neoplasm or idiopathic.[118] The aetiology is unknown in many cases, presumed to be secondary to an occult viral pericarditis and other causes of pericarditis.[118] Outside the USA, the most common cause is probably infectious. Any insult to the pericardium can progress from an acute pericarditis with pericardial effusion to a subacute stage of resorption of the effusion with organisation, and then to a chronic phase of fibrous scarring, pericardial thickening and obliteration of the pericardial cavity. Constrictive pericarditis is the condition in which a thickened, fibrotic and often calcified pericardium restricts diastolic filling of the heart. Constriction caused by neoplastic infiltration of the pericardium is most commonly secondary to carcinoma of the lung or breast, lymphoproliferative malignancies and melanoma. Pericardial constriction after mediastinal irradiation, usually performed to treat breast carcinoma or Hodgkin's disease, may occur months to years after treatment.[117] Pericardial thickening is seen in up to 88% of confirmed cases of constrictive pericarditis.[119] In the majority of cases, constrictive pericarditis involves the entire pericardium, restricting filling of all cardiac chambers. Occasionally, in particular, anterior to the right ventricle in postoperative patients, the pericardial thickening is more localised. Constrictive pericarditis and restrictive cardiomyopathy are both characterised by restriction in diastolic filling which leads to increases in diastolic pressure in all four chambers and equalisation of pressures. The clinical manifestations and findings on cardiac catheterisation and echocardiography are similar in both conditions. It is important to differentiate between these two conditions because the management approach will differ. Patients with pericardial constriction may benefit from pericardial stripping, while restrictive cardiomyopathy is managed medically or by cardiac transplantation. Diagnosing constriction often proves challenging and usually requires more than one investigation before surgery. The hallmarks of pericardial constriction are pericardial thickening, calcification and abnormal diastolic ventricular function. Although echocardiography is routinely performed and provides an excellent assessment of haemodynamic function, it is not highly accurate at depicting pericardial thickening.[120] CT and MRI are significantly more sensitive, with CT having the advantage over MRI of being able to demonstrate the presence of calcification, which is associated with pericardial constriction. Pericardial calcification can be seen in the atrioventricular groove (Fig. 4-34). Pericardial thickening of greater than 4 mm, when accompanied by clinical features of constriction, is highly suggestive of constrictive pericarditis.[119] Both CT and MRI may show the secondary effects of constriction on the central cardiovascular structures. The right ventricle tends to have a conical configuration and reduced volume. A sigmoid-shaped interventricular septum or prominent leftward convexity of the septum may be seen. The right atrium, superior and in particular inferior venae cavae and hepatic veins may be dilated. Hepatomegaly and ascites may be seen. Cardiac MRI can also be used to provide a more detailed assessment of cardiac function. Diastolic septal bounce can be seen on cardiac MR. A free-breathing sequence on cardiac MR in which a patient performs a 'sniff' while the images are acquired, which demonstrates an exaggerated septal bounce (often referred to as ventricular interdependence), is helpful in leading to the diagnosis.

Pericardial Neoplasms

Pericardial metastases are as much as 20–40 times more common than primary pericardial neoplasms. They are identified at autopsy in approximately 10% of all patients with malignancy.[121] The most common malignancies encountered are lung (Fig. 4-35), lymphoma, breast, melanoma and colon.[88]

Primary pericardial neoplasms are rare, with approximately equal incidence of benign versus malignant pericardial neoplasms. Benign tumours include teratomas, fibromas, neurofibromas, lipomas, haemangiomas and lymphangiomas. Although these patients are usually symptom free, pericardial effusion or constriction, particularly in the case of childhood teratomas, may occur.

Malignant mesothelioma is the most common primary pericardial malignancy (Fig. 4-36) and is almost

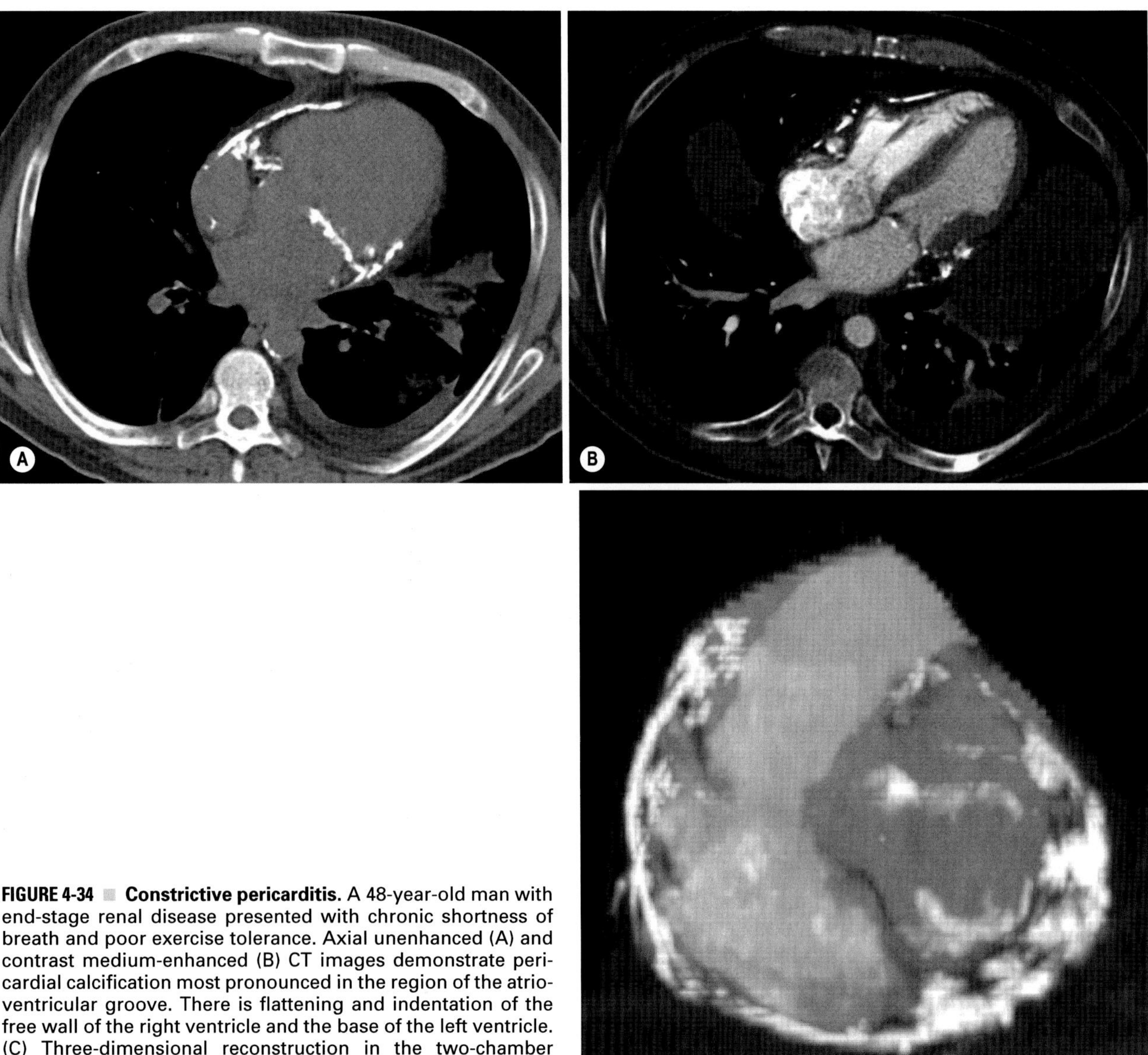

FIGURE 4-34 ■ **Constrictive pericarditis.** A 48-year-old man with end-stage renal disease presented with chronic shortness of breath and poor exercise tolerance. Axial unenhanced (A) and contrast medium-enhanced (B) CT images demonstrate pericardial calcification most pronounced in the region of the atrioventricular groove. There is flattening and indentation of the free wall of the right ventricle and the base of the left ventricle. (C) Three-dimensional reconstruction in the two-chamber short-axis plane of the heart shows the belt-like calcification surrounding the heart.

certainly related to asbestos exposure. Mesothelioma may present as a well-defined single mass, multiple nodules or diffuse plaques involving the visceral and parietal pericardium and wrapping around the cardiac chambers and great vessels. Clinically, it presents with haemorrhagic effusion and tamponade, congestive heart failure, arrhythmia and occasionally pericardial constriction. Other malignant primary tumours include lymphoma, sarcoma, paraganglioma and liposarcoma. Teratomas of the pericardium may also be malignant and are most commonly seen in children.

A pericardial effusion is the most common finding in pericardial malignancy, whether primary pericardial or metastatic. Intrapericardial neoplasms tend to *compress* and *deform* normal intrapericardial structures, whereas extrapericardial masses tend to *displace* the intrapericardial structures without compression or distortion.

Chest radiographs are often abnormal, but are nonspecific. Alteration of fat-pad contours, cardiac enlargement, mediastinal widening, hilar adenopathy or a hilar mass may be seen.

Echocardiography is usually the initial technique for evaluating a suspected pericardial neoplasm, with MRI and CT being useful for further evaluation. Both MRI and CT are excellent at providing information regarding the size, location and extent of pericardial neoplasms, but are not tissue specific. Fatty tumours (lipomas, fat-containing teratomas) are the exception, because of their typically low attenuation on CT and increased signal intensity on spin-echo T1-weighted MRI. Fatty tumours must be differentiated from the focal deposits of subepicardial fat and non-neoplastic lesions that can simulate fatty tumours, such as mesenteric fat in a hiatal hernia. Metastatic melanoma may have high signal intensity on

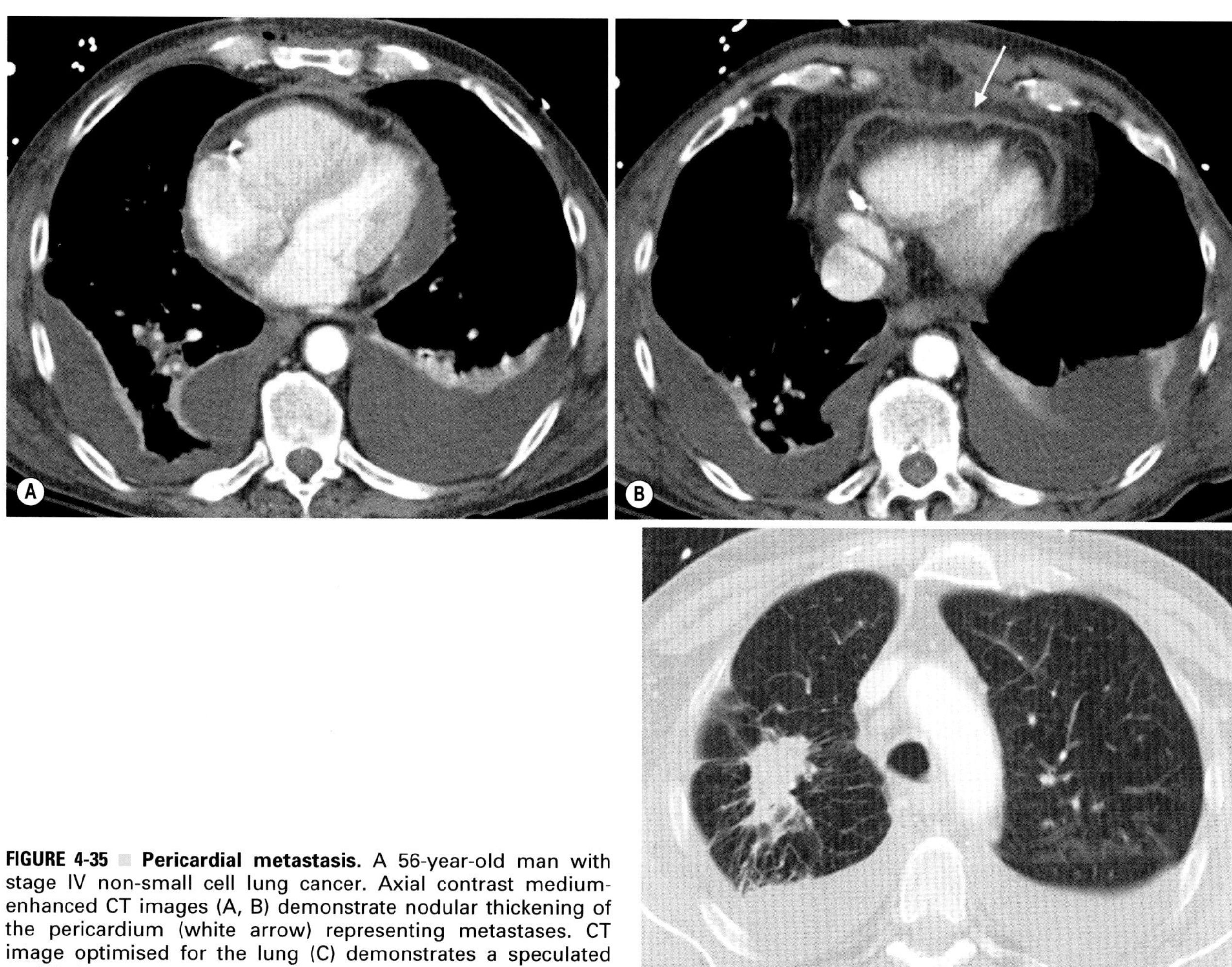

FIGURE 4-35 ■ **Pericardial metastasis.** A 56-year-old man with stage IV non-small cell lung cancer. Axial contrast medium-enhanced CT images (A, B) demonstrate nodular thickening of the pericardium (white arrow) representing metastases. CT image optimised for the lung (C) demonstrates a speculated nodule in the right upper lobe consistent with known non-small cell lung cancer.

FIGURE 4-36 ■ **Mesothelioma.** Contrast medium-enhanced CT images demonstrate confluent left pleural thickening extending into the oblique fissure caused by mesothelioma (A). Nodular pericardial thickening indicates pericardial involvement (B).

T1- and T2-weighted images,[122] a feature that may be useful in differentiating it from other metastatic neoplasms, which are frequently of low signal intensity on T1- and high signal intensity on T2-weighted images.[123] In addition to discrete masses and effusions, metastatic involvement of the pericardium may cause focal or diffuse pericardial thickening, which may be irregular and usually enhances. Primary lipoma, liposarcoma and lymphoma of the pericardium typically appear as large heterogeneous masses frequently associated with a serosanguineous pericardial effusion.

Acknowledgement

The authors acknowledge the contribution of Sharyn L. S. MacDonald to this chapter in the previous edition of the book.

REFERENCES

1. Benjamin SP, McCormack LJ, Effler DB, Groves LK. Primary tumours of the mediastinum. Chest 1972;62:297–303.
2. Wychulis AR, Payne WS, Clagett OT, Woolner LB. Surgical treatment of mediastinal tumours: a 40 year experience. J Thorac Cardiovasc Surg 1971;62:379–91.
3. Cohen AJ, Thompson LN, Edwards FH, et al. Primary cysts and tumours of the mediastinum. Ann Thorac Surg 1991;51:378–86.
4. Zylak CJ, Pallie W, Jackson R. Correlative anatomy and computed tomography: a module on the mediastinum. Radiographics 1982;2(4):555–92.
5. Friedberg JW, Chengazi V. PET scans in the staging of lymphoma: current status. Oncologist 2003;8:438–47.
6. Verboom P, van Tinteren H, Hoekstra OS, et al. Cost-effectiveness of FDG-PET in staging non-small cell lung cancer: the PLUS study. Eur J Nucl Med Mol Imaging 2003;30:1444–9.
7. Riccardo Marano MD, Carlo Liguori MD, Giancarlo Savino MD, et al. Cardiac silhouette findings and mediastinal lines and stripes radiograph and CT scan correlation. Chest 2011;139: 1186–96.
8. Whitten CR, Khan S, Munneke GJ, Grubnic S. A diagnostic approach to mediastinal abnormalities. Radiographics 2007;27: 657–71.
9. Mack E. Management of patients with substernal goiters. Surg Clin North Am 1995;75:377–94.
10. Buckley JA, Stark P. Intrathoracic mediastinal thyroid goiter. Am J Roentgenol 1999;173:471–5.
11. Glazer GM, Axel L, Moss A. CT diagnosis of mediastinal thyroid. Am J Roentgenol 1982;138:495–8.
12. Bashist B, Ellis K, Gold RP. Computed tomography of intrathoracic goiter. Am J Roentgenol 1983;140:455–60.
13. Lee VS, Spritzer CE, Coleman RE, et al. The complementary roles of fast spin-echo MR imaging and double-phase ^{99m}Tc-sestamibi scintigraphy for localization of hyperfunctioning parathyroid glands. Am J Roentgenol 1996;167:1555–62.
14. Lee VS, Spritzer CE. MR imaging of abnormal parathyroid glands. Am J Roentgenol 1998;170:1097–103.
15. Baron RL, Lee JK, Sagel SS, Peterson RR. Computed tomography of the normal thymus. Radiology 1982;142:121–5.
16. Baron RL, Sagel SS, Baglan RJ. Thymic cysts following radiation therapy for Hodgkin disease. Radiology 1981;141:593–7.
17. Hoffman OA, Gillespie DJ, Aughenbaugh GL, Brown LR. Primary mediastinal neoplasms (other than thymoma). Mayo Clin Proc 1993;68:880–91.
18. Souadjian JV, Enriquez P, Silverstein MN, Pepin JM. The spectrum of diseases associated with thymoma. Coincidence or syndrome? Arch Intern Med 1974;134:374–9.
19. Strollo DC, Rosado-de-Christenson ML. Tumors of the thymus. J Thorac Imaging 1999;14:152–71.
20. Brown LR, Muhm JR, Sheedy PF, et al. The value of computed tomography in myasthenia gravis. Am J Roentgenol 1983;140: 31–5.
21. Ellis K, Austin JH, Jaretzki A III. Radiologic detection of thymoma in patients with myasthenia gravis. Am J Roentgenol 1988;151: 873–81.
22. Chen JL, Weisbrod GL, Herman SJ. Computed tomography and pathologic correlations of thymic lesions. J Thorac Imaging 1988;3:61–5.
23. Rosado-de-Christenson ML, Galobardes J, Moran CA. Thymoma: radiologic–pathologic correlation. Radiographics 1992;12:151–68.
24. De Geer G, Webb WR, Gamsu G. Normal thymus: associated with MR and CT. Radiology 1986;158:313–17.
25. Boothroyd AE, Hall-Graggs MA, Dicks-Mireaux C, Shaw DG. The magnetic resonance appearances of the normal thymus in children. Clin Radiol 1992;45:378–81.
26. Sakai F, Sone S, Kiyono K, et al. MR imaging of thymoma: radiological-pathologic correlation. Am J Roentgenol 1991;158: 751–6.
27. Fujimoto K, Nishihara H, Abe T, et al. MR imaging of thymoma—comparison with CT, operative, and pathological findings. Nippon Igaku Hoshasen Gakkai Zasshi 1992;25:1128–38.
28. Takahashi K, Al-Janabi NJ. Computed tomography and magnetic resonance imaging of mediastinal tumors. J Magn Reson Imaging 2010;32:1325–39.
29. Lee JD, Choe KO, Kim SJ, et al. CT findings in primary thymic carcinoma. J Comput Assist Tomogr 1991;15:429–33.
30. Do YS, Im JG, Lee BH, et al. CT findings in malignant tumors of thymic epithelium. J Comput Assist Tomogr 1995;19:192–7.
31. Kushihashi T, Fujisawa H, Munechika H. Magnetic resonance imaging of thymic epithelial tumours. Crit Rev Diagn Imaging 1996;37:191–259.
32. Chaer R, Massad MG, Evans A, et al. Primary neuroendocrine tumors of the thymus. Ann Thorac Surg 2002;74:1733–40.
33. Rosado-de-Christenson ML, Pugatch RD, Moran CA, Galobardes J. Thymolipoma: analysis of 27 cases. Radiology 1994; 193:121–6.
34. Chew FS, Weissleder R. Mediastinal thymolipoma. Am J Roentgenol 1991;157:468.
35. Shirkhoda A, Chasen MH, Eftekhari F, et al. MR imaging of mediastinal thymolipoma. J Comput Assist Tomogr 1987;11: 364–5.
36. Choyke PL, Zeman RK, Gootenberg JE, et al. Thymic atrophy and regrowth in response to chemotherapy: CT evaluation. Am J Roentgenol 1987;149:269–72.
37. Kissin CM, Husband JE, Nicholas D, Eversman W. Benign thymic enlargement in adults after chemotherapy: CT demonstration. Radiology 1987;163:67–70.
38. Cohen M, Hill CA, Cangir A, Sullivan MP. Thymic rebound after treatment of childhood tumors. Am J Roentgenol 1980;135: 151–6.
39. Inaoka T, Takahashi K, Iwata K, et al. Evaluation of normal fatty replacement of the thymus with chemical-shift MR imaging for identification of the normal thymus. J Magn Reson Imaging 2005;22:341–6.
40. Inaoka T, Takahashi K, Mineta M, et al. Thymic hyperplasia and thymus gland tumors: differentiation with chemical shift MR imaging. Radiology 2007;243:869–76.
41. Moran CA, Suster S. Primary germ cell tumors of the mediastinum: I. Analysis of 322 cases with special emphasis on teratomatous lesions and a proposal for histopathologic classification and clinical staging. Cancer 1997;80:681–90.
42. Moeller KH, Rosado-de-Christenson ML, Templeton PA. Mediastinal mature teratoma: imaging features. Am J Roentgenol 1997;169:985–90.
43. Strollo DC, Rosado de Christenson ML, Jett JR. Primary mediastinal tumors. Part 1: tumours of the anterior mediastinum. Chest 1997;112:511–22.
44. Fulcher AS, Proto AV, Jolles H. Cystic teratoma of the mediastinum: demonstration of fat/fluid level. Am J Roentgenol 1990;154: 259–60.
45. Knapp RH, Hurt RD, Payne WS, et al. Malignant germ cell tumors of the mediastinum. J Thorac Cardiovasc Surg 1985;89: 82–9.
46. Shimosato Y, Mukai K. Tumors of the thymus and related lesions. In: Rosai J, editor. Tumors of the Mediastinum. 3rd ed. Washington, DC: Armed Forces Institute of Pathology; 1997. p. 33.

47. Lee K, Im J, Han M, et al. Malignant primary germ cell tumors of the mediastinum: CT features. Am J Roentgenol 1989;153: 947–51.
48. Rosado-de-Christenson ML, Templeton PA, Moran CA. From the archives of the AFIP. Mediastinal germ cell tumors: radiologic and pathologic correlation. Radiographics 1992;12:1013–30.
49. Radin DR, Baker EL, Klatt EC, et al. Visceral and nodal calcification in patients with AIDS-related *Pneumocystis carinii* infection. Am J Roentgenol 1990;154:27–31.
50. Pombo F, Rodriguez E, Mato J, et al. Patterns of contrast enhancement of tuberculous lymph nodes demonstrated by computed tomography. Clin Radiol 1992;46:13–17.
51. Landay MJ, Rollins NK. Mediastinal histoplasmosis granuloma: evaluation with CT. Radiology 1989;172:657–9.
52. Yousem DM, Scatarige JC, Fishman EK, Siegelman SS. Low-attenuation thoracic metastases in testicular malignancy. Am J Roentgenol 1986;146:291–3.
53. Hopper KD, Diehl LF, Cole BA, et al. The significance of necrotic mediastinal lymph nodes on CT in patients with newly diagnosed Hodgkin disease. Am J Roentgenol 1990;155:267–70.
54. Samuels T, Hamilton P, Shaw P. Whipple disease of the mediastinum. Am J Roentgenol 1990;154:1187–8.
55. McAdams HP, Rosado-de-Christenson M, Fishback NF, Templeton PA. Castleman disease of the thorax: radiologic features with clinical and histopathologic correlation. Radiology 1998;209: 221–8.
56. Yamashita Y, Hirai T, Matsukawa T, et al. Radiological presentations of Castleman's disease. Comput Med Imaging Graph 1993;17:107–17.
57. Suwatanapongched T, Gierada DS. CT of thoracic lymph nodes. Part II: diseases and pitfalls. Br J Radiol 2006;79:999–1006.
58. Jasmer RM, Gotway MB, Creasman JM, et al. Clinical and radiographic predictors of the etiology of computed tomography-diagnosed intrathoracic lymphadenopathy in HIV-infected patients. J Acquir Immune Defic Syndr 2002;31:291–8.
59. Haramati LB, Choi Y, Widrow CA, Austin JHM. Isolated lymphadenopathy on chest radiographs of HIV-infected patients. Clin Radiol 1996;51:345–9.
60. Zylak CJ, Eyler WR, Spizarny DL, Stone CH. Developmental lung anomalies in the adult: radiologic–pathologic correlation. Radiographics 2002;22:S25–43.
61. Strollo DC, Rosado-de-Christenson ML, Jett JR. Primary mediastinal tumors: part II. Tumours of the middle and posterior mediastinum. Chest 1997;112:1344–57.
62. Berrocal T, Madrid C, Novo S, et al. Congenital anomalies of the tracheobronchial tree, lung, and mediastinum: embryology, radiology, and pathology. Radiographics 2004;24:e17.
63. Nakata H, Nakayama C, Kimoto T, et al. Computed tomography of mediastinal bronchogenic cysts. J Comput Assist Tomogr 1982;6:733–8.
64. Mendelson DS, Rose JS, Efremidis SC, et al. Bronchogenic cysts with high CT numbers. Am J Roentgenol 1983;140:463–5.
65. Jeung M-Y, Gasser B, Gangi A, et al. Imaging of cystic masses of the mediastinum. Radiographics 2002;22:S79–93.
66. Erasmus JJ, McAdams HP, Donnelly LF, Spritzer CE. MR imaging of mediastinal masses. Magn Reson Imaging Clin North Am 2000;8:59–89.
67. Reed JC, Hallet KK, Feigin DS. Neural tumors of the thorax: subject review from the AFIP. Radiology 1978;126:9–17.
68. Bhargava R, Parham DM, Lasater OE, et al. MR imaging differentiation of benign and malignant peripheral nerve sheath tumors: use of the target sign. Pediatr Radiol 1997;27:124–9.
69. Aughenbaugh GL. Thoracic manifestations of neurocutaneous diseases. Radiol Clin North Am 1984;22:741–56.
70. Adam A, Hochholzer L. Ganglioneuroblastoma of the posterior mediastinum: a clinicopathologic review of 80 cases. Cancer 1981;47:373–81.
71. Bar-Ziv J, Nogrady MB. Mediastinal neuroblastoma and ganglioneuroma. The differentiation between primary and secondary involvement on the chest roentgenogram. Am J Roentgenol Radium Ther Nucl Med 1975;125:380–90.
72. Olson JL, Salyer WR. Mediastinal paragangliomas (aortic body tumor): a report of four cases and a review of the literature. Cancer 1978;41:2405–12.
73. Spizarny DL, Rebner M, Gross BH. CT evaluation of enhancing mediastinal masses. J Comput Assist Tomogr 1987;11:990–3.
74. van Gils AP, Falke TH, van Erkel AR, et al. MR imaging and MIBG scintigraphy of pheochromocytomas and extraadrenal functioning paragangliomas. Radiographics 1991;11:37–57.
75. Krenning EP, Kwekkeboom DJ, Bakker WH, et al. Somatostatin receptor scintigraphy with [^{111}In-DTPA-D-Phe1]- and [^{123}I-Tyr3]-octreotide: the Rotterdam experience with more than 1000 patients. Eur J Nucl Med 1993;20:716–31.
76. Miles J, Pennybacker J, Sheldon P. Intrathoracic meningocele. Its development and association with neurofibromatosis. J Neurol Neurosurg Psychiatry 1969;32:99–110.
77. Long JA Jr, Doppman JL, Nienhuis AW. Computed tomographic studies of thoracic extramedullary hematopoiesis. J Comput Assist Tomogr 1980;4:67–70.
78. Faul JL, Berry GJ, Colby TV, et al. Thoracic lymphangiomas, lymphangiectasis, lymphangiomatosis, and lymphatic dysplasia syndrome. Am J Respir Crit Care Med 2000;161:1037–46.
79. Miyake H, Shiga M, Takaki H, et al. Mediastinal lymphangiomas in adults: CT findings. J Thorac Imaging 1996;11:83–5.
80. Tecce PM, Fishman EK, Kuhlman JE. CT evaluation of the anterior mediastinum: spectrum of disease. Radiographics 1994;14: 973–90.
81. Shaffer K, Rosado-de-Christenson ML, Patz EF Jr, et al. Thoracic lymphangioma in adults: CT and MR imaging features. Am J Roentgenol 1994;162:283–9.
82. Brown LR, Reiman HM, Rosenow EC III, et al. Intrathoracic lymphangioma. Mayo Clin Proc 1986;61:882–92.
83. Glazer HS, Wick MR, Anderson DJ, et al. CT of fatty thoracic masses. Am J Roentgenol 1992;159:1181–7.
84. Whyte AM, Powell N. Mediastinal lipoblastoma of infancy. Clin Radiol 1990;42:205–6.
85. Gaerte SC, Meyer CA, Winer-Muram HT, et al. Fat-containing lesions of the chest. Radiographics 2002;22:615–78.
86. Kline ME, Patel BU, Agosti SJ. Noninfiltrating angiolipoma of the mediastinum. Radiology 1990;175:737–8.
87. Kim K, Koo BC, Davis JT, Franco-Saenz R. Primary myelolipoma of mediastinum. J Comput Tomogr 1984;8:119–23.
88. Pasricha PJ, Fleischer DE. Endoscopic perforations of the upper digestive tract: a review of their pathogenesis, prevention and management. Gastroenterology 1994;106:787–802.
89. Jolles H, Henry DA, Roberson JP, et al. Mediastinitis following median sternotomy: CT findings. Radiology 1996;201:463–6.
90. Bitkover CY, Cederlund K, Aberg B, Vaage J. Computed tomography of the sternum and mediastinum after median sternotomy. Ann Thorac Surg 1999;68:858–63.
91. Carter AR, Sostman HD, Curtis AM, Swett HA. Thoracic alterations after cardiac surgery. Am J Roentgenol 1983;140: 475–81.
92. Goodwin RA, Nickell JA, Des Prez RM. Mediastinal fibrosis complicating healed primary histoplasmosis and tuberculosis. Medicine Balt 1972;51:227–46.
93. Sherrick AD, Brown LR, Harms GF, Myers JL. The radiographic findings of fibrosing mediastinitis. Chest 1994;106:484–9.
94. Rossi SE, McAdams HP, Rosado-de-Christenson ML, et al. Fibrosing mediastinitis. Radiographics 2001;21:737–57.
95. Rodriguez E, Soler R, Pombo F, et al. Fibrosing mediastinitis: CT and MR findings. Clin Radiol 1998;53:907–10.
96. Rholl KS, Levitt RG, Glazer HS. Magnetic resonance imaging of fibrosing mediastinitis. Am J Roentgenol 1985;145:255–9.
97. Woodring JH, Loh FK, Kryscio RJ. Mediastinal hemorrhage: an evaluation of radiographic manifestations. Radiology 1984;151: 15–21.
98. Hammond DI. The 'ring-around-the-artery' sign in pneumomediastinum. J Can Assoc Radiol 1984;35:88–9.
99. Moseley JE. Loculated pneumomediastinum in the newborn: a thymic 'spinnaker sail' sign. Radiology 1960;75:788–90.
100. Levin B. The continuous diaphragm sign: a newly recognized sign of pneumomediastinum. Clin Radiol 1973;24:337–8.
101. Lillard RL, Allen RP. The extrapleural air sign in pneumomediastinum. Radiology 1965;85:1093–8.
102. Edwards ED. Applied anatomy of the heart. In: Giuliani ER, Fuster V, editors. Cardiology: Fundamentals and Practice. 2nd ed. St Louis, MO: Mosby–Year Book; 1991. pp. 47–51.
103. Bull RK, Edwards PD, Dixon AK. CT dimensions of the normal pericardium. Br J Radiol 1998;71:923–5.
104. Sechtem U, Tscholakoff D, Higgins CB. MRI of the abnormal pericardium. Am J Roentgenol 1986;147:245–52.

105. Levy-Ravetch M, Auh YH, Rubenstein WA, et al. CT of the pericardial recesses. Am J Roentgenol 1985;144:707–14.
106. Batra P, Bigoni B, Manning J, et al. Pitfalls in the diagnosis of thoracic aortic dissection at CT angiography. Radiographics 2000;20:309–20.
107. Groell R, Schaffler GJ, Rienmueller R. Pericardial sinuses and recesses: findings at electrocardiographically triggered electron-beam CT. Radiology 1999;212:69–73.
108. Spodick DH. Pericardial disease. In: Braunwald E, editor. Heart Disease: A Textbook of Cardiovascular Medicine. Philadelphia: WB Saunders; 2001. pp. 1823–76.
109. Nasser WK, Helmen C, Tavel ME, et al. Congenital absence of the left pericardium. Clinical, electrocardiographic, radiographic, hemodynamic, and angiographic findings in six cases. Circulation 1970;41:469–78.
110. Van Son JA, Danielson GK, Schaff HV, et al. Congenital partial and complete absence of the pericardium. Mayo Clin Proc 1993;68:743–7.
111. Feigin DS, Fenoglio JJ, McAllister HA, Madewell JE. Pericardial cysts. A radiologic–pathologic correlation and review. Radiology 1977;125:15–20.
112. Lane EJ Jr, Carsky EW. Epicardial fat: lateral plain film analysis in normals and in pericardial effusion. Radiology 1968;91:1–5.
113. Carsky EW, Mauceri RA, Azimi F. The epicardial fat pad sign: analysis of frontal and lateral chest radiographs in patients with pericardial effusion. Radiology 1980;137:303–8.
114. Yousem D, Traill TT, Wheeler PS, Fishman EK. Illustrative cases in pericardial effusion misdetection: correlation of echocardiography and CT. Cardiovasc Intervent Radiol 1987;10:162–7.
115. White CS. MR evaluation of the pericardium. Top Magn Reson Imaging 1995;7:258–66.
116. Tomoda H, Hoshiai M, Furuya H, et al. Evaluation of pericardial effusion with computed tomography. Am Heart J 1980;99:701–6.
117. Ling LH, Oh JK, Schaff HV, et al. Constrictive pericarditis in the modern era: evolving clinical spectrum and impact on outcome after pericardiectomy. Circulation 1999;100:1380–6.
118. Cameron J, Oesterle SN, Baldwin JC, Hancock EW. The etiologic spectrum of constrictive pericarditis. Am Heart J 1987;113:354–60.
119. Masui T, Finck S, Higgins CB. Constrictive pericarditis and restrictive cardiomyopathy: evaluation with MR imaging. Radiology 1992;182:369–73.
120. Engel PJ. Echocardiographic findings in pericardial disease. In: Fowler NO, editor. The Pericardium in Health and Disease. Armonk, NY: Futura; 1985. pp. 99–151.
121. Abraham KP, Reddy V, Gattuso P. Neoplasms metastatic to the heart: review of 3314 consecutive autopsies. Am J Cardiovasc Pathol 1990;3:195–8.
122. Mousseaux E, Meunier P, Azancott S, et al. Cardiac metastatic melanoma investigated by magnetic resonance imaging. Magn Reson Imaging 1998;16:91–5.
123. Fujita N, Caputo GR, Higgins CB. Diagnosis and characterization of intracardiac masses by magnetic resonance imaging. Am J Card Imaging 1994;8:69–80.

CHAPTER 5

Pulmonary Infection in Adults

Tomás Franquet

CHAPTER OUTLINE

Respiratory infections are the commonest illnesses occurring in humans, and pneumonia is the leading cause of death related to infectious disease and the sixth most common cause of death in the United States.[1] Pneumonia is an acute infection of the pulmonary parenchyma that is associated with at least some symptoms of acute infection, accompanied by the presence of an acute infiltrate on a chest radiograph.[2]

TYPES OF PNEUMONIAS

Currently accepted clinical classification of pneumonia differentiates community-acquired pneumonia (CAP), hospital-acquired pneumonia (HAP), ventilator-associated pneumonia (VAP), and health care–associated pneumonia (HCAP).[3]

Community-Acquired Pneumonia (CAP)

The diagnosis of CAP is based on the presence of a number of selected clinical features (e.g., cough, fever, sputum production and pleuritic chest pain) and is supported by imaging of the lung, usually by chest radiography.[4]

The spectrum of causative organisms of CAP includes Gram-positive bacteria such as *Streptoccocus pneumoniae* (pneumoccocus), *Haemophilus influenzae* and *Staphylococcus aureus*, as well as atypical organisms such as *Mycoplasma pneumoniae*, *Chlamydia pneumoniae* or *Legionella pneumophila* and viral agents such as influenza A virus and respiratory syncytial viruses. Pulmonary opacities are usually evident on the radiograph within 12 h of the onset of symptoms.[5]

Hospital-Acquired Pneumonia (HAP)

Hospital-acquired pneumonia (HAP) may be defined as one occurring after admission to the hospital that was neither present nor in a period of incubation at the time of admission. Hospital-acquired pneumonia (nosocomial) is the leading cause of death from hospital-acquired infections and occurs most commonly among intensive care unit (ICU) patients, predominately in individuals requiring mechanical ventilation.

Ventilator-Associated Pneumonia (VAP)

Microorganisms responsible for VAP may differ according to the population of patients in the ICU, the durations of hospital and ICU stays, and the specific diagnostic method(s) used. The spectrum of causative pathogens of VAP in humans includes *S. aureus*, *Pseudomonas aeruginosa* and Enterobacteriaceae.[6]

Health Care-Associated Pneumonia (HCAP)

When pneumonia is associated with health care risk factors such as prior hospitalisation, dialysis, residing in a nursing home, and immunocompromised state, it is now classified as a health care-associated pneumonia (HCAP). The number of individuals receiving health care outside the hospital setting, including home wound care or infusion therapy, dialysis, nursing homes and similar settings, is constantly increasing.

CLINICAL UTILITY AND LIMITATIONS OF CHEST RADIOGRAPHY AND CT

A clinical diagnosis of pneumonia is usually established on the basis of clinical symptoms, laboratory findings and chest radiography. Though different patterns of pneumonia are associated with certain underlying microorganisms, it has to be clearly stated that there is no specific radiological pattern of pneumonia caused by one particular microorganism. Overlap of imaging findings also with respect to course over time makes the differentiation of aetiologies based solely on the radiograph unreliable, and distinguishing pneumonia from conditions such as left heart failure and pulmonary embolism may sometimes be difficult,[1,7] especially as patients with pre-existing lung disease (severe emphysema, interstitial lung disease, etc.) who may develop very atypical patterns of pneumonia.

New emerging pathogens have been recognised such as community-acquired methicillin-resistant *S. aureus*, human metapneumovirus, avian influenza A viruses (H5N1), coronavirus associated with severe acute respiratory syndrome (SARS) and swine flu (H1N1).[8,9]

Chest radiography remains an important component of the evaluation of a patient with a suspicion of pneumonia, and usually is the first examination to be obtained.

CT, preferably with thin (<2 mm thick) slices, has been shown to be more sensitive than radiography in the detection of subtle abnormalities and may show findings suggestive of pneumonia up to 5 days earlier than chest radiographs.[10,11] CT is recommended in patients with clinical suspicion of infection and normal or non-specific radiographic findings (Fig. 5-1) and in patients with increased risk of pulmonary infection (e.g. neutropenia). CT is also indicated in patients with pneumonia and persistent or recurrent pulmonary opacities to diagnose or rule out underlying or alternative disease processes.

The presence of a radiographically visibile opacification is part of the definition of pneumonia, according to the American Thoracic Society (ATS),[12] though there might be a time delay of several hours between onset of clinical symptoms and radiographic changes, and specific conditions may further the delay or cause a negative chest radiograph.

Regression of pneumonia over time varies with the underlying organism, patient comorbidity and patient age and can take between 1 and 2 weeks or up to 2 months.

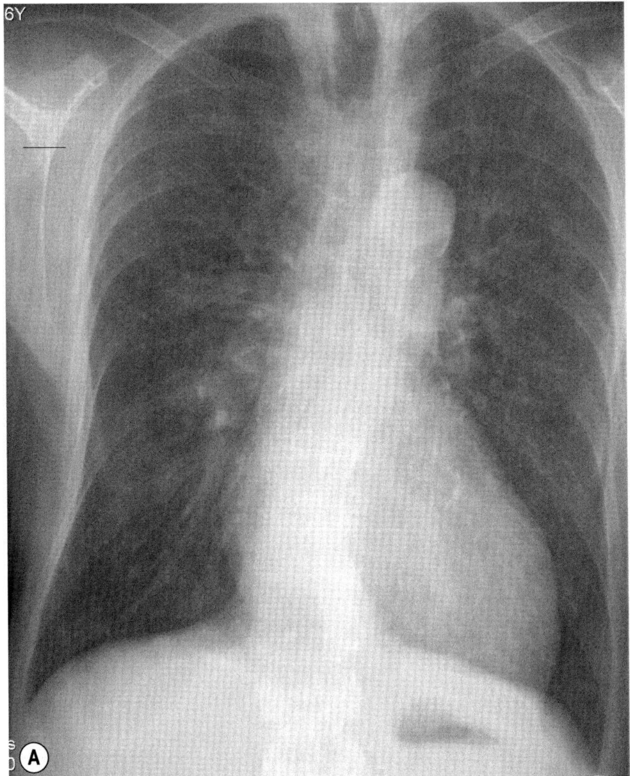

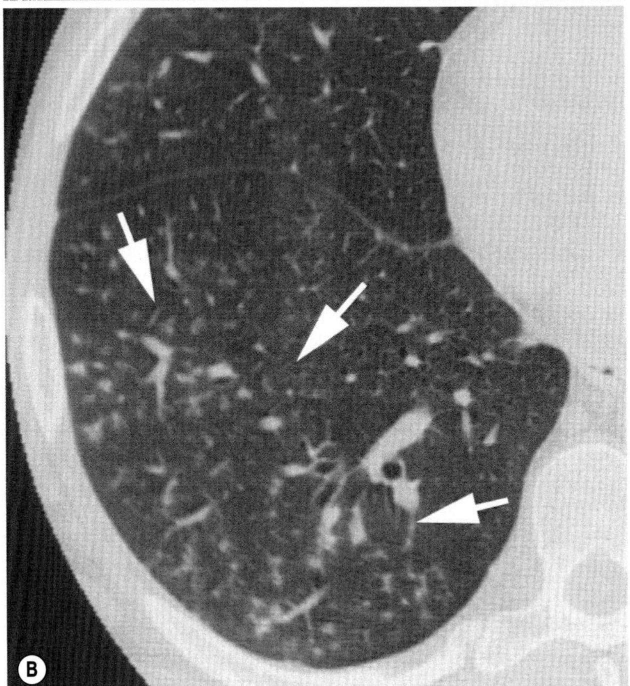

FIGURE 5-1 ■ **Cellular bronchiolitis.** A 71-year-old man with fever of 48 h duration. (A) Posteroanterior chest radiograph is normal. (B) Complementary CT shows centrilobular branching nodular and linear opacities resulting in a 'tree-in-bud' appearance (arrows). *Mycoplasma* bronchiolitis was diagnosed.

PATTERNS OF PULMONARY INFECTION

Pneumonias are usually divided, according to their chest imaging appearance, into lobar pneumonia, broncho- or lobular pneumonia and interstitial pneumonia.

In *lobar pneumonia* the inflammatory exudate begins in the distal air spaces adjacent to the visceral pleura, and then spreads via collateral air drift routes (pores of Kohn) to produce uniform homogeneous opacification of partial or complete segments of lung and occasionally an entire lobe. Occasionally, infection is manifested as a spherical focus of consolidation (Fig. 5-2). An air bronchogram is frequently seen. *S. pneumoniae* is by far the most common cause of complete lobar consolidation. Other causative agents that produce complete lobar consolidation include *Klebsiella pneumoniae* and other Gram-negative bacilli, *L. pneumophila*, *H. influenzae*, and occasionally *M. pneumoniae*.

Characteristic manifestations on CT are lobar or sublobar consolidations, sharply demarcated by the interlobar fissure.

Bronchopneumonia (lobular pneumonia) is characterised histologically by predominantly peribronchiolar inflammation. Although initially patchy, progression of disease results in lobular and segmental consolidation[13] (Fig. 5-3). An air bronchogram is usually absent. The most common causative organisms of bronchopneumonia are *S. aureus*, *H. influenzae*, *P. aeruginosa*, and anaerobic bacteria.

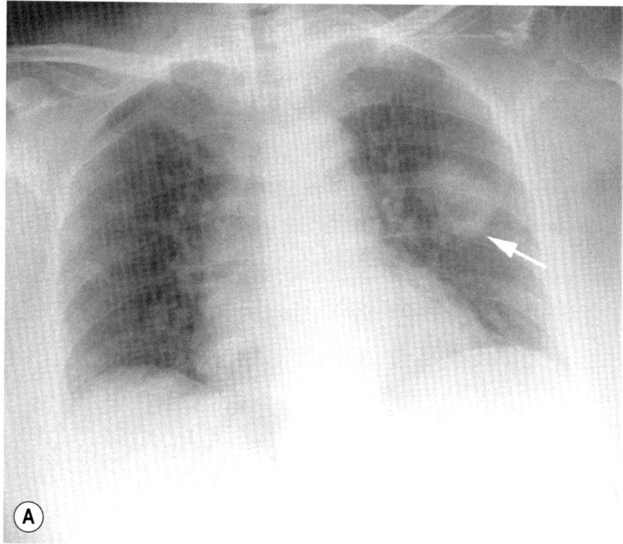
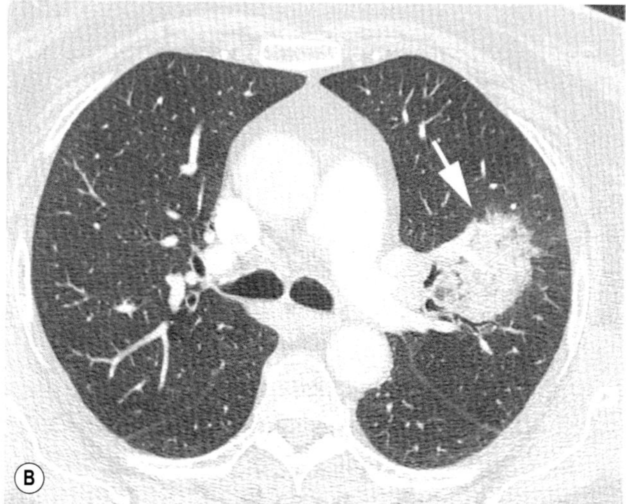

FIGURE 5-2 ■ **Round pneumonia.** A previously healthy 64-year-old man with fever and productive cough. (A) Chest radiograph shows a mass-like area of consolidation in the left upper lobe (arrow). (B) CT shows a discrete fairly well-marginated opacity in the left upper lobe containing small areas of low attenuation. The abnormality resolved following appropriate antibiotic therapy and Gram stains of sputum demonstrated *S. pneumoniae*.

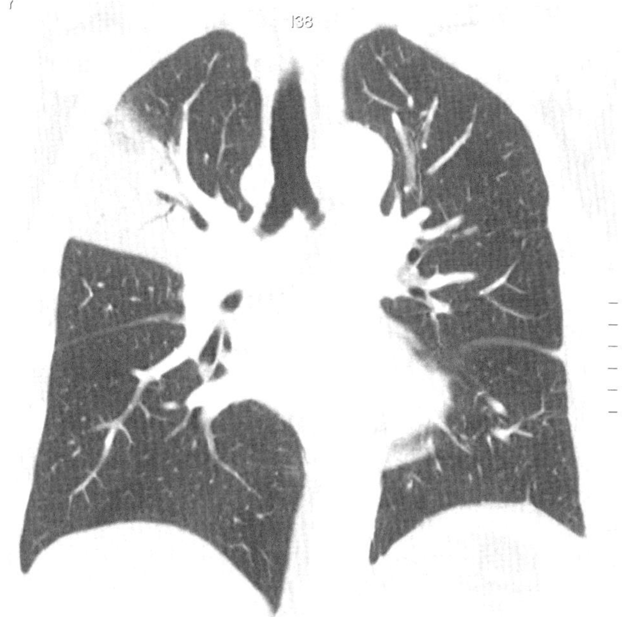

FIGURE 5-3 ■ **Lobar pneumonia.** A 36-year-old-man with *S. pneumoniae* pneumonia. Coronal reformatted CT image shows a homogeneous focal area of consolidation in the right upper lobe. Patent bronchi (air bronchograms) are seen within the area of consolidation.

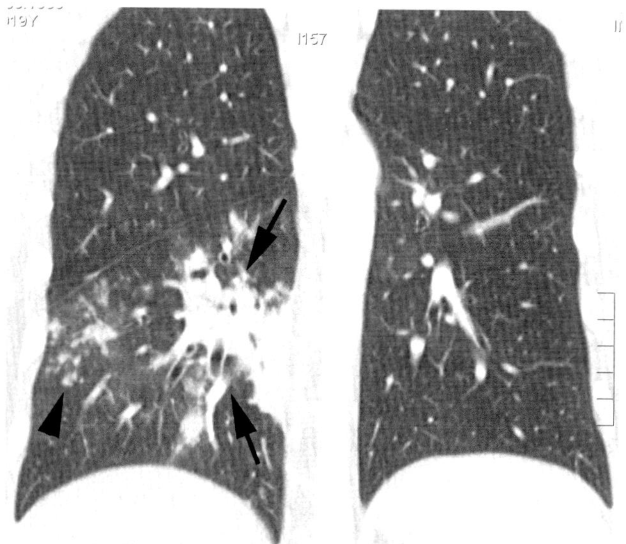

FIGURE 5-4 ■ **Bronchopneumonia caused by *H. influenzae*.** A 48-year-old man with productive cough and fever. Coronal reformatted CT shows a focal area of consolidation in the right lower lobe with visible air bronchogram and poorly defined margins (arrows). Also evident are small nodular opacities and a few 'tree-in-bud' opacities (arrowhead).

Characteristic manifestations of bronchopneumonia on CT include centrilobular ill-defined nodules and branching linear opacities, airspace nodules, and multifocal lobular areas of consolidation (Fig. 5-4).

The term **atypical pneumonia (interstitial pneumonia)** was initially applied to the clinical and radiographic appearance of lung infection not behaving or looking like that caused by *S. pneumoniae*. In the literature, the term 'atypical pneumonia' (as opposed to 'bacterial pneumonia') is still in wide usage, although technically incorrect. Many causative organisms are identified as bacteria, albeit unusual types (*Mycoplasma* is a type of bacteria without a cell wall and *Chlamydia* are intracellular parasites). It is therefore important to realise that the term 'atypical pneumonia'—if more correctly based on the underlying type of causative pathogen—does not only refer to an interstitial pattern (*Pneumocystis jiroveci* pneumonia, certain viral infections but also infections presenting with dense consolidation such as *Legionella*, *Mycoplasma*, *Chlamydia*, etc).

The usual causes of interstitial pneumonia are viral and mycoplasmal infections that radiographically present

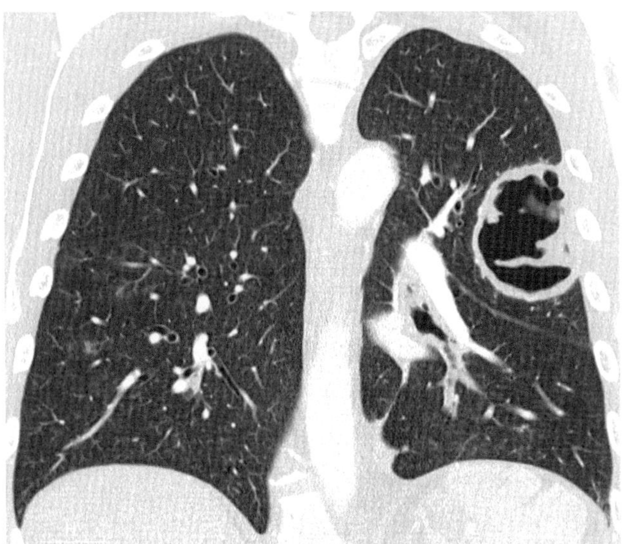

FIGURE 5-5 ■ **Lung abscess.** A 35-year-old man with high fever and large purulent sputum production with positive culture for *P. aeruginosa*. Coronal reformatted CT shows a large cavity in the left upper lobe. Note intracavitary thick septa.

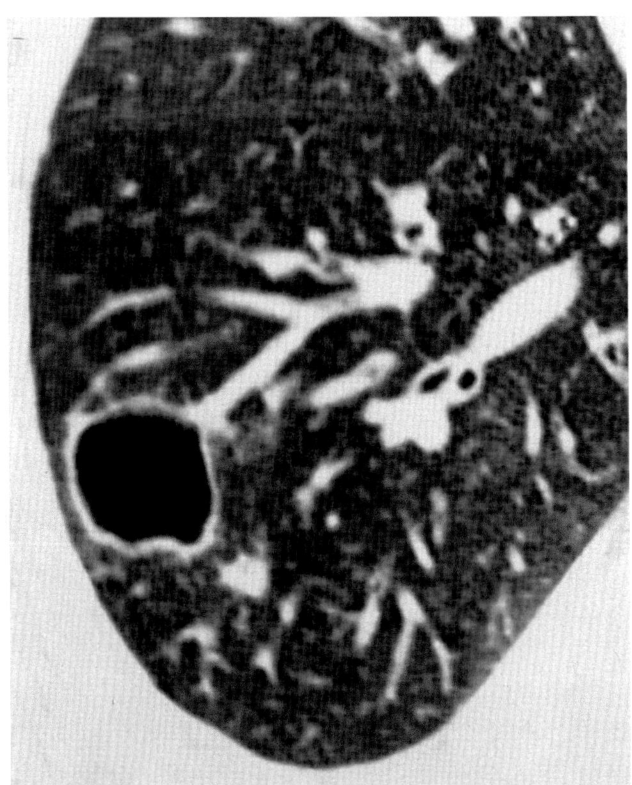

FIGURE 5-6 ■ **Pneumatocele.** A 32-year-old woman with previous *S. aureus* pneumonia. CT shows thin-walled cystic lesion (pneumatocele) in the right lower lobe.

with focal or diffuse small heterogeneous opacities uniformly distributed bilaterally in both lungs.

COMPLICATIONS OF PNEUMONIA

Lung abscess is defined as a localised necrotic cavity containing pus. The most common cause of lung abscess is aspiration.[14] They occur most commonly in the posterior segment of an upper lobe or the superior segment of a lower lobe[14] (Fig. 5-5). Common causes of lung abscess include anaerobic bacteria (most commonly *Fusobacterium nucleatum* and *Bacteroides* sp.), *S. aureus*, *P. aeruginosa* and *K. pneumoniae*.[14,15]

Pulmonary gangrene is an uncommon complication of pneumonia characterised by the development of fragments of necrotic lung within an abscess cavity (pulmonary sequestrum).[16]

Pneumatocele is a thin-walled, gas-filled space that usually develops in association with infection.[17] It presumably results from drainage of a focus of necrotic lung parenchyma followed by check-valve obstruction of the airway subtending it.[18] The complication is caused most often by *S. aureus* in infants (Fig. 5-6) and children and by *P. jiroveci* in patients who have acquired immune deficiency syndrome (AIDS) (Fig. 5-7).

Septic emboli to the lungs originate in a variety of sites, including cardiac valves (endocarditis), peripheral veins (thrombophlebitis) and venous catheters or pacemaker wires. On cross-sectional CT images the nodules often appear to have a vessel leading into them ('feeding vessel' sign)[19] (Fig. 5-8). Dependent on the underlying organism, nodules cavitate typically at different time points, resulting in the simultaneous appearance of solid nodules, and nodules with varying sizes of cavitations.

Empyema occurs in less than 5% of pulmonary infections. The pathogens traditionally associated with

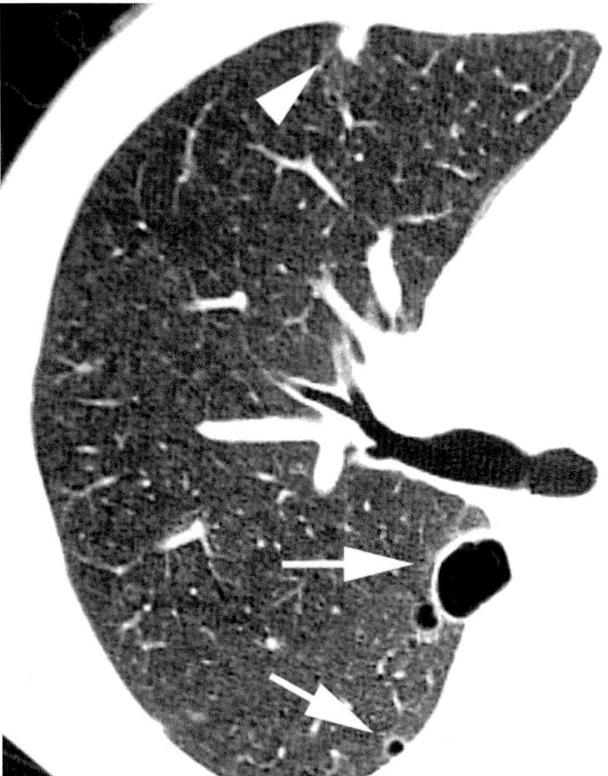

FIGURE 5-7 ■ ***Pneumocystis* pneumonia and cysts.** A 37-year-old man who had AIDS. CT at the level of the carina shows extensive ground-glass attenuation, multiple cysts (pneumatoceles) (arrows) and a nodular opacity (arrowhead). A *P. jiroveci* pneumonia was diagnosed.

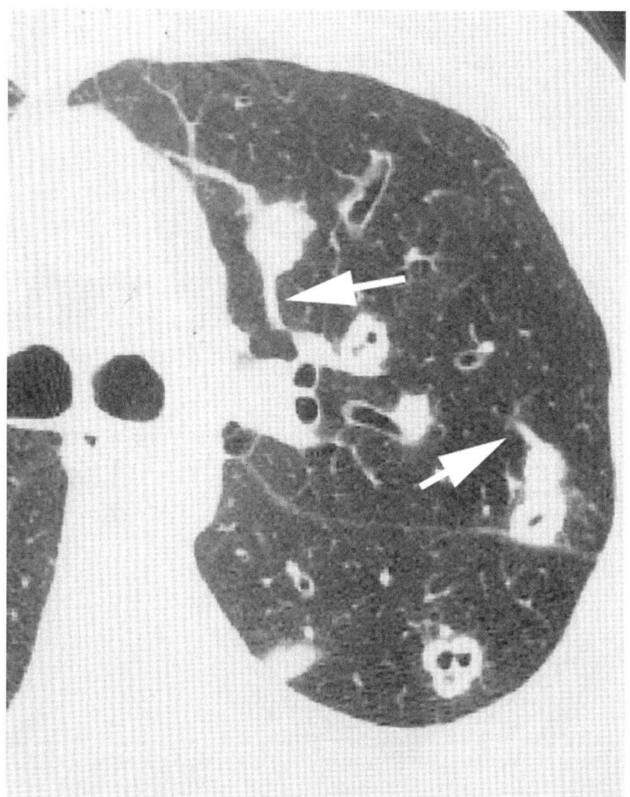

FIGURE 5-8 ■ **Septic embolism.** A 40-year-old male, intravenous drug user with fever. CT shows multiple cavitated nodules in the left upper lobe. Different vessels (arrows) course into the nodules. Blood cultures were positive for *S. aureus.*

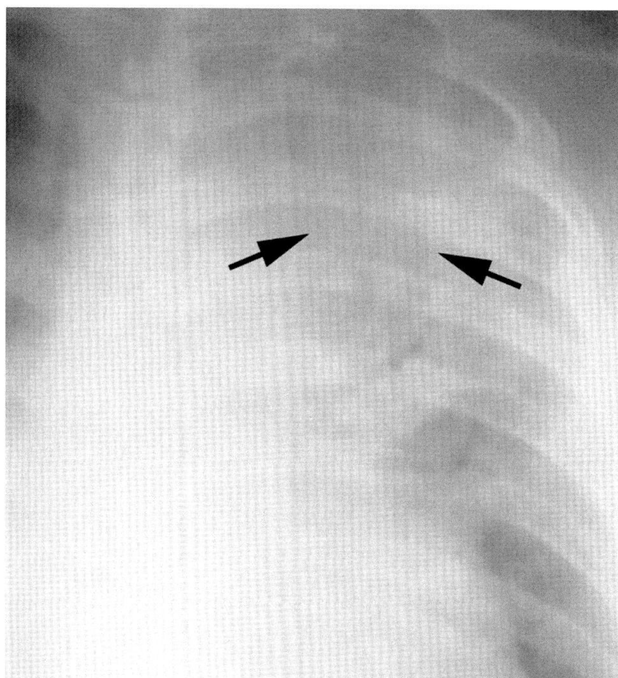

FIGURE 5-9 ■ **Lobar pneumoccocal pneumonia.** Close-up view from an anteroposterior chest radiograph shows a dense consolidation in the left upper lobe with visible air bronchogram (arrows).

empyema are *S. pneumoniae*, *Streptococcus pyogenes* and *S. aureus*. Radiographically, early signs include obliteration of the costophrenic angle. Complete opacification of an hemithorax and contralateral mediastinal displacement may occur in large effusions. CT features include (a) pleural enhancement and thickening of the parietal pleura, (b) increased density of extrathoracic fat and (c) thickening and increased density of the extrapleural subcostal fat.

Bronchopleural fistula is a sinus tract between the bronchus and the pleural space that may result from necrotising pneumonias, lung surgery, lung neoplasms and trauma. Imaging features consist of (1) increase in intrapleural air space, (2) appearance of a new air-fluid level, (3) changes in an already present air-fluid level, (4) development of tension pneumothorax and (5) demonstration of actual fistulous communication on CT scan.[20]

INTEGRATING CLINICAL AND IMAGING FINDINGS

The clinician evaluating the patient with a known or suspected diagnosis of pulmonary infection faces a diagnostic challenge because of the majority of processes presenting with similar signs and symptoms, and the radiographic findings of a pneumonia do not provide a specific aetiological diagnosis. Furthermore, radiographic manifestations of a given infectious process may be variable, depending on the immunologic status of the patient as well as the pre- or coexisting lung disease.

The most useful imaging techniques available for the evaluation of the patient with known or suspected pulmonary infection are chest radiography and computed tomography.

Lobar Pneumonia

Most Common Organisms

Streptococcus pneumoniae. *Streptoccocus pneumoniae* is responsible for approximately one-third of all cases of community-acquired pneumonia (CAP).[21] Risk factors for the development of pneumococcal pneumonia include the extremes of age, chronic heart or lung disease, immunosuppression, alcoholism, institutionalisation and prior splenectomy.

The typical radiographic appearance of acute pneumoccocal pneumonia consist of a homogeneous consolidation that crosses segmental boundaries (non-segmental) but involves only one lobe (lobar pneumonia) (Fig. 5-9). The CT 'angiogram sign', initially described in the lobar form of bronchoalveolar cell carcinoma as the enhancement of branching pulmonary vessels in a homogeneous low-attenuation consolidation of lung parenchyma, may also occur in lobar pneumonia (Fig. 5-10).[22] Occasionally, infection is manifested as a spherical focus of consolidation. Pleural effusion is common and is seen in up to half of patients.[23,24]

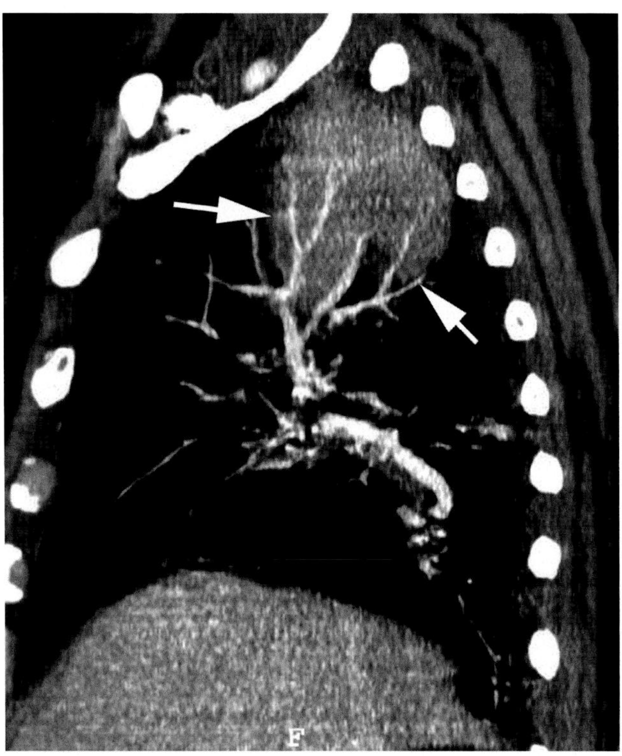

FIGURE 5-10 ■ Segmental *Pneumoccocal pneumonia* pneumonia. 48-year-old man with fever and a right upper lobe pneumonia. Sagittal reformated minimum intensity projection (MIP) image from dynamic contrast-enhanced MDCT shows a normal pattern of pulmonary vasculature within an homogeneous right upper lobe consolidation (CT angiogram sign) (arrows).

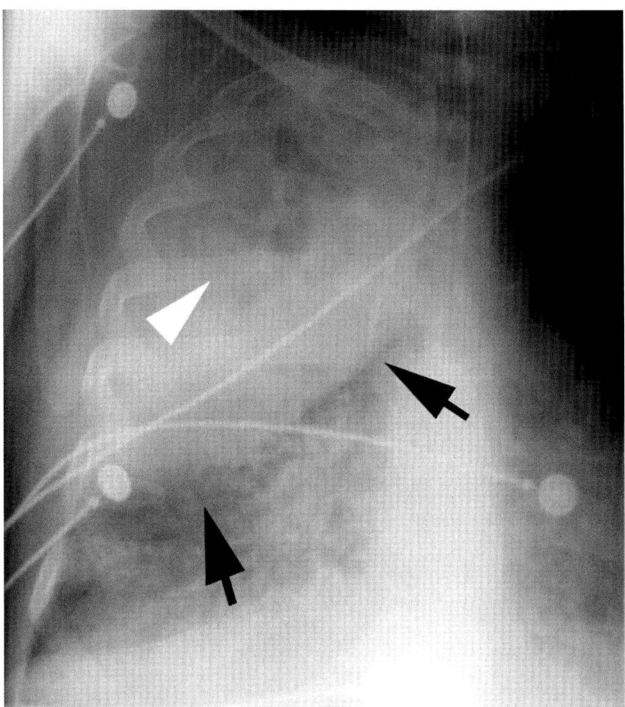

FIGURE 5-11 ■ *Klebsiella* pneumonia. A 50-year-old man with fever and a severe right pneumonia. Posteroanterior chest radiograph shows dense consolidation of the right upper lobe with visible areas of abscessification (arrowhead). Note an inferior convexity of the major fissure ('bulging fissure' sign) (arrows) characteristic of lobar expansion.

Klebsiella. *Klebsiella pneumoniae* is among the most common Gram-negative bacteria, accounting for 0.5–5.0% of all cases of pneumonia. The radiographic features include bulging fissures due to volume increase of the infected lobe, sharp margins of the advancing border of the pneumonic infiltrate and early abscess formation (Fig. 5-11). CT findings consist of ground-glass attenuation, consolidation and abscess formation.[25]

***Legionella* sp.** *Legionella* is one of the most common causes of severe CAP in immunocompetent hosts. Human infection may occur when *Legionella* contaminates water systems, such as air conditioners and condensers. Risk factors for the development of *L. pneumophila* pneumonia include immunosuppression, post-transplantation, cigarette smoking, renal disease and exposure to contaminated drinking water. Patients with *Legionella* pneumonia usually present with fever, cough, initially dry and later productive, malaise, myalgia, confusion, headaches and diarrhoea.

Imaging findings include peripheral airspace consolidation similar to that seen in acute *S. pneumoniae* pneumonia. In many cases, the area of consolidation rapidly progresses to occupy all or a large portion of a lobe (lobar pneumonia) to involve contiguous lobes or to become bilateral (Fig. 5-12). Occasionally, *Legionella* pneumonia may result in a round area of consolidation simulating a mass (round pneumonia).[26] Pleural effusion may occur in 35 to 63% of cases.

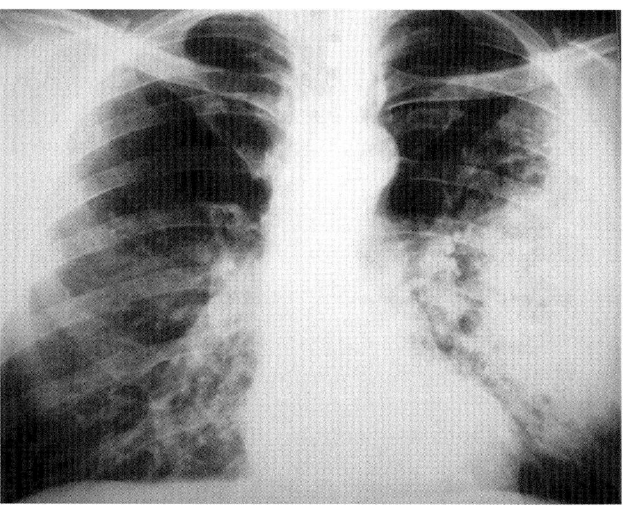

FIGURE 5-12 ■ *Legionella* pneumonia. A 51-year-old man with cough and fever. Posteroanterior chest radiograph at emergency area shows dense heterogeneous consolidation in the left lung. A community-acquired *L. pneumophila* pneumonia was diagnosed.

Chlamydia. *Chlamydia pneumoniae* (strain TWAR) is the most commonly occurring Gram-negative intracellular bacterial pathogen. It is frequently involved in respiratory tract infections and has also been implicated in the pathogenesis of asthma in both adults and children.[27,28] On CT, *C. pneumoniae* pneumonia demonstrates a wide spectrum of imaging findings that are similar to those of

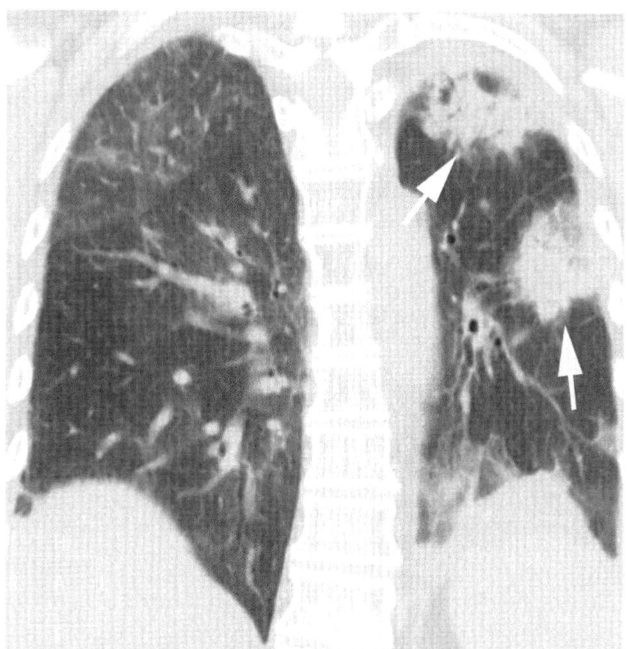

FIGURE 5-13 ■ ***Chlamydia pneumoniae* pneumonia.** A 67-year-old woman with chest pain, fever and non-productive cough. Coronal reformatted CT shows multiple ill-defined, rounded areas of consolidation in the left upper lobe with visible air bronchogram and poorly defined margins (arrows).

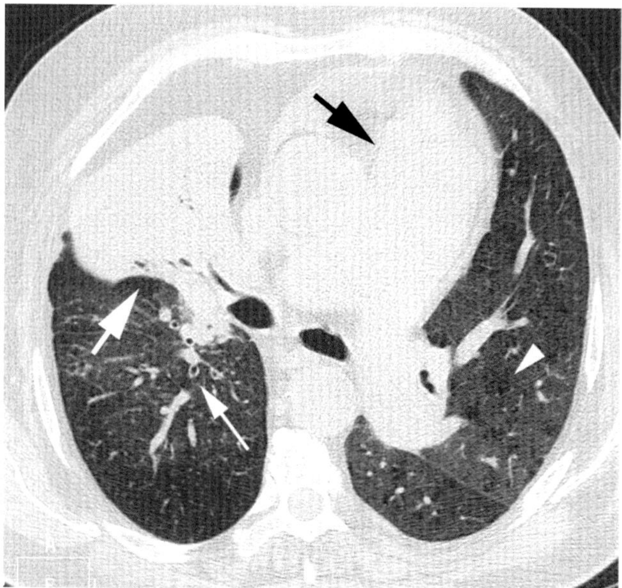

FIGURE 5-14 ■ ***Moraxella catarrhalis* pneumonia.** A 70-year-old man with fever. CT shows a complete consolidation in the middle lobe (white arrow). Note bronchial wall thickening (thin white arrow) and focal areas of ground-glass opacities in the superior segment of the right lower lobe. Also evident is a significant dilatation of the main pulmonary artery (black arrow).

S. pneumoniae pneumonia and *M. pneumoniae* pneumonia, consisting of areas of consolidation, bronchovascular bundle thickening, nodules, small pleural effusion, lymphadenopathy, reticular or linear opacities and airway dilatation (Fig. 5-13).

Moraxella catarrhalis. *Moraxella catarrhalis* (formerly known as *Branhamella catarrhalis*) is an intracellular Gram-negative coccus currently considered the third most common cause of community-acquired bacterial pneumonia (after *S. pneumoniae* and *H. influenzae*). *Moraxella catarrhalis* seldom results in pneumonia in previously healthy individuals.[29] Most patients with pneumonia (80 to 90%) have underlying COPD, and their clinical illness may be difficult to distinguish from exacerbations of lung disease by other causes. Chest radiographs show bronchopneumonia or lobar pneumonia that usually involves a single lobe (Fig. 5-14).

Immunocompromised Host

***Nocardia* sp.** *Nocardia* is a genus of filamentous Gram-positive, weakly acid-fast, aerobic bacteria that affects both immunosuppressed and immunocompetent patients. Nocardiosis usually begins with a focus of pulmonary infection and may disseminate through hematogenous spread to other organs, most commonly to the CNS. Imaging findings are variable and consist of unifocal or multifocal consolidation and single or multiple pulmonary nodules. Cavitation is common and lymphadenopathy or chest wall involvement may occur. *Nocardia asteroides* infection may complicate alveolar proteinosis[30] (Fig. 5-15).

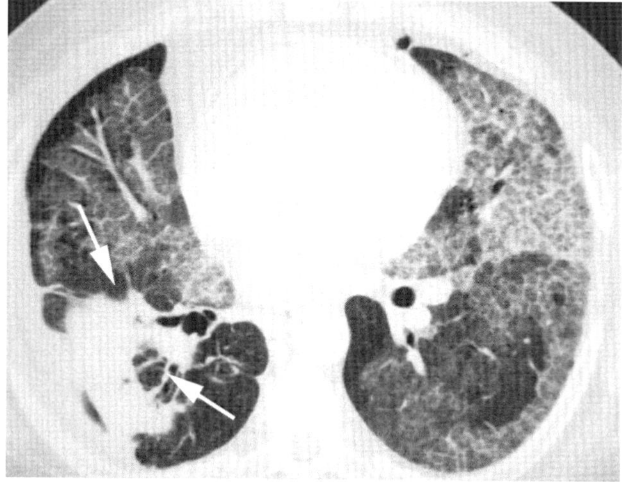

FIGURE 5-15 ■ **Alveolar proteinosis and *Nocardia* pneumonia.** A 42-year-old man with alveolar proteinosis who presented with fever. CT at the level of the lower lobes shows bilateral areas of extensive ground-glass opacities with superimposed smooth septal lines and intralobular lines, resulting in a pattern known as 'crazy-paving'. Note a localised area of consolidation (arrows) and a right pleural effusion.

***Actinomyces* sp.** Thoracic actinomycosis is a chronic suppurative pulmonary or endobronchial infection caused by *Actinomyces* species, most frequently *A. israelii*, considered to be a Gram-positive branching filamentous bacterium. Actinomycosis has the ability to spread across fascial planes to contiguous tissues without regard to normal anatomic barriers. On CT, parenchymal actinomycosis is characterised by airspace consolidation with cavitation or central areas of low attenuation and adjacent

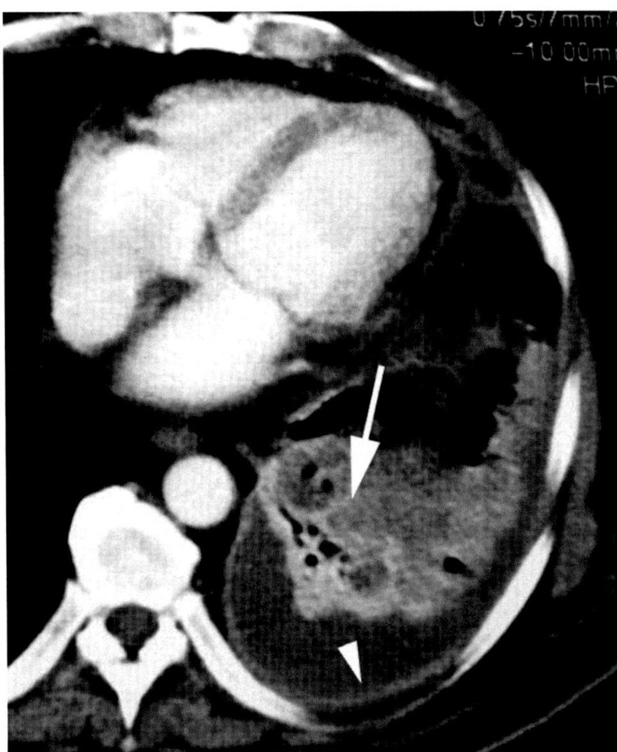

FIGURE 5-16 ■ **Pleuropulmonary actinomycosis.** A 52-year-old alcoholic man with fever, cough and left chest pain. Contrast-enhanced CT shows consolidation in the left lower lobe containing multiple areas of decreased attenuation with small air bubbles. Also evident are pleural thickening and a small pleural effusion.

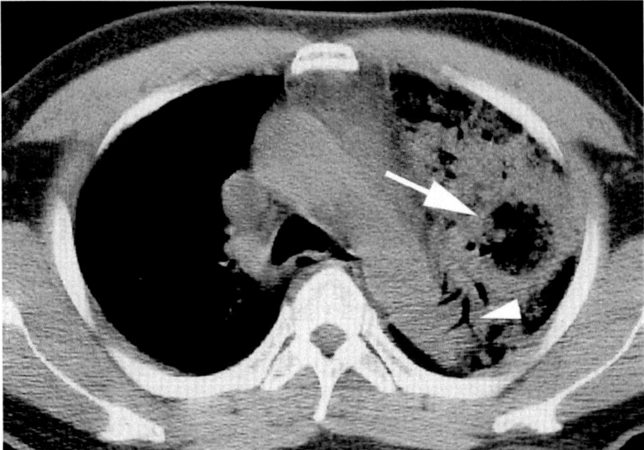

FIGURE 5-17 ■ ***Staphylococcus aureus* pneumonia.** A 13-year-old boy with fever. CT at the level of the aortic arch shows a necrotising pneumonia in the upper left lobe. A community-acquired methicillin-resistant *S. aureus* (MRSA) was diagnosed.

pleural thickening[31–33] (Fig. 5-16). Endobronchial actinomycosis can be associated with a foreign body (direct aspiration of a foreign body contaminated with *Actinomyces* organisms) or a broncholith (secondary colonisation of a pre-existing endobronchial broncholith by aspirated *Actinomyces* organisms).

Endemic in Certain Geographic Areas

***Coxiella burnetii* (Rickettsial Pneumonia).** The most common rickettsial lung infection is sporadic or epidemic Q-fever pneumonia caused by *Coxiella burnetii*, an intracellular, Gram-negative bacterium.

Infection is mainly acquired by inhalation from farm livestock or their products, and occasionally from domestic animals. Imaging findings consist of multilobar airspace consolidation, solitary or multiple nodules surrounded by a halo of 'ground-glass' opacity and vessel connection, and necrotising pneumonia.[34]

Francisella tularensis. Tularaemia is an acute, febrile, bacterial zoonosis caused by the aerobic Gram-negative bacillus *Francisella tularensis*. It is endemic in parts of Europe, Asia and North America. Primary pneumonic tularaemia occurs in rural settings.[35] Humans become infected after introduction of the bacillus by inhalation, intradermal injection or oral ingestion. Chest radiographic findings are scattered multifocal consolidations, hilar adenopathy and pleural effusion.

Bronchopneumonia

Most Common Organisms

Staphylococcus aureus. Pneumonia caused by *S. aureus* usually follows aspiration of organisms from the upper respiratory tract.[36] Risk factors for the development of staphylococcal pneumonia include underlying pulmonary disease (e.g. COPD, carcinoma), chronic illnesses (e.g. diabetes mellitus, renal failure) or viral infection. A severe pneumonia caused by community-associated methicillin-resistant *S. aureus* (MRSA) carrying genes for Panton–Valentine leukocidin has been described in healthy young adults.[37]

The characteristic pattern of presentation is as a bronchopneumonia (lobular pneumonia) that is bilateral in approximately 40% of patients[38] Other features are cavitation, pneumatoceles, pleural effusions and spontaneous pneumothorax (Fig. 5-17). Pleural effusions occur in 30 to 50% of patients and abscesses develop in 15 to 30% of patients. The CT manifestations of *S. aureus* pneumonia include centrilobular nodules and branching opacities (tree-in-bud pattern), and lobular, subsegmental, or segmental areas of consolidation with or without abscess formation.

Escherichia coli. *Escherichia coli* accounts for approximately 4% of cases of CAP and 5 to 20% of cases of HAP or HCAP. It occurs most commonly in debilitated patients.[17]

The radiographic manifestations usually are those of bronchopneumonia; rarely, a pattern of lobar pneumonia may be seen.[39] Involvement usually is multilobar and predominantely in the lower lobes (Fig. 5-18).

Pseudomonas aeruginosa. *Pseudomonas aeruginosa* is a Gram-negative bacillus that is the most common cause of nosocomial pulmonary infection.[40] It causes confluent bronchopneumonia that is often extensive and frequently cavitates. CT findings consist of multifocal, predominantly upper lobe, airspace consolidation, random large

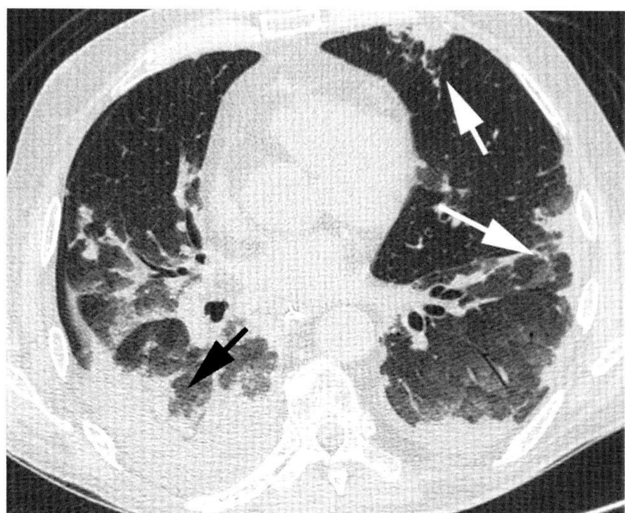

FIGURE 5-18 ■ ***Escherichia coli* pneumonia.** A 54-year-old man with fever. Minimum intensity projection CT demonstrates multiple bilateral peripheral areas of consolidation (arrows).

nodules, tree-in-bud opacities, ground-glass opacity, necrosis and pleural effusion (Fig. 5-19).

Haemophilus influenzae. *Haemophilus influenzae* is a pleomorphic, Gram-negative coccobacillus that accounts for 5 to 20% of CAP in patients in whom an organism can be identified successfully. Factors that predispose to *Haemophilus* pneumonia include COPD, malignancy, human immunodeficiency virus (HIV) infection and alcoholism. The typical radiographic appearance of *H. influenza* pneumonia consists of multilobar involvement with lobar or segmental consolidation and pleural effusion (Fig. 5-20). In 30 to 50% of patients, the pattern is that of lobar consolidation similar to that of *Streptococcus pneumoniae*.[41]

Atypical Pneumonia

Mycoplasma pneumoniae. *Mycoplasma pneumoniae* is one of the most common causes of CAP.[42] It occurs most commonly in younger persons, and infection is particularly common among military recruits. Patients with COPD appear to be more severely affected with *M. pneumoniae* than normal hosts.

The radiographic findings in *M. pneumoniae* are variable and in some cases closely resemble those seen in viral infections of the lower respiratory tract. CT findings consist of patchy segmental and lobular areas of ground-glass opacity or airspace consolidation, centrilobular nodules and thickening of the bronchovascular bundles[43,44] (Fig. 5-21).

Viral

The clinical signs and symptoms of viral pneumonia are often non-specific and the clinical course of infection will be highly dependent on the overall immune status of the host. Acute bronchiolitis is a term most often used to describe an illness in infants and children characterised

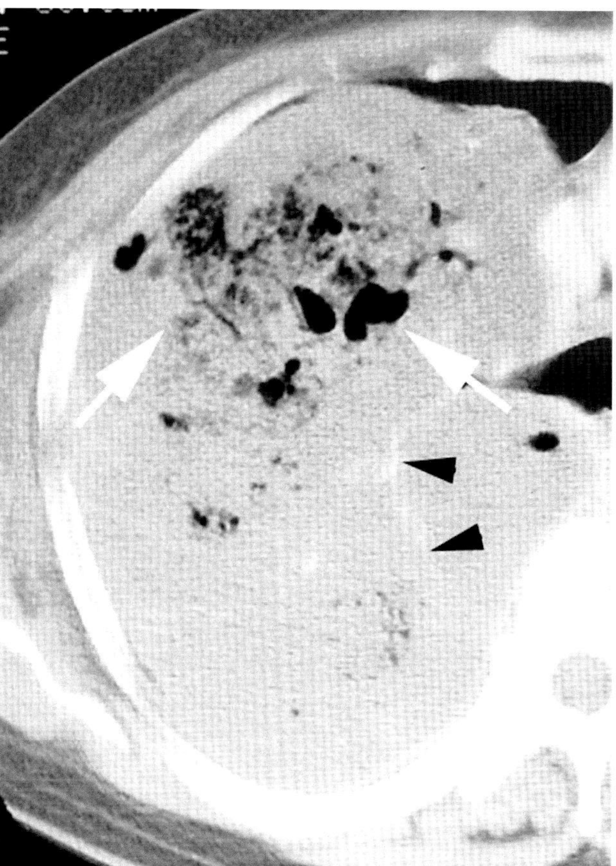

FIGURE 5-19 ■ ***Pseudomonas aeruginosa* pneumonia with abscess formation.** A 45-year-old woman with chest pain and fever. Contrast-enhanced CT shows extensive dense consolidation in the right upper lobe with associated areas of necrosis and abscessification (arrows). Note vascular structures visible within the consolidated lung (arrowheads).

by acute wheezing with concomitant signs of respiratory viral infection.

Viral infections can result in several forms of lower respiratory tract disease including tracheobronchitis, bronchiolitis and, usually, bilateral pneumonia.[45] Viral infections predispose to secondary bacterial pneumonia. Organising pneumonia, a non-specific reparative reaction, may result from a variety of causes and underlying pathological processes including viral infections.

Influenza A. Influenza type A is the most important of the respiratory viruses with respect to the morbidity and mortality in the general population. It is transmitted from person to person by aerosolised or respiratory droplets.

In recent years, both influenza and parainfluenza viruses have been recognised as a significant cause of respiratory illness in immunocompromised patients, including solid organ transplant recipients. The predominant high-resolution CT findings are widespread, bilateral ground-glass opacities, consolidation, centrilobular nodules, and branching linear opacities.[46]

Adenovirus. Adenovirus accounts for 5 to 10% of acute respiratory infections in infants and children but for less than 1% of respiratory illnesses in adults.[47]

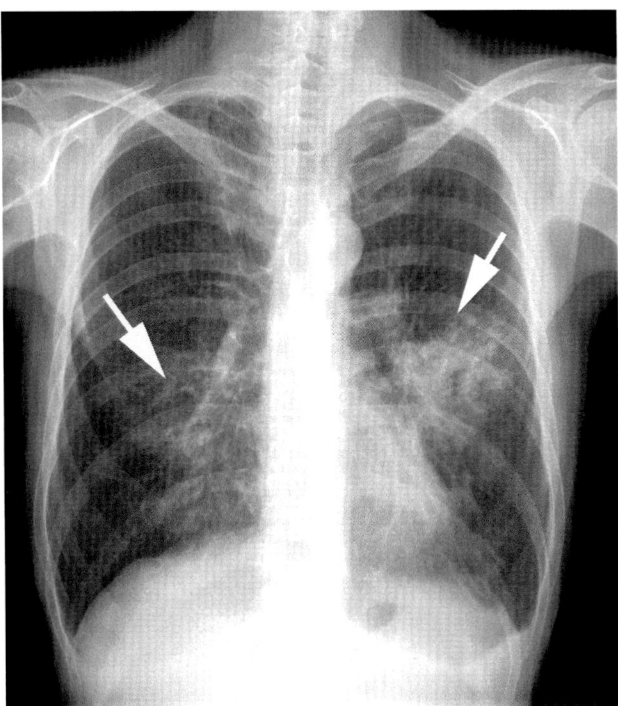

FIGURE 5-20 ■ ***Haemophilus influenzae* pneumonia.** A 49-year-old man with fever. Posteroanterior chest radiograph shows bilateral areas of consolidation with ill-defined margins. A community-acquired *H. influenzae* pneumonia was diagnosed.

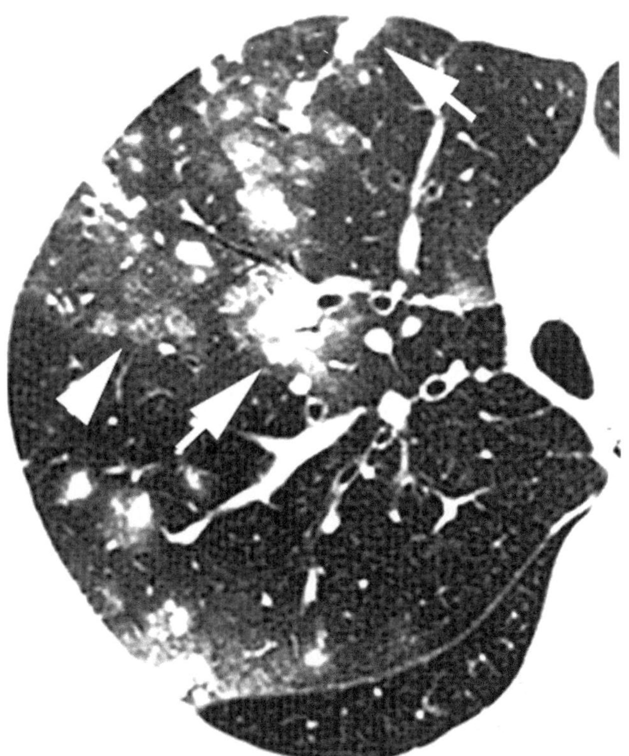

FIGURE 5-21 ■ ***Mycoplasma* pneumonia.** A 35-year-old man presents with non-productive cough and fever. CT shows airspace nodules, focal areas of lobular consolidation (arrows) and patchy ground-glass opacities (arrowhead).

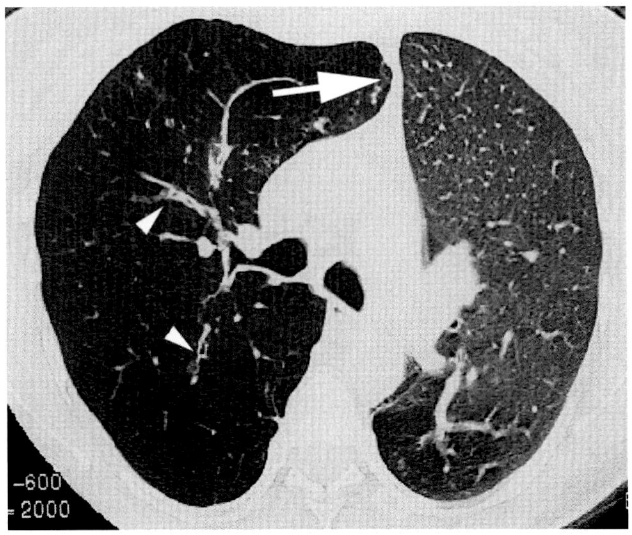

FIGURE 5-22 ■ **Swyer–James–MacLeod syndrome.** A 61-year-old woman with chronic dyspnoea. Expiratory CT shows significant air trapping in the right lung with associated bronchiectasis (arrowheads). A focal area of air trapping is also visible in the superior segment of the left lower lobe. Note the contralateral shift of the mediastinum and anterior junction line (arrow).

Swyer–James–MacLeod syndrome is considered to be a post-infectious bronchiolitis obliterans (BO) secondary to adenovirus infection in childhood.[48]

CT findings in post-infectious BO consist of sharply marginated focal areas of increased and decreased lung opacity with reduced vessel size in lucent lung regions, bronchial wall thickening and bronchiectasis. Air trapping is commonly visible on expiratory CT as lucent areas that represent regions of lung that are poorly ventilated and perfused[49] (Fig. 5-22).

Adenovirus infections in immunocompromised individuals, such as stem cell and solid organ transplant recipients, are increasingly recognised as significant causes of morbidity and mortality.

The CT findings consist of patchy bilateral areas of consolidation in a lobular or segmental distribution, centrilobular nodules, and branching linear opacities, and/or bilateral ground-glass opacities with a random distribution (Fig. 5-23).

Respiratory Syncytial Virus (RSV). Respiratory syncytial virus (RSV) is the most frequent viral cause of lower respiratory tract infection in infants. The major risk factors for severe RSV disease in children are prematurity (< 36 weeks' gestation), congenital heart disease, chronic lung disease, immunocompromised status and multiple congenital abnormalities.[45]

CT findings consist of small centrilobular nodules, airspace consolidation, ground-glass opacities and bronchial wall thickening (Fig. 5-24).

Epstein–Barr Virus (EBV). Primary infection with EBV occurs early in life and presents as infectious mononucleosis with the typical triad of fever, pharyngitis and lymph adenopathy, often accompanied by splenomegaly. Mild, asymptomatic pneumonitis occurs in about 5–10%

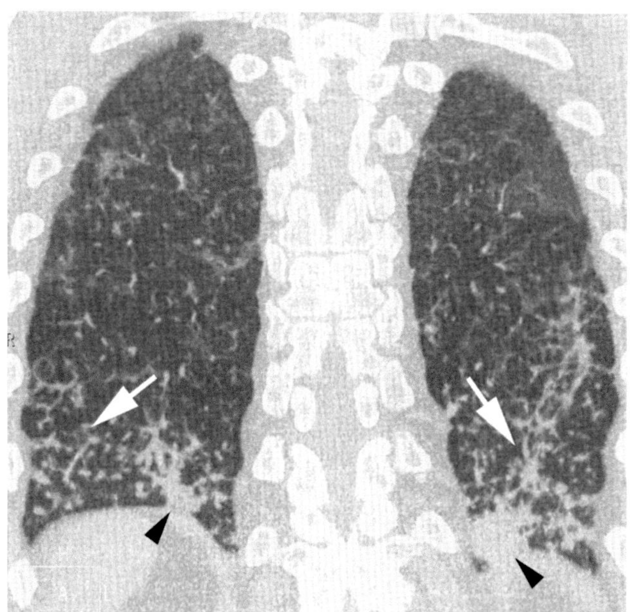

FIGURE 5-23 ■ **Adenovirus pneumonia.** A 46-year-old man with fever. Coronal reformatted CT shows bilateral multiple small branching centrilobular opacities, representing dilated peripheral bronchioles (arrows), associated with bilateral focal areas of consolidation (arrowheads).

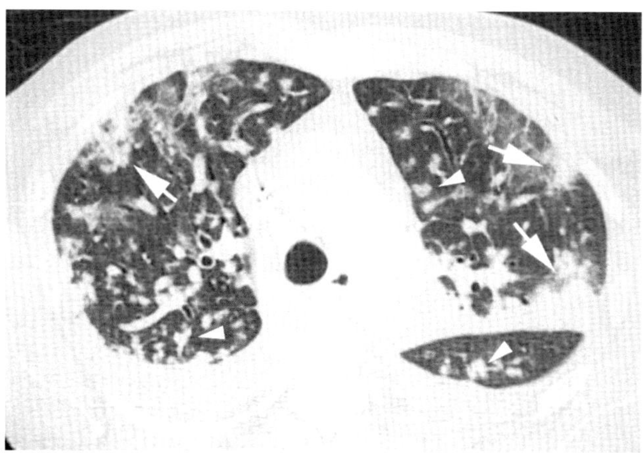

FIGURE 5-24 ■ **Respiratory syncytial virus pneumonia.** A 43-year-old man after receiving allogeneic hematopoietic stem cell transplant. CT through the upper lobes shows bilateral areas of consolidation (arrows) and multiple ill-defined nodules (arrowheads). Note bilateral pleural effusion.

of cases of infectious mononucleosis. The CT manifestations of EBV pneumonia are similar to those of other viral pneumonias.[45]

Varicella-Zoster Virus. Varicella-zoster virus is a common contagious infection in childhood with increasing incidence in adults. Clinically it presents in two forms: chickenpox (varicella) representing a primary disseminated disease in uninfected individuals and zoster (shingles) representing reactivation of latent virus (unilateral dermatomal skin eruption).

Pneumonia, although rare, is the most serious complication affecting adults with chickenpox. Varicella pneumonia is estimated to occur in one of every 400 cases of adulthood chickenpox infections, being more common in pregnant and immunosuppressed patients. The thin-section CT appearances include numerous nodular opacities measuring 5 to 10 mm in diameter (Fig. 5-25), some with a surrounding halo of ground-glass opacity, patchy ground-glass opacities and coalescence of nodules.[50] Occasionally, lesions may calcify and persist as well-defined, randomly scattered, 2- to 3-mm densely calcified nodules.

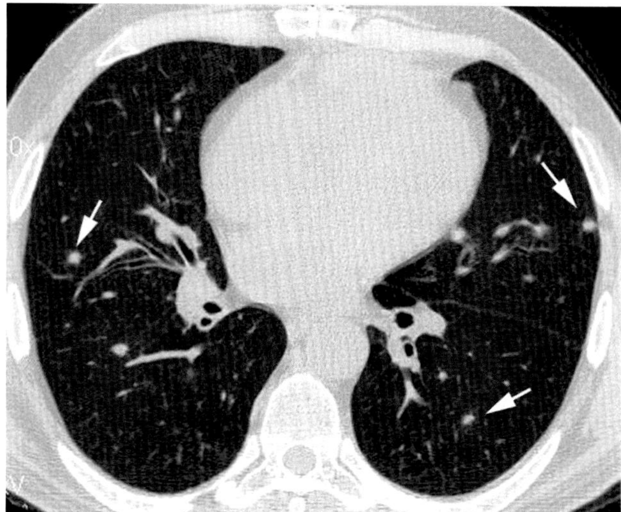

FIGURE 5-25 ■ **Varicella pneumonia.** A 30-year-old man with lymphoma and new development of fever and skin rash. CT of the lower lobes shows multiple, bilateral and randomly distributed well-defined small pulmonary nodules (arrows).

Herpes Simplex Virus Type 1 (HSV-1). Herpes simplex virus type 1 (HSV-1) pneumonia may be a life-threatening infection seen almost exclusively in immunocompromised and/or mechanically ventilated patients, usually as a component of polymicrobial infection.

CT findings consist of patchy lobular, subsegmental or segmental consolidation and ground-glass opacities; associated small centrilobular nodules and tree-in-bud pattern have been described in patients infected with herpes simplex virus type 2; nodules surrounded by a 'halo' of ground-glass opacity may also occur[51] (Fig. 5-26).

Hantaviruses. During the spring of 1993, an emerging rodent-borne zoonotic disease, characterised by a severe acute respiratory failure, rapid clinical progression and high case-fatality, occurred among healthy adults in the southwestern United States.[52]

Hantavirus infection may cause diffuse airspace disease, termed hantavirus pulmonary syndrome (HPS). The mortality rate of treated patients can approach 35%. Histologically, changes are characteristic for exudative and proliferative stages of diffuse alveolar damage.

Imaging findings may be initially normal, but progressively worsen, displaying signs of pulmonary oedema and acute respiratory distress syndrome[53,54] (Fig. 5-27). The chest radiograph findings may represent differences in

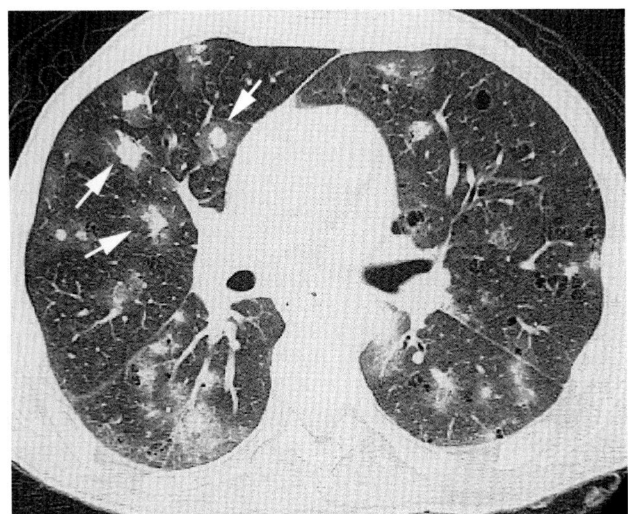

FIGURE 5-26 ■ **Herpesvirus pneumonia.** A 34-year-old severely immunocompromised patient with fever. CT at the level of the bronchus intermedius in a patient with herpesvirus infection shows multiple, bilateral and randomly distributed pulmonary nodules surrounded by a 'halo' of ground-glass opacity (arrows).

the extent of alveolar epithelial damage seen in HPS and acute respiratory distress syndrome (ARDS).

Cytomegalovirus (CMV). Cytomegalovirus pneumonia is a major cause of morbidity and mortality following hematopoietic stem cell (HSC) and solid organ transplantation and in patients with AIDS in whom CD4 cells are decreased to fewer than 100 cells/mm^3. Cytomegalovirus infection occurs in up to 70% of BMT recipients, and approximately one-third develop CMV pneumonia.[55] This complication characteristically occurs during the post-engraftment period (30–100 days after transplantation), with a median time onset of 50–60 days post-transplantation.

CT features of CMV pneumonia consist of lobar consolidation, diffuse and focal ground-glass opacities, irregular reticular opacities, and multiple miliary nodules or small nodules with associated areas of ground-glass attenuation ('halo')[55,56] (Fig. 5-28).

New Emerging Viruses

Human Metapneumovirus (hMPV). Human metapneumovirus (hMPV) is a recently identified RNA virus, genus ***Metapneumovirus***. It is usually associated with acute respiratory tract infections including upper airway disease, lower airway bronchitis and bronchiolitis, influenza-like syndrome and pneumonia.

CT findings consist of patchy areas of ground-glass attenuation, small nodules and multifocal areas of consolidation in a bilateral asymmetric distribution (Fig. 5-29). Pulmonary parenchymal involvement during the course of hMPV pneumonia infection may result in interstitial lung disease and fibrosis.[57]

Severe Acute Respiratory Syndrome Coronavirus. Severe acute respiratory syndrome (SARS) caused by SARS-associated coronavirus (SARS-CoV) is a systemic infection that clinically manifests as progressive pneumonia. Histologically, acute diffuse alveolar damage with airspace oedema is the most prominent feature in patients who die before the 10th day after onset of illness.

The imaging features of SARS-CoV infection consist of unilateral or bilateral ground-glass opacities, focal unilateral or bilateral areas of consolidation, or a mixture of both. In the areas of ground-glass opacification, thickening of the intralobular interstitium or interlobular septa may be present (Fig. 5-30).

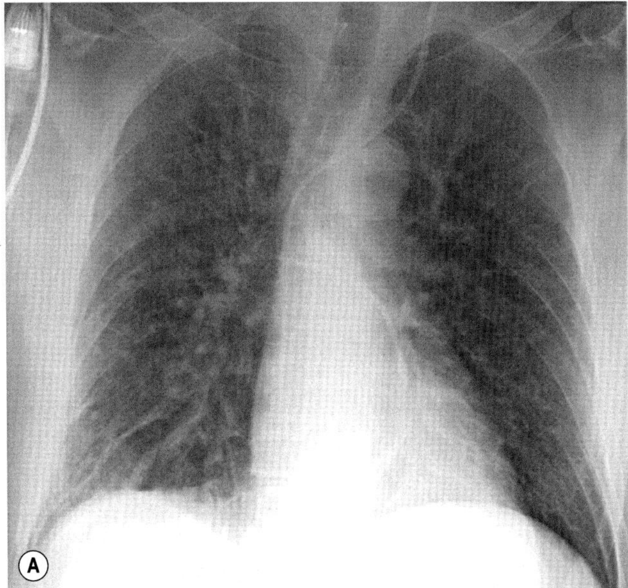

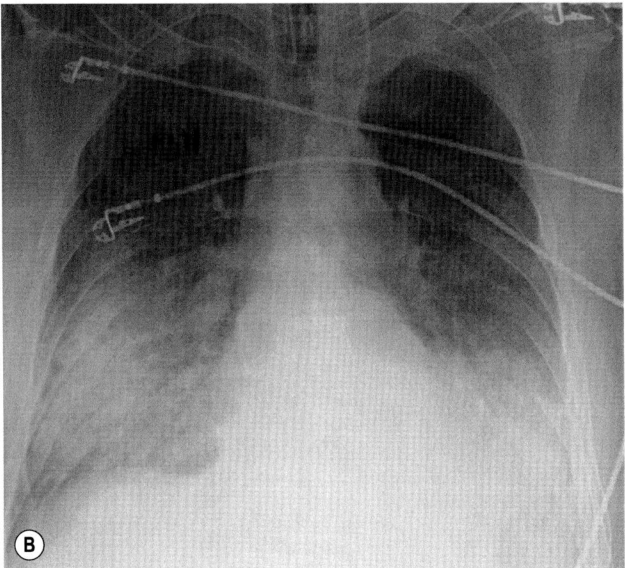

FIGURE 5-27 ■ **Hantavirus syndrome.** A 52-year-old man with severe hantavirus pulmonary syndrome. (A) Portable chest radiograph shows extensive bilateral interstitial pulmonary oedema. (B) Six hours later a frontal chest radiograph demonstrates that interstitial oedema has rapidly progressed to perihilar and bibasilar diffuse consolidations representing diffuse alveolar damage. (Courtesy of Loren Ketai, Alburquerque, NM, USA.)

Avian Flu (H5N1). Avian influenza is caused by the H5N1 subtype of the influenza A virus. Most human

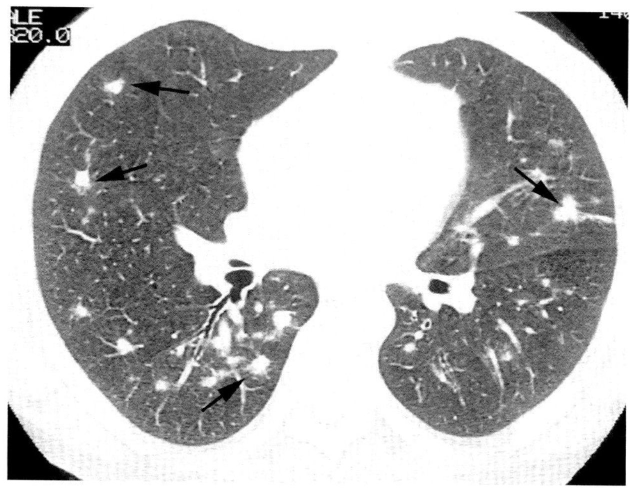
FIGURE 12-28 ■ **CMV pneumonia.** A 25-year-old man with acute myeloid leukaemia and hematopoietic stem cell transplantation. CT shows multiple scattered poorly defined nodules (arrows).

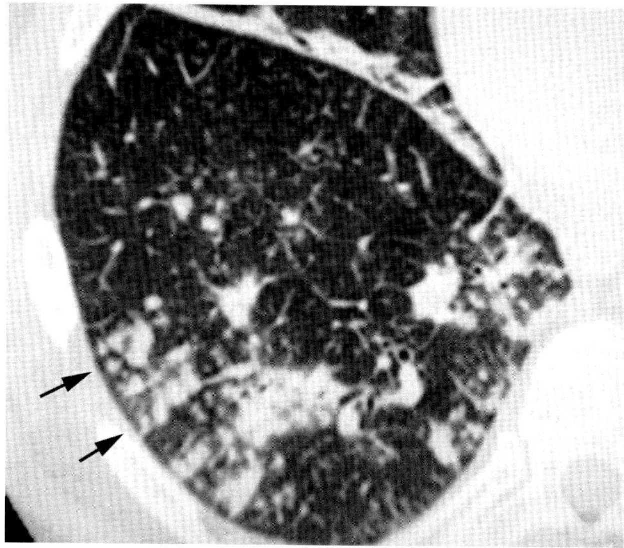
FIGURE 5-29 ■ **Metapneumovirus pneumonia.** A 34-year-old man after receiving allogeneic hematopoietic stem cell transplant. CT obtained at level of right lower lobe shows multiple centrilobular branching opacities (tree-in-bud pattern) (arrows), and focal areas of consolidation.

infections appear to be the result of close contact with infected birds, usually poultry or their products. The overall case fatality rate for H5N1 infections exceeds 60%.

Most chest radiographs are abnormal at the time of presentation, with multifocal consolidation the commonest radiographic finding. The most common CT findings consist of focal, multifocal, or diffuse ground-glass opacities or areas of consolidation.[58] Pseudocavitation, pneumatocele formation, lymphadenopathy and centrilobular nodules are often seen.

Swine Influenza (H1N1). In the spring of 2009, an outbreak of severe pneumonia was reported in

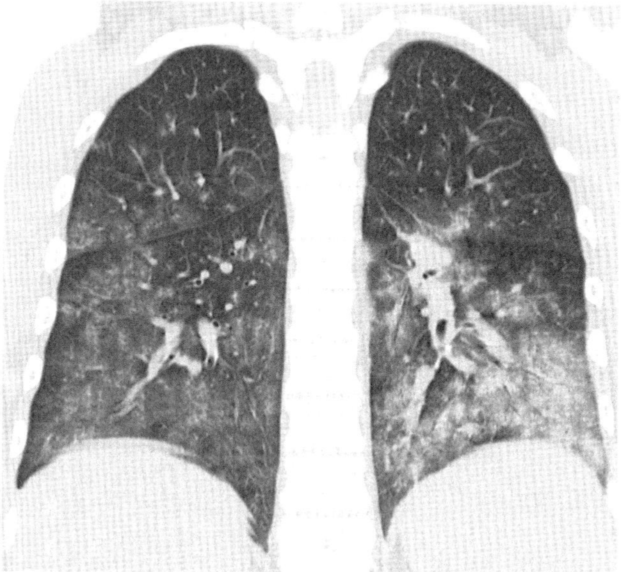
FIGURE 5-30 ■ **Severe acute respiratory syndrome (SARS).** A previously healthy 43-year-old woman with dyspnoea and fever. Coronal reformatted CT shows bilateral ground-glass opacities involving both lower lungs.

conjunction with the concurrent isolation of a novel swine-origin influenza A (H1N1) virus.[59]

On 11 June 2009, the World Health Organisation declared the first pandemic of the twenty-first century caused by swine-origin influenza virus A (H1N1). Today, the virus continues to spread globally and its transmission among humans appears to be high but its virulence is not greater than that observed with seasonal influenza. The disease has spread rapidly, with 254,206 cases having been documented worldwide as of 7 September 2009, and an estimated 2837 deaths.

The predominant CT findings are unilateral or bilateral ground-glass opacities with or without associated focal or multifocal areas of consolidation. On CT, the ground-glass opacities and areas of consolidation have a predominant peribronchovascular and subpleural distribution, resembling organising pneumonia (Fig. 5-31). Multifocal areas of air trapping may also be observed (Fig. 5-32).

CHANGING SPECTRUM OF HIV INFECTIONS: 30 YEARS LATER

Cases of HIV/AIDS increased rapidly in the developed world in the 1980s.[60] Decades later, the widespread use of anti-PCP prophylaxis, the changing demographics of the HIV-positive population, and the tremendous advancement in the management of HIV/AIDS in the developed world with the advent of highly active antiretroviral therapy (HAART) have contributed to the changing spectrum of HIV-related infections. Rates of AIDS-defining malignancies such as Kaposi's sarcoma and non-Hodgkin's lymphoma have also decreased.

In resource-limited settings, AIDS-related infectious complications such as *P. jiroveci* pneumonia and

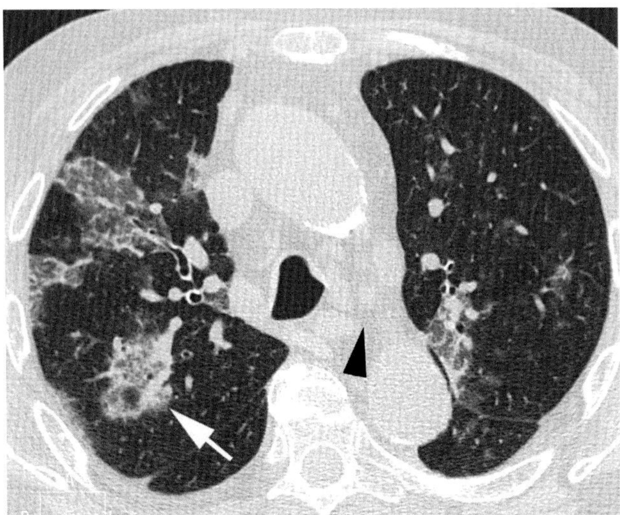

FIGURE 5-31 ■ **H1N1 pneumonia.** A previously healthy 38-year-old man with fever. CT shows patchy bilateral ground-glass opacities. Ring-like area of consolidation outline one of the ground-glass opacities (arrow) ('reverse halo' sign). The diagnosis of H1N1 was serologically confirmed.

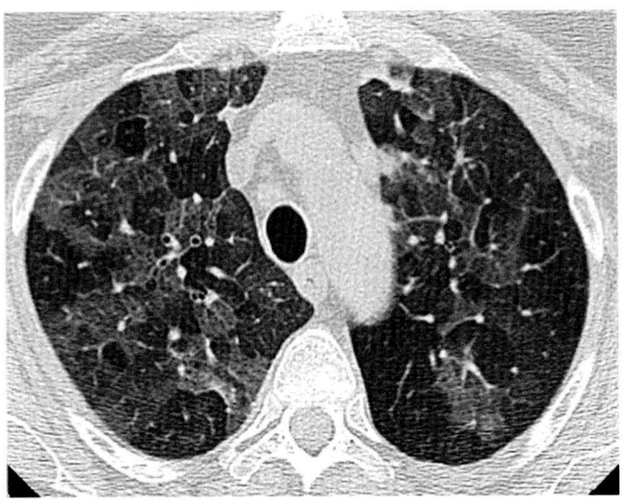

FIGURE 5-32 ■ **H1N1 obliterative bronchiolitis.** A previously healthy 53-year-old woman with dyspnoea and fever. Inspiratory CT shows extensive bilateral areas of decreased attenuation and vascularity (mosaic perfusion/attenuation pattern). Expiratory CT confirmed air trapping (not shown). (Courtesy of Dr. Amador Prieto, Oviedo, Spain.)

pulmonary tuberculosis still predominate. In the developed and developing world settings, bacterial infections have now become the commonest infectious thoracic complication in the HIV population. Aetiologically, *S. pneumoniae* predominates, followed by *H. influenzae*.

Immune reconstitution inflammatory syndrome (IRIS) in HIV-infected patients with mycobacterial infections starting highly active antiretroviral therapy is defined as an exacerbation of symptoms, signs, or radiological manifestations of a pathogenic antigen, which are not due to relapse or recurrence. Patients affected with IRIS undergo deterioration in their clinical status at a time when viral replication appears to be under control and CD4

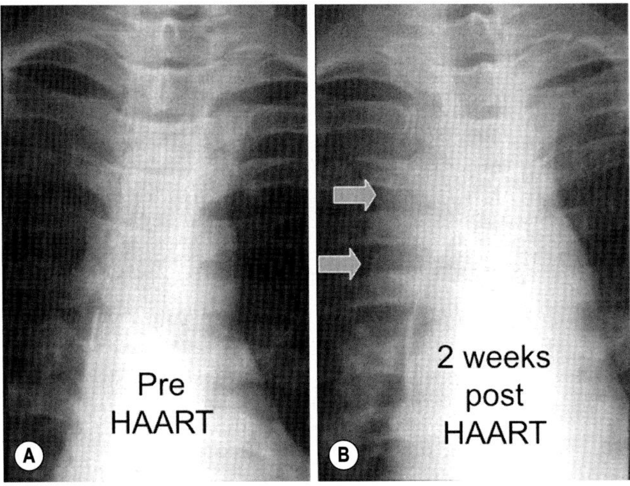

FIGURE 5-33 ■ **Immune reconstitution inflammatory syndrome (IRIS) in a patient with tuberculosis.** Posteroanterior normal chest radiograph after initiation of HAART and before onset of IRIS (A). Follow-up chest radiograph (B) obtained 14 days later shows a significant enlargement of paratracheal lymph nodes (arrows).

counts are rising, known as a paradoxical response.[61,62] These paradoxical reactions have been reported to occur in patients with both infectious and non-infectious antigens.

The most common imaging features of IRIS consist of mediastinal lymph node enlargement, with central low attenuation, diffuse and bilateral pulmonary nodules and small pleural effusions (Fig. 5-33).

Mycobacterium tuberculosis

Mycobacterium tuberculosis accounts for more than 95% of pulmonary mycobacterial infections. Other mycobacterial species, mainly *Mycobacterium kansasii* and the *Mycobacterium avium–intracellulare* complex (MAC) account for the remainder.

Factors that contribute to the large number of cases seen worldwide are HIV infection, inner-city poverty, homelessness and immigration from areas with high rates of infection. Other predisposing conditions are diabetes mellitus, alcoholism, silicosis, malignancy, immune compromise from a variety of causes and living in closed institutions.

The imaging findings of patients with tuberculosis take many forms and are best discussed as primary, reactivation and reinfection tuberculosis.

Primary Tuberculosis

This form is commonly seen in infants and children. With improved control of tuberculosis in Western societies, however, more people reach adulthood without exposure, and primary patterns of disease are being seen with increasing frequency in adulthood, representing about 23–34% of all adult cases of tuberculosis.[63]

Although primary tuberculosis typically presents with radiographic manifestations, chest radiographs may be normal in 15% of cases.[63] Lymphadenopathy is the most

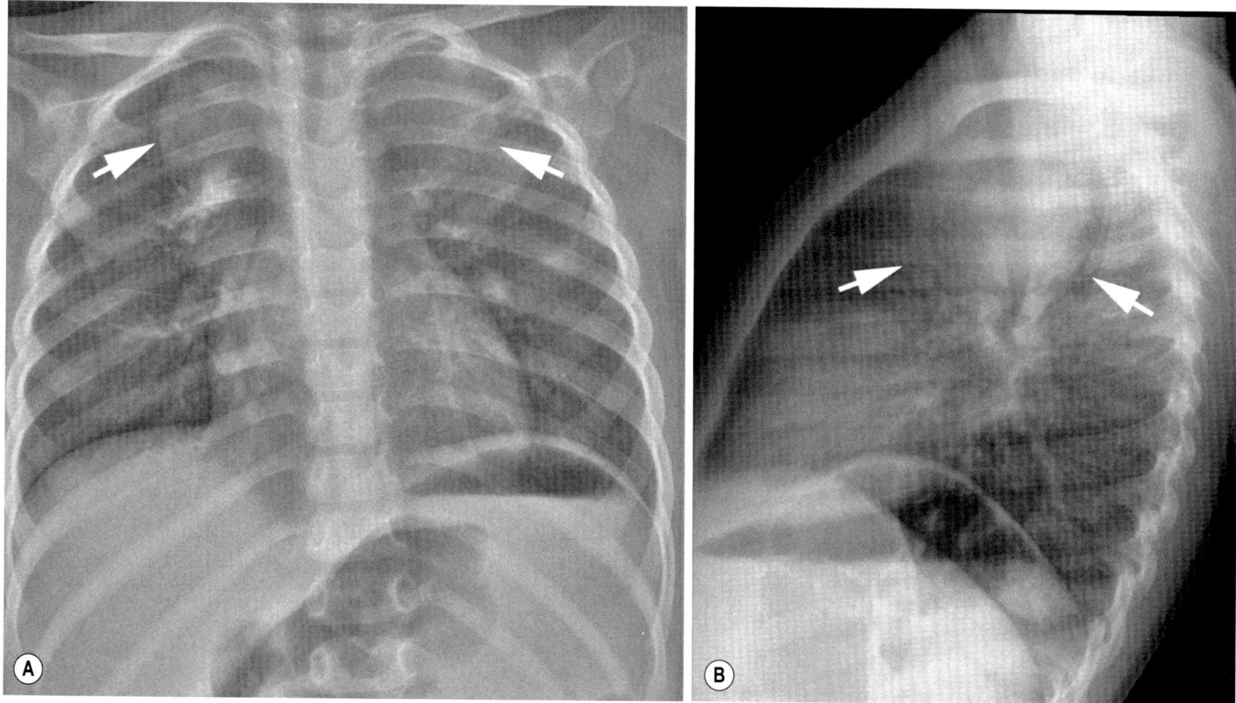

FIGURE 5-34 ■ **Primary TB.** A 2-year-old boy with stridor and fever. Anteroposterior (A) and lateral (B) chest radiographs show bilateral enlargement of mediastinal lymph nodes (arrows).

common manifestation of primary tuberculosis in children and occurs with or without pneumonia (Fig. 5-34). The effusions are often large and unilateral and residual pleural change is unusual.

Usually the primary pneumonia resolves completely. In one-third of patients a residual well-defined rounded or irregular (linear) opacity, with or without calcification remains (Ghon lesion or focus). When a Ghon lesion or focus and ipsilateral lymph node calcification are seen together the combination is termed a Ranke complex.

Reactivation and Reinfection Tuberculosis

Most cases are due to reactivation of quiescent lesions, but reinfection from an exogenous source may also occur. Pathologically, the ability of the host to respond immunologically results in a greater inflammatory reaction and caseous necrosis.

The radiological manifestations may overlap with those of primary tuberculosis, but the absence of lymph adenopathy, more frequent cavitation and a predilection for the upper lobes are more typical of reactivation and reinfection tuberculosis.

Cavitation indicates active disease and is seen in the region of abnormality in 40–80% of cases (Fig. 5-35). Air–fluid levels are unusual but have been recorded in up to 20% of cases. A Rasmussen aneurysm is a rare life-threatening complication of cavitary tuberculosis caused by granulomatous weakening of a pulmonary arterial wall (Fig. 5-36).

Endobronchial spread can occur with or without cavitary disease and is similar to that seen with primary tuberculosis, leading to the appearance of the typical images of 'tree-in-bud'[64] (Fig. 5-37).

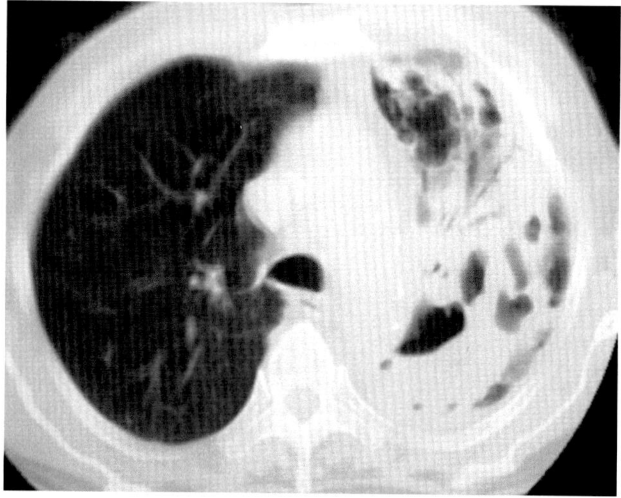

FIGURE 5-35 ■ **Reinfection tuberculosis.** A 40-year-old man presents with night sweats, non-productive cough and fever. CT shows extensive parenchymal consolidation of the left upper lobe with multiple cavities.

After antituberculous treatment healing results in scar formation, often with evidence of severe volume loss and pleural thickening. Residual thin-walled cavities may be present in both active and inactive disease.

Although classically a manifestation of primary disease, miliary tuberculosis is now more commonly seen as a post-primary process in older patients. Multiple small (1–2 mm) discrete nodules are scattered evenly throughout both lungs.[65–67] (Fig. 5-38).

A tuberculoma may occur in the setting of primary or post-primary tuberculosis and represents localised

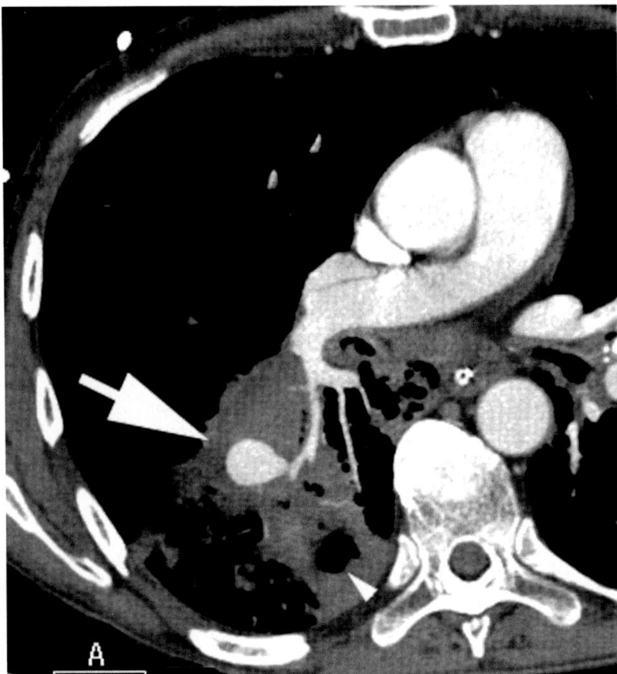

FIGURE 5-36 ■ **Rasmussen aneurysm.** A 65-year-old man with chronic destructive pulmonary tuberculosis. Contrast-enhanced CT at the level of the right pulmonary artery shows a contrast-filling aneurysm (arrow) within parenchymal consolidation in a superior segment of the right lower lobe. Note an associated parenchymal cavity (arrowhead).

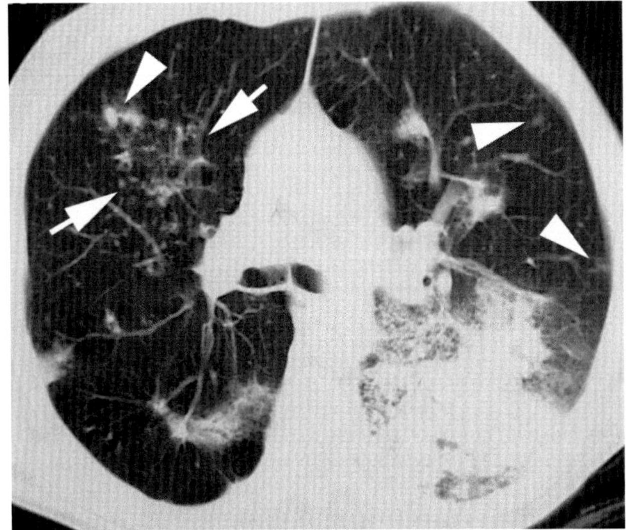

FIGURE 5-37 ■ **Endobronchial spread of tuberculosis.** A 56-year-old man with post-primary tuberculosis. CT shows a non-cavitating consolidation in the left lung. Note typical images of 'tree-in-bud' opacities (arrows) and variable-sized bilateral nodular lesions (arrowheads).

parenchymal disease that alternately activates and heals. It usually calcifies and frequently remains stable for years.

Chest wall involvement may be due to haematogenous seeding or direct spread from the lung and may affect soft tissue, rib, or costal cartilage ('empyema necessitatis').

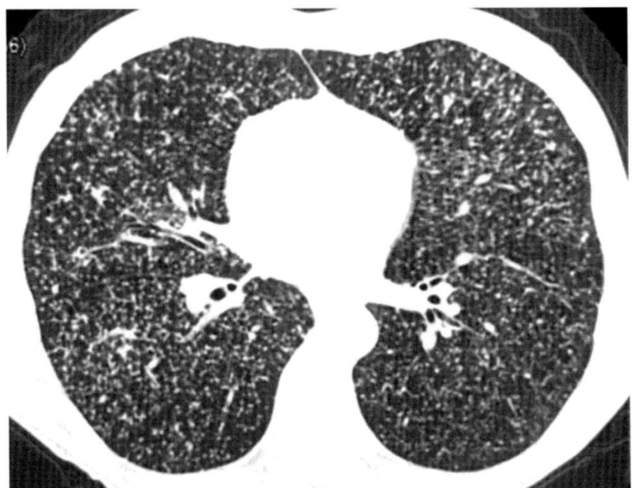

FIGURE 5-38 ■ **Miliary tuberculosis.** A 26-year-old man with fever and shortness of breath. CT shows a random distribution of multiple, discrete 1–2 mm in diameter nodules.

Pulmonary Non-Tuberculous Mycobacteria (NTMB)

As mentioned above, 1–3% of pulmonary mycobacterial infections are caused by agents other than *M. tuberculosis*: usually MAC and less commonly *M. kansasii*. These are free-living saprophytes, and infections are not acquired from human contacts but from the environment by inhalation or ingestion. The severity of disease depends on the presence of underlying lung disease and the status of immunocompetence. Clinically, MAC may be an indolent process with symptoms of cough, with or without sputum production.[68]

The radiological pattern of *M. kansasii* is generally indistinguishable from reactivation or reinfection tuberculosis and changes equivalent to primary tuberculosis are rarely described.

The most typical form of pulmonary non-tuberculous mycobacteria (NTMB) infection is frequently associated to elderly men with underlying lung disease. Another form of NTMB infection affects elderly white women without underlying lung disease.

Radiological findings consist of mild to moderate cylindrical bronchiectasis and multiple 1–3 mm diameter centrilobular nodules usually affecting the middle lobe and lingula (Fig. 5-39).

Fungal Infection

Fungi involved in pulmonary infections are either pathogenic fungi, which can infect any host, or saprophytic fungi, which infect only immunocompromised hosts. Pathogenic fungi cause coccidioidomycosis, blastomycosis and histoplasmosis. Saprophytes cause *Pneumocystis* pneumonia, candidiasis, mucormycosis and aspergillosis.

***Aspergillus* Infection.** Aspergillosis is a fungal disease caused by *Aspergillus* species, usually *A. fumigatus* that can take different forms, depending on an individual's immune response to the organism.[69] Classically,

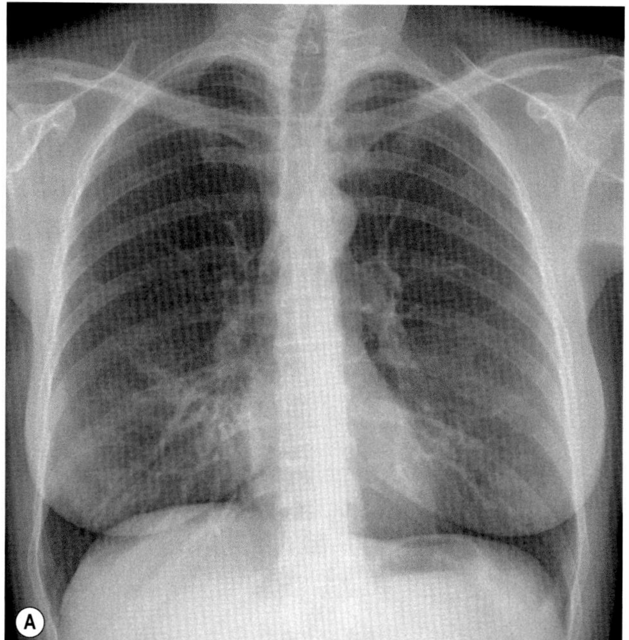

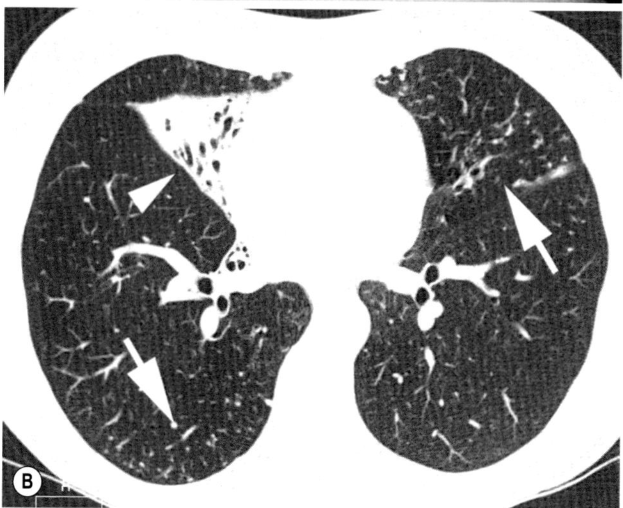

FIGURE 5-39 ■ ***Mycobacterium avium–intracellulare* complex.** A 65-year-old woman with chronic cough. (A) Posteroanterior chest radiograph shows bilateral opacities in the right middle lobe and lingula. (B) CT at the level of the inferior pulmonary veins shows complete collapse of the middle lobe containing visible bronchiectasis (arrowhead). Note the presence of small nodular opacities and few tree-in-bud opacities in the lingula and in the superior segment of the right lower lobe (arrows).

pulmonary aspergillosis has been categorised into saprophytic, allergic and invasive forms.

Aspergillus mycetomas are saprophytic growths which colonise a pre-existing cavity in the lung (e.g. from sarcoidosis or tuberculosis) usually in the upper lobes or superior segments of the lower lobes. The great majority of aspergillomas are asymptomatic. Haemoptysis is the most important complication.

At computed tomography (CT), saprophytic aspergillosis (aspergilloma) is characterised by a mass with soft-tissue attenuation within a lung cavity. The mass is typically separated from the cavity wall by an air space ('air crescent' sign) (Fig. 5-40). Bilateral involvement may occur and multiple nodules have been reported.

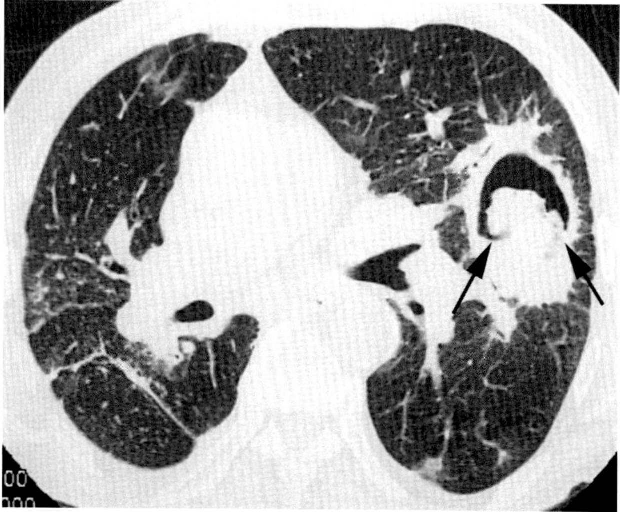

FIGURE 5-40 ■ **Intracavitary mycetoma ('fungus ball').** A 68-year-old man with chronic lung disease and mild haemoptysis. CT shows a left upper lobe cavity containing a rounded soft-tissue opacity representing a fungus ball (arrows).

Allergic bronchopulmonary aspergillosis (ABPA) describes a hypersensitivity reaction which occurs in the major airways. It is associated with asthma, an elevated serum IgE, positive serum precipitins and skin reactivity to *Aspergillus*. The radiographic appearances consist of non-segmental areas of opacity most common in the upper lobes, lobar collapse, branching thick tubular opacities due to bronchi distended with mucus and fungus ('finger-in-glove sign') and occasionally pulmonary cavitation. On CT, although the mucus plugs are generally hypodense, in up to 20% of cases they can be hyperdense[70,71] (Fig. 5-41).

Bronchial invasive aspergillosis is associated to patients with severe neutropenia and in patients with AIDS. The clinical and radiological manifestations include acute tracheobronchitis, bronchiolitis and bronchopneumonia.[72]

Angioinvasive aspergillosis is almost exclusively seen in immunocompromised hosts, mainly in patients with severe neutropenia. This form is characterised by invasion and occlusion of small-to-medium pulmonary arteries, developing necrotic haemorrhagic nodules or infarcts. The most common pattern seen in CT consists of multiple nodules surrounded by a halo of ground-glass attenuation ('halo sign') or pleural-based wedge-shaped areas of consolidation[73–75] (Fig. 5-42).

Semi-invasive or chronic necrotising aspergillosis is a form of aspergillosis that occurs in immunocompromised patients such as those with chronic illness, diabetes mellitus, malnutrition, alcoholism, advanced age, prolonged corticosteroid administration and chronic obstructive disease. Radiologically, the appearances are variable, but a common pattern is of one or more rounded poorly marginated areas of homogeneous opacification with or without air bronchograms and/or cavitation. With time, the margins may become more discrete and the lesions resemble masses.

Candidiasis. *Candida* species has been increasingly recognised as an important source of fungal pneumonia in

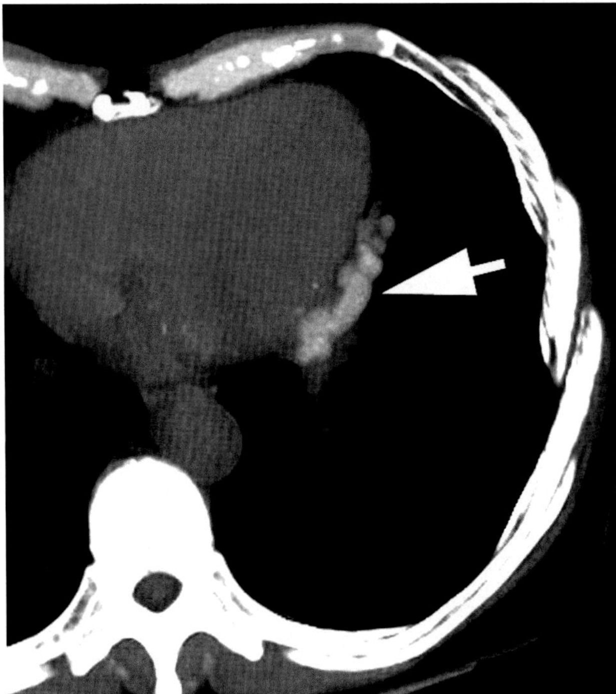

FIGURE 5-41 ■ **Allergic bronchopulmonary aspergillosis.** A 43-year-old asthmatic man with cough. Non-enhanced CT section shows a tubular opacity in the lingula containing a hyperdense mucoid impaction.

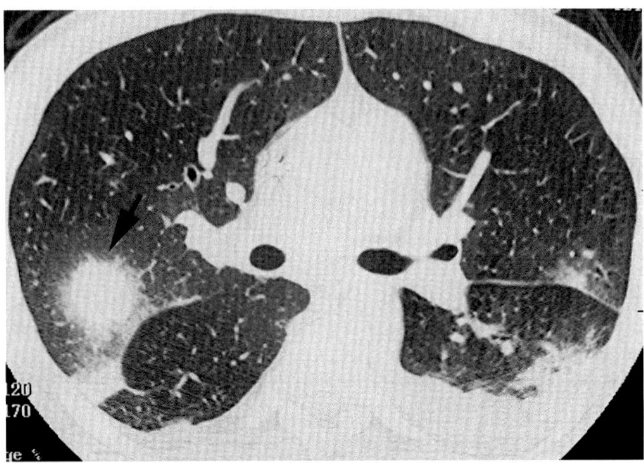

FIGURE 5-42 ■ **Angioinvasive aspergillosis.** A 65-year-old man with immunosuppression and severe neutropenia presents with fever. CT shows a nodule with surrounding ground-glass attenuation (CT halo sign) (arrow). Note also bilateral poorly marginated peripheral areas of consolidation.

immunocompromised patients, particularly in those with underlying malignancy (acute leukaemia and lymphoma), intravenous drug abuse, AIDS and following bone marrow transplantation.[76] The most common thin-section CT findings of pulmonary candidiasis consist of multiple bilateral nodular opacities often associated with areas of consolidation and ground-glass opacity (Fig. 5-43). Less common CT findings are pleural effusion, thickening of the bronchial walls and cavitation.

Pneumocystis jiroveci. *Pneumocystis jiroveci* (formerly *Pneumocystis carinii*) is a unique opportunistic fungal pathogen that causes pneumonia in immunocompromised individuals such as patients with AIDS (CD4 counts below 100 cells/mm^3), patients with organ transplants, and patients with haematological or solid organ malignancies who are undergoing chemotherapy, and in patients receiving immune-suppressive treatments, particularly systemic corticosteroids.

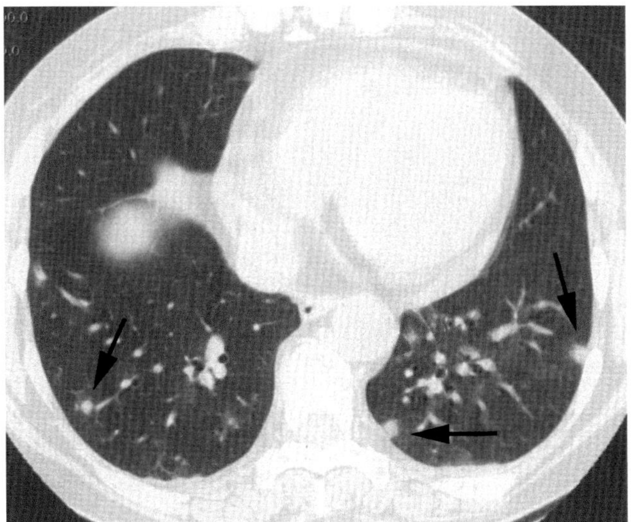

FIGURE 5-43 ■ ***Candida* pneumonia.** A 52-year-old man who underwent bone marrow transplantation. CT shows multiple ill-defined bilateral nodules (arrows).

Reportedly > 90% of patients show radiographic abnormalities, mainly the classical findings of diffuse bilateral interstitial infiltrates in a perihilar distribution, although normal radiographs do not exclude the diagnosis. In these patients, CT may be helpful in confirming the diagnosis of *Pneumocystis carinii* pneumonia (PCP) when clinical suspicion is high, typically showing images with perihilar ground-glass opacities, in a patchy or geographical distribution[77] (Fig. 5-44).

Mucormycosis. Mucormycosis is an opportunistic fungal infection of the order Mucorales, characterised by broad, non-septated hyphae that randomly branch at right angles.

The most common radiographic findings consist of lobar or multilobar areas of consolidation and solitary or multiple pulmonary nodules and masses; associated cavitation is found in 26 to 40% of cases. An air-crescent sign, highly suggestive of an invasive fungal infection, can be identified in 5 to 12.5% of cases. CT features are non-specific and consist of solitary or multiple areas of consolidation and solitary or multiples nodules surrounded by a halo of ground-glass attenuation ('halo sign') and cavitation (Fig. 5-45).

Cryptococcosis. Cryptococcosis is caused by inhaling spores of *Cryptococcus neoformans*, a fungus of worldwide distribution which is found in soil and in bird droppings. Many patients have no symptoms and the pulmonary lesions heal spontaneously.[78] Cryptococcal pneumonia is a common pulmonary infection in AIDS patients with CD4 count below 100 cells/mm^3. The most typical

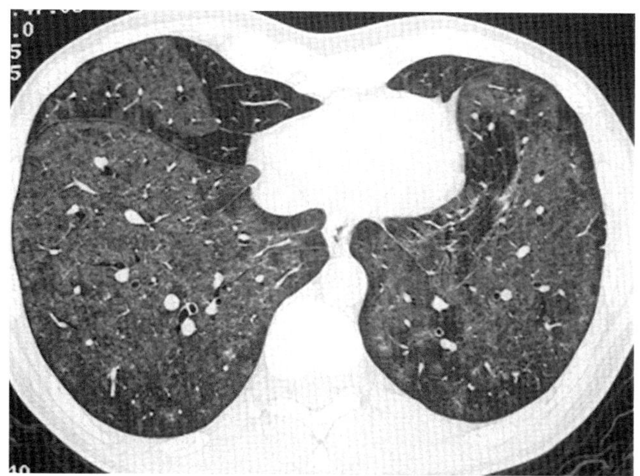

FIGURE 5-44 ■ ***Pneumocystis* pneumonia.** A 45-year-old homosexual man with severe dyspnoea. CT shows extensive bilateral ground-glass opacities. Bronchoalveolar lavage showed *P. jiroveci.*

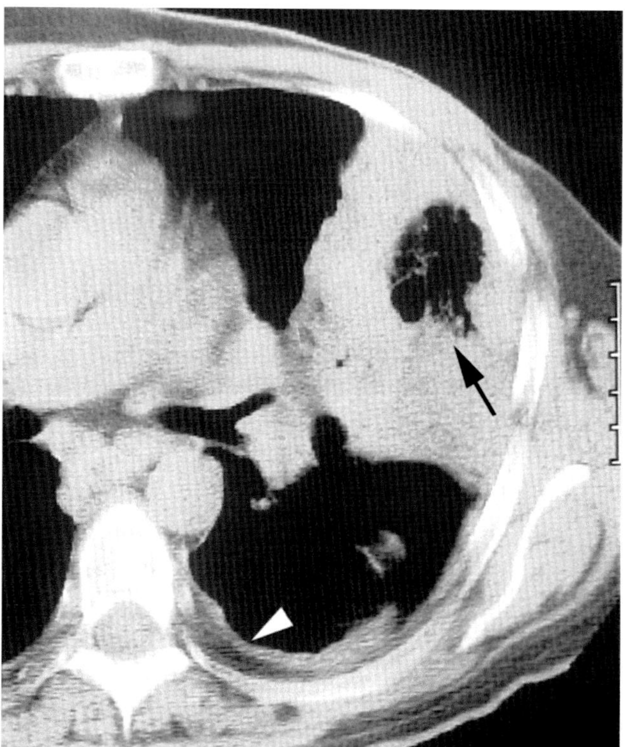

FIGURE 5-45 ■ **Mucormycosis.** A 62-year-old diabetic man with fever. A contrast-enhanced CT image shows lobar consolidation in the left upper lobe. An area of low attenuation is visible within the consolidation, consistent with abscess formation (arrow). Also note a small left pleural effusion (arrowhead).

radiographic manifestation consists of pulmonary masses, homogeneous segmental or lobar opacifications, and miliary, reticular or reticulonodular interstitial patterns (Fig. 5-46). The masses, ranging from 5 mm to very large size, usually have an ill-defined edge, may show a halo similarly to an invasive *Aspergillus* lesion and may cavitate.

Histoplasmosis. *Histoplasma capsulatum* is a fungus found in moist soil and in bird or bat excreta in many

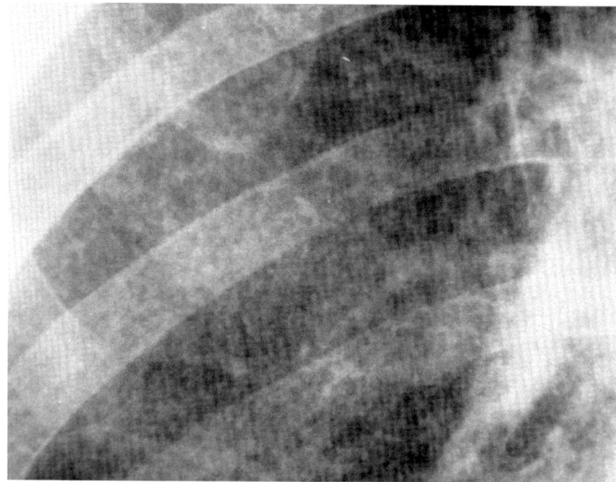

FIGURE 5-46 ■ **Cryptococcosis.** A 24-year-old HIV-positive man with dyspnoea and fever. Close-up view of a posteroanterior chest radiograph shows diffuse small ill-defined nodules.

parts of the world but human infection is endemic in areas such Ohio–Mississippi and St. Lawrence River valleys (North America).[79]

Though nodules greater than 3 cm may be seen (Fig. 5-47), the most common radiographic findings consist of diffuse nodular opacities of 3 mm or less in diameter, nodules greater than 3 mm in diameter, small linear opacities and focal or patchy areas of consolidation. As these findings are not seen on chest radiography in approximately 40% of patients with pulmonary histoplasmosis, CT is requested as a more sensitive imaging investigation. Hilar and mediastinal lymph nodes are frequently enlarged. Chronic pulmonary histoplasmosis radiologically resembles post-primary tuberculosis. In some cases, fibrosing mediastinitis may develop and can lead to constriction of mediastinal structures, including the airways, superior vena cava, pulmonary arteries and pulmonary veins.

Coccidioidomycosis. Coccidioidomycosis is caused by *Coccidioides immitis*, a fungus which is found in soil in arid regions of the southwestern United States, northern Mexico and in the semi-arid northeastern region of Brazil.

In primary coccidioidomycosis unifocal or multifocal homogeneous opacities, resembling community-acquired bacterial pneumonia, may be seen. Cavitation and hilar/mediastinal adenopathy may be seen with approximately 20% of these lesions. Primary disease almost invariably resolves spontaneously or reveals only small residual linear or nodular scars. A characteristic CT appearance consisting of a central area of soft-tissue attenuation with a surrounding halo of ground-glass attenuation may be seen around these nodules. Disseminated coccidioidomycosis may cause miliary nodules (Fig. 5-48). Chronic fibronodular cavitary disease may resemble reactivated tuberculosis.[80]

Paracoccidioidomycosis (South American Blastomycosis). Paracoccidioidomycosis (PCM), an endemic disease caused by the dimorphic fungus *Paracoccidioides*

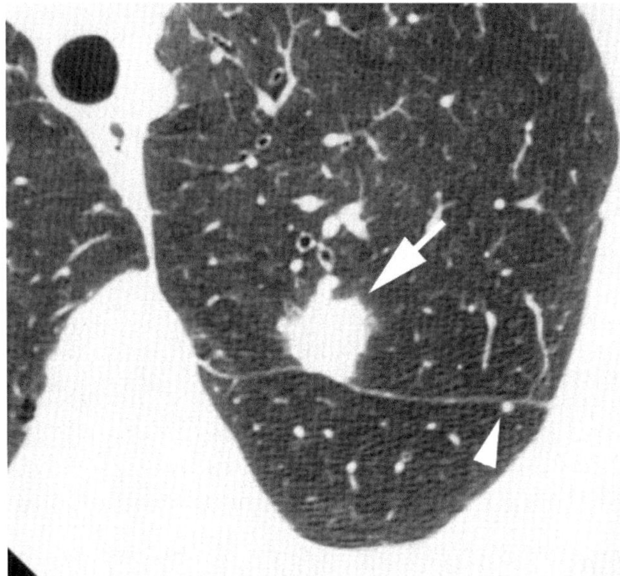

FIGURE 5-47 ■ **Histoplasmoma.** A 62-year-old asymptomatic woman living in an area endemic for histoplasmosis. An incidental nodule was found on routine chest radiography. CT shows a rounded opacity in the left upper lobe (arrow). A 3-mm nodule (arrowhead) is also seen in the superior segment of the left lower lobe.

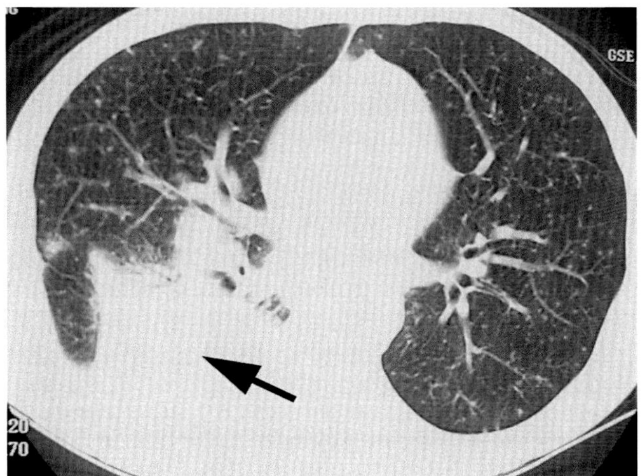

FIGURE 5-48 ■ **Coccidioidomycosis.** A 38-year-old man with vague chest pain and fever. CT shows a parenchymal consolidation in the superior segment of the right lower lobe (arrow). Note multiple miliary nodules randomly distributed through both lungs.

brasiliensis, is the most frequent systemic mycosis in Latin America, especially in Brazil. The predominant HRCT findings consist of areas of ground-glass opacities, nodules, interlobular septal thickening, airspace consolidation, cavitation and fibrosis[81] (Fig. 5-49).

North American Blastomycosis. North American blastomycosis is caused by *Blastomyces dermatitidis*. Pulmonary infection may be accompanied by infection of the skin, bones and genitourinary tract. The chest radiograph reveals homogeneous unifocal or multifocal segmental or lobar opacification indistinguishable from acute pneumonia. Cavitation occurs in approximately 15% of cases.

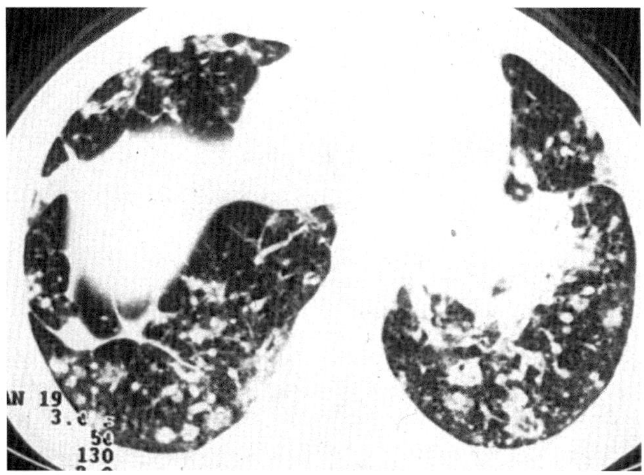

FIGURE 5-49 ■ **Paracoccidioidomycosis.** A 61-year-ol patient with cough and fever. CT at level of the lung bases shows combination of subsegmental areas of consolidation and randomly distributed bilateral ill-defined nodules of variable size. (Courtesy of Dr. Edson Marchiori, Rio de Janeiro, Brazil.)

Blastomycosis may cause miliary nodules, particularly in immunocompromised patients. A chronic fibrocavitary form of the disease is also seen.[82]

PARASITIC INFECTIONS

Parasitic infections of the lung occur worldwide among both immunocompetent and immunocompromised patients.[83] Parasitic diseases account for an increasing presence in industrialised countries because of returning travellers, immigration and mass movements as a result of political or socioeconomic reasons.

Protozoa

Amoebiasis

Pleuropulmonary amoebiasis caused by *Entamoeba histolytica* is usually secondary to liver involvement.[84] The lung is the second most common extraintestinal site of amoebic involvement after the liver. Pleuropulmonary amoebiasis is a significant complication of amoebic liver abscess. Right-sided abnormalities are found in 86% of cases and consists of hemidiaphragmatic elevation, pleural effusion or empyema, and/or thickening and plate-like atelectasis. Liver abscess can extend directly into the lung, causing pulmonary consolidation. If communication with a major bronchus occurs, haemoptysis can develop, containing the 'anchovy paste' pus coming from the amoebic abscess.

Nematodes

Dirofilariasis

Although not common in humans, dirofilariasis is occurring with increasing frequency as the canine population grows.[85] *Dirofilaria immitis*, or the dog heartworm, is a rare cause of pulmonary nodules in humans. The majority of patients with dirofilariasis are asymptomatic. *Dirofilaria immitis* is transmitted by mosquitoes from dogs to humans. An immature adult worm unable to mature in the accidental human host can reach a peripheral vein and travel in the bloodstream until it lodges in a pulmonary vein. The disease has been reported predominantly in the temperate climates of the East Coast and Southern United States, but sporadic cases have been found worldwide.[86]

Cestodes

Echinococcosis (Hydatid Disease)

Hydatid disease (echinococcosis) is caused by the larval forms of *Echinococcus granulosus*, *Echinococcus multilocularis* and *Echinococcus vogeli*. *Echinococcus granulosus* (unilocular cystic echinococcosis) is the most common form affecting man and is seen in the Mediterranean area, Eastern Europe, Africa, South America, the Middle East, Australia and New Zealand.

Humans are accidental hosts and acquire infection by ingesting ova from fomites or contaminated water and by direct contact with dogs. Cysts in the mediastinum, heart and pulmonary arteries are rare.

The clinical manifestations of pulmonary hydatidosis are non-specific. Complications occur because of cyst rupture. Hydatid cysts are usually solitary but may be multiple and/or bilateral in 10% of cases. They may be ruptured (two-thirds) or unruptured (one-third) at the time of presentation. Aggressive invasion of vascular structures such as bronchial and pulmonary arteries may result in massive haemoptysis and haemorrhage.

The radiological findings in patients with unruptured pulmonary cysts are one or more homogeneous, roughly spherical or oval, sharply demarcated mass lesions. Cyst rupture is usually associated with secondary infection and may spread into the airways or pleural space.[87]

The radiographic appearance resembles the air crescent of a mycetoma. Should there be disruption of the inner layers, a complex cavitary lesion results with one or more of the following radiographic features: an air–fluid level, a floating membrane (water lily sign, camalote sign) (Fig. 5-50), a double wall, an essentially dry cyst with crumpled membranes lying at its bottom (rising sun sign, serpent sign), and a cyst with all its contents expectorated (empty cyst sign). Secondary infection of a hydatid cyst may produce a lung abscess with or without surrounding lung opacity. Rupture into the pleural space causes an effusion or, if there is airway communication, a hydropneumothorax.[87]

Trematodes

Paragonimiasis

Pleuropulmonary paragonimiasis is a disease caused by a fluke (*Paragonimus westermani*) characterised by migration of a juvenile worm in the early stage and by formation of cysts around the worm later on.[88] Water snails and crustaceans are intermediate hosts and infestations are acquired from eating raw or incompletely cooked fresh

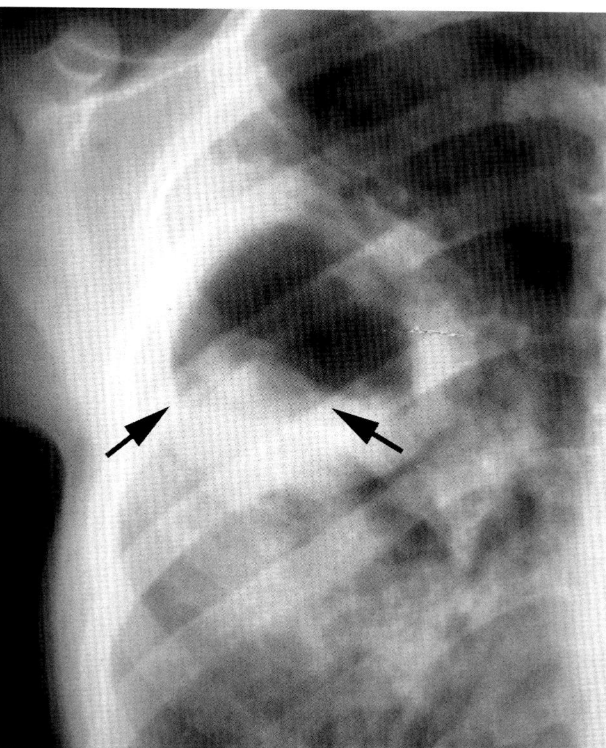

FIGURE 5-50 ■ **Ruptured hydatid cyst.** A 65-year-old male shepherd with abrupt onset of expectoration and pruritus. Close-up view of the right upper lung shows a cystic lesion surrounded by a parenchymal consolidation due to a massive aspiration of intracystic content. Note a rounded opacity immediately above the fluid level ('water lily' sign) (arrows).

water crabs and crayfish. The disease mainly occurs in the Far East, southeast Asia and Africa.

Radiological changes tend to be bilateral, including a mixture of consolidation, nodules and band, tubular and ring opacities. In the lower lobes parenchymal changes mimic bronchiectasis, and in the upper lobes, tuberculosis. The constellation of focal pleural thickening and subpleural linear opacities leading to a necrotic peripheral pulmonary nodule is another frequent CT finding of paragonimiasis.

REFERENCES

1. Franquet T. Imaging of pneumonia: trends and algorithms. Eur Respir J 2001;18(1):196–208.
2. American Thoracic Society, Infectious Diseases Society of America. 2005 Guidelines for the management of adults with hospital-acquired, ventilator-associated, and healthcare-associated pneumonia. Am J Respir Crit Care Med 2005;171(4):388–416.
3. Anand N, Kollef MH. The alphabet soup of pneumonia: CAP, HAP, HCAP, NHAP, and VAP. Semin Respir Crit Care Med 2009;30(1):3–9.
4. Mandell LA, Wunderink RG, Anzueto A, et al. Infectious Diseases Society of America/American Thoracic Society consensus guidelines on the management of community-acquired pneumonia in adults. Clin Infect Dis 2007;44(Suppl 2):S27–72.
5. Hagaman JT, Rouan GW, Shipley RT, Panos RJ. Admission chest radiograph lacks sensitivity in the diagnosis of community-acquired pneumonia. Am J Med Sci 2009;337(4):236–40.
6. Chastre J, Fagon JY. Ventilator-associated pneumonia. Am J Respir Crit Care Med 2002;165(7):867–903.
7. Franquet T, Gimenez A, Roson N, et al. Aspiration diseases: findings, pitfalls, and differential diagnosis. Radiographics 2000;20(3):673–85.

8. Valente T, Lassandro F, Marino M, et al. H1N1 pneumonia: our experience in 50 patients with a severe clinical course of novel swine-origin influenza A (H1N1) virus (S-OIV). Radiol Med 2012;117(2):165–84.
9. Muller MP, McGeer A. Severe acute respiratory syndrome (SARS) coronavirus. Semin Respir Crit Care Med 2007;28(2): 201–12.
10. Heussel CP, Kauczor HU, Heussel G, et al. Early detection of pneumonia in febrile neutropenic patients: use of thin-section CT. Am J Roentgenol 1997;169(5):1347–53.
11. Heussel CP, Kauczor HU, Heussel GE, et al. Pneumonia in febrile neutropenic patients and in bone marrow and blood stem-cell transplant recipients: use of high-resolution computed tomography. J Clin Oncol 1999;17(3):796–805.
12. Niederman MS, Mandell LA, Anzueto A, et al. Guidelines for the management of adults with community-acquired pneumonia. Diagnosis, assessment of severity, antimicrobial therapy, and prevention. Am J Resp Crit Care Med 2001;163(7):1730–54.
13. Müller NL, Fraser RS, Lee KS, Johkoh T. Diseases of the Lung: Radiologic and Pathologic Correlations. Philadelphia: Lippincott Williams & Wilkins; 2003.
14. Travis WD, Colby TV, Koss MN, et al. Non-neoplastic Disorders of the Lower Respiratory Tract. Washington, DC. 2002.
15. Mori T, Ebe T, Takahashi M, et al. Lung abscess: analysis of 66 cases from 1979 to 1991. Intern Med 1993;32(4):278–84.
16. Fraser RS, Müller NL, Colman N, Paré PD. Diagnosis of Diseases of the Chest. 4th ed. Philadelphia: Saunders; 1999.
17. Fraser RS, Colman N, Müller NL, Pare PD. Synopsis of Diseases of the Chest. Philadelphia: Elsevier Saunders; 2005.
18. Quigley MJ, Fraser RS. Pulmonary pneumatocele: pathology and pathogenesis. Am J Roentgenol 1988;150(6):1275–7.
19. Kuhlman JE, Fishman EK, Teigen C. Pulmonary septic emboli: diagnosis with CT. Radiology 1990;174(1):211–13.
20. Sarkar P, Patel N, Chusid J, et al. The role of computed tomography bronchography in the management of bronchopleural fistulas. J Thorac Imaging 2010;25(1):W10–13.
21. Falguera M, Sacristan O, Nogues A, et al. Nonsevere community-acquired pneumonia: correlation between cause and severity or comorbidity. Arch Intern Med 2001;161(15):1866–72.
22. Shah RM, Friedman AC. CT angiogram sign: incidence and significance in lobar consolidations evaluated by contrast-enhanced CT. Am J Roentgenol 1998;170(3):719–21.
23. Light RW, Girard WM, Jenkinson SG, George RB. Parapneumonic effusions. Am J Med 1980;69(4):507–12.
24. Ferrero F, Nascimento-Carvalho CM, Cardoso MR, et al. Radiographic findings among children hospitalized with severe community-acquired pneumonia. Pediatr Pulmonol 2010;45(10): 1009–13.
25. Okada F, Ando Y, Honda K, et al. Clinical and pulmonary thin-section CT findings in acute *Klebsiella pneumoniae* pneumonia. Eur Radiol 2009;19(4):809–15.
26. Pope TL Jr, Armstrong P, Thompson R, Donowitz GR. Pittsburgh pneumonia agent: chest film manifestations. Am J Roentgenol 1982;138(2):237–41.
27. Blasi F, Tarsia P, Arosio C, et al. Epidemiology of *Chlamydia pneumoniae*. Clin Microbiol Infect 1998;4(Suppl 4):S1–6.
28. Gaillat J, Flahault A, deBarbeyrac B, et al. Community epidemiology of *Chlamydia* and *Mycoplasma pneumoniae* in LRTI in France over 29 months. Eur J Epidemiol 2005;20(7):643–51.
29. Simmons WP. *Moraxella catarrhalis* pneumonia and bacteremia in an otherwise healthy child. Clin Pediatr 1999;38(9):560–1.
30. Godwin JD, Muller NL, Takasugi JE. Pulmonary alveolar proteinosis: CT findings. Radiology 1988;169(3):609–13.
31. Kwong JS, Muller NL, Godwin JD, et al. Thoracic actinomycosis: CT findings in eight patients. Radiology 1992;183(1):189–92.
32. Kim TS, Han J, Koh WJ, et al. Endobronchial actinomycosis associated with broncholithiasis: CT findings for nine patients. Am J Roentgenol 2005;185(2):347–53.
33. Kim TS, Han J, Koh WJ, et al. Thoracic actinomycosis: CT features with histopathologic correlation. Am J Roentgenol 2006; 186(1):225–31.
34. Voloudaki AE, Kofteridis DP, Tritou IN, et al. Q fever pneumonia: CT findings. Radiology 2000;215(3):880–3.
35. Feldman KA, Enscore RE, Lathrop SL, et al. An outbreak of primary pneumonic tularemia on Martha's Vineyard. N Engl J Med 2001;345(22):1601–6.
36. Stralin K, Soderquist B. *Staphylococcus aureus* in community-acquired pneumonia. Chest 2006;130(2):623.
37. Micek ST, Dunne M, Kollef MH. Pleuropulmonary complications of Panton-Valentine leukocidin-positive community-acquired methicillin-resistant *Staphylococcus aureus*: importance of treatment with antimicrobials inhibiting exotoxin production. Chest 2005; 128(4):2732–8.
38. Macfarlane J, Rose D. Radiographic features of staphylococcal pneumonia in adults and children. Thorax 1996;51(5):539–40.
39. Jaffey PB, English PW 2nd, Campbell GA, et al. *Escherichia coli* lobar pneumonia: fatal infection in a patient with mental retardation. South Med J 1996;89(6):628–30.
40. Renner RR, Coccaro AP, Heitzman ER, et al. *Pseudomonas pneumonia*: a prototype of hospital-based infection. Radiology 1972; 105(3):555–62.
41. Gomez J, Banos V, Ruiz Gomez J, et al. Prospective study of epidemiology and prognostic factors in community-acquired pneumonia. Eur J Clin Microbiol Infect Dis 1996;15(7):556–60.
42. Bochud PY, Moser F, Erard P, et al. Community-acquired pneumonia. A prospective outpatient study. Medicine (Baltimore) 2001;80(2):75–87.
43. Tanaka N, Matsumoto T, Kuramitsu T, et al. High resolution CT findings in community-acquired pneumonia. J Comput Assist Tomogr 1996;20(4):600–8.
44. Reittner P, Muller NL, Heyneman L, et al. *Mycoplasma pneumoniae* pneumonia: radiographic and high-resolution CT features in 28 patients. Am J Roentgenol 2000;174(1):37–41.
45. Franquet T. Imaging of pulmonary viral pneumonia. Radiology 2011;260(1):18–39.
46. Oikonomou A, Muller NL, Nantel S. Radiographic and high-resolution CT findings of influenza virus pneumonia in patients with hematologic malignancies. Am J Roentgenol 2003;181(2): 507–11.
47. Hsieh WY, Chiu NC, Chi H, et al. Respiratory adenoviral infections in Taiwanese children: a hospital-based study. J Microbiol Immunol Infect 2009;42(5):371–7.
48. Muller NL. Unilateral hyperlucent lung: MacLeod versus Swyer-James. Clin Radiol 2004;59(11):1048.
49. Lucaya J, Gartner S, Garcia-Pena P, et al. Spectrum of manifestations of Swyer-James-MacLeod syndrome. J Comput Assist Tomogr 1998;22(4):592–7.
50. Kim JS, Ryu CW, Lee SI, et al. High-resolution CT findings of varicella-zoster pneumonia. Am J Roentgenol 1999;172(1):113–16.
51. Gasparetto EL, Escuissato DL, Inoue C, et al. Herpes simplex virus type 2 pneumonia after bone marrow transplantation: high-resolution CT findings in 3 patients. J Thorac Imaging 2005; 20(2):71–3.
52. Duchin JS, Koster FT, Peters CJ, et al. Hantavirus pulmonary syndrome: a clinical description of 17 patients with a newly recognized disease. The Hantavirus Study Group. N Engl J Med 1994; 330(14):949–55.
53. Ketai LH, Williamson MR, Telepak RJ, et al. Hantavirus pulmonary syndrome: radiographic findings in 16 patients. Radiology 1994;191(3):665–8.
54. Ketai LH, Kelsey CA, Jordan K, et al. Distinguishing hantavirus pulmonary syndrome from acute respiratory distress syndrome by chest radiography: are there different radiographic manifestations of increased alveolar permeability? J Thorac Imaging 1998;13(3): 172–7.
55. Gasparetto EL, Ono SE, Escuissato D, et al. Cytomegalovirus pneumonia after bone marrow transplantation: high resolution CT findings. Br J Radiol 2004;77(921):724–7.
56. Franquet T, Lee KS, Muller NL. Thin-section CT findings in 32 immunocompromised patients with cytomegalovirus pneumonia who do not have AIDS. Am J Roentgenol 2003;181(4): 1059–63.
57. Franquet T, Rodriguez S, Martino R, et al. Human metapneumovirus infection in hematopoietic stem cell transplant recipients: high-resolution computed tomography findings. J Comput Assist Tomogr 2005;29(2):223–7.
58. Qureshi NR, Hien TT, Farrar J, Gleeson FV. The radiologic manifestations of H5N1 avian influenza. J Thorac Imaging 2006;21(4): 259–64.
59. Chowell G, Bertozzi SM, Colchero MA, et al. Severe respiratory disease concurrent with the circulation of H1N1 influenza. N Engl J Med 2009;361(7):674–9.

60. Centers for Disease Control and Prevention (CDC). Pneumocystis pneumonia—Los Angeles. MMWR Morb Mortal Wkly Rep 1981;30(21):250–2.
61. Shelburne SA 3rd, Hamill RJ, Rodriguez-Barradas MC, et al. Immune reconstitution inflammatory syndrome: emergence of a unique syndrome during highly active antiretroviral therapy. Medicine (Baltimore) 2002;81(3):213–27.
62. Buckingham SJ, Haddow LJ, Shaw PJ, Miller RF. Immune reconstitution inflammatory syndrome in HIV-infected patients with mycobacterial infections starting highly active anti-retroviral therapy. Clin Radiol 2004;59(6):505–13.
63. Miller WT, Miller WT Jr. Tuberculosis in the normal host: radiological findings. Semin Roentgenol 1993;28(2):109–18.
64. Aquino SL, Gamsu G, Webb WR, Kee ST. Tree-in-bud pattern: frequency and significance on thin section CT. J Comput Assist Tomogr 1996;20(4):594–9.
65. Kim JY, Jeong YJ, Kim KI, et al. Miliary tuberculosis: a comparison of CT findings in HIV-seropositive and HIV-seronegative patients. Br J Radiol 2010;83(987):206–11.
66. Jeong YJ, Lee KS. Pulmonary tuberculosis: up-to-date imaging and management. Am J Roentgenol 2008;191(3):834–44.
67. Pipavath SN, Sharma SK, Sinha S, et al. High resolution CT (HRCT) in miliary tuberculosis (MTB) of the lung: Correlation with pulmonary function tests & gas exchange parameters in north Indian patients. Indian J Med Res 2007;126(3):193–8.
68. Reich JM. Pathogenesis of Lady Windermere syndrome. Scand J Infect Dis 2012;44(1):1–2.
69. Gefter WB. The spectrum of pulmonary aspergillosis. J Thorac Imaging 1992;7(4):56–74.
70. Franquet T. Respiratory infection in the AIDS and immunocompromised patient. Eur Radiol 2004;14(Suppl 3):E21–33.
71. Agarwal R. High attenuation mucoid impaction in allergic bronchopulmonary aspergillosis. World J Radiol 2010;2(1):41–3.
72. Franquet T, Muller NL, Oikonomou A, Flint JD. Aspergillus infection of the airways: computed tomography and pathologic findings. J Comput Assist Tomogr 2004;28(1):10–16.
73. Kuhlman JE, Fishman EK, Burch PA, et al. Invasive pulmonary aspergillosis in acute leukemia. The contribution of CT to early diagnosis and aggressive management. Chest 1987;92(1):95–9.
74. Kuhlman JE, Fishman EK, Burch PA, et al. CT of invasive pulmonary aspergillosis. Am J Roentgenol 1988;150(5):1015–20.
75. Kuhlman JE, Fishman EK, Siegelman SS. Invasive pulmonary aspergillosis in acute leukemia: characteristic findings on CT, the CT halo sign, and the role of CT in early diagnosis. Radiology 1985;157(3):611–14.
76. Franquet T, Muller NL, Lee KS, et al. Pulmonary candidiasis after hematopoietic stem cell transplantation: thin-section CT findings. Radiology 2005;236(1):332–7.
77. Hidalgo A, Falco V, Mauleon S, et al. Accuracy of high-resolution CT in distinguishing between *Pneumocystis carinii* pneumonia and non-*Pneumocystis carinii* pneumonia in AIDS patients. Eur Radiol 2003;13(5):1179–84.
78. Choe YH, Moon H, Park SJ, et al. Pulmonary cryptococcosis in asymptomatic immunocompetent hosts. Scand J Infect Dis 2009; 41(8):602–7.
79. McAdams HP, Rosado-de-Christenson ML, Lesar M, et al. Thoracic mycoses from endemic fungi: radiologic-pathologic correlation. Radiographics 1995;15(2):255–70.
80. Kim KI, Leung AN, Flint JD, Muller NL. Chronic pulmonary coccidioidomycosis: computed tomographic and pathologic findings in 18 patients. Can Assoc Radiol J 1998;49(6):401–7.
81. Souza AS Jr, Gasparetto EL, Davaus T, et al. High-resolution CT findings of 77 patients with untreated pulmonary paracoccidioidomycosis. Am J Roentgenol 2006;187(5):1248–52.
82. Fang W, Washington L, Kumar N. Imaging manifestations of blastomycosis: a pulmonary infection with potential dissemination. Radiographics 2007;27(3):641–55.
83. Kunst H, Mack D, Kon OM, et al. Parasitic infections of the lung: a guide for the respiratory physician. Thorax 2011;66(6):528–36.
84. Kimura K, Stoopen M, Reeder MM, Moncada R. Amebiasis: modern diagnostic imaging with pathological and clinical correlation. Semin Roentgenol 1997;32(4):250–75.
85. Martinez S, Restrepo CS, Carrillo JA, et al. Thoracic manifestations of tropical parasitic infections: a pictorial review. Radiographics 2005;25(1):135–55.
86. Levinson ED, Ziter FM Jr, Westcott JL. Pulmonary lesions due to *Dirofilaria immitis* (dog heartworm). Report of four cases with radiologic findings. Radiology 1979;131(2):305–7.
87. Pedrosa I, Saiz A, Arrazola J, et al. Hydatid disease: radiologic and pathologic features and complications. Radiographics 2000;20(3): 795–817.
88. Im JG, Whang HY, Kim WS, et al. Pleuropulmonary paragonimiasis: radiologic findings in 71 patients. Am J Roentgenol 1992; 159(1):39–43.

CHAPTER 6

Airway Disease and Chronic Airway Obstruction

Philippe A. Grenier • Catherine Beigelman-Aubry

CHAPTER OUTLINE

INTRODUCTION

The purpose of this chapter is to review lesions involving the trachea and proximal bronchi, to describe the radiological signs of bronchiectasis and to discuss the role of imaging in obstructive lung disease, a group of diffuse lung disease associated with chronic airflow obstruction that includes chronic obstructive pulmonary disease (COPD), asthma and obliterative bronchiolitis. In obstructive lung disease, decreased expiratory flow may be related to loss of lung recoil or small airway obstruction or combination of both. The abnormality which is better correlated with loss of recoil is emphysema. The process that causes the small airway obstruction is inflammatory in nature and is characterised by thickening of all the layers of the bronchiolar walls as well as an accumulation of mucus in the airway lumen (COPD and asthma), and/or an irreversible fibrosis (COPD and obliterative bronchiolitis).

TRACHEAL DISORDERS[1–8]

The trachea may be affected by a variety of extrinsic or intrinsic processes. Extrinsic processes, particularly masses, displace and distort the trachea, while intrinsic ones cause narrowing, widening or a mass effect. Tracheal narrowing may affect a short or a long segment, and may extend to the mainstem bronchi. Tracheal disease, often initially missed on CXR, is usually evident on careful evaluation of the frontal and lateral radiographs. CT allows precise delineation of the intratracheal and extratracheal extent of the abnormality. Multidetector CT, by combining helical volumetric CT acquisition and thin collimation during a single breath-hold, provides an accurate assessment of proximal airways, allowing multiplanar reformations and 3D rendering of high quality. Complementary CT acquisition at suspended or continuous expiration allows for assessing tracheal collapsibility.

Post-Traumatic Strictures[7]

Strictures of the trachea are usually secondary to damage from a cuffed endotracheal or tracheostomy tube or to external neck trauma. The lesions consist of granulation tissue leading to dense mucosal and submucosal fibrosis associated with distortion of cartilage plates. The two principal sites of stenosis following intubation or tracheostomy are at the level of the stoma or the endotracheal balloon.

On radiography, the stenosis may be seen as a focus of circumferential or eccentric narrowing associated with a segment of increased soft tissue. The size of narrowing is usually well seen at CT and is often concentric. Post-intubation stenosis extends for several centimetres and is typically seen above the level of the thoracic inlet. Post-tracheostomy stenosis typically begins 1–1.5 cm distal to the inferior stromal margin and extends for 1.5–2.5 cm. Multiplanar reformations accurately determine the site, the length and the degree of the stenosis (Fig. 6-1). In selected cases, the degree of stenosis may also be attained by use of virtual bronchoscopy.

Infectious Tracheobronchitis[3–7]

A number of infections, both acute and more often chronic, may affect the trachea and proximal bronchi, resulting in both focal and diffuse airway disease. Subsequent fibrosis may result in localised airway narrowing. The commonest causes of infectious tracheobronchitis are bacterial tracheitis in immunocompromised patients (Fig. 6-2), tuberculosis, rhinoscleroma (*Klebsiella rhinoscleromatis*), and necrotising invasive aspergillosis. On CT,

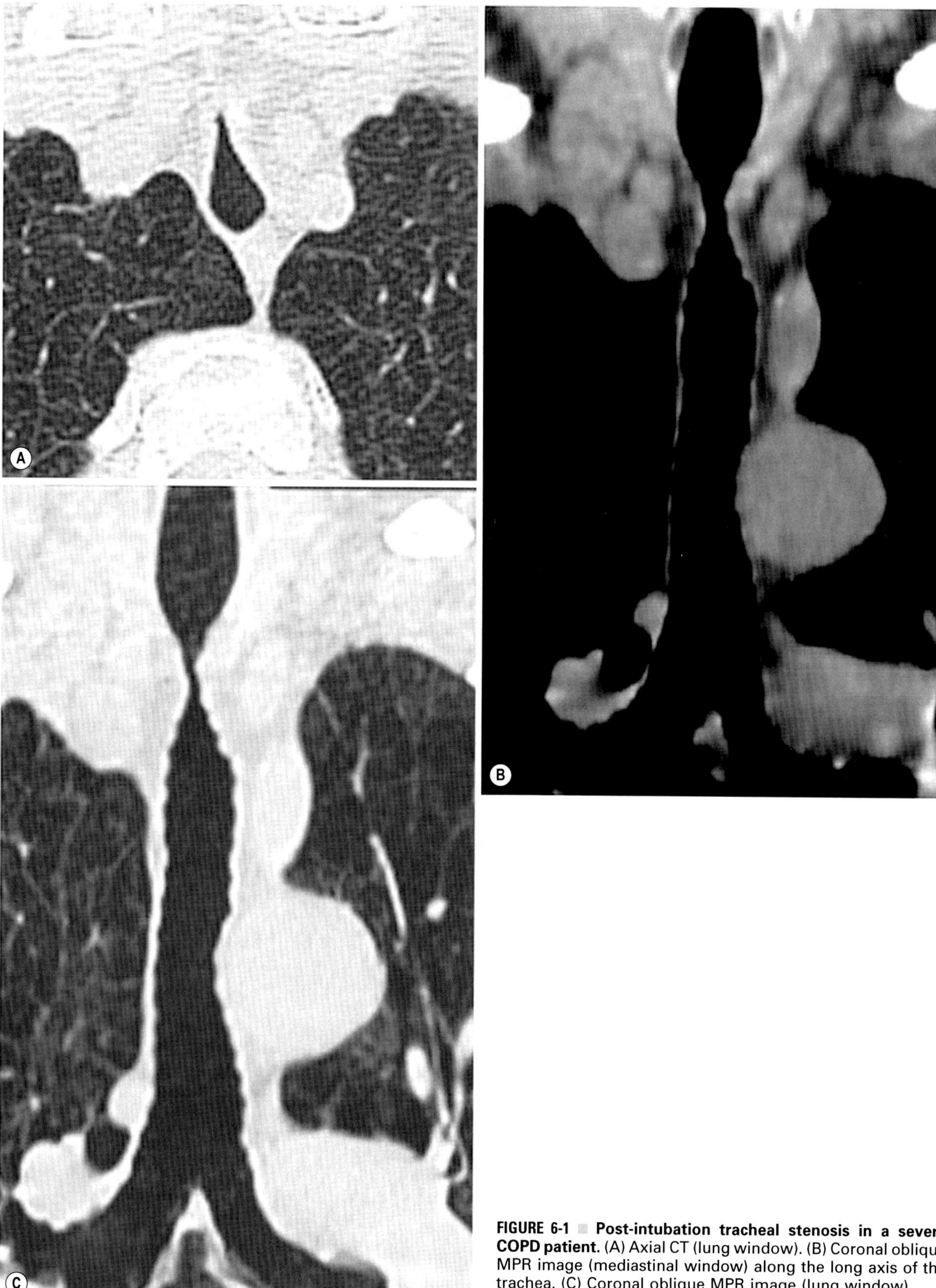

FIGURE 6-1 ■ Post-intubation tracheal stenosis in a severe COPD patient. (A) Axial CT (lung window). (B) Coronal oblique MPR image (mediastinal window) along the long axis of the trachea. (C) Coronal oblique MPR image (lung window).

Continued on following page

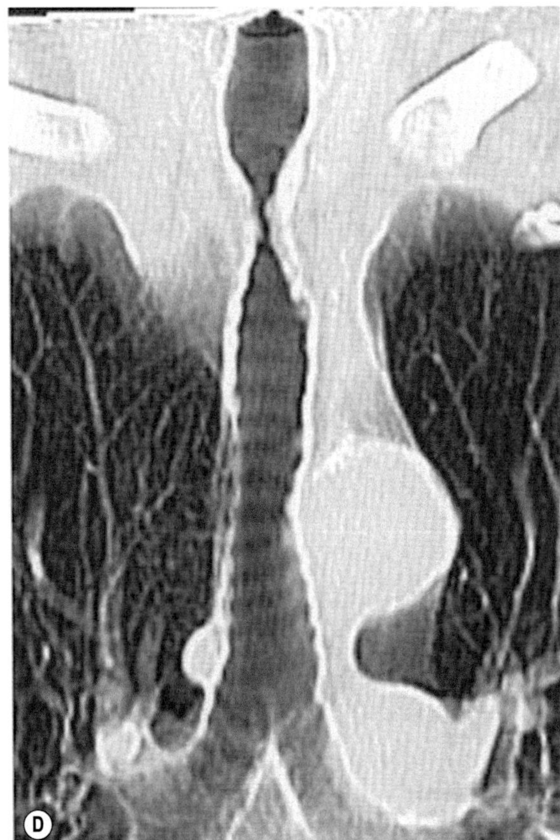

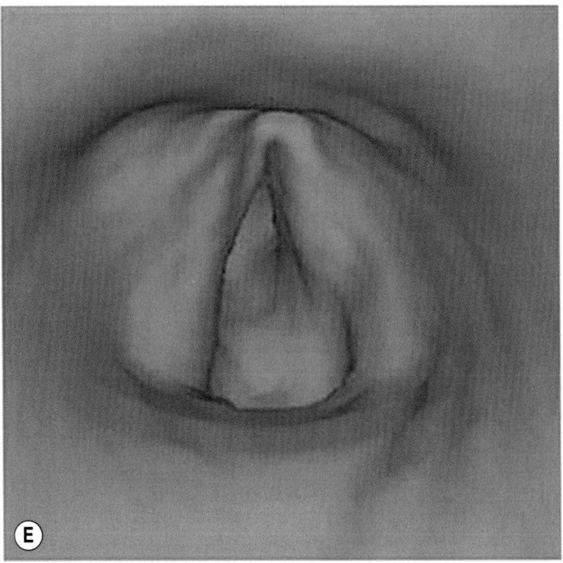

FIGURE 6-1, Continued ■ (D) Coronal oblique average image (21-mm-thick slab). Note the visibility of the ring cartilages of the trachea. (E) Endoscopic view. There is a circumferential luminal narrowing of the trachea extending along 2 cm associated with soft-tissue thickening which produces the characteristic 'hourglass' configuration, well assessed on coronal views (C, D). Note the roughly triangular shape on axial views (A, E) and the slightly irregular and nodular aspect on 3D image (E).

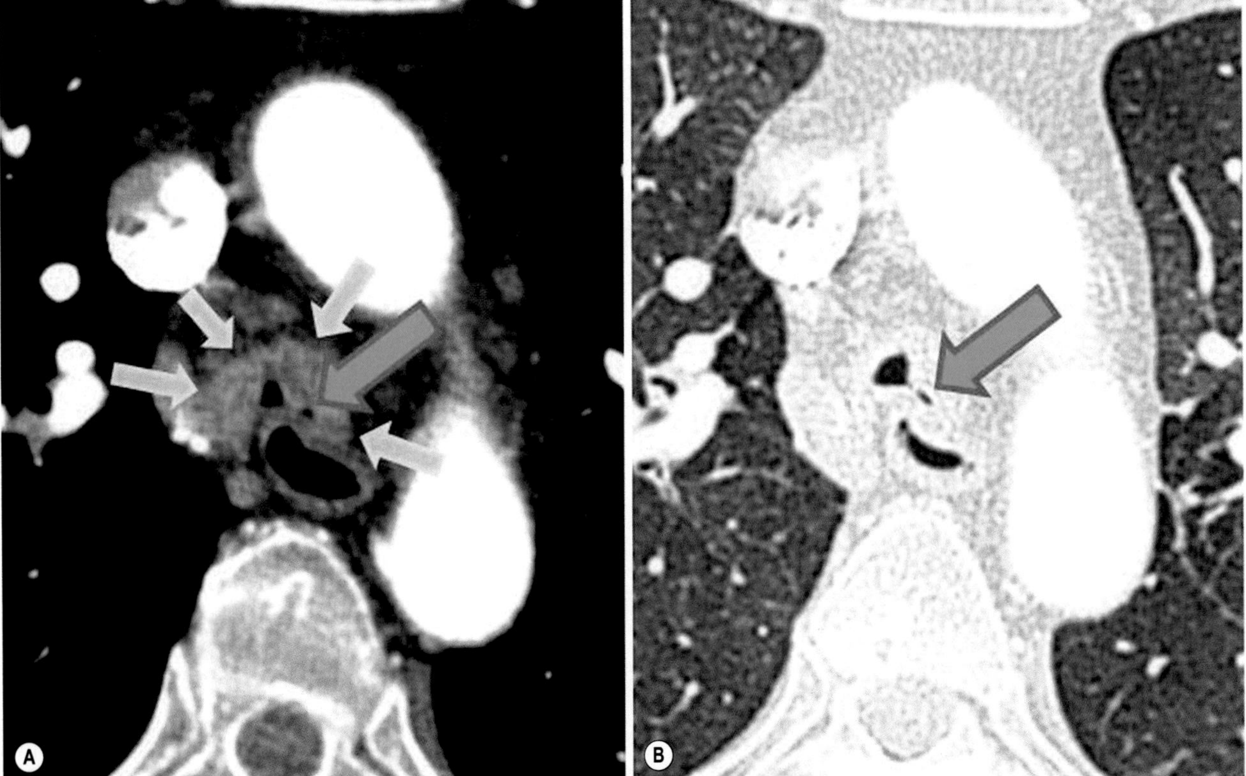

FIGURE 6-2 ■ **Infectious tracheobronchitis.** Bacterial tracheitis in a severely immunocompromised patient suffering from a rheumatoid arthritis with vasculitis. She presented with dyspnoea and cough as she was in agranulocytosis secondary to cyclophosphamide treatment. A severe stenosis of the distal trachea (orange arrows) and proximal main bronchi predominant on the left side associated with a fistulous tract (blue arrow) connecting with a paratracheal submucosal abcess was shown during bronchoscopy. This was related to *Pseudomonas aeruginosa*, *Escherichia coli* and *Streptococcus* infection. (A) Axial CT (mediastinal window) at the level of the distal part of the trachea showing the irregular thickening with a lucency on the left side (blue arrow) related to the fistulous tract. (B) Axial CT (lung window) at the same level.

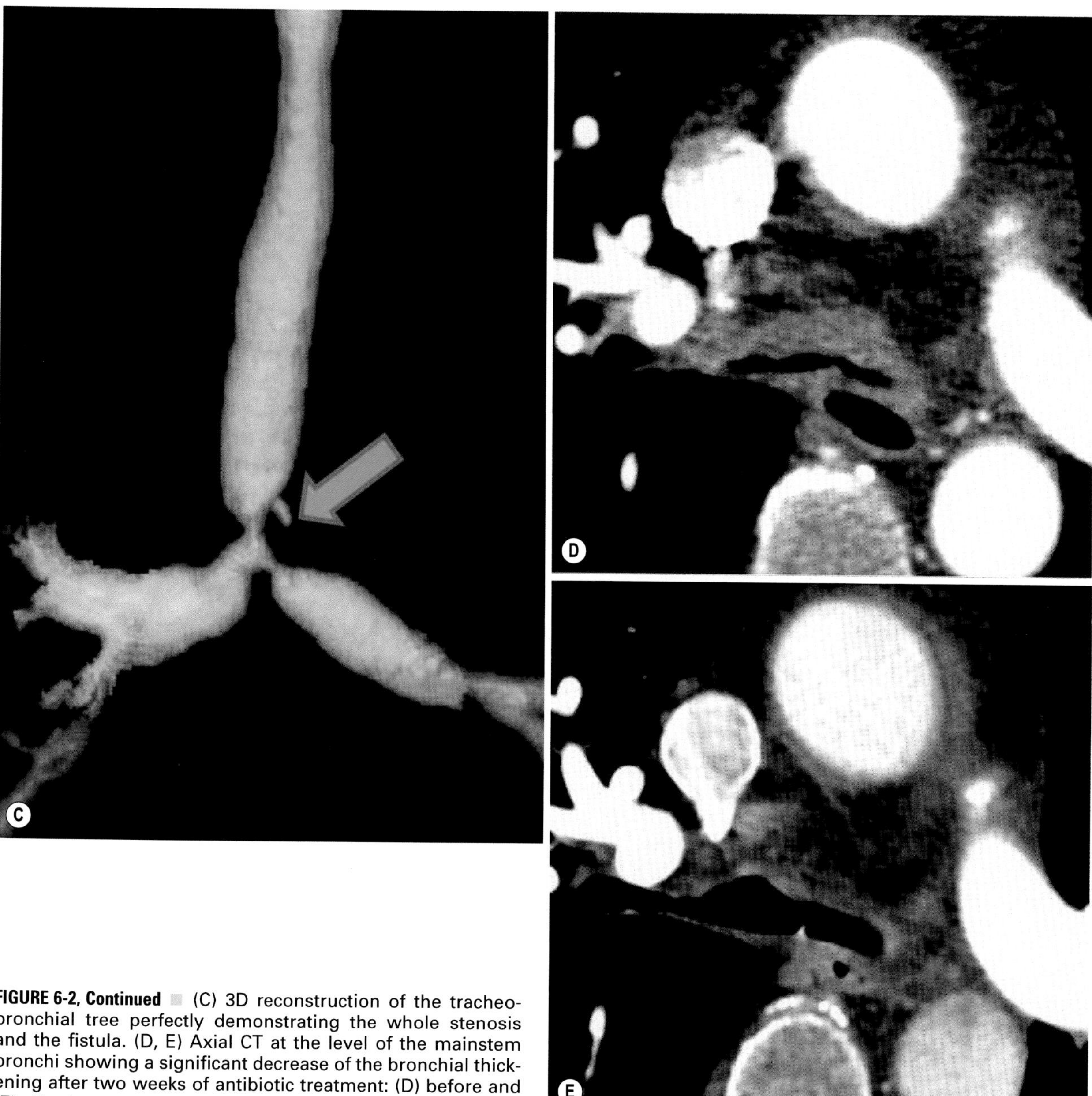

FIGURE 6-2, Continued (C) 3D reconstruction of the tracheobronchial tree perfectly demonstrating the whole stenosis and the fistula. (D, E) Axial CT at the level of the mainstem bronchi showing a significant decrease of the bronchial thickening after two weeks of antibiotic treatment: (D) before and (E) after treatment.

the extent of irregular and circumferential tracheobronchial narrowing is clearly demonstrated, with an accompanying mediastinitis (opacification of the mediastinal fat) evident in some patients. In active disease, the narrowed trachea (and frequently a main bronchus) has an irregularly thickened wall. In the fibrotic or healed phase, the trachea is narrowed but has a smooth and normal thickness wall.

Primary Malignant Neoplasms[2–4,6,8]

They are uncommon, accounting for less than 1% of all thoracic malignancies. Most are squamous cell carcinomas and adenoid cystic carcinomas (Fig. 6-3). Other neoplasms, such as mucoepidermoid carcinoma, carcinoid tumour (Fig. 6-4), lymphoma, plasmocytoma and adenocarcinoma are rare. On CT, they appear as a soft-tissue mass, usually affecting the posterior and lateral wall (Fig. 6-3A). Often sessile and eccentric, resulting in asymmetric luminal narrowing, they are occasionally circumferential. They can be polypoid and mostly intraluminal, with mediastinal extension in 30–40%. The surface of tumour is often irregular in squamous cell carcinoma, whereas it is smooth in adenoid cystic carcinoma. Multiplanar reformation and volumetric rendering images are recommended for a precise pre-therapeutic assessment of extent (Figs. 6-3B, 6-4B and 6-4D). These tumours are best treated surgically (primary resection and re-anastomosis), followed by radiation.

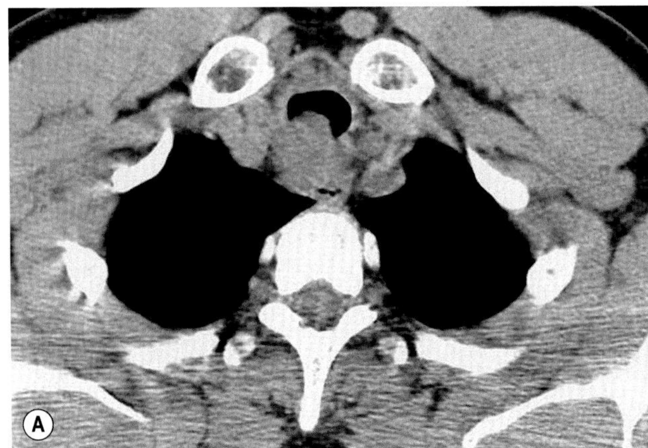

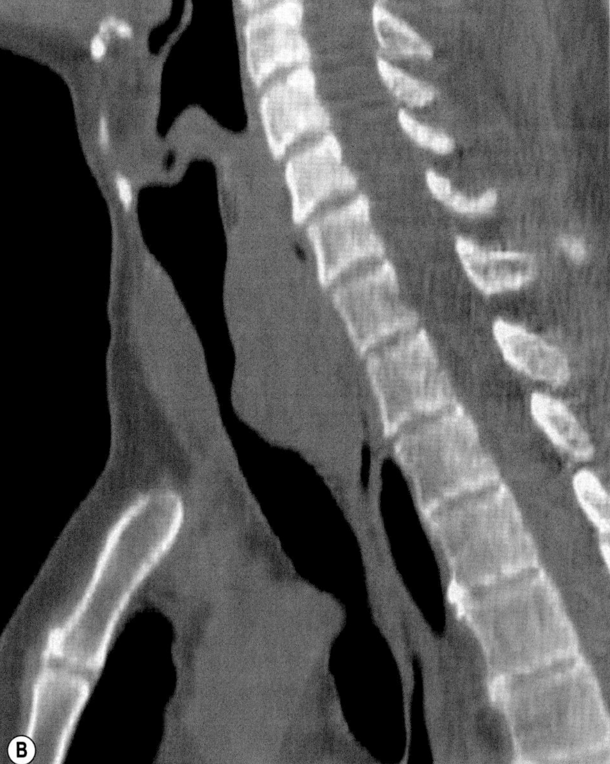

FIGURE 6-3 ■ **Adenoid cystic carcinoma of the trachea.** (A) Axial CT at the level of the supra-aortic part of the mediastinum. Soft-tissue mass arising from the posterior wall of the trachea and bulging into the lumen of the trachea. (B) Sagittal reformation showing the smooth appearance of the surface of the tumour, and the posterior extent of the extraluminal tumour growth.

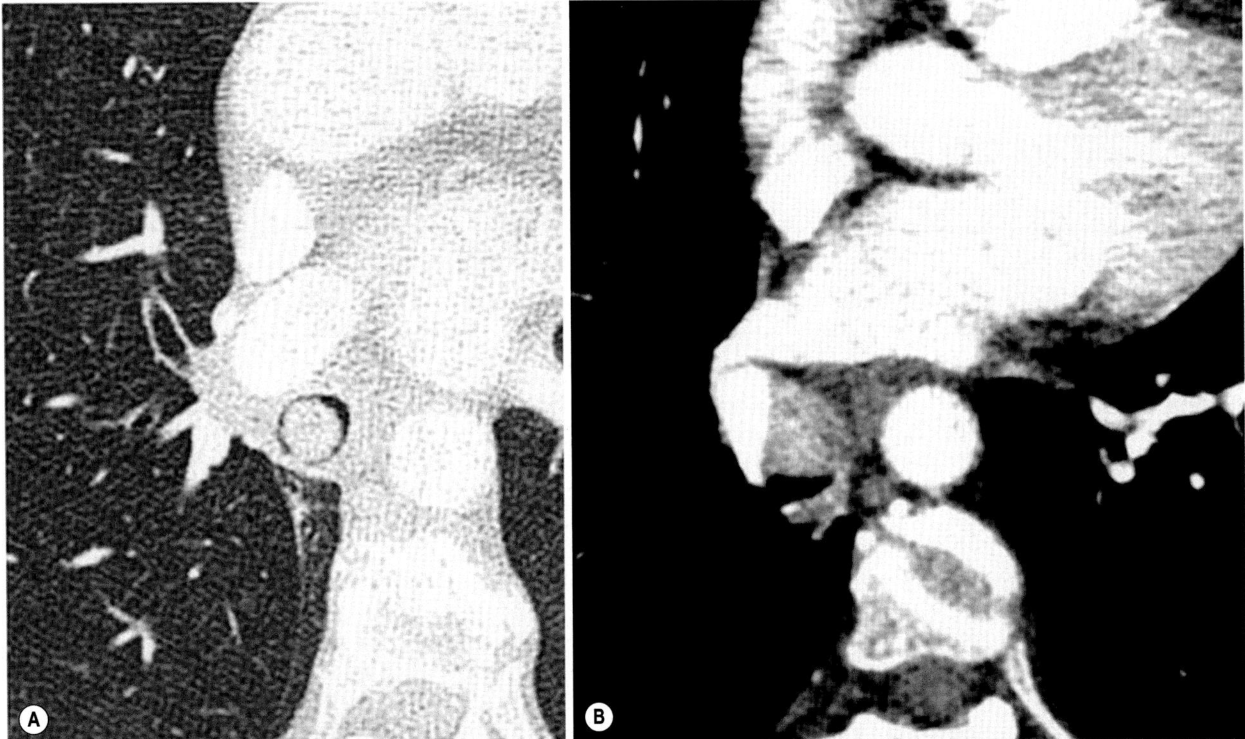

FIGURE 6-4 ■ **Atypical carcinoid tumour of the intermediate trunk.** Atypical carcinoid tumour revealed by recent recurrent haemoptysis. (A) Axial slice (lung window) showing the upper portion of the endobronchial lesion with a rounded shape. (B) Axial slice (mediastinal window) showing strong enhancement after intravenous contrast medium.

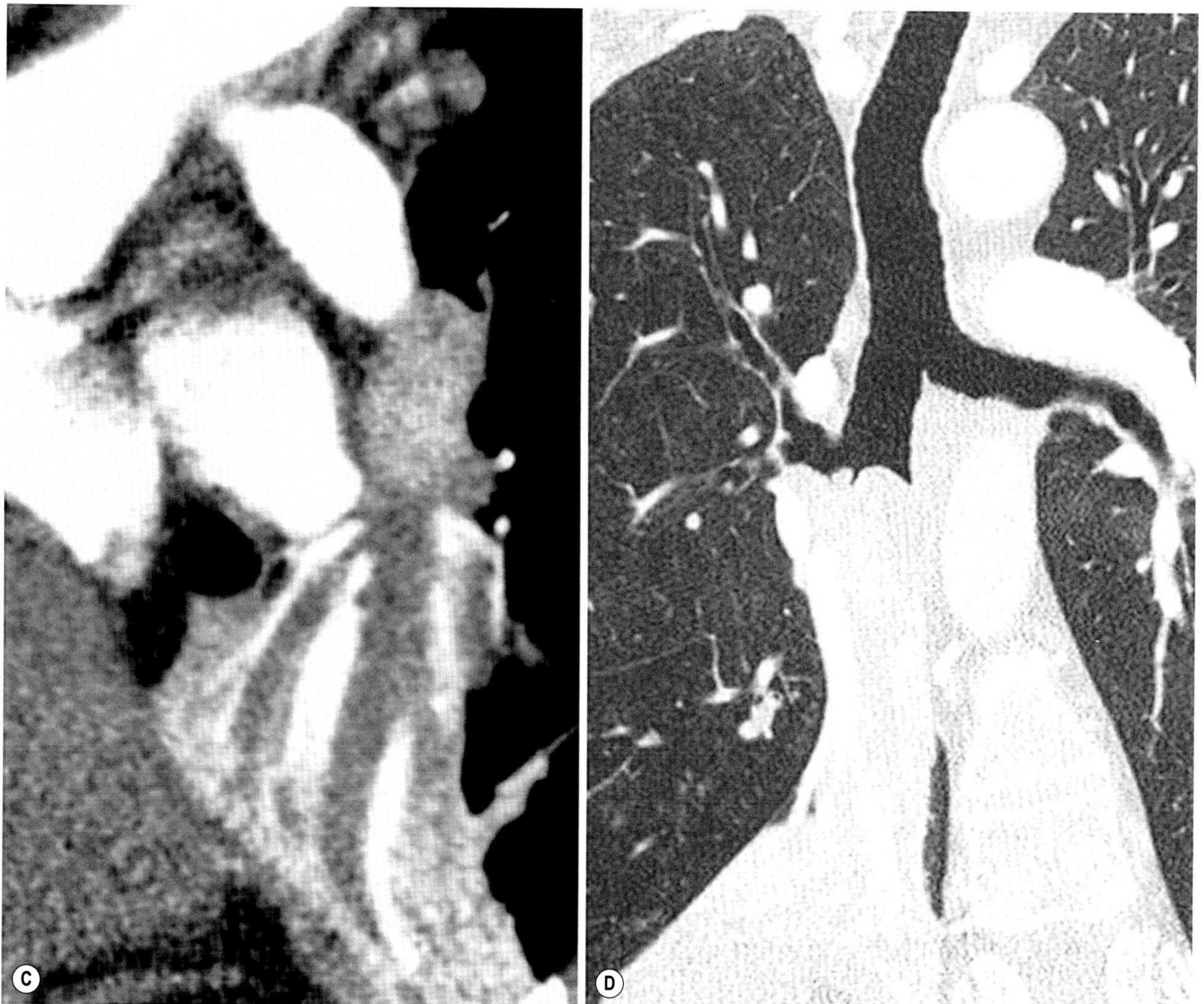

FIGURE 6-4, Continued (C) Sagittal oblique reformation (mediastinal window) demonstrating the filled bronchiectasis distally of the tumour. (D) Coronal oblique reformation (lung window) showing the upper limit of the tumour obstructing the intermediate trunk with distal atelectasis.

Secondary Malignant Neoplasms[2–4,6,8]

The large airways may be involved secondarily by malignant neoplasms as a result of either haematogenous metastasis or direct invasion from the oesophagus, thyroid, mediastinum or lung. Neoplasms that have a propensity to metastasise to the trachea and major bronchi include renal cell carcinoma and melanoma. On CT the abnormalities are usually focal and include intraluminal soft-tissue nodules and wall thickening (Fig. 6-5).

Benign Neoplasms[2–4,6,8]

The commonest benign neoplasms are hamartoma, leiomyoma, neurogenic tumour and lipoma. They are usually well demarcated, round and less than 2 cm in diameter, with typical radiological appearances of a smoothly marginated intraluminal polyp. Hamartomas and lipomas may demonstrate fat attenuation on CT.

Tracheobronchial papillomatosis is a particular entity caused by human papillomavirus infection usually acquired at birth from an infected mother. The larynx is affected most commonly; extension into the trachea and proximal bronchi occurs occasionally. Exceptionally, the infection spreads into the lung parenchyma. The typical radiological findings consist of multiple small nodules projecting into the airway lumen or diffuse nodular thickening of the airway wall. Although benign, papilloma may undergo transformation to squamous cell carcinoma.

ANCA-Associated Granulomatous Vasculitis[2,3,7]

Involvement of the large airways is a common manifestation of ANCA-associated granulomatous vasculitis (previously named Wegener granulomatosis). Inflammatory lesions may be present with or without subglottic or

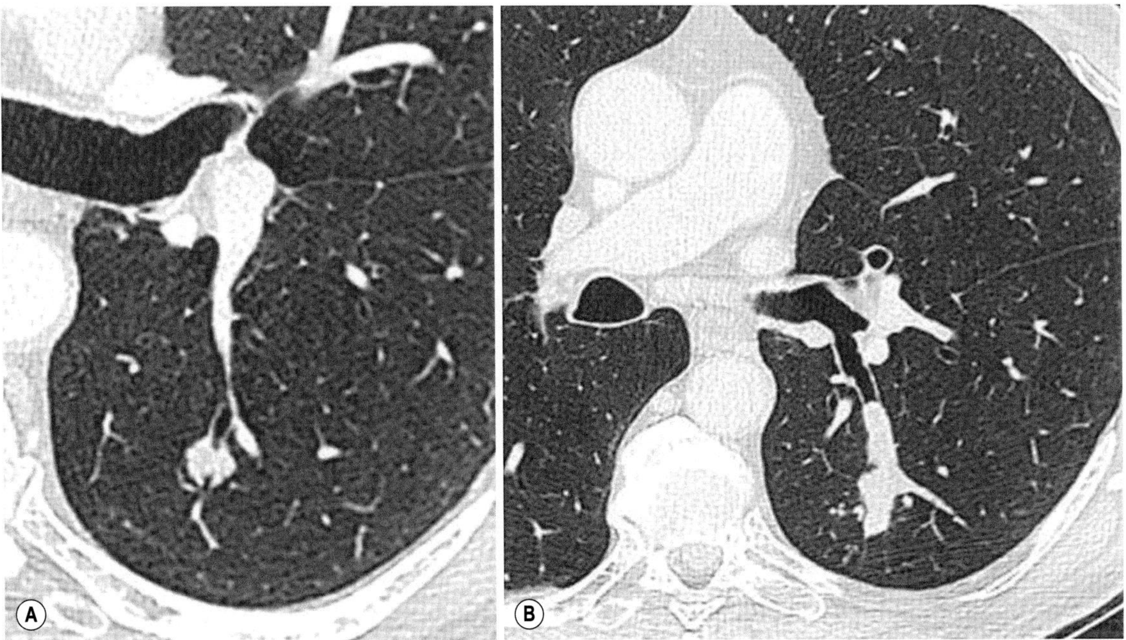

FIGURE 6-5 ■ Endobronchial metastasis. Patient suffering from lung and liver metastasis from colon carcinoma. (A) Axial slice with lung window showing the firstly appeared peribronchial metastasis. (B) Oblique reformation along the axis of the upper segmental bronchus of the left lower lobe. The enlarged and filled bronchus reflects the growth of the metastasis seen 5 months earlier.

bronchial stenosis, ulcerations and pseudotumours. Radiological manifestations include thickening of the subglottic region and proximal trachea with a smooth symmetric or asymmetric narrowing over variable length. Stenosis may also be seen on any main, lobar or segmental bronchus, sometimes causing lobar or sublobar atelectasis. Nodular or polypoid lesions may also be seen on the inner contour of the airway lumen.

Relapsing Polychondritis[2,3,7]

Relapsing polychondritis is a rare systemic disease of autoimmune pathogenesis that affects cartilage at various sites, including the ears, nose, joints, and tracheobronchial tree. Histologically, the acute inflammatory infiltrate present in the cartilages and perichondrial tissue induces progressive dissolution and fragmentation of the cartilage followed by fibrosis. Symmetric subglottic stenosis is the most frequent manifestation in the chest. As the disease progresses, the distal trachea and bronchi may be involved. CT shows smooth thickening of the airway wall associated with more or less diffuse narrowing (Fig. 6-6). In the early stage, the posterior wall of the trachea is spared but in advanced disease circumferential wall thickening occurs (Fig. 6-7). The trachea may become flaccid with considerable collapse at expiration. Gross destruction of the cartilaginous rings with fibrosis may cause stenosis.

Tracheobronchial Amyloidosis[2,3,7]

Deposition of amyloid in the trachea and bronchi may be seen in association with systemic amyloidosis or as an isolated manifestation. As a result, the amyloid forms either multifocal or diffuse submucosal plaques or masses. The overlying mucosa is usually intact. Dystrophic calcification or ossification is frequently present. CT shows focal or, more commonly, diffuse thickening of the airway wall and narrowing of the lumen. Calcification may be seen. Narrowing of the proximal bronchi can lead to distal atelectasis, bronchiectasis, or both, obstructive pneumonia.

Sarcoidosis[2,3,6,7]

Involvement of the trachea is rare, and when it occurs, it is associated with laryngeal involvement. The proximal and distal parts of the trachea may be affected and the appearance of the stenosis may be smooth, irregular and nodular, or even mass-like. Bronchial involvement is much more common as a manifestation of sarcoidosis. The commonest signs at CT are regular or nodular bronchial wall thickening reflecting the presence of granulomas and fibrous tissue in the peribronchial interstitium. This bronchial wall thickening may result in smooth or irregular bronchial narrowing, which correlates with the presence of mucosal thickening at bronchoscopy and presumably reflects prominent inflammation in this location. Obstruction of lobar or segmental bronchi may occur as a result of airway wall fibrosis, compression by granuloma or peribronchial lymph nodes, of conglomerate fibrosis or some combination of these phenomena. Bronchial stenosis may clear spontaneously or with steroid treatment.

Inflammatory Bowel Disease[2,3,7]

Ulcerative tracheitis and tracheobronchitis are rare complications and occur more often in association with

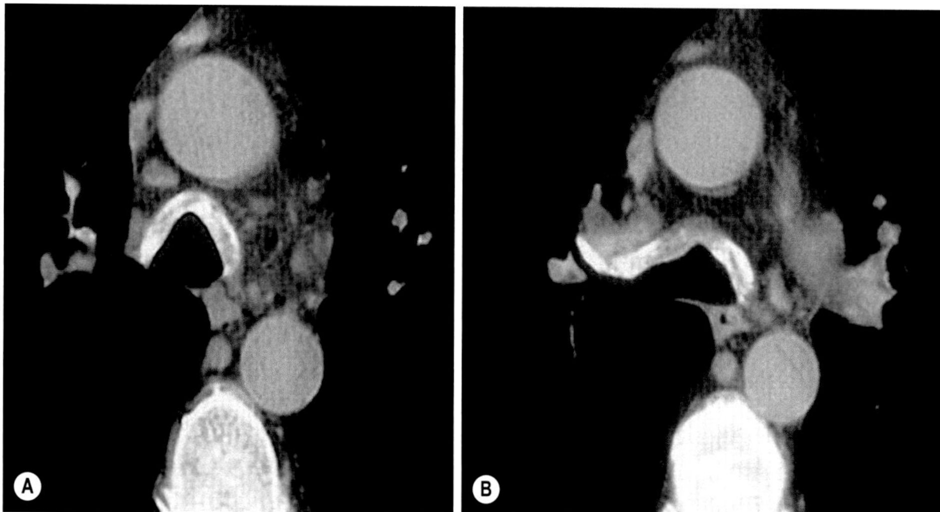

FIGURE 6-6 ■ **Relapsing polychondritis.** (A, B) Axial CT images at the levels of the distal part of the trachea and mainstem bronchi. Abnormal thickening of the anterior and lateral walls of the trachea and mainstem bronchi and right upper lobar bronchus associated with calcium deposits. The posterior membranous wall of the trachea is unaffected.

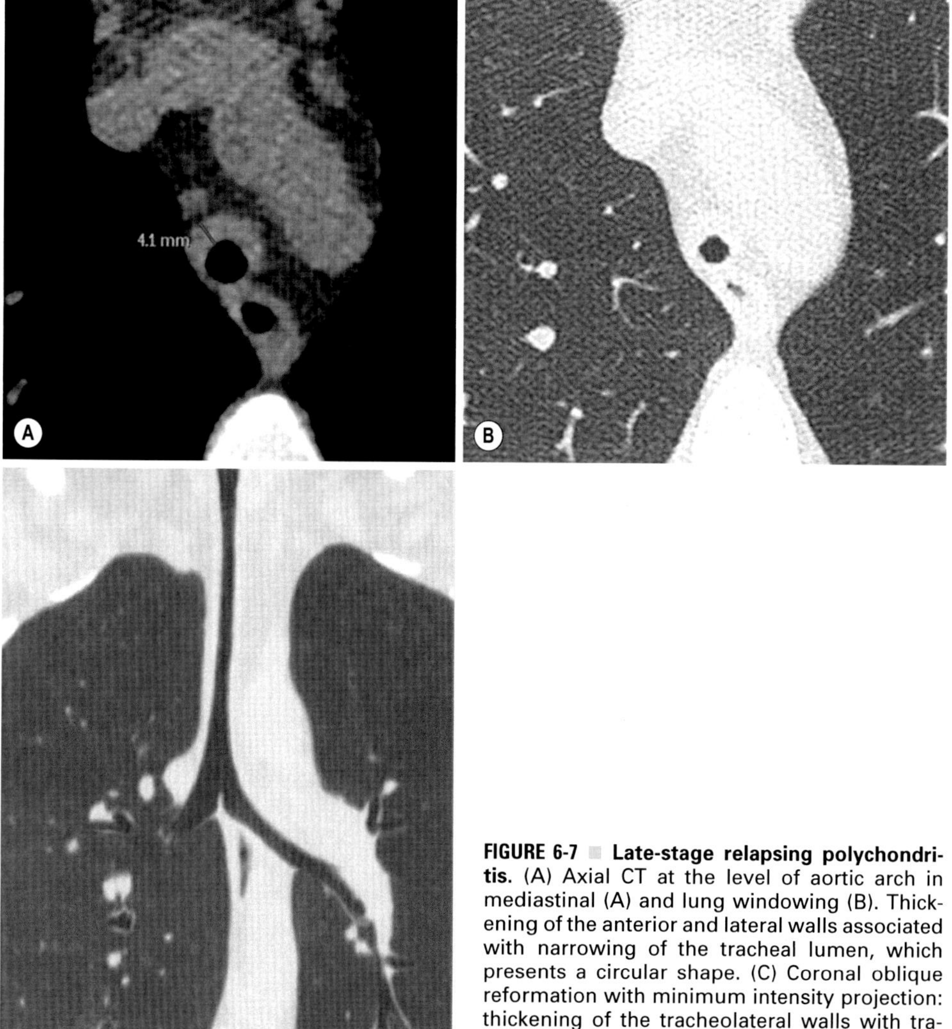

FIGURE 6-7 ■ **Late-stage relapsing polychondritis.** (A) Axial CT at the level of aortic arch in mediastinal (A) and lung windowing (B). Thickening of the anterior and lateral walls associated with narrowing of the tracheal lumen, which presents a circular shape. (C) Coronal oblique reformation with minimum intensity projection: thickening of the tracheolateral walls with tracheal luminal narrowing extending from the cervical part of the trachea to the carina.

ulcerative colitis than Crohn's disease. In most but not all cases, the diagnosis of inflammatory bowel disease precedes the presence of airway disease. Histologically, tracheobronchitis is characterised by more or less concentric mucosal and submucosal fibrosis and chronic inflammation. Ulceration and luminal narrowing may be evident. Cartilaginous plates are not destroyed. On CT, the tracheobronchial walls are thickened and produce irregular luminal narrowing (Fig. 6-8). Bronchial wall thickening and bronchiectasis also may be present with or without mucoïd impaction.

Tracheobronchopathia Osteochondroplastica[2,3]

This rare disorder is characterised by the presence of multiple cartilaginous nodules and bony submucosal nodules on the inner surface of the trachea and proximal airways. Men are more frequently involved than women and most patients are more than 50 years on age. Histologically, the nodules contain heterotopic bone, cartilage and calcified acellular protein matrix. The overlying bronchial mucosa is normal and because it contains no cartilage, the posterior wall of the trachea is spared. The chest radiograph may be normal or may demonstrate lobar collapse or infective consolidation. If the tracheal air column is clearly seen, multiple sessile nodules that project into the tracheal lumen extending over a long segment of the trachea can be appreciated. CT shows thickened tracheal cartilage with irregular calcifications. The nodules may protrude from the anterior and lateral walls into the lumen; they usually show foci of calcification (Fig. 6-9).

Sabre-Sheath Trachea[2,3,6,7]

Characterised by a diffuse narrowing involving the intrathoracic trachea, this entity is almost always associated with COPD (Fig. 6-10). The pathogenesis of the lesion is obscure, but probably it is an acquired deformity related to the abnormal pattern and magnitude of intrathoracic pressure changes in COPD. On radiographs and CT, the condition is easily recognised by noting that the internal side-to-side diameter of the trachea is decreased to half or less than the corresponding sagittal diameter. On the postero-anterior radiograph and CT multiplanar reformations, the narrowing usually affects the whole intrathoracic trachea, with an abrupt return to normal calibre at the thoracic inlet (Fig. 6-10). The trachea usually shows a smooth inner margin but occasionally has a nodular contour. Tracheal cartilage calcification is frequently evident.

Tracheobronchomegaly (Mounier–Kuhn Syndrome)[2,3,6,7]

It refers to patients who have marked dilatation of the trachea and mainstem bronchi. It is often associated with tracheal diverticulosis, recurrent lower respiratory tract infection and bronchiectasis. Atrophy affects the elastic and muscular elements of both the cartilaginous and membranous parts of the trachea. The diagnosis is based on radiological findings. The immediately subglottic trachea has a normal diameter, but it expands as it passes to the carina and this dilatation often continues into the major bronchi. Atrophic mucosa prolapses between cartilage rings and gives the trachea a characteristically corrugated outline on a plain radiograph. Corrugations may become exaggerated to form sacculations or diverticula. On CT a tracheal diameter of greater than 3 cm (measured 2 cm above the aortic arch) and diameter of 2.4 and 2.3 cm for the right and left bronchi, respectively, determine the diagnosis (Fig. 6-11). Additional findings include tracheal scalloping or diverticula (especially along the posterior membranous tracheal wall).

Tracheobronchomalacia[3,7,9]

Resulting from weakened tracheal cartilages, this abnormality may be seen in association with a number of disorders including tracheobronchomegaly, COPD, diffuse tracheal inflammation such as relapsing polychondritis, as well as following trauma. On the radiographs, a reduction by almost 75% of the sagittal diameter at expiration is an excellent indicator of the diagnosis.

The increase in compliance is due to the loss of integrity of the wall's structural components and is particularly associated with damaged or destroyed cartilages. The coronal diameter of the trachea becomes significantly larger than the sagittal one, producing a lunate configuration to the trachea.[9] The flaccidity of the trachea or bronchi is usually most apparent during coughing or forced expiration. In patients with COPD with high downstream resistance particularly high dynamic pressure gradients can be generated across the tracheal wall and it is likely that calibre changes of more than 50% can occur at expiration with normal tracheal compliance. As a result only a decrease in cross-section area of the tracheal lumen greater than 70% at expiration indicates tracheomalacia. Dynamic expiratory multislice CT may offer a meaningful alternative to bronchoscopy in patients with suspected tracheobronchomalacia[10,11] because of its possibilities to provide morphological and functional information simultaneously. Dynamic expiratory CT may show complete collapse or collapse of greater than 75% of luminal cross-section (Fig. 6-12). Involvement of the central tracheobronchial tree may be diffuse or focal. The reduction of airway may result in an oval or crescent shape. The crescent shape is due to the bowing of posterior membranous trachea.

Tracheobronchial Fistula and Dehiscence[2,3,5]

Multidetector CT (MDCT) with thin collimation is the most accurate technique for identifying peripheral bronchopleural fistula most commonly caused by necrotising pneumonia or secondary to traumatic lesions.

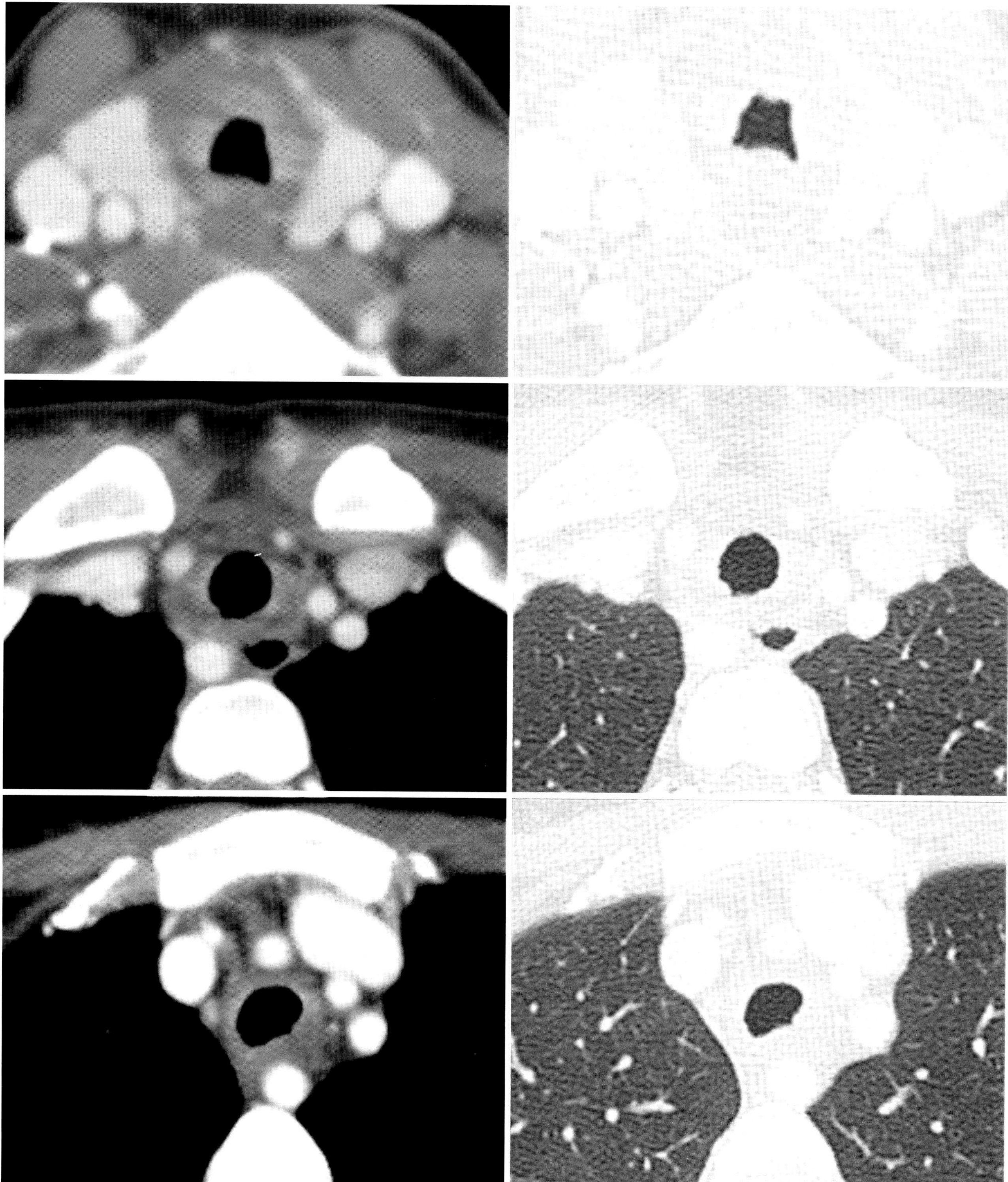

FIGURE 6-8 ■ **Tracheal involvement in Crohn's disease.** Axial CT images at the levels of subglottic and upper thoracic parts of the trachea. Circumferential thickening of the trachea walls associated with irregularities of the inner surface of the posterolateral trachea wall, and slight deformity of the tracheal lumen. Note the right aberrant retro-oesophageal subclavian artery.

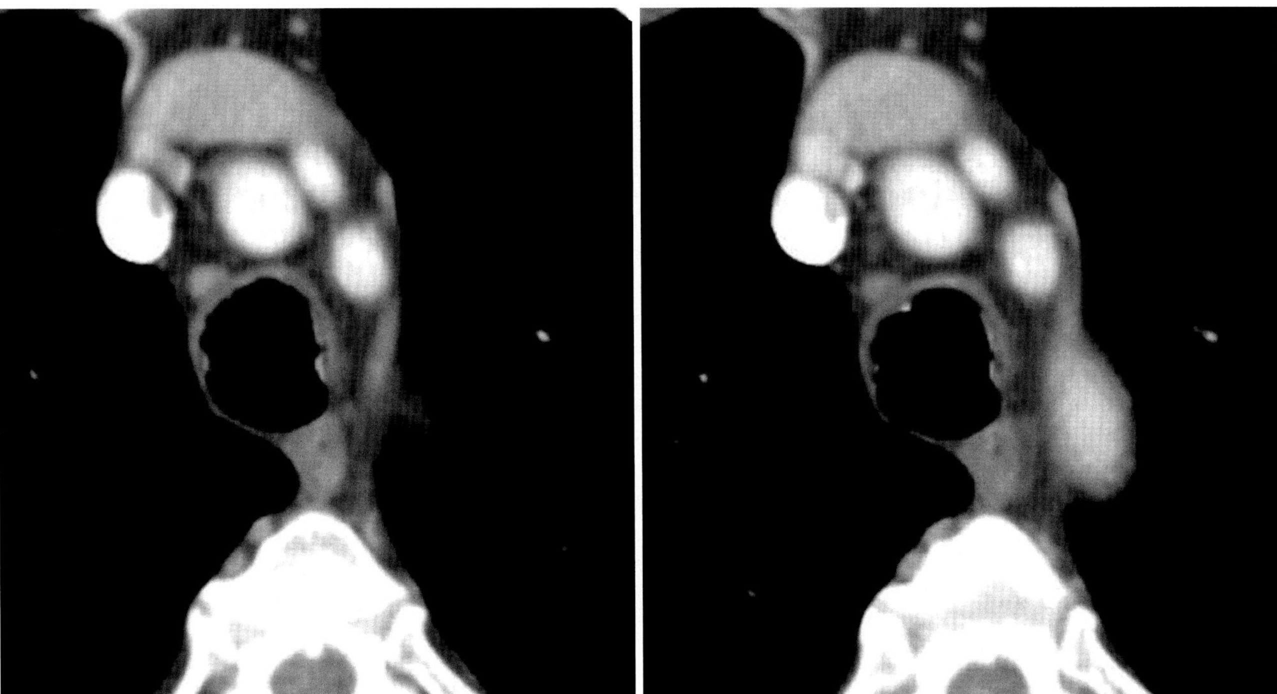

FIGURE 6-9 ■ **Tracheopathia osteochondroplastica.** Axial CT at the level of the upper part of the intrathoracic trachea. Calcified or partly calcified nodules arising from the inner surface of the trachea which protrude into the lumen.

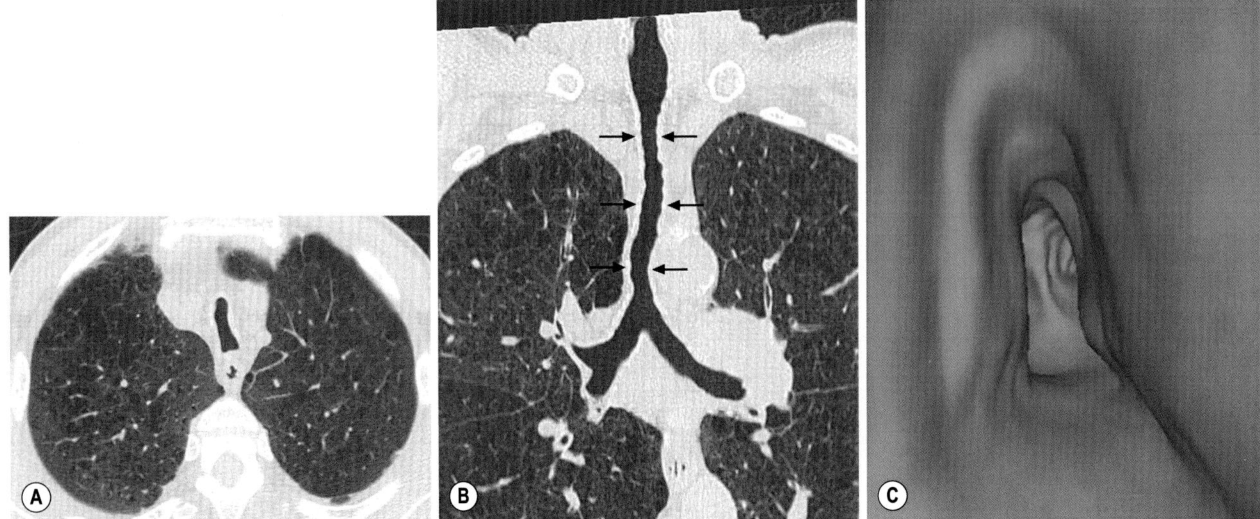

FIGURE 6-10 ■ **Saber-sheath trachea in a COPD patient.** (A) Axial CT at the level of the upper lobes shows a significant reduction of the coronal diameter of the trachea. Bilateral centrilobular and paraseptal emphysematous areas are also present in the upper lobes. (B) Coronal oblique reformation along the long axis of the trachea. Reduction of the coronal diameter of the trachea lumen (arrows). Note the upper part of the trachea above the thoracic inlet has a normal appearance. (C) Endoscopic view.

Nodobronchial and nodobroncho-oesophageal fistulas most commonly caused by *Mycobacterium tuberculosis* infection are depicted by the presence of gas in cavitated hilar or mediastinal lymph adenopathy adjacent to the airways. Tracheal diverticula and tracheobroncho-oesophageal fistula may also be diagnosed even in adults. Malignant neoplasia, particularly oesophageal, is the most common cause of tracheo-oesophageal fistulas in adults. Occasionally congenital fistulas are first manifested in adults. Infection and trauma are the most frequent non-malignant causes.

MDCT has a high degree of sensitivity and specificity for depicting bronchial anastomotic dehiscence occurring after lung transplantation. Bronchial dehiscence is

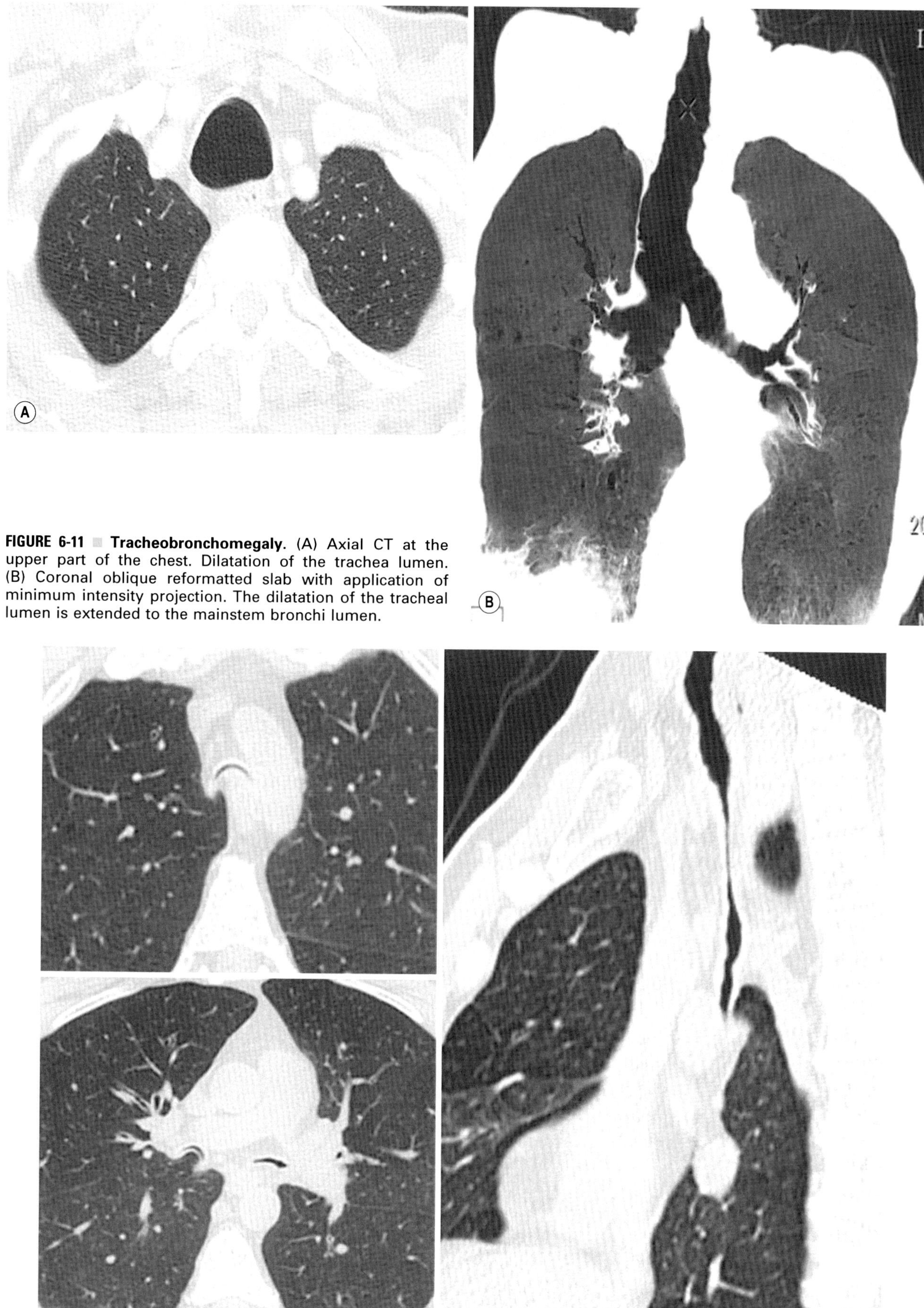

FIGURE 6-11 ■ **Tracheobronchomegaly.** (A) Axial CT at the upper part of the chest. Dilatation of the trachea lumen. (B) Coronal oblique reformatted slab with application of minimum intensity projection. The dilatation of the tracheal lumen is extended to the mainstem bronchi lumen.

FIGURE 6-12 ■ **Tracheobronchomalacia.** Axial CT and sagittal reformation acquired during dynamic expiratory manoeuvre. Almost complete collapse of the trachea, (left) mainstem and (right) intermediate bronchi lumen. The airway lumen is crescent-shaped because of the anterior bowing of the posterior membranous trachea.

seen as bronchial wall defect associated with extraluminal air collections.

BRONCHIECTASIS[2–6,12–14]

Bronchiectasis is a chronic condition characterised by local, irreversible dilatation of bronchi, usually associated with inflammation. Despite its decreased prevalence in developed countries, bronchiectasis remains an important cause of haemoptysis and chronic sputum production. Although the causes of bronchiectasis are numerous, there are three mechanisms by which the dilatation can develop: bronchial obstruction, bronchial wall damage and parenchymal fibrosis (Table 6-1). In the first two mechanisms, the common factor is the combination of mucus plugging and bacterial colonisation. Cytokines and enzymes released by inflammatory cells plus toxins from the bacteria result in a vicious cycle of increasing airway wall damage, mucus retention and bacterial proliferation. In the case of parenchymal fibrosis, the dilatation of bronchi is caused by maturation and retraction of fibrous tissue located in the parenchyma adjacent to an airway (traction bronchiectasis).

Pathologically, bronchiectasis has been classified into three subtypes, reflecting increasing severity of disease: cylindrical, characterised by relatively uniform airway dilatation; varicose, characterised by non-uniform and somewhat serpiginous dilatation; and cystic. As the extent and degree of airway dilatation increase, the lung parenchyma distal to the affected airway shows increasing collapse of fibrosis.

TABLE 6-1 **Mechanisms and Causes of Bronchiectasis**

Bronchial Obstruction
Carcinoma
Fibrous stricture (e.g. tuberculosis)
Broncholithiasis
Extensive compression (lymphadenopathy, neoplasm)
Parenchymal Fibrosis (traction bronchiectasis)
Tuberculosis
Sarcoidosis
Idiopathic pulmonary fibrosis
Bronchial Wall Injury
Childhood viral and bacterial infection
Immunodeficiency disorders
Allergic bronchopulmonary aspergillosis
Lung and bone marrow transplantation
Panbronchiolitis
Systemic disorders (rheumatoid arthritis, Sjögren syndrome, inflammatory bowel disease, yellow nail syndrome)
α_1-antitrypsin syndrom
Congenital
Williams–Campbell syndrome
Cystic fibrosis
Dyskinetic cilia syndrome

Radiographic Findings

CXR reveals abnormalities in the majority of cases. Thickened bronchial walls are visible either as single thin lines or as parallel line opacities (tramline) (Fig. 6-13).

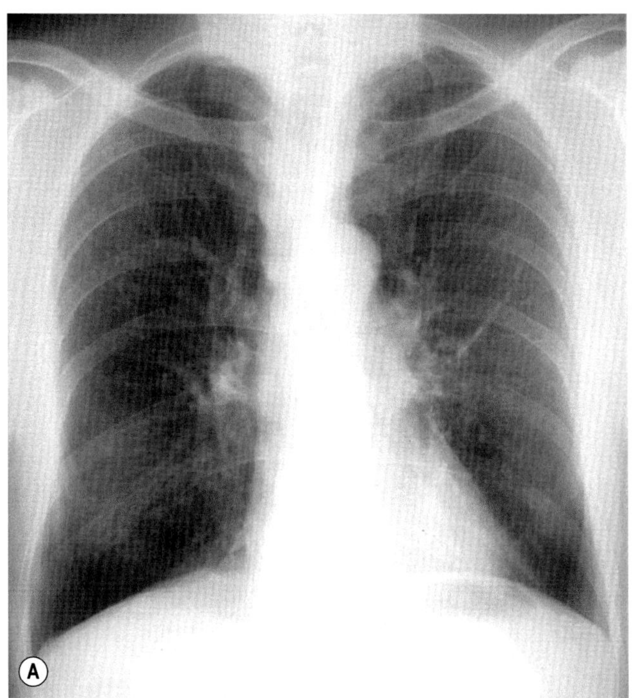

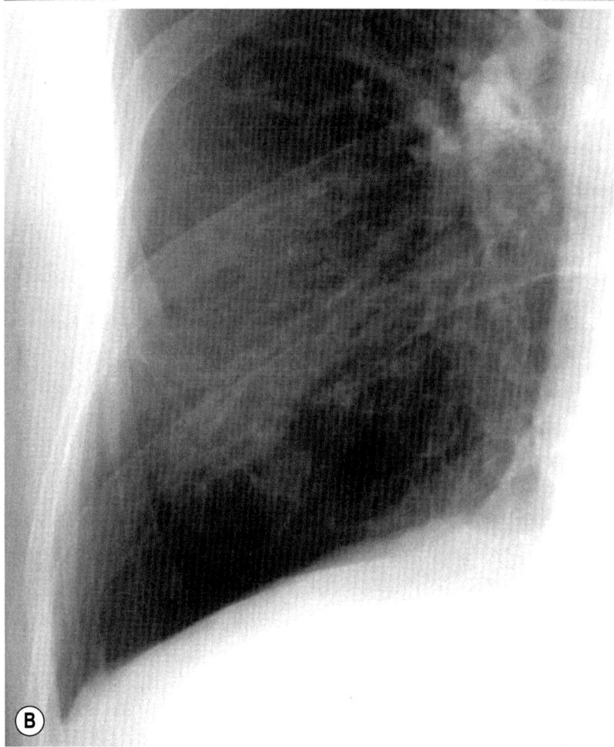

FIGURE 6-13 ■ Bronchiectasis and obliterative bronchiolitis. (A) PA chest radiograph shows oligaemia in the lung bases with pulmonary blood flow redistribution in the upper parts of the lungs, and slight overinflation of the lungs predominant on the right side. (B) Targeted image on the right lung basis in the same patient shows tramlines and ring opacities reflecting the presence of dilated and wall-thickened bronchi.

When seen end-on, bronchiectatic airway appears as poorly defined ring or curvilinear opacities. Dilated bronchi filled with mucus or pus result in tubular or ovoid opacities of variable size. Cystic bronchiectasis manifests as multiple thin-walled ring shadows often containing air–fluid levels (Fig. 6-14). Pulmonary vessels may appear increased in size and may be indistinct because of adjacent peribronchial inflammation and fibrosis. In generalised bronchiectasis, such as that associated with cystic fibrosis, overinflation is often present. Localised forms are frequently accompanied by atelectasis which may be mild and detected only because of vascular crowding, fissure displacement or obscuration of part of the diaphragm.

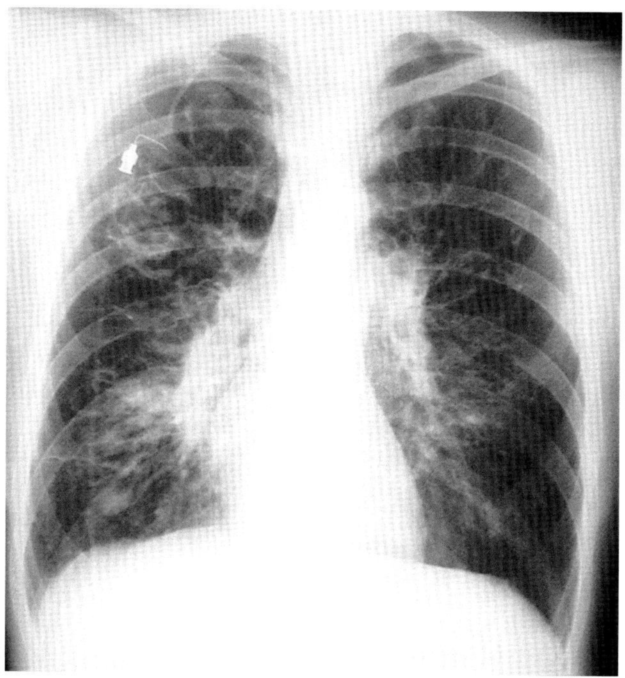

FIGURE 6-14 ■ **Cystic fibrosis.** The PA radiograph shows a slight overinflation, and the presence of multiple thin wall ring shadows in the right lung and the left upper lung, reflecting cystic bronchiectasis. Some ring shadows contain air–fluid levels.

CT Findings

The major sign of bronchiectasis on thin collimation CT (high-resolution CT, HRCT) is dilatation of the bronchi, either with or without bronchial wall thickening (Figs. 13.15–13.19). CT shows bronchial dilatation including lack of tapering of bronchial lumina (the cardinal sign of bronchiectasis), internal diameter bronchi greater than that of the adjacent pulmonary artery (signet ring sign), visualisation of bronchi within 1 cm of the costal pleura or abutting the mediastinal pleura, and mucus-filled dilated bronchi. In varicose bronchiectasis, the bronchial

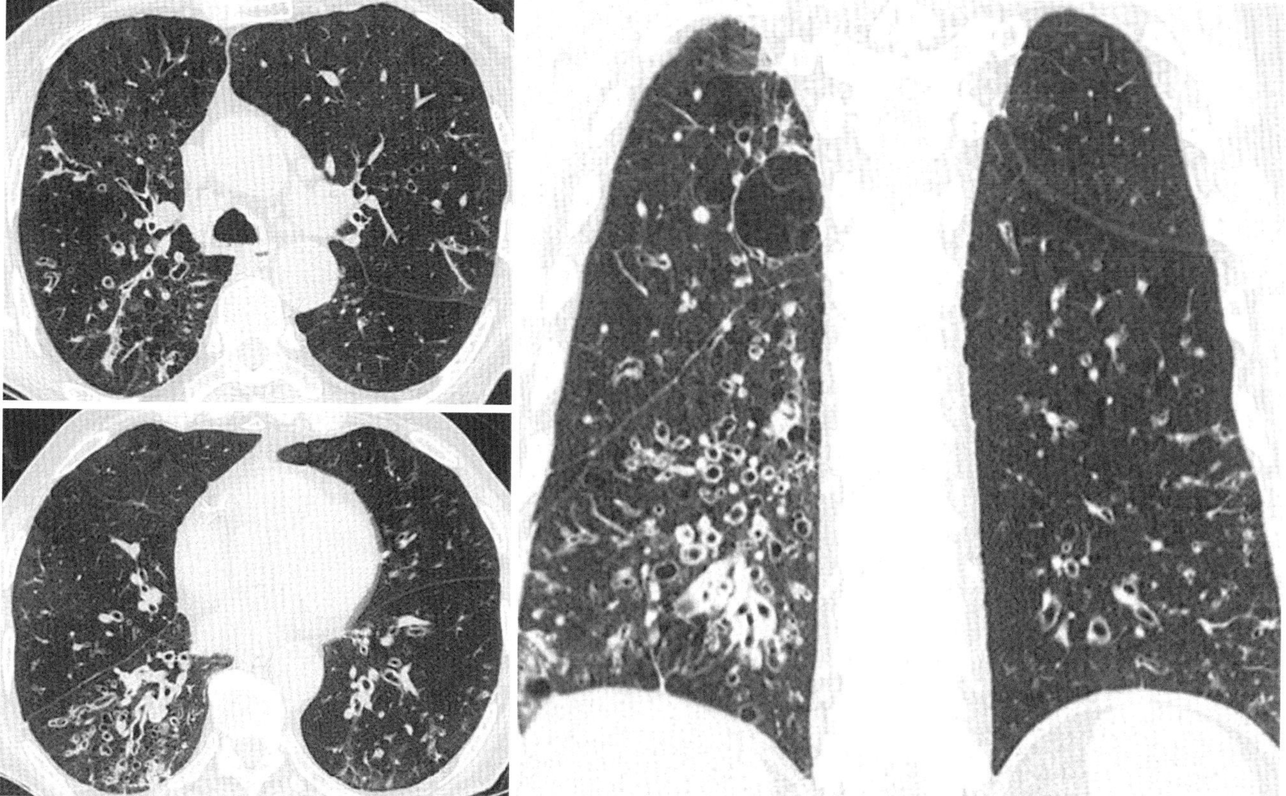

FIGURE 6-15 ■ **Post-infectious bronchiectasis.** Axial CT (left) and coronal multiplanar reformation (right). Bilateral cylindrical bronchiectasis involving the right upper and the lower lobes. Note the presence of bronchial wall thickening and mucoid impactions with slight volume loss of the right lower lobe. Note lung cyst in the posterior part of the right upper lobe.

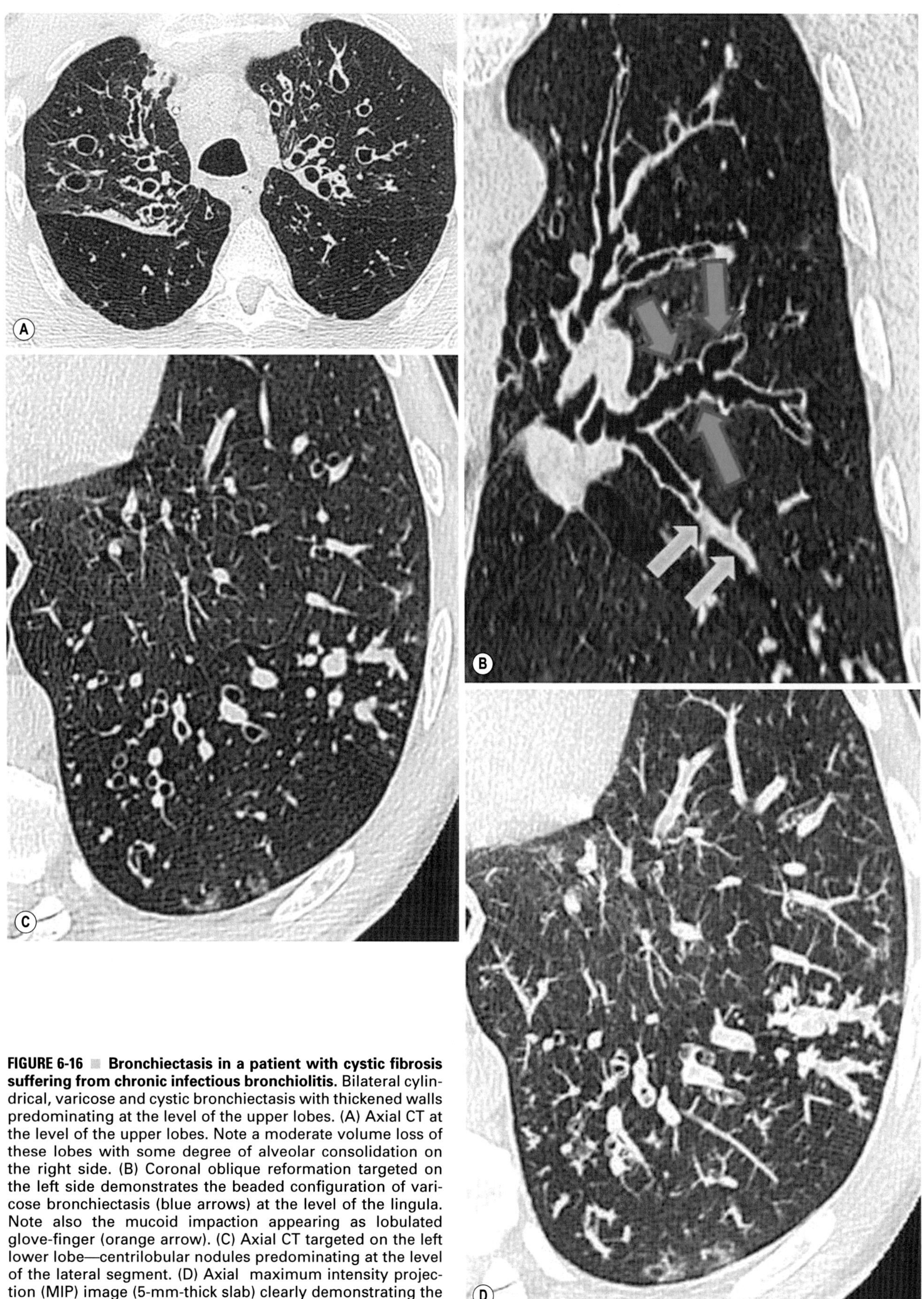

FIGURE 6-16 ■ **Bronchiectasis in a patient with cystic fibrosis suffering from chronic infectious bronchiolitis.** Bilateral cylindrical, varicose and cystic bronchiectasis with thickened walls predominating at the level of the upper lobes. (A) Axial CT at the level of the upper lobes. Note a moderate volume loss of these lobes with some degree of alveolar consolidation on the right side. (B) Coronal oblique reformation targeted on the left side demonstrates the beaded configuration of varicose bronchiectasis (blue arrows) at the level of the lingula. Note also the mucoid impaction appearing as lobulated glove-finger (orange arrow). (C) Axial CT targeted on the left lower lobe—centrilobular nodules predominating at the level of the lateral segment. (D) Axial maximum intensity projection (MIP) image (5-mm-thick slab) clearly demonstrating the tree-in-bud appearance related to infectious bronchiolitis.

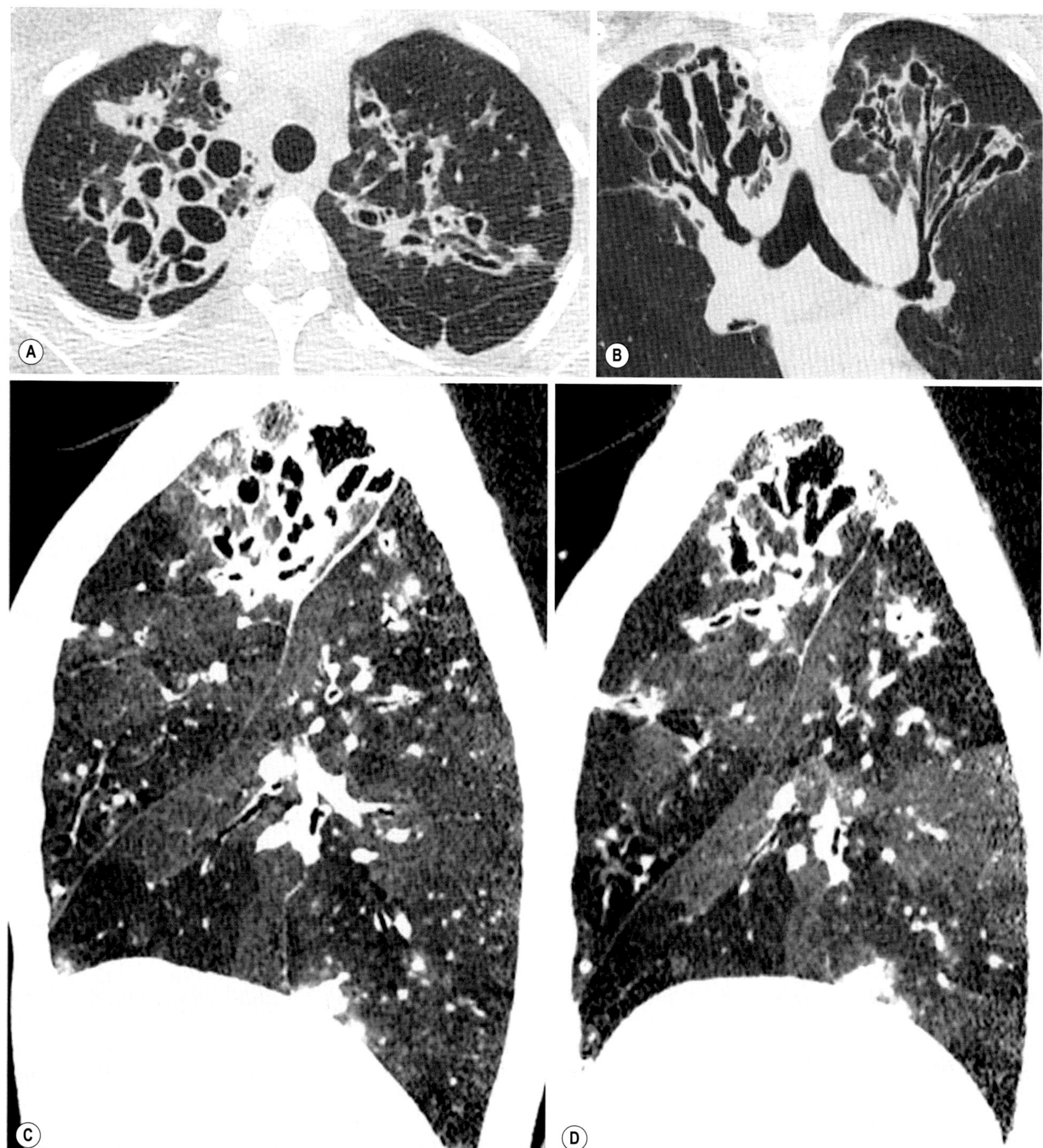

FIGURE 6-17 ■ **Cystic bronchiectasis and obliterative bronchiolitis.** Cystic fibrosis in a young female patient chronically infected with *P. aeruginosa*, *Mycobacterium abscessus* and *Aspergillus fumigatus*—low-dose CT performed on inspiration and expiration with a CTDI of, respectively, 0.66 and 0.33 mGy, resulting in a DLP of, respectively, 24 and 11 mGy/cm. (A) Axial CT at the level of the upper lobes showing alveolar consolidation with cystic lesions predominating on the right side. (B) Coronal oblique mIP image (3-mm-thick slab) perfectly assesses the varicose and cystic bronchiectatic nature of the cystic lesions. (C) Sagittal coronal oblique minimal intensity projection (mIP) image (3-mm-thick slab) targeted on the right lung on inspiration. (D) Sagittal mIP image (3-mm-thick slab) at the equivalent level on expiration. Note the multifocal air trapping on (D) perfectly matched with areas of low attenuation that reflect hypoperfusion due to hypoventilation secondary to obliterative bronchiolitis (mosaic perfusion) on (C) well assessed by adapting the window width and window level.

lumen assumes a beaded configuration. Cystic bronchiectasis is seen as a string of cysts caused by sectioning irregular dilated bronchi along their lengths, or a cluster of cysts, caused by multiple dilated bronchi lying adjacent to each other. Cluster of cysts are most frequently seen in atelectatic lobes. Air–fluid levels, caused by retained secretion may be present in the dependent portion of the dilated bronchi. Secretion accumulation within bronchiectatic airways is generally easily recognisable as lobulated glove-finger, V- or Y-shaped densities (Fig. 6-16). When oriented perpendicular to the CT slice, filled dilated bronchi are visualised as nodular opacities running alongside adjacent pulmonary arteries (whose diameters are smaller than those of the dilated bronchi). CT may show complete collapse of the lobe containing bronchiectatic airways. Subtle degrees of volume loss may be seen in lobes in early disease. This is most evident in the lower lobes on the basis of crowding of the mildly dilated bronchi and posterior displacement of the oblique fissure (Fig. 6-15).

Associated CT findings of bronchiolitis are seen in about 70% of patients with bronchiectasis. Small centrilobular nodular and linear branching opacities (tree-in-bud sign) express inflammatory and infectious bronchiolitis (Fig. 6-16). Areas of decreased attenuation and vascularity, mosaic perfusion pattern, and expiratory air trapping reflect the extent of obliterative bronchiolitis (Fig. 6-17). These abnormalities are very common in patients with severe bronchiectasis and can even precede the development of bronchiectasis. Obstructive pulmonary function patterns in bronchiectasis do not seem to be related to the degree of collapse of large airways on expiratory CT or the extent of mucus plugging, but, rather, due to obliterative bronchiolitis of the peripheral airways.[15] The CT findings about small airway disease (decreased lung attenuation, expiratory air trapping) and bronchial wall thickening in patients with bronchiectasis have proven to be the major determinants of airflow obstruction.[16] The bronchial wall thickening assessed on CT has been demonstrated to be the primary determinant of subsequent major functional decline.[17] In one study, pulmonary arterial enlargement was the best predictor of mortality and was associated with outcome, independently of CT signs of bronchiectasis. Pulmonary hypertension, reflected by pulmonary arterial enlargement on CT is a highly significant prognostic indicator in the evaluation of patients with bronchiectasis.[18]

Accuracy of CT

By combining helical volumetric CT acquisition and thin collimation, CT has gained greater advantages by circumventing the limitations of HRCT, particularly the risk of missing bronchiectasis strictly localised within the intervals between slices.[19,20] At the present time, multidetector CT with thin collimation is the highly recommended technique to assess the presence and extent of bronchiectasis. Multiplanar reformations increase the detection rate and the reader's confidence, as to the distribution of bronchiectasis, and improve agreement between observers, as to the diagnosis of bronchiectasis.[21–23] In addition maximum intensity projections improve the detection and display of both mucoid impactions and small centrilobular and linear branching opacities (tree-in-bud sign), characteristic of infectious bronchiolitis.

The reliability of CT for distinguishing among the causes of bronchiectasis is somewhat controversial. An underlying cause for bronchiectasis is found in fewer than half of patients and CT features alone do not usually allow a confident distinction between idiopathic bronchiectasis versus known cause of bronchiectasis.[5,12] Bilateral upper lobe distribution is commonly seen in patients with cystic fibrosis and allergic bronchopulmonary aspergillosis, unilateral upper lobe distribution is commonest in patients with tuberculosis, and a lower lobe distribution is most often seen in patients after childhood viral infections. However, CT remains of little value in diagnosing specific aetiologies of bronchiectasis.

Cystic Fibrosis[2,12]

Cystic fibrosis results from an autosomal recessive genetic defect in the structure of the cystic fibrosis transmembrane regulation protein which leads to abnormal chloride transport across epithelial membranes. Although the mechanisms by which this defect leads to lung disease are not entirely understood, an abnormally low water content of airway mucus is at least partially responsible for decreased mucus clearance, mucus plugging of airways, and an increased incidence of bacterial airway infection. Bronchial wall inflammation progressing to secondary bronchiectasis is always present in patients with longstanding disease.

In patients with early or mild disease, radiographic findings may quite subtle. Hyperinflation reflects the presence of obstruction of the small airways. Thickening of the wall of the upper lobar bronchi can also be seen on the lateral radiograph. In more advanced disease, radiographs can be diagnostic, showing increased lung volume, accentuated linear opacities in the upper lung areas, resulting from bronchial wall thickening or bronchiectasis, proximal bronchiectasis and mucoid impaction. Additional findings include cystic regions of the upper lobes, representing cystic bronchiectasis, healed abscess, cavities, or bullae, atelectasis, findings of pulmonary hypertension or cor pulmonale, pneumothorax or pleural effusion (Fig. 6-14). Chest radiographs are sufficient for clinical management, but it is important to know that there is usually little visible radiographic change in clinical exacerbations. Low-dose CT offers a superior alternative to routine radiography and clinical methods for monitoring disease status, as well as for assessing response to treatment. These studies consistently document close correlation between HRCT findings and both clinical and pulmonary functional evaluation of these patients.

On CT, peripheral and/or central bronchiectasis is present in all patients with advanced cystic fibrosis (Figs. 6-16 and 6-17). All lobes are typically involved, although early in the disease abnormalities are often predominantly distributed in the upper lobes, and sometimes with a right upper lobe predominance. Bronchial wall thickening and/or peribronchial interstitial thickening are also commonly present and are generally even more evident than bronchial dilatation in patients with early disease. Mucus plugging is present in about 25–50% of patients, and may be seen in all lobes. Collapse or consolidation is visible in up to 80% of patients. Lobar volume loss is often present in patients with advanced disease. Bullae may be difficult to distinguish from cystic bronchiectasis, particularly in fibrotic upper lobes. Abscesses may be difficult to distinguish from cystic bronchiectasis, particularly as both may contain air–fluid levels. Pleural thickening, often apparent on CXR, is demonstrated better by CT. Small centrilobular nodular and branching linear opacities (tree-in-bud sign) can be an early sign of disease. They reflect presence of mucous impactions in dilated bronchioles associated with peribronchiolar inflammation. Focal areas of decreased lung attenuation are frequently present, representing air trapping and mosaic perfusion due to obstruction of the small airways (obliterative bronchiolitis).

At an early stage of disease, CT can demonstrate any airway abnormalities in patients who are asymptomatic and have normal pulmonary functions and normal chest radiograph. In patients with more advanced disease, CT is superior to chest radiograph in detecting bronchiectasis and mucus plugging.

Magnetic resonance imaging has been recommended as a novel method without the use of ionising radiation and as a substitute for CT in the assessment of patients with cystic fibrosis. Although the spatial resolution of pulmonary MR is lower than that of CT, it has the advantage of being able to distinguish different aspects of tissue on the basis of different contrast media on T1- and T2-weighted images as well as enhancement after contrast media administration.

In general on MR imaging the central bronchi and central bronchiectasis are well visualised.

A high signal of the bronchial wall on T2-weighted turbo spin-echo imaging represents oedema due to active inflammation. Enhancement of the thickened bronchial wall on contrast-enhanced (CE) T1-weighted MR imaging seems to be related to inflammatory activity. Mucus plugging is well visualised on T2-weighted turbo spin-echo images even down to the small airways because of the high T2 signal of their fluid content. In addition, mucus plugs do not enhance after contrast enhancement, and, as a result, are easily differentiated from bronchial wall thickening. Pulmonary consolidation leads to a high signal on T2-weighted turbo spin-echo imaging.[24,25] With progression of the disease, complete destruction of lung segments or lobes can be assessed on T1- and T2-weighted MR images, as well as on CT images. Pulmonary MR imaging may also be used as a combined method for morphological and functional evaluation of disease severity and therapeutic responses.[25] CE perfusion MR imaging, O_2-enhanced MR imaging are able to differentiate regional functional changes in lung parenchyma of patients with cystic fibrosis. Perfusion defects, assessed by CT perfusion MR imaging, showed good correlation with the degree of tissue destruction. When O_2-enhanced MR is used in CF patients, heterogeneous signal change after 100% oxygen inhalation is generated by the heterogeneous combination of regional ventilation and perfusion.[24,25]

Allergic Bronchopulmonary Aspergillosis (ABPA)[2–4]

Hypersensitivity reaction to *Aspergillus* species, ABPA is characterised by asthma, blood, eosinophilia, radiographic pulmonary opacities and evidence of allergy to antigens of *Aspergillus* species. It may also occur in patients with cystic fibrosis. Recurrent acute episodes cause progressive lung damage that can be controlled by steroids. The radiological features can be classified as acute and transient, or chronic and permanent. The commonest acute changes are transient consolidation, mucoid impaction and atelectasis. Consolidation ranges from massive and homogeneous to lobar or segmental in configuration, or, to subsegmental or smaller. When consolidation clears, it often leaves residual bronchiectasis that creates favourable conditions for fungal recolonisation, a finding that accounts for the fact consolidation recurs often in the same area. Mucoid impaction obstructs the airway lumen, which becomes distended by retained secretions. At the same time, lung parenchyma remains aerated by collateral drift, permitting the visualisation of the impacted airway. Bronchoceles appear as opacities of a variety of shapes (linear, branched or unbranched, band-like opacities that point to the hilum, tooth-paste opacities, V- and Y-shape opacities, glove-finger opacities) (Fig. 6-16). These opacities disappear once their airway contents have been coughed up, leaving ring or parallel linear opacities. Atelectasis is subsegmental, segmental, lobar or even affects a whole lung and has a tendency to recur in the same area.

Permanent changes indicate irreversible lung damage and are the clue that an asthmatic has ABPA when he/she is in remission. Bronchiectasis is responsible for most of the permanent radiological changes. It affects lobar bronchi and the first- and second-orders segmental

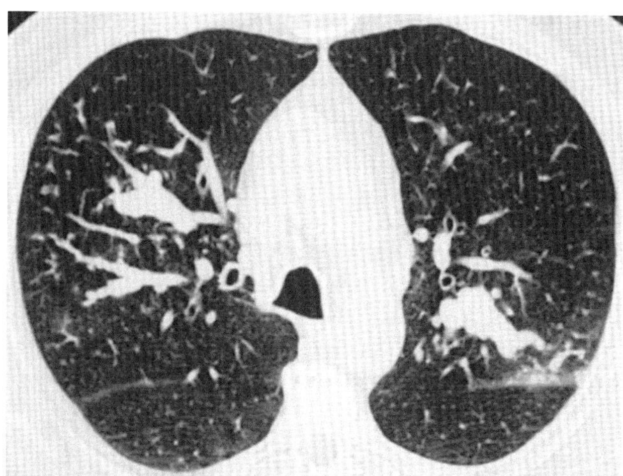

FIGURE 6-18 ■ **Allergic bronchopulmonary aspergillosis.** Axial CT in the upper lobes. Presence of mucoid impactions within segmental and subsegmental dilated bronchi of the upper lobes. Small centrilobular linear branching opacities are seen in the periphery of the right upper lobe.

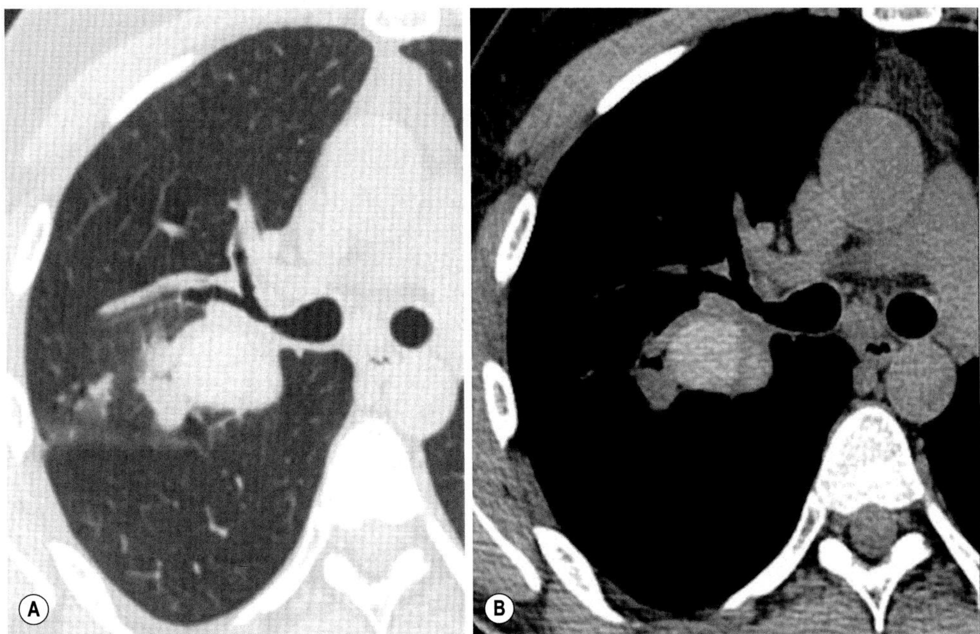

FIGURE 6-19 ■ **Allergic bronchopulmonary aspergillosis.** Axial CT targeted on the right lung at the level of the right upper lobar bronchus in lung windowing (A) and mediastinal windowing (B). The oval mass located in the posterior segment of the right upper lobe presents a hyperattenuated component, reflecting the presence of calcium into a large mucoid impaction within a dilated bronchus.

bronchi. Beyond the proximal bronchi, more distal airways remain normal and patent, though small airway abnormalities are seen on CT. These abnormalities include tree-in-bud appearance reflecting mucoid impaction in dilated bronchioles and focal areas of decreased lung attenuation and air trapping reflecting obstruction of the small airways. Compared with other bronchiectatic diseases, bronchiectasis in ABPA is more commonly centrally located, and more likely to contain cystic or varicose components. Mucus plugs within the ectatic airways are frequently seen on CT. High attenuation within the plugs is also relatively frequent, reflecting the presence of calcium concentration by the fungus (Fig. 6-19). Hyperattenuated mucus plugs may be depicted within the areas of consolidation.

Parenchymal scarring represents the fibrotic stage of the disease. It commonly follows bronchiectasis, and manifests as linear opacities and lobar shrinkage. Mirroring the distribution of bronchiectasis, these features have a strong upper zone predilection. Despite this upper lobar shrinkage, the lung volume is frequently increased, reflecting overinflation in the lower lobes due to obstruction of the small airways and the presence of bullae in cavitation in the upper lobes.

Dyskinetic Cilia Syndrome[2–4]

Resulting from a genetic abnormality having autosomal recessive transmission, dyskinetic cilia syndrome is characterised by abnormal ciliary structure and function, leading to a reduced mucociliary clearance and chronic airway infection. Bronchiectasis and sinusitis are common manifestations. About half of patients have also a situs inversus. The combination of bronchiectasis, sinusitis and situs inversus is termed Kartagener's syndrome (Fig. 6-20). Men and women are equally affected, but in men the syndrome may be associated with immotile spermatozoa and infertility. Respiratory symptoms can generally be traced back to childhood. Bronchiectasis develops in childhood and adolescence and is associated with recurrent pneumonia. Both radiographs and CT typically show bilateral bronchiectasis with a basal (lower or middle lobe) predominance. Similar to that seen in patients with other causes of post-infectious bronchiolitis, cylindrical bronchiectasis is commonest and a diffuse bronchiolitis may be present.

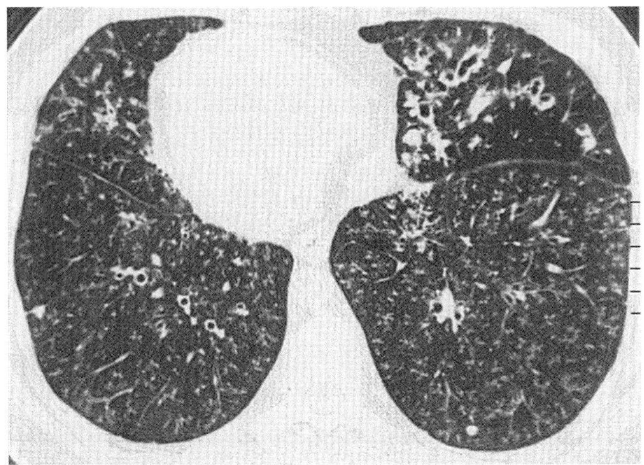

FIGURE 6-20 ■ **Dyskinetic cilia syndrome.** Axial CT at the level of the lower part of the chest. Bilateral bronchiectasis in the right middle lobe and the left lower lobe with some mucoid impactions. Note the presence of bronchial wall thickening and multiple foci of 'tree-in-bud' sign, reflecting infectious bronchiolitis. This patient also has situs inversus (Kartagener's syndrome).

BRONCHOLITHIASIS[2–4]

Broncholithiasis is a condition in which peribronchial calcified nodal disease erodes into or distorts an adjacent bronchus. The underlying abnormality is usually granulomatous lymphadenitis caused by *Mycobacterium tuberculosis* or fungi such as *Histoplasma capsulatum*. A few cases have been reported with silicosis. Calcified material in a bronchial lumen or bronchial distortion by peribronchial disease results in airway obstruction. This leads to collapse, obstructive pneumonitis, mucoid impaction or bronchiectasis. Symptoms include cough, hemoptysis, recurrent episodes of fever and purulent sputum. Broncholithiasis is more common on the right, and obstructive changes particularly affect the right middle lobe.

On chest radiographs, three major types of changes may be seen:

- Disappearance of a previously identified calcified nidus;
- Change in position of a calcified nidus; and
- Evidence of airway obstruction, including segmental or lobar atelectasis, mucoid impaction, obstructive pneumonitis, obstructive oligaemia with air trapping.

Calcified hilar or mediastinal nodes are a key feature.

CT and fibreoptic bronchoscopy complement each other in this condition. Broncholithiasis is recognised at CT by the presence of a calcified endobronchial or peribronchial lymph node, associated with bronchopulmonary complication due to obstruction (including atelectasis, pneumonia, bronchiectasis and air trapping), in the absence of an associated soft-tissue mass.

BRONCHIOLITIS

The term of bronchiolitis is often used synonymously with 'small airway disease'. Bronchiolitis includes various inflammatory diseases that affect the bronchioles (the small airways that do not contain cartilage in their walls). Acute bronchiolitis usually results from processes that cause bronchiolar injury over a short period of time such as viral infection or the inhalation of toxic gases. Chronic bronchiolitis is typically associated with prolonged injury and is characterised by bronchiolar infiltration by mononuclear cells, typically followed by the development of a fibrotic process. Bronchiolitis may occur in a variety of clinical settings (infection, toxic gas inhalation, cigarette smoking, drug reactions, collagen vascular disease, bone marrow transplantation and solid organ transplantation) or in association with large airway diseases such as bronchiectasis, or parenchymal lung disease such as hypersensitivity pneumonitis. HRCT plays a major role in the diagnosis of bronchiolitis. Certain patterns of abnormalities on HRCT imaging are highly suggestive of the diagnosis in many cases. The findings on CT often provide the first indication of presence of small airway diseases.

Although normal bronchioles cannot be visualised, bronchiolar disease may result in direct and indirect signs on HRCT images. Direct signs result from the presence of bronchiolar secretion, bronchiolar wall thickening or peribronchiolar inflammation. They include small centrilobular nodular and linear branching opacities (tree-in-bud sign) and centrilobular ill-defined nodular opacities. Indirect signs include areas of decreased attenuation and vascularity (mosaic attenuation and perfusion pattern) on inspiration imaging and areas of air trapping on HRCT imaging obtained at end-expiration.

Pathologically, bronchiolitis may be classified as a cellular bronchiolitis (infective and non-infective bronchiolitis) and obliterative bronchiolitis (luminal narrowing related to submucosal and periadventitial fibrosis).

Infective Bronchiolitis

Infective bronchiolitis results from infection of the small airways by a viral, bacterial, mycobacterial or fungal agent for which the tree-in-bud sign represents the hallmark finding on CT. Tree-in-bud may be an isolated finding, but more frequently it is associated with findings of bronchitis and/or bronchiectasis (see Chapter 5, 'Pulmonary Infection in Adults').Whatever the agent responsible, infective bronchiolitis may be reversible under treatment and/or lead to irreversible narrowing of the terminal bronchioles (obliterative bronchiolitis).

Inflammatory (Non-Infective) Bronchiolitis

Inflammation of the small airways is a common pathological disorder; however, the extent of inflammatory lesions is rarely extensive enough to cause clinical symptoms. The most common example is respiratory bronchiolitis characterised by macrophage accumulation in respiratory bronchioles occurring in smokers (see Chapter 9). Follicular bronchiolitis, another example, is characterised by lymphoid hyperplasia and occurs in connective tissue diseases and immunodeficiency syndrome. The characteristic HRCT pattern is made of ill-defined centrilobular nodular opacities having a diffuse and homogeneous distribution, often associated with CT signs of bronchitis (bronchial wall thickening) and cylindrical bronchiectasis.

Inflammation of the bronchioles may be reversible under specific or anti-inflammatory treatment or lead to subsequent scarring and obliteration (obliterative bronchiolitis).

Obliterative (Constrictive) Bronchiolitis[2–4,26]

Obliterative bronchiolitis is a condition characterised by bronchiolar and peribronchiolar inflammation and fibrosis that ultimately leads to luminal obliteration affecting membranous and respiratory bronchioles. Obliterative bronchiolitis has numerous causes and is only rarely idiopathic (Table 6-2). When a large proportion of airways are affected, patients usually present with progressive shortness of breath and functional evidence of airflow obstruction.

Pathological Features

The pattern of obliterative bronchiolitis is characterised by the development of an irreversible circumferential

TABLE 6-2 Causes of and Association with Obliterative (Constrictive) Bronchiolitis

Post-Infection
Childhood viral infection (adenovirus, respiratory syncytial virus, influenza, parainfluenza)
Adulthood and childhood (*Mycoplasma pneumoniae, Pneumocystis carinii* in AIDS patients, endobronchial spread of tuberculosis, bacterial bronchiolar infection)
Post-Inhalation (toxic fumes and gases)
Nitrogen dioxide (silo filler's disease), sulphur dioxide, ammonia, chlorine, phosgene
Hot gases
Gastric Aspiration
Diffuse aspiration bronchiolitis (chronic occult aspiration in the elderly, patients with dysphagia)
Connective Tissue Disorders
Rheumatoid arthritis
Sjögren's syndrome
Allograft Recipients
Bone-marrow transplant
Heart–lung or lung transplant
Drugs
Penicillamine
Lomustine
Ulcerative colitis
Other Conditions
Bronchiectasis
Chronic bronchitis
Cystic fibrosis
Hypersensitivity pneumonitis
Sarcoidosis
Microcarcinoid tumourlets (neuroendocrine cell hyperplasia)
Sauropus androgynus ingestion
Idiopathic

submucosal fibrosis, resulting in bronchiolar narrowing or obliteration of bronchioles in the absence of intraluminal granulation tissue polyps or surrounding parenchymal inflammation. Proliferation of fibrosis extends predominantly between the epithelium and the muscular mucosa and along the long axis of the airway, impairing collateral ventilation, and leading to airflow obstruction. The epithelium overlying the abnormal fibrosis tissue may be flattened or metaplastic and is usually intact without any ulceration. In some instances, the accompanying artery is also obliterated by the same fibrotic process.

Radiological Findings

The CXR is often normal. In a small number of patients, mild hyperinflation, subtle peripheral attenuation of the vascular makings, widespread and conspicuous abnormalities in lung attenuation, and central bronchiectasis may be seen.

Thin-section CT is superior to radiography in demonstrating the presence and extent of abnormalities and usually demonstrates areas of decreased lung attenuation associated with vessels of decreased calibre on inspiration and air trapping on expiration. Because the lesions of bronchiolar narrowing or obstruction are heterogeneously distributed throughout the lungs, redistribution of blood flow to areas of normal lung or less diseased areas results in a pattern of mosaic perfusion (Fig. 6-17). Bronchial wall thickening and bronchiectasis, both central and peripheral, are also commonly present.

Although the vessels within areas of decreased attenuation on thin-section CT may be of markedly reduced calibre, they are not distorted as in emphysema. The lung areas of decreased attenuation related to decreased perfusion can be patchy or widespread. They are poorly defined or sharply demarcated, giving a geographical outline, representing a collection of affected secondary pulmonary lobules. Redistribution of blood flow to the normally ventilated areas causes increased attenuation of lung parenchyma in these areas. The patchwork of abnormal areas of low attenuation and normal lung or less diseased areas, appearing normal in attenuation or hyperattenuated, gives the appearance of mosaic attenuation. The vessels in the abnormal hypoattenuated areas are reduced in calibre, whereas the vessels in normal areas are increased in size, and the resulting pattern is called 'mosaic perfusion'. The difference in vessel size between low- and high-attenuation areas allows one to distinguish the mosaic perfusion pattern from mosaic attenuation due to an infiltrative lung disease with patchy distribution, in which the vessels have the same calibre in both high-attenuation and normal-attenuation areas. The areas of decreased lung attenuation and perfusion may be confined to or predominant in one lung, particularly in Swyer–James or Macleod syndrome, that is a variant form of post-infectious obliterative bronchiolitis in which the obliterative bronchiolar lesions affect predominantly one lung. The regional heterogeneity of lung density usually seen at end-inspiration on thin-section CT is accentuated on images obtained at end, or during, expiration because the high-attenuation areas increase in density and the low-attenuation areas remain unchanged. In the case of more global involvement of the small airways, the lack of regional homogeneity of the lung attenuation is difficult to perceive on inspiratory CT, and as a result, mosaic perfusion becomes visible only on expiratory CT. In patients with particularly severe and widespread involvement of the small airways, the patchy distribution of hypoattenuation and mosaic pattern is lost. Inspiratory CT shows an apparent uniformity of decreased attenuation in the lungs, while end-expiration CT may appear unremarkable (Fig. 6-21). In these patients, the most striking features are a paucity of pulmonary vessels and a lack of change of cross-sectional area of the lung at comparable levels on inspiration and expiration. In such a situation, there is a risk of misdiagnoses between obliterative bronchiolitis and panlobular emphysema. Both conditions are characterised by bronchial wall thickening and generalised decreased attenuation of the lung parenchyma and bronchial dilatation. However, patients with panlobular emphysema demonstrate parenchymal destruction with higher frequency and greater extent than those with obliterative bronchiolitis. Long lines reflecting limited thickened interlobular septa were

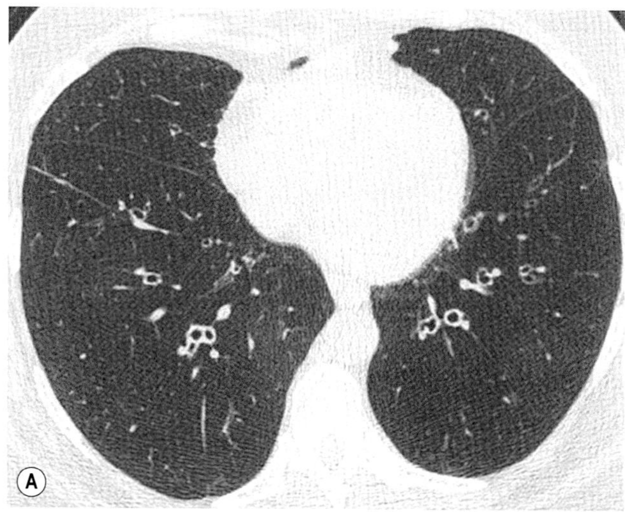

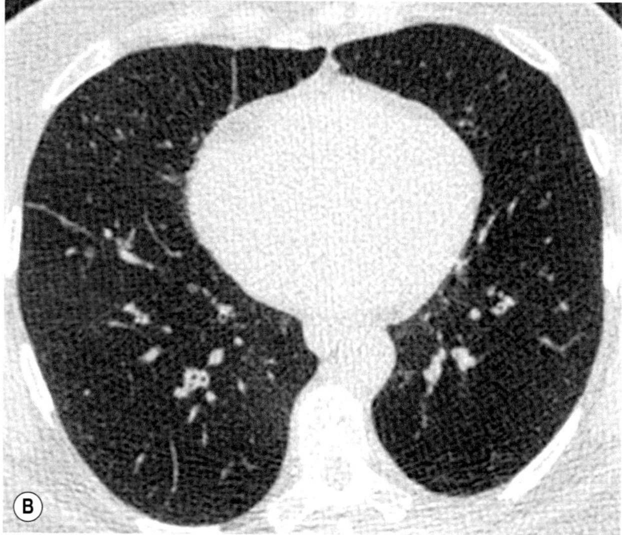

FIGURE 6-21 ■ **Post bone marrow transplantation obliterative bronchiolitis.** (A) Axial CT at the level of the lower part of the chest. Diffuse hypoattenuation of lung parenchyma. Lung vessels are reduced in number and in calibre. Note the slight dilatation of the bronchi lumens and the presence of bronchial wall thickening. (B) Low-dose axial CT performed at short suspended end-expiration at the same level as A. The absence of increase in lung attenuation and significant reduction in lung cross-sectional area reflect the presence of diffuse air trapping. The complete collapse of the bronchial lumens in the lower lobes testifies that CT was acquired at the end of a forced expiratory manoeuvre.

significantly more frequent in patients with panlobular emphysema.[27]

CT Assessment of Air Trapping

The commonest technique for the assessment of air trapping at CT is based on post-expiratory thin-section CT obtained during suspended respiration following a forced exhalation. Each post-expiratory CT image is compared with the inspiratory CT that most closely duplicates its anatomical level to detect air trapping. Dynamic expiratory manoeuvres performed during helical CT acquisition have been described; these permit a small increase in the degree of expiration, which leads to a better detection of air trapping.[28] This technique is recommended when patients have difficulty performing adequate suspended end-expiration. Ultra low dose MDCT with thin collimation over the lungs has become routine in many institutions to improve the conspicuity and the apparent extent of air trapping.

Multiplanar volume rendering slab associated with the technique of minimum intensity projection increases the contrast media between areas of normal lung attenuation and areas of lung hypoattenuation. This helps the depiction of mosaic perfusion pattern. Its applications on expiratory CT images can also facilitate assessment of the presence and extent of air trapping.

The extent of air trapping present on expiratory CT can be measured using a semiquantitative scoring system that estimates the per cent of lung that appears abnormal. In the scoring system proposed by Stern et al., estimates of air trapping were made at each level and for each lung on a four-point scale: 0, no air trapping; 1, 1–25%; 2, 26–50%; 3, 51–75%; and 4, 76–100% of cross-sectional areas of lung affected. The air trapping score is the summation of these numbers for the different level studied. This scoring system allows good interobserver and intraobserver agreement. The extent of expiratory air trapping at CT has proved to be correlated with the degree of airflow obstruction at pulmonary function tests in patients with obliterative bronchiolitis.[29]

Objective measurement of air trapping can be done using CT densitometry. In the density mask technique, all the pixels included in areas of air trapping are segmented by thresholding at –910 HU and are highlighted and automatically counted. Density changes between full inspiration and full expiration can be compared, and expiratory/inspiratory ratios can be calculated. The density mask has the advantage that it combines density measurement with the visual assessment of pathology. Using multidetector CT with thin collimation over the lungs performed at full expiration, an exhaustive assessment of the volume of air trapping may be provided as well as a 3D visualisation of distribution of air trapping.

CHRONIC OBSTRUCTIVE PULMONARY DISEASE (COPD)[4,28,30]

Characterised by functional abnormalities, COPD is a slowly progressive airway obstructive disorder resulting from an exaggerated inflammatory response to cigarette smoke or other inhaled pollutants that ultimately destroy lung parenchyma (emphysema) and induce irreversible reduction of the calibre of the small airways (obstructive bronchiolitis). Both lesions may be associated in the same patient. On the other hand, narrowing and loss of terminal bronchioles clearly precede the appearance of microscopic emphysematous destruction.[31] The use of CT in evaluation of patients with COPD has made it clear that individuals with identical severity of airflow obstruction exhibit different morphological appearances. Some have extensive emphysema while others have only a little emphysema, suggesting more significant small airway disease. These differences in morphological appearances may be related to differences in pathophysiology and genomic profile. So, as a result, CT may be employed to objectively classify individuals as having either emphysema- or airway-predominant disease. Whether this 'phenotyping' of COPD patients will help to stratify patients in clinical trials and to optimise treatment in given individuals is currently under intense investigation.

Pathological Findings[32]

Inflammatory Changes in the Airways in COPD

Inflammatory changes in the airways in COPD patients involve both small airways and large airways. Small airway disease in COPD is initially characterised by inflammatory change in the walls and around the respiratory bronchioles (respiratory bronchiolitis characterised by pigmented macrophages). In more advanced disease, inflammatory changes in respiratory bronchioles are associated or replaced by obstruction of the lumen of the small airways with plugs of inflammatory exudates and mucus. In even more advanced involvement, the lumen of the terminal bronchioles are narrowed by peribronchiolar fibrosis (obstructive bronchiolitis). Large airway disease in COPD includes inflammation and remodelling of the trachea and bronchi. Histologically, this is characterised by wall inflammation, squamous metaplasia of bronchial epithelium, slight increase of basal membrane and smooth muscle, submucosal cells, glands hyperplasia, and deficit in cartilage.

Emphysema

Emphysema is defined as a condition of the lung characterised by permanent, abnormal enlargement of airspaces distal to the terminal bronchiole, accompanied by the destruction of their walls without obvious fibrosis. The most important factor by far is cigarette smoking. There is also a causal relationship between HIV infection and the development of early emphysema. Various genetic disorders may be associated with emphysema, including α_1-antitrypsin deficiency, heritable diseases of connective tissue such as cutix laxa, Marfan syndrome and familial emphysema.

Emphysema is thought to result from the destruction of elastic fibres caused by an imbalance between proteases and protease inhibitors in the lung and from the mechanical stresses of ventilation and coughing. Proteases are normally released in low concentration by phagocytes in the lung. Protease inhibitors, mainly α_1-protease inhibitor (α_1-antitrypsin), prevent them from causing structural damage to the lung. Imbalance in the protease–antiprotease activity may result from antiprotease deficiency (α_1-antitrypsin deficiency), from excess release of protease stimulated by environmental agents, or from the defective repair of protease-induced damage. Tobacco smoke increases the number of pulmonary macrophages and neutrophils, reduces antiprotease activity and may impair the synthesis of elastin. As emphysema develops, lung destruction progresses, airspaces enlarge, and elastic recoil declines, reducing radial traction on bronchial walls and on blood vessels and allowing airways and vessels to collapse.

Emphysema is traditionally based on the microscopic region of disease within the secondary pulmonary lobule. The principal types are centrilobular, panlobular, paraseptal and irregular emphysema. *Centrilobular (centriacinar) emphysema* affects mainly the proximal respiratory bronchioles and alveoli in the central part of the acinus. The process tends to be most developed in upper parts of the lungs. It is strongly associated with cigarette smoking. Inflammatory changes in the small airways are common with plugging, mural infiltration and fibrosis leading to stenosis, distortion and destruction. *Paraseptal emphysema* selectively involves the alveoli adjacent to connective tissues septa and bronchovascular bundles, particularly at the margins of the acinus and lobule but also subpleurally and adjacent to the bronchovascular bundles. Airspaces in paraseptal emphysema may become confluent and develop into bullae, which may be large. Airway obstruction and physiological disturbance may be minor. *Panlobular (panacinar) emphysema* is characterised by a dilatation of the airspaces of the entire acinus and lobule. With progressive destruction, all that eventually remains are thin strands of deranged tissue surrounding blood vessels. It is the most widespread and severe type of emphysema. Pathological changes are distributed throughout the lungs, but they are often basely predominant. Panlobular emphysema is the type occurring in α_1-antitrypsin deficiency and in familial cases. *Irregular emphysema* is referred to as para-cicatricial emphysema or irregular airspace enlargement, and occurs in patients with pulmonary fibrosis. It is commonly seen adjacent to localised parenchymal scars, diffuse pulmonary fibrosis, and in the pneumoconiosis, particularly progressive massive fibrosis.

Radiographic Findings

Chest radiography may be normal. When radiographic abnormalities are present, they can include hyperinflation, oligaemia, bronchial wall thickening and accentuation of linear lung markings. Thickening of the bronchial walls leads to tubular and ring shadows (Fig. 6-22). Increased lung markings cause the appearance of 'dirty chest', a term widely used for describing a loss in clarity of the lung vessels (Fig. 6-22). Sabre-sheath trachea may be present. Cor pulmonale is a recognised complication which is seen most exclusively in hypoxic patients. With the onset of heart failure, the heart and hila and intermediate lung vessels become enlarged. Enlargement of vessels is present in all zones and affects particularly segmental vessels and a few divisions beyond.

Signs of overinflation are the best predictors of the presence and severity of emphysema. Signs of overinflation include the height of the right lung being greater than 29.9 cm, location of the right hemidiaphragm at or below the anterior aspect of the seventh rib, flattening of the hemidiaphragm, enlargement of the retrosternal space, widening of the sternodiaphragmatic angle, and narrowing of the transverse cardiac diameter. Alterations in lung vessels include arterial depletion, whereas vessels of normal, or occasionally increased, calibre are present in unaffected areas of the lung, absence or displacement of vessels caused by bullae, widened branching angles with

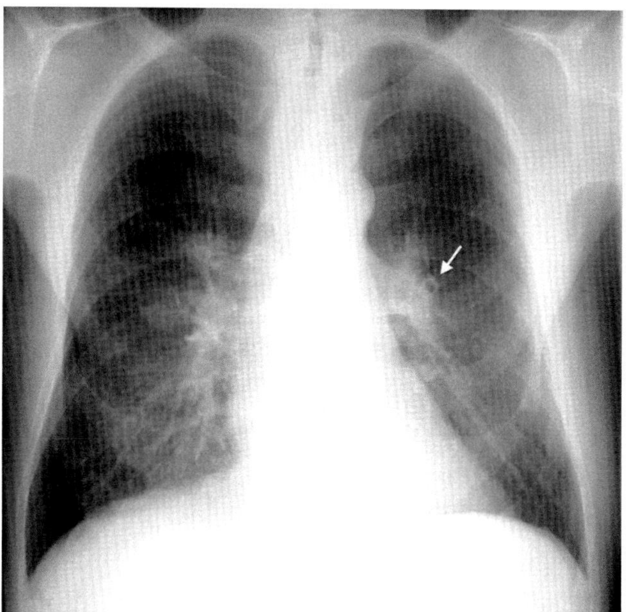

FIGURE 6-22 ■ **Chronic bronchitis and obstructive lung disease.** Postero-anterior chest radiograph shows mild overinflation. A ring shadow is visible above the left hilum (arrow), reflecting bronchial wall thickening. There is also an accentuation of linear markings in the right lung basis.

loss of side branches and vascular redistribution. With the development of cor pulmonale, or left heart failure, the radiographic appearances will alter and may become less obviously abnormal. The heart may then appear to be normal in size, or sometimes enlarged, the diaphragm becomes less flat and the pulmonary vessels less attenuated. Bullae may be as small as 1 cm in diameter or may occupy the whole hemithorax, causing marked relaxation collapse of the adjacent lung (Fig. 6-23). Bullae caused by paraseptal emphysema are much more common in the upper zones, but when they are associated with widespread panlobular emphysema, the distribution is much more even. Occasionally the wall is completely absent and in such a case bullae can be difficult to detect. The presence of emphysema associated with large bullae is referred to as *bullous emphysema* (Fig. 6-24). An entity mainly seen in young men, characterised by the presence of large progressive upper lobe bullae which occupy a significant volume of a hemithorax and are often asymmetrical, is referred as *giant bullous emphysema*, *vanishing lung syndrome* or *primary bullous disease of the lung*. Large bullae may be seen as avascular transradiant areas usually separated from the remaining lung parenchyma by a thin curvilinear wall. They can cause marked relaxation collapse of the adjacent lung and can even extend across into the opposite hemithorax, particularly by way of the anterior junction area.

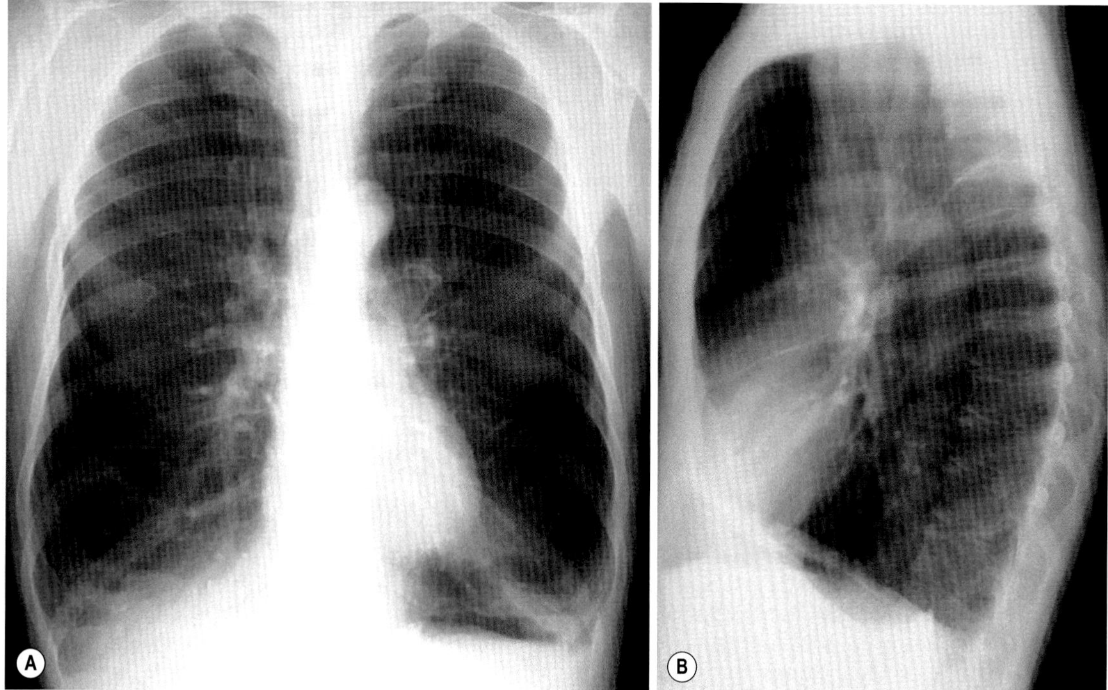

FIGURE 6-23 ■ **Severe diffuse emphysema.** Postero-anterior (A) and lateral (B) chest radiographs. The diaphragm is displaced downwards, and appears flattened. On the PA radiograph (A), the transverse cardiac diameter is reduced. The diaphragm appears irregular in contours due to an abnormal visibility of diaphragmatic insertions on the ribs. Note the depression of vessels in the periphery of the lungs. On the lateral radiograph (B), there is a widening of the sternodiaphragm angle and an increase of dimensions of the retrosternal transradiant area.

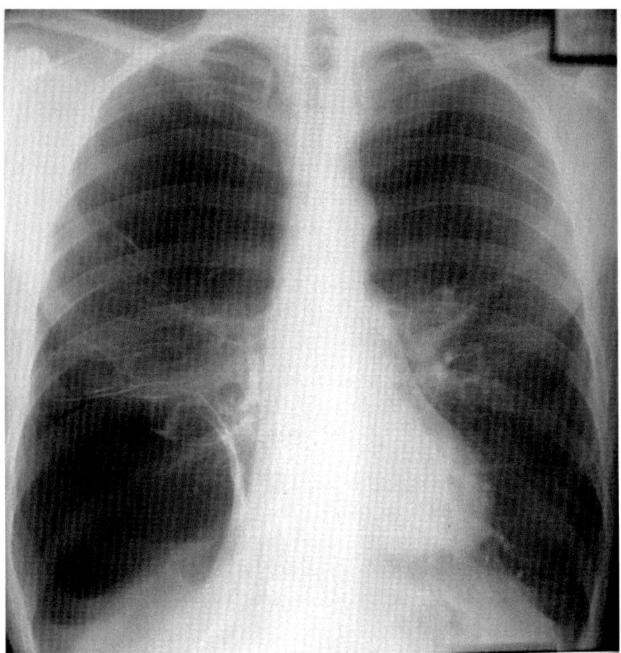

FIGURE 6-24 ■ **Giant bullous emphysema.** The PA chest radiograph shows large avascular transradiant areas in the upper and lower parts of the right lung. The bullae are marginated with thin curvilinear opacities.

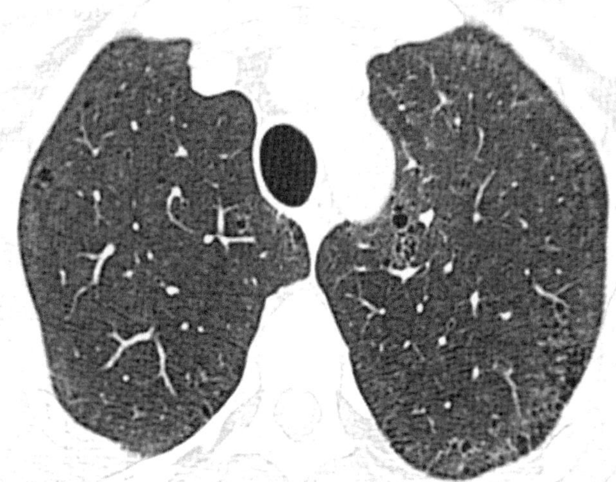

FIGURE 6-25 ■ **Respiratory bronchiolitis in heavy smoker.** Axial CT at the level of the upper lobes. Centrilobular ill-defined small nodular opacities distributed in the periphery of the upper lobes on a background of ground-glass opacities. Some small centrilobular and paraseptal emphysematous spaces are also present.

Spontaneous pneumothorax commonly occurs in association with localised areas of emphysema or bullae affecting the lung apices.

Bullae may enlarge progressively over months or years; a period of stability may be followed by a sudden expansion. Bullae may also disappear, either spontaneously or following infection or haemorrhage. The main complications of bullae include pneumothorax, infection and haemorrhage. In case of infection or haemorrhage, bullae contain fluid and develop an air–fluid level. When a bulla becomes infected the hairline wall becomes thickened and may mimic a lung abscess. Carcinoma arising in or adjacent to bullae should be suspected in case of mural nodule, mural thickening, a change in diameter of the bulla, pneumothorax and the accumulation of fluid within the bulla.

CT Findings[28,30,33]

Small Airway Disease

At the earlier stage of the disease, the inflammatory changes in the small airways are seen on CT as multiple areas of ground-glass attenuation and small centrilobular ill-defined nodular opacities (Fig. 6-25). These abnormalities, predominant in the upper lobes or sometimes more diffuse in distribution, have been reported to be present in about 22–25% of asymptomatic smokers.[34] At the later stage of the disease, the CT findings include mosaic perfusion pattern (low attenuation and low perfusion areas where the terminal bronchioles are obstructed) and expiratory air trapping in the same areas (Fig. 6-26).

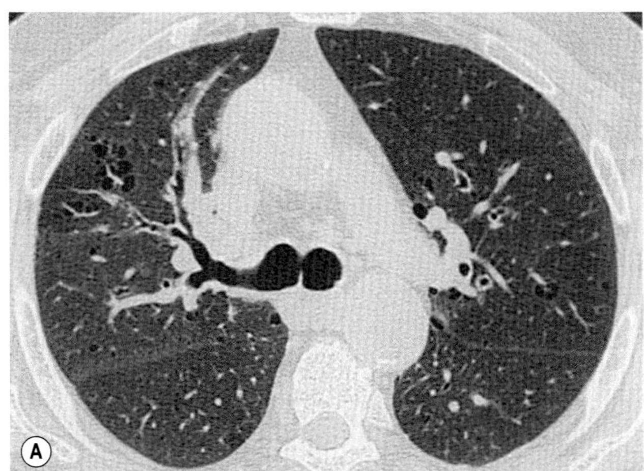

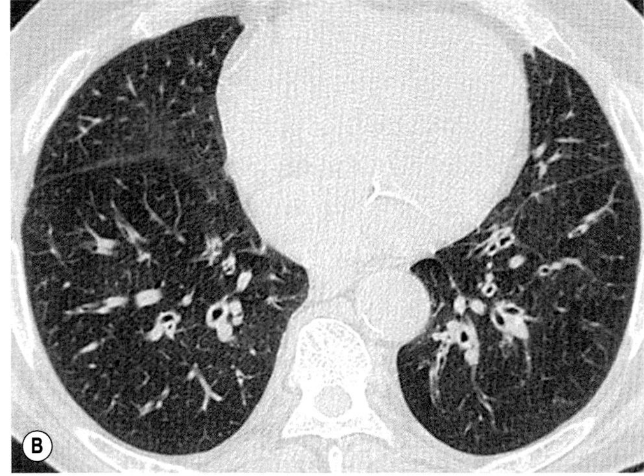

FIGURE 6-26 ■ **COPD patient with airway disease predominant phenotype.** Axial CT at the levels of the upper (A) and lower (B) parts of the chest. Few small centrilobular and paraseptal emphysematous spaces in the upper lobes. Bronchial wall thickening, slight bronchial dilatation and lung parenchyma hypoattenuation reflecting obstructive bronchiolitis in the lower lobes.

Emphysema

CT is the most accurate imaging technique to detect emphysema in vivo and to determine morphological type and extent. Emphysema is characterised by the presence of areas of abnormally low attenuation which can be easily contrasted with surrounding normal lung parenchyma if sufficiently low window values (–800 to –1000 HU) are used. Focal areas of emphysema usually lack distinct walls as opposed to lung cysts. In many patients, it is possible to classify the type of emphysema on the basis of its CT appearance, although the different types, as well as bullae, may be present in association in the same patient.

Centrilobular Emphysema (CLE). Centrilobular emphysema is recognised on CT by the presence of small well or poorly defined local lucencies surrounded by normal lung (Fig. 6-27). Small vessels, often seen traversing the hypoattenuated areas, are centrilobular pulmonary arteries or arterioles, marking the centre of each lobule. However, the pulmonary arteries appear normal in calibre. This pattern of emphysema correlates well with pathologically demonstrated centrilobular emphysema. This is the commonest type of smoking-related emphysema, and is usually upper lung predominant. Although the centrilobular location of the lucencies cannot always be recognised on CT, the presence of multiple small areas of emphysema scattered throughout the lung is diagnostic of centrilobular emphysema. As the emphysema becomes more severe, the areas of low attenuation become larger and coalescent, making the centrilobular distribution of emphysema less apparent (Fig. 6-28). Large areas of CLE may be distinguished from panlobular emphysema by the presence of a preserved rim of normal lung attenuation intervening between areas of lung destruction (Fig. 6-28). In most cases the areas of low attenuation have no visible walls; however, very thin walls may be seen, particularly when the areas of emphysema are extensive. The apparent walls in such cases probably represent atelectasis or interlobular septa adjacent to the emphysematous spaces. When the extent of emphysema increases, the distribution of low-attenuation areas may appear diffuse without predominance.

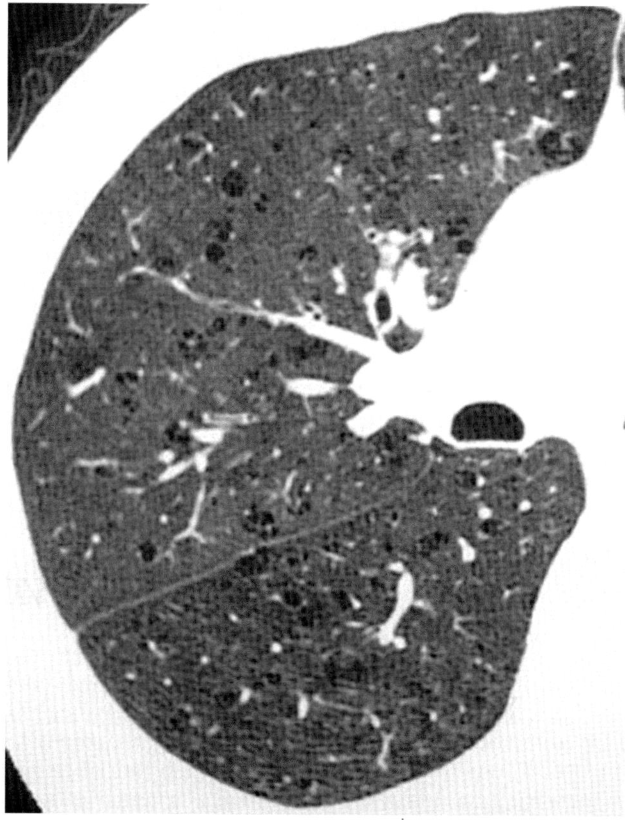

FIGURE 6-27 ■ Centrilobular emphysema. HRCT targeted on the right lung shows multiple small round areas of low attenuation distributed through the lungs, mainly around the centrilobular arteries.

Panlobular or Panacinar Emphysema (PLE). Panlobular or panacinar emphysema is manifested as a generalised decrease of attenuation of the lung parenchyma without focal lucencies. Although this pattern is classically described with α_1-antitryspin deficiency, a similar pattern may be seen with severe smoking-related emphysema. The vessels in the affected lung are usually reduced in number and in calibre, straightened and show decreased branching. The appearance of featureless decreased attenuation may sometimes be quite difficult to distinguish from severe obliterative bronchiolitis. The presence of long lines in the lower lobes reflecting fibrosis within the remaining interlobular septa in panlobular emphysema helps distinguish this entity from obliterative bronchiolitis (Fig. 6-29). Usually these abnormalities are most severe in the lower lobes. As clinical manifestations of PLE associated with α_1-protease inhibitor deficiency are often seen in cigarette smokers, focal lucencies due

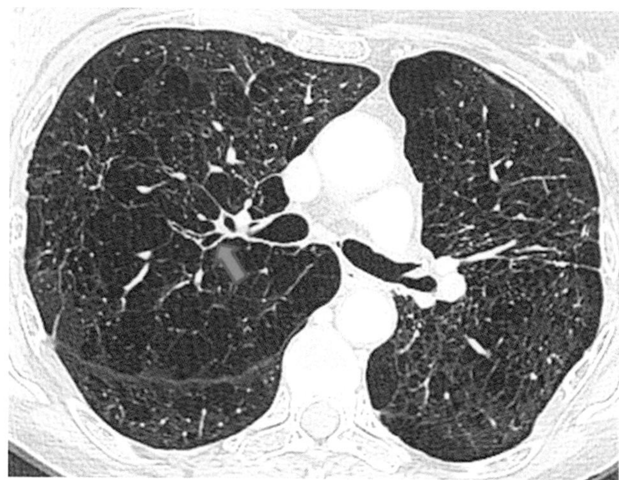

FIGURE 6-28 ■ Advanced centrilobular emphysema in a smoker. Axial CT at the level of the upper lobes shows large and coalescent areas of low attenuation with lobular margins corresponding to advanced centrilobular emphysematous spaces predominantly distributed on the right side. The patient had a history of left upper lobectomy for bronchopulmonary carcinoma. Note the thickened bronchi related to associated airway remodelling (arrow).

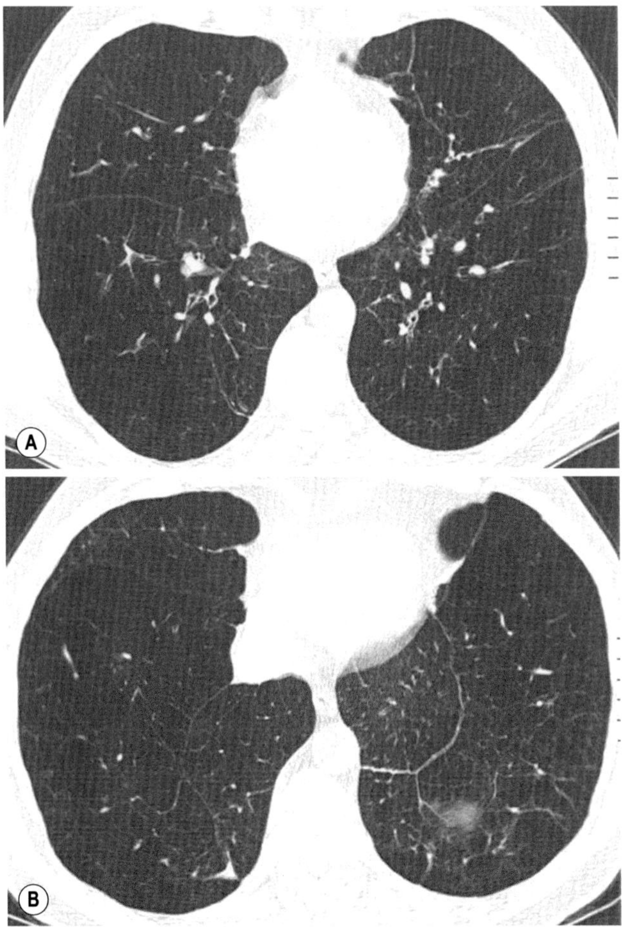

FIGURE 6-29 ■ Panlobular emphysema in a patient with α_1-antitryspin deficiency. Axial CT at the levels of the mild (A) and lower parts (B) of the lung with diffuse lung attenuation and paucity of the pulmonary vessels. The presence of multiple thin lines, particularly throughout the lung bases, reflects a distortion of the anatomical structure of the lung parenchyma and thickening of the remaining interlobular septa by lung fibrosis.

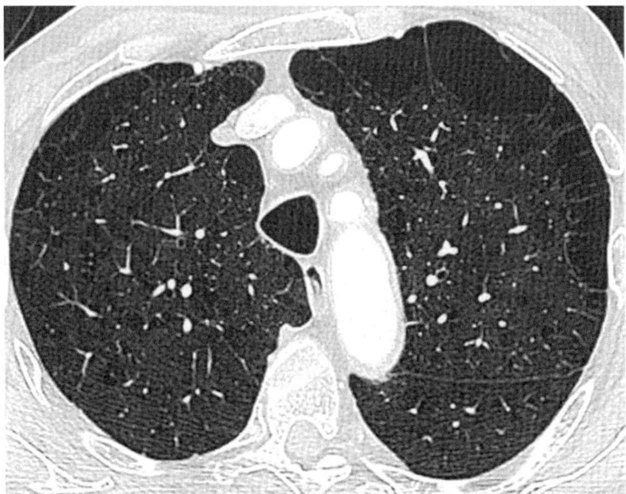

FIGURE 6-30 ■ Paraseptal emphysema. Axial CT at the level of the upper lobes. Predominant paraseptal emphysema in a COPD patient appearing as areas of low attenuation mainly distributed along the peripheral and mediastinal pleura on the left side. Note associated centrilobular emphysema.

to centrilobular emphysema may be seen in the upper lobes. Occasionally, PLE occurring in smokers is predominant in the upper lungs. Paraseptal emphysema and bullae can also be seen, but are not a major feature of the disease. In severe PLE, the characteristic appearance of extensive lung destruction and the associated paucity of vascular markings may have a diffuse distribution. On the other hand, mild and even moderately severe PLE can be very subtle and difficult to detect radiologically.

Paraseptal Emphysema (PSE). Paraseptal emphysema is characterised by subpleural and peribronchovascular regions of low attenuation separated by intact interlobular septa thickened by associated mild fibrosis (Fig. 6-30). PSE has a special predilection for peripheral subpleural lobules (along the mediastinal and peripheral pleura, and fissures) in the anterior and posterior aspect of the upper lobes and the posterior aspect of the lower lobes. It is not associated with vascular distortion. CT shows subpleural areas of low attenuation, usually with a well-defined wall. Rows of paraseptal emphysema may mimic honeycombing, but the cyst size is usually larger than honeycomb cysts, and architectural distortion is not present. In addition, as opposed to PSE, honeycombing is most often made of several layers of cysts. PSE is often associated with multifocal areas of centrilobular emphysema and CT findings of inflammatory changes in and around the small airways.

Bullae. Bullae are seen as avascular low-attenuation areas that are > 1 cm in diameter, and that can have a thin but perceptible wall. The bullae are often multiple and associated with emphysema of any type. Bullae are often located in the upper lobes in both CLE and in PSE, but are more evenly distributed in the lungs of patients with PLE. *Bullous emphysema* is a pattern characterised by multiple large avascular lucencies partly bounded by a thin wall (Fig. 6-31). Bullae may be large enough to compress the adjacent lung parenchyma. Although such compression is usually relatively mild, it may result occasionally in relaxation atelectasis appearing as a parenchymal band or a mass-like opacity. Most patients having bullous lung disease have concomitant centrilobular, panlobular or paraseptal emphysema. The term giant bullous emphysema has been used to describe the presence of bullae occupying at least once-third of a hemithorax. Giant bullae may be compressive not only on the underlying lung parenchyma but also on the diaphragm and the right atrium with the risk of tamponade.

Emphysema Associated with Interstitial Pneumonias. Emphysema associated with interstitial pneumonias, which include respiratory bronchiolitis associated with interstitial lung disease (RB-ILD), desquamative interstitial pneumonia (DIP) or other interstitial pneumonias may occur in heavy smokers, particularly those having COPD. The association of emphysema and usual interstitial pneumonia (UIP) is responsible for a specific CT pattern in which extensive emphysema involves the upper lung and honeycombing the bases. In such a

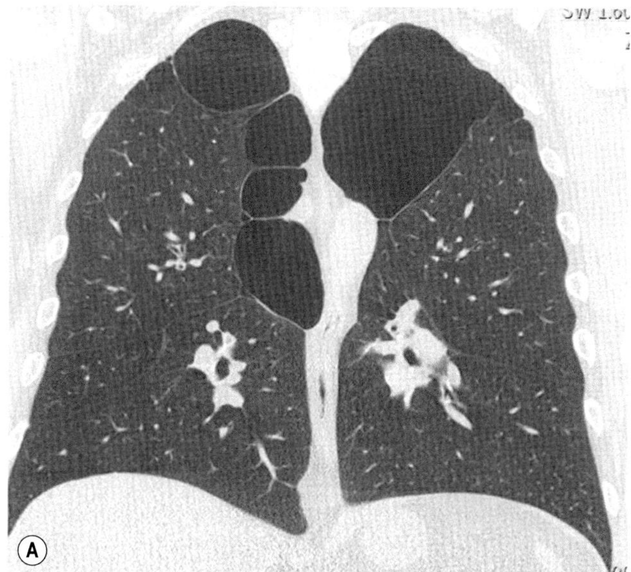

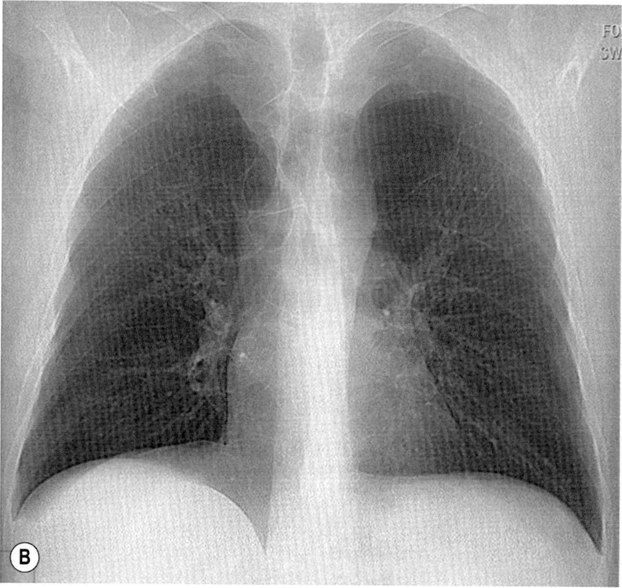

FIGURE 6-31 ■ **Bullous emphysema.** (A) Coronal reformat. (B) Coronal average image (200-mm-thick slab) giving a rendering of chest X-ray equivalent.

particular situation, restrictive and obstructive disease counteract each other, explaining why these patients present with normal or almost normal lung volumes and FEV1 despite a significant drop of diffuse capacity of carbon monoxide and a deep hypoaxemia at exercise.

Large Airway Disease[28,30,35]

The commonest CT finding of remodelling of bronchi is bronchial wall thickening, which is common in smokers, more particularly those with functional impairment, and more particularly those presenting clinical symptoms of chronic bronchitis.[36] Bronchial wall and lumen irregularities are commonly visualised on CT, reflecting remodelling and deficit in cartilage (Fig. 6-26). Evidence of moderate tubular (cylindrical) bronchiectasis (most in the lower lobes) is common (29–58%).[37] Bronchiectasis is associated with severe airflow obstruction, more severe COPD exacerbation, lower airway bacterial colonisation, and increased sputum inflammatory markers.[38] Bronchial diverticula, seen as outpouchings in addition to the lumen of mainstem and lobar bronchi, reflect fusion of multiple depressions and dilatations of bronchial gland ducts; these features are best visualised on longitudinal minimal intensity projection thick-slab reconstructions and have been reported in 12% of smokers (mostly in heavy smokers with cough, with severe functional impairment, extensive emphysema and more severe bronchial wall thickening).[39] Bronchomalacia may be demonstrated on expiratory CT as almost complete collapse of the lumen of segmental or subsegmental bronchi, mostly in the lower lobes where the deficit in cartilage is more apparent.[40]

CT Quantitative Analysis of Extent of Disease

Quantitative analysis may include extent of emphysema, measurement of airway dimensions and extent of air trapping.

The distribution and severity of emphysema may be quantified by CT. CT findings can be assessed by subjective visual methods, density measurements or by post-processing and texture analysis. The simplest method for estimating the severity of emphysema involves assigning a grade based on visual CT interpretation. Typically this approach calls for assessing individual HRCT sections, using 4- or 5-point scale, as either normal or showing mild (<25% of the lung), moderate (25–50% of the lung), marked (50–75% of the lung), or severe (75–100%) of the lung) emphysema, with the total score expressed as percentage of total lung at that level. In general, visual inspection has yielded good correlations between CT and pathological measures of the extent and severity, especially of centrilobular emphysema. However, subjective grading of emphysema appears significantly less accurate than objective CT densitometric results and visual assessment and leads to a significant overestimation of the extent of emphysema. CT densitometry provides better correlation with a morphological reference.[41] The density of emphysematous area is abnormally low. If a histogram plot is made of frequency against pixel density (HU), the emphysematous curve is shifted to the left compared with normal. Voxels with values below a certain number can be highlighted on a CT image (density mask technique) and expressed as a percentage of the total pixels included in the lung section. The use of −960/−970 HU threshold shows optimal anatomical correlation with both macroscopic and microscopic morphometry (the use of −950 HU has proved good correlations as well) and is the optimal threshold to use when evaluating 1-mm section with MDCT acquisition.[42] The percentile density is defined as the value (Hounsfield) at which a certain percentage of the voxels in the frequency distribution histogram have a lower density. Madani et al. showed that the strongest morphometric correlations were observed with using the first percentile on 1.25-mm-thick sections obtained after volumetric acquisition using MDCT.[42] It has also become feasible to apply density thresholding technique to volumetric data. Lung volume and volume of emphysema are quantified and displayed at a regional level, for better preoperative assessment in severe emphysematous patients, candidates for bullectomy, lung volume reduction surgery or lung transplantation. Some recommendations have been made in order to standardise sequential CT studies in patients with emphysema: air calibration; image reconstruction with standard reconstruction algorithms; images obtained in deep inspiration (close to total lung capacity) overcome the need for spirometric gating; and not to decrease the dose below 50 mA.

Different methods have also been proposed for quantitative analysis of air trapping extent:[43]

1. The percentage of voxels below –850 HU in expiration.
2. The percentage of voxels between –850 and –910 HU in expiration.
3. The expiration-to-inspiration ratio of mean lung density.
4. The change in relative lung volume with attenuation values from –850 to –950 HU between paired inspiratory and expiratory examinations. This latest method allows the degree of airway dysfunction after extraction of emphysema from the volume of interest.[44]

According to the literature, there is a significant association between the dimensions of the small and large airways in COPD patients, meaning that measuring airway dimension in the larger bronchi can provide an estimate of small airway remodelling.[45]

Specific software permits 3D reconstruction of the lumen of the tracheobronchial tree, followed by an automatic extraction of the central axis of the airways. On any point of the tracheobronchial tree, the software provides a cross-section of the airway at this point strictly perpendicular to the central axis. Then the algorithm permits automatic segmentation of inner and outer contours of the airways, and calculation of wall area (WA), luminal area (LA) and wall area percentage (WA%). Several investigators have used this technique in COPD patients.

Bronchial wall thickening in cigarette smokers has been related to lung function (FEV1).[46] In COPD patients, bronchial wall thickening and extent of emphysema are both the strongest determinants of FEV1.[47,48] Both bronchial wall thickening and the percentage of emphysema extent have been demonstrated to be associated with COPD exacerbation frequency.[49]

ASTHMA[3,4,50]

Asthma is a chronic inflammatory condition involving the airways. This inflammation causes a generalised increase in existing bronchial hyper-responsiveness to a variety of stimuli. This is commonly used in practice to confirm the clinical diagnosis of asthma. In susceptible individuals, this inflammation induces recurrent episodes of wheezing, chest tightness, breathlessness, and coughing usually associated with widespread but variable airflow obstruction that is often reversible either spontaneously or with treatment. The chronic inflammation process leads to structural changes, such as new vessel formation, airway smooth muscle thickening, and fibrosis, which may result in irreversible airway narrowing.

Radiographic Findings

Chest radiography is usually recommended in all asthmatic patients who are ill enough to justify admission to a hospital. Hyperinflation may be seen in both relapse and remission. The prevalence of hyperinflation is generally higher in children and in patients needing hospital admission. While hyperinflation is initially often transient, it may become a permanent change. Bronchial wall thickening is more frequent in children, but in adults when it becomes visible it is usually an irreversible phenomenon. The walls of end-on segmental airways become thickened and the normally invisible airways appear on radiographs as parallel or single line opacities which may be seen in up to two-thirds of patients. Chest radiography may depict complications including consolidation, atelectasis, mucoid impaction, pneumothorax and pneumomediastinum. Consolidation is commonly infective but, in some cases, it is due to eosinophilic consolidation probably associated with allergic aspergillosis. Collapse ranges from subsegmental to lobar and occasionally involves the whole lung. Collapse is due to mucoid impaction in large airways or more commonly mucus plugging in many small airways.

CT Findings

The clinical indications for performing CT in patients with asthma include the detection of bronchiectasis in patients with suspected allergic bronchopulmonary aspergillosis, the documentation of the presence and extent of emphysema in smokers with asthma, and the identification of conditions that may be confused with asthma, such as hypersensitivity pneumonitis, chronic eosinophilic pneumonia and Churg–Strauss syndrome.[50] In uncomplicated asthma, HRCT may show bronchial dilatation, bronchial wall thickening, mucoid impaction, decreased lung attenuation, air trapping and small centrilobular opacities. These abnormalities may or may not be reversible with steroid treatment. The prevalence of these thin-section CT abnormalities increases with increasing severity of symptoms. Considerable variation exists, however, in the reported frequency of abnormalities. This variation is related to differences in diagnostic criteria and patient selection.

Bronchial wall thickness measured on CT has proved to be prominent in patients with more severe asthma.[51–53] It is correlated with the duration and severity of disease and the degree of airflow obstruction. Peribronchial inflammation may be partly responsible for the bronchial wall thickening, but when the feature is not reversible after steroids, it reflects the development of hyperplasia and hypertrophy of smooth muscle on the bronchial wall, reflecting airway wall remodelling.[54] This observation supports the concept that quantitative assessment of bronchial wall area on CT could be used to assess airway

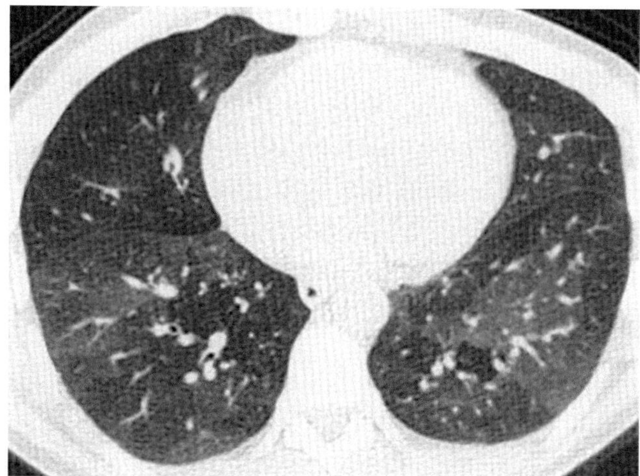

FIGURE 6-32 ■ **Mild persistent asthmatic patient.** Axial CT at suspended end-expiration. Patchy areas of air trapping involving individual lobules and segments in the lower and right middle lobes.

wall remodelling in asthmatic patients for longitudinal studies to evaluate the effects of new therapies.

Focal and diffuse areas of decreased lung attenuation seen in 20–30% of asthmatic patients are likely the results of a combination of air trapping and pulmonary oligaemia owing to alveolar hypoventilation. The areas of decreased attenuation in acute asthma almost always reflect hypoxic vasoconstriction in parts of the lung that are underventilated due to bronchospasm, and such areas of air trapping are more conspicuous and extensive on expiratory CT.

In chronic asthma, morphological features of emphysema on CT are almost variably related to cigarette smoking, rather than the asthma itself, in which the decreased attenuation areas represent small airway obstruction. Expiratory CT can show abnormal air trapping even in patients who have normal inspiratory CT findings (Fig. 6-32). In addition, CT may depict air trapping before lung function deteriorates. Abnormal expiratory air trapping has been observed in 50% of asthmatic patients.[55] This reflects the luminal obstruction of the airways and is potentially, but not always, reversible. In mild-to-moderate asthmatics, the index of air trapping may decrease significantly after 3 months' inhaled corticosteroids.[56] In patients with persistent asthma, the absence of change in air trapping scores after inhalation of bronchodilator suggests that the air trapping may reflect permanent changes resulting from small airway remodelling. The mosaic perfusion pattern is frequent in patients with moderate persistent asthma[57] (Fig. 6-33). In severe persistent asthma, diffuse decreased lung attenuation and expiratory air trapping make the pattern difficult to distinguish from that of obliterative bronchiolitis. The extent of air trapping correlates with the severity of the asthma, airflow limitation, airway hyperresponsiveness and disease duration.[58] Those with air trapping are significantly more likely to have a history of asthma-related hospitalisations, ICU visits and/or mechanical ventilation.[59]

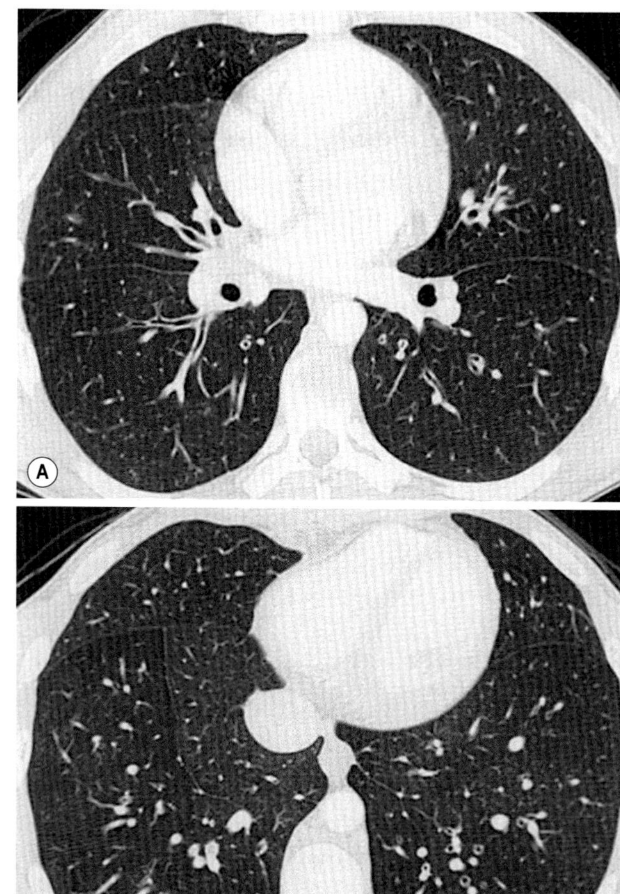

FIGURE 6-33 ■ **Moderate persistent asthmatic patient.** Axial CT at the levels of mid- (A) and lower (B) parts of the lungs. Diffuse bronchial wall thickening with mucoid impactions in the subsegmental and segmental bronchi in the basilar segments of the right lower lobe. Patchy areas of hypoattenuation in the anterior, lateral and posterobasal segments of the right lower lobe and the posterior segment of the left lower lobe, reflecting the presence of small airway remodelling.

REFERENCES

1. Beigelman-Aubry C, Brillet PY, Grenier PA. MDCT of the airways: technique and normal results. Radiol Clin North Am 2009;47:185–201.
2. Naidich DP, Webb WR, Grenier PA, et al. Imaging of the Airways. Philadelphia: Lippincott Williams & Wilkins; 2005.
3. Boiselle P, Lynch D. CT of the Airways. Humana Press; 2008.
4. Hansell DM, Armstrong P, Lynch DA, et al. Imaging of Diseases of the Chest. 4th ed. Philadelphia: Elsevier Mosby; 2005.
5. Grenier PA, Beigelman-Aubry C, Fetita C, et al. New frontiers in CT imaging of airway disease. Eur Radiol 2012;12:1022–44.
6. Kang EY. Large airway diseases. J Thorac Imaging 2011;26:249–62.
7. Grenier PA, Beigelman-Aubry C, Brillet PY. Nonneoplastic tracheal and bronchial stenoses. Radiol Clin North Am 2009;47:243–60.
8. Ferretti GR, Bithigoffer C, Righini CA, et al. Imaging of tumors of the trachea and central bronchi. Radiol Clin North Am 2009;47:227–41.
9. Lee EY, Litmanovich D, Boiselle PM. Multidetector CT evaluation of tracheobronchomalacia. Radiol Clin North Am 2009;47:261–9.
10. Baroni RH, Feller-Kopman D, Nishino M, et al. Tracheobronchomalacia: comparison between end-expiratory and dynamic expiratory CT for evaluation of central airway collapse. Radiology 2005;235:635–41.

11. Ridge CA, O'Donnell CR, Lee EY, et al. Tracheobronchomalacia: current concepts and controversies. J Thorac Imaging 2011;26: 278–89.
12. Javidan-Nejad C, Bhalla S. Bronchiectasis. Radiol Clin North Am 2009;47:289–306.
13. O'Donnell AE. Bronchiectasis. Chest 2008;134:815–23.
14. Feldman C. Bronchiectasis: new approaches to diagnosis and management. Clin Chest Med 2011;32:535–46.
15. Ooi GC, Khong PL, Chan-Yeung M, et al. High-resolution CT quantification of bronchiectasis: clinical and functional correlation. Radiology 2002;225:663–72.
16. Roberts HR, Wells AU, Milne DG, et al. Airflow obstruction in bronchiectasis: correlation between computed tomography features and pulmonary function tests. Thorax 2000;55:198–204.
17. Sheehan RE, Wells AU, Copley SJ, et al. A comparison of serial computed tomography and functional change in bronchiectasis. Eur Respir J 2002;20:581–7.
18. Devaraj A, Wells AU, Meister MG, et al. Pulmonary hypertension in patients with bronchiectasis: prognostic significance of CT signs. Am J Roentgenol 2011;196:1300–4.
19. Dodd JD, Souza CA, Müller NL. Conventional high-resolution CT versus helical high-resolution MDCT in the detection of bronchiectasis. Am J Roentgenol 2006;187:414–20.
20. Hill LE, Ritchie G, Wightman AJ, et al. Comparison between conventional interrupted high-resolution CT and volume multidetector CT acquisition in the assessment of bronchiectasis. Br J Radiol 2010;83:67–70.
21. Remy-Jardin M, Amara A, Campistron P, et al. Diagnosis of bronchiectasis with multislice spiral CT: accuracy of 3-mm-thick structured sections. Eur Radiol 2003;13:1165–71.
22. Chooi WK, Matthews S, Bull MJ, Morcos SK. Multislice helical CT: the value of multiplanar image reconstruction in assessment of the bronchi and small airways disease. Br J Radiol 2003;76:536–40.
23. Sung YM, Lee KS, Yi CA, et al. Additional coronal images using low-milliamperage multidetector-row computed tomography: effectiveness in the diagnosis of bronchiectasis. J Comput Assist Tomogr 2003;27:490–5.
24. Eichinger M, Heussel CP, Kauczor HU, et al. Computed tomography and magnetic resonance imaging in cystic fibrosis lung disease. J Magn Reson Imaging 2010;32:1370–8.
25. Ohno Y, Koyama H, Yoshikawa T, et al. Pulmonary magnetic resonance imaging for airway diseases. J Thorac Imaging 2011;26: 301–16.
26. Pipavath SN, Stern EJ. Imaging of small airway disease (SAD). Radiol Clin North Am 2009;47:307–16.
27. Copley SJ, Wells AU, Muller NL, et al. Thin-section CT in obstructive pulmonary disease: discriminatory value. Radiology 2002;223:812–19.
28. Ley-Zaporozhan J, Kauczor HU. Imaging of airways: chronic obstructive pulmonary disease. Radiol Clin North Am 2009;47: 331–42.
29. Hansell DM, Rubens MB, Padley SP, et al. Obliterative bronchiolitis: individual CT signs of small airways disease and functional correlation. Radiology 1997;203:721–6.
30. Kauczor HU, Wielpütz MO, Owsijewitsch M, Ley-Zaporozhan J. Computed tomographic imaging of the airways in COPD and asthma. J Thorac Imaging 2011;26:290–300.
31. McDonough JE, Yuan R, Suzuki M, et al. Small-airway obstruction and emphysema in chronic obstructive pulmonary disease. N Engl J Med 2011;365:1567–75.
32. Hogg JC, McDonough J. Anatomic pathology of COPD. In: Crapo JD, editor. Atlas of Chronic Obstructive Pulmonary Disease. Berlin: Springer; 2009. pp. 73–89.
33. Grenier PA, Beigelman-Aubry C. Radiological phenotypes of COPD. In: Crapo JD, editor. Atlas of Chronic Obstructive Pulmonary Disease. Berlin: Springer; 2009. pp. 65–72.
34. Remy-Jardin M, Remy J, Boulenguez C, et al. Morphological effects of cigarette smoking on airways and pulmonary parenchyma in healthy adult volunteers: CT evaluation and correlation with pulmonary function tests. Radiology 1993;186:107–15.
35. Brillet PY, Fetita CI, Saragaglia A, et al. Investigation of airways using MDCT for visual and quantitative assessment in COPD patients. Int J Chronic Obstruct Pulm Dis 2008;3:97–107.
36. Devici F, Murat A, Targut T, et al. Airway wall thickness in patients with COPD and healthy current smokers and healthy non-smokers in assessment with high-resolution computed tomographic scanning. Respiration 2004;71:602–10.
37. O'Brien C, Guest PJ, Hill SL, Stockley RA. Physiological and radiological characterisation of patients diagnosed with chronic obstructive pulmonary disease in primary care. Thorax 2000;55: 635–42.
38. Martínez-García MÁ, Soler-Cataluña JJ, Donat Sanz Y, et al. Factors associated with bronchiectasis in patients with COPD. Chest 2011;140:1130–7.
39. Sverzellati N, Ingegnoli A, Calabrò E, et al. Bronchial diverticula in smokers on thin-section CT. Eur Radiol 2010;20:88–94.
40. Matsuoka S, Kurihara Y, Yagihashi K, et al. Airway dimensions at inspiratory and expiratory multisection CT in chronic obstructive pulmonary disease: correlation with airflow limitation. Radiology 2008;248:1042–9.
41. Bankier AA, De Maertelaer V, Keyzer C, et al. Pulmonary emphysema: subjective visual grading versus objective quantification with macroscopic morphometry and thin-section CT densitometry. Radiology 1999;211:851–8.
42. Madani A, Zanen J, de Maertelaer V, Gevenois PA. Pulmonary emphysema: objective quantification at multi-detector row-CT—comparison with macroscopic and microscopic morphometry. Radiology 2006;238:1036–43.
43. Mets OM, Murphy K, Zanen P, et al. The relationship between lung function impairment and quantitative computed tomography in chronic obstructive pulmonary disease. Eur Radiol 2012;22: 120–8.
44. Matsuoka S, Kurihara Y, Yagihashi K, et al. Quantitative assessment of air trapping in chronic obstructive pulmonary disease using inspiratory and expiratory volumetric MDCT. Am J Roentgenol 2008;190:762–9.
45. Nakano Y, Wong JC, de Jong PA, et al. The prediction of small airway dimensions using computed tomography. Am J Respir Crit Care Med 2005;171:142–6.
46. Berger P, Perot V, Desbarats P, et al. Airway wall thickness in cigarette smokers: quantitative thin-section CT assessment. Radiology 2005;235:1055–64.
47. Aziz ZA, Wells AU, Desai SR, et al. Functional impairment in emphysema: contribution of airway abnormalities and distribution of parenchymal disease. Am J Roentgenol 2005;185:1509–15.
48. Nakano Y, Muro S, Sakai H, et al. Computed tomographic measurements of airway dimensions and emphysema in smokers. Correlation with lung function. Am J Respir Crit Care Med 2000; 162:1102–8.
49. Han MK, Kazerooni EA, Lynch DA, et al; COPDGene Investigators. Chronic obstructive pulmonary disease exacerbations in the COPDGene study: associated radiological phenotypes. Radiology 2011;261:274–82.
50. Woods AQ, Lynch DA. Asthma: an imaging update. Radiol Clin N Am 2009;47:317–29.
51. Aysola RS, Hoffman EA, Gierada D, et al. Airway remodeling measured by multidetector CT is increased in severe asthma and correlates with pathology. Chest 2008;134:1183–91.
52. Montaudon M, Lederlin M, Reich S, et al. Bronchial measurements in patients with asthma: comparison of quantitative thin-section CT findings with those in healthy subjects and correlation with pathological findings. Radiology 2009;253:844–53.
53. Gupta S, Siddiqui S, Haldar P, et al. Quantitative analysis of high-resolution computed tomography scans in severe asthma subphenotypes. Thorax 2010;65:775–81.
54. Niimi A, Matsumoto H, Amitani R, et al. Effect of short-term treatment with inhaled corticosteroid on airway wall thickening in asthma. Am J Med 2004;116:725–31.
55. Park CS, Muller NL, Worthy SA, et al. Airway obstruction in asthmatic and healthy individuals: inspiratory and expiratory thin-section CT findings. Radiology 1997;203:361–7.
56. Kurashima K, Kanauchi T, Hoshi T, et al. Effect of early versus late intervention with inhaled corticosteroids on airway wall thickness in patients with asthma. Respirology 2008;13: 1008–13.
57. Laurent F, Latrabe V, Raherison C, et al. Functional significance of air trapping detected in moderate asthma. Eur Radiol 2000;10:1404–10.
58. Ueda T, Niimi A, Matsumoto H, et al. Role of small airways in asthma: investigation using high-resolution computed tomography. J Allergy Clin Immunol 2006;118:1019–25.
59. Busacker A, Newell JD Jr, Keefe T, et al. A multivariate analysis of risk factors for the air-trapping asthmatic phenotype as measured by quantitative CT analysis. Chest 2009;135:48–56.

CHAPTER 7

Pulmonary Lobar Collapse: Essential Considerations

Susan J. Copley

CHAPTER OUTLINE

Collapse and atelectasis are terms which are often used synonymously and refer to loss of volume within the lung. In North America, the term collapse is often reserved to denote complete loss of volume within an entire lobe or lung.[1] Atelectasis can be described according to extent (linear, plate-like or subsegmental atelectasis, sublobar and lobar atelectasis) or due to the underlying aetiology: compression or passive atelectasis (e.g. by pleural effusion, pneumothorax or bulla) and obstructive or post-stenotoic atelectasis. Rounded atelectasis refers to a specific type of a sublobar atelectasis associated with previous (often haemorrhagic) exudative pleural effusion (e.g. post-thoracotomy, trauma and asbestos exposure). It is associated with adjacent visceral pleural thickening and has characteristic CT appearances which are described elsewhere.

MECHANISMS AND CAUSES OF LOBAR COLLAPSE

Broadly, lobar collapse can be divided into those due to endobronchial obstruction (either intrinsic or extrinsic) and those without obstruction.[2,3] The causes of lobar collapse are summarised in Table 7-1. The common causes differ slightly between adults and children. In adults the frequent causes of intrinsic obstruction are tumours and mucus plugs. In the clinical context of a middle-aged or elderly smoker, lobar collapse should always be suspected to be due to a bronchogenic carcinoma until proved otherwise. All cell types of bronchogenic carcinoma can potentially cause intrinsic large airway obstruction and produce segmental, lobar or whole lung collapse (Fig. 7-1).[2] More rarely, foreign bodies, broncholiths and focal bronchostenosis due to inflammation or trauma may be encountered. In children, causes such as inhaled foreign bodies or mucus plugs are common (Fig. 7-2), with tumours being very rare.

RADIOGRAPHIC CONSIDERATIONS

The cardinal radiographic features of lobar collapse are increased opacity of the affected lobe and volume loss. The latter can be inferred by direct and indirect signs. Direct signs of volume loss refer to displacement of interlobar fissures, pulmonary vessels and bronchi, whereas indirect signs include compensatory shifts of adjacent structures such as hyperinflation of other lobes. The effects of a lobar collapse are often maximal on immediately adjacent structures; e.g. an upper lobe collapse often results in a shift of the superior mediastinum, whereas a lower lobe collapse often demonstrates elevation of the posterior part of the diaphragm in particular. However, the general principles and fundamental radiographic signs are similar for all lobes.

A collapsed lobe appears radiographically dense due to a combination of retained secretions or fluid within the lobe and reduction in aeration of the lobe.[4] However, retained fluid is the dominant process, resulting in increased opacity of a partially collapsed lobe, as virtually complete collapse is required to displace sufficient air for the normally radiographically hyperlucent lung to appear dense.

Direct Signs of Volume Loss

Displacement of fissures is a reliable feature of lobar collapse, and is generally characteristic depending on the affected lobe.[5] The pulmonary vessels and bronchi become crowded together in the affected lobe as the lung loses volume. The sign may be one of the earliest seen in lobar collapse and can often be readily appreciated by comparison with previous radiographs.

Hilar elevation on the posteroanterior (PA) chest radiograph is a well-known sign of upper lobe collapse: the ipsilateral interlobar and lower lobe arteries remain visible as these structures are still outlined by aerated lung. It

TABLE 7-1 **Causes of Lobar Collapse**[2,3]

Lobar Collapse due to Endobronchial Obstruction
• Intrinsic
Bronchogenic carcinoma
Bronchial carcinoid
Adenoid cystic carcinoma
Metastases (e.g. breast, renal cell and colonic carcinoma, melanoma, sarcoma)
Lymphoma
Benign tumours (e.g. lipoma, hamartoma, papillomas, endometriomas)
Granulomatous diseases (e.g. sarcoidosis and tuberculosis)
Miscellaneous conditions (e.g. aspirated foreign bodies, mucus plugs, gastric contents, malpositioned endotracheal tubes, bronchial torsion or rupture, amyloidosis, Wegener's granulomatosis)
• Extrinsic
Hilar or mediastinal lymphadenopathy (commonly due to bronchogenic or breast carcinoma)
Mediastinal masses
Fibrosing mediastinitis
Aortic aneurysms and congenital vascular anomalies
Cardiac enlargement
Lobar Collapse without Endobronchial Obstruction
• Miscellaneous conditions (e.g. passive collapse due to pleural fluid or pneumothorax, radiation-induced collapse, tumour replacement (adenocarcinoma))

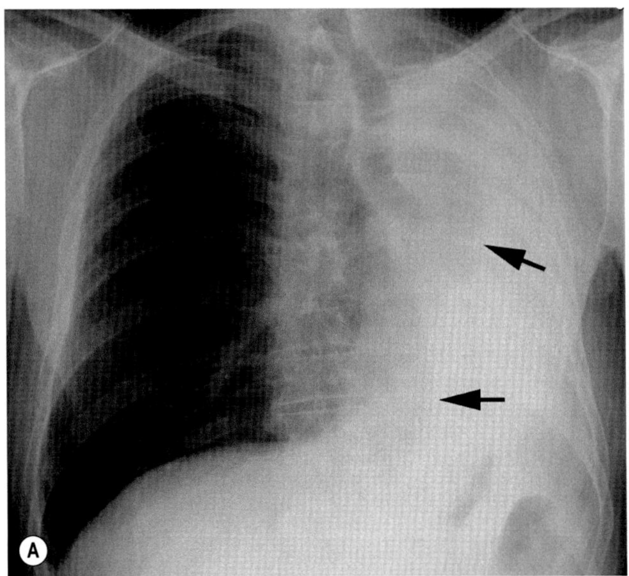

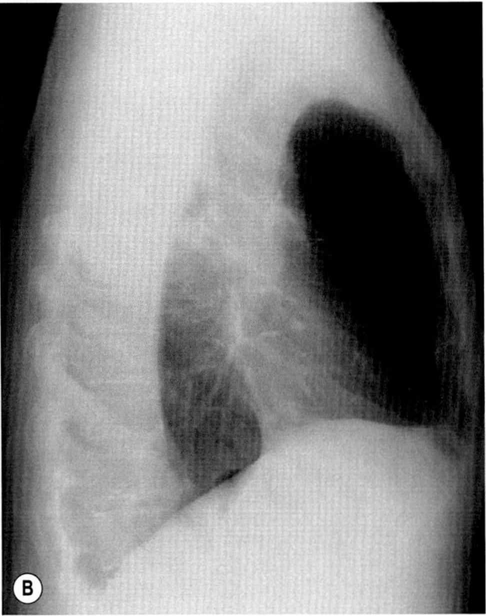

FIGURE 7-1 ■ **Total left lung collapse.** (A) Frontal and (B) lateral chest radiographs. The cause of the collapse is a bronchogenic carcinoma; the endobronchial component is visible as an abrupt cut-off of the left main bronchus. Note the marked displacement of the right lung anteriorly and posteriorly across the midline (arrows). Note the marked anterior hyperlucency of the thorax on the lateral view (B).

would seem logical to consider 'hilar depression' to be a sign of lower lobe collapse, but some authorities believe the small hilum to be a more accurate description.[5] This is due to the fact that when a lower lobe collapses, the opaque, collapsed lobe obscures the lower lobe artery that lies within it, and the interlobar artery is usually rotated so the margin is no longer in profile to the frontal X-ray beam. Consequently, it is difficult to recognise the hilum as being depressed and, instead, smaller vascular structures are noted at the expected position of the hilum. Occasionally, confusion with a central hilar mass/adenopathy can arise if the convex margin of an interlobar artery remains visible due to minimal rotation.[6]

As well as vascular reorientation, hilar bronchial alterations also occur. The central large bronchi undergo characteristic changes in position with collapse of either the upper or lower lobe. When either upper lobe collapses significantly, the ipsilateral main bronchus becomes more horizontally orientated than usual; hence the bronchus intermedius and the left lower lobe bronchus swing laterally. Conversely, when either lower lobe collapses, each main bronchus is more vertically orientated than usual, with a medial swing of the bronchus intermedius on the right and the lower lobe bronchus on the left.

Indirect Signs of Volume Loss

Compensatory hyperinflation of adjacent lobes occurs with lobar collapse, resulting in fewer vessels per unit volume of lung. It is often easier to detect a paucity of vessels, which are more widely spaced than on the unaffected side, than subtle increased radiolucency. In isolation, the sign may be due to causes other than lobar collapse and other confirmatory features should be sought before making the diagnosis. The normal lung parenchyma should expand proportionally to compensate for the degree of collapse and often the greater the degree of lobar collapse, the greater the compensatory overinflation. Therefore when small lung volumes are involved, the hyperinflation usually only involves the remainder of the ipsilateral lung, whereas with larger volumes, the contralateral lung may expand across the midline. On a frontal radiograph the lung may expand across the midline

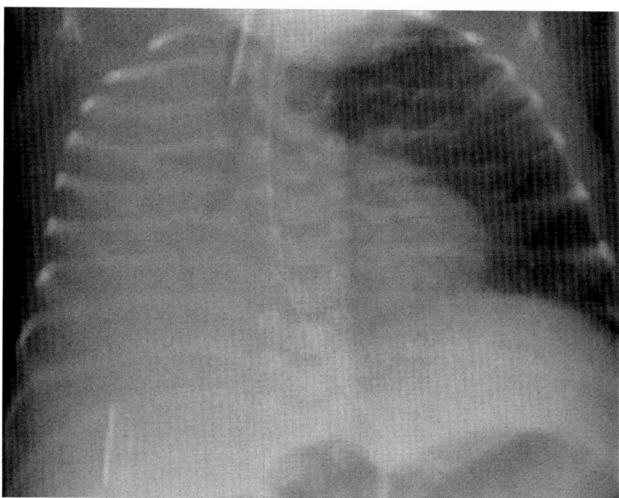

FIGURE 7-2 ■ Total right lung collapse in a neonate. The patient was ventilated for respiratory distress syndrome and the cause of the total lung collapse was a mucus plug.

superiorly, thus displacing the anterior junctional line to the contralateral side (Fig. 7-1A). On a lateral view, the anterior mediastinum appears hyperlucent (Fig. 7-1B). Displacement of the azygo-oesophageal line and posterior junctional line on the PA radiograph, which denote protrusion of contralateral lung through other weak areas between the oesophagus and vertebral column and the retrocardiac space, respectively, may be more difficult to recognise. Although the term 'mediastinal herniation' is sometimes used, some authorities emphasise that there is no actual mediastinal defect or hiatus and the sign more accurately denotes *displacement* of mediastinal structures.[7]

A divergent or parallel pattern of vascular reorientation seen near the hilum has been described in marked upper lobe collapse.[8] The pattern is seen more commonly on the left than on the right, as a result of the different degree of compensatory overinflation in the superior segment of the ipsilateral lower lobe on each side.[8] The right middle lobe can also overinflate in compensation, which further explains the lesser degree of overinflation of the superior segment of the right lower lobe. The sign of vascular reorientation can be helpful when unusual patterns of upper lobe collapse are present. Hyperexpansion may also result in a change in position of lung lesions, such as granulomas resulting in the so-called shifting granuloma sign (Fig. 7-3). Of particular note, the Luftsichel sign (from German, meaning air crescent) is due to the overinflated superior segment of the ipsilateral lower lobe occupying the space between the mediastinum and the medial aspect of the collapsed upper lobe, resulting in a paramediastinal translucency (Fig. 7-4).[9] The sign is more common on the left than on the right and is regarded as a typical appearance of left upper lobe collapse.[9] CT demonstrates the increased paramediastinal lucency to be due to a wedge shape of the collapsed upper lobe, with the apex of the V resulting from tethering of the major fissure by hilar structures (Fig. 7-4B).

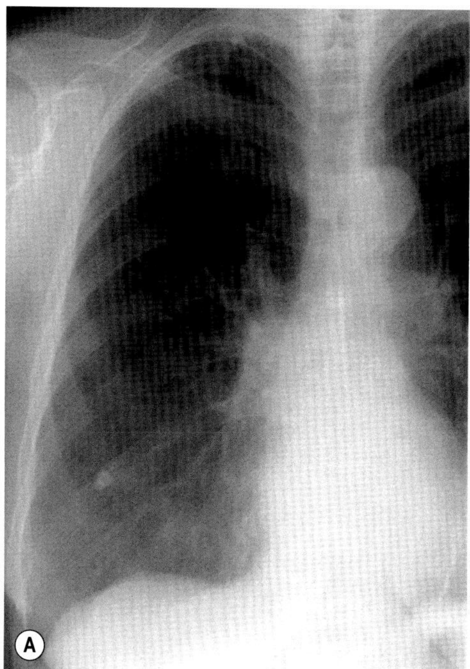

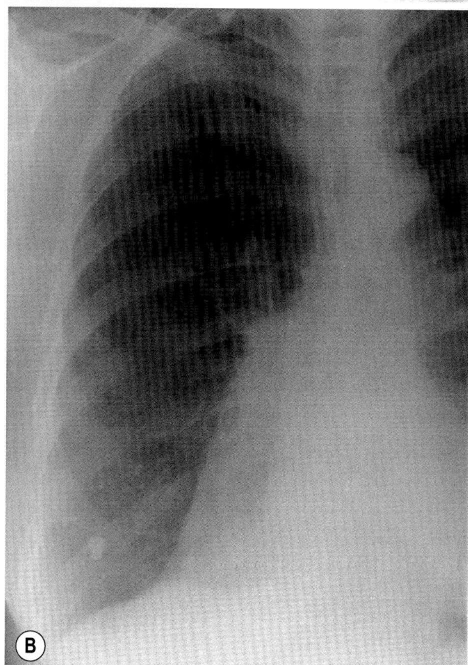

FIGURE 7-3 ■ Shifting granuloma sign. (A) Before and (B) after right lower lobe collapse.

Mediastinal shift is another indirect sign of volume loss and the degree varies according to the position of the affected lobe. Usually the least mediastinal shift occurs in right middle lobe collapse, whilst the greatest shift, particularly of the inferior mediastinum, is seen with lower lobe collapse. The amount of mediastinal shift due to upper lobe collapse is often dependent on the chronicity: in acute upper lobe collapse there is often little shift, whereas in chronic upper lobe volume loss with fibrosis, the shift may be greater. The position of the trachea may be a useful indicator of superior mediastinal shift as it should be central in the superior mediastinum between

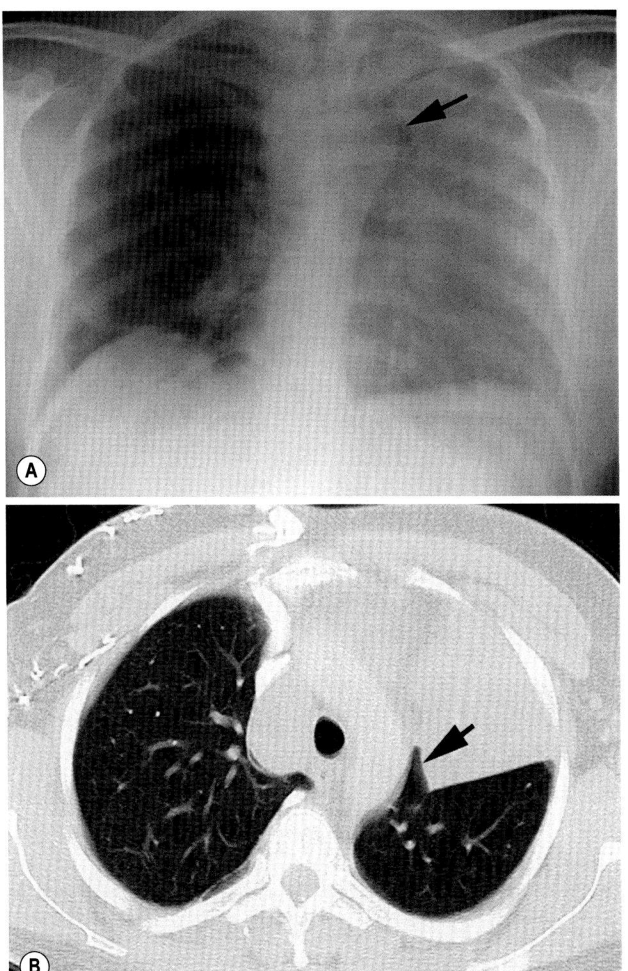

FIGURE 7-4 ■ **Luftsichel sign.** (A) A left upper lobe collapse demonstrating paramediastinal lucency (arrow). (B) CT shows interposition of aerated lung between the collapse and the mediastinum (arrow). There is also a large right paratracheal node causing some distortion of the SVC.

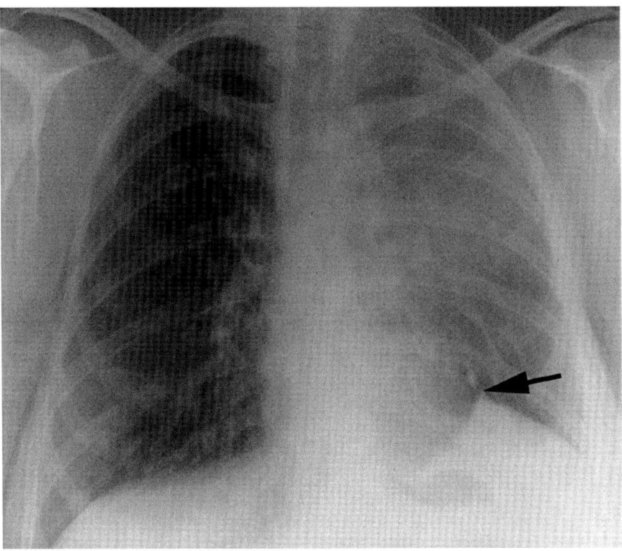

FIGURE 7-5 ■ **Juxtaphrenic peak sign.** A small triangular density (arrow) is seen in a left upper lobe collapse. The sign is due to reorientation of an inferior accessory fissure.

the anterior ends of the clavicles or slightly deviated to the right by the aortic arch. Inferiorly within the mediastinum, anywhere between one-half and one-fifth of the cardiac outline normally lies to the right of the midline and greater or lesser variations indicate mediastinal shift. However, because of the wide variation in normal subjects, displacement of the cardiac outline may be more difficult to assess than changes in position of the trachea.

The hemidiaphragms may be elevated in lobar collapse, particularly involving the left upper lobe and to a lesser extent the right upper and both lower lobes. However, the sign is of limited value because the position of the right hemidiaphragm is highly variable (0–3 cm higher than the left on the frontal chest radiograph). A useful ancillary sign of upper lobe collapse (or a combination of right upper and middle lobe collapse) is a juxtaphrenic peak of the diaphragm (Fig. 7-5).[10] The sign refers to a small triangular density at the highest point of the dome of the hemidiaphragm, due to the anterior volume loss of the affected upper lobe, resulting in traction and reorientation of an inferior accessory fissure.[11,12]

Reduction in the volume of a hemithorax may result in relative reduction of the spaces between the ribs by comparison to the unaffected side. Rib crowding or approximation may be recognisable on the frontal radiograph in cases of chronic lobar collapse, but in acute collapse it may be more difficult to appreciate. Furthermore, the sign is considered to be unreliable as patient rotation and minor degrees of scoliosis may result in apparent rib crowding.

Ancillary Features of Lobar Collapse

Occasionally the cause of a lobar collapse may be apparent and an endobronchial lesion may be clearly demonstrated radiographically (Fig. 7-1A). However, although the actual endobronchial component is often not directly visualised, lobar collapse due to a central obstructing bronchogenic carcinoma is most likely when Golden's S sign is seen (Fig. 7-6). The sign refers to the S shape (or more accurately, reverse S on the right) of the fissure due to the combination of collapse and mass centrally resulting in a focal convexity with a concave outline peripherally. Although the sign was originally described in the right upper lobe, it can be seen in any lobe.[5,13] The CT equivalent is discussed later. Generally, absence of air bronchograms within the affected lobe should also raise the suspicion of a central obstructing lesion as there is absorption of air from both the lung parenchyma and airways. The sign may be useful for distinguishing a central obstructing mass from a consolidative process such as bacterial pneumonia (Fig. 7-7). The rare important caveats are when a mass results in only partial obstruction of the airways or in cases of acute bronchopneumonia where the airways are filled with an inflammatory exudate. However, the sign is not as reliable on CT, and often distal air bronchograms are visible in part of a collapsed lobe due to a central neoplasm (Fig. 7-9).

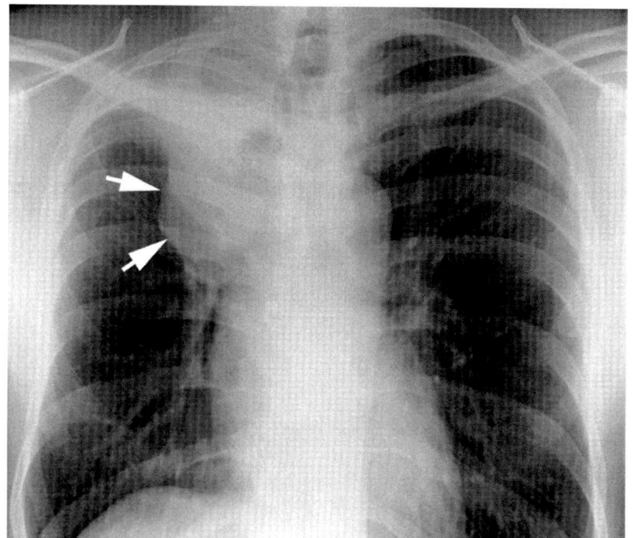

FIGURE 7-6 ■ **Golden's S sign.** A right upper lobe collapse demonstrating peripheral concavity and central convexity (arrows) due to an underlying bronchogenic carcinoma resulting in a reverse S shape.

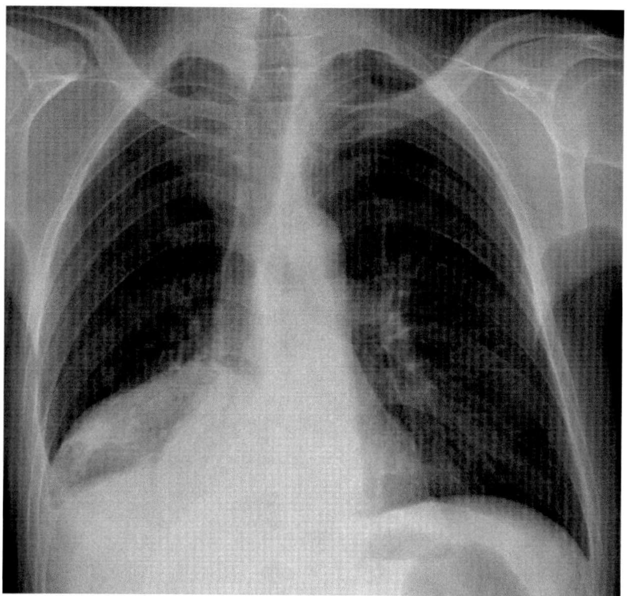

FIGURE 7-7 ■ **Air bronchograms in a collapsed and consolidated right lower lobe.** The sign can be helpful in excluding a central obstructing mass and in this case the cause was a bacterial pneumonia.

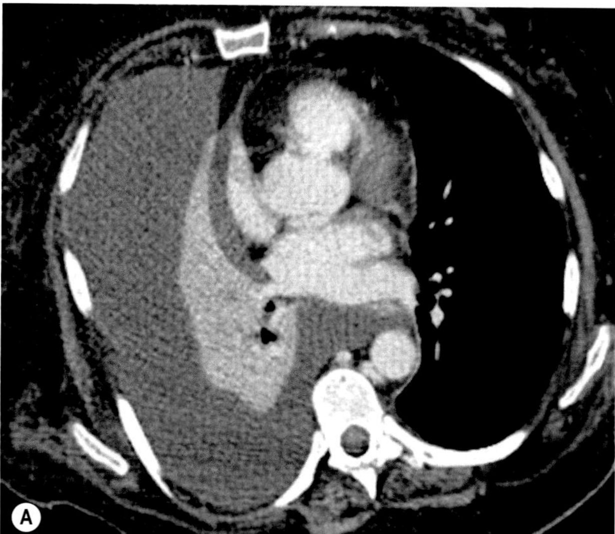

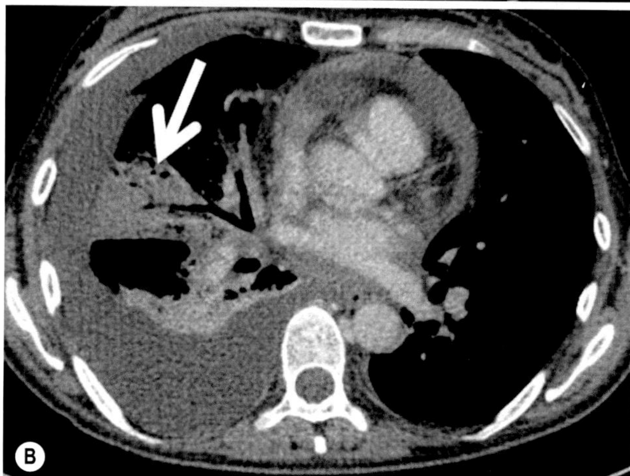

FIGURE 7-8 ■ **Enhancement of atelectatic lung versus pneumonia.** (A) Axial intravenous contrast-enhanced CT in a patient with passive atelectasis of the right lower lobe due to a large pleural effusion. Note the dense homogeneous enhancement of the collapsed right lower lobe. (B) Axial intravenous contrast-enhanced CT of a patient with right upper lobe pneumonia, right pleural effusion and pericardial effusion. Note the relative lack of enhancement of the posterior right upper lobe (arrow) resulting in less clear differentiation of pulmonary parenchyma from pleural fluid than demonstrated in (A).

COMPUTED TOMOGRAPHY OF LOBAR COLLAPSE

CT has become an invaluable method for investigating patients with lobar collapse. The obvious benefits are a lack of superimposition of overlying structures with the added advantage of demonstration of anatomical structures in the axial and, with computer reformatting, coronal and sagittal planes. Not only does CT aid the understanding of the radiographic appearances of lobar collapse but also it provides invaluable information about the cause, which may not be apparent on chest radiography. The most common indication for CT in adults with lobar collapse is to identify an endobronchial or compressing lesion.

Technique

Careful attention to CT technique is still required to accurately demonstrate an obstructing lesion resulting in lobar collapse, despite the widespread use of multidetector CT. The old recommendations using single-slice CT[14] are now outdated and reconstruction and reformatting of volumetric data now provide routine display of tracheobronchial anatomy. Three-dimensional (3D) and multiplanar (2D) images provide an extremely useful adjunct to axial images.[15]

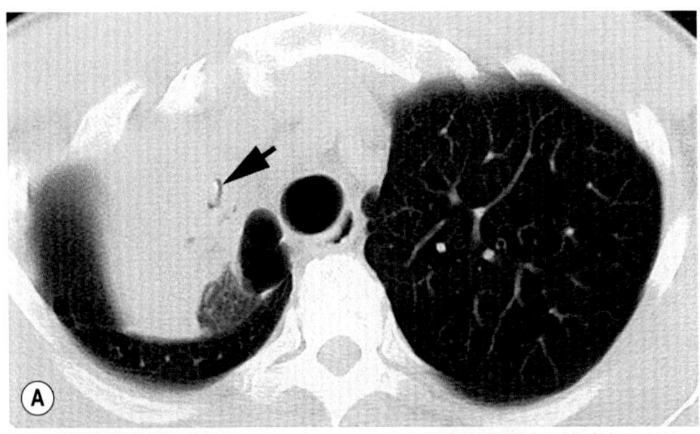

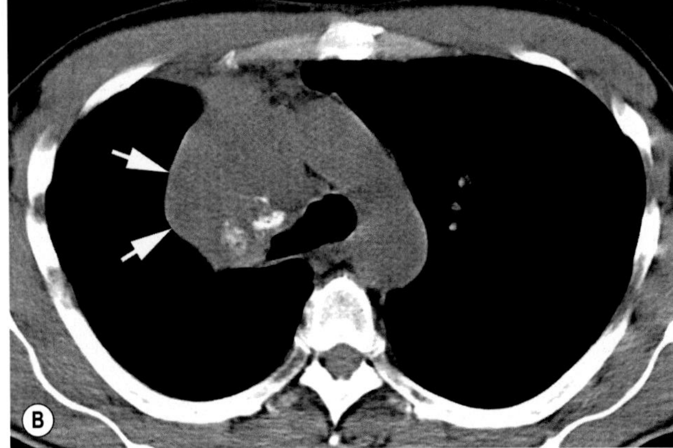

FIGURE 7-9 ■ CT of a collapsed right upper lobe due to a squamous cell carcinoma. Note the peripheral air bronchograms (arrow) in (A) despite a central obstructing mass with amorphous calcification (B). There is a convex border of the collapsed lobe (arrows) (B) which is the CT equivalent of Golden's S sign.

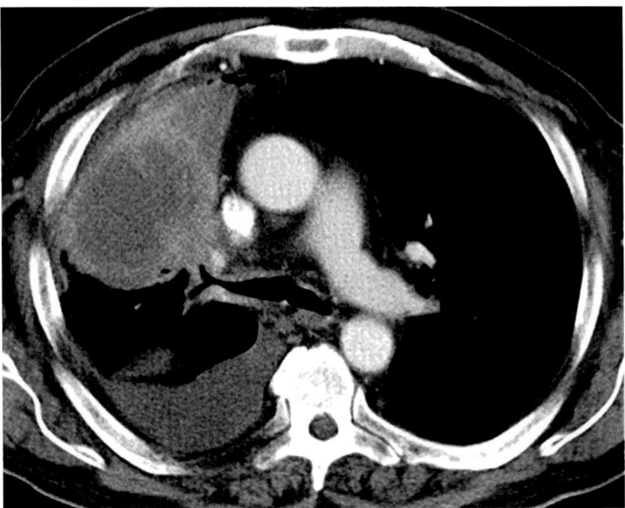

FIGURE 7-10 ■ CT of right upper lobe collapse due to bronchogenic carcinoma. Note how the attenuation of the necrotic tumour is lower than the adjacent collapsed lung which enhances with intravenous contrast medium.

Utility

In some cases, the aetiology of lobar collapse can be determined from the patient's clinical history, examination and chest radiographic features. Using fibreoptic bronchoscopy as the reference standard, CT is clearly more sensitive than chest radiography for the detection of an obstructing carcinoma.[16] Reported sensitivities for detection by CT range from 83 to 100%,[17–20] but generally, when an endobronchial lesion is sufficiently large to cause lobar collapse, CT is a reliable method for detection.[2,16] False-positive diagnoses may be due to bronchial strictures, plugs of mucus or secretions and compression by large pleural effusions.[2,3,16] CT is not histologically specific, however, as bronchogenic carcinoma, endobronchial metastases, bronchial adenomas and lymphoma may all have similar appearances.[2] The accuracy of CT is, to some extent, dependent on technique and it may be more difficult to demonstrate endobronchial lesions in the right middle lobe and lingular bronchi owing to their oblique orientation relative to the axial plane. This is much less of a problem with MDCT.

Accurate delineation of a tumour mass from a surrounding collapsed lobe may be problematic, but collapsed lung usually enhances to a greater degree than tumour with contrast-enhanced CT (Fig. 7-10).[21] The difference in attenuation value is maximal between 40 s and 2 min after a bolus injection of intravenous contrast;[21] these numbers, however, vary with contrast administration and CT technique.

Golden's S sign on chest radiography has a CT equivalent that may be helpful in identifying an obstructing tumour.[22,23] Usually, a collapsed lobe is associated with concavity of the adjacent fissure and a localised convexity is highly suggestive of an underlying mass (see Fig. 7-9). The sign is not entirely specific, but it is strongly indicative of a bronchogenic carcinoma. Unlike the frontal chest radiograph, in which the S sign is only helpful in the right upper lobe and to a lesser extent the right and left lower lobes, the S sign can be applied to all lobes on CT.

Another CT sign that is highly suggestive of an obstructing lesion causing lobar collapse is the CT mucous bronchogram sign.[24] Histopathologically, the lobar and segmental bronchi are filled with inspissated secretions and are usually dilated. The airways are optimally demonstrated as tubular, low attenuation branching structures within the enhancing collapsed lobe following intravenous contrast enhancement (Fig. 7-11).

Obstructing lesions such as bronchogenic carcinoma or benign causes, including tuberculous bronchostenosis, should be considered. The sign may also result from excessive mucus production combined with decreased mucociliary function in conditions such as allergic bronchopulmonary aspergillosis, asthma and cystic fibrosis.[25]

CT also has a role in complicated or atypical lobar collapse as their appearances may be confusing on chest radiography. In particular, combined right middle lobe and right upper lobe collapse may be difficult to diagnose on chest radiography when the collapse is nearly complete.[26] CT is useful for demonstrating mediastinal anatomy and provides information about mediastinal lymph nodes and the staging of a tumour causing lobar collapse. Additional signs of lobar collapse, such as

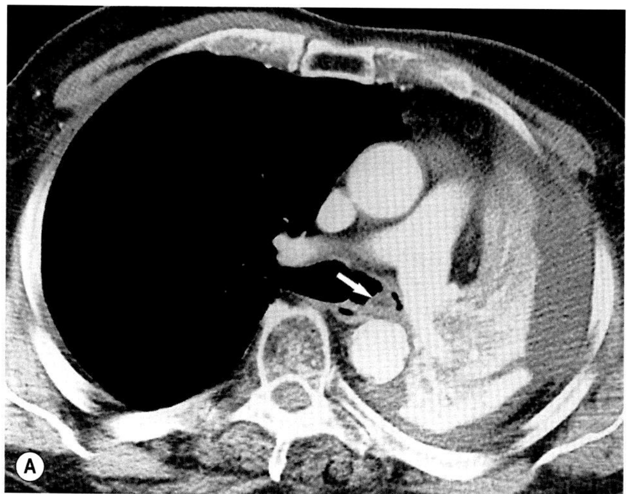

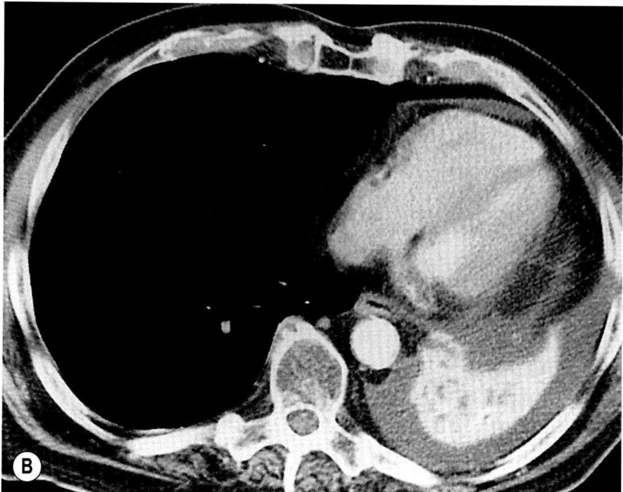

FIGURE 7-11 ■ **Left lung collapse.** (A, B) Contrast-enhanced CT sections of whole lung collapse due to a squamous cell carcinoma in the left main bronchus (arrow in A). There is also a left pleural effusion and a small pericardial effusion. Note the low-attenuation areas relative to the densely enhancing left lower lobe parenchyma (B) which represent mucus-filled airways—the CT mucous bronchogram sign.

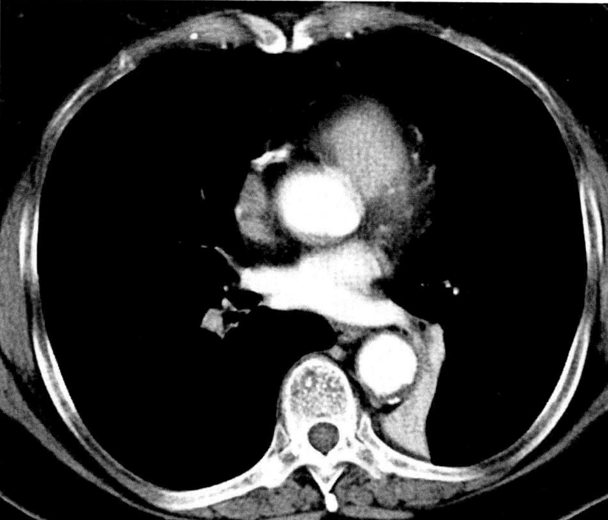

FIGURE 7-12 ■ **Left lower lobe collapse.** Contrast-enhanced CT showing a tight left lower lobe collapse. Normal mediastinal structures (particularly left-sided) may cause a focal bulge in the contour of a lobar collapse (in this case by the well-opacified descending thoracic aorta) and should not be confused with a Golden's S sign due to tumour.

compensatory overinflation and the Luftsichel sign (described above), are also well demonstrated, providing explanations for the radiographic appearances of lobar collapse.[27,28]

In addition to findings indicative of volume loss, the usually strong and homogeneous enhancement of atelectatic lung parenchyma as opposed to consolidated lung parenchyma due to inflammation provides a useful sign for discriminating pneumonia from atelectasis (Fig. 7-8).

Potential Pitfalls

The increased sensitivity of CT by comparison with radiography means that the presence of an air bronchogram within a lobar collapse does not necessarily exclude a central obstructing lesion (see Fig. 7-9).[24] In this context, an air bronchogram may be seen in the peripheral part of a collapsed lobe due to collateral air drift or tumour necrosis.[16] Similarly, a proximal obstructing lesion may not cause complete lobar collapse when a fissure is incomplete, allowing ventilation by collateral air drift.[29] Occasionally the parenchyma and airways become filled with fluid owing to the presence of a central obstructing lesion with little or no associated volume loss, and the lobe may even be expanded, giving rise to the appearance termed 'drowned lobe'. The CT equivalent of the Golden's S sign is particularly well demonstrated with right-sided lobar collapse and, on the left, care should be taken in interpretation owing to the fact that normal mediastinal structures may mimic a mass (e.g. thoracic aorta)[22] (Fig. 7-12).

The accurate determination of the reversibility and chronicity of a lobar collapse may be problematic. Relatively acute collapses may show apparent bronchiectatic dilatation of the airways and may mimic a long-standing irreversible event (Fig. 7-13); a meaningful evaluation of the airways in the context of a lobar collapse is therefore often difficult.

OTHER IMAGING TECHNIQUES IN LOBAR COLLAPSE

Previously, magnetic resonance imaging (MRI) was surpassed by CT in the investigation of lobar collapse largely due to the superior spatial resolution of lung parenchyma in the latter, but also due to cost, availability and speed of acquisition. In particular, endobronchial tumours and smaller bronchi were less well demonstrated by MRI than CT.[30] CT is still the imaging investigation of choice but some studies have investigated the ability of MRI to differentiate a tumour mass from postobstructive collapse by utilising differences in signal characteristics.[31–33]

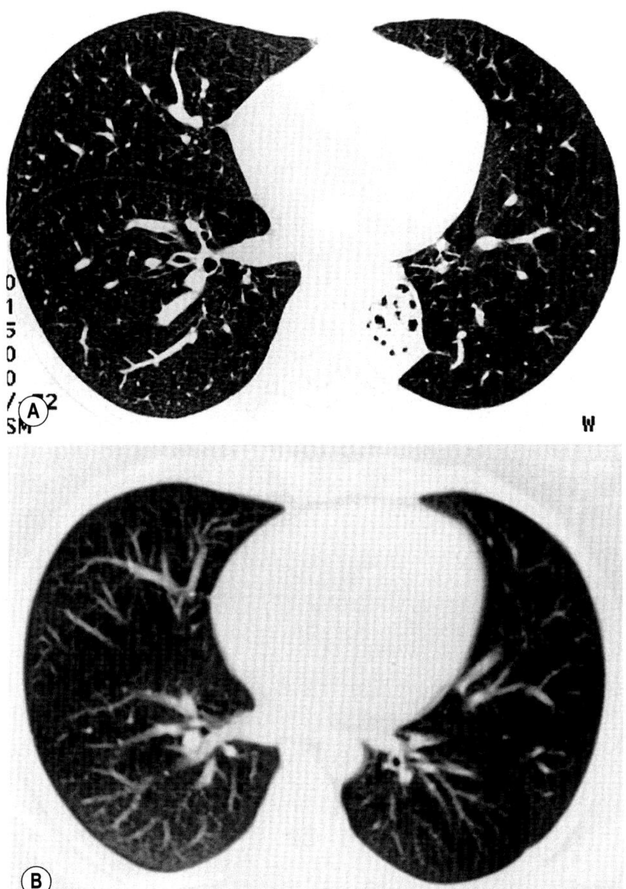

FIGURE 7-13 ■ **Resolution of left lower lobe collapse.** (A) An initial high-resolution CT of a young female patient with symptoms of recurrent respiratory tract infections shows a collapsed left lower lobe with possible bronchiectatic airways, raising the possibility of chronicity. (B) Follow-up conventional CT at the same level several months later shows complete resolution of the left lower lobe collapse and normal airways. This case illustrates the difficulty in making an accurate assessment of the airways in patients with lobar collapse.

Sometimes the distinction can be made on T1-weighted images, but it is generally accepted that T2-weighted images are superior as the tumour is of lower signal intensity than the obstructed lung which has higher water content.

On ultrasound of a large pleural effusion, the underlying collapsed lung is often visible as a hyperechoic wedge-shaped area within hypoechoic or anechoic fluid (Fig. 7-14). In practice, the main utility of ultrasound is to readily distinguish pleural effusion from a collapsed and consolidated lung when radiographic appearances are equivocal, but ultrasound may also be used to guide biopsy of a peripheral lesion within a collapsed lobe (Fig. 7-15C).

On positron emission tomography (PET), a collapsed lobe demonstrates less uptake of [^{18}F]fluorodeoxyglucose than tumour. CT PET may provide more accurate delineation of tumour from postobstructive collapsed lung than CT alone, which may be useful for guiding biopsy and treatment, e.g. radiotherapy[34] (Fig. 7-15).

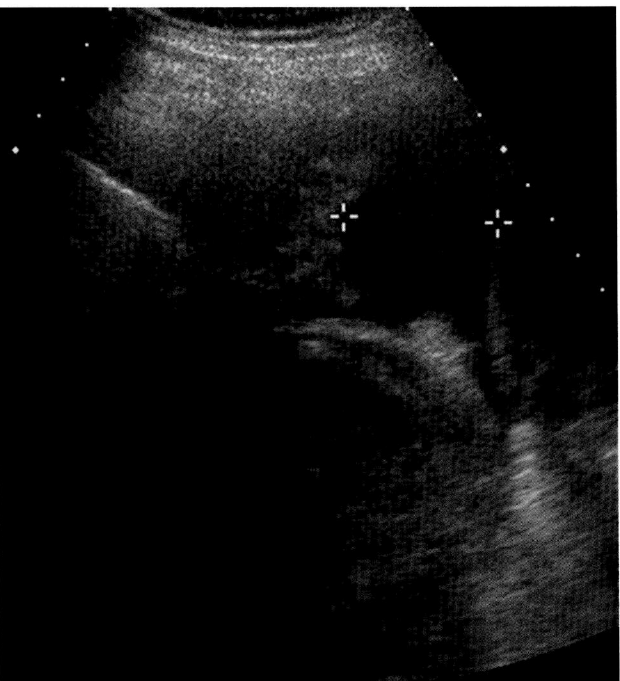

FIGURE 7-14 ■ **Ultrasound demonstrating a linear collapsed lower lobe with a large pleural effusion.** The asterisks demonstrate the distance between the collapsed lung and hemidiaphragm.

PATTERNS OF LOBAR COLLAPSE

Right Upper Lobe Collapse

On the frontal radiographic view of a right upper lobe collapse, the collapsed lobe forms increased density at the apex of the hemithorax adjacent to the right side of the mediastinum, with the elevated horizontal fissure resulting in a concave inferior outline depending on the degree of collapse (Fig. 7-16). Even in cases where there is no obstructing lesion, there is often a small convexity at the hilum due to the pulmonary veins and artery where the apex of the lobe is attached to the hilum. On the lateral view, the horizontal and oblique fissure approximate and are both displaced superiorly and medially with the collapsed lobe, forming a superior ill-defined wedge-shaped density. In cases where the collapse is very severe, the horizontal fissure parallels the mediastinum and appearances may simulate an apical cap of pleural fluid (Fig. 7-17) or mediastinal widening on the frontal radiograph (Fig. 7-18).

There is also usually compensatory hyperinflation of the right middle and lower lobes, resulting in elevation and a more horizontal course of the lower lobe pulmonary artery and right main bronchus. The vascular reorientation can be recognised on the frontal view, but the right main and lower lobe bronchial displacement can be difficult to appreciate on both the frontal and lateral view.

On CT the right upper lobe forms a triangular density with the base anteriorly against the chest wall and the apex at the hilum (Fig. 7-19). A focal bulge of the lateral

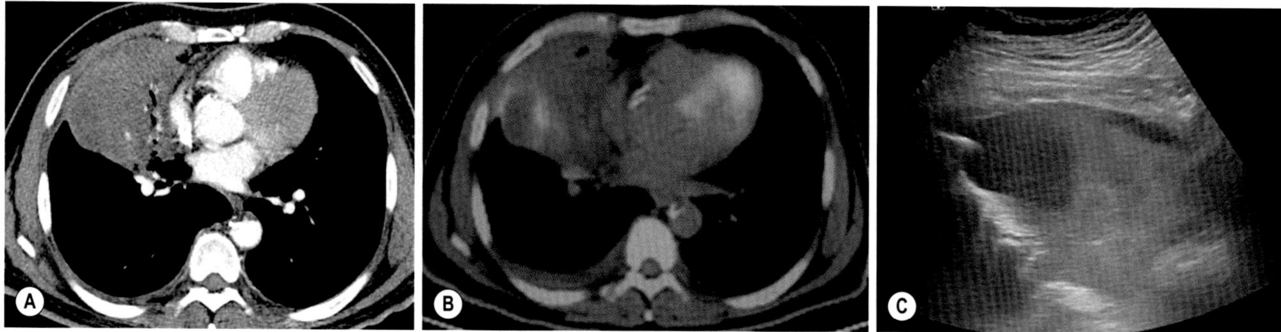

FIGURE 7-15 ■ Intravenous contrast-enhanced CT demonstrating right middle lobe collapse (A). Image from a CT PET study at the same level (B) shows increased uptake of radioisotope within the collapse. A targeted ultrasound-guided biopsy was performed (C), and bronchogenic carcinoma confirmed.

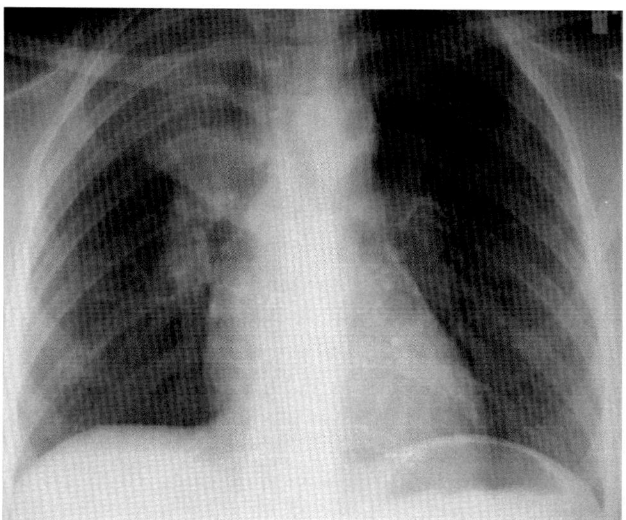

FIGURE 7-16 ■ **Right upper lobe collapse.** Typical example of a collapsed right upper lobe demonstrating the slightly concave inferior border of the opacified lung due to the horizontal fissure.

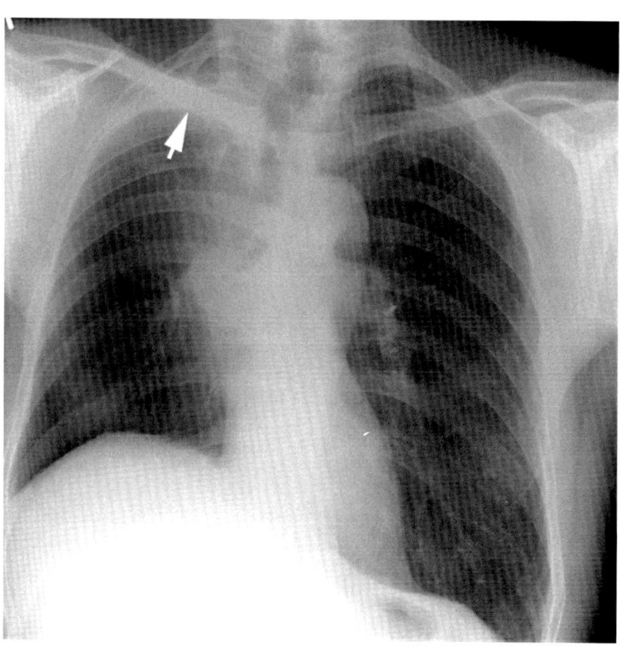

FIGURE 7-17 ■ **Right upper lobe collapse.** An example of right upper lobe collapse mimicking an apical cap of fluid (arrow).

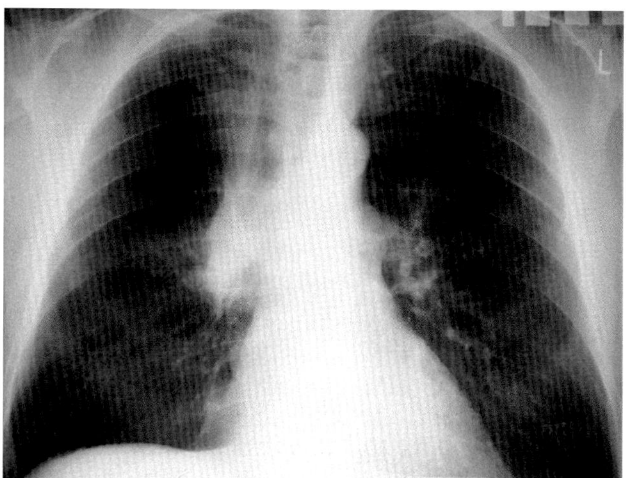

FIGURE 7-18 ■ **Tight right upper lobe collapse.** Note how the collapsed lobe (due to a central bronchogenic carcinoma) results in increased right paramediastinal density.

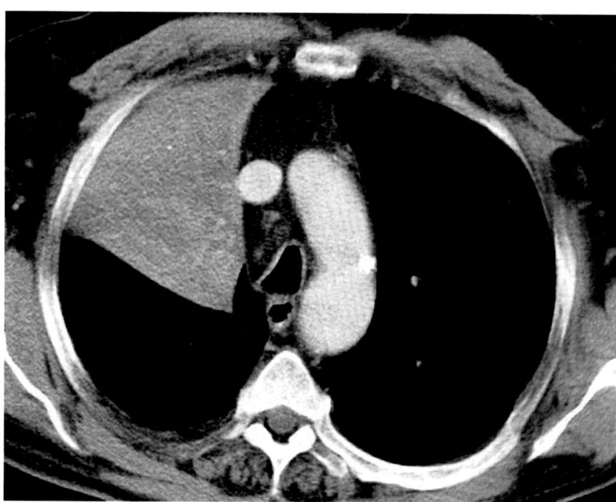

FIGURE 7-19 ■ **CT of right upper lobe collapse.** The collapsed lobe forms a triangular wedge of soft tissue anteriorly in the right hemithorax.

border usually indicates an underlying mass. Compensatory hyperinflation of not only the right middle and right lower lobes but also the left upper lobe is often more easily appreciated on CT.

Left Upper Lobe Collapse

The cardinal features of left upper lobe collapse are fundamentally different from right upper lobe collapse as there is very rarely a horizontal fissure on the left. Consequently, the main direction of volume loss is anteriorly and medially rather than superiorly, and the entire oblique fissure is displaced in that direction parallel to the chest wall on the lateral view. On the frontal view the signs may be variable, depending on the degree of collapse, but there is a 'veil-like' increased density of the whole of the affected hemithorax in most cases. The increased density is often greatest at the hilum and it gradually fades out laterally, superiorly and inferiorly without the clear inferior demarcation of the horizontal fissure as seen in right upper lobe collapse. The difference in transradiancy may be relatively subtle and therefore overlooked by the unwary. The other features that aid diagnosis on the frontal view are loss of the normal silhouette of structures adjacent to the collapse, such as the left heart border, mediastinum and aortic arch, as these structures are no longer adjacent to aerated lung. There is some variability in which outlines are obscured, depending on the degree of collapse. In cases of relatively less severe collapse, the left heart border, left mediastinal outline and aortic knuckle are obscured (see Fig. 7-5), whereas in more severe cases the apical segment of the left lower lobe is hyperexpanded superiorly adjacent to the aortic arch and somewhat paradoxically the aortic knuckle outline is therefore visible in more severe cases as it is adjacent to aerated lung (Fig. 7-20A). The Luftsichel sign (described above; see Fig. 7-4) is a particular manifestation of the hyperexpansion, and literally describes an 'air crescent' which may be seen between the aortic arch and the medial border of the collapse. On the lateral view the anterior outline of the ascending thoracic aorta can be seen with unusual clarity and this is due to compensatory hyperinflation of the right upper lobe across the midline and rotation of the mediastinum so the anterior aspect of the aorta is outlined by aerated lung tangential to the X-ray beam (Fig. 7-20B). This feature is often readily appreciated on CT (Fig. 7-21). On the frontal radiograph the left main bronchus is reorientated and has a more horizontal course than usual. The superior displacement of this structure results in angulation between the left main bronchus and the left lower lobe bronchus (Fig. 7-20A).

The CT appearances of left upper lobe collapse are similar to that of the right upper lobe with a triangular soft-tissue density, the apex at the origin of the upper lobe bronchus and the base against the anterior chest wall, adjacent to the left border of the mediastinum. However, in the left upper lobe the lingular segment is seen as a density closely opposed to the left heart border.

Rarely, left upper lobe collapse may mimic right upper lobe collapse (Fig. 7-22). The appearance is due to collapse of the apicoposterior and anterior segments of the left upper lobe with sparing of the lingular portion

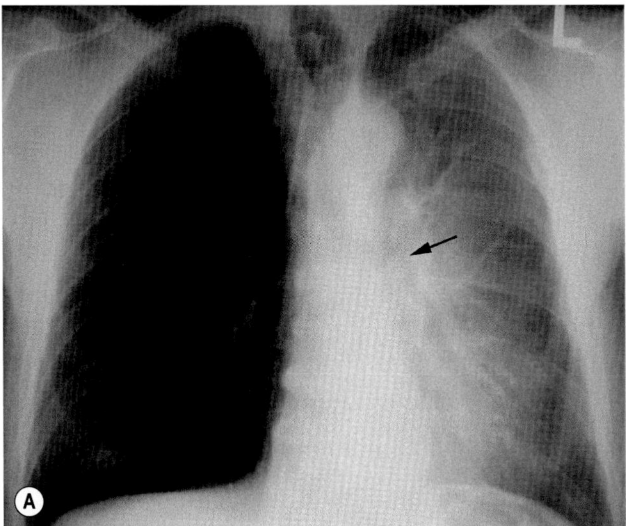

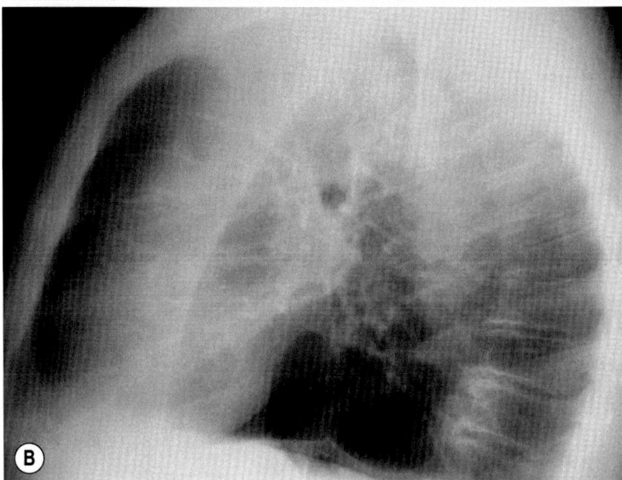

FIGURE 7-20 ■ **Left upper lobe collapse.** (A) A typical example of left upper lobe collapse demonstrating increased angulation between the left main bronchus and the lower lobe bronchus (arrow) on the frontal view. The aortic knuckle is visible in this example due to compensatory hyperinflation of the left lower lobe. (B) The lateral view demonstrates anterior displacement of the oblique fissure. Note the increased retrosternal lucency (see Fig. 7-21).

resulting in a concavity to the inferior border of the collapse, even in the absence of a left minor fissure.[5] Apart from being on the left, isolated collapse of the lingula has a very similar appearance to that of right middle lobe collapse (Fig. 7-23).

Right Middle Lobe Collapse

The features of right middle lobe collapse may be extremely subtle on the frontal view and consequently easy to overlook. The collapsed lobe lies adjacent to the right heart border and there is loss of the silhouette of this structure to a variable degree (Fig. 7-24). There may or may not be a recognisable increase in density, depending on the orientation of the collapse relative to the X-ray beam. When the collapse is orientated roughly parallel to the beam or if the patient is in a lordotic position, a triangular, sail-shaped density may be seen adjacent to the heart border (Fig. 7-25). However, if the collapsed lobe lies obliquely in the chest, more parallel with the major fissure, the only sign on the frontal radiograph may be indistinctness of a portion of the right atrial border (Fig. 7-24A). By comparison, the triangular density of the collapsed right middle lobe is relatively easy to identify on the lateral view, with approximation of the minor and inferior portion of the major fissure, the apex of the triangle being at the hilum (Fig. 7-24B). In increasingly severe collapse the triangular shape is less marked as the fissures become almost parallel with only a thin wedge of density separating them.

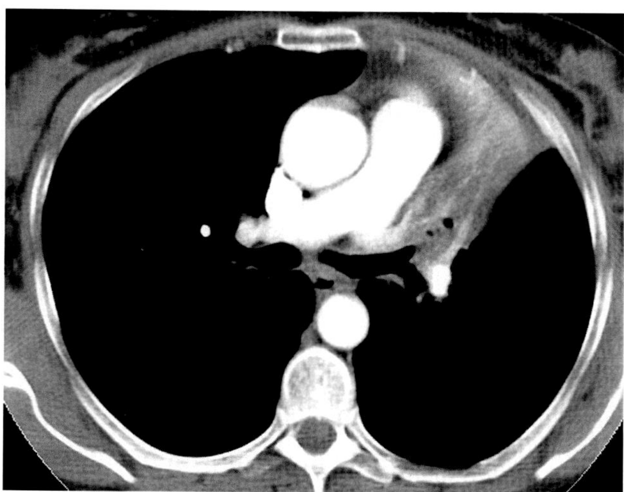

FIGURE 7-21 ■ **Left upper lobe collapse.** Intravenous contrast-enhanced CT of left upper lobe collapse shows increased wedge-shaped density of the left upper lobe adjacent to the mediastinum. Note the displacement of the right lung across the midline anteriorly, resulting in retrosternal hyperlucency and increased clarity of the anterior ascending thoracic aorta on the lateral view (see Fig. 7-20).

The CT appearances are characteristically of a triangular-shaped density of varying size adjacent to the heart border. Depending on the orientation of the collapse, only a small portion may be identified on each section as the collapse represents a relatively flat sheet of tissue. The so-called 'middle lobe syndrome' refers to a collapsed right middle lobe with bronchiectasis due to a focal bronchostenosis secondary to pulmonary tuberculosis. Although in theory any lobe may be affected, the middle lobe is the most common, resulting in characteristic CT features (Fig. 7-26).

Right and Left Lower Lobe Collapse

The features of right and left lower lobe collapse are very similar and will be considered together. In collapse of the lower lobes, the oblique fissure is displaced posteriorly and medially, and the collapsed lobe lies in the posteromedial portion of the chest, a feature readily appreciated on CT (see Fig. 7-11). On the frontal radiograph, the collapsed lower lobes usually form a triangular density behind the heart (Fig. 7-27A). The medial portion of the hemidiaphragm may be obscured as it is no longer outlined by aerated lung (Fig. 7-28), but if the inferior pulmonary ligament is incomplete and does not attach to the diaphragm, the medial contour of the diaphragm may still be visualised. On the lateral radiograph, a posterior portion of the hemidiaphragm may not be seen (Fig. 7-27B), but in more severe collapse the contour may reappear as it becomes outlined by aerated lung from the hyperexpanded upper lobe. In addition, the vertebral column appears progressively denser inferiorly in lower lobe collapse (Fig. 7-27), whereas normally the converse is true.

On the frontal radiograph the lower lobe pulmonary artery is usually not seen in lower lobe collapse as it is no longer outlined by aerated lung (Fig. 7-29). The major airways, including the right and left main bronchi, are also displaced more vertically in lower lobe collapse and

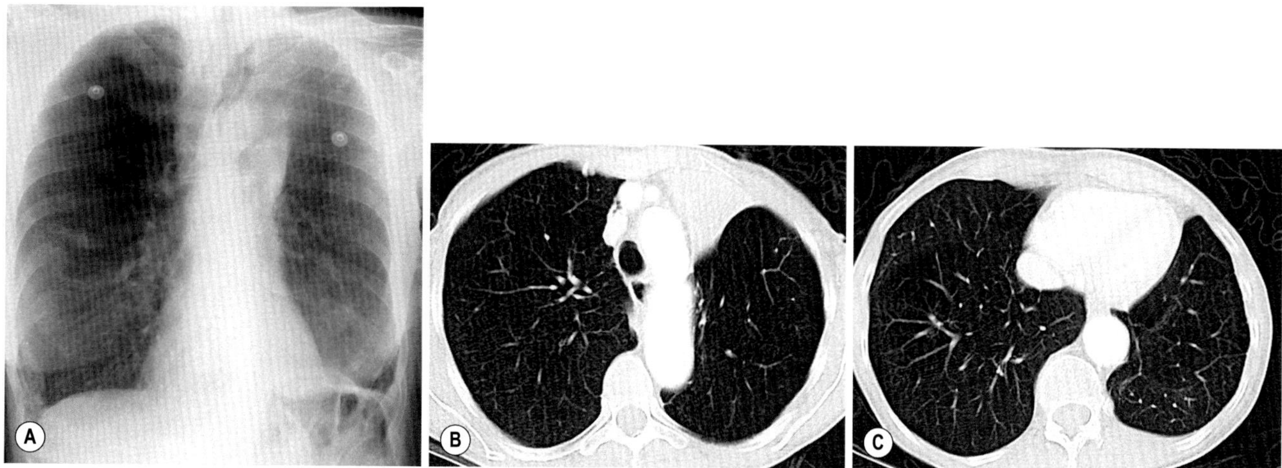

FIGURE 7-22 ■ **Atypical left upper lobe collapse.** (A) The frontal radiograph demonstrates the inferior concave border of the collapsed lobe and resembles a right upper lobe collapse. (B, C) CT images show increased triangular density to the left of the mediastinum (B), which does not extend along the left heart border (C), a feature usually seen in left upper lobe collapse. The appearance is due to sparing of the lingular segments.

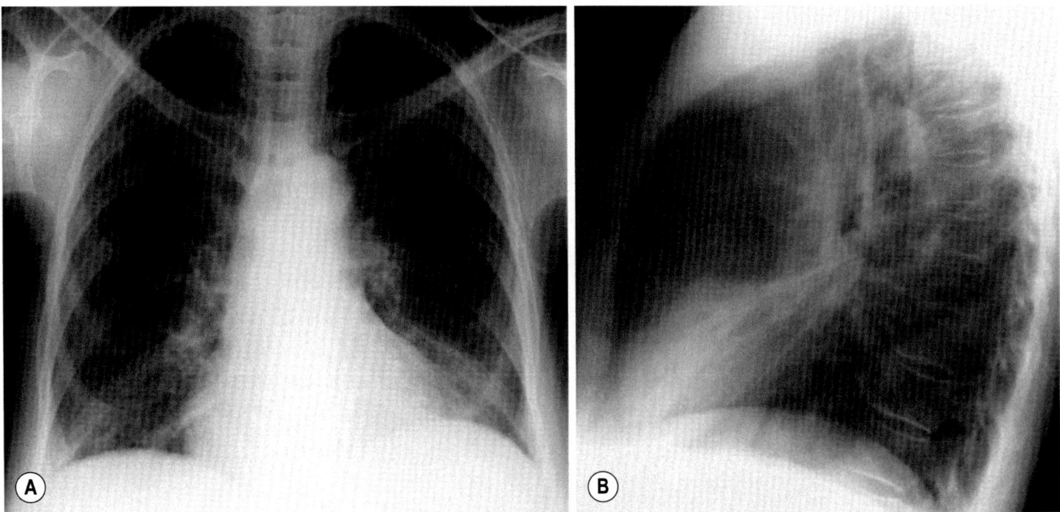

FIGURE 7-23 ■ **Lingular collapse.** (A) Frontal view of isolated collapse of the lingular segments of the left upper lobe showing loss of clarity of the left heart border and a raised hemidiaphragm. (B) The similarity to a right middle lobe collapse can be appreciated on the lateral view.

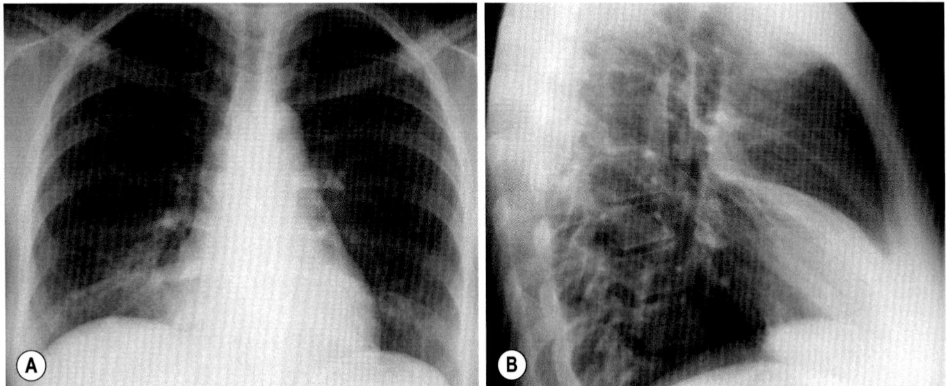

FIGURE 7-24 ■ **Right middle lobe collapse.** (A) Frontal view of a typical example showing loss of clarity of the right heart border. (B) The lateral view shows the wedge-shaped density extending anteriorly from the hilum.

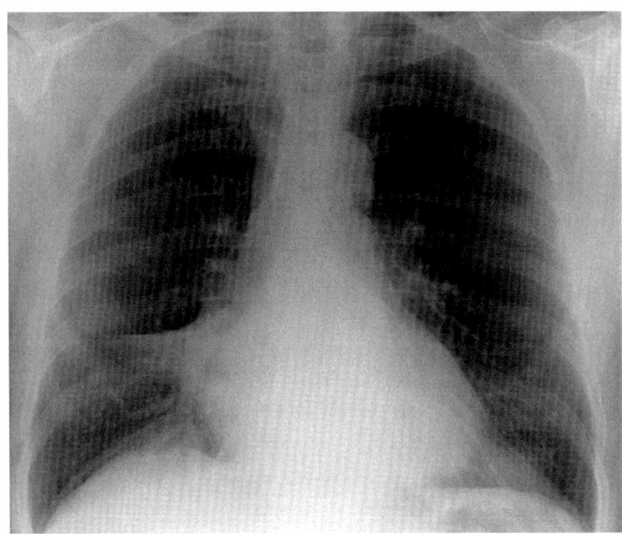

FIGURE 7-25 ■ **Right middle lobe collapse.** An example showing a triangular-shaped density adjacent to the right heart border.

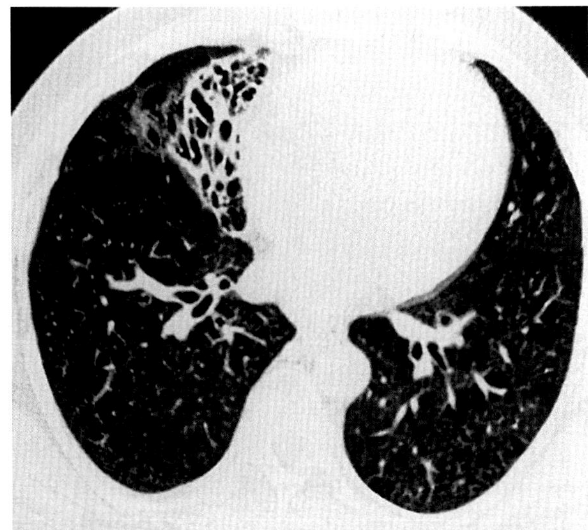

FIGURE 7-26 ■ **Middle lobe syndrome.** High-resolution CT showing right middle lobe collapse and bronchiectasis due to previous tuberculous infection.

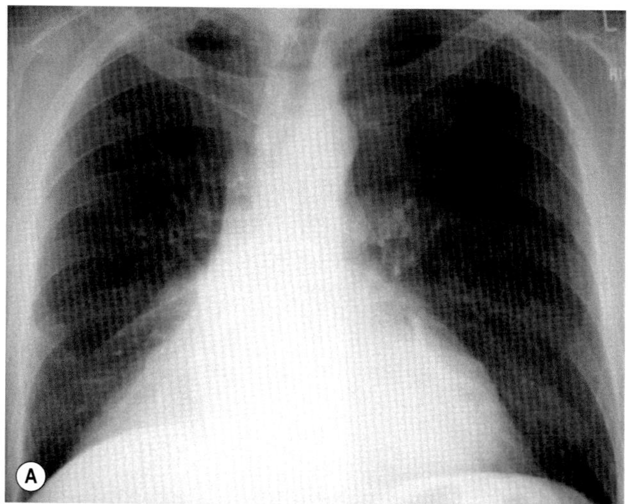

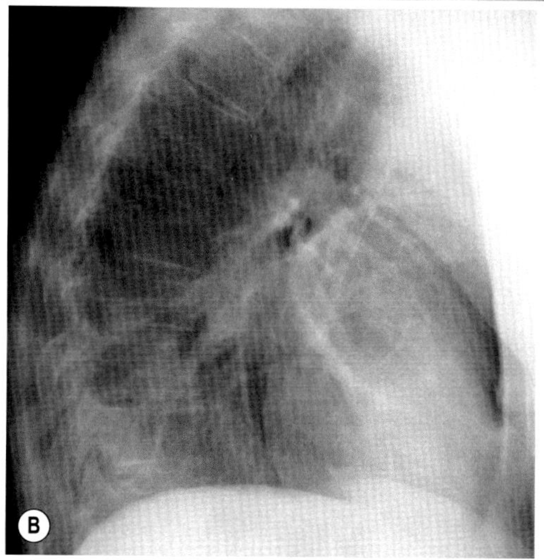

FIGURE 7-27 ■ **Right lower lobe collapse.** (A) Frontal view of an example of right lower lobe collapse demonstrating a triangular density which does not obscure the right hemidiaphragm silhouette. (B) The lateral radiograph shows the typical features of increased density of the posterior costophrenic angle and loss of the silhouette of the right diaphragm posteriorly.

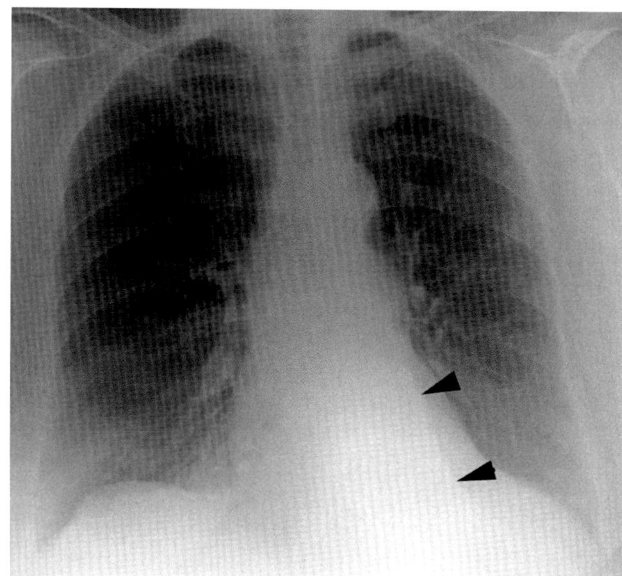

FIGURE 7-28 ■ **Left lower lobe collapse.** A typical appearance of left lower lobe collapse resulting in a triangular density behind the heart (arrowheads). The contour of the medial left hemidiaphragm is lost.

often the relevant air-containing bronchus can be identified as leading directly into the triangular density of the collapsed lobe. There are several features involving the upper mediastinum which are sometimes helpful in diagnosing lower lobe collapse.[35] The first of these is the 'superior triangle sign' and refers to a triangular density to the right of the mediastinum seen in right lower lobe collapse due to displacement of anterior junctional structures[36] (Fig. 7-29). The appearance should not be confused with right upper lobe collapse. The 'flat waist sign' is seen in extensive collapse of the left lower lobe and describes flattening of the contours of the aortic knuckle and main pulmonary artery due to cardiac rotation and displacement to the left.[37] Third, the outline of the superior aortic knuckle may be lost in severe left lower lobe collapse.[35]

On CT, the collapsed lower lobes form a triangle of soft-tissue density posteriomedially in the thorax, adjacent to the spine. On the left, the collapsed lower lobe is seen to drape over the descending aorta, giving a focal convexity to the lateral border, a feature which potentially can cause confusion with an underlying mass on an unenhanced CT (Fig. 7-11). Figure 7-30 summarises the schematic radiographic appearances of the various individual lobar collapses.

Whole Lung Collapse

Collapse of an entire lung results in complete opacification or 'white-out' of the affected hemithorax. In adults, the cause is often an obstructing neoplasm in the right or left main bronchi (see Fig. 7-1) or mucus plugging. There is marked volume loss with compensatory hyperinflation of the contralateral lung across the midline. The cardinal feature of volume loss can help discriminate between collapsed lung and a large pleural effusion, the latter usually resulting in mediastinal shift to the contralateral side. The lateral radiograph shows accentuation of the retrosternal space as the displacement of the contralateral lung is greatest anteriorly (see Fig. 7-1). By comparison, the opacity of the hemithorax is more uniform on the lateral view in large pleural effusion and may be a useful discriminating feature in equivocal cases.

Combinations of Lobar Collapse

Occasionally, various combinations of lobar collapse occur. Collapse of the right middle and right lower lobes is often due to an obstructing lesion in the bronchus intermedius (Fig. 7-31). The features are similar to right lower lobe collapse with the exception that the opacity extends laterally to the costophrenic angle on the frontal view and from the front to the back of the hemithorax on the lateral view[5] (Fig. 7-31B).

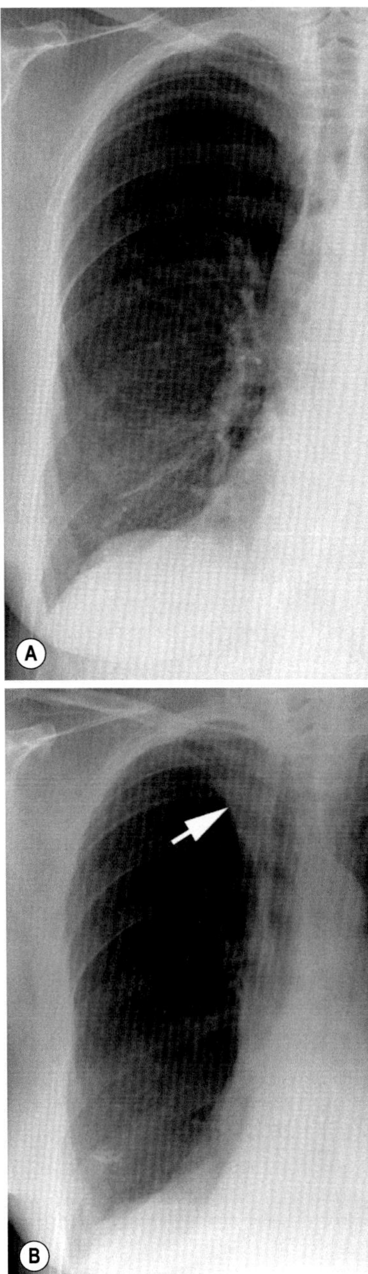

FIGURE 7-29 ■ **Superior triangle sign.** (A) An initial image shows the normal appearances (note the lower lobe artery is clearly visible). (B) The subsequent image shows a right lower lobe collapse demonstrating the superior triangle sign (arrow) (which should not be confused with a right upper lobe collapse). The lower lobe artery can no longer be seen.

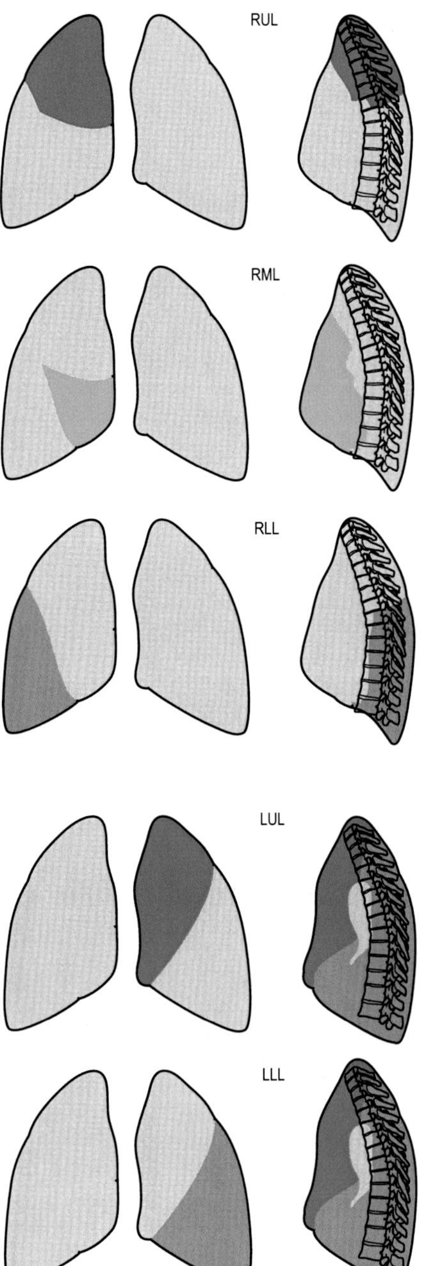

FIGURE 7-30 ■ **Schematic appearances of the various lobar collapses on frontal and lateral radiographs.** RUL, right upper lobe; RML, right middle lobe; RLL, right lower lobe; LUL, left upper lobe; LLL, left lower lobe.

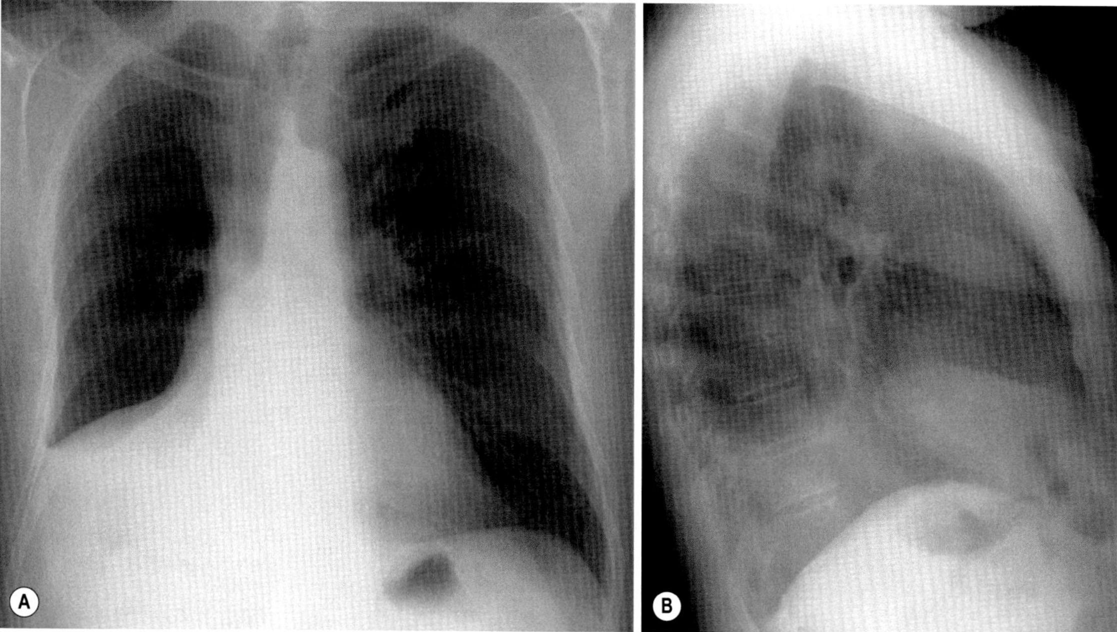

FIGURE 7-31 ■ Combined right middle and right lower lobe collapse. (A) On the frontal view the increased density extends to the right costophrenic angle. (B) On the lateral view the increased density also extends from the anterior to the posterior chest wall. The cause in this case was a bronchogenic carcinoma obstructing the bronchus intermedius.

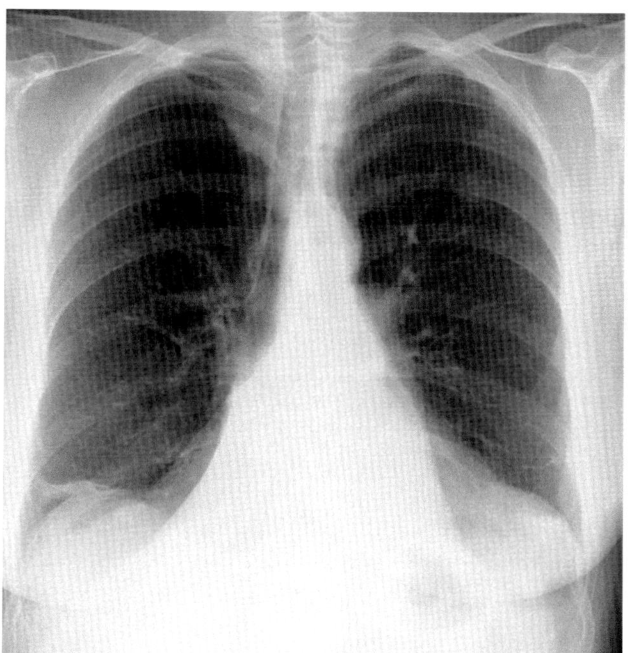

FIGURE 7-32 ■ Bilateral lower lobe collapse. Bilateral triangular densities are seen with obscuration of the medial portions of the hemidiaphragms. The cause was mucus plugging.

Collapse of the right upper and right middle lobes is more unusual as these lobes do not have a common bronchial origin which spares the lower lobe. In adults the cause is often a carcinoma which obstructs one bronchus and causes extrinsic compression of the other due to mass effect. Combined collapse of the right upper and right middle lobes results in an appearance very similar to left upper lobe collapse on both frontal and lateral radiographs and CT.[38]

Both bilateral lower lobe and upper lobe collapse are exceedingly rare and may occur as a result of metachronous bronchial neoplasms or mucus plugging (Fig. 7-32).

REFERENCES

1. Tuddenham WJ. Glossary of terms for thoracic radiology: recommendations of the Nomenclature Committee of the Fleischner Society. Am J Roentgenol 1984;143:509–17.
2. Naidich DP, McCauley DI, Khouri NF, et al. Computed tomography of lobar collapse: 1. Endobronchial obstruction. J Comput Assist Tomogr 1983;7:745–57.
3. Naidich DP, McCauley DI, Khouri NF, et al. Computed tomography of lobar collapse: 2. Collapse in the absence of endobronchial obstruction. J Comput Assist Tomogr 1983;7:758–67.
4. Stein LA, Vidal JJ, Hogg JC, Fraser RG. Acute lobar collapse in canine lungs. Invest Radiol 1976;11:518–27.
5. Proto AV, Tocino I. Radiographic manifestations of lobar collapse. Semin Roentgenol 1980;15:117–73.
6. Proto AV. The chest radiograph: anatomic considerations. Clin Chest Med 1984;5:213–46.
7. Lodin H. Mediastinal herniation and displacement studied by transversal radiography. Acta Radiol 1957;48:337–50.
8. Proto AV, Moser ES Jr. Upper lobe volume loss: divergent and parallel patterns of vascular reorientation. Radiographics 1987;7: 875–87.
9. Webber M, Davies P. The Luftsichel: an old sign in upper lobe collapse. Clin Radiol 1981;32:271–5.
10. Kattan KR, Eyler WR, Felson B. The juxtaphrenic peak in upper lobe collapse. Semin Roentgenol 1980;15:187–93.
11. Cameron DC. Juxtaphrenic peak (Katten's sign) is produced by rotation of an inferior accessory fissure. Australas Radiol 1993; 37:332–5.
12. Davis SD, Yankelevitz DF, Wand A, Chiarella DA. Juxtaphrenic peak in upper and middle lobe volume loss: assessment with CT. Radiology 1996;198:143–9.

13. Golden R. The effect of bronchostenosis upon the roentgen-ray shadows in carcinoma of the bronchus. Am J Roentgenol Radiat Ther 1925;13:21–30.
14. Naidich DP, Webb WR, Müller NL, et al. Computed tomography and magnetic resonance of the thorax. 3rd ed. Philadelphia: Lippincott–Raven; 1999.
15. LoCicero J, Costello P, Campos CT, et al. Spiral CT with multiplanar and three-dimensional reconstructions accurately predicts tracheobronchial pathology. Ann Thorac Surg 1996;62:818–22.
16. Woodring JH. Determining the cause of pulmonary atelectasis: a comparison of plain radiography and CT. Am J Roentgenol 1988; 150:757–63.
17. Henschke CI, Davis SD, Auh Y, et al. Detection of bronchial abnormalities: comparison of CT and bronchoscopy. J Comput Assist Tomogr 1987;11:432–5.
18. Webb WR, Gamsu G, Speckman JM. Computed tomography of the pulmonary hilum in patients with bronchogenic carcinoma. J Comput Assist Tomogr 1983;7:219–25.
19. Naidich DP, Lee J-J, Garay SM, et al. Comparison of CT and fibreoptic bronchoscopy in the evaluation of bronchial disease. Am J Roentgenol 1987;148:1–7.
20. Mayr B, Ingrisch H, Häussinger K, et al. Tumours of the bronchi: role of evaluation with CT. Radiology 1989;172:647–52.
21. Onitsuka H, Tsukuda M, Araki A, et al. Differentiation of central lung tumor from postobstructive lobar collapse by rapid sequence computed tomography. J Thorac Imaging 1991;6:28–31.
22. Reinig JW, Ross P. Computed tomography appearance of Golden's 'S' sign. J Comput Assist Tomogr 1984;8:219–23.
23. Khoury MB, Godwin JD, Halvorsen RA, Putman CE. CT of obstructive lobar collapse. Invest Radiol 1985;20:708–16.
24. Woodring JH. The computed tomography mucous bronchogram sign. J Comput Assist Tomogr 1988;12:165–8.
25. Glazer HS, Anderson DJ, Sagel SS. Bronchial impaction in lobar collapse: CT demonstration and pathologic correlation. Am J Roentgenol 1989;153:485–8.
26. Saida Y, Itai Y, Kujiraoka Y, et al. Bronchoarterial inversion: radiographic–CT correlation in combined right middle and lower lobe collapse. J Thorac Imaging 1997;12:59–63.
27. Flanagan JJ, Flower CD, Dixon AK. Compensatory emphysema shown by computed tomography. Clin Radiol 1982;33:553–4.
28. Blankenbaker DG. The Luftsichel sign. Radiology 1998;208: 319–20.
29. Woodring JH, Reed JC. Radiographic manifestations of lobar atelectasis. J Thorac Imaging 1996;11:109–44.
30. Mayr B, Heywang SH, Ingrisch H, et al. Comparison of CT with MR imaging of endobronchial tumors. J Comput Assist Tomogr 1987;11:43–8.
31. Shioya S, Haida M, Ono Y, et al. Lung cancer: differentiation of tumor, necrosis, and atelectasis by means of T1 and T2 values measured in vitro. Radiology 1988;167:105–9.
32. Herold CJ, Kuhlman JE, Zerhouni EA. Pulmonary atelectasis: signal patterns with MR imaging. Radiology 1991;178:715–20.
33. Bourgouin PM, McLoud TC, Fitzgibbon JF, et al. Differentiation of bronchogenic carcinoma from postobstructive pneumonitis by magnetic resonance imaging: histopathologic correlation. J Thorac Imaging 1991;6:22–7.
34. Nestle U, Walter K, Schmidt S, et al. ^{18}F-deoxyglucose positron emission tomography (FDG-PET) for the planning of radiotherapy in lung cancer: high impact in patients with atelectasis. Int J Radiat Oncol Biol Phys 1999;44:593–7.
35. Kattan KR. Upper mediastinal changes in lower lobe collapse. Semin Roentgenol 1980;15:183–6.
36. Kattan KR, Felson B, Holder LE, Eyler WR. Superior mediastinal shift in right lower lobe collapse: the 'upper triangle sign'. Radiology 1975;116:305–9.
37. Kattan KR, Wiot JF. Cardiac rotation in left lower lobe collapse: 'the flat waist sign'. Radiology 1976;118:275–9.
38. Saterfiel JL, Virapongse C, Clore FC. Computed tomography of combined right upper and middle lobe collapse. J Comput Assist Tomogr 1988;12:383–7.

CHAPTER 8

Pulmonary Neoplasms

Simon P.G. Padley • Olga Lazoura

CHAPTER OUTLINE

BRONCHOGENIC CARCINOMA

Bronchogenic carcinoma remains the most common cause of cancer death worldwide. The incidence of the disease has accelerated over the past century, closely in step with tobacco smoking, to peak towards the end of the last century. In the United States in 2011 there were almost 160,000 deaths from lung cancer, with a continuing decline in incidence in men of nearly 30% since a peak in 1990.[1] The incidence of lung cancer in females is following a different trajectory, beginning to increase rapidly in the mid-1960s with only a minimal fall since the peak in 2000. Lung cancer is a disease of the elderly: 60% of cancers are diagnosed in people of more than 65 years of age and 70% of cancer deaths occur after 65 years of age.[2]

HISTOPATHOLOGY

All types of lung cancer are related to cigarette smoking. The predominant cell types are small cell lung cancer (SCLC) and non-small cell lung cancer (NSCLC). NSCLC is divided into three main subtypes, squamous cell carcinoma, adenocarcinoma and large cell cancer. The strongest link with cigarette smoking is seen with squamous cell carcinoma.[3] Thirty years ago squamous cell carcinoma was much more common than adenocarcinoma but over the past three decades the frequency of adenocarcinoma has greatly increased and the ratio is now 1.4 to 1.[4]

GENETIC FACTORS

There have been important advances in the understanding of the genetics of different forms of lung cancer. There are a number of specific genetic mutations that can now be routinely identified and which convey prognostic and treatment implications. The best known of these is the expression of epidermal growth factor receptor (EFGR) mutations in adenocarcinomas of non-smokers.

Although a major risk factor for lung cancer development is smoking, the disease is increasingly recognised in never smokers. These patients make up as much of 25% of the lung cancer patients in some populations.[5] These patients are more commonly female with adenocarcinoma, and this type of disease is particularly common in Asian patients, with some studies reporting as many as 40% of patients to be non-smokers.[6]

Epidermal Growth Factor Receptor (EGFR)

Identification of mutations in oncogenes associated with non-squamous (NSCLC) can help guide targeted therapy. Currently the most important oncogene, which is now routinely sought with genetic profiling assays, is epidermal growth factor receptor (EGFR). This protein stimulates tyrosine kinase. EFGR overexpression and mutations in the tyrosine kinase domain of the EGFR gene can directly lead to tumour growth and progression;

therefore, EGRF has itself become a target for chemotherapy and a number of specific agents have been developed that prevent activation, block the relevant signalling pathways and improve response rates to therapy. The relevant EGFR mutations, associated with sensitivity to tyrosine kinase inhibitors, are most commonly encountered in non-smoking females with adenocarcinoma. Therefore the detection of these mutations will predict a response rate of up to 70%, making targeted therapy prescription of these relatively costly treatments more cost-effective.[7]

K-Ras

This protein stimulates signalling pathways downstream from EGFR. Specific mutations lead to the production of activated K-Ras protein, which continues to stimulate tumour growth. Although tyrosine kinase may block EGFR activation, it does not block the activity of mutated K-Ras proteins. Therefore patients with specific K-Ras mutations will not respond to tyrosine kinase inhibitors. Identification of K-Ras mutations is more common in smoking patients with adenocarcinoma, usually Caucasian rather than Asian. K-Ras mutations confer a poor prognostic outlook.

ALK

Mutations within the anaplastic lymphoma kinase (ALK) gene are associated with NSCLC (usually adenocarcinoma). Patients with ALK specific rearrangements do not benefit from tyrosine kinase inhibitors but may respond favourably to other therapies such as crizotinib, the first approved ALK inhibitor.

There are a number of other mutations of potential importance in non-cell lung cancer. These can only be identified by molecular testing, which in turn may allow targeted therapy or prediction of resistance. EGRF, K-Ras and ALK mutations are usually mutually exclusive. Application of lung cancer mutation panel tests is therefore becoming increasingly commonplace, particularly as funding for this investigation becomes more widely approved.

LUNG CANCER AND OTHER ENVIRONMENTAL FACTORS

Smoking

Smoking, by a large margin, is the major risk factor for lung cancer, and a dose relationship has been reconfirmed several times since the hallmark study of Doll and Hill.[8] Cigarettes have changed in composition since the 1950s. Cigarette smoke is complex in nature and there are up to 60 identified carcinogens in tobacco smoke. Filters are now commonplace and nicotine levels have fallen in the tobacco varieties now produced. Nicotine itself is not thought to cause tumours, but seems to promote their growth. Since nicotine is the major dependent pharmacological agent in cigarettes, lowering levels may have resulted in a habit of greater depths of inhalation and in total numbers of cigarettes consumed.

Passive Smoking

Passive smoking has received considerable attention and is now recognised as a major contributor to worldwide morbidity and mortality related to lung cancer. A number of studies have demonstrated that non-smoking spouses of smokers have a 20–30% increase in lung cancer[9] and a dose–response relationship has been demonstrated.[10]

Huge efforts have been made to reduce smoking rates, and clearly never commencing smoking is the aim. There are now almost as many former smokers as active smokers in the United States,[11] and cessation of smoking reduces all lung cancer risk, especially those most strongly associated with smoking, namely small cell lung cancer and squamous cell carcinoma. It is estimated that the risk of lung cancer will have dropped by 50% 15 years after ceasing to smoke.[12]

General Environmental Pollutants

General environmental pollutants have been suggested as a further risk factor for lung cancer development. The influence of air pollutants has been long recognised as an environmental issue. More recently, attention has been paid to air quality and particularly to the concentrations on fine particles within the air that we breathe.[13] Particles of less than 2.5 μm in diameter are strongly associated with lung cancer, especially in non-smokers. These particles are particularly associated with diesel engine exhaust.

Asbestos

Asbestos has also long been associated with increased lung cancer risk as well as being a known trigger for non-malignant lung and pleural disease. Chrysotile fibres are most closely linked with lung and pleural malignancy. The exposure to both asbestos and tobacco is particularly carcinogenic and estimates of a 15- to 50-fold increased risk of developing lung cancer are frequently quoted.[14]

Radon

Perhaps the forgotten aetiological agent is ^{222}radon, second only to smoking as a cause of bronchogenic carcinoma. Since radon is in the earth's crust, there is little that can be done to alter exposure levels. Certain geographical areas, for geological reasons, result in greater exposure levels.[3] Data related to radon risk largely come from underground workers, where levels are high.

LUNG CANCER SCREENING

Chest Radiographic Screening

There is a considerable literature on the use of chest radiography as a screening tool for early lung cancer. These trials have been of all varieties, including randomised controlled trials (RCTs). Some have been undertaken in conjunction with sputum cytology. Two early important trials were performed in Japan.[15,16] Although designed differently and coming to slightly different conclusions in large numbers of patients, these mass screening programmes concluded there was a benefit associated with chest X-ray screening and sputum cytology compared to non-screening. These studies were both case-controlled studies.

The next landmark study was the Mayo Lung Project performed between 1971 and 1983, a randomised controlled trial on nearly 11,000 patients. Rather than a case-control study, this RCT also set out to determine whether chest X-ray and sputum cytology provided an effective means of screening for lung cancer. Perhaps unusually, patients were randomised into two different screening regimes, screened annually or every 4 months for 6 years, with further follow-up. This study demonstrated a clear stage shift in the more frequently screened patients, resulting in a better 5-year survival but at 20-year follow-up there was no overall survival benefit.[17] Further large studies from the Memorial Sloane Kettering Hospital,[18] the Johns Hopkins lung project[19] and a Czechoslovakian study[20] all had insufficient statistical power to demonstrate a reduction in mortality between screened and non-screened patients. Since the question remained open to doubt, the prostate, lung, colorectal and ovarian cancer screening trial, recruiting between 1993 and 2001 at 10 screening centres across the United States, attempted to resolve whether chest X-ray could be used as an effective screening technique for lung cancer and result in subsequent reduction in mortality.[21] Unlike previous studies, many of the enrolees were never smokers (45%), or non-smokers (42%) and only about 10% were current smokers. Of the total 154,000 men and women enrolled, only 24,000 were considered to be of high risk for lung cancer. In this study, despite a slight stage shift in the screening group, there is no difference in lung cancer deaths between the screen group and the usual care group. From these various trials, providing some contradictory data, it can be reasonably concluded that chest X-ray alone has no useful role in lung cancer screening. Although lung cancers may be detected, often at a slightly earlier stage, the eventual outcome between screened and non-screened groups is almost identical.

CT Screening

More recently the debate has concentrated on lung cancer screening with CT, more recently using a low-dose technique. Again, it was the Japanese that led the way with two early trials.[22,23] These studies set the pattern of subsequent CT screening projects. High-risk patients were identified, and a volumetric CT was undertaken. Detected nodules were followed up according to protocol. Very small nodules were not followed up, intermediate-sized nodules would continue along a screening pathway and subsequent CT at varying intervals, to detect growth. Larger nodules would be immediately sampled. Subsequent studies, including the landmark Early Lung Cancer Action Project (ELCAP)[24] concluded that low-dose CT results in lung cancers being diagnosed at an earlier stage and with a higher cure rate than lung cancers detected as a result of symptoms. There has since followed at least 20 subsequent studies using CT as a screening tool.[25] A full discussion of these trials is beyond the scope of this chapter. However, some have had a greater impact than others, most importantly the National Lung Cancer Screening Trial (NLST).[26] This large and well-funded trial, by the US National Cancer Institute, enrolled 53,454 smokers or ex-smokers between the ages of 55 and 74, randomised to low-dose CT or PA chest radiography on an annual basis for 3 years. This design is slightly unusual, since there is no non-screening arm, but compares two different screening methods. There have been a number of important findings to come out of this large trial:

- Many patients have a positive screening test, either X-ray (16%) or CT (39%) at least once over the course of 3 years.
- More cancers were detected in the CT arm than the chest X-ray arm.
- Investigation of possible lung cancers resulted in complications in both the CT and chest X-ray arms, described as major complications in approximately 10% of both groups, undergoing invasive evaluation.
- Screen-detected cancers are at an earlier stage in the CT arm compared with the chest X-ray arm.
- Adenocarcinomas are more common in the screening population than in the symptomatic population.
- There is a 20% reduction in lung cancer specific mortality in the CT group.

This study, it is generally agreed, has demonstrated that CT screening applied to a carefully targeted group of patients can reduce lung cancer mortality. The cost of this approach looms large amongst the other questions that await a definitive answer. Cost-effective analyses are still underway.

This is not the end of the story—there are a number of ongoing European randomised controlled trials[25] underway or in preparation from Italy, France, Holland, Denmark and the UK.

All of these trials have been designed slightly differently, but the question, as yet unanswered, is should this form of screening be rolled out across the general at-risk population. Amongst the many other questions that require consideration are the issues around the psychological burden of telling a patient they have a small nodule that requires follow-up to exclude lung cancer, with no answer likely for at least 2 years.

CT screening techniques are not perfect and the accuracy of CT as a detection technique has resulted in considerable debate. In the early days, 10-mm contiguous slices were utilised. Technology has since evolved, with multi-detector CT being routine and the ability to produce contiguous 1-mm collimation images now being commonplace. A simple, cheap but very effective technique, now widely employed on these narrow section data sets, has been the use of maximum intensity projection image reconstructions. This technique can be used on all CT workstations and most picture archiving and communication system (PACS) workstations and has been demonstrated to greatly improve conspicuity of nodules.

There has also been considerable resource expended on the development of computer-assisted diagnosis (CAD). Scrolling through many hundreds of images in

TABLE 8-1 Fleischner Society Guidelines for Nodule Follow-up

Nodule Size (mm)	Low-Risk Patient	High-Risk Patient
<4	No follow-up needed	Follow-up CT at 12 months; if unchanged, no further follow-up
>4–6	Follow-up CT at 12 months; if unchanged, no further follow-up	Initial follow-up CT at 6–12 months, then at 18–24 months if no change
>6–8	Initial follow-up CT at 6–12 months, then at 18–24 months if no change	Initial follow-up CT at 3–6 months, then at 9–12 months if no change
>8	Follow-up at around 3, 9 and 24 months, dynamic contrast-enhanced CT, PET, biopsy	Same as for low-risk patients

Adapted from the MacMahon et al.[1]

an attempt to detect small nodules leads fairly rapidly to reader fatigue. CAD systems have been shown to augment the ability of a radiologist to detect all relevant lesions, by highlighting candidate lesions and allowing the radiologist to include or dismiss them as appropriate.[27] The corollary of CAD utilisation is high initial false-positive rates: many lesions that are highlighted by the CAD system are subsequently dismissed by the radiologist. This may not result in a faster assessment, but does improve accuracy overall.[28]

In both the screening studies and in general practice, once a nodule has been detected, typically between 5 and 8 mm in size, the usual practice is to undertake follow-up CT studies and most radiologists will follow the Fleischner guidelines for the follow-up of lung nodules (Table 8-1).[1]

The vast majority of detected lung nodules, at least 98%, will be of no clinical significance, particularly in low-risk patients. Most of these nodules will not increase in size. However, being small, reproducible measurements are potentially problematic and therefore accurate determination of genuine increase becomes of critical importance in managing further follow-up intervals. Most radiologists routinely employ 2D calibre measurements, but for small nodules this is notoriously inaccurate, and is not reproducible either across different readers or between the same readers on different occasions, and the technique also does not lend itself to non-spherical lesions. Therefore, as well as being able to assist in the detection of nodules, computer-assisted characterisation tools have also become commonplace, through automatic segmentation and volume calculation. This technique, of producing a semi-automated nodule volume, is much more reproducible than 2D calibre techniques[29] even though others have shown that the technique itself, when repeatedly measuring the same nodule, may give varying results.[30] The practice of routine volumetric assessment is, however, beginning to become routine as CT workstation vendors provide the relevant software as a standard (Fig. 8-1).

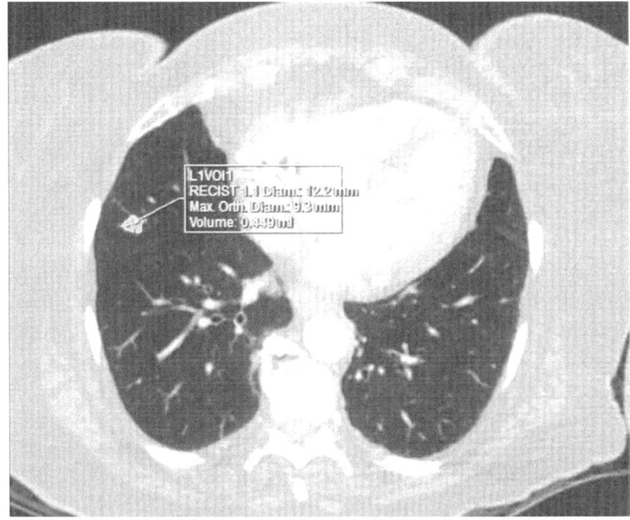

FIGURE 8-1 ■ Example of automatic segmentation and volume calculation of a middle lobe nodule.

Radiation Dose Considerations

It is important at all times, and particularly in a screening population where there is a high likelihood of detected nodules being of no significance, to reduce radiation exposure to a minimum. The use of a 'low-dose' CT technique should be automatic. This can be achieved by reducing tube current and tube voltage and increasing pitch. It is also important not to over-investigate screening or incidentally detected nodules, and to time follow-up studies appropriately. Furthermore, it is sometimes preferable to target the follow-up examination to only examine the nodule in question, rather than repeating the CT study of the entire thorax.

The Future of Screening

The NLST screening study has demonstrated a decrease in mortality from lung cancer in patients undergoing low-dose CT assessment. The resources required to roll out a CT screening programme are huge. The medical community is currently awaiting to see if the NLST trial results are confirmed by one or more of the other ongoing studies in Europe. None of these are individually as large as the NLST study, but in combination they might provide sufficient evidence to recommend screening across the general smoking population. What is not yet defined is how wide the screening net should be cast, whether the parameters used by the NLST are appropriate, and which nodules require further follow-up and further investigation. Currently, both in Europe and the United States, it is agreed that the patients undergoing screening CT should do so according to agreed guidelines. These guidelines also advise in detail about the management of screening results. The American Lung Association has also recently issued guidance on lung cancer screening to patients and physicians.[7,31,32] In the UK a recent opinion piece from the UK Lung Screening (UKLS) group neatly defines the problems that remain unresolved as psychosocial and cost-effectiveness issues, harmonisation of CT acquisition techniques, management of findings, screening frequency and subject selection.[33]

PULMONARY NODULES

Management of Small Pulmonary Nodules

Nodule detection, now an everyday occurrence in patients undergoing multi-slice CT, raises a series of management problems for the referring physician and reporting radiologist. The wildly utilised Fleischner Society Recommendations (Table 8-1) have provided clear and frequently utilised guidance since their publication in 2005.[1]

In evaluating a pulmonary nodule it is helpful to bear in mind likely causes. Assessment of nodular morphology and characteristics can also provide useful information.

Nodule Size

Small nodules are very unlikely to be due to malignancy. Indeed screening studies have demonstrated that malignancy in nodules of less than 5 mm in size (4 mm or less) is so low, and these nodules are so common, that follow-up is not generally recommended. However this does not hold true in patients with a known primary malignancy elsewhere. Most benign nodules measure less than 2 cm in diameter and the smaller the nodule is, the more likely it is to be benign.[34-36]

Location, Shape and Morphology

Perifissural nodules are a recognised entity following CT screening studies. These small subpleural nodules have been shown to frequently represent intrapulmonary lymphoid tissue or complete intraparenchymal lymph nodes.[37] Characteristic features of intraparenchymal lymph nodes (Fig. 8-2)[38] are nodules less than 15 mm from the pleural surface, being ellipsoid in shape and usually being connected to the pleural surface by a fine linear opacity.[39] Follow-up studies of nodules of this variety, detected during the Nelson Screening Trial demonstrated that no nodules with these features developed into lung cancer.[40] Nodule outline can also be helpful when other features typical of intrapulmonary lymphoid material are absent. Concave surfaces on all sides or a straight surface of contact with the pleura has also been shown to represent benign features.[41] The less spherical a nodule is, particularly on volumetric assessment, the less likely a malignant aetiology. Flat or tubular nodules are more likely to be benign than round nodules. Therefore, solid, subpleural, polygonal nodules with a low sphericity index are highly unlikely to be malignant.

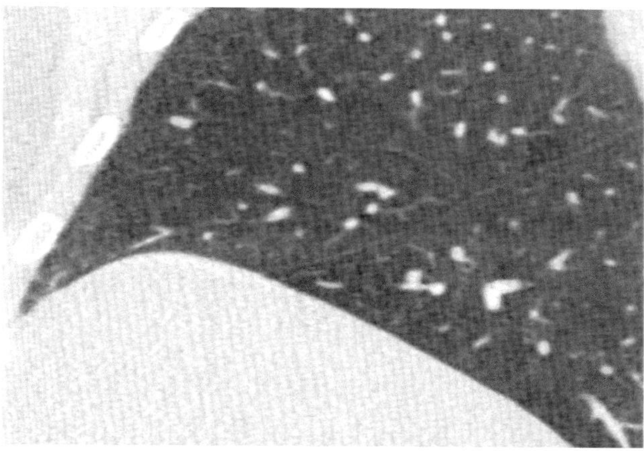

FIGURE 8-2 ■ **Intrapulmonary lymph node.** Small ellipsoid perifissural nodule with concave surfaces on CT corresponds to an intraparenchymal lymph node.

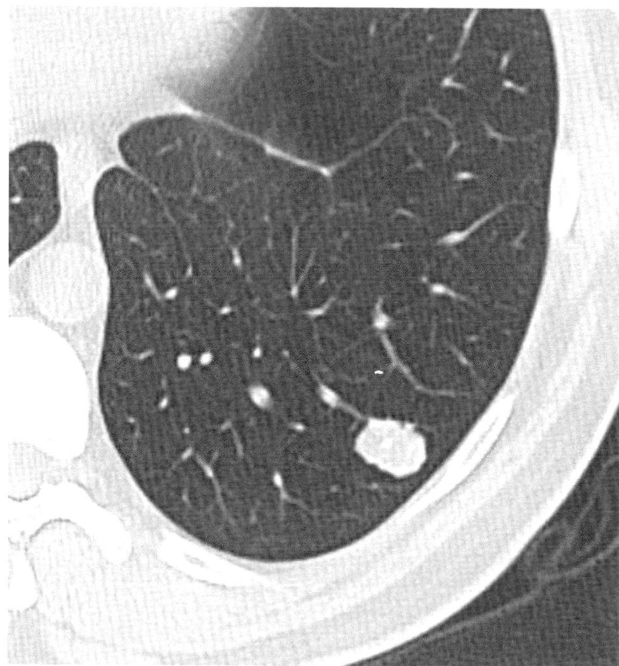

FIGURE 8-3 ■ **CT demonstrates a mildly lobulated nodule with calcification in the left lower lobe which corresponds to a hamartoma.**

Cavitation within a nodule can occur and be both benign and malignant in aetiology. Malignant cavitation is often associated with a thick and irregular internal cavity wall, compared to the more uniform cavitation associated with benign nodules, although this is not a reliable distinguishing feature.[42]

Nodule Contour

Nodules without obvious benign morphology may be smoothly marginated, lobulated or spiculated. Smoothly marginated nodules are more likely to be benign or metastatic. Lobulated nodules are more likely to be malignant[43] but there is considerable overlap (Fig. 8-3).

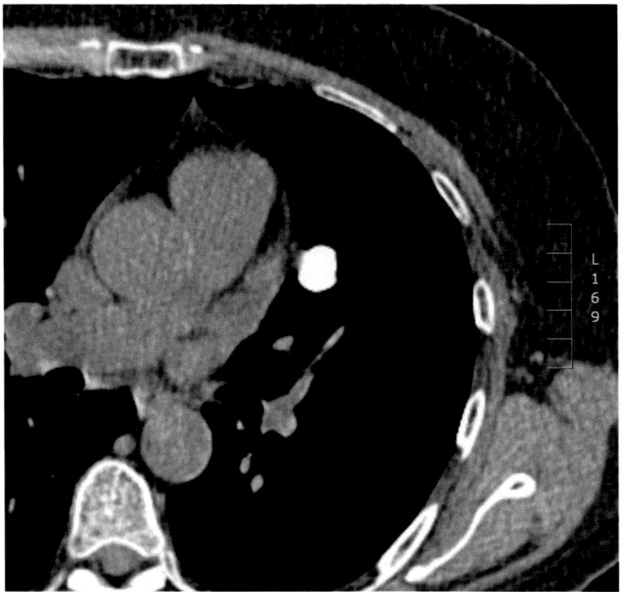

FIGURE 8-4 ■ **Granuloma.** Focal dense solid parenchymal calcification on chest CT indicates previous granulomatous infection.

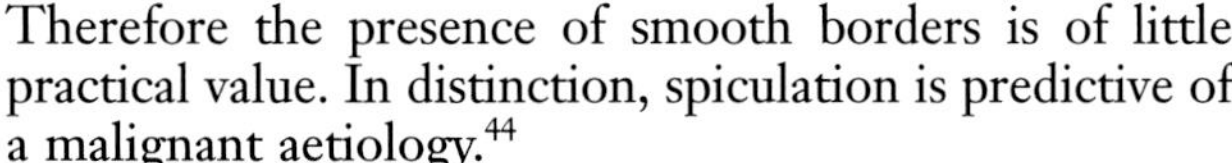

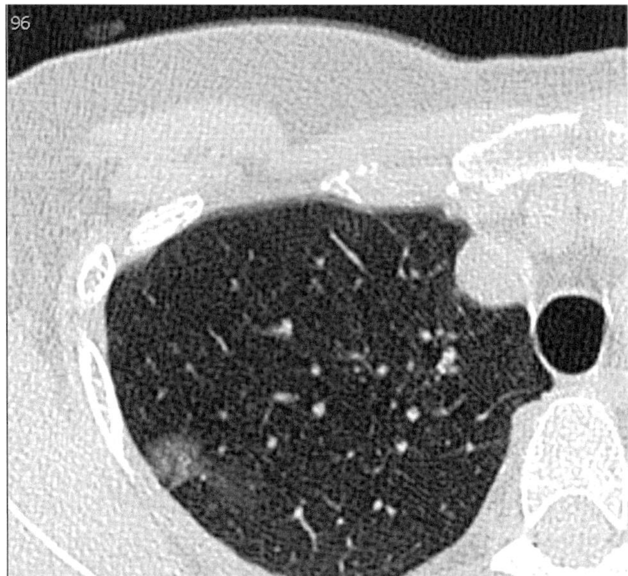

FIGURE 8-5 ■ **Pure ground-glass opacity.** A focal area of increased lung attenuation on CT through which normal structures can be discerned is termed 'pure ground-glass opacity'.

Therefore the presence of smooth borders is of little practical value. In distinction, spiculation is predictive of a malignant aetiology.[44]

The presence of central air bronchograms or soap bubble lucency centrally within a nodule has been previously evaluated. Multiple spherical areas of air may be present in adenocarcinoma, due to the lepidic growth pattern of these lesions, where tumour cells have grown along the alveolar walls and adjacent airways without filling the alveolar spaces. In comparison, the presence of air bronchograms,[45] rather than bubble-like lucencies, may also be seen in lymphoma, organising pneumonia and alveolar sarcoidosis.

Nodule Density

Certain patterns of calcification are recognised as being highly predictive of a benign aetiology. Recognised benign patterns are lamellated, solid, central and popcorn-like. Central or lamellated calcification is typically indicative of previous granulomatous disease[44] and, similarly, dense solid calcification is likely to indicate previous granulomatous infection (Fig. 8-4). Popcorn calcification usually indicates the presence of a hamartoma[46] and these lesions may also contain convincing evidence of internal fat density. When fat is present in a lesion of less than 2.5 cm in diameter, then, particularly if the lesion is PET negative, further evaluation is not required, but most hamartomas do not demonstrate this helpful characteristic. Calcification, which is eccentric or stippled within an area of soft tissue density, may be seen in malignancy. Very occasionally metastases from bone-forming or cartilage-forming tumours may present a benign pattern of calcification, but usually there is a relevant history.

Ground-Glass Nodules

A focal area of increased lung attenuation, which may be well or poorly defined but through which normal structures can still be discerned, is typically referred to as a ground-glass density. If localised, the opacity may be described as a ground-glass opacity (GGO) or ground-glass nodule (GGN) (Fig. 8-5). The term 'pure ground glass nodule' is the preferred descriptive term if there is no soft-tissue component.[46] If an area of ground-glass density includes a solid component which does obscure lung architecture, this may be termed a part-solid ground-glass nodule. In the literature both **pure ground-glass nodules** and **part-solid ground-glass nodules** may be grouped together under the term **sub-solid nodules**. The Fleischner Society have now published guidelines on the management of these sub-solid nodules, recognising that such sub-solid nodules may represent early forms of adenocarcinoma.[47] Because of the relevance of the current classification of lung adenocarcinoma to the management of sub-solid nodules the new classification will be considered here.[48] The new classification eliminates the term bronchoalveolar carcinoma and mixed subtype adenocarcinoma and now divides adenocarcinoma into the following categories:

- **Pre-malignant lesions.** This includes atypical adenomatous hyperplasia and adenocarcinoma in situ. These lesions are 3 cm or less in diameter and histology manifests pure lepidic growth with no solid components. These will appear as pure GGO on CT.
- **Malignant lesions**, divided into the following:
  - Minimally invasive adenocarcinoma, with predominantly (in distinction to pure) lepidic growth, 3 cm or less, and with invasive components of no more than 5 mm. These are generally sub-solid nodules on CT.

TABLE 8-2 **Recommendations for the Management of Sub-Solid Pulmonary Nodules Detected at CT: a Statement from the Fleishner Society**

Nodule Type	Management Recommendations	Additional Remarks
<5 mm	No CT follow-up required	Obtain contiguous 1-mm-thick sections to confirm that nodule is truly a pure GGN
>5 mm	Initial follow-up CT to confirm persistence; then annual surveillance CT for a minimum of 3 years	FDG-PET is of limited value, potentially misleading and therefore not recommended
Solitary part-solid nodules	Initial follow-up CT at 3 months to confirm persistence. If persistent and solid component <5 mm, then yearly surveillance CT for a minimum of 3 years. If persistent and solid component >5 mm, then biopsy or surgical resection	Consider PET/CT for part solid nodules >10 mm.
Multiple sub-solid nodules Pure GGNs <5 mm	Obtain follow-up CT at 2 and 4 years	Consider alternative causes for multiple GGNs <5 mm
Pure GGNs >5 mm without a dominant lesion(s)	Initial follow-up CT at 3 months to confirm persistence and then annual surveillance CT for a minimum of 3 years	FDG-PET is of limited value, potentially misleading and therefore not recommended
Dominant nodules with part-solid or solid component	Initial follow-up at 3 months to confirm persistence. If persistent, biopsy or surgical resection is recommended, especially for lesions with >5 mm solid component	Consider lung-sparing surgery for patients with dominant lesion(s) for lung cancer

Reproduced with permission from Naidich et al.[47]

Note: These guidelines assume meticulous evaluation, optimally and contiguous thin sections (1 mm) reconstructed with narrow and wide and/or lung windows to evaluate the non-solid component of nodules. If indicated, when electronic calipers are used for bi-dimensional measurements, both the solid and ground-glass components of lesions should be obtained as necessary. The use of a consistent low-dose technique is recommended, especially in cases for which prolonged follow-up is recommended, particularly in younger patients. With serial scans, always compare with the original baseline study to detect subtle indolent growth.

- Invasive adenocarcinomas, subclassified as predominantly lepidic, acinar, papillary, micropapillary and solid types.
- Invasive mucinous adenocarcinoma, an entity formerly described as mucinous bronchioalveolar carcinoma and considered as a separate group from the non-mucinous types above.

Prognosis of patients with adenocarcinoma in situ or minimally invasive adenocarcinoma (characterised on CT as pure ground-glass lesions) is excellent; these patients should have almost 100% disease-free survival.[48] Invasive adenocarcinoma has a variable outlook, and to some extent this depends on the histological subtype. Detailed discussion is beyond the scope of this chapter.

The new recommendations for the management of sub-solid pulmonary nodules detected by CT from the Fleischner Society, reflecting the new classification of adenocarcinoma, are given in Table 8-2.

In essence there are six current recommendations regarding sub-solid nodules:

- Solitary pure ground-glass nodules measuring 5 mm or less do not require follow-up surveillance.
- Solitary pure ground-glass nodules of more than 5 mm but less than 3 cm require 3 months limited follow-up to determine their persistent nature and then yearly surveillance for a minimum of 3 years if persistent but unchanged.
- Solitary part-solid ground-glass nodules, with a solid component of more than 5 mm, should be considered malignant until proven otherwise if there has been growth or no change at the 3-month follow-up study (Fig. 8-6).
- Multiple well-defined ground-glass nodules all measuring 5-mm or less should be conservatively managed with follow-up CT examinations performed at 2 and 4 years.
- In cases in which pure multiple ground-glass nodules are identified (Fig. 8-7), at least one of which is larger than 5 mm, and in the absence of a dominant lesion, an initial follow-up CT examination in 3 months is recommended followed by yearly surveillance CT examinations for at least 3 years.
- In the case of multiple sub-solid nodules in which there is a dominant lesion, the dominant lesion determines further management. After initial follow-up, a CT at 3 months to confirm persistence, an aggressive approach to diagnosis and management is recommended, especially when the solid component is larger than 5 mm (reproduced with permission).

OTHER FORMS OF NODULE ASSESSMENT

Nodule Follow-Up

Since repeat CT is a common recommendation in the management of both solid and sub-solid pulmonary nodules, it is important that subsequent CT examinations are undertaken using an identical protocol in order to accurately estimate doubling times. This is particularly so in cases of ground-glass nodules where very long doubling times are recognised in low-grade malignancies.[49]

Nodule Enhancement

Contrast-enhanced CT has been demonstrated as an effective management tool in the assessment of lung

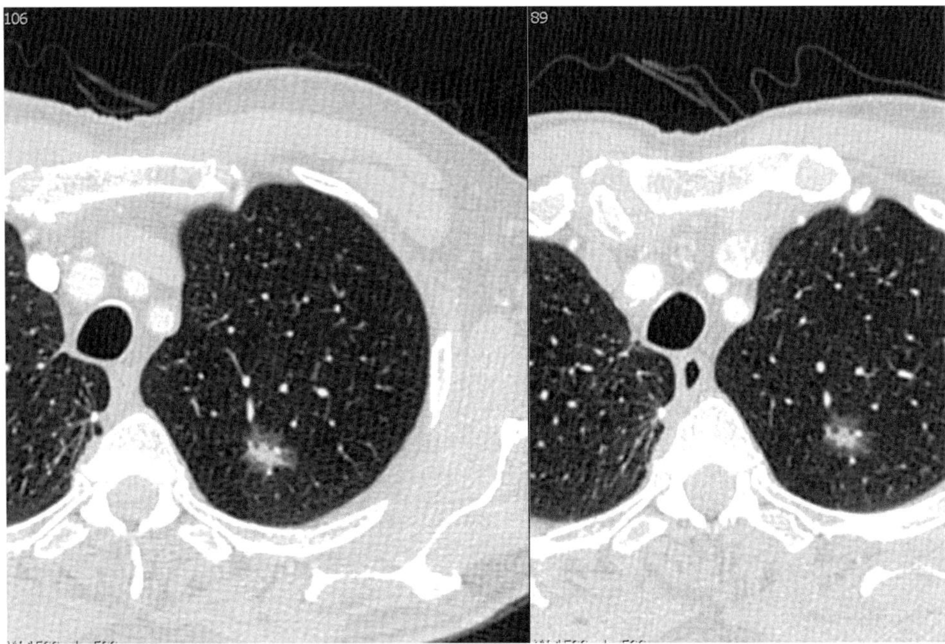

FIGURE 8-6 ■ Solitary part-solid ground-glass nodule (left) with an enlarging solid component at 3-month follow-up (right) is indicative of malignancy.

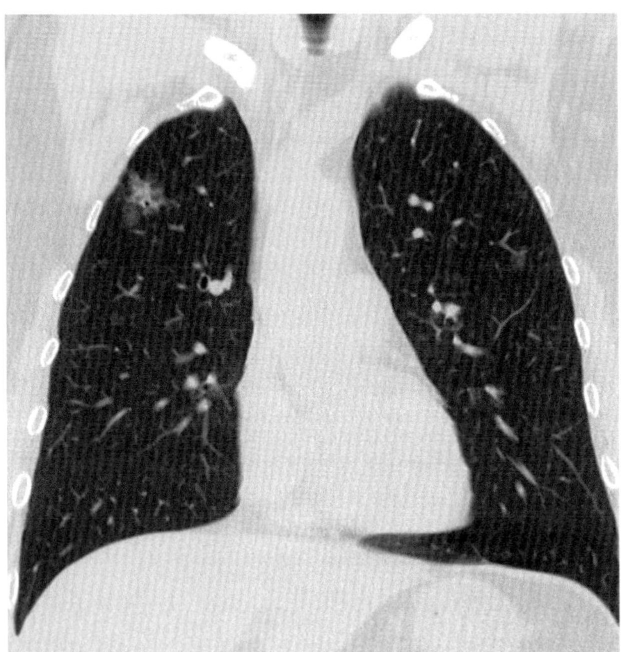

FIGURE 8-7 ■ Example of multiple pure ground-glass nodules, one of which larger than 5 mm.

nodules. In essence, malignant nodules will demonstrate enhancement, as will some benign nodules. If there is no enhancement, malignancy is effectively excluded.[50] This technique works well in soft-tissue density nodules, but is less applicable to nodules containing calcification, cavitation or ground-glass opacity. The possibility of generating a virtual non-contrast data set, using dual-energy CT, has been investigated as a means to reduce radiation exposure yet provide similar information to a pre- and post-contrast acquisition.[51] Although nodule enhancement has been demonstrated to be practical, in practice it has largely been superseded by PET/CT evaluation.

PET/CT

PET/CT is now an essential tool in the management and the work-up of patients with possible pulmonary malignancy. It forms part of the standard staging in patients with proven or suspected lung cancer but is also a frequently utilised tool in the work-up of patients with an indeterminate lung nodule. The commonest isotope utilised is 2-deoxy-2-[^{18}F]fluoro-D-glucose, a glucose analogue, with the positron-emitting radioactive isotope fluorine-18 substituted for the normal hydroxyl group at the 2′ position in the glucose molecule, commonly referred to as FDG. The technique relies on increased uptake in neoplastic nodules (Fig. 8-8). Increased uptake also occurs within many inflammatory processes. Nevertheless, the utility of PET/CT has been documented, in a number of studies,[52] to have sensitivities of 90% and specificities of 83% for a diagnosis of malignancy. However, in the context of small nodules, FDG results must be interpreted with some caution, since nodules of less than 1 cm are more likely to result in a false-negative interpretation, particularly with certain lower-grade adenocarcinoma subtypes[53] and carcinoid tumours. The application of PET/CT for nodules of less than 6 mm is currently not justified. In the context of lung disease, sarcoidosis, granulomatous infection and a number of inflammatory processes are recognised as resulting in significant PET FDG avidity.

Tissue Sampling

Tissue sampling of nodules which are both accessible and of a size, shape and morphology to suggest the possibility

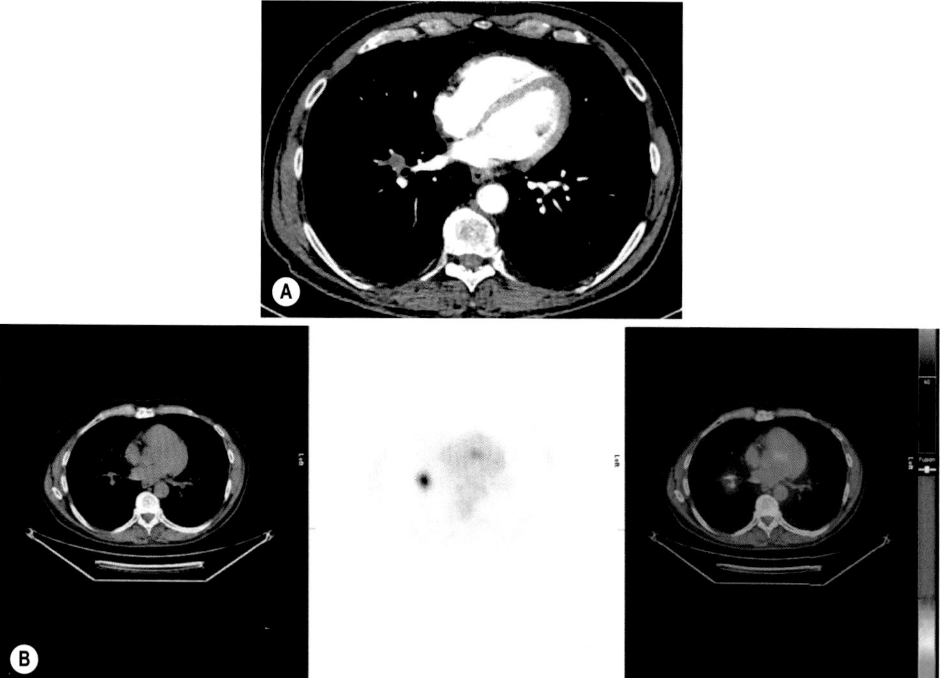

FIGURE 8-8 ■ Axial image from a contrast enhanced CT and CT image, FDG PET image and fused image from a CT PET study, demonstrating a PET positive right lung nodule. (A) Lung nodule close to the right hilum with (B) increased uptake on PET/CT corresponding to lung cancer.

of malignancy, may be undertaken transbronchially, surgically or percutanously with radiological guidance. Central lesions may be amenable to bronchoscopic biopsy but even perihilar nodules, in the absence of an endoluminal component, remain very challenging for bronchoscopic diagnosis.[54] Bronchoscopic biopsy of peripheral lung cancer using conventional techniques is also highly problematic.[55] Percutaneous fine needle or cutting needle biopsy has been demonstrated as an accurate technique for the identification of malignancy, but not all nodules are suitable for this approach. When a final diagnosis of lung cancer is eventually established, a previous aspiration biopsy has a 90% likelihood of providing confirmation of a malignant diagnosis. There is a very low false-positive rate but there is a recognised and troubling false-negative rate. Transthoracic needle biopsy remains an essential tool in the management part of indeterminate nodules. Multidisciplinary team discussion of the relative merits of a follow-up strategy, further imaging, percutaneous or bronchoscopic diagnostic procedures or surgical resection for an individual lung nodule remains the ideal management step in this common problem.

Decisions regarding further investigation of pulmonary nodules can also be helpfully guided by the pre-test probability of malignancy: most importantly, previous known malignancy, patient age and smoking history. The use of risk management modelling has been previously studied,[56,57] incorporating various risk factors, but all methods reported to date confirm that a significant current or previous smoking history in an elderly patient with a nodule diameter of more than 1 cm are all highly suggestive of a malignant aetiology. It should be remembered that 99% of all nodules of 4 mm or less in diameter will turn out to be benign on follow-up or resection. These lesions are so frequently seen on CT that follow-up is no longer recommended in the low-risk patient and a single follow-up CT is required in the high-risk patient. Between 4 and 8 mm in size, surveillance CT is the recommended approach, with the goal of demonstrating stability over a 24-month period. The frequency of interval CT will depend on the initial size of the lesion and the patient's malignant risk (see Table 8-1). A more aggressive approach, including contrast enhancement CT, PET/CT, needle biopsy or resection is adopted for lesions of more than 8 mm.

LUNG CANCER STAGING—THE 7TH EDITION OF THE TNM STAGING SYSTEM FOR LUNG CANCER

The new 7th edition of the TNM staging system is based on a much larger database of patients than previously available, comprised of over 100,000 cases from 45 centres in 20 countries of which more than 80,000 had sufficient information to contribute to the analysis. The 7th edition was published in 2009.[58] Radiologists are divided as to whether it is desirable to give a TNM description in radiology staging reports, but if this information is provided then an intimate understanding of the TNM staging system is required. TNM staging is now an essential part of the multidisciplinary team decision process. The changes to the previous staging system are highlighted below.

The T descriptor not only describes the absolute size of the tumour but also assesses local invasion. The criteria for local invasion were not revised due to insufficient patient numbers and lack of validation. The main discrimination to be made is between T3 and T4 disease. Chest wall invasion, parietal pleural invasion, mediastinal pleural invasion and parietal pericardial invasion all remain T3 descriptors. Visceral pleural invasion remains a T2 descriptor. Even a tumour of less than 3 cm with parietal pleural invasion is described as a T3 lesion and this is important since these patients will receive adjuvant chemotherapy following resection.[59] Lesions that invade across a fissure into an adjacent lobe have remained as T2 lesions.[60] Assessment of pleural and chest wall invasion has long been recognised as a difficult task for CT analysis. Where there is obvious soft-tissue extension into the intercostal muscles or bone destruction, the issue is easily resolved. More subtle chest wall parietal pleural invasion is more difficult to define and, as in the past, local chest wall pain is known to be more specific than CT findings for chest wall and parietal pleural involvement.[61] Efforts to more clearly define the presence or absence of pleural invasion have included MRI imaging, high-resolution targeted ultrasound and even diagnostic artificial pneumothorax.[62] Invasion of the diaphragm is classified in the same manner as parietal pleural invasion and is a T3 descriptor.

Direct extension into the heart, great vessels, trachea, oesophagus, vertebral body and mediastinal fat are all T4 descriptors. Phrenic nerve involvement is a T3 descriptor but recurrent laryngeal nerve involvement, indicating direct mediastinal infiltration, is a T4 descriptor. Pancoast's (superior sulcus) tumours are individually staged according to the involved tissues. For example an apical tumour with parietal pleural involvement is defined as a T3 lesion, but a similar tumour extending into a vertebral body or involving subclavian vessels becomes a T4 lesion. Because of the importance of this differentiation, the utility of multiplanar reformatted images on CT and targeted MRI examination has been highlighted. As in the 6th edition, bronchogenic lesions extending into a mainstem bronchus, but more than 2 cm from the carina, remain T2 lesions, less than 2 cm from the carina T3 lesions and invading the carina T4 lesions. An airway lesion causing peripheral atelectasis is now classified as T2a or b (depending on the size of the primary lesion) if less than the whole lung is involved and T3 if the whole lung is involved.

Additional Pulmonary Nodules in the Presence of Lung Cancer

Previously, a nodule in the same lobe as the primary tumour confirmed T4 status and if in a different lobe M1 status. This has been revised in the 7th edition (see Table 8-3). Improved outcomes for patients in this situation led to reclassification of nodules in the same lobe as the primary tumour as a T3 status, and for similar reasons a nodule in the ipsilateral lung but in a different lobe, whilst predicting a poor 5-year survival, confirms a slightly better outlook than M1 disease of other types. Therefore the combination of a primary lesion with a further nodule within an ipsilateral different lobe is now described as T4 disease in the 7th edition.

N Descriptors

Nodes are described as either N0 (no involvement), N1 (nodes up to and including hilar stations), N2 (ipsilateral

TABLE 8-3 **Overall Stage Groupings with Respect to the TNM Description in the 7th Edition of the TNM Staging of Lung Cancer**

6th Edition T/M Descriptor	7th Edition T/M Descriptor	N0	N1	N2	N3
T1 (<2 cm)	T1a	IA	IIA	IIIA	111B
T1 (>2–3 cm)	T1b	1A	IIA	IIIA	111B
T2 (5 cm)	T2a	1B	IIA (6th edn 11B)	IIIA	111B
T2 (>5–<7 cm)	T2b	11A (6th edn 1B)	11B	11A	111B
T2 (>7 cm)	T3	11B (6th edn IB)	111A (6th edn 11B)	111A	111B
T3 (invasion)	T3	11B	111A	111A	111B
T4 (same lobe nodules)	T3	11B (6th edn 111B)	111A (6th edn 111B)	11A (6th edn 111B)	111B
T4 (extension)	T4	111A (6th edn 111B)	111A (6th edn 111B)	111B	111B
M1 (ipsilateral lobe nodule)	T4	111A (6th edn IV)	111A (6th edn IV)	111B (6th edn IV)	111B (6th edn IV)
T4 (pleural dissemination)	M1a	IV (6th edn 111B)	IV (6th edn 111B)	IV (6th edn 111B)	IV (6th edn 111B)
M1 (contralateral lung nodule)	M1a	IV	IV	IV	IV
M1 (distant metastasis)	M1b	IV	IV	IV	IV

Note: Changes to 6th edition in parentheses, highlighted stage groups are potential operative candidates. For each stage, the prognoses, or estimated 5-year survival rates, in Europe are as follows:

- Stage IA—60%
- Stage IB—38%
- Stage IIA—34%
- Stage IIB—24%
- Stage IIIA—13%
- Stage IIB—5% (Stage IIB and IV lesions are non-resectable.)
- Stage IV—<1%

TABLE 8-4 **Nodal Zones**

Supraclavicular zone	Station 1—Low cervical, supraclavicular and sternal notch nodes
Upper zone	Station 2—Upper tracheal nodes Station 3—Prevascular and retro-tracheal nodes Station 4—Lower paratracheal nodes
AP zone	Station 5—Subaortic nodes (aortopulmonary window) Station 6—Para-aortic nodes (ascending aorta or phrenic)
Subcarinal zone	Station 7—Subcarinal nodes
Lower zone	Station 8—Paraoesophageal nodes (below carinal) Station 9—Pulmonary ligament nodes
Hilar/interlobular zone	Station 10—Hilar nodes Station 11—Interlobular nodes
Peripheral zone	Station 12—Lobar nodes Station 13—Segmental nodes Station 14—Subsegmental nodes

mediastinal nodes) or N3 (contralateral mediastinal or more distant nodes). Before the 7th edition, there were two different nodal maps in common usage. These were largely similar but there were some important discrepancies, particularly with regard to subcarinal lymph nodes. These discrepancies have been resolved with the production of a new nodal map with anatomically defined borders. Relevant changes are supraclavicular and sternal notch nodes being designated station 1 and the shift of the midline for right and left level 2 and level 4 nodes from the midline of the trachea to the left lateral border of the trachea. Therefore a lymph node lying directly anterior to the trachea using the 7th edition nodal map would be designated as a right paratracheal lymph node.

This work has also led to the proposal of lymph node zones (Table 8-4), not incorporated into the current staging nomenclature but likely to be used in future iterations.[63] Potential advantages are to facilitate description of large nodal masses crossing nodal stations. This nodal zonal concept also allowed an analysis to be undertaken of the significance of skip metastases where an N2 node is involved without evidence of N1 disease. This nuance has revealed that the presence of station 5 (aortopulmonary) nodes in association with a left upper lobe tumour but without N1 disease confers a better outcome status than other forms of N2 disease. The same was not found for right paratracheal (N2) nodes with right upper lobe tumours. The zonal mapping system also demonstrated better outcomes with patients of single zone N1 disease compared to multiple zone N1 disease and, similarly, single zone N2 disease confers a better 5-year survival than multiple zone N2 disease. The outcome of this proposal is the definition of three distinct groups of patients with progressively worse outcomes: namely, single zone N1 disease, multiple-zone N1 or single-zone N2 disease and multiple-zone N2 disease. These changes have not been incorporated into the 7th edition.

M Descriptors

M disease is now divided into M1a, indicating additional tumour nodules in the contralateral lung, previously staged as M1. M1a disease now also includes patients with pleural or pericardial dissemination, previously described as T4 disease. M1b disease (previously M1) indicates the presence of distant metastases. These staging changes are related to more comprehensive examination of survival patterns, a direct result of the large database from which the 7th edition has been derived.

Small Cell Lung Cancer

Small cell lung cancer (SCLC) presents a different phenotype to non-small cell lung cancer. It is relatively common (up to 20% of all lung cancers). The disease is characterised by rapid growth rate, early metastatic spread and an association with smoking. Characteristically these tumours are initially responsive to radiation and chemotherapeutic treatment but are also associated with early recurrence. In the 7th edition of the lung cancer TMN staging, SLCLC has been divided simply into limited disease and extensive disease groups. Limited disease indicates disease confined to one hemithorax but includes contralateral mediastinal and supraclavicular nodes and malignant pleural effusions. Patients with disease beyond these parameters are described as having extensive disease. Patients with limited disease typically receive chemotherapy and possibly radiotherapy. Patients with extensive disease will have chemotherapy alone.

Bronchopulmonary Carcinoid Tumour

Bronchopulmonary carcinoid tumours are now classified under the 7th edition TMN staging. Carcinoid tumours are potentially malignant neuroendocrine tumours. The spectrum of disease ranges from low-grade typical carcinoids, through atypical carcinoids to higher-grade large cell and small cell carcinomas. The distinction between these neuroendocrine tumours is based on pathological analysis. The field is also slightly complicated by the relatively small numbers available for analysis and the phenomenon of a preinvasive lesion of diffuse idiopathic pulmonary neuroendocrine-cell hyperplasia (DIPNECH), to be distinguished from genuine metastatic disease.[48,64] The presence of multiple small nodules of less than 5 mm in size in association with mosaic attenuation pattern within the lungs in the setting of a known carcinoid tumour should now raise the possibility of DIPNECH.[65]

Bronchial carcinoids are uncommon, constituting less than 5% of pulmonary tumours. The peak age at diagnosis is in the fifth decade, but the age range is wide and includes children. Two forms of bronchial carcinoid are described: typical (85–90%) and atypical (10–15%). Typical carcinoids most commonly arise in central airways. Atypical carcinoids usually arise in the lung periphery. Bronchial carcinoids can invade locally and may metastasise to hilar and mediastinal lymph nodes as well as to the brain, liver and bone. The atypical carcinoids have histological and clinical features intermediate between typical bronchial carcinoid and small cell carcinoma of the lung and have a poorer prognosis.

Bronchial carcinoid may present with wheeze, pneumonia, or haemoptysis. Even when small, tumours may

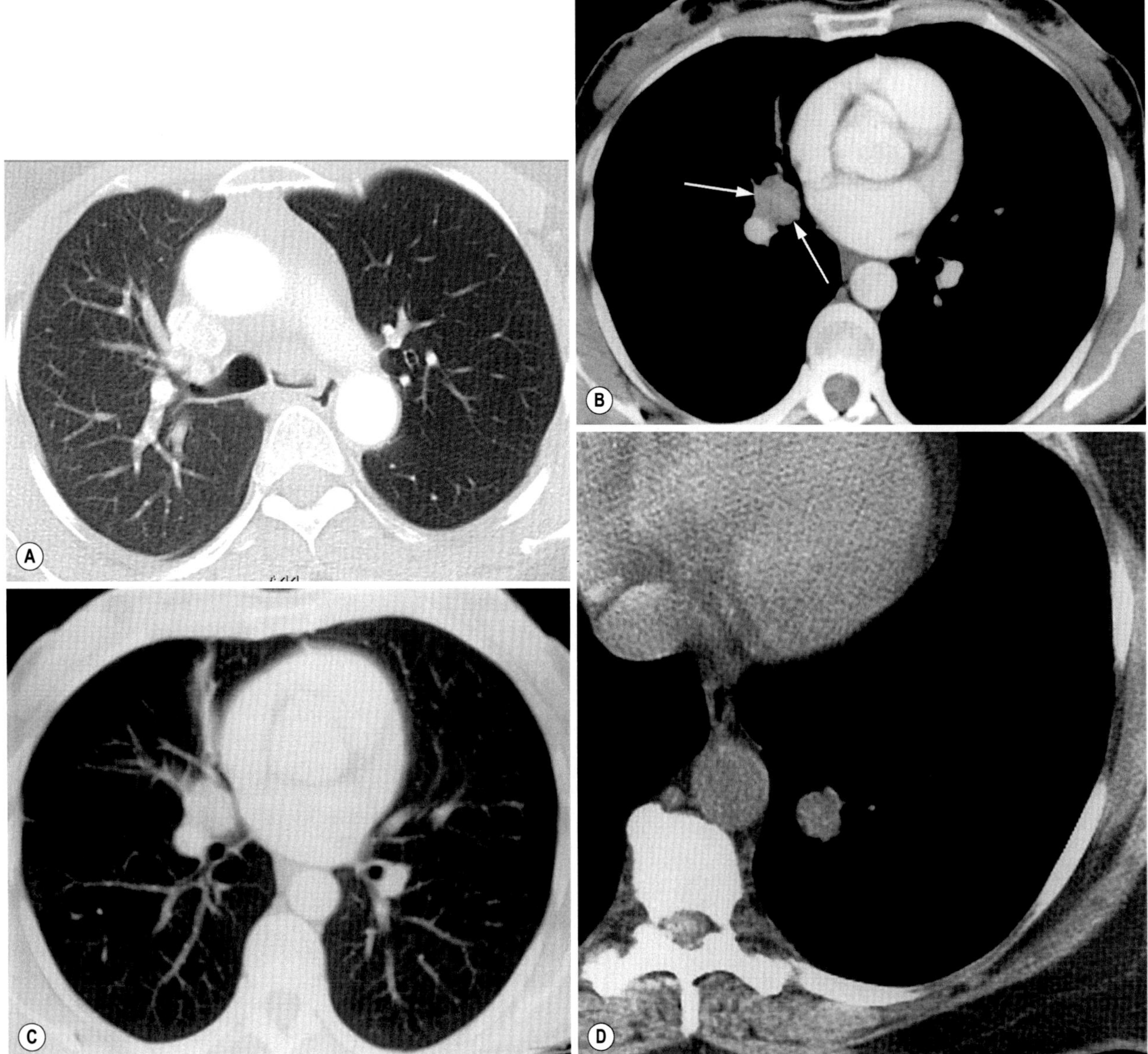

FIGURE 8-9 ■ **Carcinoid tumour.** (A) A tumour is partially occluding the left main bronchus. (B) A well-defined perihilar carcinoid tumour (arrows) is demonstrated anterior to the artery to the right lower lobe. (C) On lung windows there is only a small band of atelectasis in the middle lobe. (D) A small peripheral carcinoid tumour indistinguishable from a number of other causes of a solitary pulmonary nodule.

secrete adrenocorticotrophic hormone (ACTH) in sufficient quantities to cause Cushing's syndrome. Carcinoid syndrome is very rare if the tumour is still confined to the lung.

Radiographic appearances vary with location of the tumour. There is no lobar predilection and on rare occasions carcinoids may arise in the trachea. Bronchial carcinoids, particularly those located centrally, may calcify and occasionally ossify. Calcification is seen on CT in up to one-third of cases, but is only occasionally visible on chest radiography.[66] Marked contrast enhancement may be seen on CT.

Carcinoids arising in central bronchi (80–90% of cases) often show a larger mass external to the bronchus than within the lumen ('iceberg' lesions), and the extrabronchial component may be visible as a hilar mass (Fig. 8-9). Central lesions usually produce partial or complete bronchial obstruction, resulting in atelectasis with or without pneumonia. Central bronchial obstruction may be complicated by development of distal bronchiectasis or lung abscess. Occasionally, a bronchial carcinoid in a segmental or subsegmental bronchus may obstruct bronchial secretions, thereby causing a mucocele.

Peripheral lesions (10–20% of carcinoids) present as solitary spherical or lobular nodules, 2–4 cm in diameter, with a well-defined smooth edge (Fig. 8-9). Noncalcified peripheral bronchial carcinoid tumours closely resemble bronchial carcinomas, both radiologically and cytologically, and are therefore frequently removed surgically in the belief that they are carcinomas.

Summary

The use of the TMN staging system in NSCLC, SCLC and bronchopulmonary carcinoid informs the stage grouping system that guides treatment choices (see Table 8-3). Since the adoption of the 7th edition TMN descriptors, the group staging has become more complex, with T2b N0 M0 cases moving from a Ib to a IIa status, T2a N1 M0 cases moving from a IIb to a IIa status and T4 N0 or N1 M0 cases moving from a IIIb to a IIIa status. These stage groupings are of relatively little importance for the thoracic radiologist in day-to-day practice but will have a significant effect in some patients in determining treatment options and trial eligibility. Perhaps the most important change to underline is the presence of additional tumour nodules in the same lobe as the primary tumour. This no longer confers T4 status and therefore these patients become surgical candidates. Patients with tumour nodules in a different lobe of the same lung may also be reclassified from stage IIIb to stage IIIa. Since it is widely excepted that patients with stage IIIa disease and below may be surgical candidates and the patients with stage IIIb disease and above non-surgical candidates, these stage group changes may open surgical options up to a significant number of patients.

IMAGING PROTOCOLS FOR LUNG CANCER STAGING

Clinical features vary with cell type and extent of disease. Approximately 25% of patients are asymptomatic at the time of diagnosis, following the discovery of an abnormality on chest radiograph or computed tomography. Pneumonia is the other common presentation. Cough, wheeze, haemoptysis, symptoms of pneumonia and paraneoplastic syndromes, such as the inappropriate secretion of antidiuretic hormone or a peripheral neuropathy, are the cardinal symptoms at a stage when lobectomy or pneumonectomy may be curative. Hoarseness, chest pain, brachial plexus neuropathy and Horner's syndrome (Pancoast's tumour), superior vena caval obstruction, dysphagia and the problems of pericardial tamponade indicate invasion of the mediastinum or chest wall and a poorer prognosis.

The chest radiograph will remain the initial investigation in all patients suspected of lung cancer. As the lung cancer screening studies have shown, the ability of a chest radiograph to detect all lung cancers is distinctly limited. Therefore the mainstay of staging investigation for a patient with suspected lung cancer (in distinction to patients undergoing lung cancer screening) is contrast-enhanced CT supplemented by PET/CT and MR when required. In certain circumstances ultrasound assessment of peripheral tumours and supraclavicular lymph nodes adds further useful information.

The Current Standards of CT Technology

The current standard of CT technology is a multi-slice (usually 64 detector row) CT system, able to acquire sub-millimetre collimation images through the thorax in a short breath-hold. The decision to include abdominal, pelvic and intracranial assessment varies from centre to centre. However, a comprehensive brain, chest, abdomen and pelvis acquisition can be undertaken in very short order and the main rate-limiting steps are now patient identification, preparation and documentation rather than the acquisition of the data sets. Most institutions will routinely use intravenous contrast, although this is not mandatory. Not infrequently, difficulty with venous access, asthma, allergy or previous contrast reaction and impaired renal function will prevent contrast administration. A standard thoracic CT will be undertaken with the patient in supine position and the arms elevated. Imaging planning and dose reduction optimisation require an AP, and sometimes a lateral scout projection. If contrast medium is administered, then image acquisition is timed to optimise opacification of central pulmonary vasculature (usually 20–30 s). If an abdominal and pelvic study is also undertaken, this component is best acquired during the portal venous phase of contrast enhancement (65 s). This will require two short breath-holds and two preplanned acquisition ranges with some overlap at the lung bases.

The ability to produce isotropic voxels allows multiplanar reformatting to be undertaken as a routine, either by the radiographic staff or at the time of reporting by the radiologist.

The PET/CT technique is similar for the CT acquisition of the study, usually obtained from skull base to upper thigh. If the patient is also undergoing a conventional CT, the CT acquisition for PET co-registration can be of a low-dose non-contrast variety. Since the PET component of the acquisition takes considerably longer than the CT acquisition, in this situation the non-contrast low-dose CT will usually be undertaken during gentle respiration, to allow optimum co-registration with the PET data. Usually the PET acquisition takes between 5 and 7 bed couch positions, with each position taking up to 5 min, and therefore the whole study may take up to 35 min to acquire. More modern systems achieve the entire study in considerably less time.

MRI of the thorax is usually undertaken to answer a particular question as a problem-solving tool. In the context of lung cancer staging, the MR study is often to assess superior sulcus tumours, chest wall or thoracic invasion or to assess the integrity of the diaphragm. Usually triplanar examinations are untaken with respiratory gating and T1 and T2 weighting. A variety of more refined techniques, including dynamic contrast-enhanced MR sequences for evaluation of lung nodules, have been described. Furthermore, dynamic ultra-fast acquisitions can be utilised to assess fixation of a peripheral tumour to chest wall or mediastinal structures.

IMAGING FEATURES OF BRONCHOGENIC CARCINOMA

The thoracic imaging features of bronchial carcinoma are discussed under three headings: peripheral tumours; central tumours (arising in a large bronchus at or close

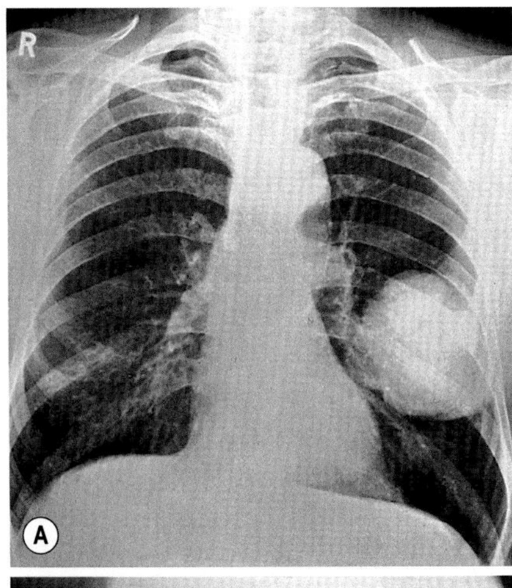

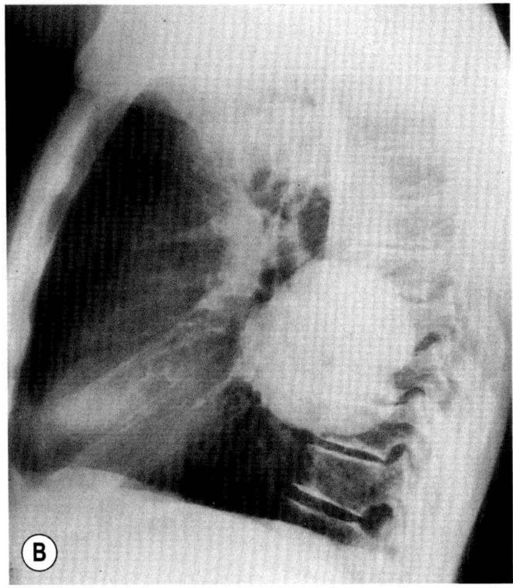

FIGURE 8-10 ■ (A, B) Bronchial carcinoma in the left lower lobe showing typical rounded, slightly lobular configuration. The mass shows a notch posteriorly.

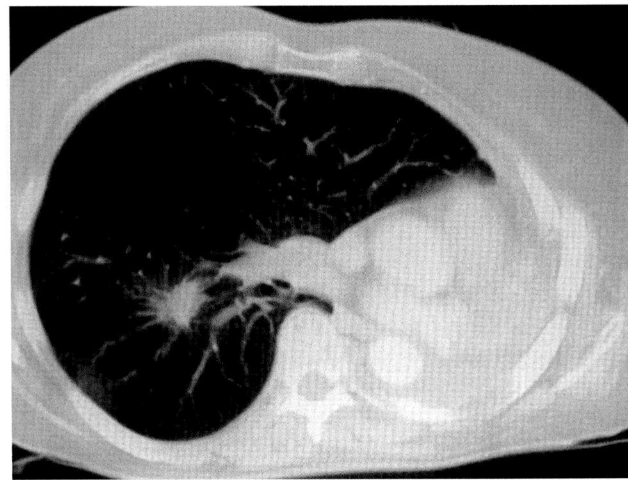

FIGURE 8-11 ■ CT demonstrating a second primary bronchogenic carcinoma in the right lung. The patient had undergone a previous left pneumonectomy 7 years earlier. The new tumour has spiculated edges, infiltrating into the adjacent lung (corona radiata).

to the hilum); and staging intrathoracic spread of bronchial carcinoma.

Peripheral Tumours

Approximately 40% of bronchial carcinomas arise beyond the segmental bronchi, and in 30% a peripheral mass is the sole radiographic finding[67] (Fig. 8-10).

Tumour Shape and Margins

Tumours at the lung apex (Pancoast's tumours, superior sulcus tumours) may resemble apical pleural thickening; however, the majority of peripheral lung cancers are approximately spherical or oval in shape. Lobulation, a sign that indicates uneven growth rates in different parts of the tumour, is common. Occasionally, a dumb-bell shape is encountered or two nodules are seen next to one another.

The term 'corona radiata' is used to describe numerous fine strands radiating into the lung from a central mass, sometimes with transradiant lung parenchyma between these strands. While not specific, this sign is highly suggestive of bronchial carcinoma (Fig. 8-11). Absolutely spherical, sharply defined, smooth-edged nodules due to carcinoma of the lung are rare. A peripheral line shadow or 'tail' may be seen between a peripherally located mass lesion and the pleura, a phenomenon that occurs in both benign and malignant lesions. When associated with carcinoma of the lung, the 'tail' probably represents either plate-like atelectasis secondary to bronchial obstruction beyond the mass or septal oedema due to lymphatic obstruction.

Although the edges of a tumour are frequently well defined, some peripheral cancers, notably some types of adenocarcinoma, have ill-defined edges similar to pneumonia (Fig. 8-12).

Cavitation

Cavitation may be identified in tumours of any size (Fig. 8-13) and is best demonstrated by CT (Fig. 8-14). Squamous cell carcinoma is the most likely cell type to show cavitation. The walls of the cavity are of irregular thickness and may contain tumour nodules, but sometimes the wall has smooth inner and outer margins. The cavity wall is usually 8-mm thick or greater. Fluid levels are common.

Calcification

Calcification within bronchogenic carcinomas is rarely seen on chest radiography but is identified on CT in 6–10% of cases. Some foci of calcification represent pre-existing calcified granulomatous disease engulfed by tumour (Fig. 8-15). However, amorphous or cloud-like calcification consistent with dystrophic tumour calcification is still seen in a small proportion of cases (<10%) (Fig. 8-16).[68,69] Most calcified tumours are large, with a diameter of 5 cm or more, but calcification can also be seen in small peripheral tumours.

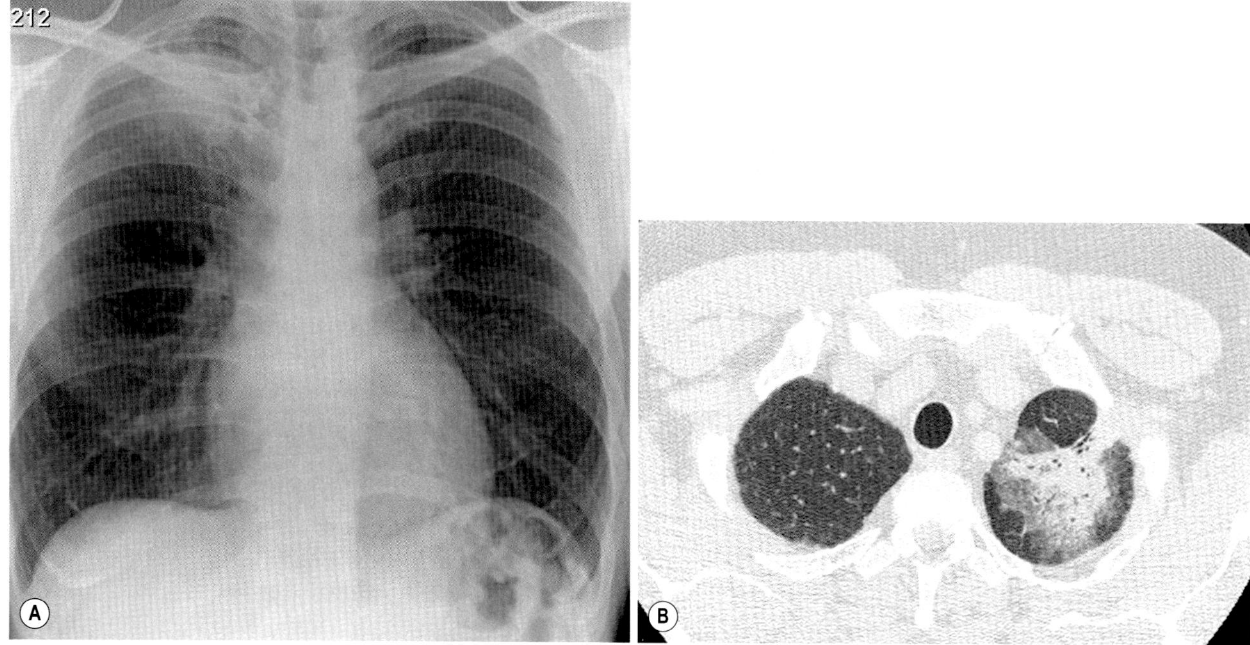

FIGURE 8-12 ■ Lung cancer mimicking pneumonia. (A) Squamous cell carcinoma resembling pneumonia. The entire opacity seen in the right upper zone on this radiograph is due to the carcinoma itself. (B) Apical adenocarcinoma of the left upper lobe of a different patient with ground-glass attenuation margins and an air bronchogram.

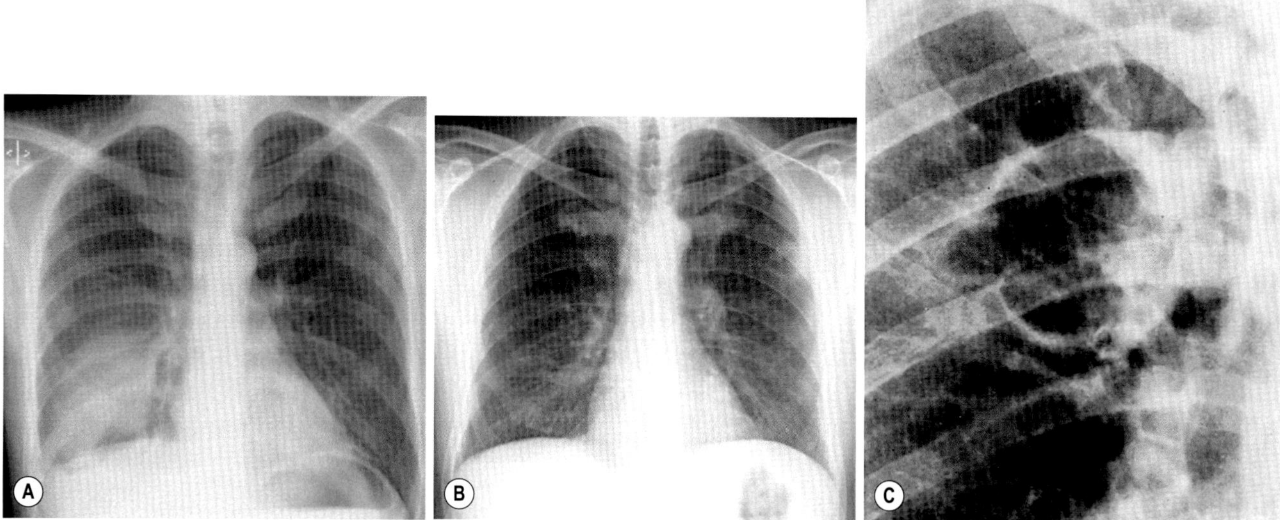

FIGURE 8-13 ■ Examples of neoplastic cavitation on chest radiography. (A) The cavity is eccentric (large cell undifferentiated carcinoma). (B) The inner wall of the cavity is irregular (squamous cell carcinoma). (C) The cavity wall is very thin (squamous cell carcinoma).

Other Findings

Air bronchograms and bubble-like lucencies or pseudocavitation may be seen within lung cancers, in particular with adenocarcinoma.[36] Occasionally, dilated mucus-filled bronchi (bronchocele, mucocele, mucoid impaction) are seen distal to a carcinoma obstructing a segmental or subsegmental bronchus. Ground-glass attenuation may be seen as a component of nodules and is associated with a greater risk of malignancy than that of purely solid nodules. It is more commonly associated with adenocarcinoma,[70] which may present as a purely ground-glass opacity.

Central Tumours

The cardinal imaging signs of a central tumour are collapse/consolidation of the lung beyond the tumour and the presence of hilar enlargement, signs that may be seen in isolation or in conjunction with one another.

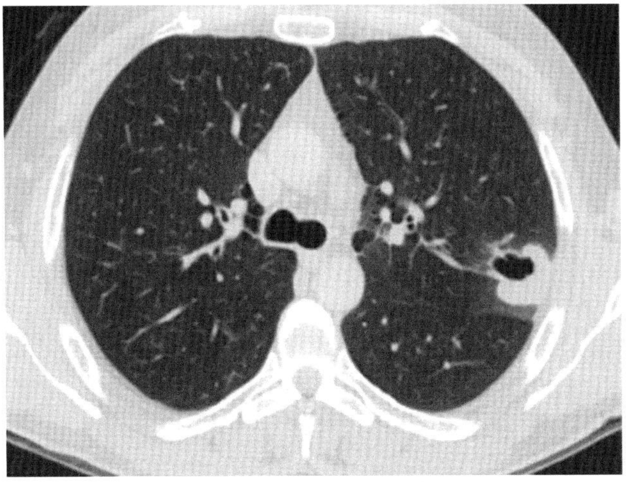

FIGURE 8-14 ■ CT showing a cavitating squamous cell carcinoma in the left lung. The wall of the cavity is variable in thickness.

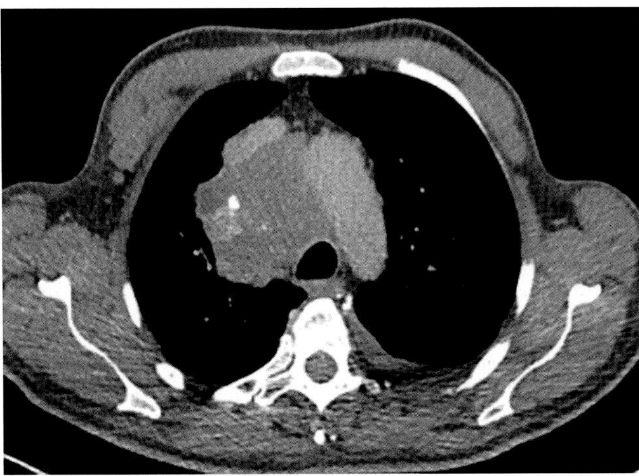

FIGURE 8-16 ■ Tumour calcification. Large bronchial carcinoma invading the mediastinum demonstrates coarse and cloud-like calcification.

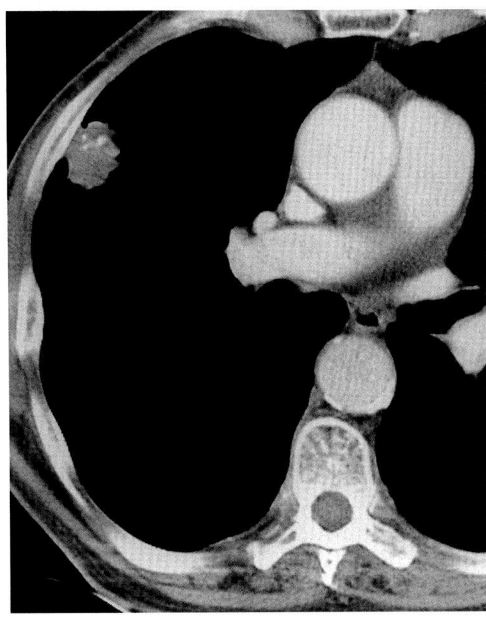

FIGURE 8-15 ■ Calcified infectious granuloma engulfed by lung cancer. CT shows a cluster of densely calcified small nodules almost at the centre of a small carcinoma.

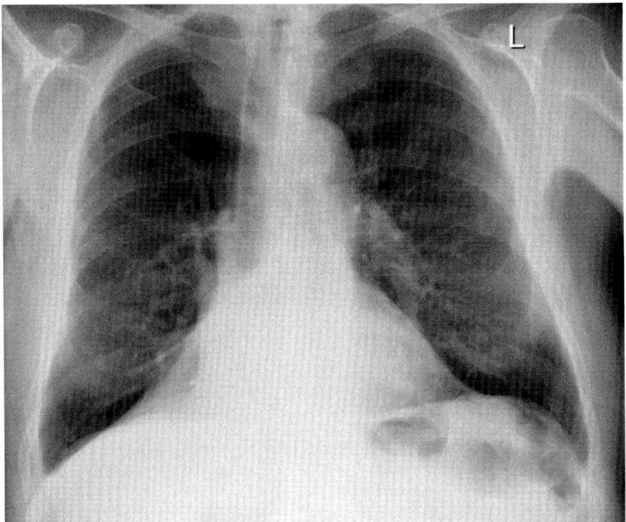

FIGURE 8-17 ■ Lobar collapse. The tumour in the bronchus intermedius is causing partial middle and lower lobe collapse.

Collapse/Consolidation in Association with Central Tumours

Obstruction of a major bronchus often leads to a combination of atelectasis and retention of secretions with consequent pulmonary opacity, but collateral air drift may partially or completely prevent these postobstructive changes. Secondary infection may occur beyond the obstruction.

The following features suggest that pneumonia is secondary to an obstructing neoplasm:

1. The shape of the collapsed or consolidated lobe may be altered because of the bulk of the underlying tumour. In cases with lobar collapse due to a central tumour mass, the fissure in the region of the mass is unable to move in the usual manner and, therefore, the fissure may show a bulge (the Golden S sign if involving the right upper lobe).[71] The description now seems to have become extended to include the CT equivalent appearance of a hilar mass and collapsed distal lobe and also to describe the phenomenon in other lobes (Fig. 8-17).
2. The presence of pneumonia in an at-risk patient, confined to one lobe (or more lobes if there is a common bronchus) that persists unchanged for longer than 2–3 weeks, or a pneumonia that recurs in the same lobe, particularly if the lobe shows loss of volume and no air bronchograms. Simple pneumonia often clears or spreads to other segments within a few weeks. In practice, complete resolution of pneumonia virtually excludes an obstructing neoplasm as a cause of infection. Although consolidation may improve partially on appropriate antibiotic therapy, it almost never resolves completely if secondary to an underlying carcinoma. Occasionally, the opacified lobe may

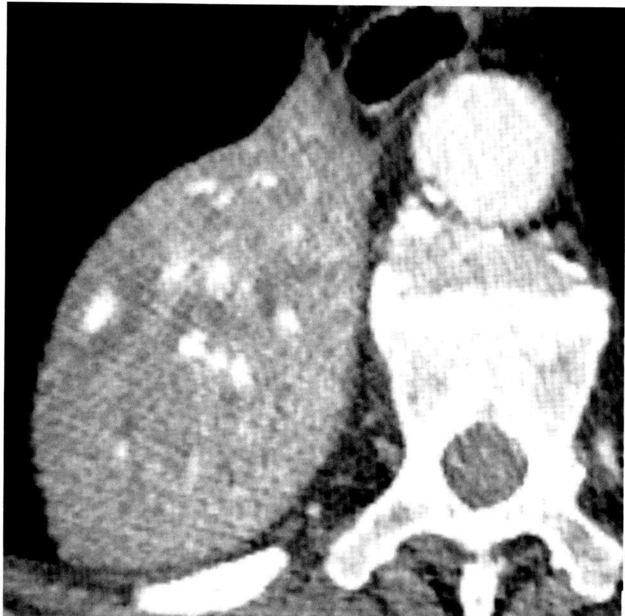

FIGURE 8-18 ■ Fluid-filled dilated bronchi beyond a central obstructing carcinoma are visible in this collapsed and consolidated right lower lobe.

appear larger than normal because of the build-up of infected secretions beyond the obstructing carcinoma, an appearance that has been labelled the 'drowned lobe'.

3. A visible mass with irregular stenosis of a mainstem or lobar bronchus. Careful analysis of CT images may demonstrate the presence of an obstructing tumour when there is obstructive atelectasis.[42]
4. Simple pneumonia rarely causes radiographically visible hilar adenopathy, though enlarged central nodes may be seen on CT or MRI. Lung abscess can occasionally be confused with bronchial carcinoma because it may result in hilar or mediastinal adenopathy.[72]
5. Mucus-filled dilated bronchi may be visible within collapsed lobes on a CT examination as branching, tubular low-density structures, and when seen should prompt a search for a centrally obstructing tumour (Fig. 8-18).

Staging Intrathoracic Spread of Bronchial Carcinoma

Hilar Enlargement

Hilar enlargement is a common presenting feature in patients with bronchial carcinoma. It may reflect a proximal tumour, lymphadenopathy, consolidated lung, or a combination of these phenomena.

A mass superimposed on the hilum may lead to increased density of the hilum, owing to summation of the opacity of the mass and that of the normal hilar shadows (Fig. 8-19). This sign may be the only indication of lung cancer on a frontal chest radiograph; when suspected, it is essential to inspect the lateral radiograph with care.

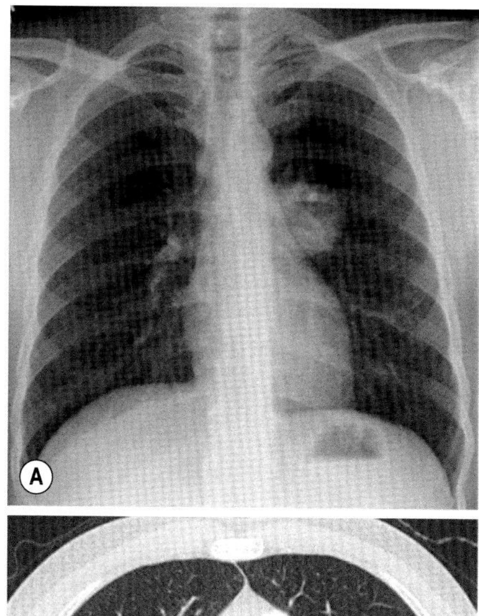

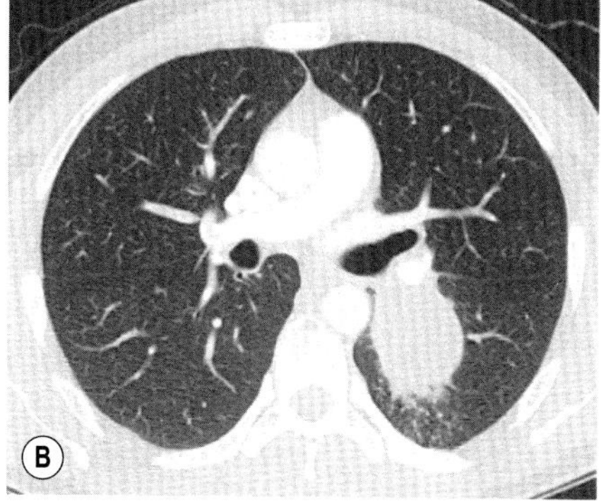

FIGURE 8-19 ■ Dense hilum. (A) The left hilum is dense, owing to a mass superimposed directly over it. (B) Corresponding axial CT image demonstrates the mass lying behind the left hilum. The mass proved to be a squamous cell carcinoma.

Mediastinal Invasion

Plain radiograph evidence of mediastinal invasion relies on demonstrating phrenic nerve paralysis. Caution is needed, however, before deciding that a high hemidiaphragm is caused by phrenic nerve invasion, because lobar collapse can also lead to elevation of a hemidiaphragm, a subpulmonary effusion may mimic it, and diaphragmatic eventration is common.

The major CT and MRI signs of mediastinal invasion include the demonstration of visible tumour deep within the mediastinal fat, particularly if tumour surrounds the mediastinal vessels, oesophagus, or proximal mainstem bronchi (Fig. 8-20). Associated pneumonia or atelectasis may make it very difficult to determine whether or not mediastinal contact is present. Even clear-cut contact with the mediastinum is not enough for the diagnosis of invasion, and the apparent interdigitation of tumour with mediastinal fat can be a misleading sign on both CT and MRI. Glazer et al. showed that the presence of (A) less than 3 cm of contact with the mediastinum, (B) less than 90° of circumferential contact with the aorta, or (C) a visible mediastinal fat plane between the mass and any vital mediastinal structures indicated a very high likelihood of technical resectability, even if the tumour had crossed into the mediastinum, and that most tumours in their series conforming to this description had no mediastinal invasion at surgery.[73] When the question is turned round to enquire as to the criteria for unresectability, however, the answer is less certain.[74] Tumours that obliterate fat planes or show greater contact than that described above are not necessarily unresectable, though the greater the degree of invasion and the extent of contact, the more likely it is that there is significant mediastinal involvement.[75]

MRI does not appear to offer any advantages over CT for the routine diagnosis of mediastinal invasion, its role being limited to problem solving in specific cases. Before the advent of multidetector CT (MDCT), the multiplanar capabilities of MRI could be used to advantage to identify involvement of major mediastinal blood vessels (Fig. 8-21) and the tracheal carina. MDCT has largely obviated the need to proceed to MRI to take advantage of multiplanar imaging alone; however, MRI sequences optimised for evaluation of the heart and vessels may still offer advantages where there is concern about invasion of hilar or mediastinal vessels, the heart or pericardium.

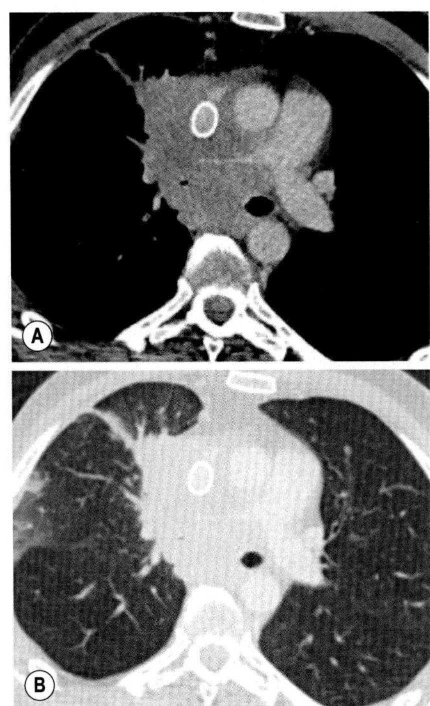

FIGURE 8-20 ■ **Mediastinal invasion.** CT image (A) displayed on mediastinal windows and (B) displayed on lung windows of deep mediastinal invasion by non-small cell lung cancer. The tumour is obstructing the right main bronchus and compressing the right main pulmonary artery; it is also encasing the stented superior vena cava and the aorta. Some postobstructive atelectasis is noted on lung window.

Chest Wall Invasion

The presence of chest wall invasion alone does not preclude surgical resection, though it does adversely affect prognosis.[76] The necessarily more extensive surgery is associated with increased morbidity and mortality and it therefore helps the surgeon to know the extent of any chest wall invasion preoperatively.

The diagnosis of chest wall involvement adjacent to a tumour is unreliable on CT, unless there is clear-cut bone destruction or a large soft-tissue mass (Fig. 8-22). Local chest wall pain remains the single most specific indicator of whether or not the tumour has spread to the parietal pleura or chest wall.[77] Contact with the pleura on CT examination, even if the pleura is thickened, does not necessarily indicate invasion, though the greater the degree of contact and the greater the pleural thickening, the more likely it is that the parietal pleura has been invaded, particularly if the extrapleural fat plane is obliterated. A definite extrapleural mass that is not explicable by previous chest trauma is likely to be the result of invasion by tumour, but even this sign may be misleading

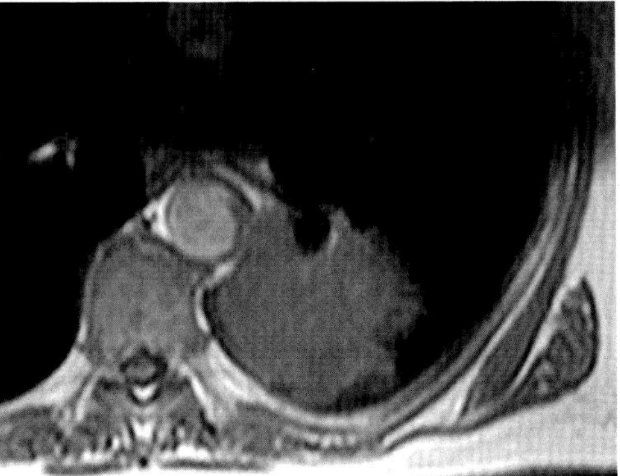

FIGURE 8-21 ■ **MRI of a left lower lobe tumour that has directly invaded the aortic wall, which has altered signal adjacent to the tumour.**

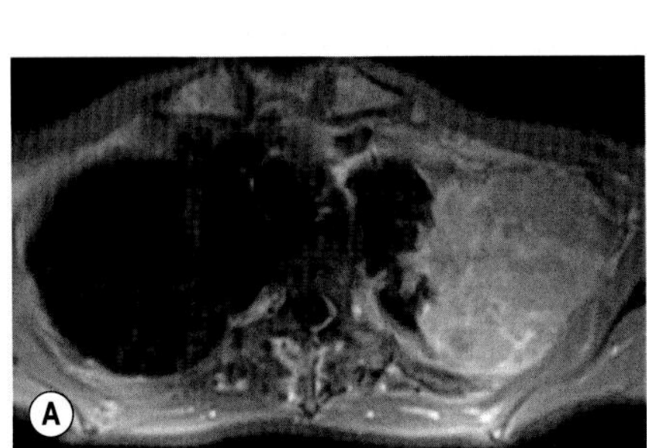

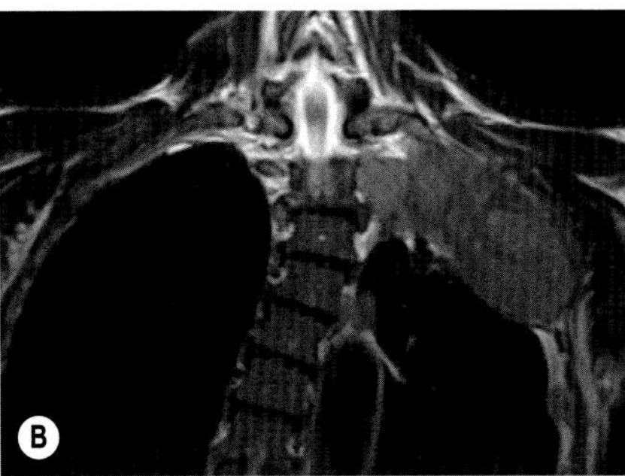

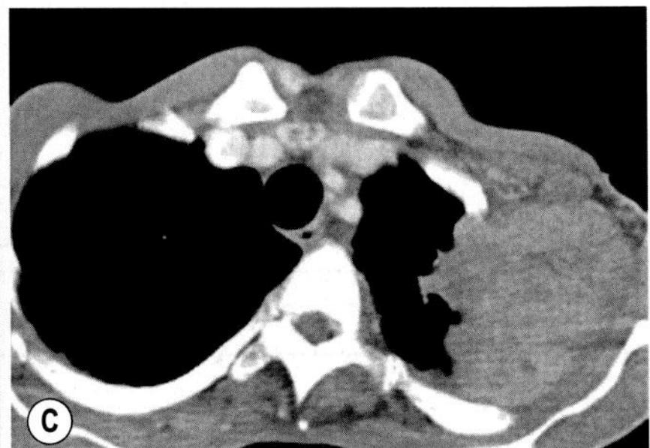

FIGURE 8-22 ■ **Chest wall invasion by a Pancoast's tumour.** Involvement of the soft tissues of the chest wall and the left second rib is appreciated on the (A) axial T1-, (B) coronal T2-weighted MRI and (C) CT images.

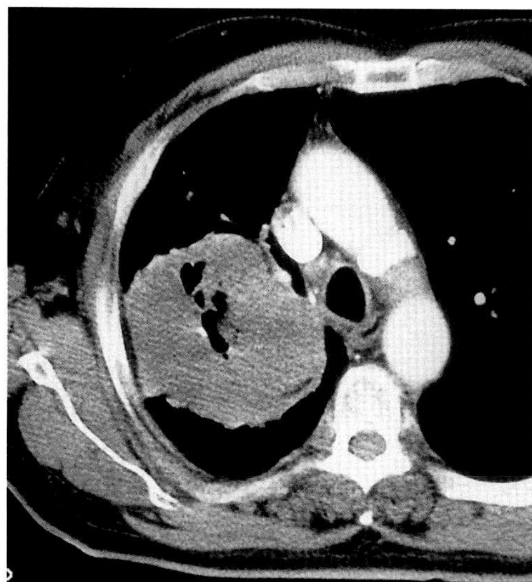

FIGURE 8-23 **Cavitating bronchogenic carcinoma.** There is preservation of the extrapleural fat plane at the point of contact with the chest wall. Although the pleura may be involved, the chest wall is likely to be otherwise spared.

since soft-tissue swelling may be due to inflammation and fibrosis rather than neoplasm.[78] Conversely, a clear extrapleural fat plane adjacent to the mass may be helpful, but again not definitive, in excluding chest wall invasion[79] (Fig. 8-23).

Previously, in selected cases, MRI proved to be better than CT in demonstrating chest wall and diaphragmatic invasion. MRI was regarded as the optimal technique for demonstrating the extent of superior sulcus tumours (Pancoast's tumour) (Fig. 8-22), reliably diagnosing mediastinal invasion, extension into the root of the neck and involvement of vascular and neural structures. With the ability of CT to provided routine multiplanar reformatted images, routine MRI assessment is not usually required.[80]

Transthoracic ultrasound can identify chest wall invasion with a high degree of accuracy; however, in many centres the technique is rarely used.[81]

^{99m}Tc radionuclide skeletal scintigraphy is a sensitive technique with which to assess bone invasion and it may be positive when the plain radiograph still shows no bony abnormality. However, as discussed above, PET/CT is now the examination of choice for detection of distant spread (outside the CNS) and has been shown to provide assessment of skeletal as well as soft-tissue spread.

Generally, chest radiography is insensitive for nodal staging. However, the presence of enlarged hilar or paratracheal nodes has been shown to be specific (92%) for N2–N3 disease.[82]

Lymph node assessment on CT and MRI is limited to size, shape and location, with size being the major criterion used to predict metastatic involvement (Fig. 8-24).

Normal mediastinal lymph node size on CT or MRI varies according to the location of the nodes within the mediastinum, but a simple and reasonably accurate rule is that nodes with a short-axis diameter of less than 10 mm fall within the 95th percentile and nodes above this size should, therefore, be considered enlarged.

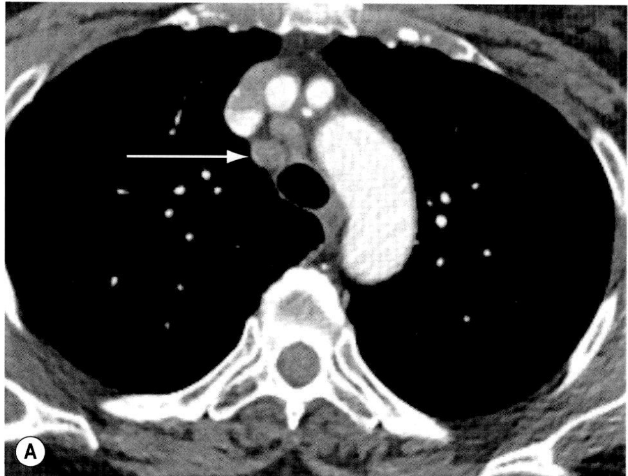

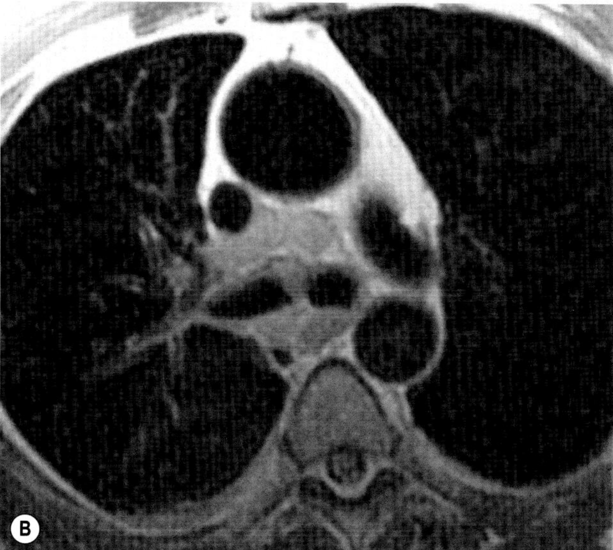

FIGURE 8-24 (A) True-positive CT for metastatic lymphadenopathy. There are several enlarged nodes in the right paratracheal area. The largest measured 14 mm in its short-axis diameter (arrow). The primary tumour was a bronchial carcinoma in the right lung. (B) MRI of involved mediastinal nodes in a patient with a right lower lobe non-small cell lung cancer.

The problem with using size as the only criterion for malignant involvement is that intrathoracic lymph node enlargement has many non-malignant causes, including previous tuberculosis, histoplasmosis, pneumoconiosis, sarcoidosis and, most importantly, reactive hyperplasia to the tumour (Fig. 8-25) or associated pneumonia/atelectasis: it has repeatedly been shown that one-half to two-thirds of enlarged nodes draining postobstructive pneumonia/atelectasis are free of tumour. Conversely, microscopic involvement by tumour can be present in normal-sized nodes. It will, therefore, be clear that there is no measurement above which all nodes can be assumed to be malignant and below which all can be considered to be benign. The sensitivity and specificity of CT for diagnosing metastatic involvement of mediastinal lymph nodes vary greatly in different published series, reflecting different size criteria and the methods used to confirm or exclude lymph node metastases. A reasonable

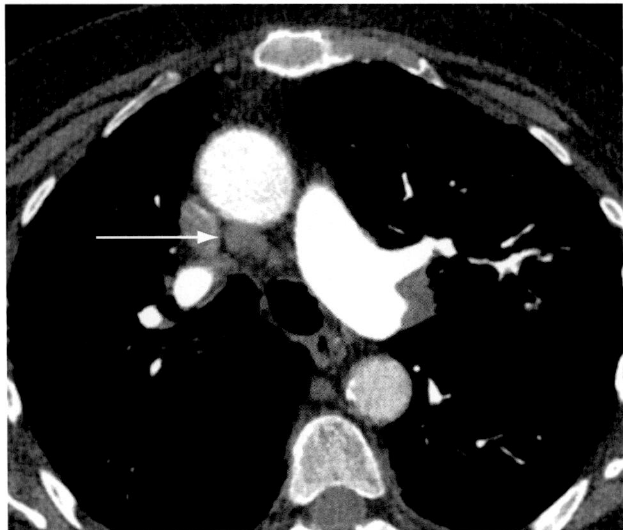

FIGURE 8-25 ■ False-positive CT for metastatic mediastinal lymphadenopathy. The largest of the right paratracheal nodes (arrow) is 15 mm in its short-axis diameter. This node proved to be free of malignant tumour at thoracotomy. The enlargement was due to reactive hyperplasia. The primary tumour was in the right lower lobe.

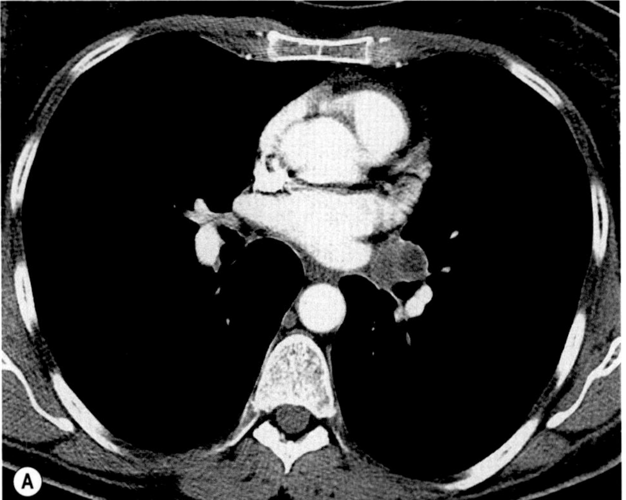

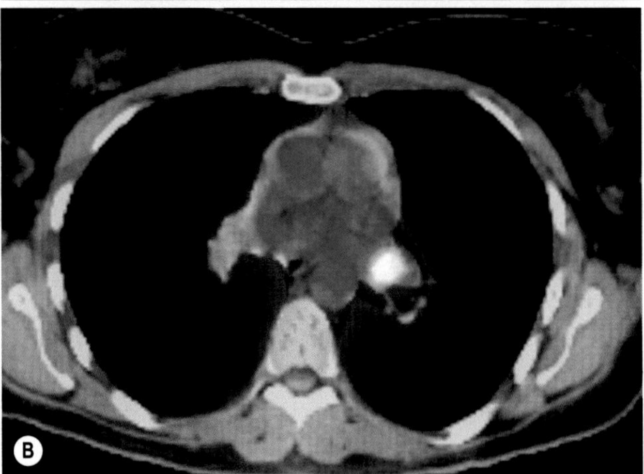

FIGURE 8-26 ■ Recurrent malignant left hilar lymph nodes from a small peripheral non-small cell lung cancer. (A) CT demonstrates nodes at the left hilum. (B) The PET/CT image confirms high FDG uptake in keeping with malignant involvement.

generalisation in the USA (where fungal infection is endemic) is that both sensitivity and specificity are in the 50 to low 60% range when the cut-off point for normal is a short-axis diameter of 1 cm.[82–84] Better specificity figures have been obtained in Europe[85] and Japan,[86] probably because the prevalence of coincidental histoplasmosis is much lower than in the USA. The positive predictive value for nodal metastatic disease may be improved (to up to 95%) by ensuring that nodes draining the tumour are larger than nodes elsewhere in the mediastinum.[85]

The accuracy of MRI, despite its improved contrast resolution, is limited by the same constraint as for CT of overlap of features of benign and malignant causes of node enlargement. Although it is generally considered that the MRI signal within nodes is not a useful predictor of involvement, it has been reported that STIR imaging produces sufficient signal difference between normal and pathological nodal tissue to detect metastases with 93% sensitivity and 87% specificity.[87] The previously cited advantage of MRI over CT in nodal detection because of its ability to distinguish small nodes from vessels without intravenous enhancement has been effectively negated by the advantages of MDCT.[88]

Endoscopic ultrasound (EUS) can be used to assess the size and morphology of, and to guide fine needle aspiration (FNA) of, aortopulmonary, subcarinal and posterior mediastinal nodes, achieving greater sensitivity and specificities for nodal involvement than CT and PET in some series.[89] Ultrasound assessment (± FNA) of supraclavicular lymph nodes improves sensitivity for detection of supraclavicular lymph node involvement; its routine use has been suggested as a method to improve the accuracy of preoperative staging.[90]

PET imaging with fluorodeoxyglucose (FDG) is increasingly used for staging lung carcinoma, with published studies consistently demonstrating greater accuracy compared to CT and MRI in the detection of nodal disease (Fig. 8-26). False-positive results still occur, most commonly due to inflammation and reactive hyperplasia. Fused PET/CT imaging provides registration of FDG metabolic activity with the anatomical detail of CT (Fig. 8-26).[52,74,88,91] Decision analysis studies have shown that PET can be incorporated into the work-up of lung cancer in a cost-effective manner, with savings derived from identifying inoperable patients before thoracotomy.[92]

Mediastinoscopy and mediastinotomy remain the most widely employed techniques for mediastinal lymph node sampling. They have high sensitivity and specificity for detecting malignant disease and, although invasive, are indicated prior to thoracotomy when other forms of imaging suggest nodal involvement.

Current practice has struck a balance between PET/CT and tissue sampling for the assessment of mediastinal nodes. In essence,

- When the CT assessment and PET assessment are negative, the patient is offered resection without preoperative nodal sampling.

- When the CT is negative but the PET is positive, the mediastinal nodes will require sampling by endobronchial US (EBUS) or mediastinoscopy to assess resectability or guide presurgical therapy with a view to downstaging and reassessement.
- When CT and PET are positive, tissue confirmation is required, assuming there are no distant metastatic sites.

Pleural Involvement

Pleural involvement may occur as a result of direct spread, lymphatic involvement, or tumour emboli. On occasion, adenocarcinoma takes the form of a sheet of lobular pleural thickening indistinguishable from malignant mesothelioma.

A pleural effusion in association with a primary lung cancer designates the tumour as being M1a. The exception is the few patients who have clinical evidence of another cause for the effusion (e.g. heart failure) and in whom cytology examinations of multiple pleural fluid samples are negative for tumour cells, in which case the effusion can be disregarded as a staging criterion. Attempts to characterise the nature of the pleural fluid based on density measurements at CT or signal intensities at MRI have not so far proven useful. Several studies suggest PET may have a role in the evaluation of pleural effusion in patients with lung cancer.[93]

Summary

Staging the intrathoracic extent of lung cancer is a multidisciplinary process utilising imaging, bronchoscopy and biopsy. Chest radiography, CT and PET (where available) are currently the routine imaging procedures for assessing intrathoracic spread and determining resectability, with MRI and ultrasound reserved for specific indications.

The essential points to establish when staging the intrathoracic extent of non-small cell cancers are: (A) whether the tumour has spread to hilar or mediastinal nodes; (B) if it has, which nodal groups are involved; (C) whether the tumour has invaded the chest wall or mediastinum; and (D) if it has, whether it is still potentially curable surgically.

If chest radiography and CT ± PET show no evidence of spread beyond the lung (other than to ipsilateral hilar nodes) in a patient who is suitable for surgery, and in whom bronchoscopy shows the tumour to be resectable, then that patient should be offered surgical resection without further preoperative invasive procedures. Spread to ipsilateral nodes, whilst not necessarily precluding surgical resection, has a significantly adverse effect on prognosis and even if surgery is undertaken, it is performed with the understanding that 5-year survival rates are poor.

The poor specificity of CT in determining nodal involvement must be appreciated. Nodal enlargement, whilst probably due to metastatic carcinoma, may also be due to coincidental benign disease, reactive hyperplasia to the presence of the tumour, or to any associated obstructive consolidation/atelectasis. Thus, biopsy confirmation of neoplastic nodal involvement by mediastinoscopy, mediastinotomy, or needle aspiration is usually essential before a patient is denied surgery. Positive PET findings for nodal involvement do not obviate the need for histological confirmation of nodal involvement. However, in patients with no enlarged lymph nodes on CT and normal findings on PET, the likelihood of nodal involvement is so low that mediastinoscopy can be omitted.

For lung cancers that have invaded the mediastinum or chest wall, it is important to decide whether the tumour is nevertheless resectable for possible cure, again recognising that the prognosis will be poorer than for tumours confined to the lung. CT may show definitively that the tumour is too extensive for resective surgery (i.e. that it is a T4 lesion).[83] Alternatively, CT may leave the issue in doubt and MRI may then help to solve the problem.

Extrathoracic Staging of Lung Cancer

Lung cancer is commonly associated with widespread haematogenous dissemination at the time of presentation. Sites of spread include the adrenal glands, bones, brain, liver and more distant lymph nodes. Detection of metastatic disease precludes surgical resection of the primary tumour. In most centres chest CT is extended to include the liver and adrenals (with appropriate timing for portal venous enhancement). Further imaging is usually only undertaken if there are clinical features suggesting metastatic disease. In many European countries it is now routine to undertake PET/CT in any patient who is to be offered radical therapy for lung cancer. In patients initially selected for curative resection using standard tumour staging, PET/CT has been reported to detect occult metastatic disease in 11–14% of patients, and to alter management in up to 40%.[74]

PULMONARY SARCOMA AND OTHER PRIMARY MALIGNANT NEOPLASMS

The majority of pulmonary sarcomas in the lungs are metastases from extrathoracic primary tumours. Primary pulmonary sarcomas are rare, the most common primary forms being fibrosarcoma and leiomyosarcoma. Chondrosarcoma, fibroleiomyosarcoma, rhabdomyosarcoma, malignant fibrous histiocytoma, carcinosarcoma, liposarcoma and osteosarcoma are among the other sarcomas that may occasionally arise as primary airway or pulmonary tumours. All the above neoplasms present as a solitary pulmonary nodule or as a tracheal or endobronchial

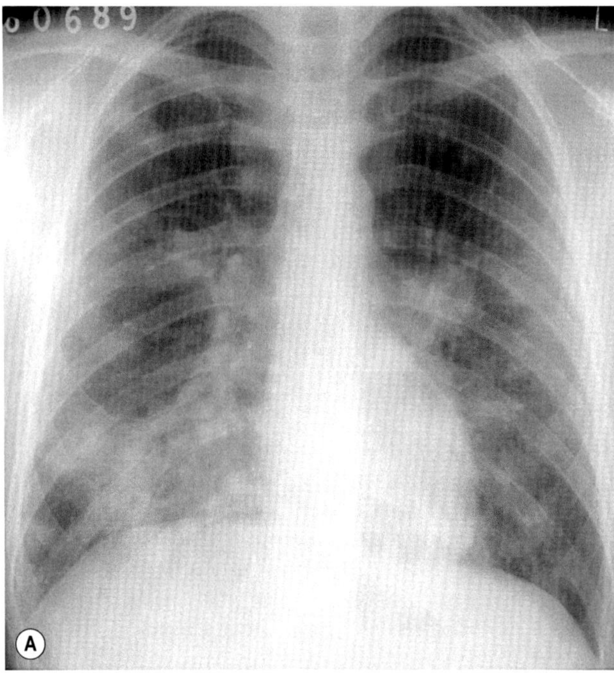

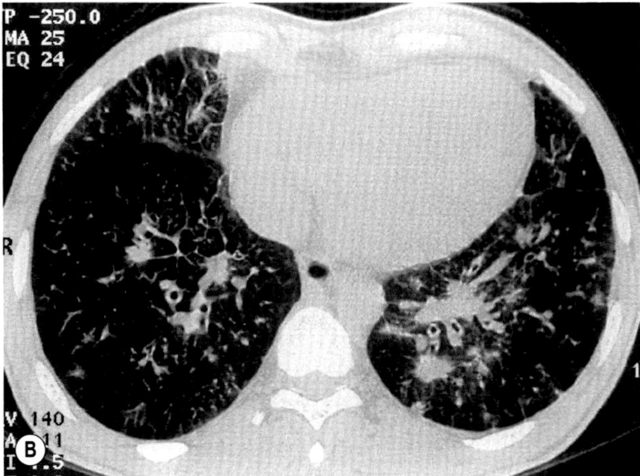

FIGURE 8-27 ■ **Kaposi's sarcoma in two patients with AIDS.** (A) Plain chest radiograph showing extensive pulmonary shadowing consisting of a mixture of ill-defined rounded and band-like shadows maximal in the perihilar regions and lower zones. (B) CT showing the peribronchial distribution of the ill-defined pulmonary nodules. There is interlobular septal thickening, a feature also frequently identified on the chest radiograph.

mass indistinguishable radiologically from bronchial carcinoma. Angiosarcomas of the pulmonary artery extend or arise intravascularly.

The acquired immunodeficiency syndrome (AIDS) epidemic led to an increased number of cases of Kaposi's sarcoma involving the lung, a situation largely redressed by effective anti-retroviral therapy. Kaposi's sarcoma in the respiratory tract is rare in the absence of cutaneous involvement. Coincidental involvement of the tracheobronchial tree is relatively frequent but parenchymal involvement may occur in the absence of endobronchial disease. Imaging may show the disease to be focal or widespread.[94–96] Focal segmental or lobar opacities are usually due to the tumour itself, but endobronchial Kaposi's sarcoma may result in atelectasis or postobstructive pneumonia. Radiographically widespread disease is the more frequent pattern, with a tendency to perihilar predominance of linear, rounded, or reticulonodular shadowing, reflecting a bronchocentric distribution of the lesions[95] (Fig. 8-27). The pulmonary opacities of Kaposi's sarcoma do not fluctuate in severity, whereas the major differential diagnoses—pulmonary oedema and opportunistic infections—may do so. Intrathoracic hilar/mediastinal lymphadenopathy has been detected in 25–60% of cases in some series.[94,95,97] Pleural involvement is frequent pleural effusions which are most commonly bilateral and may on occasion be large.[94]

Other rare malignant pulmonary neoplasms include haemangiopericytoma, pulmonary blastoma, plasmacytoma, choriocarcinoma, teratoma and Askin tumours.

BENIGN PULMONARY TUMOURS

There are a variety of relatively rare lesions that may present as an asymptomatic solitary pulmonary mass (Table 8-5). Imaging plays a key part in the characterisation of these lesions and will guide the need for further investigation or surgery.

HAMARTOMA

Hamartomas are tumour-like malformations composed of an abnormal mixture of mature tissues normally found in the organ in which the tumour occurs. Pulmonary hamartomas consist predominantly of masses of cartilage, with clefts lined by bronchial epithelium, and may contain large collections of fat. Malignant transformation is either non-existent or extremely rare. Pulmonary hamartomas are very occasionally multiple. A triad of pulmonary chondroma(s) (often multiple), gastric epithelioid leiomyosarcoma (leiomyoblastoma) and functioning extra-adrenal paragangliomas, known as Carney's triad, has been reported, as has a form with just pulmonary chondromas and gastric smooth muscle tumours.[98,99]

The age range for hamartoma is from young adulthood to old age, with presentation peaking in the seventh decade; they are only occasionally seen in children.

The distribution of pulmonary hamartomas is opposite to that seen with bronchial carcinoid: 90% are peripheral and present as a solitary pulmonary nodule,

TABLE 8-5 **Causes and Mimics of a Solitary Pulmonary Mass**

Causes
Bronchial carcinoma
Bronchial carcinoid
Granuloma
Hamartoma
Metastasis
Chronic pneumonia or abscess
Hydatid cyst
Pulmonary haematoma
Bronchocele
Fungus ball
Massive fibrosis in coal workers
Bronchogenic cyst
Sequestration
Arteriovenous malformation
Pulmonary infarct

Mimics
Extrathoracic artefacts
Cutaneous masses
Bony lesions
Pleural tumours or plaques
Encysted pleural fluid
Pulmonary vessels

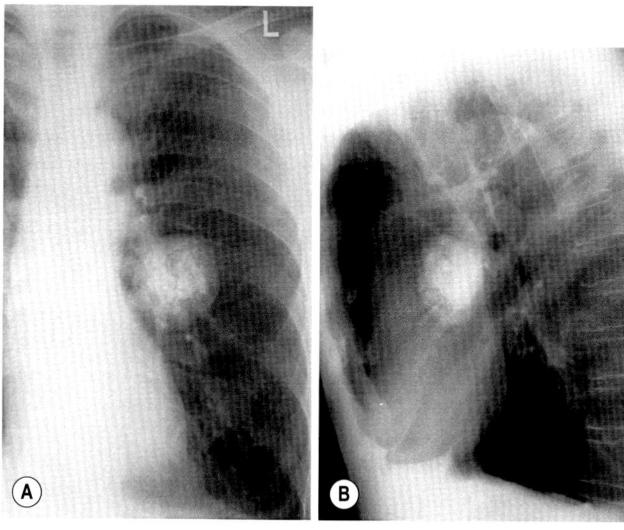

FIGURE 8-28 ■ **Hamartoma of the lung.** (A, B) Round, completely smooth, hamartoma in a 57-year-old asymptomatic man. There is typical coarse popcorn calcification in this lesion, which is unusually large.

while the remaining 10% arise within a major bronchus. Central lesions may lead to major airway obstruction and the features are then identical to those seen with bronchial carcinoids.

On plain chest radiography[100,101] the tumour is seen as a spherical or slightly lobulated, well-defined nodule, usually less than 4 cm in size, with normal surrounding lung (Fig. 8-28). Some hamartomas show calcification, which may be spotty or linear or show the characteristic 'popcorn' configuration associated with calcification in cartilage (Fig. 8-28). The frequency of calcification increases significantly with the size of the lesion. Popcorn calcification, if present, is virtually diagnostic of a hamartoma (the only differential diagnosis is a chondrosarcoma). Central fat density on CT is another important finding, which, if present, establishes the diagnosis.[102] The lesions grow slowly, usually much more slowly than carcinoma of the bronchus, and cavity formation is almost unknown.

OTHER BENIGN PULMONARY NEOPLASMS

Fibroma, chondroma, lipoma, haemangioma, benign clear cell tumours, neurogenic tumours, chemodectoma and granular cell myoblastoma are benign neoplasms that are occasionally encountered in the trachea, bronchi, or lungs. The plain radiograph and CT findings vary with the size and location of the tumour mass, but no features distinguish any one of these lesions from any other, and therefore the specific diagnosis has to be made histologically. They are indistinguishable radiologically from carcinoid tumour and solitary metastasis.

Leiomyoma

Leiomyoma of the lung may be a solitary lesion, radiographically indistinguishable from the other benign connective tissue neoplasms. Multiple leiomyomas present as multiple discrete nodules in the lungs. They are given a wide variety of names, including benign metastasising leiomyoma. In women these tumours may be very slow-growing metastases from a uterine leiomyoma; women with multiple pulmonary leiomyomas often have a history of previous hysterectomy for uterine fibroids.

Intrapulmonary teratomas are very unusual. Most are benign, though malignant lesions are occasionally encountered. Radiographically, and on CT, intrapulmonary teratomas appear as lobulated masses that may show calcification or cavitation.[103]

Plasma Cell Granuloma

Plasma cell granuloma of the lung (inflammatory pseudotumour) is the name given to a lesion that is presumed to be reactive inflammatory granulomatous tissue. The age range is wide and includes children. Most patients present with an asymptomatic solitary pulmonary nodule. Cavitation and calcification have both been described. These lesions are PET positive and mimic bronchogenic carcinomas.

Sclerosing Haemangioma

Sclerosing haemangioma is a benign neoplasm,[104,105] which almost always presents as an asymptomatic solitary pulmonary mass. Calcification may be seen.

Squamous Papillomas

Squamous papillomas of the trachea, bronchi and lungs are most commonly associated with laryngeal papillomatosis, a disease that usually commences in childhood and is believed to be viral in origin. Rarely, these papillomas are also present in the lung and are seen on plain chest radiography or CT as multiple, small, widely scattered and well-defined, round pulmonary nodules, frequently showing cavitation.[106]

BENIGN LYMPHOPROLIFERATIVE DISORDERS

LYMPHOCYTIC INTERSTITIAL PNEUMONIA

Lymphocytic interstitial pneumonia (LIP) is an uncommon non-neoplastic lymphoproliferative disorder characterised by diffuse infiltration of the pulmonary parenchymal interstitium by lymphocytes and plasma cells. Histological differentiation between benign proliferation and low-grade lymphoma can be difficult. LIP may occur as an isolated entity (it is included in the classification of idiopathic interstitial pneumonias); however, this is rare. It is more commonly seen in association with an underlying immunological abnormality such as Sjögren's syndrome and AIDS. The main imaging findings are of bilateral areas of ground-glass opacification and thin-walled cysts.[107]

FOLLICULAR BRONCHIOLITIS

Follicular bronchiolitis, also known as diffuse lymphoid hyperplasia, is characterised by hyperplasia of bronchial mucosa-associated lymphoid tissue (MALT) in relation to airways. Reticular or reticular nodular shadowing with centrilobular nodules and ground-glass opacity and occasionally bronchial wall thickening, bronchial dilatation, interlobular septal thickening and peribronchovascular air-space consolidation is seen.[108]

MALIGNANT LYMPHOPROLIFERATIVE DISORDERS

LYMPHOMA

Only pulmonary parenchymal involvement by lymphoma is considered in this chapter. Pulmonary parenchymal involvement can be broadly divided into that occurring in association with existing or previously treated nodal disease, and that due to primary lymphoma of the lung (Hodgkin's or non-Hodgkin's). Parenchymal involvement is comparatively rare at initial presentation (10–15% of cases[109]), but it becomes considerably more common as the disease progresses. It is particularly frequent in patients who relapse after treatment.[110] Involvement of the lung appears to be three times as frequent in Hodgkin's lymphoma as it is in non-Hodgkin's lymphoma.[109] In Hodgkin's lymphoma the lung disease is almost invariably accompanied by visible intrathoracic adenopathy, whereas in the non-Hodgkin's lymphomas, isolated pulmonary involvement is not uncommon. If the mediastinal and hilar nodes have been previously irradiated, then recurrence confined to the lungs may be seen in both Hodgkin's and non-Hodgkin's lymphoma.

The radiographic appearances of lung involvement in malignant lymphoma vary.[110,111] The usual patterns are (1) one or more areas of pulmonary consolidation resembling pneumonia (Fig. 8-29), (2) multiple pulmonary nodules (Fig. 8-30) and, occasionally, (3) miliary nodulation or reticulonodular shadowing resembling lymphangitis carcinomatosa (Fig. 8-31).

The areas of pulmonary consolidation, which may contain air bronchograms, may be segmental or lobar in shape, but often they radiate from the hila or mediastinum without conforming to segmental anatomy, in keeping with the concept that extension into the lungs is by direct invasion from involved hilar or mediastinal nodes. Peripheral subpleural masses or areas of consolidation without any visible connection to enlarged nodes in the mediastinum and hila are, however, common in both Hodgkin's disease and non-Hodgkin's lymphoma. Very rapid increase in the size of lymphomatous deposits in the lung, so rapid that the disease may be confused with pneumonia, has been reported with high-grade non-Hodgkin's lymphoma.[112]

Primary lymphoma of the lung (Fig. 8-29) (i.e. lymphoma isolated to the lung at initial presentation) is very uncommon, non-Hodgkin's lymphoma of MALT type, being the most frequently encountered form. These are low-grade B-cell lymphomas of MALT (also called bronchus-associated lymphoid tissue or BALT), which consist of mucosal lymphoid follicles located in distal bronchi and bronchioles, particularly at airway bifurcations. The second most common primary tumour, known as angiocentric immunoproliferative lesion or lymphoid granulomatosis, is high grade and may have B- or T-cell phenotype.[113] Primary pulmonary Hodgkin's disease is notably rare.

The imaging features of MALT[114,115] lymphomas are solitary or multifocal, round or segmental areas of pulmonary consolidation. There is no lobar predilection and the consolidations may be placed centrally or peripherally in the lung parenchyma. Air bronchograms are frequently visible and may be a striking feature. A few of the lesions show cavitation, but calcification does not occur. MALT lymphomas are relatively rarely associated with pleural effusions despite contact with the pleura.

Other Findings in Pulmonary Lymphoma

Lobar atelectasis caused by endobronchial lymphoma is occasionally encountered, but, somewhat surprisingly, atelectasis as a result of extrinsic compression by enlarged

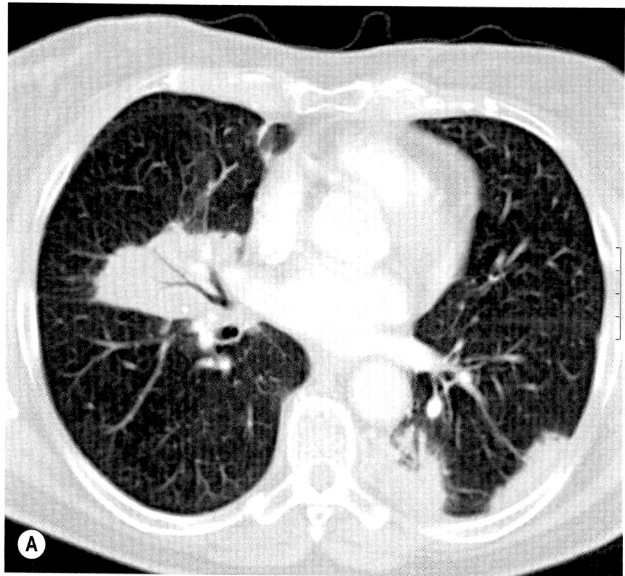

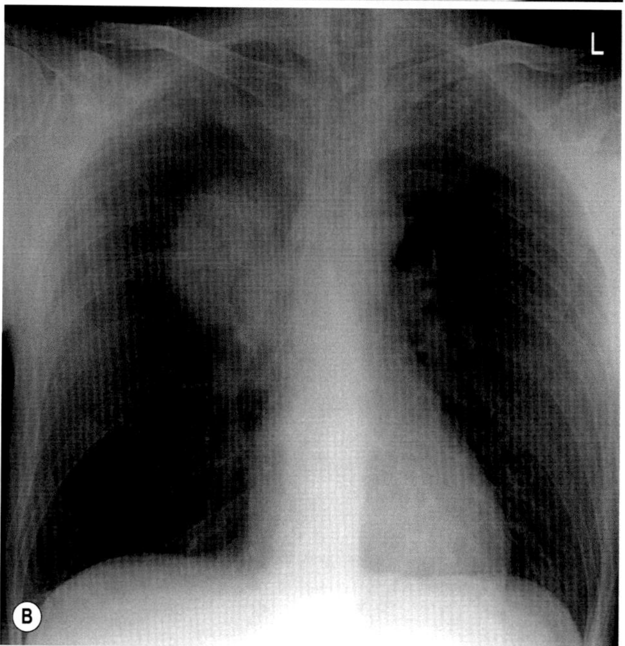

FIGURE 8-29 ■ **Primary pulmonary lymphoma.** (A) CT imaging demonstrates multiple areas of consolidation. This appearance had been very slowly progressive over several years. (B) Chest X-ray shows an area of consolidation in the right upper lung zone in a patient with primary pulmonary Hodgkin's lymphoma.

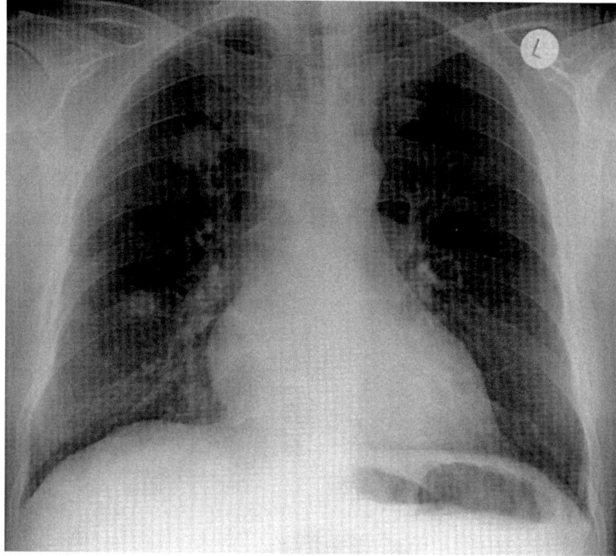

FIGURE 8-30 ■ **Pulmonary involvement by lymphocytic lymphoma showing multiple pulmonary masses.**

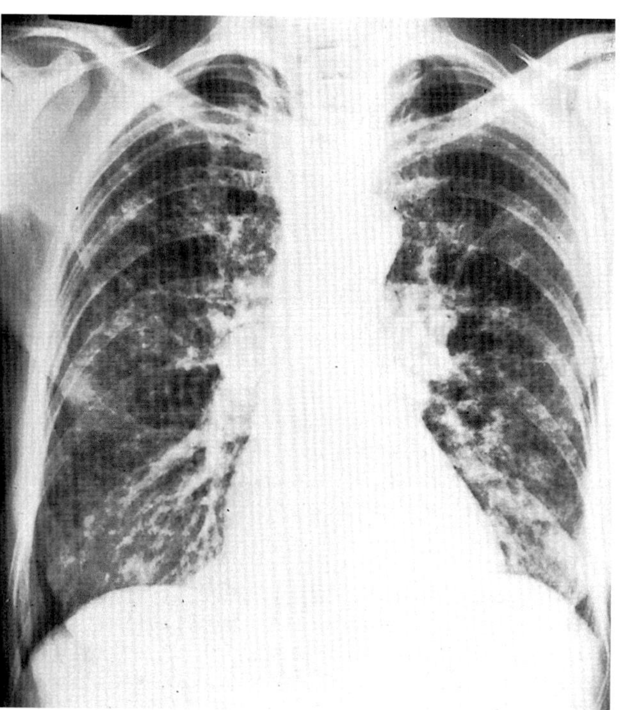

FIGURE 8-31 ■ **Pulmonary involvement by non-Hodgkin's lymphoma.** This appearance closely resembles lymphangitis carcinomatosa, with widespread nodules and thickened septal lines.

lymph nodes is rare, with encasement rather than obstruction being the usual pattern of disease.

Pleural effusions are common except in MALT lymphoma. They are usually unilateral and accompanied by visible intrathoracic adenopathy. They frequently disappear once the mediastinal nodes have been irradiated; in such cases they are probably due to venous or lymphatic obstruction rather than neoplastic involvement of the pleura.

The usual radiographic problem is in deciding whether the pulmonary abnormality is due to involvement by lymphomatous tissue, infection or a complication of therapy. It should be remembered that the pattern of pulmonary infection in patients with lymphoma is modified because they are immunocompromised hosts, owing either to their disease or, more often, to the drugs used for treating the disorder. In many instances, a biopsy is the only way to establish the precise diagnosis. Since Hodgkin's disease is believed to spread from nodal sites, a useful guideline is that if a patient presents with Hodgkin's lymphoma and a pulmonary opacity, but no evidence of hilar or mediastinal disease, it is more likely that the opacity represents something other than Hodgkin's lymphoma. A caveat here is that the patient should not previously have received radiation therapy to the mediastinum.

LEUKAEMIA

The incidence of leukaemic infiltration of the lungs, mediastinal lymph nodes and pleura varies with the course of the disease. Pulmonary infiltration by leukaemic cells is found at autopsy in nearly two-thirds of patients who have leukaemia. However, provided those patients with leukostasis (see below) are considered separately, leukaemic infiltration of the lungs, though very common pathologically, is usually asymptomatic and is rarely a cause of significant pulmonary opacity on a chest radiograph. When respiratory impairment is present, pulmonary infection, oedema or haemorrhage are more likely causes of the patient's symptoms.[116] Imaging features include diffuse bilateral reticulation and patterns resembling interstitial oedema; lymphangitic carcinomatosis, small nodules, ground-glass opacification and consolidation have also been described.[117]

Radiographically visible hilar and/or mediastinal lymph node enlargement may be present and pleural effusions are common, though it is not possible to state the cause of the effusion with any confidence. The distribution of nodal enlargement closely resembles that of the lymphomas. T-cell leukaemias may show massive mediastinal adenopathy that responds rapidly to chemotherapy or radiation treatment. Huge mediastinal masses of T-cell leukaemia may disappear within a few days following appropriate treatment.

Pleural thickening due to a mass of leukaemic cells in patients with myeloid leukaemia, so-called granulocytic sarcoma or chloroma formation (because of its green appearance), may be encountered on rare occasions.[118]

Leukostasis is seen in patients with acute myeloid leukaemia with very high white blood cell counts in the order of 100,000–300,000 cells mm^{-3}. The patients may be dyspnoeic because of the obliteration of their small pulmonary blood vessels by the leukaemic cells.[118] The chest radiograph may be normal or show air-space shadowing, which is probably due to pulmonary oedema rather than directly to the accumulation of leukaemic cells in the lungs.[119,120]

METASTASES

Pulmonary metastases[121] in adults are usually from breast, gastrointestinal tract, kidney, testes, head and neck tumours or from a variety of bone and soft-tissue sarcomas. The basic sign of haematogenous pulmonary metastasis is one or more discrete pulmonary nodules (Fig. 8-32), usually in the outer portions of the lungs, a distribution that is most evident on CT (Fig. 8-33). The nodules are usually spherical and well defined, but they may be almost any shape and can occasionally have a very irregular edge. Such irregular edges are seen particularly with metastases from adenocarcinomas (Fig. 8-34). Cavitation is occasionally seen in pulmonary metastases; it is a particular feature of squamous cell carcinoma.[122] Calcification is very unusual except in osteosarcoma and chondrosarcoma. Even if the primary tumour shows calcification, e.g. in breast and colon, visible calcification in the pulmonary metastases is rare. The rate of growth of metastases is highly variable; in some choriocarcinomas and osteosarcomas, for example, it may be explosive and double the volume of the lesions in less than 30 days.[123] Alternatively, metastases can remain unchanged in size for a long time, as in some cases of thyroid carcinoma.[124]

A solitary pulmonary metastasis may be the presenting feature in a patient without a known primary tumour. However, a metastasis is a rare cause of the asymptomatic pulmonary nodule in patients who do not have a known extrathoracic primary neoplasm, comprising no more than 2–3% of most series.

The simplest technique for diagnosing pulmonary metastases is the plain posteroanterior (PA) and lateral chest radiograph. High-kV techniques are often used routinely, since substantial portions of the lungs are obscured on low-kV radiographs by overlying structures such as the diaphragm, heart, mediastinum, hila and ribs. Such radiographs will detect most lung metastases above 1 cm in diameter. Increasing sensitivity can be obtained with CT, in particular MDCT. The increase in sensitivity for small nodules is, however, at the cost of decreasing specificity. On CT, lesions smaller than 1 cm are regularly demonstrated, together with most lesions above 3 mm in diameter. Below 1 cm, and particularly below 6 mm, the differential diagnosis from granulomas due to

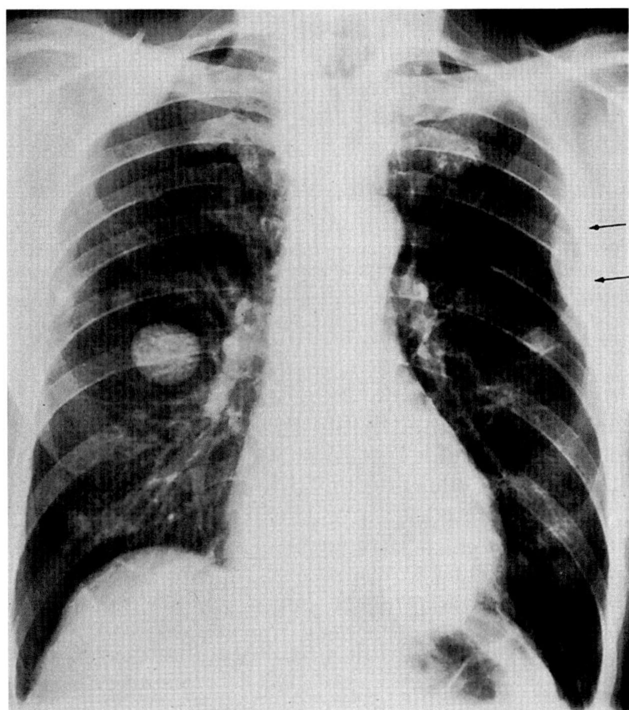

FIGURE 8-32 ■ Typical pulmonary metastases. Multiple well-defined spherical nodules in the lungs. Rib metastases with associated soft-tissue swelling are also present (arrows). In this case the primary tumour was a synovial cell carcinoma.

tuberculosis, histoplasmosis, or other fungi becomes difficult. Where calcification can be identified, metastases (except from osteogenic sarcoma or chondrosarcoma) can effectively be dismissed from consideration. If the nodules are not calcified, the best that can be done in most instances is to give a statistical probability of the nodules being metastases. With a plain chest radiograph showing multiple non-calcified nodules, the probability is high, well over 90%, even in areas endemic for fungus granulomas, and approaches 100% in areas where fungus granulomas are rare or non-existent. With the smaller lesions detectable on CT, this probability diminishes.

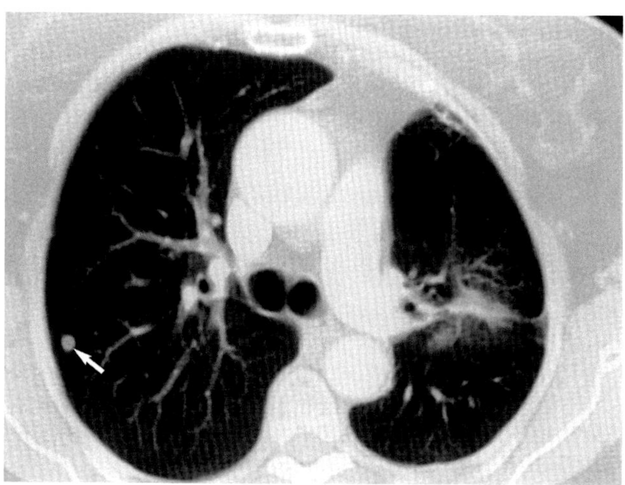

FIGURE 8-33 ■ **Pulmonary metastases.** CT demonstrating a single peripheral metastasis (arrow). There were multiple lesions at other levels. The volume loss and scarring in the left lung is secondary to previous resection of the primary bronchogenic carcinoma.

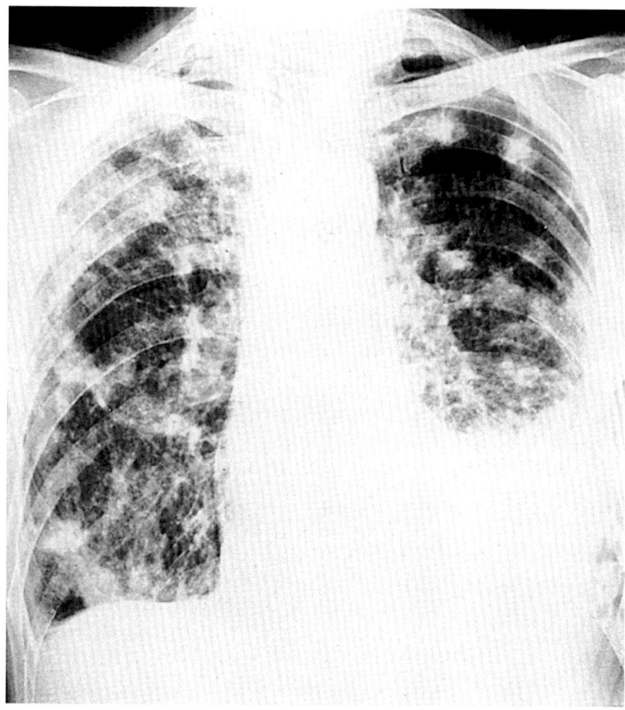

FIGURE 8-34 ■ **Irregular pulmonary metastases.** Metastatic adenocarcinoma from an unknown primary. The nodules are irregular in outline. A large left pleural effusion is also present.

Depending on the prevalence of infectious granulomas in the community and the likelihood of a particular tumour metastasising to the lung, the probability that a pulmonary nodule seen solely on CT is indeed a metastasis may drop to as low as 50%.

LYMPHANGITIC CARCINOMATOSIS

Lymphangitic carcinomatosis is the name given to permeation of pulmonary lymphatics and/or their adjacent interstitial tissue by neoplastic cells. The most common tumours that spread in this manner are carcinomas of the bronchus, breast, stomach and prostate.[125] Lymphangitic carcinomatosis may develop secondary to blood-borne emboli lodging in smaller pulmonary arteries and subsequently spreading through the vessel walls into the perivascular interstitium and lymphatic vessels. Such spread tends to give rise to bilateral symmetric pulmonary abnormality. Alternatively, lymphangitic carcinomatosis may result from direct extension of tumour from hilar lymph nodes into peribronchovascular interstitium, from the pleura into adjacent interlobular septa, or from a primary carcinoma of the lung into the adjacent peribronchovascular interstitium. Tumour spreading by these mechanisms tends to be more localised.

The radiological findings are fine reticulonodular shadowing and/or thickened septal lines (Figs. 8-35 and 8-36). These signs occur because of a combination of dilated lymphatics and interstitial oedema, together with shadows due to the tumour cells themselves along with any desmoplastic response which may have been induced by the tumour.[125] Another useful sign of lymphangitis carcinomatosa is subpleural oedema resulting from lymphatic obstruction by tumour cells, a feature that is most readily visible as thickening of the fissures. Pleural effusion is common, and is seen in about 30%.

As would be expected, CT is more sensitive than plain radiography in the detection of lymphangitic spread and

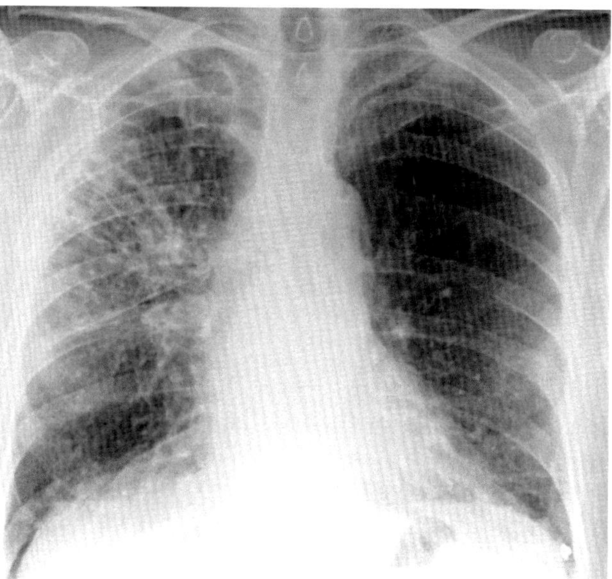

FIGURE 8-35 ■ **Unilateral lymphangitic carcinomatosis.** Carcinoma of the bronchus, showing thickened septal lines and nodules confined to the right lung.

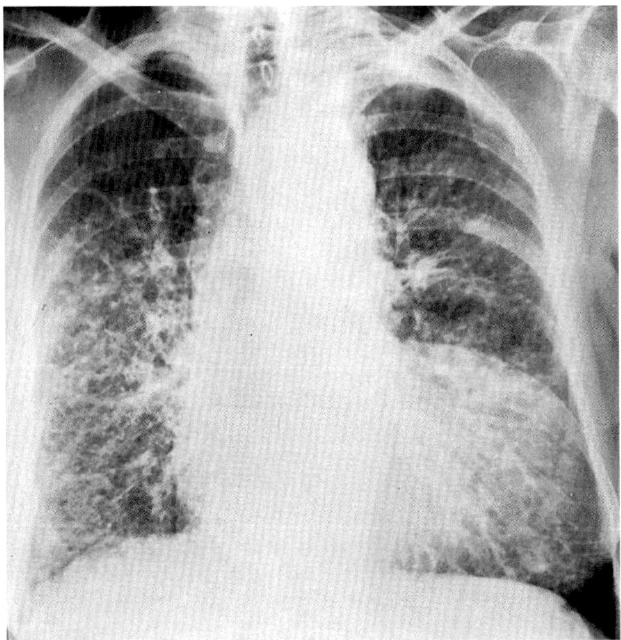

FIGURE 8-36 ■ **Bilateral lymphangitic carcinomatosis.** Bilateral thickened septal lines, together with widespread nodulation of the lungs, are seen. The primary tumour in this 71-year-old woman was presumed to be a bronchial carcinoma (a diagnosis based on sputum cytology).

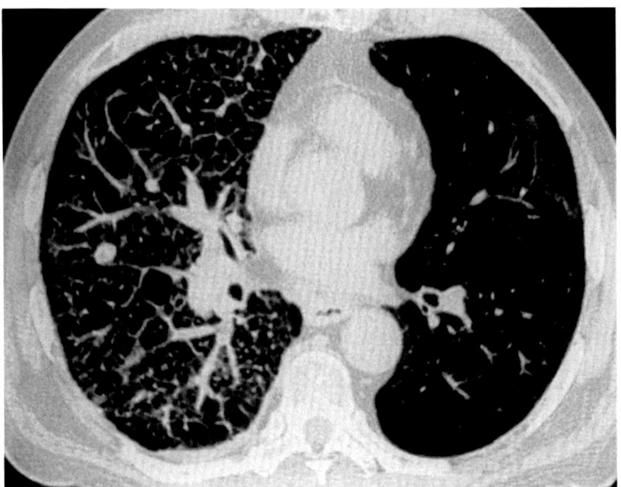

FIGURE 8-37 ■ **High-resolution CT of lymphangitic carcinomatosis.** Note the variable thickening of the interlobular septa and the enlargement of the bronchovascular bundle in the centre of the secondary pulmonary lobules. The polygonal shape of the walls (septa) of the secondary pulmonary lobules is particularly well shown anteriorly. The pulmonary nodule is due to a discrete metastasis, a relatively frequent finding in this condition.

may show changes in patients whose chest radiograph is normal. CT, particularly high-resolution CT,[126–128] shows non-uniform, often nodular, thickening of the interlobular septa and irregular thickening of the bronchovascular bundles in the central portions of the lungs (Fig. 8-37). Small, peripherally located, wedge-shaped densities are sometimes seen as well; these may represent volume averaging of the thickened septa. There is often patchy airspace shadowing, but an important differential diagnostic feature from pulmonary oedema is that many of the acini subtended by thickened interlobular septa are normally aerated. Nodular shadows may be seen scattered through the parenchyma. The abnormalities may involve all zones of both lungs or they may be centrally or peripherally predominant; sometimes, particularly when lymphangitis is due to bronchial carcinoma, they are confined to a lobe or one lung. Hilar lymph node enlargement is seen in only some of the patients.

UNUSUAL PATTERNS OF METASTATIC CANCER

Endobronchial Metastases

Endobronchial metastases are most unusual. Melanoma and renal, colorectal and breast carcinomas are the primary tumours that most frequently give endobronchial submucosal metastases.[129] In such cases the effect of airway obstruction is the dominant feature.

Miliary Metastases

Occasionally, innumerable tiny nodules closely resembling miliary tuberculosis are seen throughout both lungs, with no large masses and no evidence of lymphatic obstruction, such as is seen in lymphangitis carcinomatosa. Metastases are, however, one of the rarest causes of this pattern. The primary tumours that are most likely to produce miliary nodulation of the lungs are thyroid and renal carcinomas, bone sarcomas and choriocarcinoma.

Tumour Emboli

Radiologically recognisable pulmonary arterial hypertension may occur on rare occasions as a result of tumour emboli blocking small pulmonary arteries.[106] Many tumours can embolise in this fashion, particularly hepatoma, carcinoma of the breast, kidney, stomach, and prostate and choriocarcinoma.

REFERENCES

1. MacMahon H, Austin JH, Gamsu G, et al. Guidelines for management of small pulmonary nodules detected on CT scans: a statement from the Fleischner Society. Radiology 2005;237(2): 395–400.
2. Siegel R, Ward E, Brawley O, Jemal A. Cancer statistics, 2011: the impact of eliminating socioeconomic and racial disparities on premature cancer deaths. CA Cancer J Clin 2011;61(4): 212–36.
3. de Groot P, Munden RF. Lung cancer epidemiology, risk factors, and prevention. Radiol Clin North Am 2012;50(5):863–76.
4. Yang P, Cerhan J, Vierkant R, et al. Adenocarcinoma of the lung is strongly associated with cigarette smoking: further evidence from a prospective study of women. Am J Epidemiol 2002;156(12): 1114–22.
5. Hoffmann D, Djordjevic MV, Hoffmann I. The changing cigarette. Prev Med 1997;26:427–34.
6. Torok S, Hegedus B, Laszlo V, et al. Lung cancer in never smokers. Future Oncol 2011;7(10):1195–211.
7. National Comprehensive Cancer Network (NCCN). Clinical Practice Guidelines in Oncology: Non-small cell lung cancer. Available at <https://subscriptions.nccn.org/gl_login.aspx?ReturnURL=http://www.nccn.org/professionals/physician_gls/pdf/nscl.pdf> 2012.

8. Doll R, Hill AB. The mortality of doctors in relation to their smoking habits. Br Med J 1954;1(4877):1451.
9. Öberg M, Jaakkola MS, Woodward A, et al. Worldwide burden of disease from exposure to second-hand smoke: a retrospective analysis of data from 192 countries. Lancet 2011;377(9760): 139–46.
10. Lai HK, Hedley AJ, Repace J, et al. Lung function and exposure to workplace second-hand smoke during exemptions from smoking ban legislation: an exposure–response relationship based on indoor PM2.5 and urinary cotinine levels. Thorax 2011;66(7): 615–23.
11. Patel JD. Lung cancer in women. J Clin Oncol 2005;23(14): 3212–18.
12. Khuder SA, Mutgi AB. Effect of smoking cessation on major histologic types of lung cancer. Chest 2001;120(5):1577–83.
13. Pope CA III, Burnett RT, Thun MJ, et al. Lung cancer, cardiopulmonary mortality, and long-term exposure to fine particulate air pollution. JAMA 2002;287(9):1132–41.
14. Cruz D, Tanoue LT, Matthay RA. Lung cancer: epidemiology, etiology, and prevention. Clin Chest Med 2011;32(4):605–44.
15. Sagawa M, Tsubono Y, Saito Y, et al. A case-control study for evaluating the efficacy of mass screening program for lung cancer in Miyagi Prefecture, Japan. Cancer 2001;92(3):588–94.
16. Nishii K, Ueoka H, Kiura K, et al. A case-control study of lung cancer screening in Okayama Prefecture, Japan. Lung Cancer 2001;34(3):325–32.
17. Fontana RS, Sanderson DR, Taylor WF, et al. Early lung cancer detection: results of the initial (prevalence) radiologic and cytologic screening in the Mayo Clinic study. Am Rev Respir Dis 1984;130(4):561–5.
18. Melamed M, Flehinger B, Zaman M, et al. Screening for early lung cancer. Results of the Memorial Sloan-Kettering study in New York. Chest 1984;86(1):44.
19. Frost J, Ball W Jr, Levin M, et al. Early lung cancer detection: results of the initial (prevalence) radiologic and cytologic screening in the Johns Hopkins study. Am Rev Respir Dis 1984;130(4):549.
20. Kubik A, Polak J. Lung cancer detection results of a randomized prospective study in Czechoslovakia. Cancer 1986;57(12): 2427–37.
21. Oken MM, Hocking WG, Kvale PA, et al. Screening by chest radiograph and lung cancer mortality. JAMA 2011;306(17): 1865–73.
22. Nawa T, Nakagawa T, Mizoue T, et al. A decrease in lung cancer mortality following the introduction of low-dose chest CT screening in Hitachi, Japan. Lung Cancer 2012;78(3):225–8.
23. Nawa T, Nakagawa T, Kusano S, et al. Lung cancer screening using low-dose spiral CT: results of baseline and 1-year follow-up studies. Chest 2002;122(1):15–20.
24. Henschke CI, McCauley DI, Yankelevitz DF, et al. Early Lung Cancer Action Project: overall design and findings from baseline screening. Lancet 1999;354:99.
25. Schmidlin EJ, Sundaram B, Kazerooni EA. Computed tomography screening for lung cancer. Radiol Clin North Am 2012; 50(5):877–94.
26. Aberle D, Adams A, Berg C, et al. Reduced lung-cancer mortality with low-dose computed tomographic screening. N Engl J Med 2011;365(5):395.
27. Das M, Mühlenbruch G, Heinen S, et al. Performance evaluation of a computer-aided detection algorithm for solid pulmonary nodules in low-dose and standard-dose MDCT chest examinations and its influence on radiologists. Br J Radiol 2008; 81(971):841–7.
28. Yuan R, Vos PM, Cooperberg PL. Computer-aided detection in screening CT for pulmonary nodules. Am J Roentgenol 2006; 186(5):1280–7.
29. Van de Wiel J, Wang Y, Xu D, et al. Neglectable benefit of searching for incidental findings in the Dutch–Belgian lung cancer screening trial (NELSON) using low-dose multidetector CT. Eur Radiol 2007;17(6):1474–82.
30. Gietema HA, Wang Y, Xu D, et al. Pulmonary nodules detected at lung cancer screening: interobserver variability of semiautomated volume measurements. Radiology 2006;241(1):251–7.
31. American Lung Association. Providing guidance on lung cancer screening to patients and physicians. 2012.
32. NCCN. NCCN Clinical Practice Guidelines in Oncology: Lung Cancer Screening. Available at <https://subscriptions.nccn.org/gl_login.aspx?ReturnURL=http://www.nccn.org/professionals/physician_gls/pdf/lung_screening.pdf>; 2012.
33. Field JK, Baldwin D, Brain K, et al. CT screening for lung cancer in the UK: position statement by UKLS investigators following the NLST report. Thorax 2011;66(8):736–7.
34. Gurney JW, Swensen SJ. Solitary pulmonary nodules: determining the likelihood of malignancy with neural network analysis. Radiology 1995;196(3):823–9.
35. Takashima S, Sone S, Li F, et al. Small solitary pulmonary nodules (≤ 1 cm) detected at population-based CT screening for lung cancer: reliable high-resolution CT features of benign lesions. Am J Roentgenol 2003;180(4):955–64.
36. Zwirewich C, Vedal S, Miller R, Müller N. Solitary pulmonary nodule: high-resolution CT and radiologic-pathologic correlation. Radiology 1991;179(2):469–76.
37. Bankoff MS, McEniff NJ, Bhadelia RA, et al. Prevalence of pathologically proven intrapulmonary lymph nodes and their appearance on CT. Am J Roentgenol 1996;167(3):629–30.
38. Sykes AG, Swensen SJ, Tazelaar HD, Jung S. Computed tomography of benign intrapulmonary lymph nodes: retrospective comparison with sarcoma metastases. Mayo Clin Proc 2002;77(4): 329–33.
39. Hyodo T, Kanazawa S, Dendo S, et al. Intrapulmonary lymph nodes: thin-section CT findings, pathological findings, and CT differential diagnosis from pulmonary metastatic nodules. Acta Medica Okayama 2004;58:235–40.
40. Ahn MI, Gleeson TG, Chan IH, et al. Perifissural nodules seen at CT screening for lung cancer. Radiology 2010;254(3):949–56.
41. Edey AJ, Hansell DM. Incidentally detected small pulmonary nodules on CT. Clin Radiol 2009;64(9):872–84.
42. Woodring JH, Fried AM. Significance of wall thickness in solitary cavities of the lung: a follow-up study. Am J Roentgenol 1983; 140(3):473–4.
43. Xu DM, van Klaveren RJ, de Bock GH, et al. Limited value of shape, margin and CT density in the discrimination between benign and malignant screen detected solid pulmonary nodules of the NELSON trial. Eur J Radiol 2008;68(2):347–52.
44. Winer-Muram HT. The solitary pulmonary nodule. Radiology 2006;239(1):34–49.
45. Erasmus JJ, Connolly JE, McAdams HP, Roggli VL. Solitary pulmonary nodules: part I: Morphologic evaluation for differentiation of benign and malignant lesions. Radiographics 2000; 20(1):43–58.
46. Hamper U, Khouri N, Stitik F, Siegelman S. Pulmonary hamartoma: diagnosis by transthoracic needle-aspiration biopsy. Radiology 1985;155(1):15–18.
47. Naidich DP, Bankier AA, MacMahon H, et al. Recommendations for the management of subsolid pulmonary nodules detected at CT: a statement from the Fleischner Society. Radiology 2013; 266(1):304–17.
48. Travis WD, Brambilla E, Noguchi M, et al. International Association for the Study of Lung Cancer/American Thoracic Society/European Respiratory Society: international multidisciplinary classification of lung adenocarcinoma executive summary. Proc Am Thor Soc 2011;8(5):381–5.
49. Kakinuma R, Ohmatsu H, Kaneko M, et al. Progression of focal pure ground-glass opacity detected by low-dose helical computed tomography screening for lung cancer. J Comput Assist Tomogr 2004;28(1):17–23.
50. Swensen SJ, Viggiano RW, Midthun DE, et al. Lung nodule enhancement at CT: multicenter study. Radiology 2000;214(1): 73–80.
51. Chae EJ, Song J, Seo JB, et al. Clinical utility of dual-energy CT in the evaluation of solitary pulmonary nodules: initial experience. Radiology 2008;249(2):671–81.
52. Rohren EM, Turkington TG, Coleman RE. Clinical applications of PET in oncology. Radiology 2004;231(2):305–32.
53. Higashi K, Ueda Y, Seki H, et al. Fluorine-18-FDG PET imaging is negative in bronchioloalveolar lung carcinoma. J Nucl Med 1998;39(6):1016–20.
54. Saita S, Tanzillo A, Riscica C, et al. Bronchial brushing and biopsy: a comparative evaluation iu diagnosing visible bronchial lesions. Eur J Cardiothorac Surg 1990;4:270–2.
55. Rivera MP, Mehta AC. Initial diagnosis of lung cancer: ACCP evidence-based clinical practice guidelines (2nd edition). Chest 2007;132(3 Suppl):131S–48S.

56. Gurney J, Lyddon D, McKay J. Determining the likelihood of malignancy in solitary pulmonary nodules with Bayesian analysis. Part II. Application. Radiology 1993;186(2):415–22.
57. Gurney J. Determining the likelihood of malignancy in solitary pulmonary nodules with Bayesian analysis. Part I. Theory. Radiology 1993;186(2):405–13.
58. UICC. TNM Classification of Malignant Tumors, 7th ed. Chichester: Wiley Blackwell; 2009.
59. Tsuboi M, Ohira T, Saji H, et al. The present status of postoperative adjuvant chemotherapy for completely resected non-small cell lung cancer. Ann Thorac Cardiovasc Surg 2007;13(2):73.
60. Travis WD, Brambilla E, Rami-Porta R, et al. Visceral pleural invasion: pathologic criteria and use of elastic stains: proposal for the 7th edition of the TNM classification for lung cancer. J Thorac Oncol 2008;3(12):1384–90.
61. Glazer H, Duncan-Meyer J, Aronberg D, et al. Pleural and chest wall invasion in bronchogenic carcinoma: CT evaluation. Radiology 1985;157(1):191–4.
62. Akata S, Kajiwara N, Park J, et al. Evaluation of chest wall invasion by lung cancer using respiratory dynamic MRI. J Med Imaging Radiat Oncol 2008;52(1):36–9.
63. Raptis CA, Bhalla S. The 7th Edition of the TNM staging system for lung cancer: what the radiologist needs to know. Radiol Clin North Am 2012;50(5):915–33.
64. Travis WD, Giroux DJ, Chansky K, et al. The IASLC Lung Cancer Staging Project: proposals for the inclusion of bronchopulmonary carcinoid tumors in the forthcoming (seventh) edition of the TNM Classification for Lung Cancer. J Thorac Oncol 2008;3(11):1213–23.
65. Gorshtein A, Gross DJ, Barak D, et al. Diffuse idiopathic pulmonary neuroendocrine cell hyperplasia and the associated lung neuroendocrine tumors. Cancer 2012;118(3):612–19.
66. Zwiebel B, Austin J, Grimes M. Bronchial carcinoid tumors: assessment with CT of location and intratumoral calcification in 31 patients. Radiology 1991;179(2):483–6.
67. Auerbach O, Garfinkel L. The changing pattern of lung carcinoma. Cancer 1991;68(9):1973–7.
68. Grewal RG, Austin JH. CT demonstration of calcification in carcinoma of the lung. J Comput Assist Tomogr 1994;18(6): 867–71.
69. Stewart JG, MacMahon H, Vyborny CJ, Pollak ER. Dystrophic calcification in carcinoma of the lung: demonstration by CT. Am J Roentgenol 1987;148(1):29–30.
70. Henschke CI, Yankelevitz DF, Mirtcheva R, et al. CT screening for lung cancer frequency and significance of part-solid and nonsolid nodules. Am J Roentgenol 2002;178(5):1053–7.
71. Gupta P. The golden S sign. Radiology 2004;233(3):790–1.
72. Rohlfing BM, White EA, Webb WR, Goodman PC. Hilar and mediastinal adenopathy caused by bacterial abscess of the lung. Radiology 1978;128(2):289–93.
73. Glazer H, Kaiser L, Anderson D, et al. Indeterminate mediastinal invasion in bronchogenic carcinoma: CT evaluation. Radiology 1989;173(1):37–42.
74. Dougherty B, Jersmann HP, Robinson PC, Nguyen P. Staging the mediastinum: what is current best practice? Lung Cancer Management 2013;2(2):153–62.
75. Herman SJ, Winton TL, Weisbrod GL, et al. Mediastinal invasion by bronchogenic carcinoma: CT signs. Radiology 1994; 190(3):841–6.
76. Allen MS, Mathisen DJ, Grillo HC, et al. Bronchogenic carcinoma with chest wall invasion. Ann Thorac Surg 1991;51(6): 948–51.
77. Ratto G, Piacenza G, Frola C, et al. Chest wall involvement by lung cancer: computed tomographic detection and results of operation. Ann Thorac Surg 1991;51(2):182–8.
78. Pearlberg JL, Sandier MA, Beute GH, et al. Limitations of CT in evaluation of neoplasms involving chest wall. J Comput Assist Tomogr 1987;11(2):290–3.
79. Scott I, Müller N, Miller R, et al. Resectable stage III lung cancer: CT, surgical, and pathologic correlation. Radiology 1988;166(1): 75–9.
80. Pauls S, Schmidt SA, Juchems MS, et al. Diffusion-weighted MR imaging in comparison to integrated [^{18}F]-FDG PET/CT for N-staging in patients with lung cancer. Eur J Radiol 2012;81(1): 178–82.
81. Suzuki N, Saitoh T, Kitamura S. Tumor invasion of the chest wall in lung cancer: diagnosis with US. Radiology 1993;187(1): 39–42.
82. Webb W, Gatsonis C, Zerhouni E, et al. CT and MR imaging in staging non-small cell bronchogenic carcinoma: report of the Radiologic Diagnostic Oncology Group. Radiology 1991;178(3): 705–13.
83. Primack SL, Lee KS, Logan PM, et al. Bronchogenic carcinoma: utility of CT in the evaluation of patients with suspected lesions. Radiology 1994;193(3):795–800.
84. McLoud T, Bourgouin P, Greenberg R, et al. Bronchogenic carcinoma: analysis of staging in the mediastinum with CT by correlative lymph node mapping and sampling. Radiology 1992; 182(2):319–23.
85. Buy J, Ghossain MA, Poirson F, et al. Computed tomography of mediastinal lymph nodes in nonsmall cell lung cancer: a new approach based on the lymphatic pathway of tumor spread. J Comput Assist Tomogr 1998;12(4):545.
86. Ikezoe J, Kadowaki K, Morimoto S, et al. Mediastinal lymph node metastases from nonsmall cell bronchogenic carcinoma: reevaluation with CT. J Comput Assist Tomogr 1990;14(3):340–4.
87. Koyama H, Ohno Y, Seki S, et al. Magnetic resonance imaging for lung cancer. J Thorac Imaging 2013;28(3):138–50.
88. Jeon TY, Lee KS, Chin AY, et al. Incremental value of PET/CT over CT for mediastinal nodal staging of non-small cell lung cancer: comparison between patients with and without idiopathic pulmonary fibrosis. Am J Roentgenol 2010;195(2):370–6.
89. Gilbert C, Yarmus L, Feller-Kopman D. Use of endobronchial ultrasound and endoscopic ultrasound to stage the mediastinum in early-stage lung cancer. J Natl Compr Canc Netw 2012; 10(10):1277–82.
90. Kalemkerian GP, Gadgeel SM. Modern staging of small cell lung cancer. J Natl Compr Canc Netw 2013;11(1):99–104.
91. Caulo A, Mirsadraee S, Maggi F, et al. Integrated imaging of non-small cell lung cancer recurrence: CT and PET-CT findings, possible pitfalls and risk of recurrence criteria. Eur Radiol 2012;22(3):588–606.
92. Gambhir S, Hoh C, Phelps M, et al. Decision tree sensitivity analysis for cost-effectiveness of FDG-PET in the staging and management of non-small-cell lung carcinoma. J Nucl Med 1996;37(9):1428–36.
93. Alkhawaldeh K, Biersack H, Henke A, Ezziddin S. Impact of dual-time-point F-18 FDG PET/CT in the assessment of pleural effusion in patients with non-small-cell lung cancer. Clin Nucl Med 2011;36(6):423.
94. Davis S, Henschke C, Chamides B, Westcott J. Intrathoracic Kaposi sarcoma in AIDS patients: radiographic-pathologic correlation. Radiology 1987;163(2):495–500.
95. Sivit CJ, Schwartz AM, Rockoff S. Kaposi's sarcoma of the lung in AIDS: radiologic-pathologic analysis. Am J Roentgenol 1987; 148(1):25–8.
96. Naidich D, Tarras M, Garay S, et al. Kaposi's sarcoma. CT-radiographic correlation. Chest 1989;96(4):723–8.
97. Zibrak JD, Silvestri RC, Costello P, et al. Bronchoscopic and radiologic features of Kaposi's sarcoma involving the respiratory system. Chest 1986;90(4):476–9.
98. Carney JA. The triad of gastric epithelioid leiomyosarcoma, pulmonary chondroma, and functioning extra-adrenal paraganglioma: a five-year review. Medicine 1983;62(3):159–69.
99. Mazas-Artasona L, Romeo M, Felices R, et al. Gastro-oesophageal leiomyoblastomas and multiple pulmonary chondromas: an incomplete variant of Carney's triad. Br J Radiol 1988;61(732): 1181–4.
100. Poirier T, Van Ordstrand HS. Pulmonary chondromatous hamartomas: report of seventeen cases and review of the literature. Chest 1971;59(1):50–5.
101. Bateson EM, Abbott EK. Mixed tumours of the lung, or hamartochondromas: A review of the radiological appearances of cases published in the literature and a report of fifteen new cases. Clin Radiol 1960;11(4):232–46.
102. Siegelman S, Khouri N, Scott W, et al. Pulmonary hamartoma: CT findings. Radiology 1986;160(2):313–17.
103. Morgan DE, Sanders C, McElvein RB, et al. Intrapulmonary teratoma: a case report and review of the literature. J Thorac Imaging 1992;7(3):70.

104. Katzenstein AA, Gmelich JT, Carrington CB. Sclerosing hemangioma of the lung: a clinicopathologic study of 51 cases. Am J Surg Pathol 1980;4(4):343–56.
105. Sugio K, Yokoyama H, Kaneko S, et al. Sclerosing hemangioma of the lung: radiographic and pathological study. Ann Thorac Surg 1992;53(2):295–300.
106. Park CM, Goo JM, Lee HJ, et al. Tumors in the tracheobronchial tree: CT and FDG PET features. Radiographics 2009;29(1): 55–71.
107. Pipavath SJ, Lynch DA, Cool C, et al. Radiologic and pathologic features of bronchiolitis. Am J Roentgenol 2005;185(2):354–63.
108. Howling SJ, Hansell DM, Wells AU, et al. Follicular bronchiolitis: thin-section CT and histologic findings. Radiology 1999; 212(3):637–42.
109. Abdulqadhr G, Molin D, Åström G, et al. Whole-body diffusion-weighted imaging compared with FDG-PET/CT in staging of lymphoma patients. Acta Radiol 2011;52(2):173–80.
110. Au V, Leung AN. Radiologic manifestations of lymphoma in the thorax. Am J Roentgenol 1997;168(1):93–8.
111. Lee KS, Kim Y, Primack SL. Imaging of pulmonary lymphomas. Am J Roentgenol 1997;168(2):339–45.
112. Dunnick NR, Parker BR, Castellino RA. Rapid onset of pulmonary infiltration due to histiocytic lymphoma. Radiology 1976; 118(2):281–5.
113. Muller NL, Fraser RS, Lee KS, Johkoh T. Diseases of the Lung: Radiologic and Pathologic Correlations. Philadelphia: Lippincott Williams and Wilkins; 2003.
114. King L, Padley S, Wotherspoon A, Nicholson A. Pulmonary MALT lymphoma: imaging findings in 24 cases. Eur Radiol 2000;10(12):1932–8.
115. Lee DK, Im J, Lee KS, et al. B-cell lymphoma of bronchus-associated lymphoid tissue (BALT): CT features in 10 patients. J Comput Assist Tomogr 2000;24(1):30–4.
116. Maile CW, Moore AV, Ulreich S, Putman CE. Chest radiographic–pathologic correlation in adult leukemia patients. Invest Radiol 1983;18(6):495–9.
117. Heyneman LE, Johkoh T, Ward S, et al. Pulmonary leukemic infiltrates: high-resolution CT findings in 10 patients. Am J Roentgenol 2000;174(2):517–21.
118. Siegel M, Shackelford G, McAlister W. Pleural thickening. An unusual feature of childhood leukemia. Radiology 1981;138(2): 367–9.
119. Van Buchem M, Wondergem J, Kool L, et al. Pulmonary leukostasis: radiologic–pathologic study. Radiology 1987;165(3): 739–41.
120. Vernant J, Brun B, Mannoni P, Dreyfus B. Respiratory distress of hyperleukocytic granulocytic leukemias. Cancer 1979;44(1): 264–8.
121. Coppage L, Shaw C, Curtis AM. Metastatic disease to the chest in patients with extrathoracic malignancy. J Thorac Imaging 1987;2(4):24–37.
122. Chaudhuri MR. Primary pulmonary cavitating carcinomas. Thorax 1973;28(3):354–66.
123. Ishihara T, Kikuchi K, Ikeda T, Yamazaki S. Metastatic pulmonary diseases: biologic factors and modes of treatment. Chest 1973; 63(2):227–32.
124. Schaner EG, Chang AE, Doppman JL, et al. Comparison of computed and conventional whole lung tomography in detecting pulmonary nodules: a prospective radiologic-pathologic study. Am J Roentgenol 1978;131(1):51–4.
125. Janower ML, Blennerhassett JB. Lymphangitic spread of metastatic cancer to the lung: a radiologic–pathologic classification. Radiology 1971;101(2):267–73.
126. Munk P, Müller N, Miller R, Ostrow D. Pulmonary lymphangitic carcinomatosis: CT and pathologic findings. Radiology 1988; 166(3):705–9.
127. Ren H, Hruban RH, Kuhlman JE, et al. Computed tomography of inflation-fixed lungs: the beaded septum sign of pulmonary metastases. J Comput Assist Tomogr 1989;13(3):411.
128. Stein M, Mayo J, Müller N, et al. Pulmonary lymphangitic spread of carcinoma: appearance on CT scans. Radiology 1987;162(2): 371–5.
129. Baumgartner WA, Mark JB. Metastatic malignancies from distant sites to the tracheobronchial tree. J Thorac Cardiovasc Surg 1980;79(4):499–503.

CHAPTER 9

High-Resolution Computed Tomography of Interstitial and Occupational Lung Disease

Nicola Sverzellati • Zelena A. Aziz • David M. Hansell

CHAPTER OUTLINE

The pulmonary interstitium is the network of connective tissue fibres that supports the lung. It includes the alveolar walls, interlobular septa and the peribronchovascular interstitium. The term interstitial lung disease (ILD) is used to refer to a group of disorders that mainly affects these supporting structures. Although the majority of these disorders also involve the air spaces, the *predominant* abnormality is usually thickening of the interstitium which may be due to the accumulation of fluid, cells, or fibrous tissue.

The chest radiograph remains part of the initial assessment of ILD, but the radiographic pattern is often non-specific, observer variation is considerable and it is relatively insensitive to early ILD.[1,2] High-resolution computed tomography (HRCT) has revolutionised the imaging of ILD as it enables early detection of disease, allows a histospecific diagnosis to be made in certain cases, and provides insights into disease reversibility and prognosis.

HIGH-RESOLUTION COMPUTED TOMOGRAPHY PATTERNS OF DIFFUSE LUNG DISEASE

Before considering the individual HRCT patterns related to each ILD, an understanding of normal lung anatomy is needed. In addition, radiologists should refer to a common terminology outlined in the Fleischner Glossary to describe HRCT abnormalities.[3] Diffuse abnormalities of the lung on HRCT may be broadly classified into one of the following four patterns: (A) reticular or linear; (B) nodular; (C) ground-glass opacity through to consolidation; and (D) areas of decreased lung attenuation.

Reticular Pattern

A reticular pattern on CT almost always represents significant ILD. Morphologically, a reticular pattern may be caused by thickened interlobular or intralobular septa or honeycomb (fibrotic) destruction. Numerous thickened interlobular septa indicate an extensive interstitial abnormality and causes include infiltration by fibrosis (interstitial fibrosis), abnormal cells (lymphangitis carcinomatosa), or fluid (pulmonary oedema). Although thickened interlobular septa can be a consequence of infiltration by fibrosis, this feature is not a frequent finding in idiopathic pulmonary fibrosis (IPF). Interlobular septal thickening is usually described as smooth (seen in pulmonary oedema and alveolar proteinosis) or irregular (e.g. lymphangitic spread of tumour), but the distinction is not always easily made. Sarcoidosis causes nodular septal thickening, although this pattern is not usually the dominant feature of parenchymal involvement.[4]

In some diseases, a perilobular distribution may give the spurious impression of thickening of the interlobular septa. However, such a pattern reflects a pathologic process that is 'smeared' around the internal lobular surface and is most frequently associated with organising pneumonia.[3,5]

Intralobular septal thickening manifests as a fine reticular pattern on HRCT and is seen in all ILDs but most commonly in IPF. Often, the intralobular septal thickening may be so fine that HRCT does not demonstrate discrete intralobular opacities but a generalised increase in lung density (ground-glass opacification). Severe pulmonary fibrosis usually results in a coarse reticular pattern made up of interlacing irregular linear opacities. The reticular pattern of end-stage fibrotic (honeycomb) lung is characterised by cystic air spaces surrounded by irregular walls. The certain identification of honeycombing, as opposed to other forms of reticulation, is not always straightforward but is of particular relevance as it may directly impact patient care.[3] The distortion of normal lung morphology by extensive fibrosis results in irregular dilatation of segmental and subsegmental airways (traction bronchiectasis/bronchiolectasis); in the periphery of the lung, it can be difficult to distinguish dilated airways from true honeycomb destruction.

Nodular Pattern

A nodular pattern is a feature of both interstitial and airspace diseases. The distribution and density of nodules may help narrow what can be a lengthy differential diagnosis.[6] Nodules within the lung interstitium, especially those related to the lymphatic vessels, are seen in the interlobular septa, subpleural and peribronchovascular regions; this distribution is seen most frequently in sarcoidosis but also in lymphangitis carcinomatosa. Centrilobular nodules are seen in several conditions (Table 9-1). Distinguishing between subacute hypersensitivity pneumonitis and respiratory bronchiolitis–interstitial lung disease can be difficult, because both cause relatively low-density, poorly defined centrilobular nodules which may look identical on HRCT. A random distribution of very small well-defined nodules is seen in patients with haematogenous spread of tuberculosis, pulmonary metastases, pneumoconiosis and rarely sarcoidosis.

Ground-Glass Pattern

A ground-glass pattern on HRCT is defined as a generalised increase in opacity that does not obscure pulmonary vessels.[3] At a microscopic level, the changes responsible for ground-glass opacity are complex and include partial filling of the air spaces, considerable thickening of the interstitium, or a combination of the two. Ultimately though, the pattern of ground-glass opacity on HRCT results from displacement of air from the lungs. Indeed, ground-glass opacity may be found in many conditions, either as the predominant or as an ancillary pattern. A predominant ground-glass pattern may be seen in subacute hypersensitivity pneumonitis, acute respiratory distress syndrome (ARDS), acute interstitial pneumonia (AIP), non-specific interstitial pneumonia (NSIP) and some infections, notably viral pneumonias, and *Pneumocystis jiroveci*.

TABLE 9-1 Conditions Characterised by Profuse Centrilobular Nodules on HRCT

- Subacute hypersensitivity pneumonitis
- Respiratory bronchiolitis–interstitial lung disease
- Diffuse panbronchiolitis
- Endobronchial spread of tuberculosis or bacterial pneumonia
- Cryptogenic organising pneumonia (unusual pattern)

Mosaic Attenuation Pattern

The term 'mosaic attenuation pattern', or more simply mosaic pattern, refers to regional attenuation differences demonstrated on HRCT. The attenuation of a given area of lung depends on the amount of blood, parenchymal tissue and air in that area, and thus the sign of a mosaic attenuation pattern is non-specific. It is the dominant abnormality in three completely different types of diffuse pulmonary disease: small airways disease, chronic occlusive vascular disease and infiltrative lung disease. In the first two processes, the decreased attenuation ('black') lung is abnormal; in infiltrative lung disease it is the 'grey' lung that is abnormal. In a study of 70 patients in whom a mosaic attenuation pattern was the dominant abnormality, Worthy et al. showed that small airways disease and infiltrative lung disease were correctly identified but the mosaic attenuation pattern caused by occlusive vascular disease was frequently misinterpreted.[7] Bronchial abnormalities and, to a lesser extent, the presence of air trapping on expiratory CT are the most useful discriminatory features in identifying small airways disease as the cause of mosaic attenuation. However, the phenomenon of hypoxic bronchodilatation in chronic occlusive vascular disease, and the fact that air trapping may be seen on expiratory CT in chronic thromboembolic disease, complicates interpretation.[8] Nevertheless, the differentiation between the three basic causes of a mosaic attenuation pattern is usually easily made when clinical and physiological information is taken into account.

IDIOPATHIC INTERSTITIAL PNEUMONIAS

The term idiopathic interstitial pneumonia (IIP) is applied to a group of disorders with no known cause, and with more or less distinct histological and radiological appearances.[9] In the updated American Thoracic Society (ATS)/European Respiratory Society (ERS) consensus classification of the IIPs, the overall architecture of the classification is preserved (Table 9-2), but the clinical entity, rather than the histopathological label, is given pre-eminence. In addition, an entity termed idiopathic pleuroparenchymal fibroelastosis (IPPFE) is included.[10,11] The authors of the updated classification again recommend a multidisciplinary and dynamic approach to the diagnosis of the IIPs which encourages interaction between clinicians, radiologists and pathologists.

Usual Interstitial Pneumonia/Idiopathic Pulmonary Fibrosis

The term idiopathic pulmonary fibrosis (IPF) is applied to patients with a histologic and/or computed tomography (CT) pattern of usual interstitial pneumonia (UIP)

TABLE 9-2 **Histological and Clinical Classification of the Idiopathic Interstitial Pneumonias**

Clinico-Radiological-Pathological Criteria	Histological Pattern	HRCT Features
Idiopathic pulmonary fibrosis	Usual interstitial pneumonia	Reticular opacities Honeycombing Areas of ground-glass opacity associated with traction bronchiectasis
Non-specific interstitial pneumonia	Non-specific interstitial pneumonia	Areas of ground-glass opacity ± traction bronchiectasis Honeycombing minimal
Cryptogenic organising pneumonia	Organising pneumonia	Peripheral or peribronchial consolidation Areas of ground-glass opacity Perilobular pattern (increasingly recognised)
Acute interstitial pneumonia	Diffuse alveolar damage	Consolidation (dependent lung) Areas of ground-glass opacity Traction bronchiectasis (organising phase)
Respiratory bronchiolitis–interstitial lung disease (RB–ILD)	RB–ILD	Poorly defined centrilobular nodules Areas of ground-glass opacity Bronchial wall thickening Limited emphysema
Desquamative interstitial pneumonia (DIP)	DIP	Areas of ground-glass opacity Features of interstitial fibrosis
Lymphoid interstitial pneumonia (LIP)	LIP	Areas of ground-glass opacity Centrilobular nodules Thickened interlobular septa Thin-walled discrete cysts

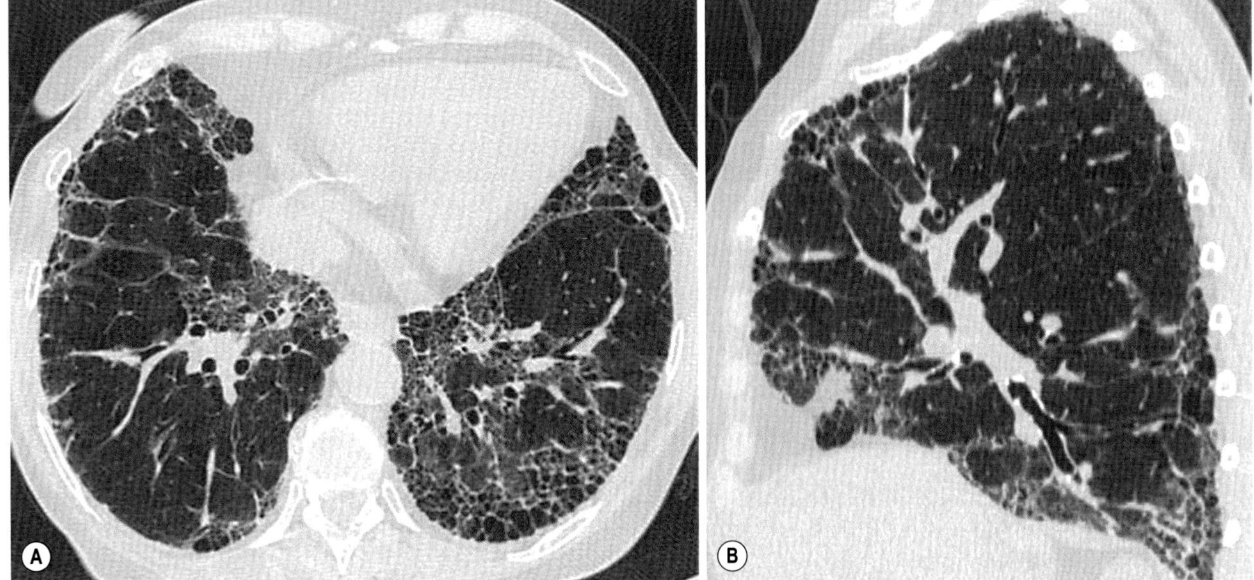

FIGURE 9-1 ■ **Usual interstitial pneumonia.** (A) HRCT abnormalities predominate in the posterior, subpleural regions of the lower lobes and comprise patchy honeycombing and traction bronchiectasis within the abnormal lung. (B) Sagittal reformation shows the abnormalities creeping up the periphery into the anterior zones of the upper lobes.

and compatible clinical and imaging features.[12] Other causes of a UIP-type pattern on histology include chronic hypersensitivity pneumonitis, asbestosis, connective tissue disease and rarely drugs. The pathological features of UIP are the presence of fibroblastic foci, normal areas, dense fibrosis and honeycombing; the crucial finding is of areas of fibrosis at different stages of maturity. The characteristic and virtually pathognomonic appearance of UIP on HRCT is of a predominantly subpleural bibasal reticular pattern within which there are areas of honeycomb destruction. As the disease progresses, it often appears to 'creep' around the periphery of the lung to involve the anterior aspects of the upper lobes (Fig. 9-1). The presence of ground-glass opacification is not a dominant feature and, when present, there is usually obvious traction bronchiectasis and bronchiolectasis.[13] Mediastinal lymphadenopathy (up to approximately 2.5 cm) unrelated to infection or malignancy is a frequent accompaniment.[14]

In the appropriate clinical setting, the presence of a classical UIP pattern on HRCT is sufficient for the diagnosis of IPF, without the need for surgical biopsy. Therefore, the primary role of HRCT is to separate patients with UIP from those with non-UIP pattern as they may have a substantially different prognosis. A confident HRCT diagnosis of UIP is not usually made unless

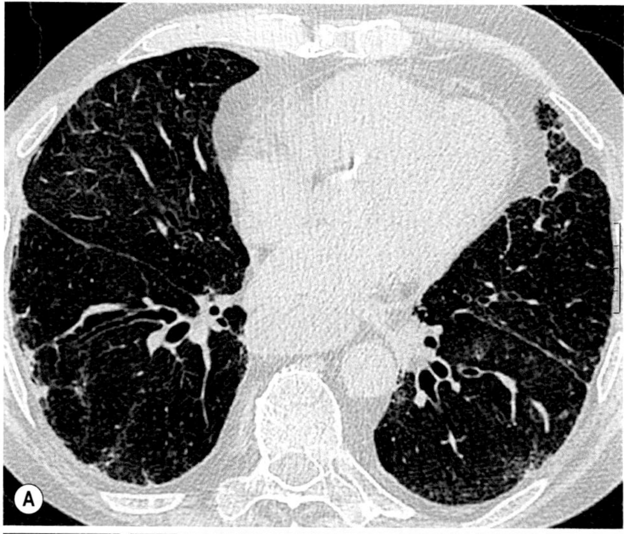

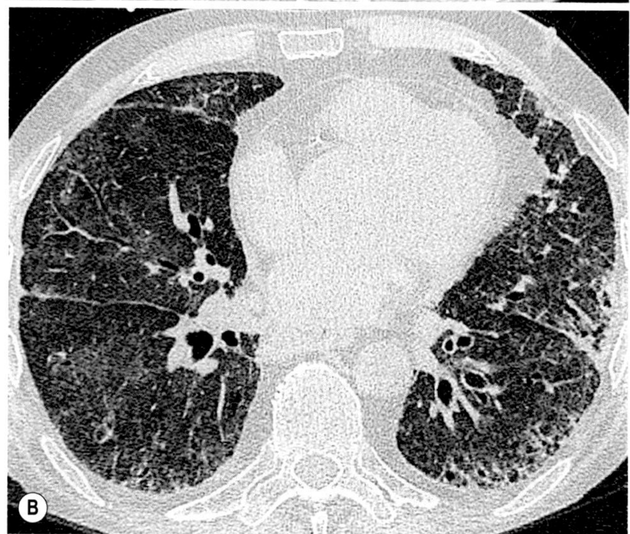

FIGURE 9-2 ■ **Biopsy-proven usual interstitial pneumonia.** HRCT performed (A) before and (B) after clinical deterioration in a biopsy-proven usual interstitial pneumonia associated with a HRCT pattern more akin with non-specific interstitial pneumonia. HRCT obtained during the accelerated phase of the disease demonstrates a generalised increase in lung attenuation and progression of both the reticular and honeycomb patterns.

honeycombing is present. If honeycombing is absent, but the imaging features otherwise meet criteria for UIP (especially when the pattern is characterised by reticular opacities in predominantly peripheral and basal distribution), the imaging features are regarded as representing possible UIP, and surgical lung biopsy is necessary to make a definitive diagnosis.[12] However, in patients whose HRCT does not demonstrate either a classical or a possible UIP pattern, the surgical lung biopsy may still demonstrate UIP pattern on histopathology. The majority of these atypical UIP cases are usually characterised by predominant ground-glass opacity. Thus, their HRCT appearances frequently mimic non-specific interstitial pneumonia (NSIP) (Fig. 9-2).[15,16] HRCT has also a role in predicting survival. A study by Flaherty et al. suggested that patients with histological UIP who had definite UIP by HRCT criteria had a worse prognosis than

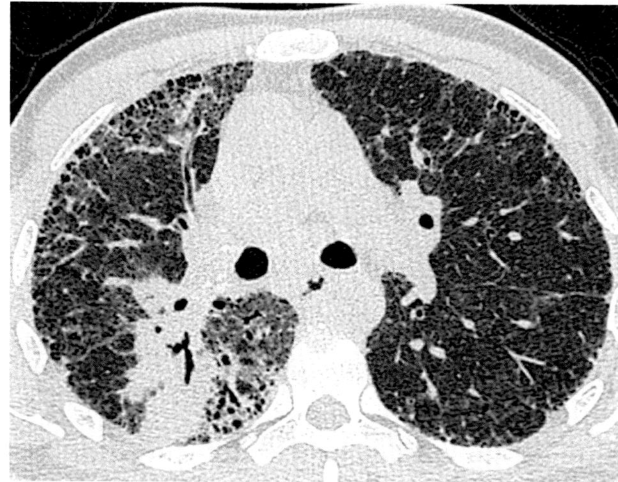

FIGURE 9-3 ■ **Tuberculosis on a background of usual interstitial pneumonia.** Biopsy of the area of consolidation in the right lower lobe confirmed tuberculosis.

those who had interdeterminate (or atypical) HRCT findings.[15] The extent of fibrosis, traction bronchiectasis and honeycombing on HRCT are also predictive of both survival and mortality in IPF.[13,17]

The rapid development of a diffuse increase in the attenuation of lung parenchyma in patients with IPF should raise the possibility of an accelerated phase (also known as an acute exacerbation) of the disease (Fig. 9-2), concurrent pulmonary oedema, or rarely an atypical infection.[12,18] Other complications include lung cancer and pulmonary tuberculosis (Fig. 9-3); the latter usually has atypical appearances on CT caused by the presence of underlying lung fibrosis.[19,20]

Classic HRCT Findings

- Subpleural basal honeycombing
- Ground-glass opacity not predominant
- Subpleural disease in the upper lobes (if present) tends to be anterior

Non-Specific Interstitial Pneumonia

Non-specific interstitial pneumonia (NSIP) is characterised by varying degrees of interstitial inflammation and fibrosis without the specific features that allow a diagnosis of UIP.[21] While NSIP may have significant fibrosis, it is usually temporally uniform (in comparison to UIP), and fibroblastic foci and honeycombing are absent or scanty. Although the clinical features of idiopathic NSIP resemble those of UIP, prognosis is considerably better. Non-idiopathic NSIP is most often found on lung biopsy in patients with connective tissue disease and may be the predominant histopathological pattern in some cases of drug-induced lung disease and chronic hypersensitivity pneumonitis. On HRCT, ground glass with or without associated distortion of airways is usually the dominant pattern (Fig. 9-4). Reticular abnormalities are common, but honeycombing is sparse or absent even when other signs of fibrotic changes are evident. Abnormalities are

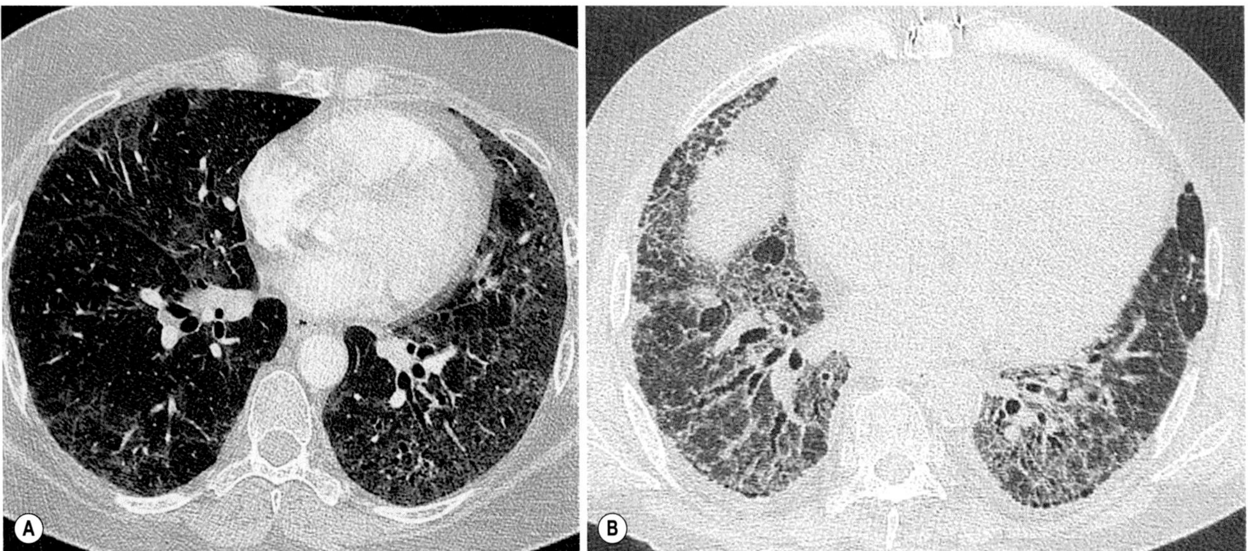

FIGURE 9-4 ■ **Non-specific interstitial pneumonia.** (A) The predominant abnormality is patchy, bilateral ground-glass opacification, mild reticulation and traction bronchiectasis. (B) In this fibrotic form, reticulation is more extensive and traction bronchiectasis more severe. However, there is no frank honeycombing destruction.

usually peribronchovascular or peripheral, although they may sometimes spare the subpleural lung.[21] In general, NSIP may be distinguished from UIP on CT by a more prominent component of ground-glass attenuation and a finer reticular pattern in the absence of honeycombing.[22] However, the variability of CT appearances reflects the heterogeneity of the pathological processes encompassed by NSIP and a confident diagnosis of NSIP based on CT alone is less readily made than in cases of UIP. Consolidation is reportedly a highly variable feature (0–98%) and this discrepancy probably reflects the fact that some patients with non-idiopathic NSIP have significant amounts of histological organising pneumonia, making classification of individual cases difficult.[23]

Classic HRCT Findings

- Bilateral ground-glass opacities and superimposed fine reticulation
- Predominantly peripheral, but also patchy or band-like
- Honeycomb pattern minimal or absent
- Traction bronchiectasis and bronchiolectasis

Cryptogenic Organising Pneumonia

This is considered in the section on airspace disease.

Respiratory Bronchiolitis–Interstitial Lung Disease and Desquamative Interstitial Pneumonia

These two entities are considered together because of their strong association with cigarette smoking. All cigarette smokers have, to some degree, inflammation around their small airways ('respiratory bronchiolitis') but this is clinically unimportant and not considered further here.

Patients with respiratory bronchiolitis–interstitial lung disease generally present with an insiduous onset of dyspnoea and cough. The chest radiograph is relatively insensitive for the detection of RB–ILD and desquamative interstitial pneumonia (DIP) and a normal chest radiograph has been reported in up to 20% of patients with RB–ILD and 25% in DIP.[24,25]

On HRCT, the features of RB–ILD include areas of patchy ground-glass opacification (resulting from macrophage accumulation within alveolar spaces and alveolar ducts) and poorly defined low-attenuation centrilobular nodules (Fig. 9-5). In addition, upper lobe centrilobular emphysema, usually of very limited extent, and areas of air trapping may be present, the latter reflecting the bronchiolitic element of this entity.[26] Some patients may show scattered thickening of the interlobular septa and features of interstitial fibrosis, but this is not the dominant pattern.[27]

Ground-glass opacification is the dominant feature seen in DIP (Fig. 9-6). The distribution is typically lower zone, peripheral and may be patchy or geographic.[28] In some patients there are HRCT features of established fibrosis (in the form of architectural distortion with dilatation of some bronchi), usually of limited extent. The majority of patients with DIP or RB–ILD have a relatively stable clinical course. Smoking cessation is an important part of the management of patients, but the influence of smoking on the clinical course of these patients has not been fully delineated; some patients have persistent abnormalities on HRCT even with smoking cessation and corticosteroid therapy. Because of the significant overlap between the clinical, imaging and histological features of DIP and RB–ILD and to a lesser extent between these two patterns and Langerhans cell histiocytosis (LCH) and interstitial fibrosis, the global term 'smoking related-interstitial lung disease' (SR-ILD) has been proposed to encompass DIP, RB–ILD, LCH and interstitial fibrosis (Fig. 9-7).[27,29]

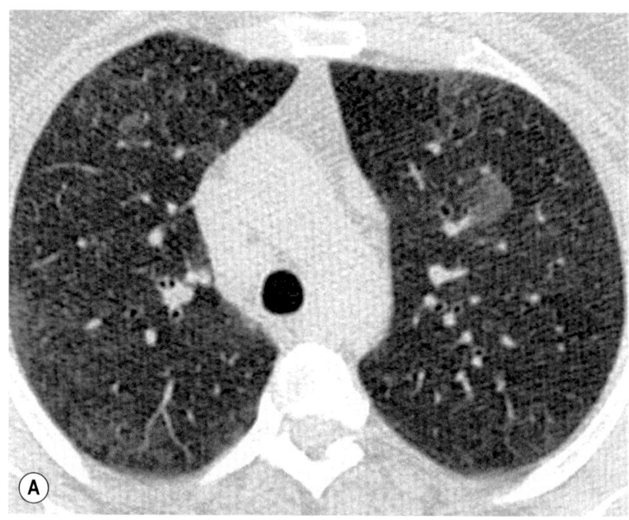

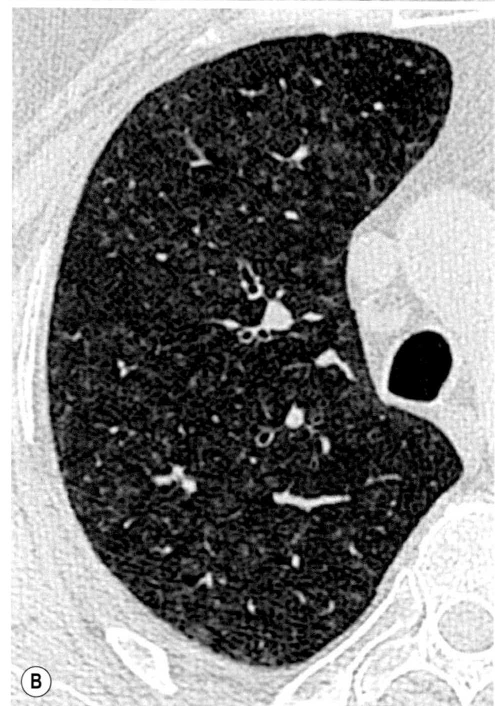

FIGURE 9-5 ■ **Respiratory bronchiolitis–interstitial lung disease.** HRCT shows (A) subtle areas of ground-glass opacification and (B) ill-defined centrilobular nodules.

Classic HRCT Findings

- Inconspicuous poorly defined centrilobular nodules of ground-glass opacification in symptomatic smokers are suggestive of RB–ILD
- Non-specific extensive ground-glass opacities, usually lower zone, with or without associated mild reticulation, are typical features of DIP

Acute Interstitial Pneumonia/Diffuse Alveolar Damage

Acute interstitial pneumonia can be regarded as an idiopathic form of ARDS and is histologically (and clinically) distinct from the other interstitial pneumonias.[9] The histological pattern seen in AIP is that of diffuse alveolar damage (DAD), which is also found in infection, connective tissue disease, drug toxicity and toxic fume inhalation. DAD has an acute exudative phase and a subsequent organising and fibrotic phase. Lung biopsy shows diffuse involvement with temporal homogeneity, which implies lung injury due to a single event. The chest radiograph shows bilateral patchy airspace opacification.[30] HRCT demonstrates a combination of ground-glass opacification, consolidation, bronchial dilatation and architectural distortion.[31] Ground-glass opacification on HRCT is found in all three phases of AIP, but coexistent traction bronchiectasis probably reflects the early incorporation of established fibrosis.[32] Follow-up CT shows reticular opacities consistent with residual fibrosis. Anterior non-dependent fibrotic damage in survivors secondary to barotrauma has also been reported.[33]

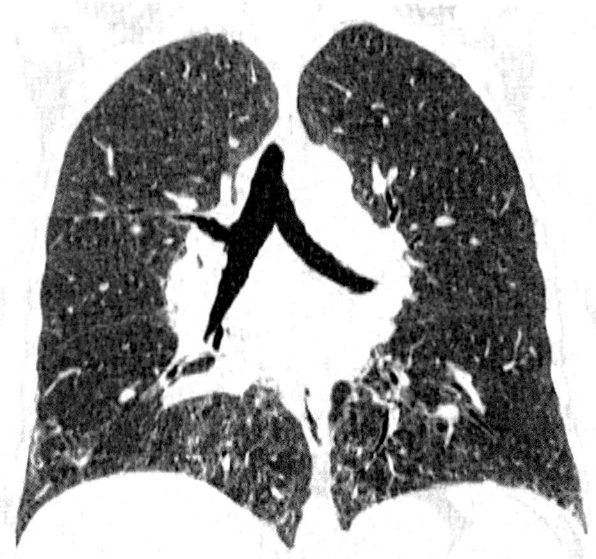

FIGURE 9-6 ■ **Biopsy-proven DIP.** Several areas of non-specific reticulation and ground-glass opacification in both lower lobes.

Classic HRCT Findings

- Patchy or diffuse ground-glass opacities and consolidation/collapse (the latter mainly in dependent lung)
- Traction bronchiectasis and reticulation may become evident after several days

Lymphoid Interstitial Pneumonia

The term ‘lymphoid interstitial pneumonia’ (LIP) was proposed by Liebow and Carrington to describe a disease entity characterised by a widespread interstitial lymphoid infiltrate of the lung, resembling lymphoma but with a clinical course more akin to a chronic interstitial pneumonia. Although in the past LIP has been considered by some to be a pulmonary lymphoproliferative disorder, evolution to frank lymphoproliferative disease is rare and thus LIP remains within the group of interstitial pneumonias.[9,34] Classically, LIP occurs in association with

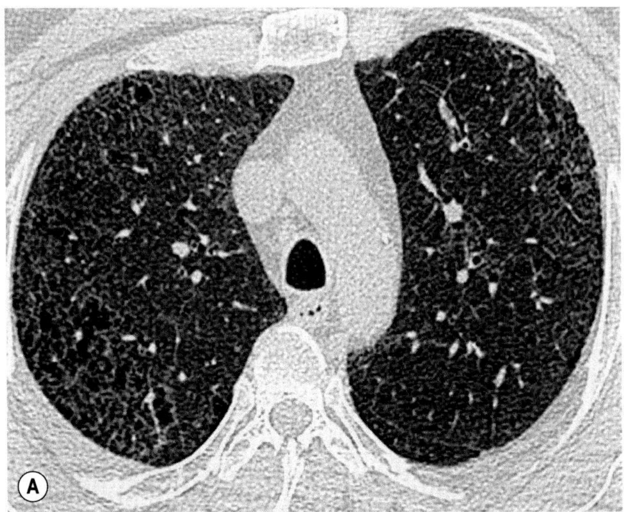

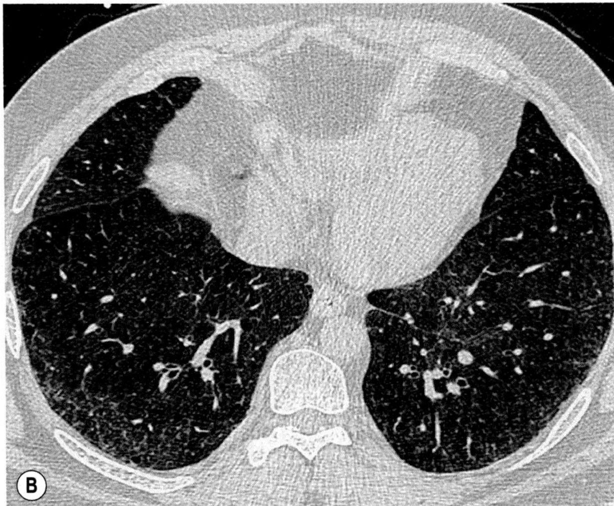

FIGURE 9-7 ■ **Smoking related-interstitial lung disease.** (A) Upper and (B) lower lobes of a 42-year-old man with a 25 pack-year smoking history and dyspnoea. The combination of a fine reticular pattern representing fibrosis and ground-glass opacification on a background of emphysema suggests a diagnosis of smoking related-interstitial lung disease.

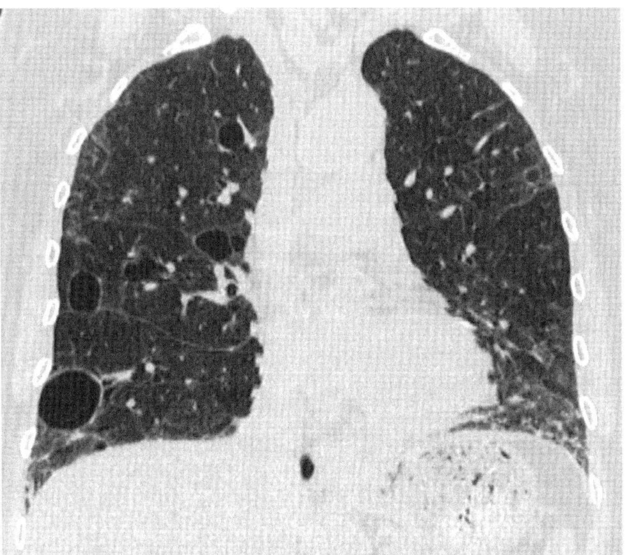

FIGURE 9-8 ■ **Lymphoid interstitial pneumonitis.** There are patchy ground-glass opacities and a few thin-walled cystic air spaces in the right lung.

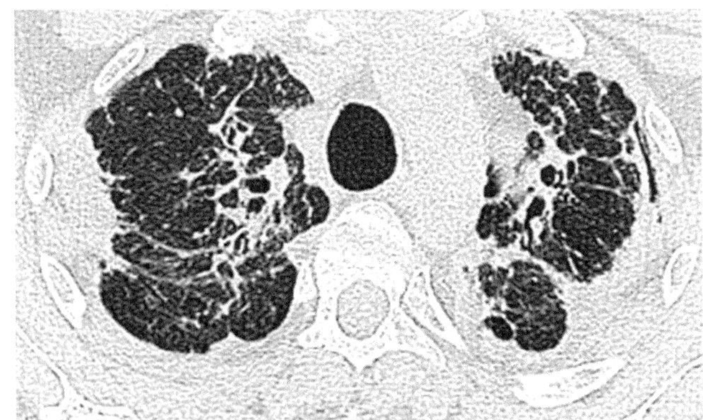

FIGURE 9-9 ■ **Idiopathic pleuroparenchymal fibroelastosis.** HRCT through the upper lobes shows bilateral irregular pleural thickening and a subjacent reticular pattern consistent with fibrosis.

autoimmune diseases, most often Sjögren's syndrome. Other diseases associated with LIP include dysproteinaemias, autologous bone marrow transplantation and viral, mycobacterial and human immunodeficiency virus (HIV) infections.[34] LIP is approximately twice as frequent in women and symptoms of progressive cough and dyspnoea usually predominate. Common HRCT findings are nodules of varying sizes (which may be ill-defined), areas of ground-glass opacification, thickened bronchovascular bundles, interlobular septal thickening and thin-walled cysts (1–30 mm) (Fig. 9-8).[35] Airspace disease, large nodules and pleural effusions are rare in these patients. The cysts in LIP are usually discrete, sometimes clustered and tend not to be subpleural.[36]

Classic HRCT Findings

- Patchy ground-glass opacities, indistinct nodules and thin-walled cysts

Idiopathic Pleuroparenchymal Fibroelastosis

Little is known regarding aetiology of idiopathic pleuroparenchymal fibroelastosis, but recurrent infections are a feature in some patients and a few cases have been reported in association with previous bone marrow or lung transplantation.[37] IPPFE is characterised by dense established intra-alveolar fibrosis containing prominent elastosis, and dense fibrous thickening of the visceral pleura; these changes have a striking upper zone predominance.[10,11] HRCT appearances consist of irregular pleural thickening and 'tags' in the upper zones that merge with fibrotic changes in the subjacent lung (Fig. 9-9; Table 9-3).[10]

Classic HRCT Findings

- Bilateral upper lobe irregular pleural thickening and subjacent reticular pattern

TABLE 9-3 **Causes of Bilateral Upper Lobe Fibrosis**

- Tuberculosis (including atypical mycobacterial infections)
- Sarcoidosis
- Histoplasmosis
- Allergic bronchopulmonary aspergillosis
- Chronic extrinsic allergic alveolitis
- Ankylosing spondylitis
- Progressive massive fibrosis (distinctive mass-like opacities)
- Idiopathic pleuroparenchymal fibroelastosis

SARCOIDOSIS

Sarcoidosis is a multisystem granulomatous disorder of unknown aetiology. As a consequence, the diagnosis of this syndrome is defined by the presence of characteristic clinical and radiological data along with histological evidence of non-caseating granuloma. Granulomas in the lung have a characteristic distribution along the lymphatics in the bronchovascular sheath and, to a lesser extent, in the interlobular septa and subpleural lung regions. Sarcoidosis is a disease of young adults, with a peak incidence in the second to fourth decades. The hilar and mediastinal nodes and the lungs are affected clinically much more commonly than any other organ or system. They are followed in decreasing order of frequency by the skin (26%), peripheral lymph nodes (22%), eyes (15%), spleen (6%), central nervous system (4%), parotid glands (4%) and bones (3%).[38]

Pulmonary involvement accounts for most of the morbidity and mortality associated with sarcoidosis. Sarcoidosis is traditionally staged according to its appearance on the chest radiograph: stage I, lymphadenopathy; stage II, lymphadenopathy with parenchymal opacity; stage III, parenchymal opacity alone.[39] Low stages at presentation are reported to have a better prognosis than high stages, although the precision and clinical usefulness of such 'staging' is questionable.

Lymphadenopathy

Sarcoidosis is characterised by bilateral, symmetrical hilar and paratracheal lymphadenopathy. Some degree of lymphadenopathy is evident on a chest radiograph in about 70–80% of patients at some time during the course of the condition. Hilar lymph node enlargement ranges from the barely detectable to the massive and gives the hila a lobulated and usually well-demarcated outline. Occasionally hilar lymphadenopathy appears to be asymmetrical or, in 1–5% of cases, may even be strictly unilateral although this is distinctly unusual.[40,41]

Paratracheal lymphadenopathy may be bilateral or unilateral and in the latter instance is usually right-sided. The most common manifestation of left-sided lymphadenopathy is enlargement of the aortopulmonary window nodes—a common and characteristic feature on the chest radiograph. Other mediastinal nodes (anterior prevascular, posterior and subcarinal) are often not identified as being enlarged on the chest radiograph but on CT are seen to be affected in about half of patients.[42] In 90% of patients with lymphadenopathy, nodal enlargement is maximal on the first radiograph and usually disappears within 6–12 months. Recurrence of lymphadenopathy is exceedingly rare.[43]

The affected lymph nodes may calcify, sometimes in a characteristic eggshell fashion. This latter feature is shared by only a few conditions such as silicosis and histoplasmosis. The calcification is of variable intensity but may be relatively light, and the affected lymph nodes are usually small in volume and evenly distributed throughout the mediastinum and hila (very different from calcified nodes due to tuberculous infection which usually follow a drainage path).[44] About 40% of patients presenting with nodal enlargement will develop parenchymal opacities, usually within a year, and of these about one-third will go on to have persistent (fibrotic) shadowing. Nodal enlargement does not develop after parenchymal opacities have appeared.

Parenchymal Changes

Parenchymal changes probably occur histologically in the majority of patients but are only detected on the chest radiograph in 50–70% of cases. Characteristically, parenchymal abnormalities appear as the nodal enlargement is subsiding (in lymphoma such abnormalities tend to progress in unison). The most common radiographic pattern, seen in 75–90% of patients with parenchymal opacities, is of rounded or irregular nodules 2–4 mm in diameter, which are usually well defined. Smaller or larger opacities are not uncommon, though they rarely exceed 5 mm. All zones can be affected but there is usually a mid and upper zonal predominance. The second most common pattern, seen in 10–20% of patients with parenchymal opacity, is patchy airspace consolidation. Opacities sometimes contain air bronchograms and have ill-defined margins that commonly break up into a nodular pattern. They tend to involve predominantly the peribronchovascular regions of the middle and upper lung zones, although they may be diffuse or, occasionally, have a subpleural predominance.

The parenchymal opacities described above will clear completely in about two-thirds of cases and progress to fibrosis in one-third. Permanent fibrotic shadowing is unusually coarse, with a mid and upper zone predominance. The radiographic pattern consists of coarse linear opacities with evidence of volume loss and ring shadowing caused by bullae or traction bronchiectasis. Occasionally a conglomerate opacity develops, resembling progressive massive fibrosis. Pulmonary hypertension, bullous disease with or without mycetoma formation, and pneumothorax are all recognised complications of this fibrotic stage.

High-Resolution Computed Tomography Features

Despite the better delineation of parenchymal disease on HRCT, it is not recommended as part of the initial diagnostic work-up in patients with suspected sarcoidosis; its greatest use is in patients who present with an atypical

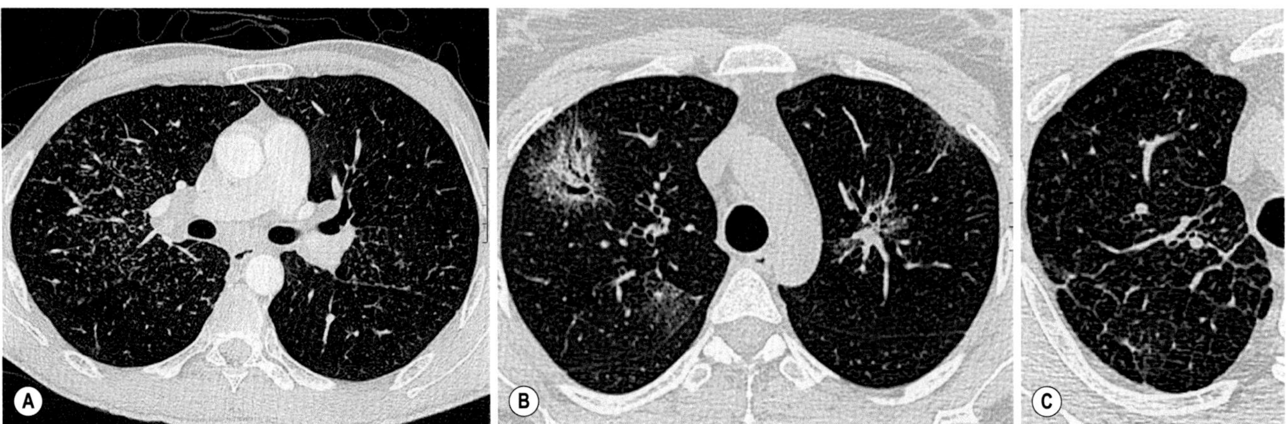

FIGURE 9-10 ■ **Sarcoidosis.** Typical HRCT features are (A) nodular opacities which (B) may become confluent, and (C) interlobular septal thickening.

chest radiograph.[45] Parenchymal opacities are well demonstrated on HRCT (Fig. 9-10) and HRCT appearances have a high sensitivity and specificity for the diagnosis of sarcoidosis.[45,46] The most consistent pulmonary parenchymal abnormality is the presence of nodular opacities (1–5 mm) distributed in a perilymphatic fashion, predominantly along the bronchovascular bundles and subpleurally and, to a lesser extent, along interlobular septa.[46] Other findings include irregular and beaded interfaces, larger ill-defined nodules with/without an air bronchogram, patchy ground-glass opacities and occasional interlobular septal thickening. In advanced disease there is evidence of fibrosis, predominantly in the perihilar regions of the middle and upper lung zones.[47] Air trapping is a common HRCT feature of sarcoidosis and its presence shows a good correlation with indices of small airways disease on pulmonary function tests.[48] Less common parenchymal changes seen in sarcoidosis evolve if the small nodules are confluent to form larger nodules (nodular sarcoidosis, galaxy sign) or if the nodules are so small, being below the resolution of the HRCT, that they appear as areas of ground glass (alveolar sarcoidosis).

Previous HRCT studies have shown that areas of parenchymal consolidation and ground-glass opacity are usually reversible, whereas resolution is not expected in patients showing reticulation and architectural distortion.[49,50] Classic fibrotic changes include linear opacities (radiating laterally from the hilum), fissural displacement, bronchovascular distortion (bronchiectasis) and honeycombing concentrated in the upper zones (Fig. 9-11).[51]

Despite this distinction between reversible and irreversible disease on HRCT, studies comparing HRCT assessment of disease activity to clinical, scintigraphic and bronchoscopic findings have yielded contradictory results.[52] Hence, HRCT is not generally used to guide prognosis in patients with sarcoidosis.

Classic HRCT Findings

- Well-defined, smooth or irregular nodules, measuring 2–4 mm, in a perilymphatic distribution (i.e. mainly along interlobar fissures, peribronchovascular interstitium and interlobular septa), most extensive in the upper lobes
- Bilateral hilar and mediastinal enlarged lymph nodes
- Fibrosis may occur and typically involves the upper lobes

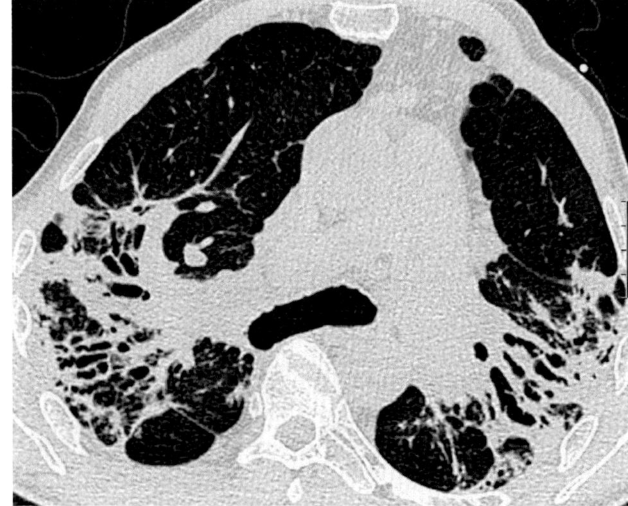

FIGURE 9-11 ■ **Fibrotic sarcoidosis.** There are areas of conglomerate fibrosis in a perihilar distribution with associated bronchial distortion and volume loss. The appearances superficially mimic progressive massive fibrosis seen in the pneumoconioses.

HYPERSENSITIVITY PNEUMONITIS

Hypersensitivity pneumonitis (HP), also known as extrinsic allergic alveolitis (EAA), is an immunologically mediated lung disease characterised by an inflammatory reaction to specific antigens contained in a variety of organic dusts. Common causes include avian proteins (e.g. bird breeder's lung) and thermophilic bacteria present in mouldy hay (farmer's lung), mouldy grain

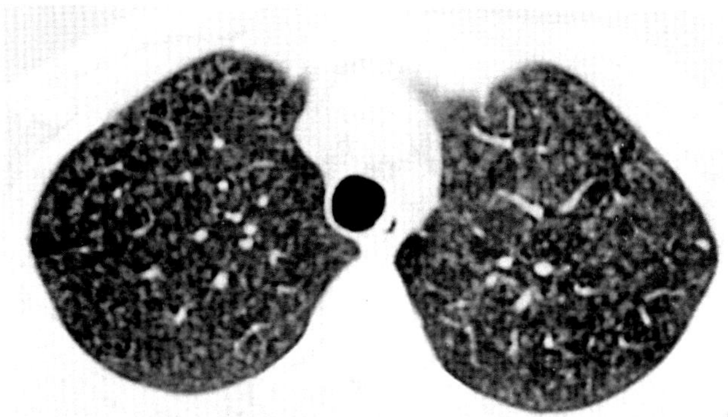

FIGURE 9-12 ■ Subacute extrinsic allergic alveolitis. HRCT shows numerous poorly defined, relatively low-attenuation nodules and ground-glass opacification in the upper lobes.

(grain handler's lung), or heated water reservoirs (humidifier or air conditioner lung).[53] These antigens reach the alveoli where they provoke an immunological reaction that includes both type III (immune complex response) and type IV (cell-mediated) mechanisms. The cell-mediated response results in a delayed hypersensitivity reaction and the presence of granulomatous inflammation within the pulmonary interstitium. Interestingly, several studies have shown that cigarette smoking has a suppressive effect that interferes with the immunopathological process that ultimately leads to HP.[54]

The clinical features of hypersensitivity pneumonitis are characteristic. Approximately 6 h after exposure the patient develops fever, chills, dyspnoea and cough. There is no eosinophilia, and wheeze is not a prominent feature. The radiological findings are influenced by the stage of the disease. Typical HRCT findings include centrilobular nodules, which are typically poorly defined, < 5 mm in diameter, centrilobular and seen throughout the lung, although a mid to lower lung zone predominance has been variably reported (Fig. 9-12).[53,55] Ground-glass opacity is most common in the acute phase but may also be a feature of subacute and chronic HP, especially if there is ongoing exposure.[56] A mosaic attenuation pattern is common in HP; the presence of lobular areas of decreased vascularity that show air trapping on expiratory HRCT reflect the coexisting bronchiolitis caused by antigen deposition in the small airways (Fig. 9-13).[57] The combination on HRCT of features of infiltrative (ill-defined nodules and ground-glass opacity) and small airways disease may be remarkably similar to that seen in patients with RB–ILD; however, the distinction can usually be made with knowledge of the smoking history. The presence of thin-walled lung cysts is also an occasional feature in subacute HP. Cysts range in size from 3 to 25 mm and resemble those seen in lymphoid interstitial pneumonia, although their pathogenesis remains uncertain.[58] Emphysema is a reported sequela of farmer's lung and a study has demonstrated that in hypersensitivity caused by farmer's lung, emphysema was a more prominent feature than honeycombing/fibrosis (even in never smokers) and was seen in approximately one-third of patients.[59] This is in comparison to pigeon breeder's disease, where lung fibrosis is the major complication.

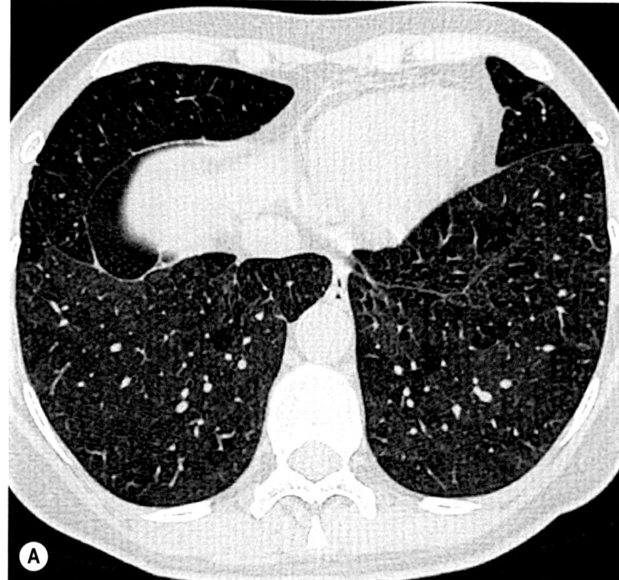

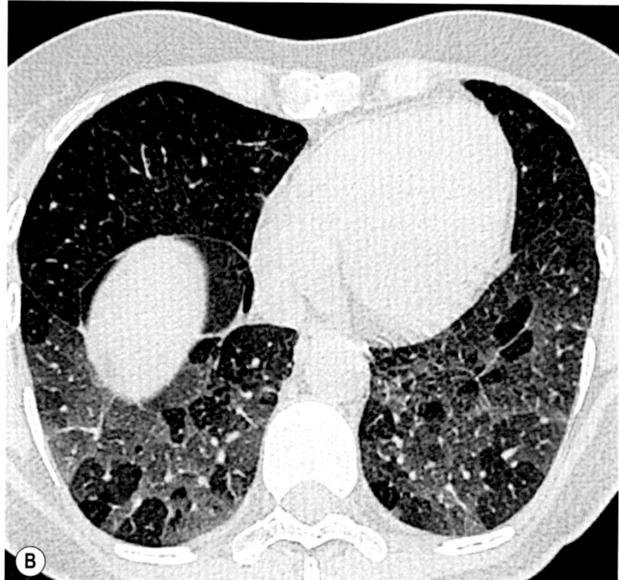

FIGURE 9-13 ■ Hypersensitivity pneumonitis. (A) Inspiratory image shows patchy density differences, reflecting both the interstitial infiltrate of subacute hypersensitivity pneumonitis and coexisting small airways disease. (B) End-expiratory image enhances the density differences, revealing several secondary pulmonary lobules of decreased attenuation.

The chronic stage of HP is characterised by fibrosis, although evidence of active disease is often present. HRCT findings include intralobular and interlobular interstitial thickening, traction bronchiectasis and honeycomb destruction (Fig. 9-14).[60,61] In some cases, there is a mid-zone predominance, but the fibrotic appearance may be seen in the upper or lower lobes.[53,61] Patients with HP may exhibit histological and imaging features of NSIP or UIP, and thus should be considered as a differential diagnosis when either IPF or NSIP is being considered on HRCT appearances.[61,62] Imaging features that favour hypersensitivity pneumonitis over IPF include an upper- or mid-zone predominance, the presence of

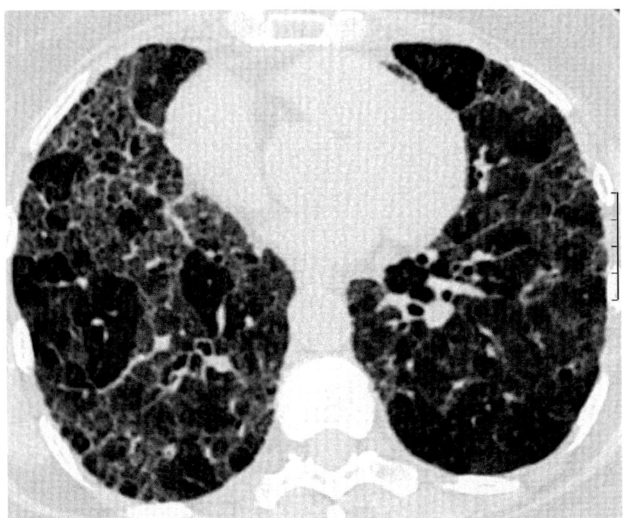

FIGURE 9-14 ■ **Chronic hypersensitivity pneumonitis.** The reticular pattern with distortion of the lung parenchyma indicates established fibrosis in this case of chronic hypersensitivity pneumonitis.

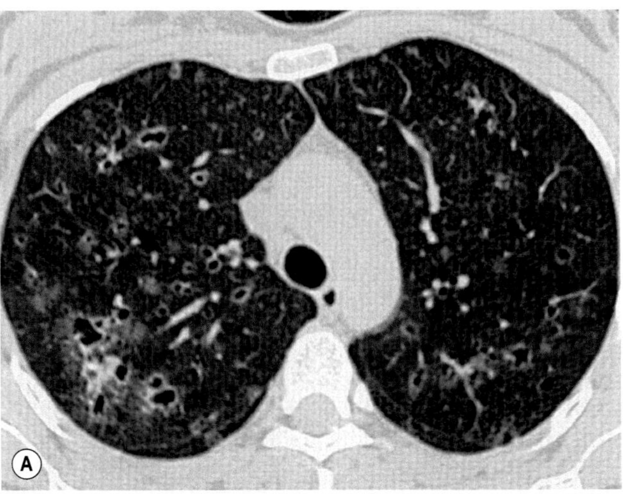

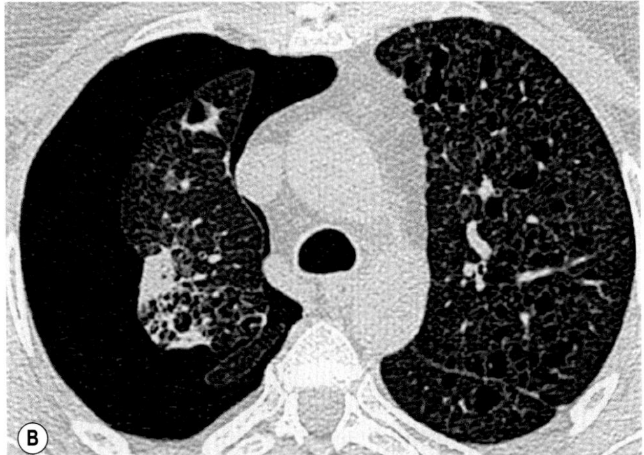

FIGURE 9-15 ■ **Langerhans cell histiocytosis.** (A) The characteristic combination of thin-walled cysts and poorly defined nodules, some of which are just beginning to cavitate. (B) Image from a patient with more advanced disease. There are numerous irregularly shaped cysts bilaterally and a pneumothorax on the right.

ground-glass opacity, centrilobular nodules and air trapping.[61,62]

Classic HRCT Findings

- In the subacute phase, poorly defined centrilobular nodules, background ground-glass opacification and lobular areas of air trapping are the main findings
- Chronic HP results in a pattern of fibrosis which may resemble NSIP or UIP; ancillary findings such as coexisting areas of air trapping, and upper lobe predominant disease may suggest the diagnosis of chronic HP

LANGERHANS CELL HISTIOCYTOSIS

Langerhans cell histiocytosis (LCH) is a granulomatous disorder characterised histologically by the presence of large histiocytes containing rod- or racket-shaped organelles (Langerhans cells).[63] The male-to-female ratio is about 4:1, and the vast majority of adult patients are cigarette smokers. In the earliest stages, patients are often asymptomatic. Others present with dyspnoea, cough, constitutional symptoms or a spontaneous pneumothorax. Pulmonary involvement is widespread, bilateral and usually symmetrical. At presentation, usually because of dyspnoea or a pneumothorax, the chest radiograph is abnormal. Typical appearances are of reticulonodular shadowing in the mid and upper zones of the lungs that are of normal or increased volume. The nodules vary in size from micronodular to approximately 1 cm in diameter and, although histopathological examination will often demonstrate cavitation, this feature is often difficult to appreciate on chest radiography.[64,65]

The classical appearances of LCH on HRCT are nodules (ranging in size from a few millimetres to 2 cm), several of which show cavitation (this feature often clinches the diagnosis), finally becoming cysts, often with bizarre shapes (Fig. 9-15).[66] At this stage of the disease, there are no obvious features of fibrosis. The distribution of disease is a useful diagnostic pointer and the typical sparing of the extreme lung bases and anterior tips of the right middle lobe and lingula is preserved even in end-stage disease. The typical nodules of LCH tend to show a predictable progression through the following stages: cavitation of the nodules, thin-walled cystic lesions, and finally emphysematous and fibrobullous destruction.[67]

Classic HRCT Findings

- Progression from ill-defined nodules which cavitate to a combination of cysts and nodules, these lesions spare the costophrenic recesses even in advanced disease

LYMPHANGIOLEIOMYOMATOSIS

Lymphangioleiomyomatosis (LAM) is a disease characterised histologically by two key features: cysts and proliferation of atypical smooth muscle cells (LAM cells) of the pulmonary interstitium, particularly in the bronchioles, pulmonary vessels and lymphatics.[68] LAM is a rare disease seen almost exclusively in women, the vast majority of cases being diagnosed during childbearing age. However, there are reports of women developing LAM after the menopause, including women in their eighth decade.[69] LAM can occur with or without evidence of other disease, such as tuberous sclerosis complex.[68,69]

The most commonly described radiographic manifestation of LAM is a pattern of generalised, symmetrical, reticular, or reticulonodular opacities with normal or increased lung volumes.[70,71] Pleural effusions (chylous) occur in 10–40% of patients (these may be unilateral or bilateral) and pneumothoraces in approximately 50% of cases.[72–74] The CT manifestations of LAM are distinctive, characterised by numerous thin-walled cysts randomly distributed throughout the lungs with no zonal predilection (Fig. 9-16).[75] Imaging features that help distinguish LAM from LCH include a more diffuse distribution of cysts, typically with no sparing of the bases, more regularly shaped spherical cysts and normal intervening lung parenchyma.[76] Occasionally HRCT may demonstrate interlobular septal thickening (attributed to dilatation of lymphatic channels secondary to obstruction of pleuropulmonary lymphatics and/or septal veins) or patchy areas of ground-glass attenuation (presumably the result of pulmonary haemorrhage).[75]

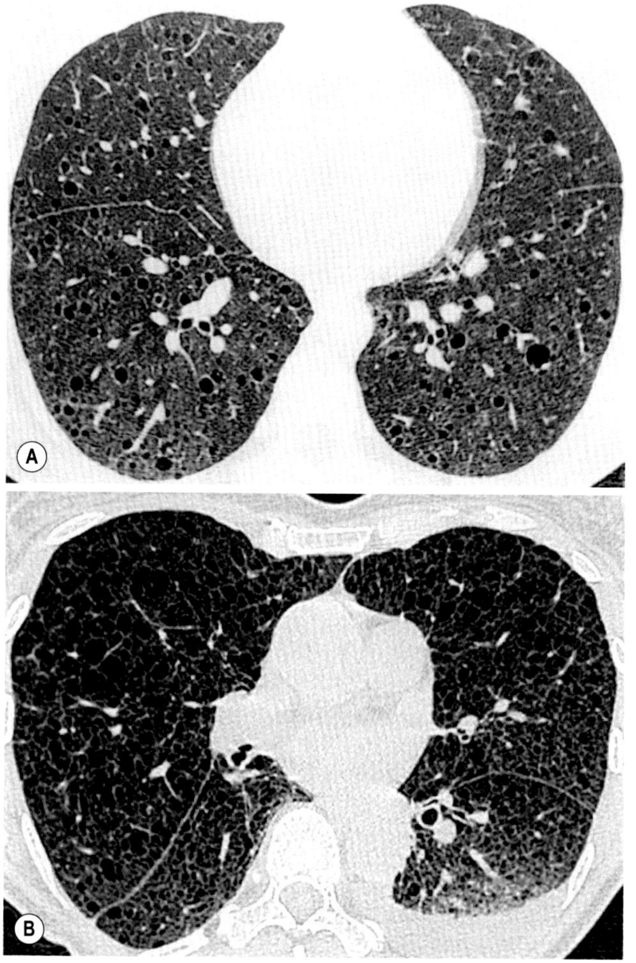

FIGURE 9-16 ■ **Lymphangioleiomyomatosis.** (A) There is a profusion of thin-walled cystic air spaces scattered evenly throughout the lungs. The cysts are relatively uniform in size. (B) In a more advanced case of LAM, note the small left pleural effusion.

Classic HRCT Findings

- Diffuse thin-walled cysts throughout the lungs with no zonal predominance

CONNECTIVE TISSUE DISEASES

The connective tissue diseases form a heterogeneous group of chronic inflammatory and immunologically mediated disorders, all of which affect the lung and pleura to a variable extent. Although the lung is a particularly vulnerable target organ, the frequency of pleuropulmonary involvement varies widely within the spectrum of disease and also in each disease separately, depending upon whether imaging, physiological, or histological criteria are used to judge involvement. Although the radiographic and HRCT appearances are not specific for any of the collagen vascular disorders, they frequently provide good corroborative evidence in substantiating what is often a difficult clinical diagnosis.

Rheumatoid Disease

Rheumatoid arthritis (RA) is associated with a broad spectrum of pleural and pulmonary disease. In a significant minority of patients with RA, pleuropulmonary disease antedates the development of arthritis and, in general, pleuropulmonary involvement is not related to the severity of the arthritis.[77]

The most frequently encountered manifestations of rheumatoid disease in the chest are listed in Table 9-4. Pleural involvement, either manifesting as effusions or thickening, is common. Pleural effusions can be unilateral or bilateral, are usually small or moderate in size, and the majority resolve spontaneously.[77]

ILD in RA is more common in men, particularly cigarette smokers, with seropositive disease. The most common histopathological patterns in RA-associated ILD are UIP and NSIP with HRCT features that are indistinguishable from idiopathic cases (Fig. 9-17).[78]

TABLE 9-4 **Intrathoracic Manifestations of Rheumatoid Disease**

- Pleural effusion or thickening
- Interstitial fibrosis (most frequently usual interstitial pneumonia type)
- Constrictive obliterative bronchiolitis
- Bronchiectasis
- Organising pneumonia
- Follicular bronchiolitis
- Drug-induced lung disease (methotrexate)
- Necrobiotic nodules/Caplan's syndrome

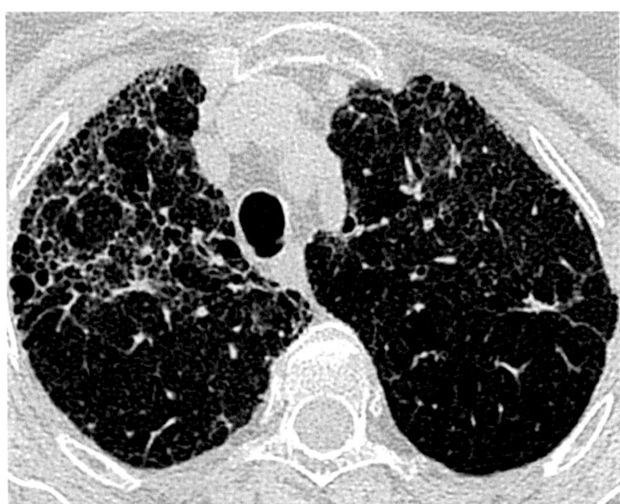

FIGURE 9-17 ■ **Rheumatoid arthritis with a usual interstitial pneumonia (UIP)-type pattern.** In this case the HRCT appearances of peripheral reticular abnormality and honeycombing are indistinguishable from that of UIP.

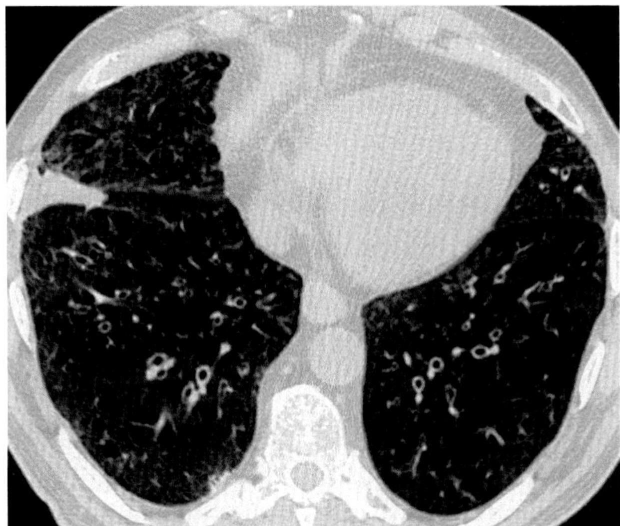

FIGURE 9-18 ■ **Rheumatoid arthritis.** HRCT demonstrates both mild cylindrical bronchiectasis and constrictive obliterative bronchiolitis (reflected by areas of low attenuation in which there is a reduction in the number of vessels present) in this patient with rheumatoid arthritis.

However, UIP is more prevalent than in the other connective tissue diseases. Although data are still controversial, it is thought that the prognosis for RA–ILD is better than for idiopathic cases.[79] Other pulmonary abnormalities seen in RA include follicular bronchiolitis, bronchiectasis (in up to 30% of cases) (Fig. 9-18), obliterative bronchiolitis (this can occur in patients who are on penicillamine, gold or no treatment), methotrexate-induced pneumonitis and organising pneumonia.[78,80–83] Obliterative bronchiolitis (causing extensive air trapping on HRCT) can cause considerable respiratory functional impairment requiring lung transplantation.[83]

Acute exacerbations may also occur in RA and differential diagnosis, for example between DAD and other conditions (e.g. opportunistic infections, pulmonary oedema), may be problematic for radiologists.

Rheumatoid (necrobiotic) pulmonary nodules are an uncommon feature of the disease. They are usually associated with the presence of subcutaneous nodules, and like them may wax and wane. They may be single or multiple, vary in size from a few millimetres to several centimetres, are well circumscribed and may cavitate; if they are subpleural they may cause a pneumothorax.[82] They show increased FDG uptake on PET, which should not be misinterpreted as metastatic disease. They are usually asymptomatic and may occur in association with pulmonary fibrosis and pleural changes.

Follicular bronchiolitis (discussed here because of its frequent association with rheumatoid disease) is part of the spectrum of lymphoproliferative disease and is characterised histologically by a diffuse peribronchiolar proliferation of hyperplastic lymphoid follicles and mild, if any, alveolar interstitial inflammation.[84] Clinically, the patients usually present during young adulthood or middle age with insidious dyspnoea. Most cases of follicular bronchiolitis are associated with connective tissue disease, especially RA and Sjögren's syndrome, but it is also seen in association with immuno deficiency syndromes including AIDS, pulmonary infections, or ill-defined hypersensitivity reactions. The cardinal features of follicular bronchiolitis on HRCT consist of centrilobular nodules measuring 1–12 mm in diameter, variably associated with peribronchial nodules and patchy areas of ground-glass opacity.[85,86] Nodules and ground-glass opacities are generally bilateral and diffuse in distribution. Mild bronchial dilatation with wall thickening and a tree-in-bud pattern are less frequent findings.[87]

Classic HRCT Findings

- Pleural effusions are common
- UIP is more frequent than NSIP
- Other findings include, organising pneumonia, bronchiectasis and evidence of small airways disease

Sjögren's Syndrome

Sjögren's syndrome (SjS) is a chronic autoimmune inflammatory disease characterised by a triad of clinical features: dry mouth (xerostomia), dry eyes (keratoconjunctivitis sicca) and arthritis.[88] SjS can occur alone as primary SjS or in association with other autoimmune diseases—secondary SjS. One study evaluating the radiological and pathological manifestations of lung diseases associated with primary SjS found that NSIP was the most common entity; other pathologies included bronchiolitis, lymphoma, amyloid and atelectasis.[89] HRCT studies have demonstrated LIP in patients with Sjögren's syndrome, the imaging findings of which are described under the section on the IIPs.[90,91] The association of LIP and amyloidosis (manifesting on HRCT as multiple irregular nodules with cysts) in patients with SjS is recognised (Fig. 9-19), but as these patients are also at increased risk of pulmonary lymphoma, the finding of LIP on HRCT in conjunction with multiple nodules in

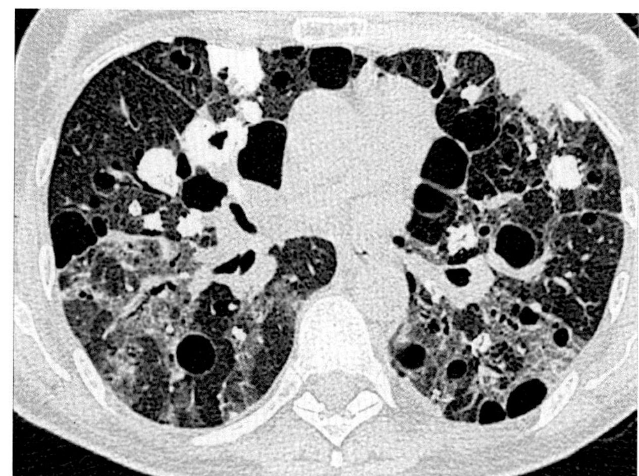

FIGURE 9-19 ■ **Sjögren's syndrome.** Lymphoid interstitial pneumonia and amyloid. There are numerous thin-walled cysts in association with multiple irregular solid nodules, some of which are heavily calcified. Histopathological examination showed marked thickening of the interstitium with an infiltrate of small, mature lymphocytes and plasma cells. Multiple deposits of amyloid were seen throughout the specimen and there was no evidence of malignancy.

a patient with SjS should at least prompt the consideration of a neoplastic process.[90,91]

Classic HRCT Findings

- The most frequent interstitial pneumonias in SjS are NSIP and LIP
- Mild bronchiectasis is common
- Lymphoproliferative disease may occur on a background of LIP

Progressive Systemic Sclerosis (Scleroderma)

Progressive systemic sclerosis (SSc) is a collagen vascular disease characterised by the deposition of excessive extracellular matrix with vascular occlusion involving several organs. It commonly affects the skin (scleroderma), peripheral vasculature, kidneys, oesophagus and lungs. ILD is common in patients with SSc and causes considerable morbidity and mortality. The interstitium and pulmonary vasculature are the predominant sites that are affected.[92,93] The HRCT findings of interstitial fibrosis in SSc include peripheral reticular opacities, ground-glass attenuation associated with traction bronchiectasis and occasionally honeycomb destruction (Fig. 9-20).[84,94,95] Thus, at microscopy, fibrotic NSIP is the most prevalent histological pattern in patients with SSc, whereas the UIP pattern is thought to occur in 5–10% of cases.[96,97] The finding of pulmonary arterial enlargement out of proportion to the severity of the lung fibrosis may indicate an independent vasculopathy akin to primary pulmonary hypertension, and a markedly dilated oesophagus is a frequent accompaniment.

Pleural disease is much less common in SSc than in other connective tissue diseases; pleural thickening is seen on HRCT in approximately 10% of patients.[84] As

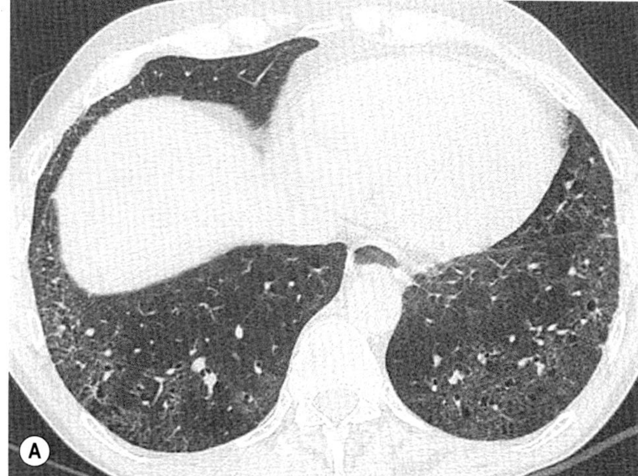

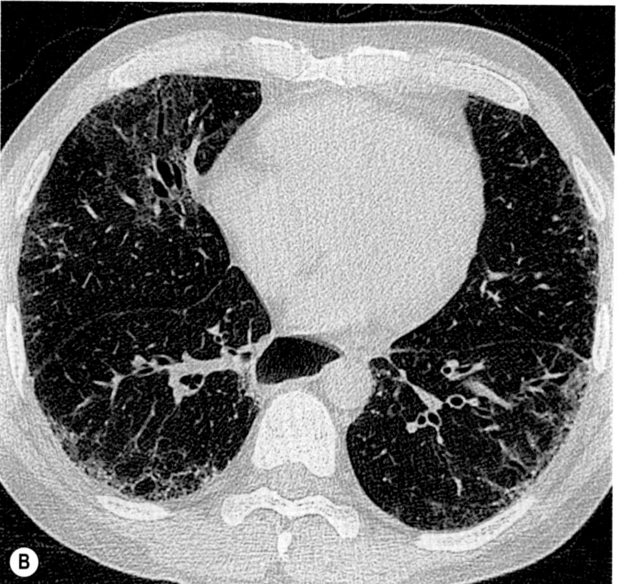

FIGURE 9-20 ■ **Scleroderma.** (A) In this case, ground-glass opacification admixed with fine reticular opacities are associated with mild traction bronchiectasis. Note the mild dilatation of the oesophagus. (B) In a more advanced case, reticulation and traction bronchiectasis are more severe but still closest to an NSIP pattern; the oesophagus is also more dilated.

in other diffuse fibrosing lung diseases, enlarged mediastinal lymph nodes (which histologically show reactive hyperplasia) are a frequent finding on CT.[98]

Classic HRCT Findings

- Appearance compatible with fibrotic NSIP is the most common pattern of lung involvement
- Dilated oesophagus is usual
- Signs of pulmonary hypertension, often without fibrotic interstitial lung disease

Polymyositis/Dermatomyositis

Polymyositis (PM) is an idiopathic autoimmune inflammatory myopathy that results in proximal muscle weakness. Dermatomyositis (DM) is similar, except that it is accompanied by a skin rash. Pulmonary complications of

PM/DM are important determinants of the clinical course with aspiration pneumonia owed to respiratory muscle weakness being an important pulmonary complication due to its prevalence as well as its associated morbidity and mortality. ILD in PM/DM occurs in an estimated 5–47% of patients. Initial clinical presentation is with cough, dyspnoea and fever, prior to musculoskeletal manifestations of arthralgia, myalgia and weakness in 30%, with simultaneous occurrence in only 20%.[99] NSIP and OP are the most common histological patterns seen in PM/DM.[99] The ILD can be acute and aggressive, similar to AIP, with some series reporting up to 10.5% mortality, or more slowly progressive. In some, the lung disease is responsive to steroids and immunosuppression.[100,101] At presentation, the most common HRCT features of PM/DM are linear opacities with a lower lung predominance, ground-glass opacities, irregular interfaces and areas of consolidation (Fig. 9-21). Honeycombing is less frequently observed.[100]

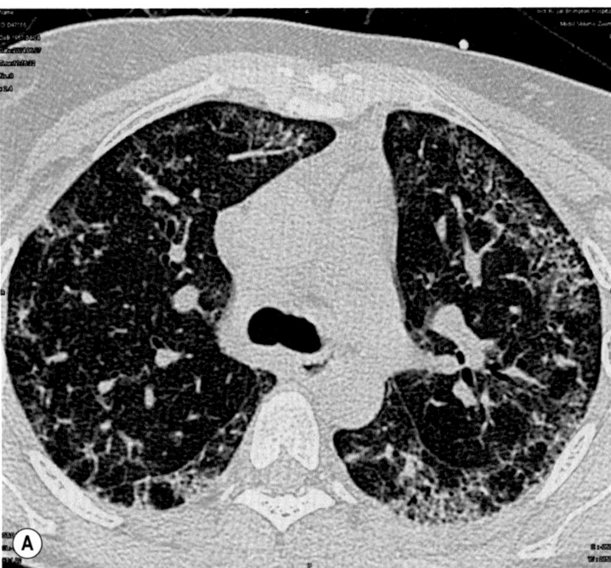

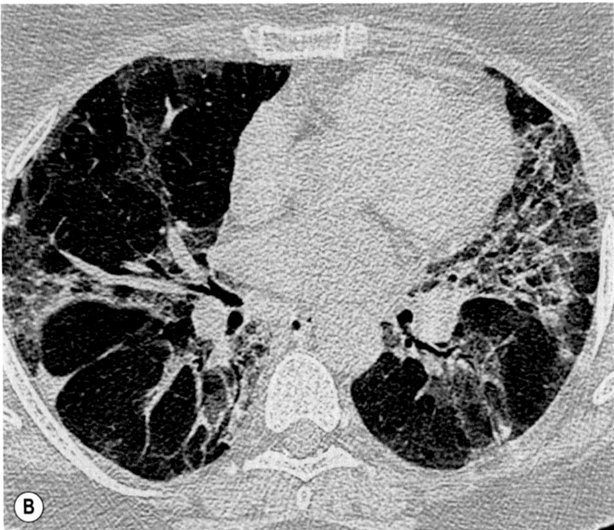

FIGURE 9-21 ■ **Polymyositis/dermatomyositis.** HRCT features include (A) reticular opacities and (B) areas of ground-glass opacification. The appearance of (B) is compatible with organising pneumonia being incorporated as fibrosis.

Histologically, organising pneumonia is the correlate of consolidation and ground-glass opacification seen on HRCT. DAD is demonstrated in some cases and is associated with widespread involvement, dense dependent consolidation and extensive diffuse ground-glass opacification. Organising pneumonia in PM/DM can also be admixed with interstitial fibrosis with a predominance of reticular elements and architectural distortion, traction bronchiectasis and honeycombing, and this overlap entity is associated with a poor prognosis.[102]

Classic HRCT Findings

- Diffuse ground-glass opacities may represent either NSIP or DAD
- Consolidation is common and represents organising pneumonia frequently admixed with NSIP and DAD patterns

Systemic Lupus Erythematosus

Pleuropulmonary disease will occur in more than half of patients with SLE at some point during the course of their illness.[103] Although pleuritis is the most common manifestation of SLE, diverse thoracic manifestations which range from diaphragmatic dysfunction (shrinking lung syndrome) to life-threatening pneumonitis or pulmonary haemorrhage are encountered. A list of the other pulmonary complications may be found in Table 9-5.

Pleural effusions are the most common radiographic abnormality. They are frequently bilateral, usually only small in volume and, unlike those in rheumatoid disease, are often associated with pleuritic pain. Thick horizontal band shadows at the lung bases due to linear atelectasis may be secondary to the pleurisy or, more likely, restricted diaphragmatic movement. Pulmonary consolidation in patients with SLE may cause diagnostic difficulty as it may be a consequence of infection (the incidence of respiratory tract infection in patients with SLE is high due to the immunological abnormalities, immunosuppression from steroids and respiratory muscle weakness), pulmonary oedema, lupus pneumonitis, or pulmonary haemorrhage. Acute lupus pneumonitis is a well-recognised but rare manifestation of the disease that is characterised by fever, severe hypoxaemia and diffuse pulmonary infiltrates. Radiological features are typically patchy

TABLE 9-5 Intrathoracic Manifestations of Systemic Lupus Erythematosus

- Pleural effusion
- Segmental or subsegmental collapse
- Lupus pneumonitis
- Pulmonary infection
- Pulmonary oedema
- Diaphragmatic dysfunction
- Interstitial fibrosis (rare)
- Pericardial effusion
- Pulmonary vascular disease
- Pulmonary arterial hypertension
- Vasculitis/capillaritis
- Pulmonary embolism
- Pulmonary veno-occlusive disease

consolidation and focal atelectasis seen predominantly in the lower lung zones with concomitant pleural effusions. Histological findings are not diagnostic but include alveolar wall damage, inflammatory cell infiltration and haemorrhage.[104]

Compared with many other collagen vascular diseases, SLE is not commonly associated with chronic diffuse ILD. When present, reported HRCT findings include irregular linear and band-like opacities (in part atelectasis), ground-glass opacities and interlobular septal thickening. Honeycombing which can resemble IPF is extremely rare.[84] Diffuse alveolar haemorrhage is a rare but dramatic complication of SLE, which manifests radiologically as widespread ground-glass opacity and consolidation. SLE is associated with increased risk of malignancy, with lymphoma being the most common.[95,105]

Classic HRCT Findings

- Pleural abnormalities and decreasing lung volumes ('shrinking lung syndrome')
- Chronic interstitial lung disease is less frequent than other connective tissue diseases
- Diffuse ground-glass opacities may represent diffuse alveolar damage or pulmonary haemorrhage

SYSTEMIC VASCULITIDES

A number of disorders are characterised histologically by a systemic vasculitis in which the primary pathogenetic mechanism is the deposition of immune complexes in the walls of blood vessels. The systemic vasculitides that most commonly affect the lung are Wegener's granulomatosis (ANCA-associated granulomatous vasculitis), Churg–Strauss syndrome and Behçet's disease. Since Wegener's granulomatosis will be considered in Chapter 11, 'Airspace Diseases', only Churg–Strauss syndrome will be covered in this section.

Churg–Strauss Syndrome

Churg–Strauss syndrome is characterised histologically by the presence of necrotising vasculitis and extravascular granulomatous inflammation rich in eosinophils, and clinically by the presence of asthma, fever, blood eosinophilia and peripheral neuropathy. HRCT appearances largely reflect the eosinophilic infiltrate and are largely non-specific.[84,106] Features include ground-glass opacities, areas of airspace consolidation, centrilobular nodules and airways abnormalities attributable to asthma (Fig. 9-22).[107] Histologically the airspace disease is due to eosinophilic infiltrate or organising pneumonia.[107] Interlobular septal thickening may be seen as a result of interstitial pulmonary oedema secondary to cardiac involvement. However, a significant proportion (up to 25%) of patients with Churg–Strauss syndrome have few or no imaging abnormalities and imaging is often of little help in making this somewhat elusive diagnosis. Even when HRCT abnormalities exist, they are not specific and the diagnostic accuracy for Churg–Strauss syndrome was less than 50% in one study.[108]

Classic HRCT Findings

- Non-specific patchy ground-glass opacities or consolidation
- Interlobular septal thickening (particularly with cardiac involvement)
- Pleural and pericardial effusion

DRUG-INDUCED LUNG DISEASE

The lung is less commonly the site of drug-induced disease than other organs such as the skin and gastrointestinal tract. Nevertheless, many drugs can cause injury to the lungs, and the list of drugs and patterns of involvement continues to increase. Respiratory disease secondary to drugs may be the result of the pharmacological action of the drug in normal or excessive dosage, or caused by an allergic or idiosyncratic reaction. The radiological manifestations of drug-induced ILD, although heterogeneous and non-specific, enable many alternative diagnoses to be excluded. There is no specific radiological pattern of parenchymal change associated with drug-induced lung disease and in the early stages of disease, patients with symptoms secondary to drug reaction may have a normal chest radiograph. Furthermore, data based on a small number of cases suggest that the different histological patterns of drug reaction are not always reflected by characteristic HRCT findings.[109] Despite these limitations, it is reasonable to understand the radiological manifestations of drug-induced lung disease through an appreciation of the underlying histological patterns of drug-induced disease.[110] The most common histological manifestations are diffuse alveolar damage, chronic interstitial pneumonia (a vague term used by histopathologists which incorporates drug-induced lung disease with histological features that resemble either NSIP or less commonly UIP), hypersensitivity pneumonitis, organising pneumonia and eosinophilic pneumonia.[110] Most drugs typically cause more than one type of histological pattern. Table 9-6 lists the drugs associated with the different histological patterns.

Diffuse Alveolar Damage

Chemotherapeutic drugs such as busulfan, cyclophosphamide, carmustine (BCNU) and bleomycin constitute the largest group of drugs associated with this pattern of lung toxicity.[109] DAD usually develops a few weeks or months after initiating therapy and disease onset is heralded by progressive dyspnoea. The corresponding radiological features, not surprisingly, are similar to those found in ARDS with bilateral patchy or homogeneous airspace consolidation involving mainly the middle and lower lung zones. HRCT demonstrates extensive bilateral ground-glass opacities and dependent areas of airspace consolidation (Fig. 9-23).[111] In most circumstances there are no histological features that allow separation of drug toxicity from other potential causes of DAD and the diagnosis of drug-induced lung disease requires vigorous exclusion of other potential aetiologies, most importantly opportunistic infection.

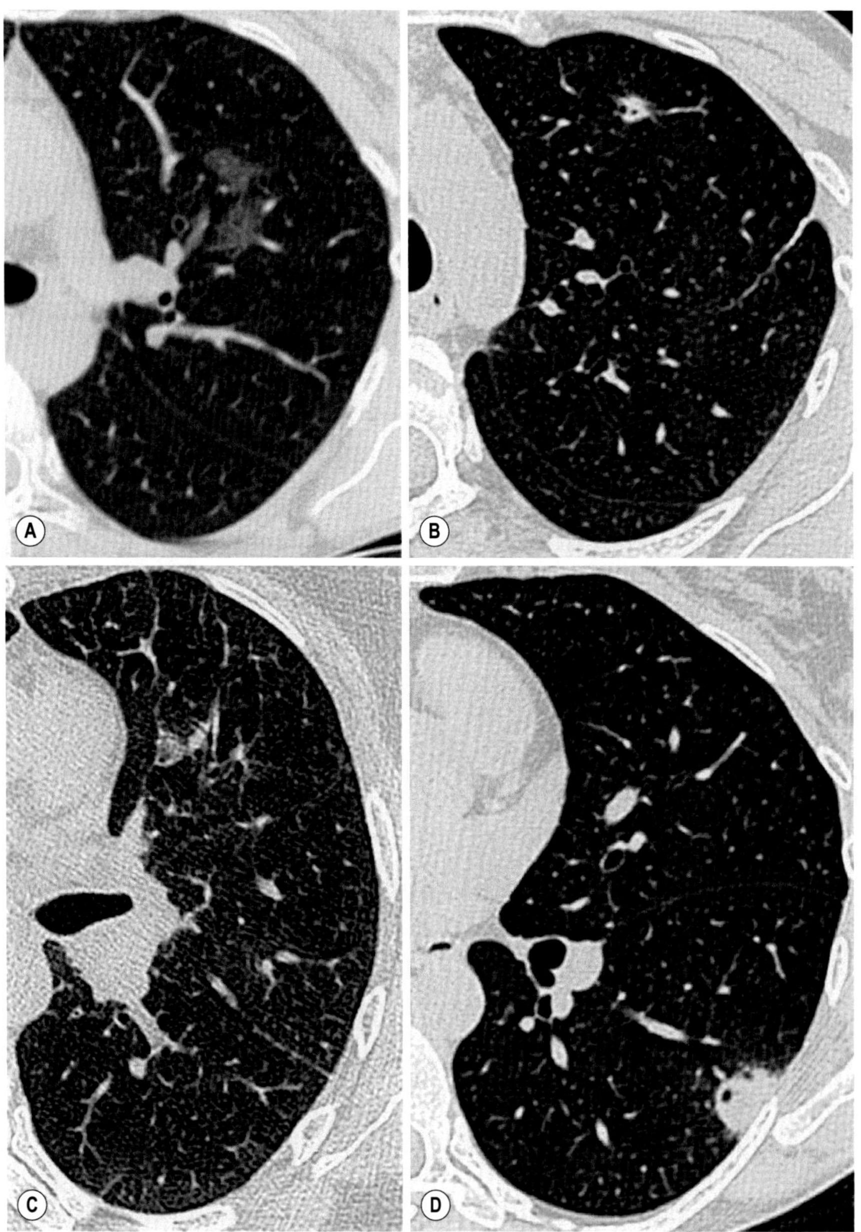

FIGURE 9-22 ■ **Churg–Strauss syndrome.** Spectrum of HRCT features: (A) areas of ground-glass opacification, (B) small cavitating nodules, (C) thickened interlobular septa and (D) an area of airspace opacification, likely to be a peripheral infarct.

TABLE 9-6 **Histological Pattern of Drug-Induced Lung Disease**

Diffuse Alveolar Damage	Diffuse Alveolar Haemorrhage	Interstitial Pneumonia	Organising Pneumonia	Eosinophilic Pneumonia
Amiodarone	Anticoagulants	Amiodarone	Amiodarone	Nitrofurantoin
	Amphotericin B		Bleomycin	Non-steroidal anti-inflammatory drugs
			Cyclophosphamide	Para-aminosalicylic acid
				Penicillamine
				Sulfasalazine
Bleomycin	Cyclophosphamide	Carmustine	Gold salts	
Cyclophosphamide	Cytosine arabinoside	Chlorambucil	Penicillamine	
Methotrexate	(ara-C)	Cyclophosphamide		
		Methotrexate	Methotrexate	
		Nitrofurantoin		
	Penicillamine		Nitrofurantoin	
Mitomycin			Sulfasalazine	
Mephalan				
Gold salts				

Interstitial Pneumonia

A variety of patterns, in particular NSIP and OP, are associated with drug-induced lung disease. Of these, the NSIP pattern is the most common. Drugs reported to cause an NSIP-type pattern include amiodarone, busulfan, carmustine, methotrexate, phenytoin and simvastatin.[110] Descriptions of HRCT findings are available for a limited number of agents, but demonstrate the same range of abnormalities described in patients with the idiopathic form of NSIP (Fig. 9-24).[111] With disease progression, there may be evidence of fibrosis with development of a reticular pattern and traction bronchiectasis. The fibrosis is patchy in distribution and predominantly peribronchovascular, a pattern sometimes seen in patients receiving nitrofurantoin. In some cases, however, HRCT features suggestive of irreversible fibrosis may show complete resolution on cessation of nitrofurantoin.[112] NSIP is the most common manifestation of amiodarone-induced lung disease. HRCT features that have been described with amiodarone-induced lung disease include ground-glass opacities in association with fine intralobular reticulation seen predominantly in a peripheral distribution. Foci of consolidation have also been described, and represent areas of organising pneumonia.[113,114] The diagnosis of amiodarone toxicity can occasionally be made on HRCT by virtue of the high-attenuation values of amiodarone deposited in the lung.[114]

Organising Pneumonia

An organising pneumonia-like reaction has been reported most frequently in association with methotrexate, cyclophosphamide, gold, nitrofurantoin, amiodarone, bleomycin and busulfan.[109] The chest radiograph shows patchy bilateral areas of consolidation, masses or nodules, which may be asymmetric. HRCT shows patchy ground-glass opacity and areas of consolidation which often have a predominantly peripheral or peribronchiolar distribution (Fig. 9-25).[115]

Eosinophilic Pneumonia

Eosinophilic pneumonia is characterised histologically by the accumulation of eosinophils in the alveolar air spaces and infiltration of the adjacent interstitial space by eosinophils and variable numbers of lymphocytes and plasma

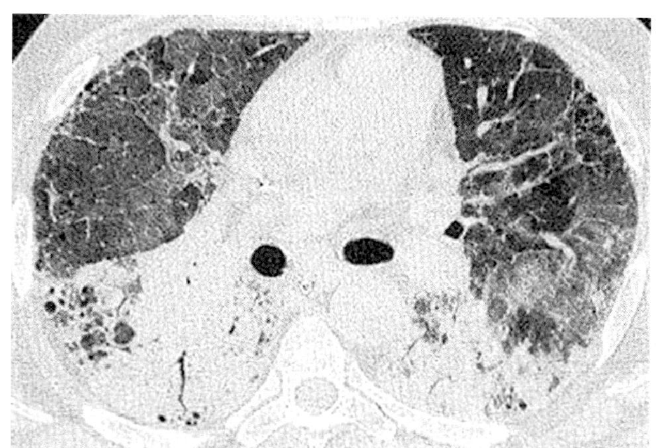

FIGURE 9-23 ■ Diffuse alveolar damage secondary to amiodarone. There is extensive bilateral ground-glass opacification and airspace consolidation.

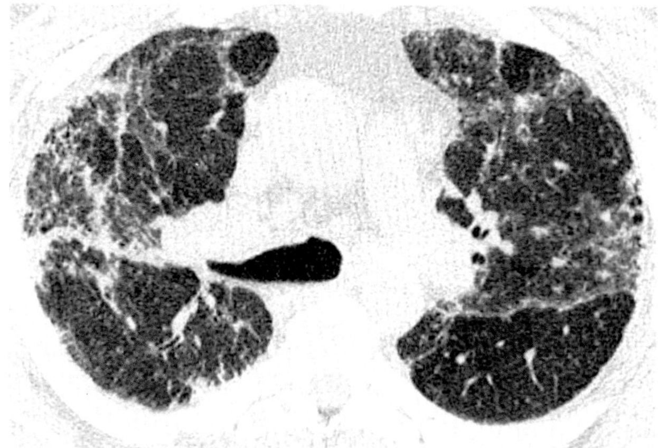

FIGURE 9-24 ■ Non-specific interstitial pneumonia secondary to bleomycin. The dominant abnormality is ground-glass opacification in association with a fine reticular pattern. The pattern of fibrosis most closely resembles non-specific interstitial pneumonia.

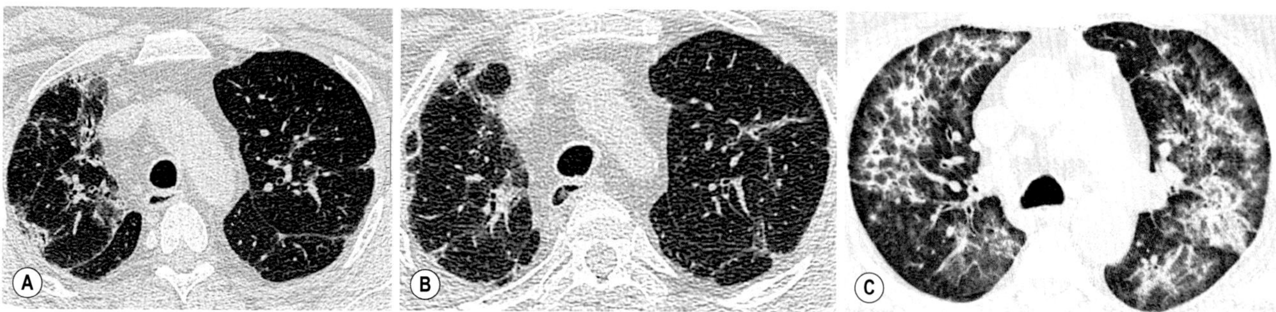

FIGURE 9-25 ■ Organising pneumonia secondary to (A, B) nitrofurantoin and (C) amiodarone. The HRCT features of ground-glass opacification and consolidation (A, C) and a perilobular pattern (B) are in keeping with organising pneumonia. The areas of consolidation in (C) are both peribronchial and perilobular in distribution.

cells. Peripheral blood eosinophilia is present in around 40% of patients. Eosinophilic pneumonia secondary to drug reaction is seen most commonly in association with methotrexate, sulfasalazine, para-aminosalicylic acid, nitrofurantoin and non-steroidal anti-inflammatory drugs. Chest radiography and HRCT show bilateral air-space consolidation, which tends to involve mainly the peripheral lung regions and the upper lobes.[111]

The diagnosis of drug-induced disease will be missed unless specifically sought as a cause of unexplained diffuse pulmonary shadowing in patients at known risk with clinical symptoms of lung disease. It is particularly important, though often difficult, to differentiate between drug-induced disease, infections (particularly of the opportunistic variety) and metastatic malignancy in patients who are susceptible to these processes.

Classic HRCT Findings

- Imaging findings of most drug reactions are non-specific and mimic those of various acute and chronic lung diseases
- A drug-specific diagnosis is rarely possible
- The main role of HRCT in this setting is the exclusion of other diseases

OCCUPATIONAL LUNG DISEASE

Diseases of the lung caused by workplace and environmental exposures are common throughout both developed and developing worlds, and as industrial techniques continue to evolve, new occupational diseases will be recognised.

The following section highlights the imaging features of the main pneumoconioses—silicosis, coal worker's pneumoconiosis and asbestos-related pulmonary disease. Table 9-7 summarises some of the other main occupational lung diseases. Hypersensitivity pneumonitis is covered in the preceding section on ILD. Work-related asthma is one of the most frequently reported occupational lung diseases in a number of industrialised countries but as these patients are not frequently imaged (and the contribution of imaging is negligible), this topic is not further discussed.

The International Labour Office Classification

The International Labour Office (ILO) International Classification of Radiographs for the Pneumoconioses is a system used for the recording of chest radiographic abnormalities related to the inhalation of dusts.[116] In the ILO system, the size, shape and profusion of opacities on radiographs are classified in a detailed manner by trained observers using a set of standard radiographs. Rounded or nodular opacities are graded as p (< 1.5 mm diameter), q (1.5–3 mm), or r (3–10 mm). Irregular opacities are classified as s, t, or u, using the same size criteria. Large opacities (> 10 mm) are graded as A, B and C based on the combined dimensions of all large opacities present. The classification also scores the extent and thickness of plaques, pleural thickening, fissural thickening and calcified nodules. Profusion of the opacities is classified into four categories (0–3); category 0 indicates that there is no excess of small opacities above normal. The use of two profusion categories is useful when appearances lie between those of the standard radiographs. Despite acknowledged limitations and problems with the ILO classification (interobserver variability, the presence of background opacities that are unrelated to dust exposure, the relative insensitivity of the chest radiograph to early disease, and the misuse of the classification in legal settlements for compensation), it remains a useful shorthand whose meaning is widely understood for epidemiological studies.

Silicosis/Coal Worker's Pneumoconiosis

Silica causes three distinct clinical patterns of lung disease which are related to both level and duration of exposure. The earliest radiographic changes of silicosis and coal worker's pneumoconiosis (CWP) are nearly identical. Typical appearances are a profusion of small (1–3 mm) round nodules distributed in the posterior aspects of the upper two-thirds of the lung.[117] Radiologically, the only difference between simple CWP and simple silicosis is that the nodules in CWP are often smaller. With advancing disease, the nodules increase in size and number to involve all lung zones. The nodules are sometimes calcified. Hilar and mediastinal lymph

TABLE 9-7 **Examples of Occupational Exposures that cause Lung Pathology**

Occupational Lung Disease	Disease	Radiology
Flock worker's lung	Lymphocytic bronchiolitis	Ground-glass opacities with centrilobular nodules
Flavour worker's lung (flavouring agents used in microwave popcorn)	Obliterative bronchiolitis	Mosaic attenuation pattern, air trapping, bronchial wall thickening
Berylliosis	Non-caseating granulomas (indistinguishable from sarcoidosis) accompanied by mononuclear cell infiltrates and interstitial fibrosis	Nodules with a similar distribution to sarcoidosis, ground-glass opacities, thickened interlobular septa, reticular opacities and honeycombing (rare). Mediastinal adenopathy is less common than in sarcoidosis. Conglomerate masses are seen in advanced disease
Hard metal pneumoconiosis (alloys of tungsten carbide and cobalt, titanium and tantalum)	Giant cell interstitial pneumonia	Ground-glass attenuation and consolidation. Cysts and reticular abnormality may also occur

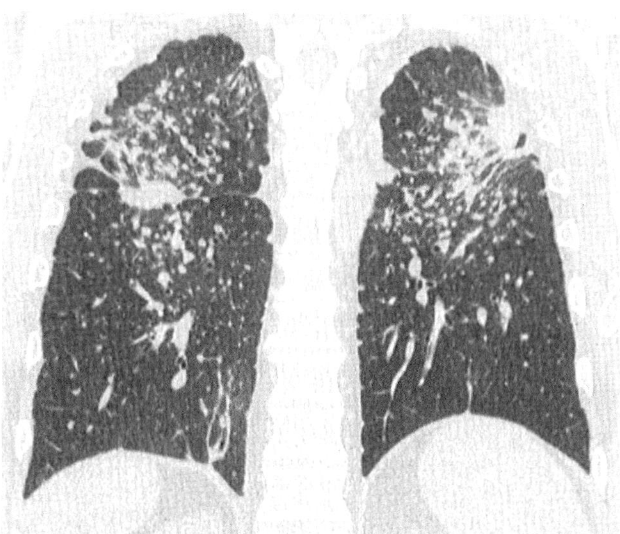

FIGURE 9-26 Progressive massive fibrosis in coalworker's pneumoconiosis. Mass-like opacities are seen bilaterally in the upper lobes in association with multiple small nodules and calcified mediastinal lymphadenopathy.

node enlargement with calcification of the eggshell type is not uncommon and may be seen on the chest radiograph or CT. On CT, the micronodules are sharply defined and distributed throughout the lungs but are frequently most numerous in the upper lung zones. The nodules may be centrilobular or subpleural in location; the subpleural micronodules may become confluent, forming a 'pseudo-plaque'.[118]

Progressive massive fibrosis (PMF) refers to the coalescence of large nodules and is much more common in silicosis than in CWP. On the chest radiograph, PMF is seen as mass-like opacities, typically in the posterior upper lobes and associated with contraction of the upper lobes and hilar elevation. Sequential evaluation of these masses often demonstrates migration towards the hila, leaving a peripheral rim of cicatricial emphysema.[119] The outer margins of PMF often parallel the contour of the adjacent chest wall. CT confirms the architectural distortion associated with PMF (Fig. 9-26). Large lesions (>5 cm) often show irregular low-attenuation regions on CT indicative of necrosis. Frank cavitation is a less frequent finding and when present should always raise the suspicion of tuberculosis (conventional or atypical). Unilateral or asymmetric PMF may be distinguished from lung cancer by the presence of lobar volume loss and peripheral emphysema.

Classic HRCT Findings

- Well-defined dense centrilobular and subpleural nodules, concentrated in the upper zones posteriorly
- Hilar and mediastinal lymph node enlargement, with or without calcification, is frequent
- Upper lobe irregular masses characterise progressive massive fibrosis

Asbestos-related Disease

Asbestos is the generic term for a group of fibrous silicates that share the property of heat resistance. They are classified into two groups: the serpentines and the amphiboles. The only serpentine asbestos used commercially is chrysolite, which accounts for more than 90% of the asbestos used in the USA. The pathological hallmark of asbestos exposure is the asbestos body consisting of an asbestos fibre usually 2–5 μm in width. These bodies can be identified in tissue sections in interstitial fibrous tissue and intra-alveolar macrophages in bronchoalveolar lavage (BAL) fluid. The effects of asbestos on the lung are diverse and clinical manifestations of these abnormalities typically do not appear until 20 years or more after initial exposure, apart from asbestos-related pleural effusions which may be present as early as 5 years post exposure.

Benign Pleural Effusions

The exact prevalence of benign pleural effusions is unknown, as many are subclinical. The effusions are typically haemorrhagic exudates of mixed cellularity and usually do not contain asbestos bodies. Their diagnosis is therefore reliant largely on the exclusion of other causes of effusions in an asbestos-exposed patient. The development of effusions is thought to be exposure-dependent.[120] The effusions are often small, may be persistent or recurrent and may be simultaneously or sequentially bilateral.[121] Diffuse pleural thickening, with or without areas of subjacent folded lung, is the usual consequence.

Pleural Plaques

The most common manifestation of asbestos exposure is the presence of pleural plaques which, macroscopically, are discrete foci of pearly white fibrous tissue, usually 2–5 mm thick. They involve the parietal pleura almost exclusively and are classically distributed under the anterior ends of the upper ribs, the paravertebral gutters and the diaphragmatic surface. Calcification is reported in 10–15% of cases.[122] CT is undoubtedly more sensitive for the detection of pleural plaques. Only 50–80% of cases of documented pleural thickening are detected by chest radiography; on chest radiography, pleural plaques were most commonly missed in the paravertebral and posterior regions of the costal pleura.[123] Studies have suggested that pleural plaques are not associated with significantly impaired lung function.[124,125]

Diffuse Pleural Thickening

The frequency of diffuse pleural thickening increases with time from first exposure and is thought to be dose-related. It results from thickening and fibrosis of the visceral pleura, which leads to fusion with the parietal pleura and may be caused by extension of interstitial fibrosis to the visceral pleura, consistent with the pleural migration of asbestos fibres. Diffuse pleural thickening superimposed on circumscribed plaques has been observed, often after a pleural effusion. CT is more sensitive and specific than chest radiography in the detection of diffuse pleural thickening and can make the distinction between mild pleural disease and extrapleural fat.[126]

Round Atelectasis

Round atelectasis, also known as folded lung, is a form of parenchymal collapse that occurs in association with pleural thickening, most commonly in the peripheral lung in the dorsal regions of the lower lobes. Pathological examination shows pleural fibrosis overlying the abnormal parenchyma as well as invaginations of fibrotic pleura into the region of collapse.

Because of the pathogenetic association with fibrosis, the areas of atelectasis are always seen adjacent to the visceral pleura. A characteristic finding is the presence of crowding of bronchi and blood vessels that extend from the border of the mass to the hilum ('comet tail' sign).[127] In most cases, the collapsed lung has a rounded or oval shape; however, wedge- and irregularly-shaped masses can also occur (Fig. 9-27). Volume loss of the affected lobe is a key sign.[128] Serial examinations show a relatively stable appearance, and the differentiation from a lung neoplasm is usually straightforward on CT by characteristic findings such as the subpleural location, comet tail sign and the strong and homogeneous enhancement after intravenous contrast medium, the latter indicative of atelectasis rather than tumour.

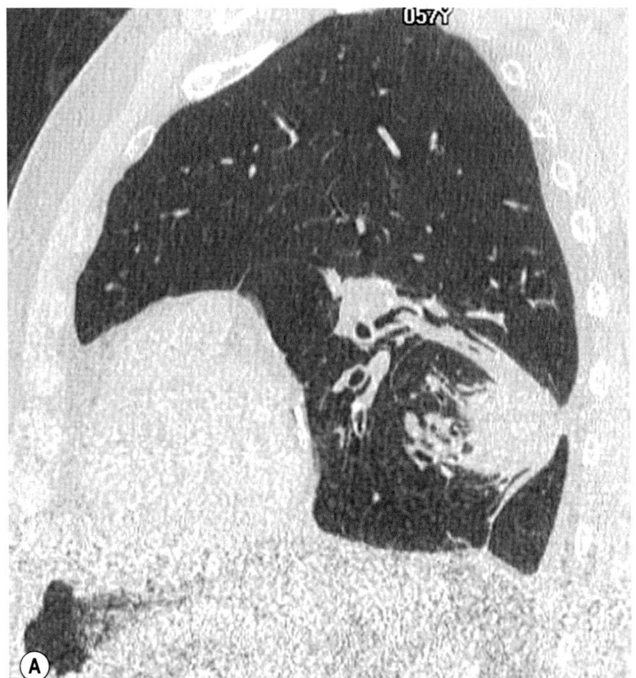

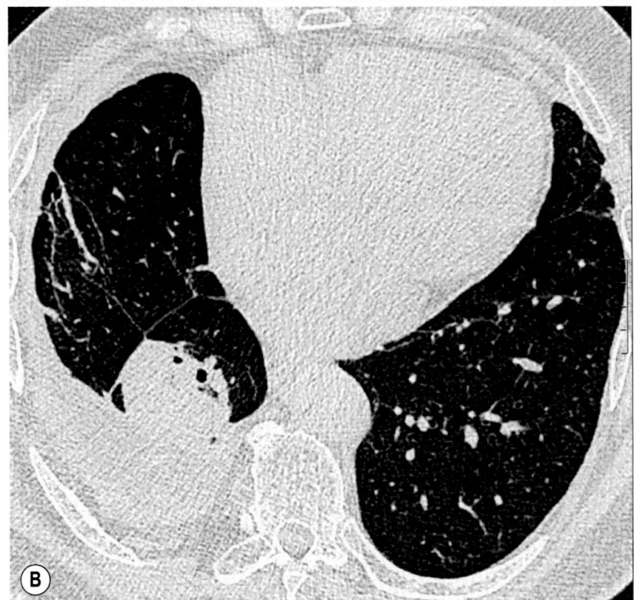

FIGURE 9-27 ■ **Atelectasis.** Two examples of rounded atelectasis in association with (A) pleural thickening and (B) a pleural effusion. In both cases, there is evidence of lobar volume loss as evidenced by displacement of fissures. The most common location of rounded atelectasis is in the lower lobes.

Asbestosis

Asbestosis is defined as pulmonary parenchymal fibrosis secondary to inhalation of asbestos fibres. The lag between exposure and onset of symptoms is usually 20 years or longer. Histologically, fibrosis is first seen in the interstitium of respiratory bronchioles, particularly in the lower lobes adjacent to the visceral pleura. With advancing disease, the fibrous tissue extends into the adjacent alveolar septa, eventually involving the entire lobule.[129] In the most severe cases there is diffuse interstitial fibrosis associated with parenchymal remodelling and honeycombing. Asbestos bodies are almost always identifiable microscopically in the fibrous tissue or macrophages in residual air spaces. Early CT changes indicative of asbestosis are the presence of subpleural curvilinear lines and dots, pleural-based nodular irregularities, parenchymal bands and septal lines.[130] The fine reticulation eventually progresses to a coarse linear pattern with honeycombing (Fig. 9-28). These abnormalities are usually most severe in the subpleural regions of the lower lobes. HRCT–pathological correlation studies have shown that subpleural dots and branching structures correspond to peribronchiolar fibrosis.[131] The sensitivity of HRCT over the chest radiograph for the identification of early fibrosis in asbestos-exposed individuals is well established; however, sensitivity is not 100% and a histopathological diagnosis of asbestosis can be present in patients with normal or near-normal HRCTs.[132] The diagnosis of asbestosis has significant implications for the patient in terms of prognosis, work ability and the possibility of receiving legal compensation. Although both the chest radiograph and HRCT can confirm previous exposure, the diagnosis of asbestosis is largely inferential and based on demonstrating a compatible structural lesion, critically an appropriate exposure history, and the exclusion of other plausible conditions. One of the problems in interpreting the presence of interstitial fibrosis, whether on chest radiography or HRCT, is the fact that asbestos-exposed individuals are as likely as the rest of the population to develop other causes of fibrosis such as IPF. Distinguishing asbestosis from IPF is also desirable, as

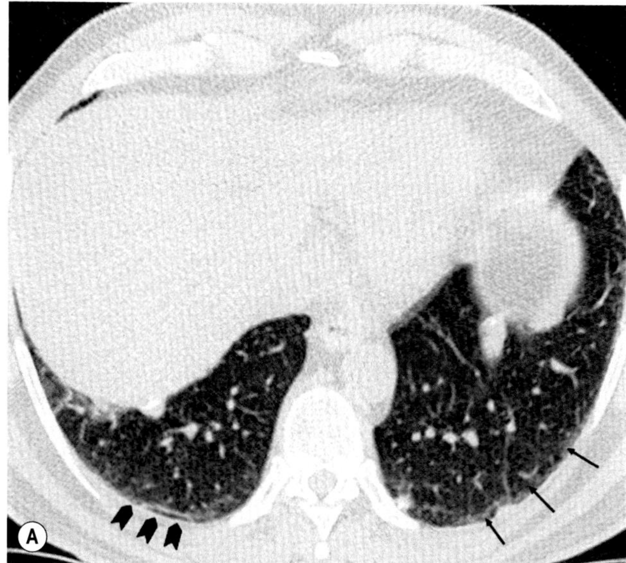

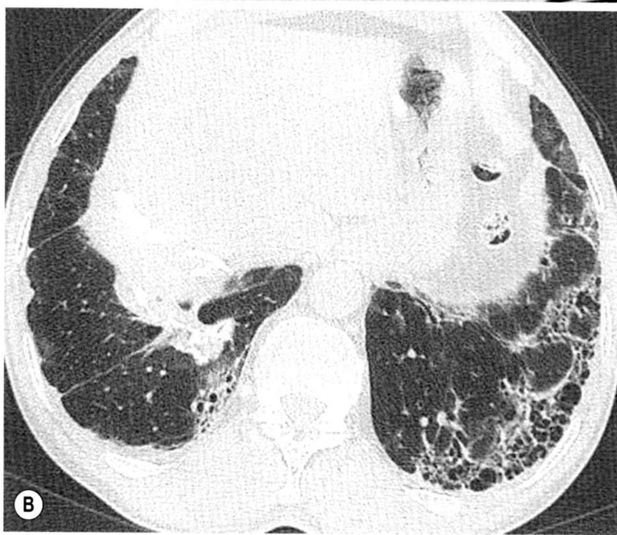

FIGURE 9-28 ■ **Asbestosis.** (A) HRCT features of early asbestosis include subpleural lines (arrowheads) and fine reticulation (arrows). These subtle abnormalities persisted on prone sections. (B) In more advanced disease, a coarse reticular pattern with honeycombing, often indistinguishable from usual interstitial pneumonia on HRCT, is seen in the left lower lobe. Note the calcified pleural plaques in both examples.

asbestosis is associated with a much slower rate of progression and hence a better prognosis. Discrimination between the two by HRCT appearances is usually impossible. However, pleural disease may be a crude discriminator: in Akira et al's study, pleural disease was found in 83% (66/80) of patients with asbestosis but only in 4% (3/80) of patients with IPF.[133] Copley et al found no statistically significant differences in the coarseness of fibrosis between individuals with asbestosis and a cohort of individuals with biopsy-proven UIP, although the CT findings of asbestosis were strikingly different from NSIP; the quality of fibrosis was coarser, there was a lower proportion of ground-glass opacification, and a higher likelihood of a basal and subpleural distribution.[134]

Classic HRCT Findings

- Asbestos-related benign pleural disease consists of either parietal pleural plaques in characteristic locations or diffuse visceral pleural thickening
- The presence of such pleural disease in individuals with HRCT findings compatible with UIP/NSIP pattern suggests the diagnosis of asbestosis in patients with an appropriate exposure history

REFERENCES

1. Collins CD, Wells AU, Hansell DM, et al. Observer variation in pattern type and extent of disease in fibrosing alveolitis on thin section computed tomography and chest radiography. Clin Radiol 1994;49(4):236–40.
2. Gaensler EA, Carrington CB. Open biopsy for chronic diffuse infiltrative lung disease: clinical, roentgenographic, and physiological correlations in 502 patients. Ann Thorac Surg 1980;30(5): 411–26.
3. Hansell DM, Bankier AA, MacMahon H, et al. Fleischner Society: glossary of terms for thoracic imaging. Radiology 2008;246(3): 697–722.
4. Hawtin KE, Roddie ME, Mauri FA, Copley SJ. Pulmonary sarcoidosis: the 'Great Pretender'. Clin Radiol 2010;65(8): 642–50.
5. Ujita M, Renzoni EA, Veeraraghavan S, et al. Organizing pneumonia: perilobular pattern at thin-section CT. Radiology 2004; 232(3):757–61.
6. Raoof S, Amchentsev A, Vlahos I, et al. Pictorial essay: multinodular disease: a high-resolution CT scan diagnostic algorithm. Chest 2006;129(3):805–15.
7. Worthy SA, Muller NL, Hartman TE, et al. Mosaic attenuation pattern on thin-section CT scans of the lung: differentiation among infiltrative lung, airway, and vascular diseases as a cause. Radiology 1997;205(2):465–70.
8. Remy-Jardin M, Remy J, Louvegny S, et al. Airway changes in chronic pulmonary embolism: CT findings in 33 patients. Radiology 1997;203(2):355–60.
9. American Thoracic Society/European Respiratory Society International Multidisciplinary Consensus Classification of the Idiopathic Interstitial Pneumonias. This joint statement of the American Thoracic Society (ATS), and the European Respiratory Society (ERS) was adopted by the ATS board of directors, June 2001 and by the ERS Executive Committee, June 2001. Am J Respir Crit Care Med 2002;165(2):277–304.
10. Frankel SK, Cool CD, Lynch DA, Brown KK. Idiopathic pleuroparenchymal fibroelastosis: description of a novel clinicopathologic entity. Chest 2004;126(6):2007–13.
11. Becker CD, Gil J, Padilla ML. Idiopathic pleuroparenchymal fibroelastosis: an unrecognized or misdiagnosed entity? Mod Pathol 2008;21(6):784–7.
12. Raghu G, Collard HR, Egan JJ, et al. An official ATS/ERS/JRS/ALAT statement: idiopathic pulmonary fibrosis: evidence-based guidelines for diagnosis and management. Am J Respir Crit Care Med 2011;183(6):788–824.
13. Sumikawa H, Johkoh T, Colby TV, et al. Computed tomography findings in pathological usual interstitial pneumonia: relationship to survival. Am J Respir Crit Care Med 2008;177(4):433–9.
14. Souza CA, Muller NL, Flint J, et al. Idiopathic pulmonary fibrosis: spectrum of high-resolution CT findings. Am J Roentgenol 2005;185(6):1531–9.
15. Flaherty KR, Thwaite EL, Kazerooni EA, et al. Radiological versus histological diagnosis in UIP and NSIP: survival implications. Thorax 2003;58(2):143–8.
16. Sverzellati N, Wells AU, Tomassetti S, et al. Biopsy-proved idiopathic pulmonary fibrosis: spectrum of nondiagnostic thin-section CT diagnoses. Radiology 2010;254(3):957–64.
17. Lynch DA, Godwin JD, Safrin S, et al. High-resolution computed tomography in idiopathic pulmonary fibrosis: diagnosis and prognosis. Am J Respir Crit Care Med 2005;172(4):488–93.
18. Collard HR, Moore BB, Flaherty KR, et al. Acute exacerbations of idiopathic pulmonary fibrosis. Am J Respir Crit Care Med 2007;176(7):636–43.

19. Kishi K, Homma S, Kurosaki A, et al. High-resolution computed tomography findings of lung cancer associated with idiopathic pulmonary fibrosis. J Comput Assist Tomogr 2006;30(1):95–9.
20. Chung MJ, Goo JM, Im JG. Pulmonary tuberculosis in patients with idiopathic pulmonary fibrosis. Eur J Radiol 2004;52(2): 175–9.
21. Travis WD, Hunninghake G, King TE Jr, et al. Idiopathic nonspecific interstitial pneumonia: report of an American Thoracic Society project. Am J Respir Crit Care Med 2008;177(12): 1338–47.
22. MacDonald SL, Rubens MB, Hansell DM, et al. Nonspecific interstitial pneumonia and usual interstitial pneumonia: comparative appearances at and diagnostic accuracy of thin-section CT. Radiology 2001;221(3):600–5.
23. Johkoh T, Muller NL, Colby TV, et al. Nonspecific interstitial pneumonia: correlation between thin-section CT findings and pathologic subgroups in 55 patients. Radiology 2002;225(1): 199–204.
24. Carrington CB, Gaensler EA, Coutu RE, et al. Natural history and treated course of usual and desquamative interstitial pneumonia. N Engl J Med 1978;298(15):801–9.
25. Park JS, Brown KK, Tuder RM, et al. Respiratory bronchiolitis-associated interstitial lung disease: radiologic features with clinical and pathologic correlation. J Comput Assist Tomogr 2002;26(1): 13–20.
26. Nakanishi M, Demura Y, Mizuno S, et al. Changes in HRCT findings in patients with respiratory bronchiolitis-associated interstitial lung disease after smoking cessation. Eur Respir J 2007;29(3): 453–61.
27. Wells AU, Nicholson AG, Hansell DM. Challenges in pulmonary fibrosis. 4: smoking-induced diffuse interstitial lung diseases. Thorax 2007;62(10):904–10.
28. Hartman TE, Primack SL, Swensen SJ, et al. Desquamative interstitial pneumonia: thin-section CT findings in 22 patients. Radiology 1993;187(3):787–90.
29. Attili AK, Kazerooni EA, Gross BH, et al. Smoking-related interstitial lung disease: radiologic-clinical-pathologic correlation. Radiographics 2008;28(5):1383–96; discussion 1396–88.
30. Primack SL, Hartman TE, Ikezoe J, et al. Acute interstitial pneumonia: radiographic and CT findings in nine patients. Radiology 1993;188(3):817–20.
31. Johkoh T, Muller NL, Taniguchi H, et al. Acute interstitial pneumonia: thin-section CT findings in 36 patients. Radiology 1999; 211(3):859–63.
32. Howling SJ, Evans TW, Hansell DM. The significance of bronchial dilatation on CT in patients with adult respiratory distress syndrome. Clin Radiol 1998;53(2):105–9.
33. Desai SR, Wells AU, Rubens MB, et al. Acute respiratory distress syndrome: CT abnormalities at long-term follow-up. Radiology 1999;210(1):29–35.
34. Swigris JJ, Berry GJ, Raffin TA, Kuschner WG. Lymphoid interstitial pneumonia: a narrative review. Chest 2002;122(6):2150–64.
35. Johkoh T, Muller NL, Pickford HA, et al. Lymphocytic interstitial pneumonia: thin-section CT findings in 22 patients. Radiology 1999;212(2):567–72.
36. Ichikawa Y, Kinoshita M, Koga T, et al. Lung cyst formation in lymphocytic interstitial pneumonia: CT features. J Comput Assist Tomogr 1994;18(5):745–8.
37. Reddy T, Tominaga M, Hansell DM. Pleuroparenchymal fibroelastosis: a spectrum of histopathological and imaging phenotypes. Eur Respir J 2012;40(2):377–85.
38. James DG, Neville E, Siltzbach LE. A worldwide review of sarcoidosis. Ann N Y Acad Sci 1976;278:321–34.
39. DeRemee RA. The roentgenographic staging of sarcoidosis. Historic and contemporary perspectives. Chest 1983;83(1):128–33.
40. Kirks DR, McCormick VD, Greenspan RH. Pulmonary sarcoidosis. Roentgenologic analysis of 150 patients. Am J Roentgenol Radium Ther Nucl Med 1973;117(4):777–86.
41. Conant EF, Glickstein MF, Mahar P, Miller WT. Pulmonary sarcoidosis in the older patient: conventional radiographic features. Radiology 1988;169(2):315–19.
42. Hamper UM, Fishman EK, Khouri NF, et al. Typical and atypical CT manifestations of pulmonary sarcoidosis. J Comput Assist Tomogr 1986;10(6):928–36.
43. Siltzbach LE, James DG, Neville E, et al. Course and prognosis of sarcoidosis around the world. Am J Med 1974;57(6):847–52.
44. Gawne-Cain ML, Hansell DM. The pattern and distribution of calcified mediastinal lymph nodes in sarcoidosis and tuberculosis: a CT study. Clin Radiol 1996;51(4):263–7.
45. Brauner MW, Grenier P, Mompoint D, et al. Pulmonary sarcoidosis: evaluation with high-resolution CT. Radiology 1989;172(2): 467–71.
46. Criado E, Sanchez M, Ramirez J, et al. Pulmonary sarcoidosis: typical and atypical manifestations at high-resolution CT with pathologic correlation. Radiographics 2010;30(6):1567–86.
47. Nishino M, Lee KS, Itoh H, Hatabu H. The spectrum of pulmonary sarcoidosis: variations of high-resolution CT findings and clues for specific diagnosis. Eur J Radiol 2010;73(1):66–73.
48. Davies CW, Tasker AD, Padley SP, et al. Air trapping in sarcoidosis on computed tomography: correlation with lung function. Clin Radiol 2000;55(3):217–21.
49. Brauner MW, Lenoir S, Grenier P, et al. Pulmonary sarcoidosis: CT assessment of lesion reversibility. Radiology 1992;182(2): 349–54.
50. Murdoch J, Muller NL. Pulmonary sarcoidosis: changes on follow-up CT examination. Am J Roentgenol 1992;159(3): 473–7.
51. Abehsera M, Valeyre D, Grenier P, et al. Sarcoidosis with pulmonary fibrosis: CT patterns and correlation with pulmonary function. Am J Roentgenol 2000;174(6):1751–7.
52. Leung AN, Brauner MW, Caillat-Vigneron N, et al. Sarcoidosis activity: correlation of HRCT findings with those of 67Ga scanning, bronchoalveolar lavage, and serum angiotensin-converting enzyme assay. J Comput Assist Tomogr 1998;22(2):229–34.
53. Hirschmann JV, Pipavath SN, Godwin JD. Hypersensitivity pneumonitis: a historical, clinical, and radiologic review. Radiographics 2009;29(7):1921–38.
54. Baldwin CI, Todd A, Bourke S, et al. Pigeon fanciers' lung: effects of smoking on serum and salivary antibody responses to pigeon antigens. Clin Exp Immunol 1998;113(2):166–72.
55. Silva CI, Churg A, Muller NL. Hypersensitivity pneumonitis: spectrum of high-resolution CT and pathologic findings. Am J Roentgenol 2007;188(2):334–44.
56. Cormier Y, Brown M, Worthy S, et al. High-resolution computed tomographic characteristics in acute farmer's lung and in its follow-up. Eur Respir J 2000;16(1):56–60.
57. Hansell DM, Wells AU, Padley SP, Muller NL. Hypersensitivity pneumonitis: correlation of individual CT patterns with functional abnormalities. Radiology 1996;199(1):123–8.
58. Franquet T, Hansell DM, Senbanjo T, et al. Lung cysts in subacute hypersensitivity pneumonitis. J Comput Assist Tomogr 2003;27(4):475–8.
59. Erkinjuntti-Pekkanen R, Rytkonen H, Kokkarinen JI, et al. Long-term risk of emphysema in patients with farmer's lung and matched control farmers. Am J Respir Crit Care Med 1998;158(2): 662–5.
60. Sahin H, Brown KK, Curran-Everett D, et al. Chronic hypersensitivity pneumonitis: CT features comparison with pathologic evidence of fibrosis and survival. Radiology 2007;244(2): 591–8.
61. Silva CI, Muller NL, Lynch DA, et al. Chronic hypersensitivity pneumonitis: differentiation from idiopathic pulmonary fibrosis and nonspecific interstitial pneumonia by using thin-section CT. Radiology 2008;246(1):288–97.
62. Zompatori M, Calabro E, Chetta A, et al. [Chronic hypersensitivity pneumonitis or idiopathic pulmonary fibrosis? Diagnostic role of high resolution computed tomography (HRCT)]. Radiol Med 2003;106(3):135–46.
63. Vassallo R, Ryu JH, Colby TV, et al. Pulmonary Langerhans'-cell histiocytosis. N Engl J Med 2000;342(26):1969–78.
64. Travis WD, Borok Z, Roum JH, et al. Pulmonary Langerhans cell granulomatosis (histiocytosis X). A clinicopathologic study of 48 cases. Am J Surg Pathol 1993;17(10):971–86.
65. Caminati A, Harari S. Smoking-related interstitial pneumonias and pulmonary Langerhans cell histiocytosis. Proc Am Thorac Soc 2006;3(4):299–306.
66. Brauner MW, Grenier P, Mouelhi MM, et al. Pulmonary histiocytosis X: evaluation with high-resolution CT. Radiology 1989;172(1):255–8.
67. Brauner MW, Grenier P, Tijani K, et al. Pulmonary Langerhans cell histiocytosis: evolution of lesions on CT scans. Radiology 1997;204(2):497–502.

68. Ryu JH, Moss J, Beck GJ, et al. The NHLBI lymphangioleiomyomatosis registry: characteristics of 230 patients at enrollment. Am J Respir Crit Care Med 2006;173(1):105–11.
69. Johnson SR. Lymphangioleiomyomatosis. Eur Respir J 2006;27(5): 1056–65.
70. Sherrier RH, Chiles C, Roggli V. Pulmonary lymphangioleiomyomatosis: CT findings. Am J Roentgenol 1989;153(5):937–40.
71. Lenoir S, Grenier P, Brauner MW, et al. Pulmonary lymphangiomyomatosis and tuberous sclerosis: comparison of radiographic and thin-section CT findings. Radiology 1990;175(2):329–34.
72. Templeton PA, McLoud TC, Muller NL, et al. Pulmonary lymphangioleiomyomatosis: CT and pathologic findings. J Comput Assist Tomogr 1989;13(1):54–7.
73. Muller NL, Chiles C, Kullnig P. Pulmonary lymphangiomyomatosis: correlation of CT with radiographic and functional findings. Radiology 1990;175(2):335–9.
74. Kitaichi M, Nishimura K, Itoh H, Izumi T. Pulmonary lymphangioleiomyomatosis: a report of 46 patients including a clinicopathologic study of prognostic factors. Am J Respir Crit Care Med 1995;151(2 Pt 1):527–33.
75. Abbott GF, Rosado-de-Christenson ML, Frazier AA, et al. From the archives of the AFIP: lymphangioleiomyomatosis: radiologic-pathologic correlation. Radiographics 2005;25(3):803–28.
76. Koyama M, Johkoh T, Honda O, et al. Chronic cystic lung disease: diagnostic accuracy of high-resolution CT in 92 patients. Am J Roentgenol 2003;180(3):827–35.
77. Tanoue LT. Pulmonary manifestations of rheumatoid arthritis. Clin Chest Med 1998;19(4):667–85, viii.
78. Lee HK, Kim DS, Yoo B, et al. Histopathologic pattern and clinical features of rheumatoid arthritis-associated interstitial lung disease. Chest 2005;127(6):2019–27.
79. Kim EJ, Elicker BM, Maldonado F, et al. Usual interstitial pneumonia in rheumatoid arthritis-associated interstitial lung disease. Eur Respir J 2010;35(6):1322–8.
80. Remy-Jardin M, Remy J, Cortet B, et al. Lung changes in rheumatoid arthritis: CT findings. Radiology 1994;193(2): 375–82.
81. Akira M, Sakatani M, Hara H. Thin-section CT findings in rheumatoid arthritis-associated lung disease: CT patterns and their courses. J Comput Assist Tomogr 1999;23(6):941–8.
82. Gamsu G. Radiographic manifestations of thoracic involvement by collagen vascular diseases. J Thorac Imaging 1992;7(3):1–12.
83. Devouassoux G, Cottin V, Liote H, et al. Characterisation of severe obliterative bronchiolitis in rheumatoid arthritis. Eur Respir J 2009;33(5):1053–61.
84. Primack SL, Muller NL. Radiologic manifestations of the systemic autoimmune diseases. Clin Chest Med 1998;19(4):573–86, vii.
85. Gibson M, Hansell DM. Lymphocytic disorders of the chest: pathology and imaging. Clin Radiol 1998;53(7):469–80.
86. Howling SJ, Hansell DM, Wells AU, et al. Follicular bronchiolitis: thin-section CT and histologic findings. Radiology 1999; 212(3):637–42.
87. Franquet T. High-resolution CT of lung disease related to collagen vascular disease. Radiol Clin North Am 2001;39(6):1171–87.
88. Cain HC, Noble PW, Matthay RA. Pulmonary manifestations of Sjogren's syndrome. Clin Chest Med 1998;19(4):687–99, viii.
89. Ito I, Nagai S, Kitaichi M, et al. Pulmonary manifestations of primary Sjogren's syndrome: a clinical, radiologic, and pathologic study. Am J Respir Crit Care Med 2005;171(6):632–8.
90. Desai SR, Nicholson AG, Stewart S, et al. Benign pulmonary lymphocytic infiltration and amyloidosis: computed tomographic and pathologic features in three cases. J Thorac Imaging 1997; 12(3):215–20.
91. Franquet T, Gimenez A, Monill JM, et al. Primary Sjogren's syndrome and associated lung disease: CT findings in 50 patients. Am J Roentgenol 1997;169(3):655–8.
92. Young RH, Mark GJ. Pulmonary vascular changes in scleroderma. Am J Med 1978;64(6):998–1004.
93. Silver RM, Miller KS. Lung involvement in systemic sclerosis. Rheum Dis Clin North Am 1990;16(1):199–216.
94. Minai OA, Dweik RA, Arroliga AC. Manifestations of scleroderma pulmonary disease. Clin Chest Med 1998;19(4):713–31, viii–ix.
95. Lynch DA. Lung disease related to collagen vascular disease. J Thorac Imaging 2009;24(4):299–309.
96. Fujita J, Yoshinouchi T, Ohtsuki Y, et al. Non-specific interstitial pneumonia as pulmonary involvement of systemic sclerosis. Ann Rheum Dis 2001;60(3):281–3.
97. Bouros D, Wells AU, Nicholson AG, et al. Histopathologic subsets of fibrosing alveolitis in patients with systemic sclerosis and their relationship to outcome. Am J Respir Crit Care Med 2002;165(12):1581–6.
98. Garber SJ, Wells AU, duBois RM, Hansell DM. Enlarged mediastinal lymph nodes in the fibrosing alveolitis of systemic sclerosis. Br J Radiol 1992;65(779):983–6.
99. Douglas WW, Tazelaar HD, Hartman TE, et al. Polymyositis-dermatomyositis-associated interstitial lung disease. Am J Respir Crit Care Med 2001;164(7):1182–5.
100. Ikezoe J, Johkoh T, Kohno N, et al. High-resolution CT findings of lung disease in patients with polymyositis and dermatomyositis. J Thorac Imaging 1996;11(4):250–9.
101. Mino M, Noma S, Taguchi Y, et al. Pulmonary involvement in polymyositis and dermatomyositis: sequential evaluation with CT. Am J Roentgenol 1997;169(1):83–7.
102. Akira M, Hara H, Sakatani M. Interstitial lung disease in association with polymyositis-dermatomyositis: long-term follow-up CT evaluation in seven patients. Radiology 1999;210(2): 333–8.
103. Murin S, Wiedemann HP, Matthay RA. Pulmonary manifestations of systemic lupus erythematosus. Clin Chest Med 1998; 19(4):641–65, viii.
104. Carmier D, Marchand-Adam S, Diot P, Diot E. Respiratory involvement in systemic lupus erythematosus. Rev Mal Respir 2010;27(8):e66–78.
105. Zamora MR, Warner ML, Tuder R, Schwarz MI. Diffuse alveolar hemorrhage and systemic lupus erythematosus. Clinical presentation, histology, survival, and outcome. Medicine (Baltimore) 1997;76(3):192–202.
106. Jeong YJ, Kim KI, Seo IJ, et al. Eosinophilic lung diseases: a clinical, radiologic, and pathologic overview. Radiographics 2007;27(3): 617–37; discussion 637–19.
107. Silva CI, Muller NL, Fujimoto K, et al. Churg-Strauss syndrome: high resolution CT and pathologic findings. J Thorac Imaging 2005;20(2):74–80.
108. Johkoh T, Muller NL, Akira M, et al. Eosinophilic lung diseases: diagnostic accuracy of thin-section CT in 111 patients. Radiology 2000;216(3):773–80.
109. Cleverley JR, Screaton NJ, Hiorns MP, et al. Drug-induced lung disease: high-resolution CT and histological findings. Clin Radiol 2002;57(4):292–9.
110. Myers JL, Limper AH, Swensen SJ. Drug-induced lung disease: a pragmatic classification incorporating HRCT appearances. Semin Respir Crit Care Med 2003;24(4):445–54.
111. Rossi SE, Erasmus JJ, McAdams HP, et al. Pulmonary drug toxicity: radiologic and pathologic manifestations. Radiographics 2000;20(5):1245–59.
112. Sheehan RE, Wells AU, Milne DG, Hansell DM. Nitrofurantoin-induced lung disease: two cases demonstrating resolution of apparently irreversible CT abnormalities. J Comput Assist Tomogr 2000;24(2):259–61.
113. Vernhet H, Bousquet C, Durand G, et al. Reversible amiodarone-induced lung disease: HRCT findings. Eur Radiol 2001;11(9): 1697–703.
114. Silva CI, Muller NL. Drug-induced lung diseases: most common reaction patterns and corresponding high-resolution CT manifestations. Semin Ultrasound CT MR 2006;27(2):111–16.
115. Ellis SJ, Cleverley JR, Muller NL. Drug-induced lung disease: high-resolution CT findings. Am J Roentgenol 2000;175(4): 1019–24.
116. Vallyathan V, Brower PS, Green FH, Attfield MD. Radiographic and pathologic correlation of coal workers' pneumoconiosis. Am J Respir Crit Care Med 1996;154(3 Pt 1):741–8.
117. Bergin CJ, Muller NL, Vedal S, Chan-Yeung M. CT in silicosis: correlation with plain films and pulmonary function tests. Am J Roentgenol 1986;146(3):477–83.
118. Remy-Jardin M, Beuscart R, Sault MC, et al. Subpleural micronodules in diffuse infiltrative lung diseases: evaluation with thin-section CT scans. Radiology 1990;177(1):133–9.
119. Ferreira AS, Moreira VB, Ricardo HM, et al. Progressive massive fibrosis in silica-exposed workers. High-resolution computed tomography findings. J Bras Pneumol 2006;32(6):523–8.

120. Epler GR, McLoud TC, Gaensler EA. Prevalence and incidence of benign asbestos pleural effusion in a working population. JAMA 1982;247(5):617–22.
121. Hillerdal G. Non-malignant asbestos pleural disease. Thorax 1981;36(9):669–75.
122. Peacock C, Copley SJ, Hansell DM. Asbestos-related benign pleural disease. Clin Radiol 2000;55(6):422–32.
123. Friedman AC, Fiel SB, Fisher MS, et al. Asbestos-related pleural disease and asbestosis: a comparison of CT and chest radiography. Am J Roentgenol 1988;150(2):269–75.
124. Van Cleemput J, De Raeve H, Verschakelen JA, et al. Surface of localized pleural plaques quantitated by computed tomography scanning: no relation with cumulative asbestos exposure and no effect on lung function. Am J Respir Crit Care Med 2001;163(3 Pt 1):705–10.
125. Sette A, Neder JA, Nery LE, et al. Thin-section CT abnormalities and pulmonary gas exchange impairment in workers exposed to asbestos. Radiology 2004;232(1):66–74.
126. al Jarad N, Poulakis N, Pearson MC, et al. Assessment of asbestos-induced pleural disease by computed tomography—correlation with chest radiograph and lung function. Respir Med 1991;85(3):203–8.
127. Schneider HJ, Felson B, Gonzalez LL. Rounded atelectasis. Am J Roentgenol 1980;134(2):225–32.
128. Lynch DA, Gamsu G, Ray CS, Aberle DR. Asbestos-related focal lung masses: manifestations on conventional and high-resolution CT scans. Radiology 1988;169(3):603–7.
129. Craighead JE, Mossman BT. The pathogenesis of asbestos-associated diseases. N Engl J Med 1982;306(24):1446–55.
130. Oksa P, Suoranta H, Koskinen H, et al. High-resolution computed tomography in the early detection of asbestosis. Int Arch Occup Environ Health 1994;65(5):299–304.
131. Akira M, Yamamoto S, Yokoyama K, et al. Asbestosis: high-resolution CT-pathologic correlation. Radiology 1990;176(2):389–94.
132. Akira M, Yokoyama K, Yamamoto S, et al. Early asbestosis: evaluation with high-resolution CT. Radiology 1991;178(2):409–16.
133. Akira M, Yamamoto S, Inoue Y, Sakatani M. High-resolution CT of asbestosis and idiopathic pulmonary fibrosis. Am J Roentgenol 2003;181(1):163–9.
134. Copley SJ, Wells AU, Sivakumaran P, et al. Asbestosis and idiopathic pulmonary fibrosis: comparison of thin-section CT features. Radiology 2003;229(3):731–6.

CHAPTER 10

Thoracic Trauma and Related Topics

John H. Reynolds • Hefin Jones

CHAPTER OUTLINE

THORACIC TRAUMA

Introduction

The thorax contains the organs most essential to basic life, namely the heart, lungs and the largest and most important of the blood vessels. The alveoli of the lungs allow exchange of oxygen and carbon dioxide and the heart and great vessels circulate nutrients, oxygen and carbon dioxide to and from all organs and tissues. Traumatic injury to these structures, more than many others, can precipitate death and extra-thoracic organ injury. Even relatively minor injuries to the chest's musculoskeletal system can lead to morbidity, such as hypoventilation and subsequent pneumonia, secondary to rib fracture.

In developed nations, trauma is the leading cause of death in the under-50 age group, of which 20% are directly related to thoracic injuries and up to 50% may be indirectly related to thoracic injuries.[1] Significant thoracic trauma, requiring hospitalisation, is thought to have an incidence of 4 per million per day worldwide.[2] Major thoracic trauma rarely occurs in isolation and other areas of injury may be present, particularly in the head, spine, abdomen and pelvis. The main cause of chest trauma is road traffic collisions (RTC) (75%); violent assault and falls are other relatively common aetiologies but with slightly different patterns of injury.[3]

Major trauma patients are assessed and treated according to the Advanced Trauma Life Support (ATLS) protocol,[3–6] which assumes a trimodal pattern of mortality, with peaks at the time of the incident, after several hours and delayed (>1 week); the protocol was designed to reduce patient mortality in survivors of the initial injury.

The initial (primary) radiological assessment includes an anteroposterior (AP) chest and AP pelvic plain radiograph but in many trauma centres, if a major injury is suggested and the patient is relatively stable, these plain radiographs may be omitted with the patient undergoing a 'trauma series' multidetector computed tomography (MDCT) examination.[7]

Experience gained in dealing with military casualties has provided a challenging cohort of patients and has helped evolve civilian medical practice in emergency departments, aided by developments such as helicopter retrieval and emergency transfer and the development of regional 'Level I' trauma centres in many developed countries (RCR). With advanced paramedical practice, many patients will arrive at the hospital intubated and will sometimes have prophylactic chest drains inserted, particularly if transferred via helicopter, and the primary survey will have often been completed prior to arrival. Focused assessment with sonography for trauma (FAST) can be performed in transit and with competent operators; this can also detect the presence of pleural and pericardial fluid before arrival in the emergency department.[8]

Once in the trauma centre, fast helical MDCT is the most useful imaging investigation in the acute setting, given its rapidity, availability and familiarity by the interpreting radiologist. Full anaesthetic and monitoring equipment can now be found in most emergency CT units, allowing even relatively unstable patients the opportunity for acute diagnostic CT. Cardiac-gated CT does reduce movement artefact of the heart and thoracic aorta but its benefits are not yet thought to outweigh the complexities of acquisition in the acute setting, particularly as there may be a decrease in image quality for assessment of lung and bone injury.[9] In cases of diagnostic uncertainty, repeat cardiac-gated CT or MRI can be performed when the patient has stabilised.

Protocols vary but all should include an unenhanced CT head and a contrast-enhanced thorax and abdomen, including full spine and pelvic imaging.[10]

Some trauma centres advocate a two-phase intravenous contrast-enhanced single CT data acquisition from the skull base to mid-femur, with more dilute contrast seen in the portovenous phase and a delayed high concentration contrast agent injected later, providing an arteriographic image within the same examination. Further advances include the use of radiolucent spinal boards or higher kilovoltage (kV) techniques to avoid the need to unnecessarily move patients with suspected spinal injuries.[10]

A disadvantage of modern CT is the large number of images for the radiologist to review with the potential for subsequent delay in provision of report. One solution is for the radiologist to complete a quick provisional pro-forma, with 'tick-box' entry for each injury-free body part and space for a brief description of any injuries seen, a copy of which is given to the emergency physician within 15 min, allowing early decision-making regarding immediate procedures or surgery. Subsequent, less pressured and more detailed analysis of the images can then take place in preparation of the final report.[10] Radiation doses can be of concern, particularly if there is poor patient selection but a well-protocolled single CT can prevent repeated attendances for plain radiography or angiography.[11]

Recent evidence suggests that due to modern, urban implementation of ATLS guidelines and an increase in availability of access to acute CT imaging, the previously recognised trimodal mortality pattern may be changing.[12]

Types of Injury

Thoracic injury can be broadly divided into blunt and penetrating but in any individual, one or both types can be present. Blunt trauma imparts kinetic energy to the point(s) of impact, causing both direct damage at these and at more distant sites. Shearing injuries can occur in sudden deceleration, for example, such as at the aortic isthmus, the right main bronchus or within the lung parenchyma. Penetrating trauma, such as knife, gunshot or shrapnel, also imparts kinetic energy into the tissues involved. The kinetic energy imparted is related to the square of the projectile velocity, which illustrates why high-velocity missiles, such as rifle bullets and shrapnel, are associated with more injury than their mass alone would suggest.

Penetrating missiles are associated with both a permanent cavity and a surrounding temporary cavity formation, created by the shock wave of impact, proportional in size to the velocity of the projectile. This temporary cavitation causes more damage in less elastic tissues, such as liver, than in the lung parenchyma. An appreciation of this, often initially occult, penumbra of damage is vital to understanding the likely outcomes of differing injuries. Further injury can be caused by fragmentation of the missile, external armour or bone fragments, dispersing velocity but increasing the area of injury and number of projectiles.[13]

If the missile passes through the air-filled cavity of the lungs, and does not come into contact with a solid organ, in particular, bone, then there is a high chance of the projectile not being retained. Even so, entry and exit points may be visualised by 'smears' of lead remaining at hard surface borders, such as bone, suggesting a likely trajectory.[14] Given its high density and radiographic attenuation, even the smallest traces left may be seen on CT. The estimated trajectory can suggest structures, such as nerves, which may have been damaged but not clinically apparent in the unconscious patient. Sometimes the site of entry wound is clinically apparent but radiographically occult, particularly an issue with long sharp weapons, such as stilettos and screwdrivers, and one solution is to ensure a radio-opaque marker is applied to the dressing overlying each suspected entry wound.

A retained projectile of high-attenuation material leads to 'beam-hardening' artefact, which can make visualisation of surrounding injury difficult. Techniques such as high kV CT and altering the angle of acquisition, either in relation to gantry or by position of patient, may be of value in this situation.

Similar problems of 'blooming' are encountered with magnetic resonance imaging (MRI), and although most bullets are composed of lead, and sometimes copper, thus ostensibly MRI compatible, their pathway may include non-MRI compatible material, particularly when there has been fragmentation.

Ultrasound can be used for peripheral objects, to assess musculoskeletal damage and can be used for a quick estimation of injury but often is unable to confidently aid initial diagnosis otherwise. Superficial wound-related collections are a major cause for re-imaging the septic patient and such collections can be easily assessed using ultrasound. This also allows imaging, and where necessary drain insertion, to be performed in the ICU setting.

A further type of injury is blast injury, caused by sudden, rapid pressure changes in either air pressure or transmitted through water to submerged areas of the body, usually as a result of an explosion. This is associated with marked damage at the air–tissue interface with air blast injuries, causing alveolar, bowel and tympanic rupture. Although the pressure wave rapidly dissipates with distance from explosion, it may be funnelled or amplified in enclosed spaces and should be considered in any indoor explosion injury.[15] Generally, however, those patients more than 6 metres from the explosion source at time of injury are unlikely to suffer from significant blast injury.[16]

Diagnostic Approach

Those patients with less severe clinical presentations and those too unstable for CT should undergo plain radiography in the ED resuscitation room as part of standard ATLS procedure and be assessed for immediate surgery or subsequent CT when resuscitated. All major traumatic presentations, stable enough to attend CT, should directly undergo trauma series CT.[10,17]

It seems prudent to seek those injuries likely to cause most serious and immediate morbidity and mortality to the patient. This requires analysis of the heart, looking for signs of cardiac injury, pericardial effusion and the more serious finding of traumatic cardiac tamponade. This is not specific for cardiac injury, as aortic root injury can also lead to this finding.

Assessment of the remainder of the mediastinum should seek evidence of mediastinal haemorrhage, in particular related to aortic injury, and the aorta should be assessed from root to below the diaphragm. Mediastinal displacement or compression by tension pneumothorax can cause haemodynamic compromise and it is this, rather than the pneumothorax itself, which represents the most immediate danger. Rapid enlargement can occur under positive pressure ventilation, leading to acute deterioration, resistant to alteration in tidal pressures. Tracheobronchial injury is relatively rare and is either seen directly or suggested by a combination of pneumothorax and pneumomediastinum.

Lung parenchymal opacification is likely to represent pulmonary contusion and this may initially obscure the more serious injury of pulmonary laceration. Pulmonary contusion is usually associated with rib fractures, which generally serve as an indirect marker of further thoracic and extra-thoracic injury, rather than significant injuries in themselves. One important finding is of multiple fractures in three or more contiguous ribs, resulting in a 'flail chest', associated with marked contusion, atelectasis and impaired ventilation, with associated increased mortality.

Diaphragmatic injuries can be often overlooked but their diagnosis and subsequent repair can prevent later bowel strangulation.[18] Herniated stomach can be misdiagnosed as pneumothorax and attempted chest drain insertion can result in contamination of the pleural space.

Spinal injury should be assessed both for direct consequences and as a marker of severe thoracic injury, particularly when associated with sternal fracture. Thoracic injury patterns can be suggestive of occult abdominal and neck injuries. In particular, diaphragmatic involvement is commonly associated with splenic and hepatic injury.

Specific Thoracic Injuries Following Trauma

Heart

The myocardium is more commonly affected by blunt rather than penetrating trauma, in those patients still alive on arrival to hospital. As with all blunt chest trauma, RTCs account for the vast majority but specific injuries to the heart include cardiopulmonary resuscitation.

Injury occurs usually due to crushing or deceleration but cardiac damage can occur due to overdistension due to excessive hydrostatic pressure, and this, combined with a reduced myocardial mass and anterior position, is likely to explain the increased incidence of right atrial and ventricular rupture.[19] Injuries can range from asymptomatic contusions and arrhythmias, to coronary artery injury, regional wall motion abnormalities, pericardial tears, papillary rupture and valve dysfunction, with the most severe septal and free wall rupture seen as perimortal findings. Acute imaging with CT may only show a pericardial effusion or haemopericardium—suggested by a higher attenuation effusion (Fig. 10-1A). It may be possible to demonstrate a focal area of hypo-enhancement of myocardium, representing contusion, but this may not be appreciated on non-cardiac-gated studies. The major differential is myocardial infarction and clinical features, ECG and biochemical markers are similar for both entities. Given a suitable history of trauma, hypotension, cardiac contusion should be suspected, particularly with evidence of mediastinal injuries or sternal fracture. Cardiac-gated CT can be performed once the patient is stable and this can demonstrate presence or absence of coronary artery occlusion.

Pericardial injury is usually associated with increased pericardial fluid, with even small effusions well demonstrated on CT. Pneumopericardium is an important sign of pericardial injury and differentiated from pneumothorax by its extent limited to the reflections at the roots of the great vessels.

Cardiac herniation is referred to as luxation and this can be associated with torsion of the great vessels and represents the most important, if rare, complication of pericardial injury (Fig. 10-2).

Sudden increases in endocardial pressure can result in traumatic papillary muscle, chordae tendinae and mitral valve leaflet tears. Increased intra-aortic pressure can cause injury to the aortic valve, with consequent aortic regurgitation. These valvular injuries may present immediately or after several years.[19]

Acute Traumatic Aortic Injury (ATAI)

The majority of cases of acute traumatic aortic injury (ATAI), around 80%,[20,21] occur as a result of RTCs. ATAI is present in 0.5–2% of all non-fatal RTCs and accounts for 10–20% of all high-speed deceleration fatalities.[22,23] In a recent Scottish study, 4% of blunt ATAI cases were dead on arrival and 19% died during triage; 68% were unsuitable for repair, with a mortality of 65%; 28% underwent open aortic repair and 4% underwent endovascular repair, with similar mortality rates of between 18 and 19%.[21] Studies have suggested mortality rates of up to 94% within 1 hour and 99% at 24 hours, if untreated.[20] This emphasises the importance of early diagnosis and appropriate patient triage.[24]

The majority of ATAI cases seen on imaging are located at the aortic isthmus, around 2 cm distal to the origin of the left subclavian artery. Other sites such as the aortic root (5% of clinical cases) and distal aorta (1% of clinical cases) are seen more frequently in post-mortem series due to the high mortality in injury at such sites. An aortic root disruption, for example, may lead to rapid death due to exsanguination, pericardial haemorrhage and tamponade, or myocardial infarction. The isthmic preponderance is thought to be related to multiple factors, including relative tethering at this site by the ligamentum arteriosum. Tethering is also thought to contribute to the increased numbers of injuries to the aortic root (5%) and as the aorta crosses the diaphragm (1%).

The mechanism of injury is thought to be multifactorial. A major factor is thought to be the relative movement of the heart and relatively mobile aorta arch relative to the more tethered descending aorta. 'Osseous pinch' is a term used to describe the mechanical compression of the aortic arch and branch vessels between the thoracic spine and the sternoclavicular junction. Increased intravascular pressure within the aorta, also known as the 'water hammer' effect, as a direct result of compression, has been suggested to cause injuries at the isthmus and root.[18,22]

Injuries may be divided into transections and non-full thickness tears, the latter being more commonly seen in

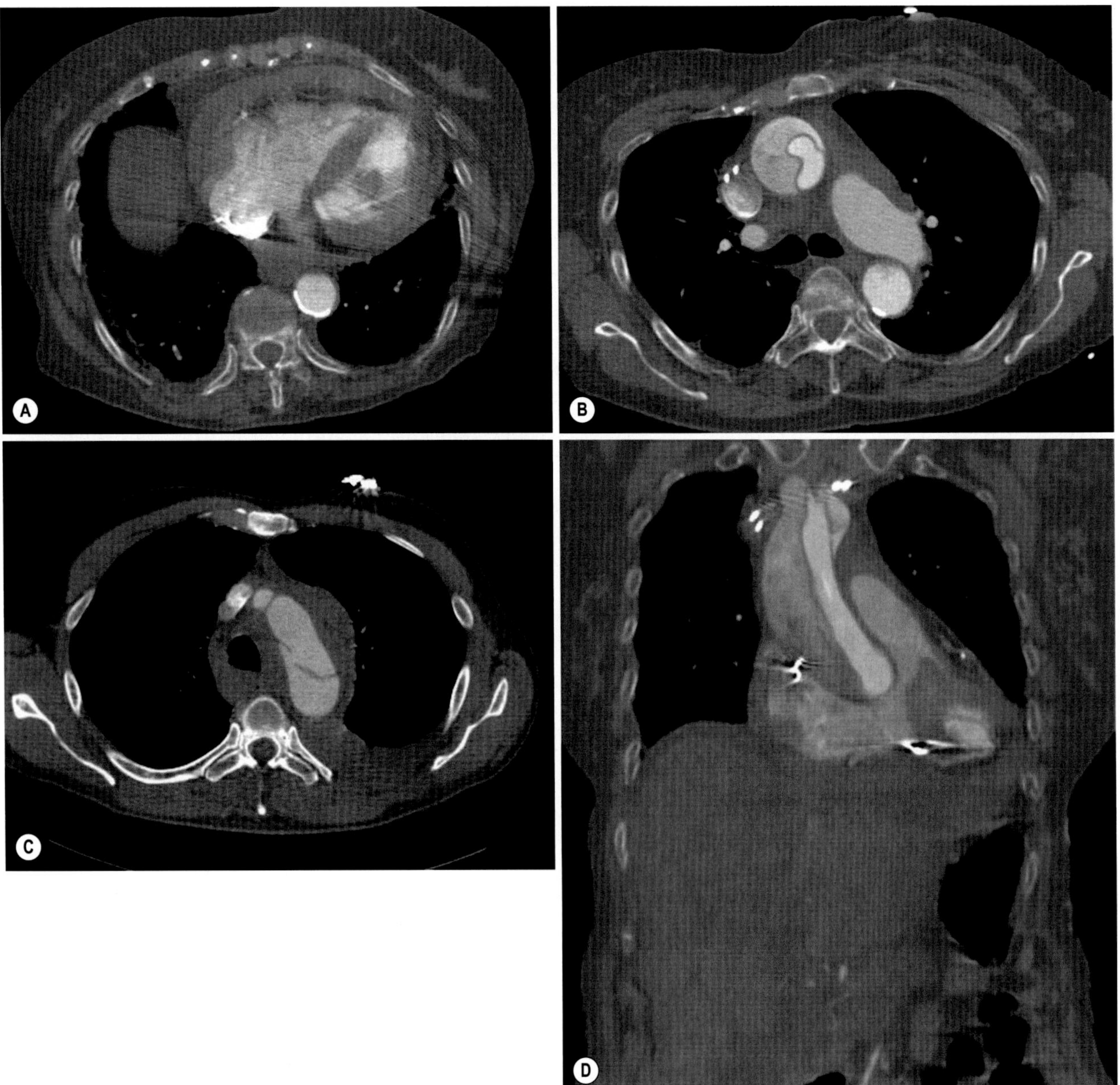

FIGURE 10-1 ■ Haemopericardium and acute traumatic aortic injury. CT image following blunt trauma with a haemopericardium (A). The patient also sustained an acute traumatic injury with a dissection visible on axial images (B, C) and on a coronal reformatted image (D).

survivors, as transections result in rapid exsanguination. Tears commonly involve the intima and media, leaving the adventitia intact but with overall weakening of the aorta and at risk of subsequent rupture and pseudoaneurysm.

The chest radiographic signs are related to the associated mediastinal haematoma and include: mediastinal widening, with a ratio of >25% of the chest width being a useful guide; blurring of the contours of the aortic arch and loss of definition of the aortopulmonary window; left apical pleural fluid; deviation of the trachea or NG tube; and widening of the paratracheal stripe and paravertebral contours (Fig. 10-3). However, given the relative poor negative predictive value of the chest X-ray, upon which 7% of ATAI may be occult, any abnormality, in the presence of a likely history, should be further investigated, usually with contrast-enhanced MDCT, particularly as ATAI only rarely occurs in isolation.[25] MDCT for ATAI has sensitivity and specificity around 98% and is generally considered the gold standard and first-line investigation.[22] Direct CT signs of ATAI includes intimal flaps, pseudoaneurysms and contained ruptures, an abnormal aortic contour and a sudden change in aortic calibre (pseudocoarctation).[26] True traumatic dissection is less common but is seen (Figs. 10-1B–D).

The presence of mediastinal haematoma but with well-defined aortic borders should be assumed to represent non-aortic bleeding from small mediastinal veins. Periaortic haematoma, without evidence of other aortic injury, should be assumed to be due to occult intimal

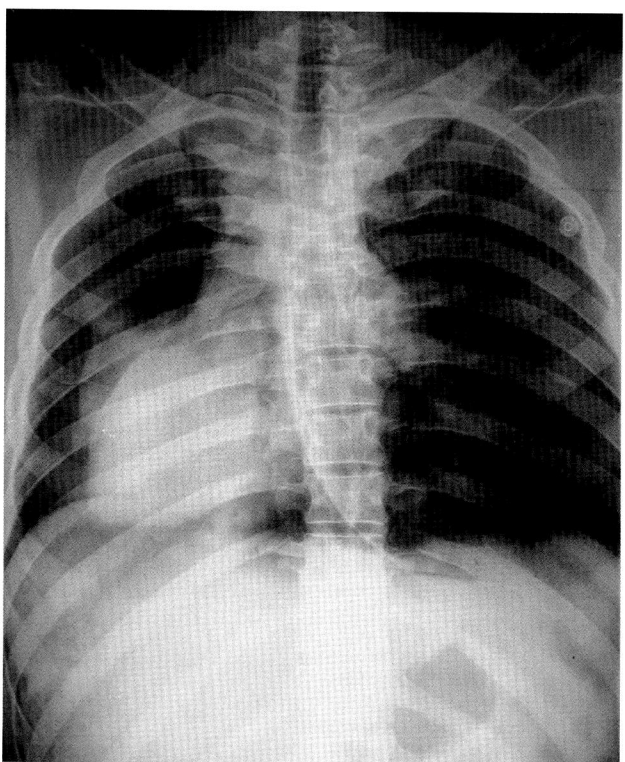

FIGURE 10-2 ■ **Cardiac herniation.** Chest radiograph following a fall from a height which resulted in traumatic pericardial rupture with herniation of the heart into the right hemithorax. Other injuries including rib and spinal fractures are present.

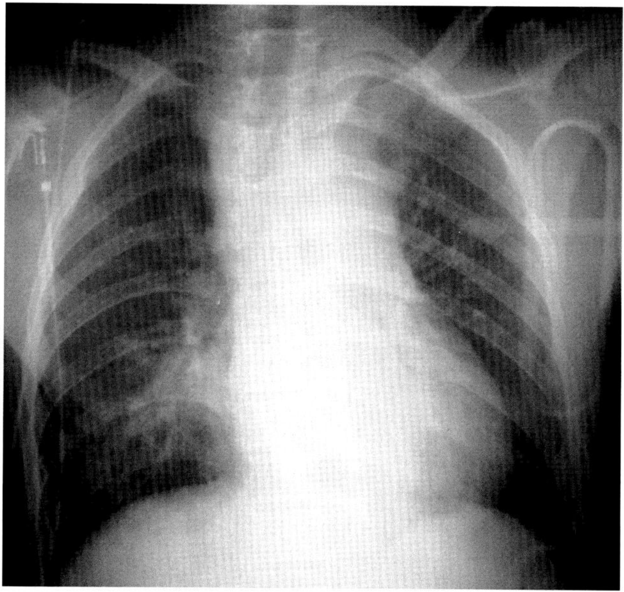

FIGURE 10-3 ■ **Aortic injury with mediastinal haematoma.** Chest radiograph in a patient with a post-traumatic aortic rupture and mediastinal haematoma. Features present include a widened mediastinum, filling in of the aortopulmonary bay and the development of a left apical pleural cap. (Courtesy of Dr L. C. Morus, Birmingham, UK.)

injury and should be followed up with further imaging depending on the patient's status. The term minimal aortic injury has been used to describe these lesions and those of intramural haematoma and intimal thrombus. Repeat CT aortography, MR aortography or trans-oesophageal ultrasound should be considered over the subsequent few days but there is no consensus as to the importance of these minimal aortic injuries. The role of diagnostic catheter angiography in these cases is limited in the acute setting, as it is estimated that 50% of these injuries are not detected via this technique.[27] Some centres advocate the use of intravascular ultrasound for these indeterminate abnormalities, particularly as a problem-solving adjunct to CT.[28]

In all cases multiplanar reformat (MPR) review should be performed, as the signs are often subtle and difficult to appreciate on axial imaging. Further difficulties arise from cardiac motion, particularly affecting the ascending aorta, which can falsely suggest intimal flap formation and from anatomical variants, such as infundibula at the origins of the branch vessels. Most centres would not require a subsequent catheter aortogram before surgical treatment and this would now be performed only as part of endovascular repair.

Mediastinum

Pneumomediastinum occurs in up to 10% of cases of blunt chest trauma, most commonly as a result of alveolar rupture, either due to trauma or positive pressure ventilation, with peribronchovascular tracking of the air into the mediastinum. Rarely, pneumomediastinum may occur as a result of tracheobronchial or oesophageal disruption. Findings on chest X-ray are of a lucency outlining the mediastinum and its structures, often extending into the neck, features better demonstrated with CT[29] (Fig. 10-4).

Trachiobronchial injury is seen in up to 2% of blunt chest trauma,[30] mainly bronchial, right-sided and within 2.5 cm of the carina, and is associated with an overall mortality of around 30%.[31] The proposed mechanism is of increased intrathoracic pressure, against a closed glottis.[17] Direct signs are of trachiobronchial disruption, with surrounding extra-luminal gas.[30] Indirect signs are of pneumomediastinum, and, pneumothorax, which is classically resistant to treatment with a chest drain. The 'fallen lung sign', where the lung parenchyma is displaced dependently indicates a complete rupture of (usually the right) main bronchus[18] (Fig. 10-5).

Traumatic oesophageal rupture is mostly iatrogenic in origin and may provide only indirect evidence of its presence, via pneumomediastinum and a left-sided pleural effusion. The use of oral water-soluble contrast agent will reveal the presence and site of rupture on either CT or fluoroscopic examination in over 90% of cases, allowing for prompt treatment to avoid development of mediastinitis, which is associated with greatly increased mortality.[32]

Pleura

Pneumothorax occurs in 30% of all chest trauma and although it may be caused by increased intrathoracic

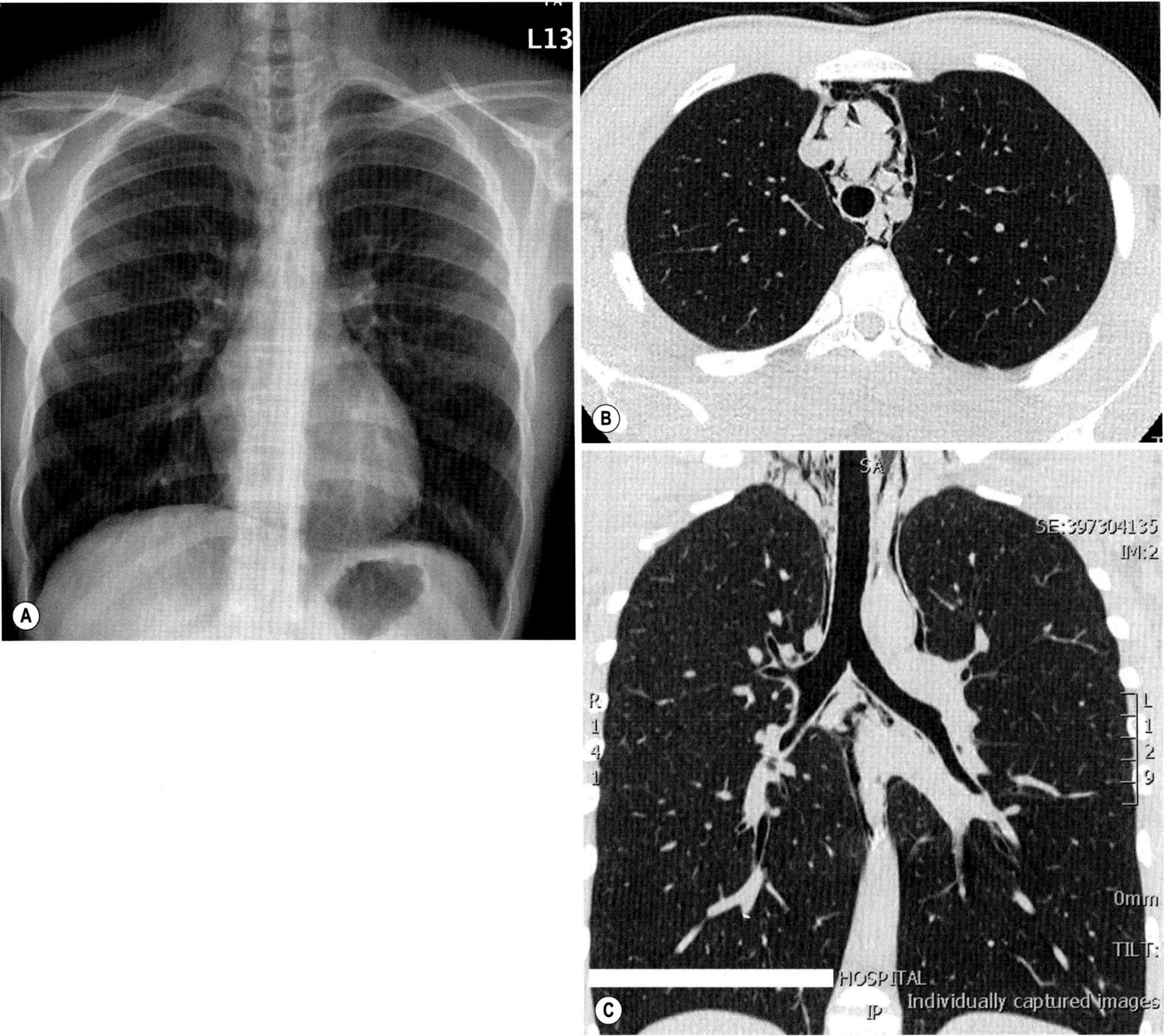

FIGURE 10-4 ■ **Pneumomediastinum.** Chest radiograph (A) with axial (B) and coronal reformatted CT (C) images demonstrating pneumomediastinum following blunt chest trauma.

pressure causing alveolar rupture into the pleural space, it is most commonly caused by either a foreign object or fractured ribs lacerating the pleural surfaces. A tension pneumothorax occurs when there is a 'flutter valve' allowing unidirectional flow of air into the pleural space, resulting in an increasing volume and pressure of pleural gas. This can result in displacement of mediastinal structures, leading to cardiovascular compromise which is a clinical emergency. Features on imaging reflect this displacement and can be identified on 'scout' views before formal CT.

The phenomenon of the occult pneumothorax arises from the inherent difficulties of interpreting the supine chest radiograph, where the pleural gas accumulates in the unfamiliar, anteromedial aspect of the pleural cavity. One study demonstrated an occult pneumothorax rate of 55%.[33] Signs on the supine chest radiograph include a deep costophrenic sulcus, hyperlucency over the hemidiaphragm and an abnormally well-defined mediastinal or cardiac border (Fig. 10-6).

CT has a sensitivity and specificity for pneumothorax of almost 100%, with the only diagnostic difficulty arising from differentiating pneumomediastinum from medial pneumothorax, when identification of the mediastinal septation is key. Communication across the chest wall of the pleural space and the extra-corporeal space can lead to a specific type of pneumothorax, colloquially referred to as a 'sucking chest wound'. This arises from the flutter-valve effect occurring through the chest wall. On CT, this type of injury can be suggested by the presence of a large pneumothorax, resistant to chest drain insertion and evidence of a chest wall defect or large penetrating wound.

Haemothorax can be found in around 50% of all chest trauma, with the haemorrhagic source ranging from ribs, intercostal vessels, lung parenchyma, great vessels or heart and pericardium. Arterial haemothorax can

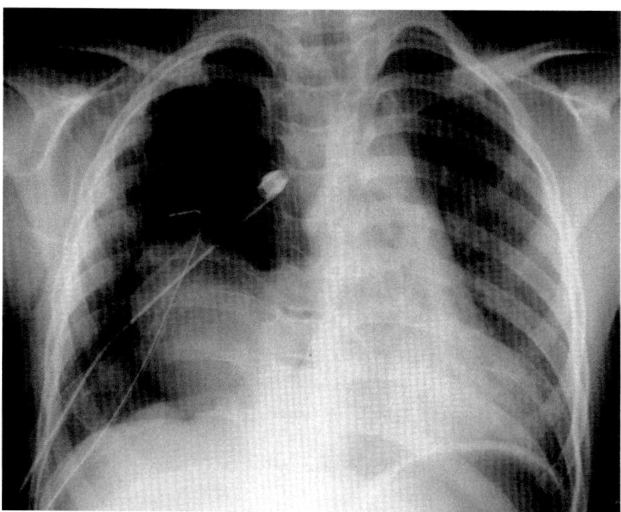

FIGURE 10-5 ■ **'Fallen lung sign'.** Chest radiograph in a boy with complete rupture of the right main bronchus following blunt chest trauma. The right lung is seen sagging to the floor of the right hemithorax.

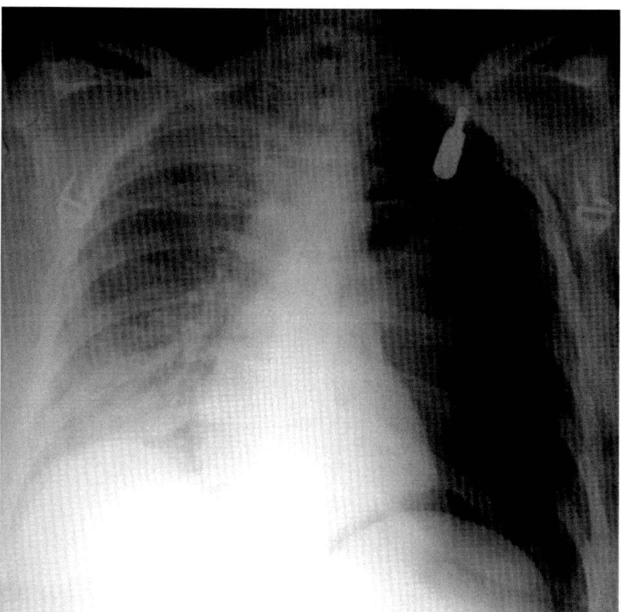

FIGURE 10-6 ■ **Pneumothorax on supine chest radiograph.** Left-sided pneumothorax seen on a supine chest radiograph demonstrating the deep sulcus sign and an unusually sharp left heart border.

accumulate rapidly and cause both lung collapse and haemodynamic compromise. The supine chest X-ray may only show increased opacification of the affected hemithorax or a subtle lamellar effusion. On CT, haemorrhage can be identified by its increased attenuation (i.e. greater than 30 HU) compared to water and may even demonstrate layering of blood products. Careful inspection of the great vessels, branch vessels and pericardium should be performed in the presence of a haemothorax.

Chylous pleural effusions usually occur secondary to penetrating injury and thoracic surgery. Features on imaging are of evidence of penetrating trauma in the region of the thoracic duct and a pleural effusion.

Lung Parenchyma

The most common parenchymal injury is of pulmonary contusion, seen in up to 70%.[34] It occurs primarily at sites of change in tissue density, such as adjacent to the thoracic spine, ribs or heart (Fig. 10-7). There is often a delay of up to 6 hours before the contusion may manifest itself on chest radiograph, although immediate detection is possible with CT. Consolidation should become maximal before 24 hours and resolve within 3–10 days. Opacification that appears after 24 hours or fails to resolve as expected, may be related to infection, aspiration, fat embolism or acute respiratory distress syndrome (ARDS).

Pulmonary laceration is a more severe injury, which results from compression, shearing or penetration. The lung tissue undergoes elastic recoil, creating a space, which can fill with air, creating a pneumatocele or with blood, creating a pulmonary haematoma. Both are more clearly demonstrated on CT and may initially be occult on the chest radiograph due to surrounding contusion (Figs. 10-8 and 10-9).

Lung herniation is a rare consequence of chest trauma, where lung parenchyma herniates through a defect in the chest wall, such as in multiple comminuted rib fractures. Generally, it can be treated conservatively but its diagnosis is important as the volume of herniated tissue can increase with positive pressure ventilation (Fig. 10-10).

The term 'blast lung' describes a condition seen in survivors of near-proximity explosions in which there is an acute lung injury causing alveolar rupture and haemorrhage that may manifest itself as large air embolism or pulmonary oedema/haemorrhage. The classic blast lung characteristics are those of hypoxia, respiratory distress and haemoptysis, radiologically manifested as bilateral diffuse pulmonary infiltrates, in a butterfly pattern on the chest radiograph.[35] Delayed lung injury may have a similar picture to acute respiratory distress syndrome,[36] but it is thought that any lung injury should be apparent within 2 hours and delayed deterioration is rare.[37] The pleura and mediastinum may be disrupted and contain air or blood and the chest wall and spine may be injured by blast debris fragments.

Chest Wall

Rib fractures are common in chest trauma, occurring in around 50% of patients but around half of these are likely to remain unidentified on the chest radiograph due to superimposition and tangential orientation. Solitary rib fractures are not of direct acute concern but can be indicative of further occult injury. Of more concern are multiple fractures in three contiguous ribs, creating a section of chest wall which can move in a paradoxical manner, in relation to the surrounding chest wall. This is related to hypoventilation of the underlying lung, is indicative of likely parenchymal contusion, increased mortality, and increased likelihood of requiring surgical treatment.[38] Rib fractures may be associated with haemothorax or more localised extra-pleural haematoma (Fig. 10-11).

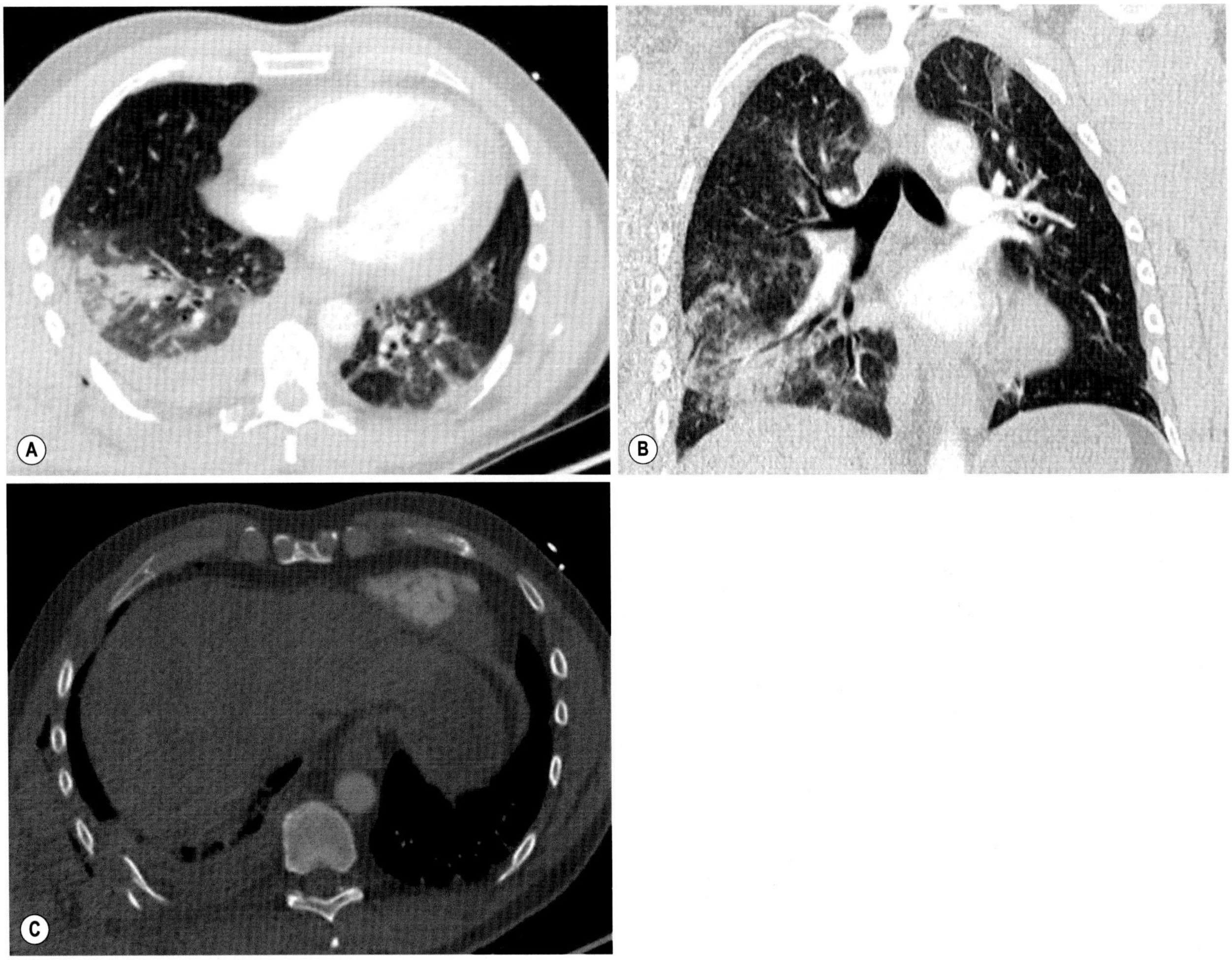

FIGURE 10-7 ■ **Lung contusion, haemothorax and rib fractures.** Axial (A) and coronal reformatted (B) CT images demonstrating air-space opacity due to post-traumatic contusion. Also seen is an associated haemothorax and axial bone window images reveal associated rib fractures (C).

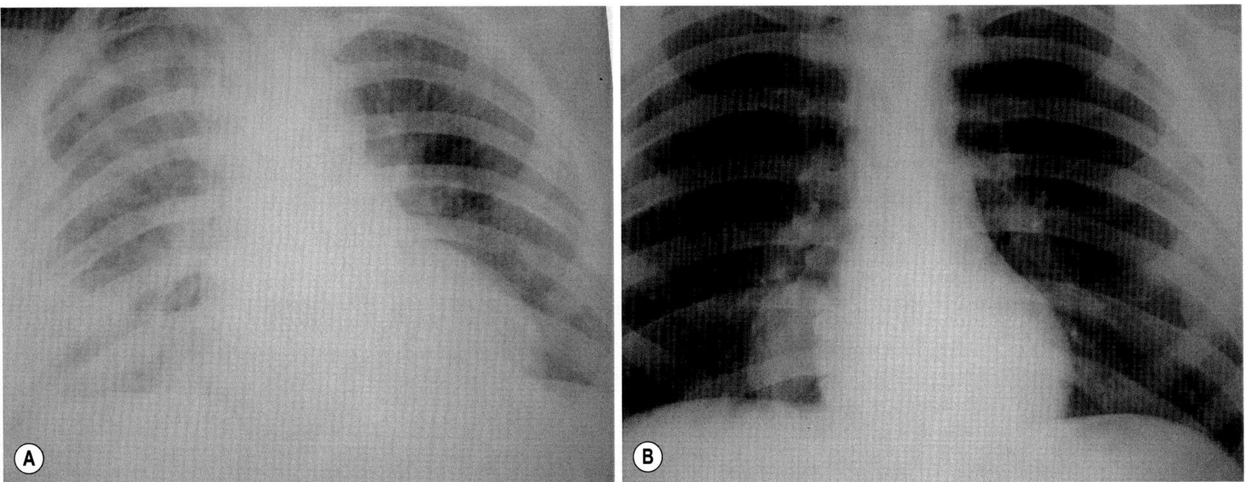

FIGURE 10-8 ■ **Pulmonary haematoma.** Chest radiograph demonstrating extensive contusion in the right lung (A). A repeat radiograph one week later (B) reveals clearing of the contusion along with a right lower zone pulmonary haematoma.

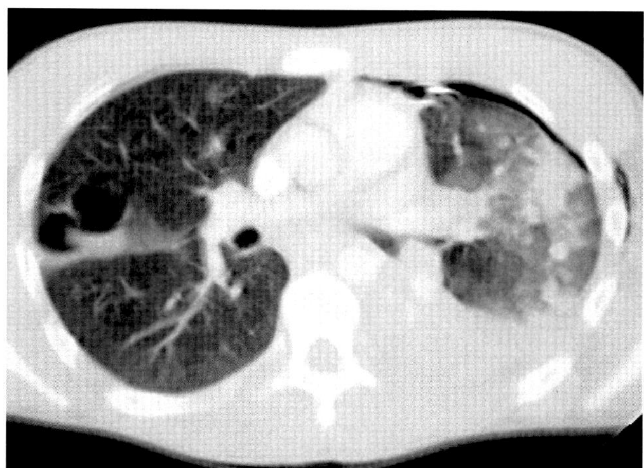

FIGURE 10-9 ■ **Traumatic pneumatocele.** Axial CT image in a patient who sustained a blunt injury to the left side of the chest with bilateral contusion and a left-sided haemothorax and pneumothorax. There are post-traumatic pneumatoceles in the right lung which occurred as a contrecoup injury.

Injuries to the most superior three ribs are associated with severe trauma and, specifically, injury to the brachial plexus, subclavian vessels, trachea and spine.[39] Scapular fractures serve as a similar indirect marker of severe trauma. Injuries to the inferior four ribs are associated with visceral injuries to the upper abdomen, left-sided with splenic and right-sided with hepatic.[18]

Rib fractures in children are rare and the possibility of non-accidental injury should be considered, particularly if the posterior aspects are involved. Children and adolescents demonstrate a greater elasticity in their ribs and subsequently may have more severe internal thoracic injuries, in the absence of rib fractures.[18]

Sternal fractures are associated with increased cardiac and ascending aortic injury[17] and sternoclavicular joint dislocations, particularly the less common posterior dislocation, are associated with injury and compression of the brachiocephalic vessels.

Spinal fractures are not only of consequence to the spinal canal and surrounding neural structures, where 62% will be associated with a neurological deficit,[40] but are also an indicator of severe trauma. Spinal fractures are commonly occult on plain radiographs and, if suspected, CT should be performed to assess further.[40]

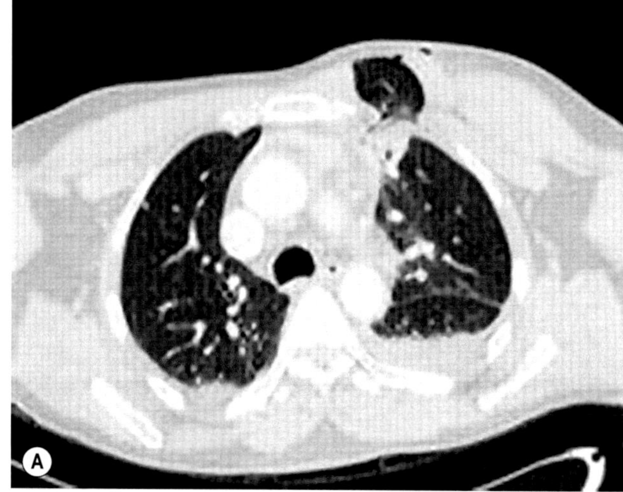

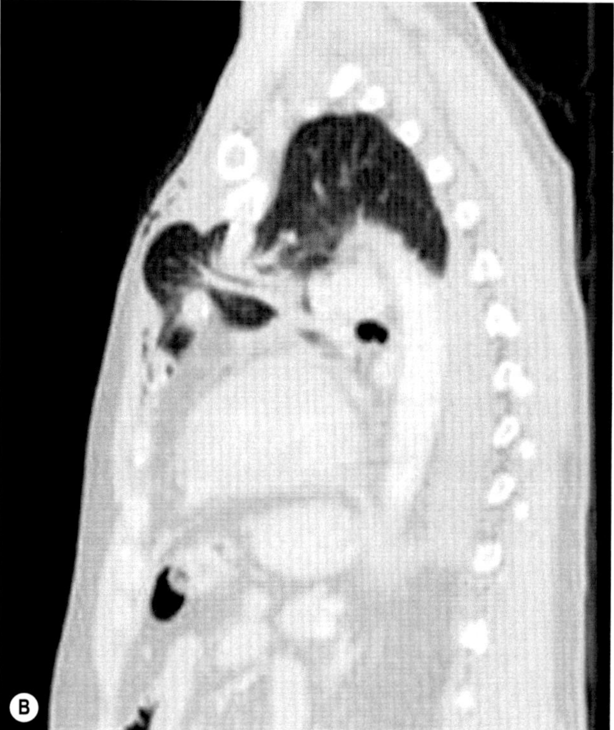

FIGURE 10-10 ■ **Lung herniation.** CT image following blunt trauma to the left side of the chest demonstrating an anterior lung herniation. This can be seen on axial (A) and coronal reformatted (B) images.

Diaphragm

The diaphragm can be injured by both penetrating and blunt trauma, particularly abdominal blunt trauma, due to a sudden increase in intra-abdominal pressure. This usually leads to a radial tear in the weaker, posterolateral tendinous insertion. Left-sided tears are more commonly seen on imaging and in surgical practice[41] and this was thought to be due to a 'protective' effect of the liver but autopsy series have demonstrated an almost equal distribution of rupture and it seems that the right-sided defects are not identified or appear to be clinically less important.[18]

Penetrating defects are generally associated with either upper abdominal or chest wall injuries and are suggested by these injury patterns and the likely trajectories. Up to 70% of diaphragmatic ruptures are missed on initial assessment and prompt surgical repair is essential to avoid subsequent bowel herniation, strangulation and rupture, with an estimated 30% mortality from delayed diagnosis.[42]

Chest radiographic signs may be delayed in appearance but include loss of clarity of the diaphragm, herniation of abdominal contents into the chest and displacement of the mediastinum away from the affected side (Fig. 10-12). Key features of diaphragmatic rupture on CT are discontinuity of the diaphragm, best demonstrated on sagittal and coronal MPR; herniation of viscera or bowel

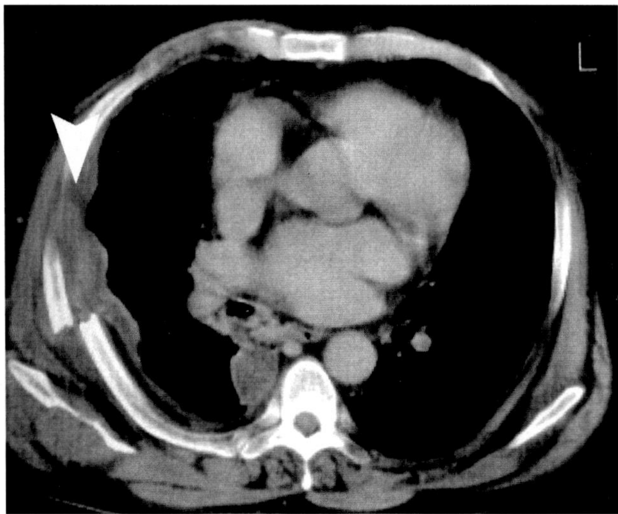

FIGURE 10-11 ■ **Extra-pleural haematoma.** CT image demonstrating extra-pleural haematoma in association with right-sided rib fractures (arrowhead).

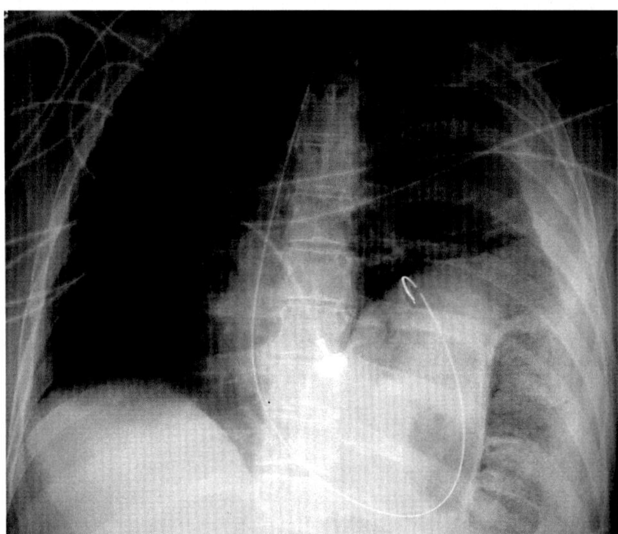

FIGURE 10-12 ■ **Diaphragmatic rupture.** Chest radiograph showing a left-sided diaphragmatic rupture. Bowel can be seen herniating into the left hemithorax, the mediastinum is displaced to the right and there is a nasogastric tube seen coiled within an intrathoracic stomach. (Courtesy of Dr. L.C. Morus, Birmingham, UK.)

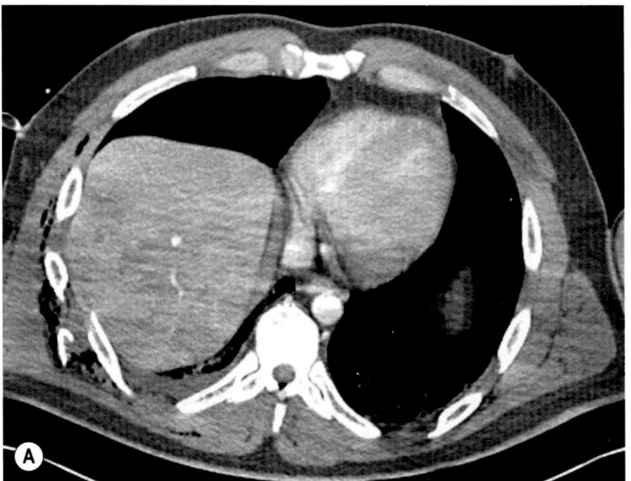

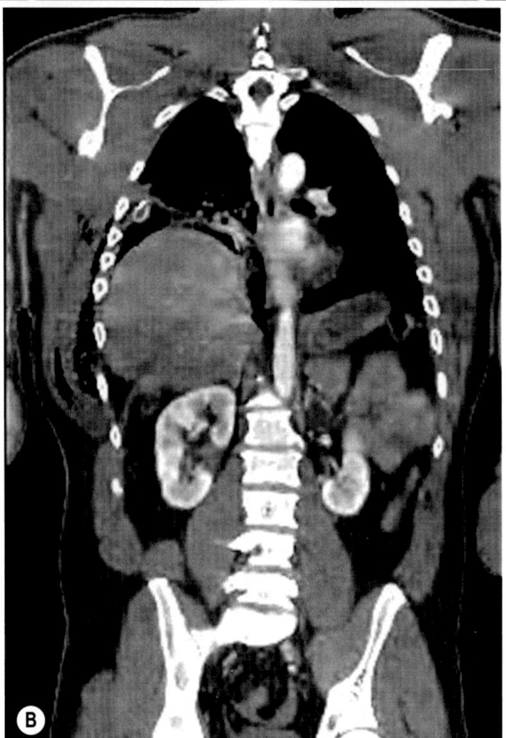

FIGURE 10-13 ■ **Right hemidiaphragmatic rupture.** Axial (A) and coronal reformatted (B) CT images demonstrating rupture of the right hemidiaphragm following blunt trauma. The liver herniates into the right hemithorax. Rib fractures and low-density regions in the liver indicating hepatic contusion are also noted on the axial image.

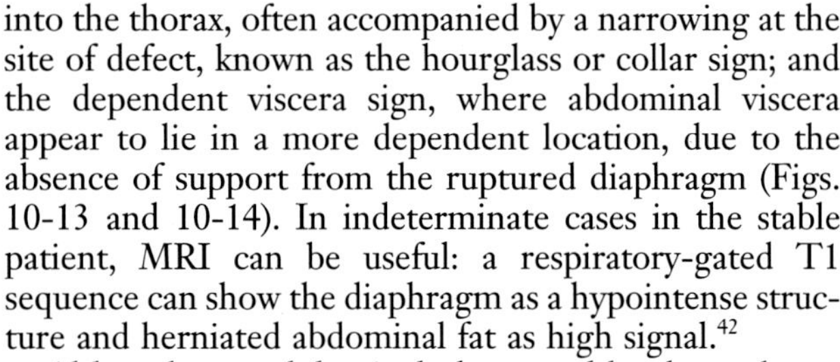

into the thorax, often accompanied by a narrowing at the site of defect, known as the hourglass or collar sign; and the dependent viscera sign, where abdominal viscera appear to lie in a more dependent location, due to the absence of support from the ruptured diaphragm (Figs. 10-13 and 10-14). In indeterminate cases in the stable patient, MRI can be useful: a respiratory-gated T1 sequence can show the diaphragm as a hypointense structure and herniated abdominal fat as high signal.[42]

Although transabdominal ultrasound has been shown to be able to diagnose diaphragmatic rupture, its use has not gained acceptance, possibly due to the difficulties associated with concomitant injuries and dressings and operator dependency.

THORACIC IMAGING IN THE INTENSIVE CARE PATIENT

Introduction

Chest radiography remains the most frequently performed chest imaging technique in the postoperative and critically ill patient. It is inexpensive and readily available

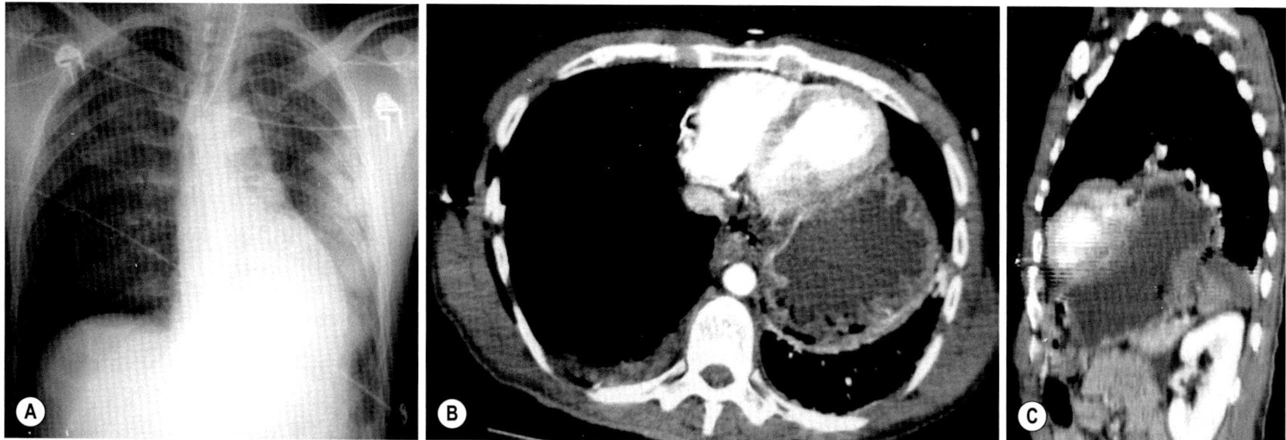

FIGURE 10-14 ■ **Left hemidiaphragmatic rupture.** Rupture of the left hemidiaphragm following blunt trauma due to a road accident. The chest radiograph reveals left mid-zone contusion (A). CT images in the axial plane (B) and a sagittal reformatted image (C) reveal a ruptured diaphragm on the left side with the stomach herniating through into the thorax. The stomach is constricted as it passes through the diaphragmatic tear—the so-called 'collar sign'.

and involves a small radiation dose of around 0.02 mSv. However, interpretational difficulties can be encountered in chest radiography in such patients and sensitivity and specificity values tend to be low.[43] The clinical problems are often complex and rapidly changing.[44] There may be more than one cardiopulmonary problem present and these may progress or regress independently. Many cardiopulmonary problems appear radiographically similar.[44] The anteroposterior (AP) projection, short tube–film distance and less than full inspiration lead to lack of sharpness and particular difficulty in assessing the cardiac shadow and lung bases. The use of computed radiography and of grids can improve image quality but interpretation remains challenging. The chest radiograph may be normal or near normal in patients with significant pulmonary insufficiency in a variety of situations such as neuromuscular disorders, pulmonary embolism and severe chronic obstructive pulmonary disease.[44] Yet, the chest radiograph remains central to the diagnostic assessment.

Ultrasound is a safe bedside procedure that can readily identify conditions such as pleural effusion. However, practical problems may occur in dealing with wound dressings, drains, subcutaneous emphysema, obesity, etc.

There has been a tendency over many years for intensive care units to request daily, 'routine' chest radiographs on all of their patients. A number of studies have evaluated this practice in recent years and most conclude that 'on-demand' rather than daily, routine chest radiography have no adverse impact and do not affect the need for additional investigations.[45]

Computed tomography, and particularly MDCT, has become an accepted investigation for the thorax for ICU patients but has potential limitations in terms of cost, risks of transfer from ICU to the radiology department, extra workload related to the transfer and there are risks related to the use of iodinated contrast medium, namely reactions and impairment of renal function. In younger patients the radiation dose would also be a consideration. In a study from an ICU in Finland it was found that of 82 MDCT examinations performed, 50 (61%) resulted in a new treatment or intervention, in 20 (24%) no additional treatment or investigations were instigated but the study was still thought to be of value while in 12 patients (15%) the MDCT study did not contribute useful additional information. The decision to proceed to CT therefore needs to be carefully considered.[43]

Cardiopulmonary Disease

Atelectasis

Atelectasis is a common finding in the critically ill patient and represents areas of non-aerated lung. Retained secretions are the most common cause. The extent can vary from linear bands of subsegmental atelectasis through to more extensive opacification to lobar collapse.[46] Air bronchograms may be visible. Atelectasis is usually basal with a particular predominance in the left lower lobe following cardiac surgery.[47] Though differentiating atelectasis from pneumonia on the bedside radiograph can be difficult, if not impossible, potential imaging clues may be available. Atelectasis is usually more sharply defined, homogeneous and associated with volume loss. In pneumonia the opacity tends to be patchy and heterogeneous and located in non-dependent areas of lung. Pneumonia tends to change more slowly over time than either atelectasis or oedema.[44]

Aspiration

Factors which predispose to aspiration include a reduced conscious level and the presence of a nasogastric tube which disrupts the function of the oesophagogastric sphincter.

Radiographic infiltrates normally appear within a few hours of aspiration of gastric contents and often progress for 24 to 48 hours. There is usually more pronounced

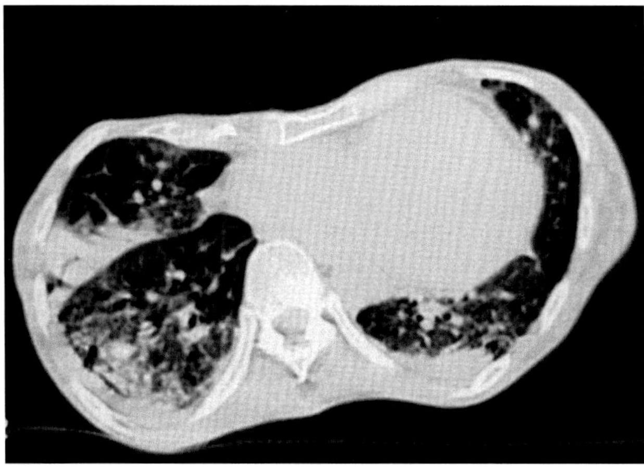

FIGURE 10-15 ■ **Aspiration.** CT image of multifocal air-space opacity due to aspiration.

TABLE 10-1 Comparison of Radiographic Appearances in Cardiac versus Non-Cardiac Oedema

Signs	Cardiac	Renal	ARDS
Cardiomegaly	Present	Present	Absent
Vascular redistribution	Present	Present	Absent
Widened vascular pedicle	Present	Present	Absent
Interstitial lines	Present	Present	Absent
Peribronchial cuffing	Present	Present	Absent
Air-space opacification	Diffuse perihilar	Central perihilar	Patchy, peripheral
Pleural effusions	Present	Present	Absent

radiological abnormality when acidic gastric contents are aspirated—pH-neutral fluids such as blood may produce little or no abnormality. When present, the infiltrates are usually patchy and diffuse. They are usually bilateral or mainly right sided and are most commonly seen in the bases or superior segments of the lower lobes. Most cases show evidence of regression after 72 hours. Persistent or increasing radiographic shadowing after this time raises the possibility of complicating infection or retained secretions. Any CT on an ICU patient showing dependent consolidation should raise the possibility of aspiration or infection (Fig. 10-15).[46] When the consolidation does not respond to appropriate treatment, the possibility of abscess formation should be considered.[44]

Pulmonary Oedema

Pulmonary oedema in the ICU patient may be due to a number of causes, the most common being cardiac failure and overhydration.[46]

With cardiac failure the heart is typically enlarged and pleural effusions are common. Upper lobe blood diversion is a normal finding on a supine radiograph so this sign, useful in the erect situation, cannot be used. Cardiogenic pulmonary oedema results in diffuse air-space opacity in association with interstitial lines (Kerley A and B lines) and peribronchial cuffing. An enlarged (more than 7 cm) or enlarging (more than 1 cm over time) vascular pedicle (the width of the mediastinum just above the aortic arch) may also be seen.[46]

Overhydration oedema may be radiologically indistinguishable from cardiogenic oedema. Overhydration features a more central distribution of oedema and a wider vascular pedicle compared with cardiogenic oedema.[46] A comparison of the key radiographic features of cardiogenic versus non-cardiogenic oedema is provided in Table 10-1.[47]

Pneumonia

Nosocomial, or hospital-acquired, pneumonia is estimated to occur in about 10% of ICU patients and the commonest infecting organisms are Gram-negative bacteria, *Staphylococcus aureus* and fungi.[48] The infection may be difficult to detect as the clinical features of out-patient pneumonia such as fever, leucocytosis or sputum production may not be present.[44] The radiological appearances of pneumonia in the intensive care patient are non-specific.[48] There may be lobar or segmental consolidation containing air bronchograms. Consolidation without loss of lung volume is particularly suggestive of infection. Some patients may have more diffuse consolidation with air bronchograms that may be symmetrical or asymmetrical and may be indistinguishable from pulmonary oedema.

The development of a cavity within an area of consolidation increases the likelihood of the presence of infection with necrosis or abscess formation. An associated pleural effusion may be parapneumonic. Loculation of pleural fluid would be suggestive of an empyema.[49]

Infection in the ICU patient may result from haematogenous spread with the development of septic emboli. Radiographically, these manifest as multiple rounded areas of consolidation which typically have a peripheral and basal predominance. The areas of consolidation typically cavitate—this is generally easier to appreciate on CT than on plain radiographs.[46]

Pulmonary haemorrhage can produce consolidation that may mimic infection. This may occur following trauma or following surgical or other interventional procedures.

Pulmonary Embolism

Pulmonary embolism is a common cause of morbidity and mortality in the ICU patient. Trauma patients are particularly susceptible to this complication. Predisposing factors include prolonged immobilisation and the frequency of surgical procedures. The clinical signs are non-specific. The chest radiograph is of limited value. It may be normal or reveal non-specific atelectasis. A peripheral area of more or less wedge-shaped consolidation may indicate associated infarction (the so-called 'Hampton's hump'). Regional oligaema with sharp cut-off of pulmonary arteries may be seen (the Westermark sign). Traditional investigations have included ventilation perfusion scintigraphy and pulmonary angiography, but CT pulmonary angiography (CTPA) has now become the preferred technique for confirming or excluding the presence of pulmonary embolism in the ICU patient even though the CTPA in the ICU patient may be suboptimal for a number of reasons, including cooperation issues, altered cardiac output and pre-existing lung disease.[44] The possibility of a false-negative study should be considered in an ICU patient with a high clinical probability of a pulmonary embolus.[44] CTPA may identify other causes for the patient's symptoms such as an undetected pneumothorax.[50] The CTPA examination should be reviewed for signs of right ventricular strain, which are more common in the ICU setting, such as right ventricular enlargement, interventricular septum shift to the left, retrograde flow of contrast medium into the inferior vena cava, and enlargement of the central pulmonary arteries.[44,51]

Haemorrhage

Bleeding can occur following thoracic surgery or other thoracic interventional procedures. The coagulation disturbances that are part of cardiopulmonary bypass predispose to a certain amount of postoperative bleeding, which normally results in a small quantity of blood passing out from mediastinal drains. More extensive bleeding may produce radiographic abnormality depending on its location. Haemorrhage into the mediastinum may produce a widened mediastinum on the chest radiograph with displacement of drains or tubes. Haemorrhage into a lung will produce consolidation that can mimic a pneumonia.[52]

Diffuse alveolar haemorrhage can occur as a complication of bone marrow transplantation. This typically produces bilateral air-space opacity on the chest radiograph, similar to that seen in pulmonary oedema.[53]

Acute Respiratory Distress Syndrome (ARDS)

A variety of direct and indirect insults to the lung can result in increased permeability of the pulmonary microvasculature, allowing protein-rich fluid to pass into the alveolar spaces of the lung at normal hydrostatic pressures. Such patients may go on to develop the clinical syndrome of acute respiratory distress syndrome, which is characterised by respiratory failure refractory to oxygen administration, diminished pulmonary compliance, normal pulmonary capillary wedge pressure and diffuse parenchymal infiltrates on the chest radiograph.[31,54] The terms ARDS and acute lung injury (ALI) describe essentially the same clinico-pathological process. The difference is merely one of severity, with ALI being defined as a ratio of arterial versus inspired fraction of oxygen of less than 300 mmHg, while ARDS is the more severe form of the disease, with the value of the ratio less than 200 mmHg.[55] The common causes of ARDS are summarised in Table 10-2.[55]

TABLE 10-2 Summary of Causes of Acute Respiratory Distress Syndrome (ARDS)

Pulmonary Causes	Extra-Pulmonary Causes
Pulmonary contusion	Non-pulmonary injury (accidental and following surgery)
Aspiration of gastric acid contents	Burns
Smoke inhalation	Hypovolaemia
Near drowning	Hypoperfusion
Pneumonia	Massive blood transfusion
Fat embolism	Systemic sepsis

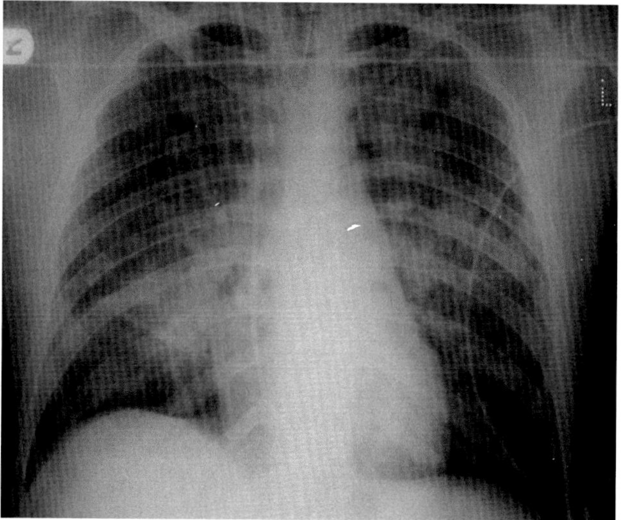

FIGURE 10-16 ■ Acute respiratory distress syndrome (ARDS). Chest radiograph showing bilateral air-space opacity in a patient with ARDS related to trauma.

Pathologists describe the changes within the lung in patients within ARDS as *diffuse alveolar damage*. Broadly speaking this can be divided into three phases. Initially there is an exudative phase, characterised by interstitial oedema, capillary congestion, and air-space filling with oedema and red blood cells. Pulmonary vascular abnormalities, including microvascular thromboses, are also common. This phase is followed by the proliferative phase, which occurs 7 to 14 days after initial injury and is characterised by organisation of the air-space exudates by macrophages and fibroblasts. Cellular proliferation is accompanied by synthesis and deposition of collagen. If sufficient collagen is deposited, the patient may enter a fibrotic phase with parenchymal fibrosis, though in many patients much of the lung abnormality resolves with little or no residual histopathological or functional abnormality.[54]

The earliest radiographic findings in the exudative phase of ARDS are those of patchy, ill-defined air-space opacities in both lungs (Fig. 10-16). Interstitial oedema is variably present.[54] The patchy opacities may progress to more diffuse consolidation. The air-space opacities tend to have a more peripheral distribution than those seen in relation to cardiogenic pulmonary oedema and pleural effusions are seldom seen on the supine radiographs obtained from such patients.[54] After a week or so, reticular opacities can be seen, corresponding to the fibrosis observed pathologically.

Computed tomography findings in ARDS are characterised by diffuse ground-glass opacity and gravity-dependent atelectasis. It has emerged that there are tendencies towards different patterns of CT abnormality, depending on the underlying cause of the lung injury. Injuries that may lead to ARDS can be subdivided into direct causes such as pneumonia, aspiration and near drowning and indirect (or extra-pulmonary) causes such as sepsis, hypovolaemic shock, acute pancreatitis and non-thoracic trauma. A study of 33 patients with ARDS using CT found that ground-glass opacity was the dominant abnormality in patients with ARDS due to extra-thoracic causes, whilst with direct pulmonary injury, ground-glass opacity and consolidation were equally prevalent. Direct injury tended to cause asymmetrical consolidation, whereas extra-pulmonary causes tended to result in symmetrical ground-glass opacity. Air bronchograms were almost universal in both groups and small pleural effusions were seen in about a half of the patients.[56]

A review of the CT appearances of 41 patients with ARDS found that *typical* appearance of ARDS occurred more frequently in cases with an extra-pulmonary cause.[57] The so-called typical features of ARDS, more strongly associated with an extra-pulmonary cause, consist of consolidation in the dependent, posterior parts of the lung with the density reducing more anteriorly. The reduction in density is usually gradual with consolidation merging with areas of ground-glass opacity with normal lung in the most anterior portion of the chest. With ARDS from pulmonary causes, the overall extent of consolidated lung and ground-glass opacity is about the same, but the opacities tend to be patchily distributed throughout the lungs, without the gradation from dependent to non-dependent areas (Fig. 10-17). Cystic spaces were a feature of the atypical appearance of ARDS.

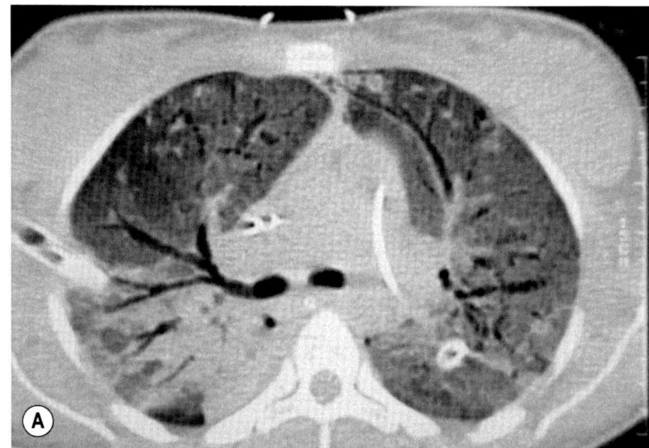

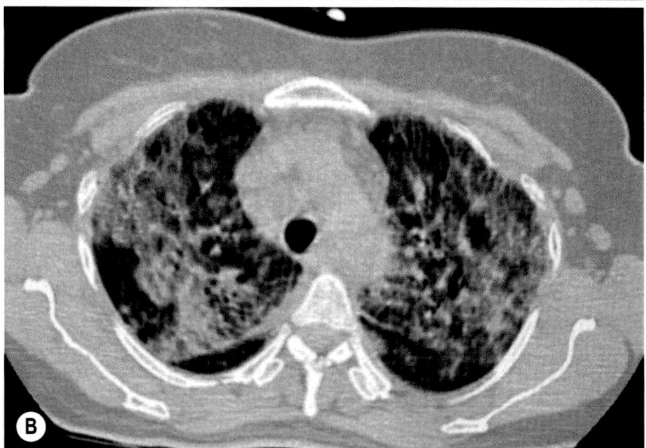

FIGURE 10-17 ■ **CT findings in ARDS.** CT images of two patients with acute respiratory distress syndrome (ARDS). In the first image (A) the patient's ARDS was due to an extra-pulmonary cause and the CT shows increased opacification in the posterior, dependent portions of the lungs and ground-glass opacity more anteriorly. A right-sided intercostal tube is also present and part of a Swan–Ganz catheter can be seen in the left main pulmonary artery. In the second patient (B) whose ARDS was related to pulmonary infection there is patchy air-space opacity present with no gradation from dependent to non-dependent lung being seen.

It is thought that the areas of dependent consolidation or opacification in ARDS represent areas of atelectatic lung which is compressed by overlying oedematous parenchyma.[57] Non-dependent pulmonary opacities (seen primarily from pulmonary causes of ARDS) are likely to represent simple consolidation. The patterns of air-space opacity noted in the studies comparing pulmonary with extra-pulmonary causes of ARDS can serve as a useful guide to the clinician but may not allow a specific cause to be identified. In many patients the causes of ARDS are multifactorial, with a combination of pulmonary and extra-pulmonary causes being present.

The commonest abnormality in long-term survivors is a reticular pattern (indicating fibrosis) and that usually has a striking anterior distribution (Fig. 10-18).[58] A suggested explanation for this anterior distribution is that the more dependent collapsed and consolidated lung is protected from injury due to barotrauma related to mechanical ventilation.

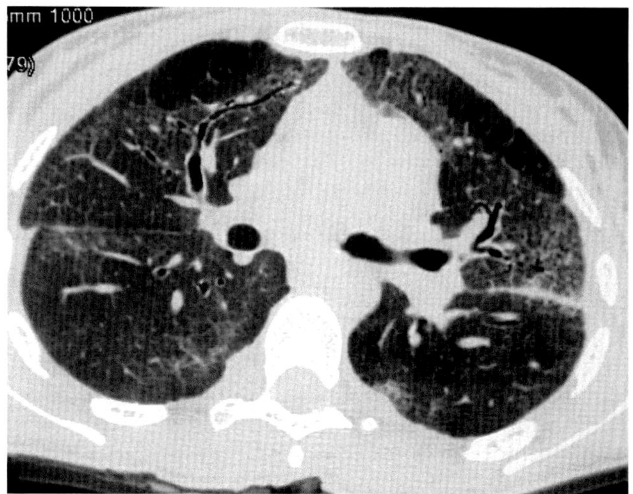

FIGURE 10-18 ■ **Post-recovery ARDS.** CT image following recovery from ARDS. Reticular opacities and traction bronchiectasis can be seen anteriorly indicating fibrosis.

Extra-Pulmonary Air

Air may escape from the normal airways in the lung due to blunt or penetrating trauma. In the ICU setting, alveolar disruption from barotrauma may lead to an air leak. Surgery and other medical procedures are another cause of extra-pulmonary air. Possible locations for extra-pulmonary air are:

- interstitial pulmonary spaces
- the mediastinum
- the pleural space
- the pericardium
- subcutaneous tissues.

Interstitial pulmonary air in adults is difficult to recognise radiographically. Escaped air dissects along bronchovascular structures towards the mediastinum. The appearance may superficially appear as air bronchograms, but, unlike air bronchograms, the lucencies do not branch or taper towards the lung periphery.[59]

Pneumomediastinum results in linear streaking of air density within the mediastinum (Fig. 10-5). Depending on the amount of air present, normal anatomical structures may become visible. The thymus may be visible; air may be seen anterior to the pericardium (best appreciated on a lateral radiograph); air surrounding the pulmonary arteries can produce a ring-like lucency; air on either side of a bronchial wall results in unusually sharp delineation of the wall—the double bronchial wall sign; and air over the diaphragmatic surface leads to the continuous diaphragm sign.[60]

As has been discussed in the previous section on thoracic trauma, diagnosing a pneumothorax on a supine anteroposterior chest radiograph can be challenging. The classical appearance of a lung edge with absent lung markings beyond may well not be present. In the supine position, air preferentially accumulates anterior to the lungs and abuts the mediastinal structures. Unusually sharp demarcation of a heart border or mediastinal vascular structure such as the superior vena cava may be the only indication on the film of a pneumothorax. An unusually deep costophrenic sulcus (the 'deep sulcus sign') is another indicator of pneumothorax on an AP radiograph (Fig. 10-6).[59] With a subpulmonary pneumothorax there may be a hyperlucent upper quarter of the abdomen and a sharply demarcated diaphragmatic surface.[59] Thoracic ultrasound is also used in the post-trauma and intensive care settings to detect pneumothorax. The ultrasound diagnosis of pneumothorax depends on the absence of the 'sliding lung' and 'comet tail' appearance that is seen in relation to a normal lung–pleural interface.[61,62] Ultrasound has been shown to be more sensitive than radiography and as sensitive as CT and, assuming the expertise is available, may allow detection of a pneumothorax without the need for the transfer of the patient to the CT unit.

Pneumopericardium may result as a consequence of barotrauma in children but in adults is more likely to be a consequence of a cardiothoracic surgical procedure. Features indicating pneumopericardium rather than pneumomediastinum include outlining of the superior pericardial reflection around the great vessels with air and visualisation of the main pulmonary artery.[59]

Pleural Effusion

Pleural effusions are common in the ICU setting and may be related to trauma, congestive cardiac failure, fluid overload, pneumonia or surgery. In the erect patient an effusion manifests as blunting of the costophrenic angle with increased basal radiographic density. In the supine patient, pleural fluid, when free rather than loculated, tends to collect in a posterobasal location. This results in a diffuse, hazy increase in density over the lower lungs through which bronchovascular markings may still be seen. Fluid in a subpulmonary location may cause apparent elevation of the hemidiaphragm.[46] In cases of uncertainty both CT and ultrasound can be of value in detecting radiographically occult effusions. When performing ultrasound on the intensive care unit it is important to evaluate the posterior, dependent aspect of the hemithorax in question in order that effusions are not overlooked—this will usually involve some manoeuvring of the patient.

Support and Monitoring Apparatus

Airway

Monitoring the presence and position of the various tubes and catheters used in the critically ill patient is an important aspect of reading an ICU chest radiograph.[63]

Endotracheal tubes are inserted to maintain an airway and administer oxygen. The ideal position for the tip is in the mid-trachea about 5 cm above the carina. This allows for a degree of upward or downward movement, which can occur when the head is moved. A tube positioned too inferiorly will tend to enter the right main bronchus leading to impaired ventilation and, ultimately, collapse of the left lung.[64]

For longer periods of intubation a tracheostomy tube is likely to be employed. These have the advantage of not moving with movement of the head. The tip of the tube should lie between half and two-thirds of the distance between the stoma and the carina. The cuff should fill but not distend the trachea wall.[64]

Intravascular

Catheters are commonly inserted to monitor central venous pressure (CVP). On the chest radiograph the tip of the catheter should be projected between the medial end of the first rib, at the junction of the brachiocephalic vein and superior vena cava or within the superior vena cava itself. Peripherally inserted central catheters (PICC) have a small calibre and can be left in place for longer durations to allow completion of a course of intravenous therapy. Ideally, PICC lines should terminate within the superior vena cava.[64]

Monitoring of left-sided cardiac pressures using pulmonary capillary wedge pressure (PCWP) is critical for maintaining accurate blood volume. The Swan–Ganz catheter normally used for this purpose is introduced into the pulmonary artery about 5 cm distal to the main pulmonary artery bifurcation. A balloon is then inflated to allow the catheter to float into the wedge position. The

TABLE 10-3 **Lines and Tubes Encountered on an ICR Chest Radiograph**

Appliance	Function	Optimum Location of Tip
Endotracheal tube	Ventilatory support	3 to 8 cm above carina
Swan–Ganz catheter	Wedge and right heart pressures	Right or left pulmonary artery
Central venous pressure catheter	Central venous pressure	Superior vena cava
Left atrial catheter	Left atrial pressure	Left atrium
PICC line	Intravenous therapy	Superior vena cava
Mediastinal drains	Mediastinal fluid evacuation	Anterior mediastinum or posterior pericardium
Pleural tubes	Pleural space evacuation	In pleural space via mid axillary line, 6th to 8th rib spaces. Directed anteriorly for pneumothorax and posteriorly for effusion
Temporary pacing wires	Cardiac pacing	Over right heart
Nasogastric tube	Gastric evacuation	Left upper quadrant of abdomen, with side-holes in stomach

catheter, when in use, should not extend beyond the proximal interlobar arteries on the chest radiograph—more distal positioning increases the risk of associated pulmonary infarction.[64]

Other devices that may be encountered include intra-aortic balloon counterpulsation devices, transvenous and epicardial pacing wires, thoracostomy tubes and nasogastric tubes. The main tubes and lines encountered on ICU images are summarised in Table 10-3.[47,52]

POST-SURGICAL IMAGING IN THE CHEST

Introduction

This section will briefly consider aspects of postoperative imaging in patients who have undergone pneumonectomy, lung transplantation and lung volume reduction surgery.

Post-Pneumonectomy

Complications may be seen following major thoracic interventions such as lobectomy and pneumonectomy. Initial chest radiographs after a pneumonectomy should demonstrate a midline position of the trachea, slight congestion in the remaining lung, and a post-pneumonectomy space that contains gas and fluid. The rate of accumulation of fluid in the post-pneumonectomy space is variable, but in most cases approximately half the space is filled with fluid after around 4 to 5 days. After the first week the air–fluid level gradually rises. Total obliteration of the pneumonectomy space usually takes weeks to months. Complications following pneumonectomy are traditionally divided into early and late.[65]

Early postoperative complications include the following:

- *Pulmonary oedema*: post-pneumonectomy pulmonary oedema is a life-threatening complication with a reported prevalence of around 2.5 to 5.0% and an associated mortality of 80 to 100%. The diagnosis is primarily one of exclusion. There should be no clinical or radiographic evidence of aspiration pneumonia, bacterial pneumonia, heart failure, thromboembolism or other possible causes of ARDS. On serial radiographs post-pneumonectomy pulmonary oedema appears as increased opacity, as seen in ARDS. Less severe cases my resemble hydrostatic pulmonary oedema with septal lines, peribronchial cuffing and loss of clarity of pulmonary vessels.
- *Bronchopleural fistula*: bronchopleural fistula is a potentially fatal complication of pneumonectomy although its incidence is declining. The most common cause of death associated with this condition is aspiration pneumonia with consequent ARDS. Radiographic features of bronchopleural fistula include failure of the pneumonectomy space to fill, persistent pneumothorax despite adequate tube drainage, progressive subcutaneous or mediastinal emphysema, a 2-cm drop in the air–fluid level with shift of the mediastinum towards the opposite side and consolidation in the opposite lung due to transbronchial spill (Figs. 10-19 and 10-20). As increased air and decreased fluid are cardinal signs of bronchopleural fistula, it is important to monitor changes in the air–fluid level in patients who have undergone a pneumonectomy.
- *Empyema*: improved surgical techniques have led to a reduced incidence of postoperative empyema though it remains a potentially fatal complication of pneumonectomy. The infection may develop early in the postoperative period or may develop months or even years after surgery. Postoperative empyema is characterised on the CT images by an expansion of the post-pneumonectomy space, with a mass effect; with a convexity or straightening of the normally concave mediastinal border of the pneumonectomy space; irregularly increased thickening of the residual parietal pleura; and bronchopleural or oesophagopleural fistula, which may cause or coexist with empyema (Fig. 10-21).
- *ARDS and acute lung injury*: post-pneumonectomy acute lung injury is a recognised complication with a likely fatal outcome. The overall incidence is approximately 5%. Patients who develop ARDS post-pneumonectomy have a high mortality of around 80% compared with 65% for all patients with ARDS. Serial chest radiographs show the rapid

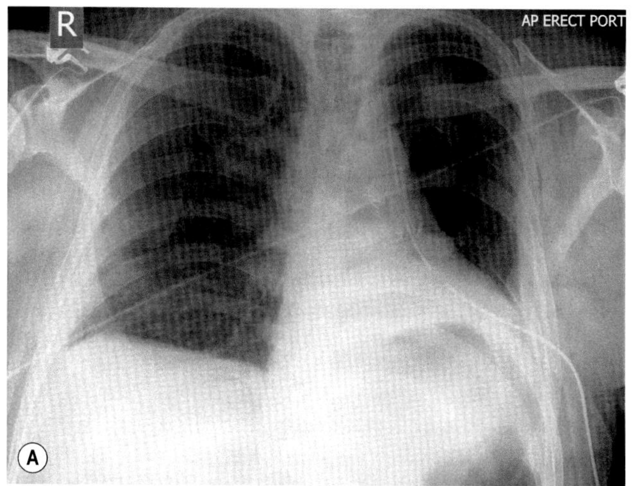

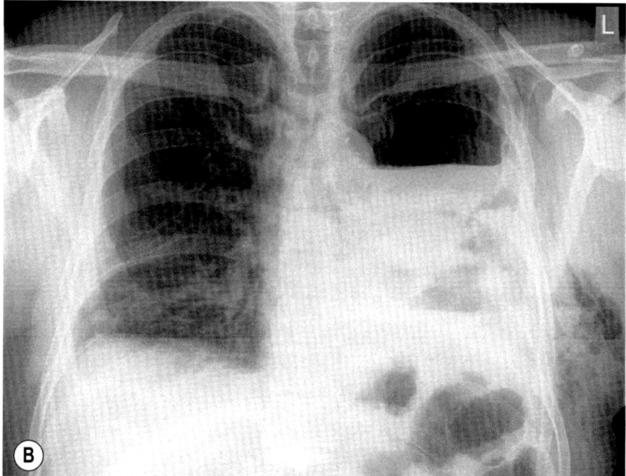

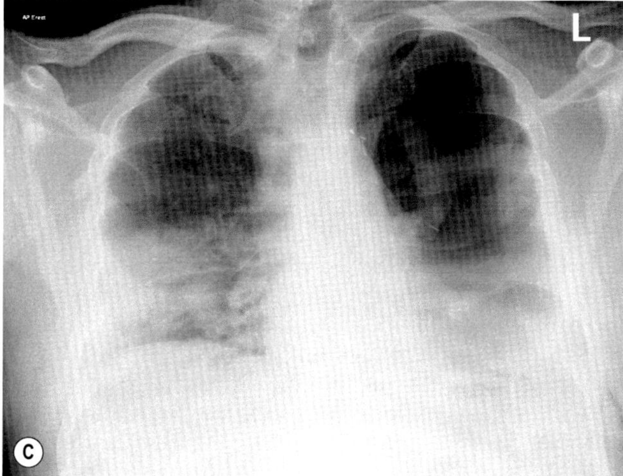

FIGURE 10-19 ■ **Bronchopleural fistula.** A chest radiograph series (A–C) in sequential order showing an initial rise in the air–fluid level in the left hemithorax following pneumonectomy but then a sudden fall due to the development of a postoperative bronchopleural fistula.

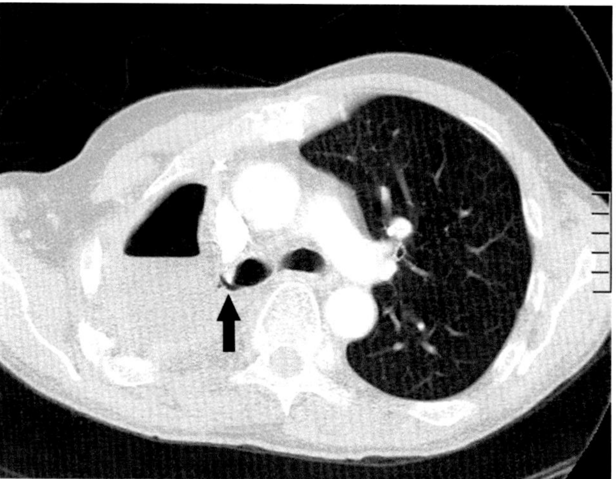

FIGURE 10-20 ■ **Bronchopleural fistula.** CT image demonstrating a right-sided bronchopleural fistula following a pneumonectomy. A track of air close to the right main bronchus can be seen due to the presence of the fistula (arrow).

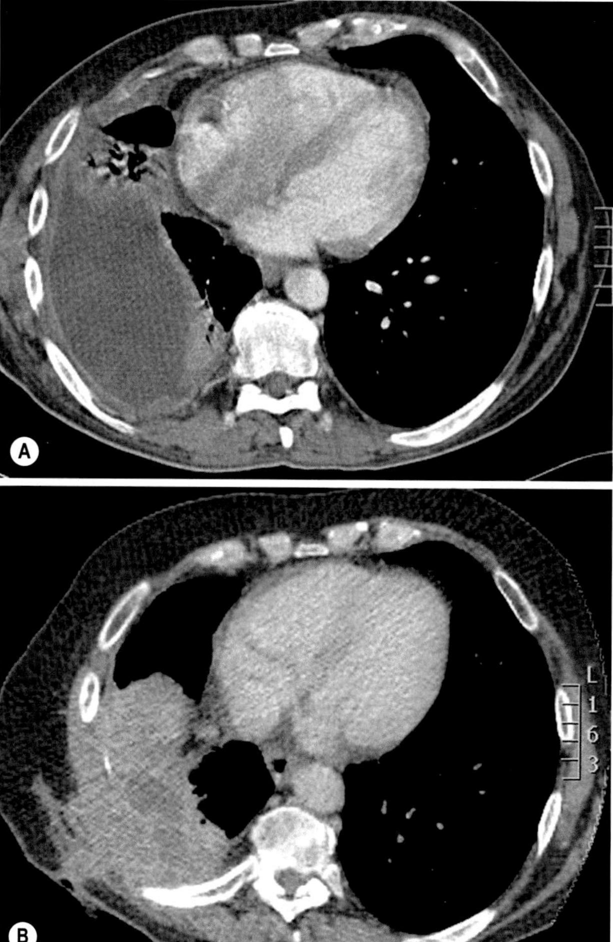

FIGURE 10-21 ■ **Post-lobectomy infection.** A postoperative CT image demonstrates a pleural fluid collection with pleural thickening and contrast enhancement indicating a postoperative empyema (A). The infection progressed and invaded the chest wall (B).

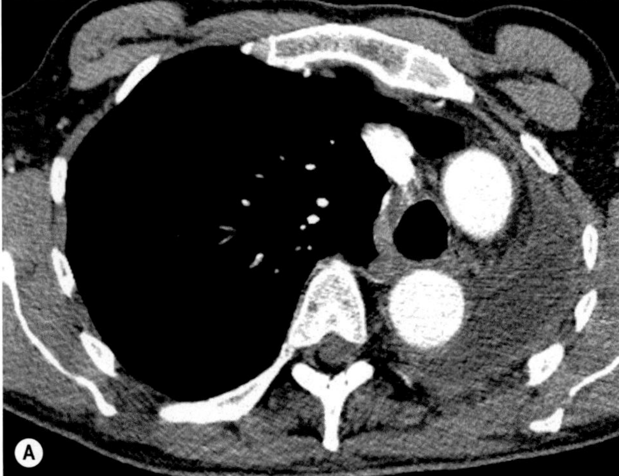

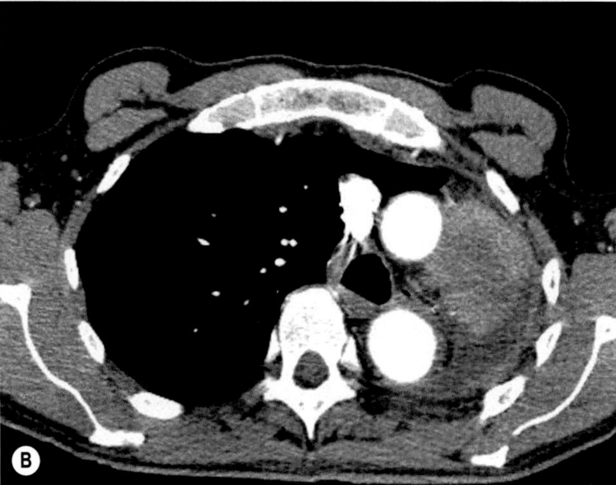

FIGURE 10-22 ■ **Recurrence of original disease.** An early CT image following a left pneumonectomy for non-small cell lung cancer demonstrates a normal post-pneumonectomy space (A). On a later follow-up examination there is a soft-tissue mass within the pneumonectomy space, which was shown by biopsy to represent recurrent tumour (B).

development of diffusely increased opacity in the remaining lung. CT depicts ground-glass opacity, visibility of interlobular septa, and an anteroposterior gradient to the lung density. ARDS may develop in conjunction with other post-pneumonectomy complications such as bronchopleural fistula, with or without empyema.

Late complications can include bronchopleural fistula, oesophageal fistula and post-pneumonectomy syndrome. Pneumonia or empyema presentation may also be delayed. There may also be recurrence of the primary disease such as tumour or tuberculosis[65] (Fig. 10-22).

Imaging, and particularly MDCT, has a role in the postoperative assessment of patients who have undergone cardiac surgery. After coronary artery bypass graft surgery, for example, chest pain is common. This can have a variety of aetiologies, including recurrent angina secondary to graft occlusion, sternal infection, pleural or pericardial effusion, and less commonly, serious complications such as pulmonary embolism or pseudoaneurysm formation. In this setting, MDCT can offer a rapid and non-invasive means of discerning the correct underlying diagnosis.[66]

Lung Transplantation

Lung transplantation is widely accepted as a form of therapy for a range of end-stage lung and pulmonary vascular diseases. Surgical options include heart-lung, single lung or bilateral lung transplantation.

Single lung transplantation has the advantage of increasing the overall number of patients who can potentially receive a lung and is the preferred method in cases of non-suppurative lung disease such as emphysema, ideopathic pulmonary fibrosis, sarcoidosis or lymphangioleiomyomatosis. Bilateral sequential lung transplantation is performed for suppurative lung diseases such as cystic fibrosis and bronchiectasis, and also for severe pulmonary hypertension. Heart-lung transplantation is performed in cases of combined heart and lung disease.[67]

Aspects of imaging in relation to lung transplantation can be subdivided into preoperative, perioperative and postoperative.

Preoperative Imaging

Typical imaging procedures performed before lung transplantation include the posteroanterior and lateral chest radiograph, chest CT and quantitative ventilation-perfusion scintigraphy. Preoperative imaging can help choose the optimum side for a single lung transplant procedure and screen for potential lung cancer. The chest radiograph can also be used for donor–recipient size matching.[67]

Perioperative Imaging

Most patients are extubated within 24 to 48 hours of transplantation. In some cases, complications such as infection or early graft dysfunction may necessitate a longer period of ventilation in which case the patient usually undergoes a tracheostomy.

Reperfusion Oedema. Reperfusion oedema (also known as the re-implantation syndrome) is caused by increased capillary permeability. Causes include interruption of lymphatic drainage in the donor lung, underlying donor lung injury, surfactant deficiency, and ischaemic damage to pulmonary capillaries.[67] In the series reported by Kundu et al., reperfusion oedema was found to be nearly universal, occurring in 44 out of 45 patients.[68] Radiographic signs were non-specific but appeared most commonly as air-space opacity in the mid and lower zones. Linear or reticular radiographic shadowing was also commonly seen. Anderson et al. found radiographic signs of reperfusion oedema in 97% of a series of 105 lung transplant patients.[69] There is poor correlation between the degree of radiographic abnormality and physiological measurements.[68] Peak radiographic shadowing usually occurs around day 4 and in most patients the shadowing will have cleared by the 10th postoperative day.[67]

Early Graft Dysfunction. Early graft dysfunction is a general term that describes a range of early injuries including reperfusion oedema, acute respiratory distress syndrome and graft failure. Although potentially related to a range of underlying problems, patients show a common clinical pattern of presentation which includes radiographic abnormalities, poor oxygenation, and biopsies, if performed, demonstrate diffuse alveolar damage or organising pneumonia.[67] Radiographic abnormalities range from mild changes of air-space opacity associated with reperfusion oedema through to complete lung opacification.

Postoperative Imaging

Infection. The lung transplant patient is particularly vulnerable to infection due to a variety of causes such as immunosuppressive therapy, lost cough reflex, and impaired mucociliary function in the denervated transplanted lung. Organisms that may infect the post-transplant lung include bacterial, viral, fungal, mycobacterial and mycoplasma species. In a review of patients with post-transplant infection, the commonest infecting organisms were cytomegalovirus, pseudomonas and aspergillus. The commonest CT findings were consolidation, ground-glass opacity, septal thickening, multiple or single nodules and pleural effusion. No significant difference in the prevalence of the CT signs was seen between the different groups of infecting organism—imaging may identify signs of infection but does not allow the specific organism to be recognised.[70]

Acute Rejection. Some degree of acute rejection occurs in virtually all transplanted lungs and usually within the first three months. The diagnosis is confirmed histopathologically with a transbronchial biopsy which typically demonstrates perivascular and interstitial mononuclear infiltrates. The rejection is graded from 0 to 4, depending on the severity of the biopsy changes and the majority of cases respond to intravenous methylprednisolone therapy.[67]

Radiographic findings are non-specific and include new or persisting air-space opacities 5 to 10 days following transplantation, pleural effusions and interstitial lines without other signs of heart failure. HRCT signs are similarly non-specific though ground-glass opacity and septal lines may be the predominant findings when acute rejection occurs after the first postoperative month.[67]

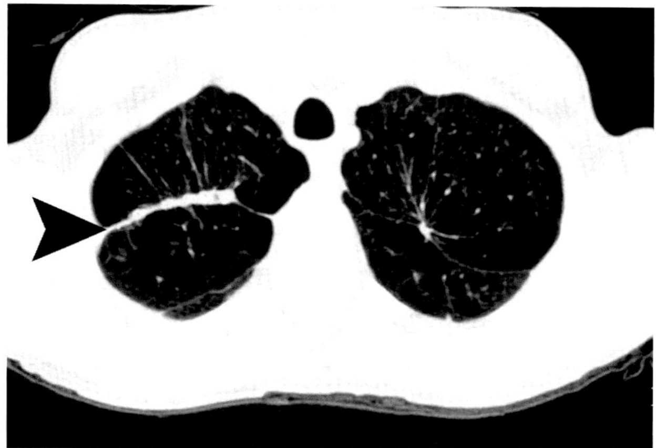

FIGURE 10-23 Appearances following lung volume reduction surgery. Postoperative CT image after lung volume reduction surgery. The staple line with bovine pericardium buttresses can be seen (arrowhead).

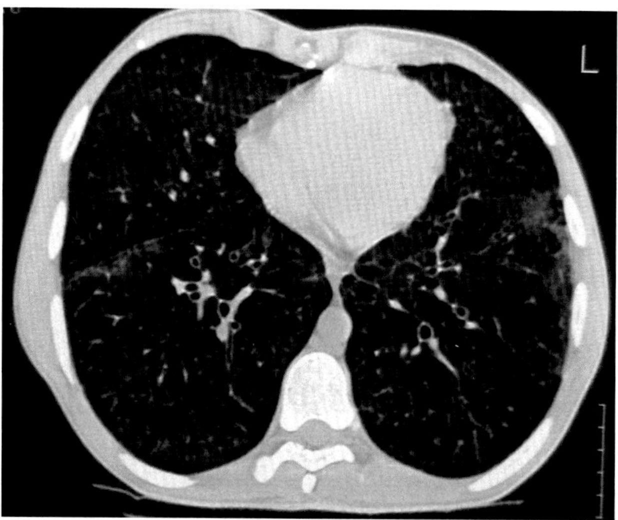

FIGURE 10-24 Post-lung transplant obliterative bronchiolitis. The lungs are overinflated with mild cylindrical bronchiectasis and attenuation of pulmonary vessels. Areas of patchy ground-glass opacity in the periphery of the lung were thought to be due to cytomegalovirus pneumonitis. The patient died within a month of this examination.

Bronchial Anastomotic Complications. The bronchial anastamoses following transplantation may be complicated by dehiscence or stenosis (Fig. 10-23). Dehiscence (or separation of the two airway ends) tends to occur in the first few months following transplantation and may be associated with infection.[67] Factors which contribute to airway problems include ischaemia, acute allograft rejection, low cardiac output and prolonged postoperative ventilation.[67]

Obliterative Bronchiolitis. Long-term survival following lung transplantation is limited primarily by the development of obliterative bronchiolitis (OB). OB is characterised histopathologically by the presence of fibrosis in small airways associated with intimal thickening and sclerosis of vessels. The process is thought to represent chronic allograft rejection.[67] Episodes of acute rejection increase the likelihood of developing OB. Although it can occur as early as 2 months following transplantation, most cases are diagnosed 6 to 12 months following surgery.

The chest radiograph on OB may be normal in the early stages though as the disease progresses signs of lung overinflation and subtle attenuation of peripheral airways may become apparent.[71] High-resolution CT findings include areas of decreased lung attenuation associated with vessels of decreased calibre. Images acquired at end-expiration can reveal air trapping (Fig. 10-24).[72] Air trapping on expiratory CT is the most sensitive and may be the only radiological sign of OB.[73] Redistribution of pulmonary blood flow to more normal areas of lung may lead to a mosaic attenuation pattern.[72] Bronchiectasis is commonly present.[72,74]

Post-transplantation Malignant Disease. Post-transplantation lymphoproliferative disease (PTLD) occurs in 5–20% of lung transplant recipients, usually in the first year after transplantation.[67] Histological findings may range from benign hyperplasia of lymphocytes through to malignant lymphoma. PTLD is thought to be caused by proliferation of donor B lymphocytes infected with the Epstein–Barr virus.[75] The most common CT manifestations are of multiple nodules, frequently in a predominantly peribronchovascular or subpleural distribution.

Disease Recurrence. Recurrence of the primary disease has been described with a number of conditions, with sarcoidosis being the disease that recurs most commonly.[76]

Surgical Treatment of Emphysema

Emphysema is defined as 'a condition of the lung characterised by abnormal, permanent enlargement of the air spaces distal to the terminal bronchioles, accompanied by destruction of their walls and without obvious fibrosis'. Over the last century a number of surgical procedures have been used to attempt to relieve the distressing symptoms of advanced emphysema. Many of these have not stood the test of time but three procedures are in current use. These are bullectomy, transplantation and lung volume reduction surgery (LVRS).

Bullectomy

Bullectomy consists of the excision of a large bulla or bullae by thoracostomy or by video-assisted thoracoscopic surgery (VATS). Bullectomy is considered in patients with a single or several large bullae identified on the chest radiograph and CT, usually with compression of adjacent lung parenchyma. The technique is usually reserved for patients with dyspnoea or recurrent pneumothoraces.[77]

Lung Transplantation

Lung transplantation can offer a marked improvement in the quality of life of the patient with advanced emphysema but the limited availability of donor organs is a major disadvantage. Transplantation is usually reserved for younger patients of below 60 to 65 years of age and such patients will normally have resting hypoxia, hypercapnoea and be dependent on supplementary oxygen. Patient selection is based primarily on clinical and physiological criteria. The main role of imaging in the preoperative patient is to assess whether alternative treatment such as LVRS might be more appropriate and to exclude incidental lung cancer.

Lung Volume Reduction Surgery

Lung volume reduction surgery involves the removal of the most severely emphysematous portions of lung in the upper lobes. Typically about 30% of each lung is removed using either a median sternotomy or a video-assisted thoracoscopic technique. Air leaks from the lung can be a problem following LVRS. The use of bovine pericardial strips to buttress the staple line and the use of a 'pleural tent' to cover the staple line have kept this problem at an acceptable level.[78]

Imaging plays a pivotal role in patient selection for LVRS. CT is the preferred method of assessing patients for LVRS but the chest radiograph remains a useful first-line investigation. The majority of patients will have a radiograph demonstrating hyperinflation with flattening of the hemidiaphragms.

CT allows for more sensitive detection of emphysema and a more accurate assessment of disease distribution. LVRS is best suited to patients with a heterogeneous distribution of emphysema, with the disease being most prevalent in the upper zones of the lungs with relatively well-preserved lung parenchyma in the mid and lower zones. Incidental lung cancers will also be more readily detected—such cancers do not preclude LVRS as, depending on their location, they may be removed by wedge excision at the same time as the volume reduction surgery.[79]

Perfusion scintigraphy can provide useful information about regional perfusion differences in the lung reflecting the distribution of emphysema. Although there is generally good correlation between CT and scintigraphy, a combination of the two provides the best preoperative assessment of disease heterogeneity.[80]

In clinical practice, chest radiographs are routinely performed following LVRS but CT is only used to deal with specific clinical problems. Complications following LVRS are generally the same as those following any thoracic surgical procedure but particular attention needs to be given to the possibility of prolonged air leak. The staple line with pericardial buttress is always seen on CT and sometimes on the postoperative chest radiograph and this may cause some confusion in interpretation (Fig. 10-23). If a pleural tent has been performed then this may be mistaken for a pneumothorax in the early postoperative period. Aside from air leaks, other complications can include pneumonia and cardiac arrhythmias.[81,82]

A number of studies have performed quantitative analyses of lungs following LVRS using CT. Lung volumes measured with CT typically reduce by around 25% following LVRS and the average lung parenchymal density increases by around 25 HU.[83]

The key roles of imaging in possible LVRS cases can be summarised as follows:

- Confirming that the patient does have emphysema and identifying the subtype.
- Assessing the distribution of emphysema. Means of assessment and criteria for surgery have varied from study to study but in practice the emphysema needs to be primarily of the centrilobular type with an upper zone predominance. There should be

complete or relative sparing of the lower zones. As a useful rule of thumb, the emphysema should be twice as severe in the upper zones as in the lower zones before a patient can be considered for possible LVRS.

- Identifying incidental cancers. Depending on their location, these may not necessarily preclude LVRS.
- Excluding other lung diseases which could lead to intraoperative or postoperative problems and thus may represent absolute or relative contraindications to surgery. These include severe bronchiectasis and diffuse parenchymal lung diseases such as idiopathic pulmonary fibrosis.
- Postoperative assessment. This includes routine assessment with chest radiography and CT when there are specific clinical questions to be addressed.

Emphysema is a common problem worldwide and LVRS can provide improved physiology, lung function and survival in certain patients. The emphysema distribution that is most favourable is that of upper lobe predominance and in practice this means centrilobular emphysema related to cigarette smoking—there is currently no role for LVRS in lower zone predominant emphysema related to α_1-antitrypsin deficiency. Only a minority of patients referred for consideration of LVRS will ultimately prove suitable for the technique.[81]

REFERENCES

1. Centre for Disease Control and Prevention. Accidents/Unintentional Injuries. Hyattsville, MD: National Center for Health Statistics; 2008.
2. Boot DA. Epidemiology of accidents. In: Alpar EK, Gosling P, editors. Trauma: A Scientific Basis for Care. London: Edward Arnold; 1999. pp. 1–19.
3. Veysi V, Nikolaou V, Paliobeis C, et al. Prevalence of chest trauma, associated injuries and mortality: a level I trauma centre experience. Int Orthop 2009;33:1425–33.
4. Advanced Trauma Life Support. Chicago: American College of Surgeons; 2012.
5. Besson A, Saegessor F. A Colour Atlas of Chest Trauma and Associated Injuries. The Netherlands: Wolfe Medical, Weert; 1982.
6. Gustavo Parreira J, Coimbra R, Rasslan S, et al. The role of associated injuries on outcome of blunt trauma patients sustaining pelvic fractures. Injury 2000;31(9):677–82.
7. Exadaktylos AK, Sclabas G, Schmid SW, et al. Do we really need routine computed tomographic scanning in the primary evaluation of blunt chest trauma in patients with 'normal' chest radiograph? J Trauma 2001;51(6):1173–6.
8. Scalea TM, Rodriguez A, Chiu WC, et al. Focused assessment with sonography for trauma (FAST): results from an international consensus conference. J Trauma 1999;46(3):466–72.
9. Schertler T, Glucker T, Wildermuth S, et al. Comparison of retrospectively ECG-gated and nongated MDCT of the chest in an emergency setting regarding workflow, image quality, and diagnostic certainty. Emerg Radiol 2005;12(1):19–29.
10. Royal College of Radiologists. Standards of Practice and Guidance for Trauma Radiology in Severely Injured Patients. London: Royal College of Radiologists; 2011.
11. Rivas LA, Fishman JE, Munera F, Bajayo DE. Multislice CT in thoracic trauma. Radiol Clin North Am 2003;41:599–616.
12. Demetriades D, Kimbrell B, Salim A, et al. Trauma deaths in a mature urban trauma system: is 'trimodal'? distribution a valid concept? J Am Coll Surg 2005;201(3):343–8.
13. US Department of Defense. Missile caused wounds. In: Emergency War Surgery, Part I: Types of Wounds and Injuries. Washington, DC: US Government Printing Office; 2001.
14. Jeffery AJ, Rutty GN, Robinson C, Morgan B. Computed tomography of projectile injuries. Clin Radiol 2008;63(10):1160–6.
15. Leibovici D, Gofrit ON, Stein M, et al. Blast injuries: bus versus open-air bombings—a comparative study of injuries in survivors of open-air versus confined-space explosions. J Trauma 1996;41(6):1030–5.
16. Stein M, Hirshberg A. Medical consequences of terrorism: the conventional weapon threat. Surg Clin North Am 1999;79(6):1537–52.
17. Oikonomou A, Prassopoulos P. CT imaging of blunt chest trauma. Insights Imaging 2011;2(3):281–95.
18. Dee P. The radiology of chest trauma. Radiol Clin North Am 1992;30:291–306.
19. Co SJ, Yong-Hing CJ, Galea-Soler S, et al. Role of imaging in penetrating and blunt traumatic injury to the heart. Radiographics 2011;31(4):E101–E115.
20. Williams JS, Graff JA, Uku JM, Steinig JP. Aortic injury in vehicular trauma. Ann Thorac Surg 1994;57(3):726–30.
21. Tambyraja AL, Scollay JM, Beard D, et al. Aortic trauma in Scotland: a population based study. Eur J Vasc Endovasc Surg 2006;32(6):686–9.
22. Steenburg SD, Ravenel JG, Ikonomidis JS, et al. Acute traumatic aortic injury: imaging evaluation and management. Radiology 2008;248(3):748–62.
23. Burkhart HM, Gomez GA, Jacobson LE, et al. Fatal blunt aortic injuries: a review of 242 autopsy cases. J Trauma 2001;50(1):113–15.
24. Arthurs ZM, Starnes BW, Sohn VY, et al. Functional and survival outcomes in traumatic blunt thoracic aortic injuries: An analysis of the National Trauma Databank. J Vasc Surg 2009;49(4):988–94.
25. Fabian TC, Richardson JD, Croce MA, et al. Prospective study of blunt aortic injury: multicenter trial of the American Association for the Surgery of Trauma. J Trauma 1997;42(3):374–80.
26. Cleverley JR, Barrie JR, Raymond GS, et al. Direct signs of aortic injury on contrast enhanced CT in surgically proven traumatic aortic injury: a multi-centre review. Clin Radiol 2002;57:281–6.
27. Malhotra AK, Fabian TC, Croce MA, et al. Minimal aortic injury: a lesion associated with advancing diagnostic techniques. J Trauma 2001;51(6):374–80.
28. Lee DE, Arslan B, Queiroz R, Waldman DL. Assessment of inter- and intraobserver agreement between intravascular US and aortic angiography of thoracic aortic injury. Radiology 2003;227(2):434–9.
29. Bevjan SM, Godwin JD. Pneumomediastinum: old and new signs. Am J Roentgenol 1996;166:1041–8.
30. Chen JD, Shanmuganathan K, Mirvis SE, et al. Using CT to diagnose tracheal rupture. Am J Roentgenol 2001;176(5):1273–80.
31. Goodman LR. Congestive heart failure and adult respiratory distress syndrome: new insights using computed tomography. Radiol Clin North Am 1996;34:33–46.
32. de Lutio di Castelguidone E, Merola S, Pinto A, et al. Esophageal injuries: spectrum of multidetector row CT findings. Eur J Radiol 2006;59(3):344–8.
33. Ball CG, Kirkpatrick AW, Laupland KB, et al. Incidence, risk factors, and outcomes for occult pneumothoraces in victims of major trauma. J Trauma 2005;59(4):917–24.
34. Gavelli GG, Canini RC, Bertaccini PB, et al. Traumatic injuries: imaging of thoracic injuries. Eur Radiol 2002;12(6):1273–94.
35. Hare SS, Goddard I, Ward P, et al. The radiological management of bomb blast injury. Clin Radiol 2007;62(1):1–9.
36. Chaloner E. Blast injuries in enclosed spaces. Br Med J 2005;331:119–20.
37. Avidan V, Hersch M, Armon Y, et al. Blast lung injury: clinical manifestations, treatment, and outcome. Am J Surg 2005;190(6):945–50.
38. Wanek S, Mayberry J. Blunt thoracic trauma: flail chest, pulmonary contusion and blast injury. Crit Care Clin 2004;20(1):71–81.
39. Gupta A, Jamshidi M, Rubin JR. Traumatic first rib fractures: is angiography necessary? Cardiovasc Surg 1997;5:48–53.
40. van Beek EJR, Been HD, Ponsen KJ, Maas M. Upper thoracic spinal fractures in trauma patients—a diagnostic pitfall. Injury 2000;31(4):219–23.
41. Dirican A, Yilmaz M, Unal B, et al. Acute traumatic diaphragmatic ruptures: a retrospective study of 48 cases. Surg Today 2011;41(10):1352–6.
42. Mirvis S, Shanmuganagthan K. Imaging hemidiaphragmatic injury. Eur Radiol 2007;17(6):1411–21.

43. Ahvenjarvi LK, Laurila J, Jartti A, et al. Multi-detector computed tomography in critically ill patients. Acta Anaesthesiol Scand 2008; 52(4):547–52.
44. Goodman LR. Imaging the intensive care patient. In: Hodler J, Schulthess GK, Zollikofer C, editors. Diseases of the Heart and Chest, Including Breast 2011–2014. Milan: Springer; 2011. pp. 66–9.
45. Kröner A, Binnekade JM, Graat ME, et al. On-demand rather than daily-routine chest radiography prescription may change neither the number nor the impact of chest computed tomography and ultrasound studies in a multidisciplinary intensive care unit. Anesthesiology 2008;108(1):40–5.
46. White CS, Pugatach RD. Thoracic imaging in the intensive care unit. In: Mirvis SE, Shanmuganathan K, editors. Imaging in Trauma and Critical Care. 2nd ed. Philadelphia: Saunders; 2003. pp. 725–40.
47. Trotman-Dickenson B. Radiography in the critical care patient. In: McLeod TC, editor. Thoracic Radiology: The Requisites. 1st ed. St. Louis: Mosby; 1998. pp. 151–72.
48. Lipchik RJ, Kuzo RS. Nosocomial pneumonia. Radiol Clin North Am 1996;34:47–58.
49. Reynolds JH, Mcdonald G, Alton H, Gordon SB. Pneumonia in the immunocompetent patient. Br J Radiol 2010;83(996): 998–1009.
50. Remy-Jardin M, Mastora I, Remy J. Pulmonary embolus imaging with multislice CT. Radiol Clin North Am 2003;41:507–19.
51. Ghaye B, Ghuysen A, Bruyere P-J, et al. Can CT pulmonary angiography allow assessment of severity and prognosis in patients presenting with pulmonary embolism? What the radiologist needs to know. Radiographics 2006;26(1):23–39.
52. Henry DA. Radiologic evaluation of the patient after cardiac surgery. Radiol Clin North Am 1996;34:119–35.
53. Winer-Muram HT, Gurney JW, Bozeman PM, Krance RA. Pulmonary complications after bone marrow transplantation. Radiol Clin North Am 1996;34:97–118.
54. Muller NL, Fraser RS, Kyung SL, Johkoh T. Pumonary edema. In: Muller NL, Fraser RS, Kyung SL, Johkoh T, editors. Diseases of the Lung: Radiologic and Pathologic Correlations. 1st ed. Philadelphia: Lippincott, Williams and Wilkins; 2003. pp. 255–65.
55. Sutcliffe AJ. ARDS: pathophysiology related to cardiorespiratory management. In: Alpar EK, Gosling P, editors. Trauma: A Scientific Basis for Care. London: Edward Arnold; 1999. pp. 142–52.
56. Goodman LR, Fumagalli R, Tagliabue P, et al. Adult respiratory distress syndrome due to pulmonary and extrapulmonary causes: CT, clinical, and functional correlations. Radiology 1999;213(2): 545–52.
57. Desai SR, Wells AU, Suntharalingam G, et al. Acute respiratory distress syndrome caused by pulmonary and extrapulmonary injury: a comparative CT study. Radiology 2001;218(3):689–93.
58. Desai SR, Wells AU, Rubens MB, et al. Acute respiratory distress syndrome: CT abnormalities at long-term follow-up. Radiology 1999;210(1):29–35.
59. Tocino I, Westcott JL. Barotrauma. Radiol Clin North Am 1996;34:59–81.
60. Zylak CM, Standen JR, Barnes GR, Zylak CJ. Pneumomediastinum revisited. Radiographics 2000;20(4):1043–57.
61. Rowan KR, Kirkpatrick AW, Liu D, et al. Traumatic pneumothorax detection with thoracic US: correlation with chest radiography and CT. Initial experience. Radiology 2002;225(1):210–14.
62. Galbois A, Ait-Oufella H, Baudel JL, et al. Pleural ultrasound compared with chest radiographic detection of pneumothorax resolution after drainage. Chest 2010;138(3):648–55.
63. Hunter TB, Taljanovic MS, Tsau PH, et al. Medical devices of the chest. Radiographics 2004;24(6):1725–46.
64. Henschke CI, Yankelevitz DF, Wand A, et al. Accuracy and efficacy of chest radiography in the intensive care unit. Radiol Clin North Am 1996;34:21–31.
65. Chae EJ, Seo JB, Kim SY, et al. Radiographic and CT findings of thoracic complications after pneumonectomy. Radiographics 2006;26(5):1449–68.
66. Frazier AA, Qureshi F, Read KM, et al. Coronary artery bypass grafts: assessment with multidetector CT in the early and late postoperative settings. Radiographics 2005;25(4):881–96.
67. Collins J. Imaging of the chest after lung transplantation. J Thorac Imaging 2002;17:102–12.
68. Kundu S, Herman SJ, Winton TL. Reperfusion edema after lung transplantation: radiographic manifestations. Radiology 1998; 206(1):75–80.
69. Anderson DC, Glazer HS, Semenkovich JW, et al. Lung transplant edema: chest radiography after lung transplantation—the first 10 days. Radiology 1995;195(1):275–81.
70. Collins J, Muller NL, Kazerooni EA, Paciocco G. CT findings of pneumonia after lung transplantation. Am J Roentgenol 2000; 175(3):811–18.
71. Skeens JL, Fuhrman CR, Yousem SA. Bronchilitis obliterans in heart-lung transplantation patients: radiologic findings in 11 patients. Am J Roentgenol 1989;153:253–6.
72. Leung AN, Fisher K, Valentine V, et al. Bronchiolitis obliterans after lung tranplantation: detection using expiratory HRCT. Chest 1998;113:365–70.
73. Webb WR. Radiology of obstructive pulmonary disease. Am J Roentgenol 1997;169:637–47.
74. Worthy SA, Muller NL, Kim JS, et al. Bronchiolitis obliterans after lung transplantation: high resolution CT findings in 15 patients. Am J Roentgenol 1997;169:673–7.
75. Collins J, Muller NL, Leung AN, et al. Epstein-Barr-virus-associated lymphoproliferative disease of the lung: CT and histologic findings. Radiology 1998;208(3):749–59.
76. Collins J, Hartman MJ, Warner TF, et al. Frequency and CT findings of recurrent disease after lung transplantation. Radiology 2001;219(2):503–9.
77. Snider GL, Kleinerman J, Thurlbeck WM. The definition of emphysema: report of a National Heart, Lung and Blood Institiute, Division of Lung Disease Workshop. Am Rev Respir Dis 1985; 132:182–5.
78. Cooper JD. The history of surgical procedures for emphysema. Ann Thorac Surg 1997;63:312–19.
79. McKenna RJ Jr, Fischel RJ, Brenner M, Gelb AF. Combined operations for lung volume reduction surgery and lung cancer. Chest 1996;110:885–90.
80. Cederlund K, Hogberg S, Jorfeldt L, et al. Lung perfusion scintigraphy prior to lung volume reduction surgery. Acta Radiol 2003; 44:246–51.
81. Fishman A, Martinez F, Naunheim K, et al. A randomised trial comparing lung-volume-reduction surgery with medical therapy for severe emphysema. N Engl J Med 2003;348(21):2059–73.
82. Slone RM, Gierada D, Yusen RM. Preoperative and postoperative imaging in the surgical management of pulmonary emphysema. Radiol Clin North Am 1998;36:57–89.
83. Screaton NJ, Reynolds JH. Lung volume reduction surgery for emphysema: what the radiologist needs to know. Clin Radiol 2005;61(3):237–49.

CHAPTER 11

AIRSPACE DISEASES

Nicola Sverzellati • Sujal R. Desai

CHAPTER OUTLINE

INTRODUCTION

Diseases that principally involve the airspaces are common but the radiological approach to diagnosis is potentially daunting since opacification of the air spaces is a non-specific sign (Table 11-1). Any pathological process that displaces air from the alveoli will be depicted as airspace opacification but this pattern is most commonly seen when either fluid accumulates (as in pulmonary oedema) or there are inflammatory cells (as with infection) in the airspaces. This chapter considers some of the common and a few of the more unusual causes of airspace opacification in clinical practice. Airspace diseases caused by infection and cancer are considered in detail elsewhere (see Chapters 5 and 8).

AN APPROACH TO THE RADIOLOGICAL DIAGNOSIS OF AIRSPACE DISEASES

The plain chest radiograph is often the first investigation clinicians will request. With experience, the radiologist can usually offer a sensible diagnosis or, at worst, a limited list of differential diagnoses. For this, an appreciation of the clinical background, the distribution of radiographic abnormalities and changes, if any, on serial examination are invaluable. It perhaps goes without saying that the imaging appearances must be considered in the clinical context and this may be diagnostic in some patients. For instance, lobar opacification in a patient with pyrexia and a productive cough is most likely to be caused by infection (Fig. 11-1). Alternatively, when there is known left ventricular dysfunction the likely cause of bilateral airspace opacification is pulmonary oedema. The distribution of airspace opacities on plain radiographs may be a differentiating feature: in cryptogenic organising pneumonia (COP), areas of consolidation tend to be more pronounced in the periphery and lower zones (Fig. 11-2).[1] By contrast, in chronic eosinophilic pneumonia, the typical finding is of upper zone infiltrates which parallel the chest wall.[2] A review of serial radiographs is an important part of the radiologist's routine. Rapid clearing—occurring over a period of hours or, at most, a few days—suggests oedema fluid (Fig. 11-3) or pulmonary haemorrhage as the likely cause as opposed to, say, pneumonia. Opacities that are transient and migratory, in a patient with constitutional symptoms, should at least make the radiologist think about a diagnosis of an eosinophilic pneumonia.

Computed tomography (CT) is frequently requested in patients with airspace disease and, occasionally, the CT features will be characteristic. One possible example is the so-called 'crazy-paving' pattern, which, in its classical form, is virtually diagnostic of alveolar proteinosis.[3,4] However, in other instances, the radiologist may only be able to limit the list of diagnostic possibilities despite the additional information from CT (e.g. cavitation that may not have been evident on plain radiographs is only shown by CT). Therefore, except certain circumstances, the advantages of CT over plain radiography in the diagnosis of airspace diseases are not clearly defined.[5]

Anatomical Considerations

The air spaces are defined as the air containing part of the lung which includes the respiratory but not the terminal bronchioles. The latter are the last purely conducting airways of the bronchial tree and the region of lung subtended by a terminal bronchiole is the acinus.[6] Important pathways of collateral ventilation (the pores of Kohn)

TABLE 11-1 **Causes of Airspace Opacification**

- Cardiogenic oedema (cardiogenic, non-cardiogenic)
- Pneumonia
- Inflammatory
  - Organising pneumonia (cryptogenic or other aetiologies)
  - Diffuse alveolar damage
  - Vasculitides (e.g. Wegener's granulomatosis)
- Haemorrhage
  - Idiopathic pulmonary haemosiderosis
  - Antibasement membrane antibody disease
  - Systemic lupus erythematosus
- Neoplasm
  - Adenocarcinoma with lepidic growth pattern (former bronchoalveolar cell carcinoma)
  - Lymphoma (MALToma)
- Miscellaneous causes
  - Eosinophilic pneumonia
  - Alveolar proteinosis
  - Alveolar microlithiasis
  - Sarcoidosis

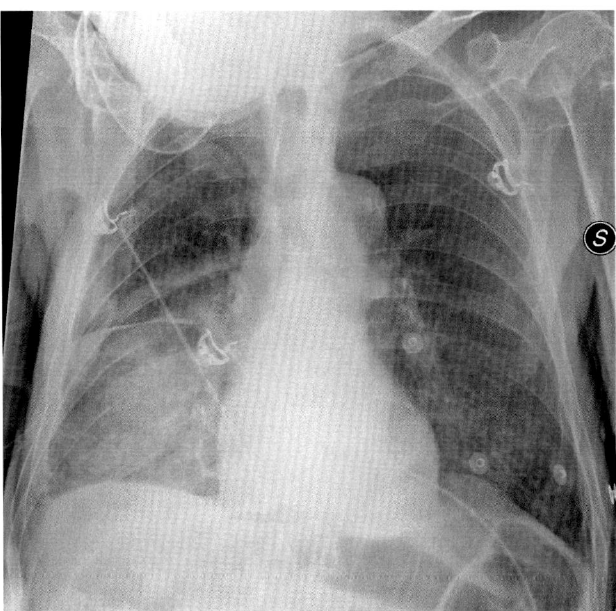

FIGURE 11-1 ■ Chest radiograph in a young male patient with pneumonia. The presence of focal consolidation in a patient with pyrexia and a productive cough should prompt a radiological diagnosis of infection as opposed to another cause of airspace opacification.

link different alveolar units and can help to maintain lung inflation in the presence of proximal airway obstruction.[7] These normal collateral pathways also facilitate the spread of certain diseases (most notably infections) into adjacent alveolar units.

Another important unit of lung structure is the pulmonary lobule, defined as the smallest unit of lung bounded by connective tissue septa.[8] Individual lobules are irregular polyhedrons, best seen subpleurally, measuring between 5 and 30 mm in diameter, and incorporating between 3 and 24 acini;[9] the lobular bronchiole and adjacent artery form the core structures. Normal centrilobular arteries (with a maximum diameter of 0.2 mm) can be seen on high-resolution computed tomography (HRCT), but the wall of the accompanying bronchiole is too thin to be resolved[10] (Fig. 11-4). The corollary is that bronchioles visible within the 2-cm subpleural space indicate wall thickening, dilatation and/or endobronchiolar filling. Infiltration of the interlobular septa by oedema fluid or malignant cells or thickening caused by fibrosis will render individual pulmonary lobules visible on HRCT[11] (Fig. 11-5).

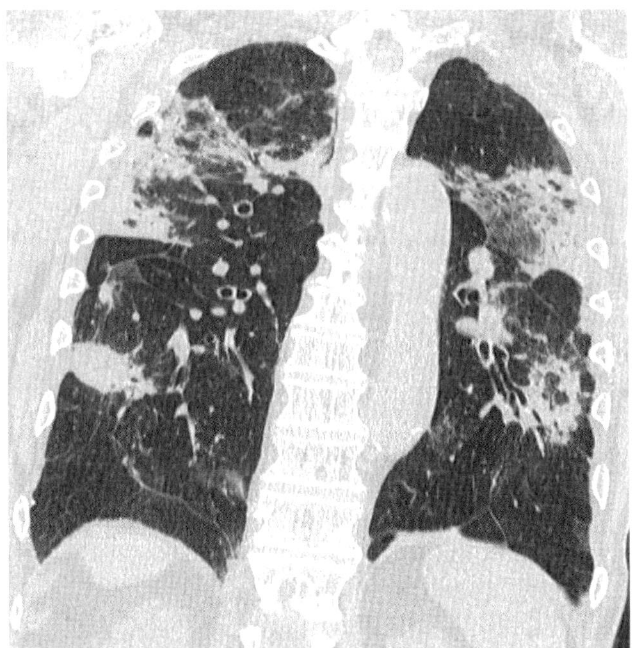

FIGURE 11-2 ■ (Non-infective) organising pneumonia. Coronal HRCT image demonstrates areas of consolidation in a subpleural and peribronchial distribution in association with areas of ground-glass opacification in the upper lobes. In the left lower lobe, a ring-shaped focus of consolidation surrounding with a central area of ground glass (the reverse halo or Atoll sign) is shown.

Radiological Signs of Airspace Disease

One of the principal limitations of imaging studies is that a multitude of pathological processes in the air spaces manifest in only a limited number of ways: thus, for most airspace diseases, a modular pattern, ground-glass opacification and consolidation represent the range of radiological abnormalities.

1. A *nodular pattern* as a sole manifestation of airspace disease is relatively uncommon. Historically, the term 'acinar nodules' or 'acinar rosettes' has been used to describe the appearance of poorly defined infiltrates on chest radiography and HRCT.[12,13] The diagnostic value of localising disease to the acinus has been questioned; in pathological studies, the acinar pattern on plain radiographs does not correspond to the filling of acini as defined anatomically.[14] This notwithstanding, the so-called acinar pattern is most frequently encountered in

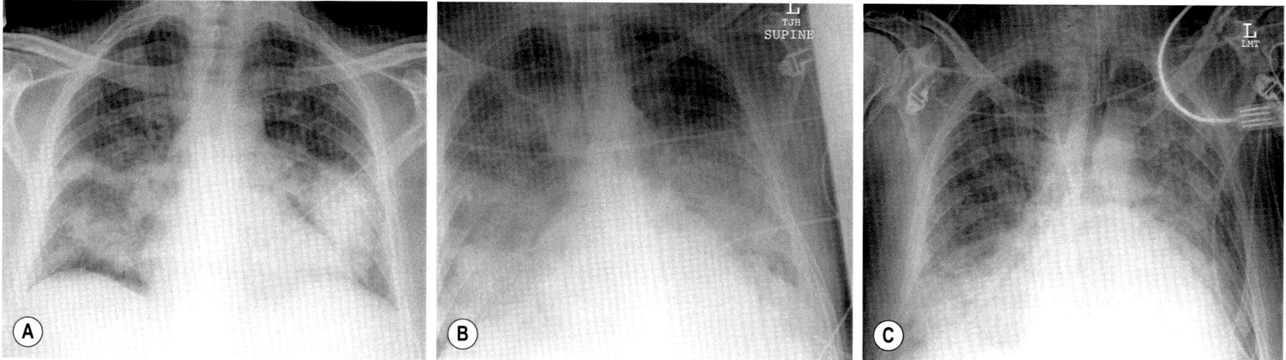

FIGURE 11-3 (A–C) Rapid changes in radiographic appearances in pulmonary oedema. Serial chest radiographs over roughly a 48-h period show striking changes in the extent/severity of airspace opacification, reflecting relatively rapid shifts of fluid between the intravascular compartment and the air spaces/interstitium.

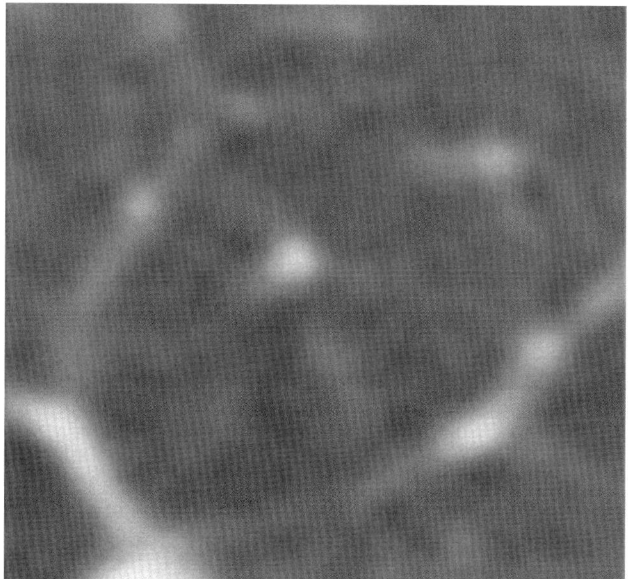

FIGURE 11-4 Magnified view of a pulmonary lobule on HRCT: under normal conditions, the three basic components of the lobule—the interlobular septa and septal structures (veins), the central lobular region (effectively the centrilobular artery alone), and the lobular parenchyma—can be identified on HRCT. The centrilobular bronchioles and lymphatic vessels are not resolved on HRCT.

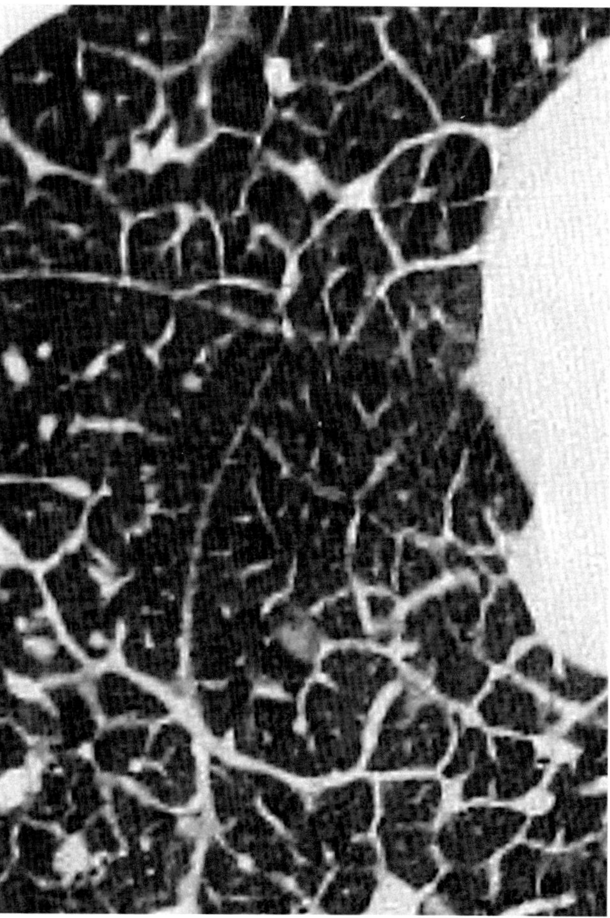

FIGURE 11-5 HRCT appearance of interstitial infiltration caused by interstitial oedema. Interlobular septal thickening can be seen in the right lung delineating several secondary pulmonary lobules.

the context of bacterial infection or pulmonary haemorrhage (Fig. 11-6).[15]

2. *Ground-glass opacification* is a relatively common sign of airspace disease. On plain radiography, ground-glass opacification is seen as hazy increased lung opacity, usually extensive, in which the margins of pulmonary vessels may be indistinct.[13] Because of the greater contrast resolution, ground-glass opacification on CT appears as a hazy increase in lung attenuation but *without* obscuration of bronchial and vascular markings (Fig. 11-7).[13] It is important to remember that ground-glass opacification is a non-specific sign that can be a manifestation of airspace and/or interstitial disease (Fig. 11-8).[16] On occasion, ground-glass opacification on CT may be barely perceptible. In such cases, a noticeable difference between the density of air in the lumen of an airway and that in the adjacent lung (the 'black bronchus' sign) may be the clue needed to confirm suspicion of lung infiltration: normally, the two densities will be roughly equal (Fig. 11-9).
3. *Consolidation* refers to the increase in lung density on chest radiography or CT in which the margins of vessels and airways are obscured (Fig. 11-10). An air bronchogram may be seen. This radiological

pattern occurs when air in the air spaces is replaced by any pathological process (e.g. inflammatory cells, blood or tumour). In some patients, a characteristic perilobular distribution (giving the spurious impression of thickened interlobular septa) may be seen (Fig. 11-11). On thin-section CT, a perilobular pattern manifests as curvilinear opacities (of greater thickness and less well-defined than interlobular septa), producing an arcade-like appearance.[13,17] This distribution reflects a pathological process that is 'smeared' around the margins of the lobule as is seen in organising pneumonia.

PULMONARY OEDEMA

Pulmonary oedema—defined as an excess of extravascular lung water—may be due to an increase in hydrostatic pressure (sometimes called cardiogenic oedema) or vascular permeability (termed non-cardiogenic oedema) (Table 11-2). Despite the attraction of simplicity, the clinical utility of this dichotomous classification of pulmonary oedema has been questioned.[18,19] This notwithstanding, hydrostatic oedema occurs when there is a shift of fluid out of the vascular compartment caused by an increase in venous/capillary pressure. A common cause of increased hydrostatic pressure is left heart failure but, rarely, a reduction in plasma osmotic pressure (e.g. in hypoalbuminaemic patients) will lead to pulmonary oedema. Non-cardiogenic pulmonary oedema occurs in conditions where the permeability of the alveolar–capillary barrier is increased. The archetypal example of increased permeability oedema is acute respiratory distress syndrome (ARDS).

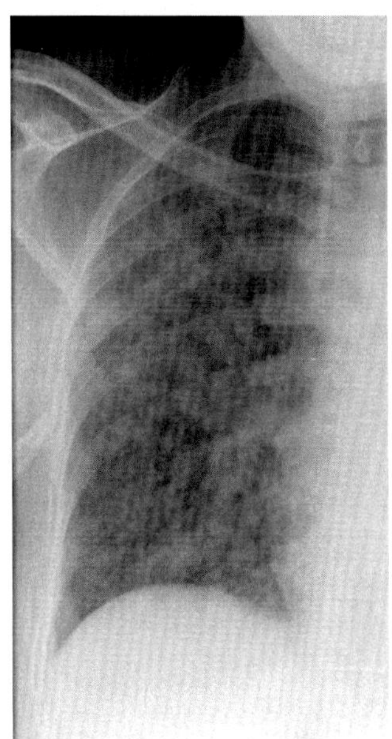

FIGURE 11-6 ■ Nodular airspace opacities on HRCT. Targeted image of the right lung showing numerous ill-defined nodules in a patient with disseminated pulmonary tuberculosis.

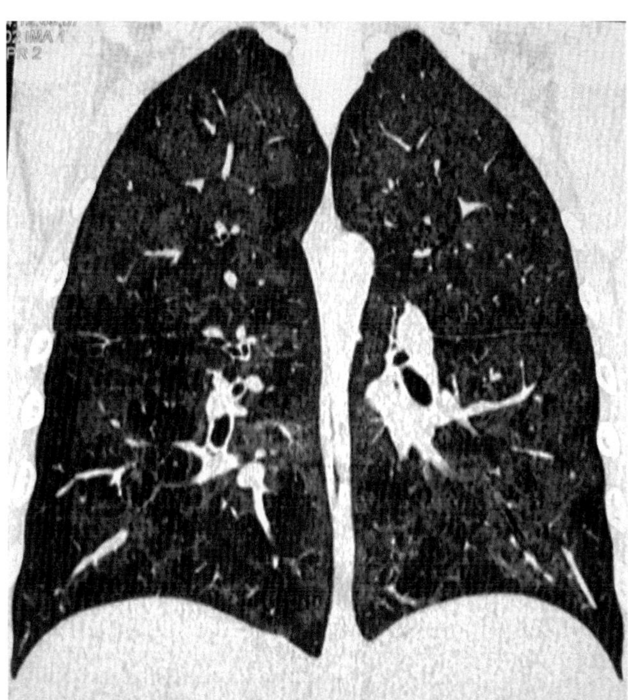

FIGURE 11-7 ■ Ground-glass opacification on CT in an immunocompromised patient with *Pneumocystis jiroveci* infection.

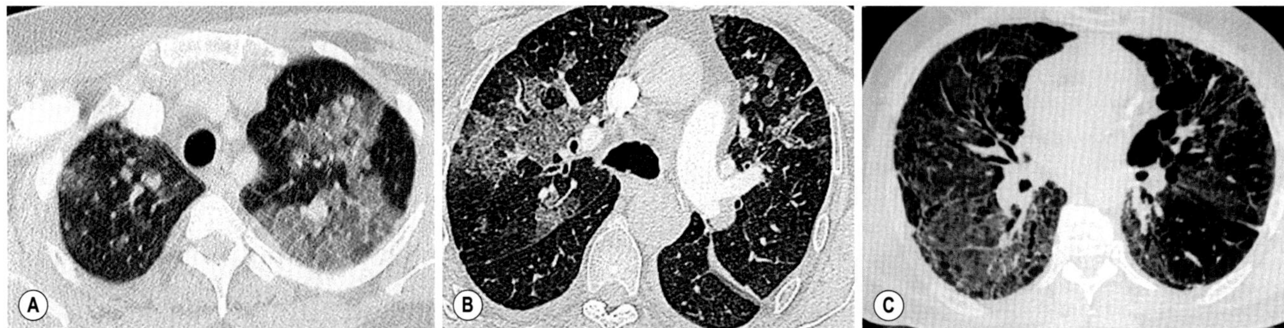

FIGURE 11-8 ■ Variable causes of ground-glass opacification on CT caused by airspace and/or interstitial processes. (A) Diffuse pulmonary haemorrhage in a patient with disseminated cancer. (B) Ground-glass opacification and thickened inter- and intralobular septa in a patient with pulmonary oedema. (C) Ground-glass opacification caused a predominant interstitial lung disease; there are dilated segmental and subsegmental airways ('traction bronchiectasis') in areas of ground-glass opacification indicating fine fibrosis.

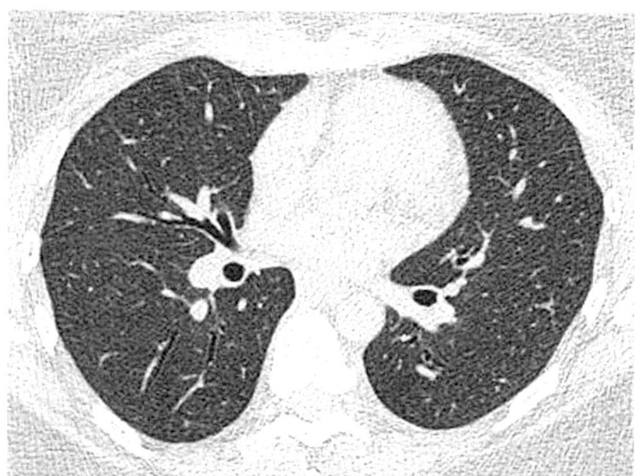

FIGURE 11-9 ■ 'Black bronchus' sign on CT. There is an almost imperceptible increase in lung density. However, air within the segmental bronchi is clearly of lower attenuation than the surrounding parenchyma.

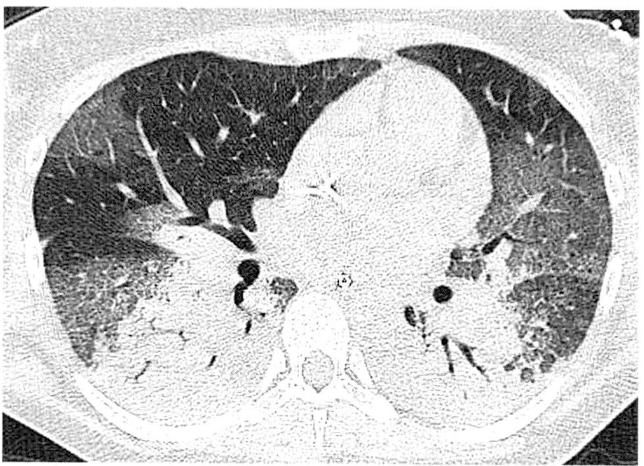

FIGURE 11-10 ■ Consolidation on CT in a patient with acute respiratory distress syndrome. Compared with areas of ground-glass opacification, there is obscuration of bronchovascular markings by areas of dense parenchymal opacification in the dependent lung.

Chest Radiography in Pulmonary Oedema

Plain chest radiography is more sensitive than clinical examination for the early detection of pulmonary oedema.[20] Because there is a roughly predictable sequence, with fluid first passing into the interstitium and then into the alveoli, the radiographic changes of interstitial oedema generally precede frank airspace opacification.[21] In the following sections, the radiographic features of pulmonary oedema are considered; for clarity the vascular, interstitial and intra-alveolar changes are discussed separately.

Vascular Changes

The signs of raised pulmonary venous pressure on chest radiography are well documented, although the mechanisms underlying blood flow redistribution are not entirely clear. Signs of vascular redistribution (from bases to apex), namely balanced flow or inverted flow, often suggest elevation of the pulmonary venous pressure (Fig. 11-12). Both vascular dilation and redistribution are more appreciable in chronic or, at least, subacute left heart dysfunction.[19,22] The ratio of the diameter of adjacent pulmonary arteries and bronchi seen end-on, particularly at the level of the upper lobes, aids in determining whether vessels are abnormally enlarged.[23]

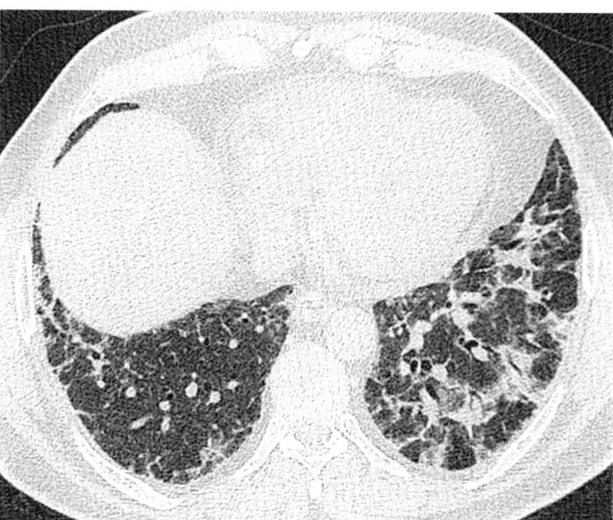

FIGURE 11-11 ■ Perilobular pattern of cryptogenic organising pneumonia in a young female patient. CT through the lung bases shows a striking 'arcade-like' distribution of consolidation.

TABLE 11-2 **CT Signs of Pulmonary Oedema**

Common Findings
- Ground-glass opacification (patchy or diffuse) ± consolidation
- Smooth interlobular septal thickening
- Peribronchovascular thickening
- Vascular dilatation

Ancillary Findings
- Pleural effusions
- Enlargement of mediastinal lymph nodes/'hazy' opacification of mediastinal fat (in heart failure)—reversible

Interstitial Oedema

One of the classical radiographic manifestations of interstitial oedema is thickening of the interlobular septa. The characteristic Kerley B lines, which represent fluid in the interlobular septa (typically 1–2 mm wide and 30–60 mm long), are only really seen in the subpleural lung, perpendicular to the pleural surface (Fig. 11-13). By comparison, Kerley A lines are longer (up to 80–100 mm), occasionally angulated and cross the inner two-thirds of the lung in varying directions but tend to point medially towards the hilum. In left heart failure, septal lines become visible as they distend with extravascular fluid. Naturally, the visualisation of oedematous septal lines will be hampered if neighbouring alveoli are also

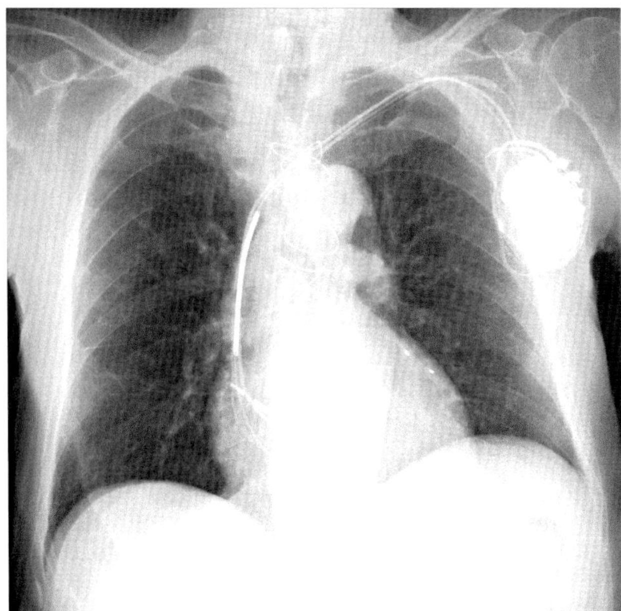

FIGURE 11-12 ■ Upper lobe blood diversion. Vessels in the upper zones are prominent in comparison to those in the lower lung zones.

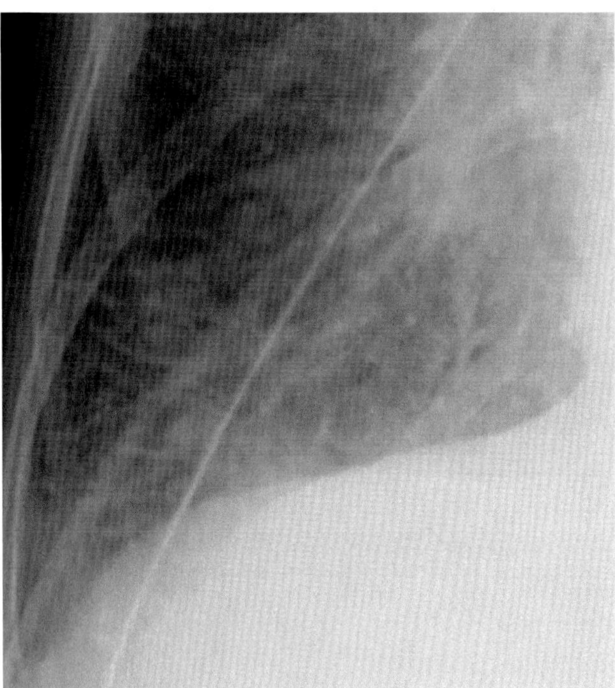

FIGURE 11-13 ■ Magnified view of the left costophrenic region demonstrating multiple interstitial (Kerley B) lines. Each line is roughly perpendicular to the chest wall and extends to the pleural surface.

opacified. It should also be remembered that the demonstration of thickened interlobular septa is *not* diagnostic of pulmonary oedema; fibrosis and malignant infiltration (as in lymphangitis carcinomatosa) will also increase the conspicuity of interlobular septa.

Another sign of interstitial oedema on frontal chest radiographs is peribronchial cuffing in which the

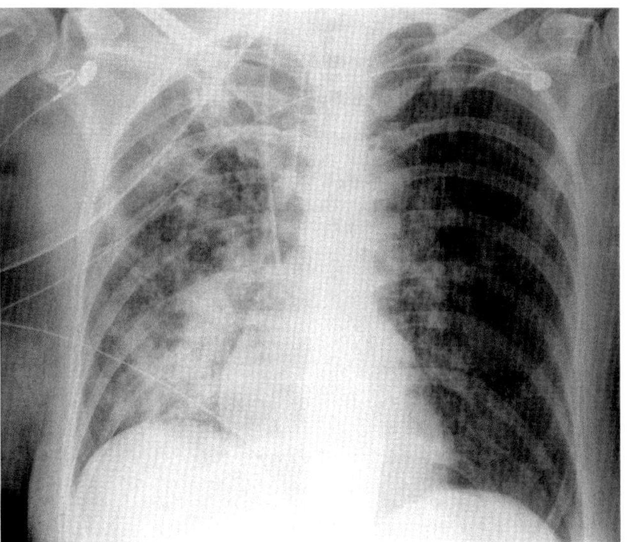

FIGURE 11-14 ■ Asymmetrical distribution of airspace opacification in a patient with pulmonary oedema. There is patchy opacification in the right lung with relative sparing of the left.

normally thin and well-defined wall of the airway appears thickened and indistinct. A loss of conspicuity of the central pulmonary vessels (termed a perihilar haze) also occurs and, as with peribronchial cuffing, is assumed to be caused by oedema of the perivascular interstitium. Oedema fluid can also collect in the potential space between the visceral pleura and lung; on chest radiography this may be seen as thickening of the interlobar fissures or as a lamellar 'effusion' in the costophrenic recesses. The latter, despite the name, indicates fluid between the lung and visceral pleura.[24]

Alveolar Oedema

Airspace opacification becomes visible on the chest radiographs as oedema fluid passes from the interstitium into the alveoli. The distribution of changes is variable but bilateral opacification is the norm. However, an asymmetric distribution (Fig. 11-14) or oedema apparently confined to one lung on chest radiographs also occurs.[25] There may be sparing of the apices and extreme lung bases. On occasion, the central lungs are more affected, producing the so-called 'bat's wing' distribution (Fig. 11-15).[26] As oedema progresses, opacities coalesce to produce a general 'white-out'. An air bronchogram or alveologram may be seen when there is intra-alveolar oedema. The severity of airspace opacification caused by pulmonary oedema can change relatively quickly; indeed, the speed of change (i.e. sometimes over hours as opposed to days or weeks) is a useful pointer to the diagnosis of oedema fluid rather than another airspace pathology.

In specific settings, the radiographic appearances of intra-alveolar oedema will be modified. For instance, the distribution of pulmonary oedema can vary with posture so that in patients lying on one side for a prolonged period, the dependent lung becomes more oedematous and there is unilateral airspace opacification.[27] Coexisting diseases such as emphysema will also affect

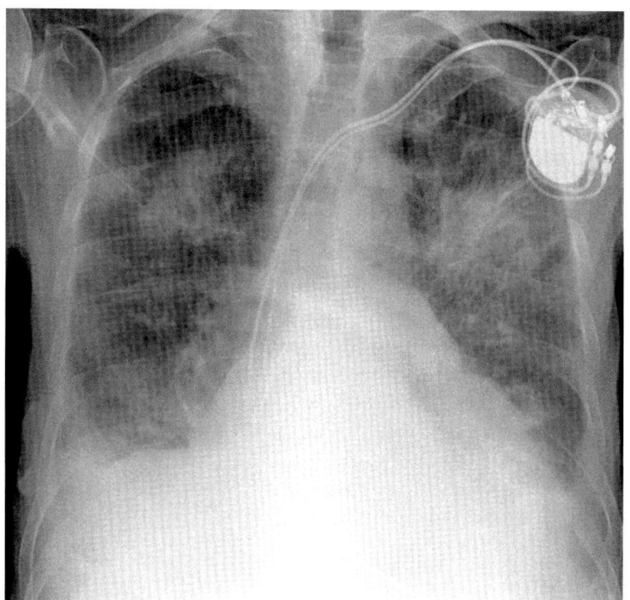

FIGURE 11-15 ■ Pulmonary oedema on chest radiography demonstrating the characteristic 'bat's wing' distribution with air-space opacification principally within the central lung.

the distribution and appearance of oedema fluid. Similarly, in patients with pulmonary fibrosis, there may be more rapid fluid accumulation in the alveolar spaces than within the interstitium.[28]

Radiographic Differentiation of Cardiogenic and Non-Cardiogenic Pulmonary Oedema

Making the distinction between hydrostatic and permeability oedema is of clinical value. In this regard, chest radiography is more reliable than physical examination.[29] However, whether chest radiography can consistently differentiate between cardiogenic and non-cardiogenic oedema is doubtful.[30,31] In one early study, the distribution of blood flow (i.e. upper zone versus lower zone) and oedema (i.e. peripheral versus central) together with the width of the vascular pedicle were considered to be discriminatory.[30] In 50% of patients with hydrostatic oedema there was upper lobe blood diversion. By contrast, in patients with non-cardiogenic oedema caused by ARDS, only 10% showed this inverted pattern: normal or 'balanced' flow was the more common finding.[30] A peripheral distribution of oedema was strikingly absent in patients with hydrostatic oedema but was the most common pattern in patients with ARDS. Based on these findings and some ancillary features, the authors claimed an overall accuracy for chest radiography of 86–89%.[30] Over time, this conclusion has been questioned:[31,32] although there is high specificity for the finding of patchy or peripherally distributed oedema in increased permeability oedema, Aberle et al. concluded that the sensitivity was below 50%.[31] Similarly, the discriminatory value of signs of interstitial fluid accumulation and pleural effusions has been questioned.[31,33] In summary, analysis of the radiographic pattern will sometimes allow a distinction to be made but the inconsistency of radiographic signs suggests that radiographic distinction between the various forms of pulmonary oedema is unreliable.

CT in Pulmonary Oedema

CT is more sensitive to small changes in lung water than chest radiography: CT may reveal clinically silent oedema or help to differentiate oedema from other disease processes. The latter may be of value in critically ill patients with multiple comorbidities.[34] The typical CT signs of pulmonary oedema are summarised in Table 11-2. However, the appearances of pulmonary oedema on CT are variable. Because of excellent contrast resolution, CT may detect abnormalities before the transudation of fluid into the interstitium and air spaces: in an animal model of fluid overload there was an increase in background lung attenuation, attributed to an expansion of intracapillary volume.[35] Vascular dilatation, particularly in the perihilar regions, may be observed in association with other CT abnormalities, before the development of frank pulmonary oedema.[35,36] The CT equivalent of radiographic upper lobe blood diversion may be seen with preferential dilatation of vessels in the anterior (non-dependent) lung.[37] Although not systematically evaluated, it is likely that the earliest detectable findings associated with enlarged vessels are scant thickened interlobular septa and ground-glass opacification. Smooth septal lines are often limited to the lung apices reflecting engorged septal veins.[38] With more florid transudation of oedema fluid, peribronchovascular cuffing, prominent interlobular septa, ground-glass opacification and consolidation become more obvious (Figs. 11-5 and 11-16). The absence of distortion of lung parenchyma and the more linear, smooth septal thickening should differentiate cardiogenic interstitial oedema from other causes including lymphangitis carcinomatosis and sarcoidosis.

As with chest radiography, the changes on CT are usually bilateral but, occasionally, confined to one lung and the appearances may be modified by coexistent disease such as emphysema. A perihilar distribution (producing a 'bat's wing' appearance) may be seen in some patients but this is by no means invariable. Such a distribution is not specific and is seen in other diseases including pulmonary alveolar proteinosis or pulmonary haemorrhage. An interesting ancillary finding in congestive heart failure is the enlargement of mediastinal lymph nodes and a hazy increase in the attenuation of mediastinal fat.[37,39,40] Overall, around one-half of patients with heart failure have nodal enlargement on CT and this prevalence rises in patients with significantly lower (e.g. <35%) ejection fraction.[37,39,40] Enlarged lymph nodes may have blurred margins. With medical therapy, a significant reduction in the volume of nodes occurs, often within days.[39]

DIFFUSE PULMONARY HAEMORRHAGE

Bleeding into the lungs is a relatively common—albeit sometimes subclinical—event. It is known, for instance,

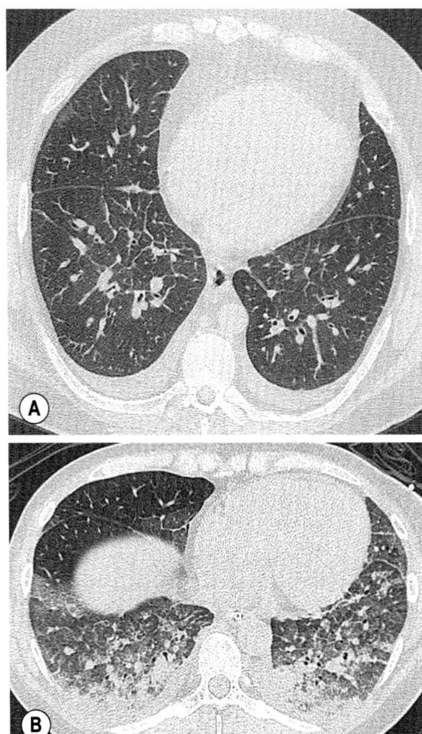

FIGURE 11-16 ■ (A) Pulmonary oedema on CT: there is subtle ground-glass opacification, smooth thickening of multiple interlobular septa and peribronchovascular cuffing. Bilateral pleural effusions are also seen. (B) More conspicuous ground-glass opacification and consolidation as the severity of oedema increases.

TABLE 11-3 Proposed Classification of Causes of Diffuse Pulmonary Haemorrhage

Immunocompetent Patients
- Immunologically-mediated
  - Antibasement membrane antibody disease (Goodpasture's syndrome)
- Disorders with a presumed immune aetiology, with or without nephropathy
  - Connective tissue diseases
    - *Systemic lupus erythematosus*
    - *Rheumatoid arthritis*
    - *Mixed connective tissue disease*
    - Systemic sclerosis
  - ANCA-associated vasculitis
    - *Wegener's granulomatosis*
    - *Churg–Strauss syndrome*
    - *Microscopic polyangiitis*
  - Anti-phospholipid syndrome
  - Pauci-immune glomerulonephritis
  - Henoch–Schönlein purpura
  - Cryoglobulinaemia
- Diseases with no known immune aetiology
  - Idiopathic pulmonary haemosiderosis
  - Rapidly progressive glomerulonephritis without immune complexes
  - Drug-induced (anticoagulants, trimellitic anhydride, cocaine)
  - Valvular heart disease
  - Disseminated intravascular coagulation
  - Diffuse alveolar damage
  - Tumours

Immunocompromised Patients
- Blood dyscrasias
- Infection
- Tumours

Adapted from Lara and Schwarz,[41] Miller[42] and Lee and D'Cruz.[49]

that patients with pneumonia and lung cancer frequently aspirate blood into the air spaces. However, because the bleeding tends to be localised and there is often an established underlying cause, the diagnosis is generally straightforward. In addition to these more common clinical settings there are a number of pulmonary haemorrhage syndromes characterised by diffuse intra-alveolar bleeding.[41] The severity of haemorrhage is highly variable, ranging from small subclinical episodes to catastrophic, life-threatening haemorrhage.

One scheme for classifying diffuse pulmonary haemorrhage (DPH) categorises syndromes according to whether the patient is immunocompromised (Table 11-3).[42] In the immunocompetent DPH may be definitely immunologically mediated (e.g. antiglomerular basement membrane disease), have a presumed immunological basis (e.g. systemic lupus erythematosus, Wegener's granulomatosis), or unrelated to immunological mechanisms (e.g. idiopathic pulmonary haemosiderosis, drug reactions). By contrast, in immunocompromised patients, infection, tumours and blood dyscrasias account for most cases.

The clinical presentation of the DPH syndromes varies[43] but recurrent haemoptyses, dyspnoea and chronic cough are typical. Non-specific clinical features include intermittent pyrexia, headache, lethargy, basal crackles on auscultation and clubbing. On histopathological examination alveolar blood and haemosiderin-laden macrophages are the cardinal findings. With repeated episodes there is thickening of alveolar septa due to fibrosis, which is occasionally florid.[44,45]

The radiographic and CT changes of diffuse pulmonary haemorrhage are stereotypical and differentiation between different causes of DPH, on the basis of radiological findings alone, is generally not possible. Following acute bleeding the chest radiograph is usually, but not invariably, abnormal. On chest radiography there may be small acinar nodules or patchy consolidation and ground-glass opacification. The changes tend to be more pronounced in the perihilar region of the mid and lower zones. A useful diagnostic clue is that, compared with other causes of airspace opacification (with the notable exception of pulmonary oedema), the changes of diffuse intra-alveolar haemorrhage typically clear over a few days because of the relatively efficient removal of blood by lung macrophages (Fig. 11-17). With repeated episodes, ill-defined nodular or reticulonodular opacities are seen and there may be enlargement of hilar lymph nodes.

CT may show poorly defined centrilobular acinar nodules and patchy ground-glass opacities in the face of a normal chest radiograph. Abnormal thickening of interlobular septa may be present and, in some patients, a combination of ground-glass opacities with thickening of inter- and intralobular septa (the crazy-paving pattern) is seen.[3,4]

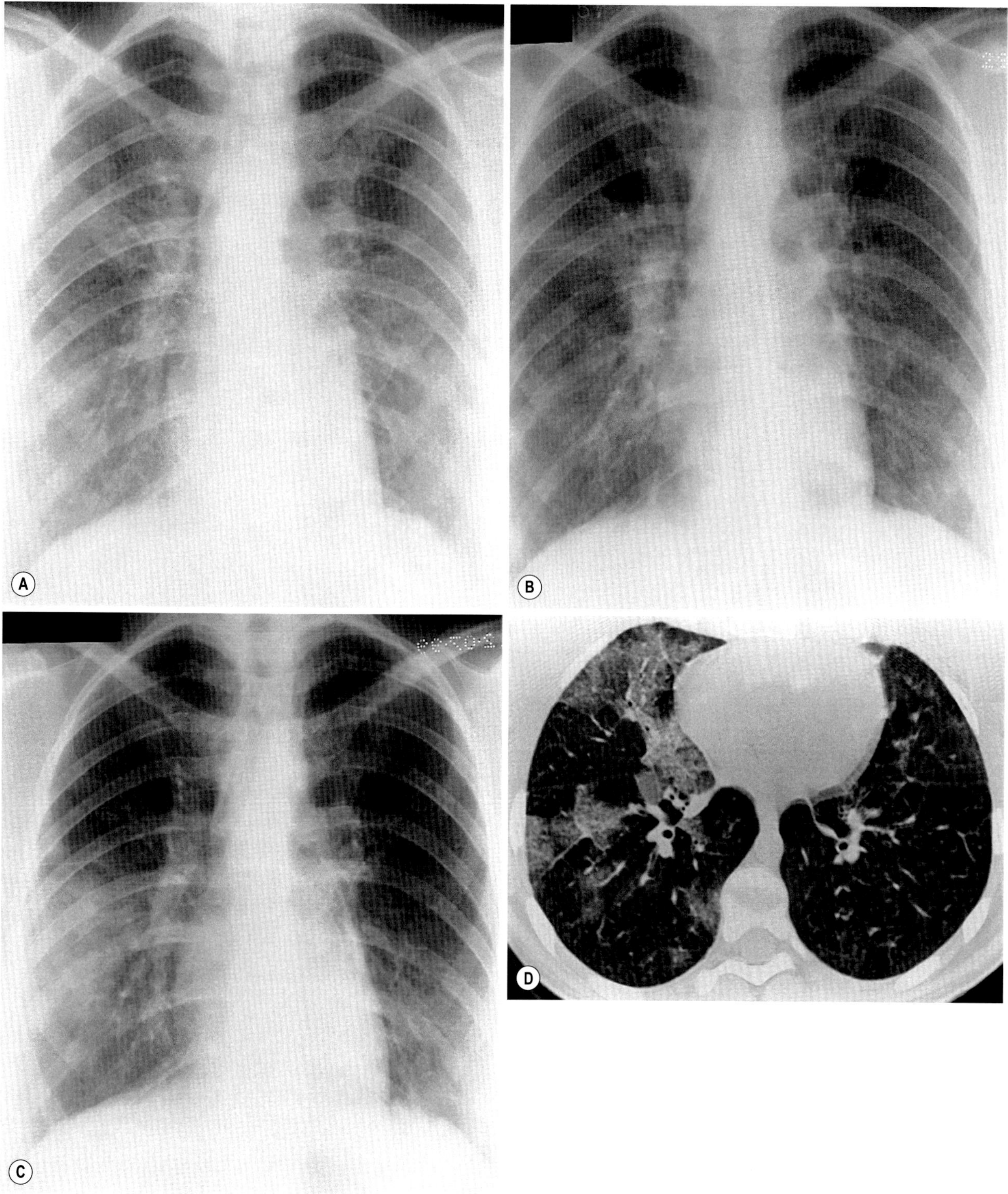

FIGURE 11-17 ■ (A–C) Chest radiographs and (D) HRCT in a patient with idiopathic pulmonary haemosiderosis. (A) There is diffuse ground-glass opacification with no zonal predilection during an acute hospital admission with haemoptysis. (B) Radiograph taken 4 days later shows striking (but incomplete) resolution of airspace opacities. There is residual opacification around the right hilum. (C) Chest radiograph obtained 1 month following admission demonstrates ground-glass opacification in the right mid zone. (D) HRCT through the lower zones (concurrent with the radiograph in (A)) shows patchy ground-glass opacification with a somewhat unusual geographical distribution; there are thickened interlobular septa in areas of ground-glass opacification.

Of the many DPH syndromes, idiopathic pulmonary haemosiderosis and antiglomerular basement membrane antibody disease (Goodpasture's syndrome) are the best documented. These two entities are considered briefly below.

Idiopathic Pulmonary Haemosiderosis

Idiopathic pulmonary haemosiderosis (IPH) is a rare disorder of unknown aetiology. The majority of patients are children (typically in the first decade)[44] although sporadic cases in older subjects have been recorded.[46] The clinical picture is that of episodic intra-alveolar haemorrhage, haemoptyses, iron-deficiency anaemia and airspace opacification on chest radiographs. Repeated bouts of bleeding may lead to lung fibrosis. The outlook for patients with IPH varies: survival may range from a few days (following massive haemorrhage) to years. The pathogenesis of IPH is not clear although a number of hypotheses have been proposed.[47] The imaging findings are non-specific and, as for other haemorrhage syndromes, the clue to the diagnosis may only come from a review of the clinical features (i.e. age, a history of haemoptysis and anaemia) together with the exclusion of other causes of widespread pulmonary haemorrhage.

Antibasement Membrane Antibody Disease (Goodpasture's Syndrome)

The link between renal disease and diffuse intra-alveolar bleeding was recognised in the twentieth century.[48] Although the historical title Goodpasture's syndrome (referring to glomerulonephritis with circulating serum antibodies directed against components of basement membrane in the lungs and kidneys) is in common use, the more pathogenetically accurate term antibasement membrane (anti-BM) antibody disease is preferred. Anti-BM antibody disease typically affects young men, with a male : female ratio of around 3 : 1. The pulmonary manifestations of anti-BM antibody disease often dominate the clinical presentation, though evidence of renal disease is present in the majority of cases.[49]

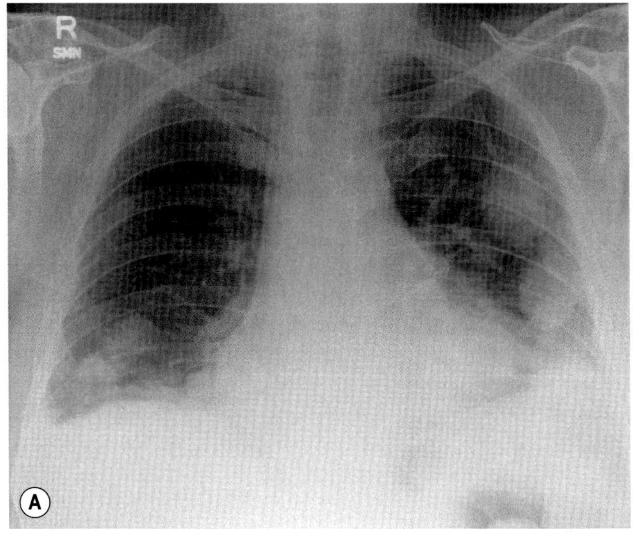

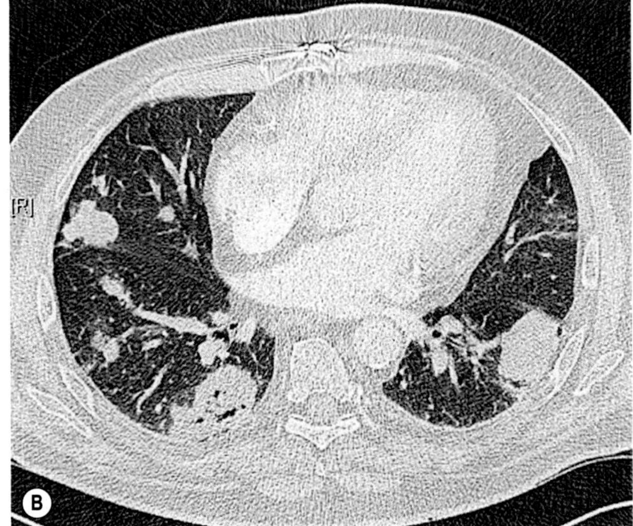

FIGURE 11-18 ■ **Wegener's granulomatosis.** (A) Multiple intrapulmonary nodules within both lungs on chest radiograph in a patient with elevated c-ANCA titres. (B) CT through the lower zones also demonstrates multiple pulmonary nodules. However, there is clear evidence of cavitation (not seen on the chest radiograph) in one of the lesions in the right lower lobe.

WEGENER'S GRANULOMATOSIS (ANCA-ASSOCIATED GRANULOMATOUS VASCULITIS)

Wegener's granulomatosis (together with microscopic polyangiitis, Churg–Strauss syndrome and isolated pauci-immune pulmonary capillaritis) is best classified as one of the primary (idiopathic) small vessel vasculitides.[50] There is multisystem disease, characterised histologically by necrotising granulomatous inflammation of small vessels in the upper and lower respiratory tracts. There is an equal gender predilection and a wide age range of presentation (from childhood to over 70 years). The lungs are affected in around 90% of patients with Wegener's granulomatosis.[51] The majority of patients present with symptoms referable to the nose, paranasal sinuses or chest; in some patients, the disease manifests solely in the respiratory tract and is termed 'limited' Wegener's granulomatosis.[52] Chest symptoms include cough, dyspnoea, pleuritic chest pain and haemoptysis. The aetiology of Wegener's granulomatosis is unknown but there is a strong link with a cytoplasmic-staining pattern of anti-neutrophil cytoplasmic antibodies (c-ANCA) directed against proteinase-3 (PR3-ANCA).

The spectrum of morphological abnormalities in Wegener's granulomatosis is wide. Multiple nodules or masses are the most prevalent finding, seen in 70–90% of patients.[53] Nodules range in size from a few millimetres up to 10 cm in diameter, are frequently multiple and can increase in size and number as the disease progresses (Fig. 11-18). Nodules are usually bilateral (in 75% of cases), have no predilection for any lung zone and cavitate usually when over 2 cm in diameter.[54] On CT, a halo of

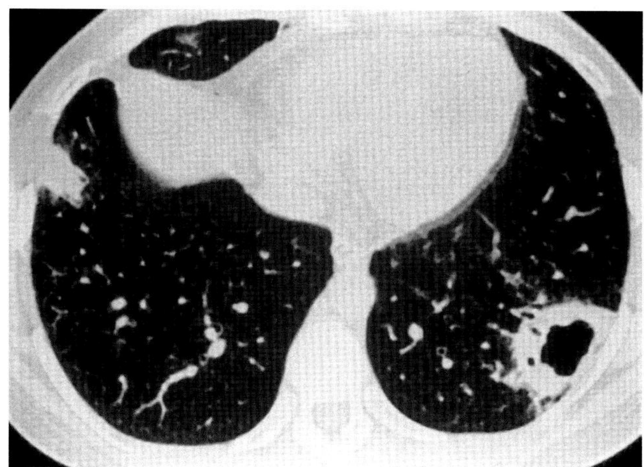

FIGURE 11-19 ■ HRCT through the lower lobes in a patient with biopsy-proven Wegener's granulomatosis. There is multifocal consolidation and a thick-walled cavity in the left lower lobe.

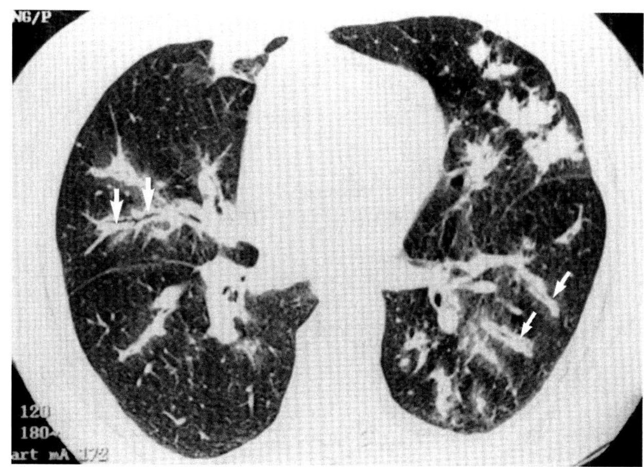

FIGURE 11-20 ■ Bronchocentric disease in Wegener's granulomatosis. Many of the segmental and subsegmental bronchi are thick walled (arrows). (Courtesy of Dr Kate Pointon, Nottingham City Hospital, UK.)

ground-glass opacification (believed to reflect surrounding haemorrhage) may be seen around nodules. In some patients there may be a 'feeding' vessel, leading to a nodule; linear bands, spiculation and pleural tags may also be seen.[55] With treatment, nodules generally regress, but the chest radiograph may not return to normal for up to a month after treatment starts.[56] There may be residual parenchymal scarring on CT despite resolution of nodules and pulmonary consolidation.[57] Cavitation is generally regarded as the classical radiological finding in pulmonary Wegener's granulomatosis and the demonstration of this sign is a useful pointer to the diagnosis (Fig. 11-19). However, cavitation is by no means invariable feature and, the absence of this sign does not preclude a diagnosis of Wegener's granulomatosis. Interestingly, the converse is apparently true in children, in whom nodules are seen less frequently.[58]

Consolidation and ground-glass opacities are recognised features on CT but are less common than nodules. The distribution of consolidation is variable and might include peripheral wedge-shaped foci abutting the pleura (mimicking pulmonary infarcts),[59] a peribronchovascular predilection (Fig. 11-20),[59] a 'reverse halo' pattern,[60] or multifocal areas of consolidation with or without cavitation.

It is important to remember airway involvement in Wegener's granulomatosis. Stenoses of large airways causing subglottic, tracheal or bronchial narrowing are well documented. Bronchiectasis is an additional feature in Wegener's granulomatosis, occurring in up to 40% of cases.[61] CT has also highlighted some of the less common features of Wegener's granulomatosis including areas of lobar or segmental atelectasis, pleural effusions or thickening and, rarely, hilar and mediastinal lymph node enlargement.[61]

ORGANISING PNEUMONIA

Cryptogenic organising pneumonia (COP) was first recognised as a clinical entity by Davison and colleagues in 1983.[62] In their paper, the authors reported the case studies of eight patients presenting with an illness of insidious onset characterised by cough, night sweats, generalised malaise and weight loss. Chest radiographs showed bilateral patchy areas of consolidation. At biopsy there were buds of fibrous connective tissue ('bourgeons conjunctifs') in the alveoli and alveolar ducts and, crucially, only occasionally in the airways.[62] Despite thorough investigation—specifically for infections—no cause was found but an important clinical message was the striking response to treatment with steroids. The authors recognised that organising pneumonia *per se* is simply a histological pattern and that the label 'cryptogenic' applies only when other potential causes of an organising pneumonia pattern have been excluded.[63] There were features pointing to a background of connective tissue disease in a subset of patients reported by Davison and colleagues. A pattern of organising pneumonia is known to occur in a variety of clinical contexts (Table 11-4). The more confusing term 'idiopathic brochiolitis obliterans

TABLE 11-4 Recognised Causes of Organising Pneumonia and Associations with Other Conditions

- Unknown (cryptogenic organising pneumonia)
- Infections (bacterial, viral)
- Toxic fume exposure
- Drugs (antibiotics, chemotherapeutic, anti-inflammatory, etc.)
- Connective tissue diseases (particularly polymyositis dermatomyositis, rheumatoid arthritis, Sjögren's syndrome, etc.)
- Vasculitis (particularly Churg–Strauss disease, Wegener's granulomatosis, etc.)
- Immunological disorders (common variable immunodeficiency syndrome, essential mixed cryoglobulinaemia)
- Organ transplantation (bone marrow, lung, renal)
- Radiation pneumonitis
- Neoplasms (particularly lymphoma)

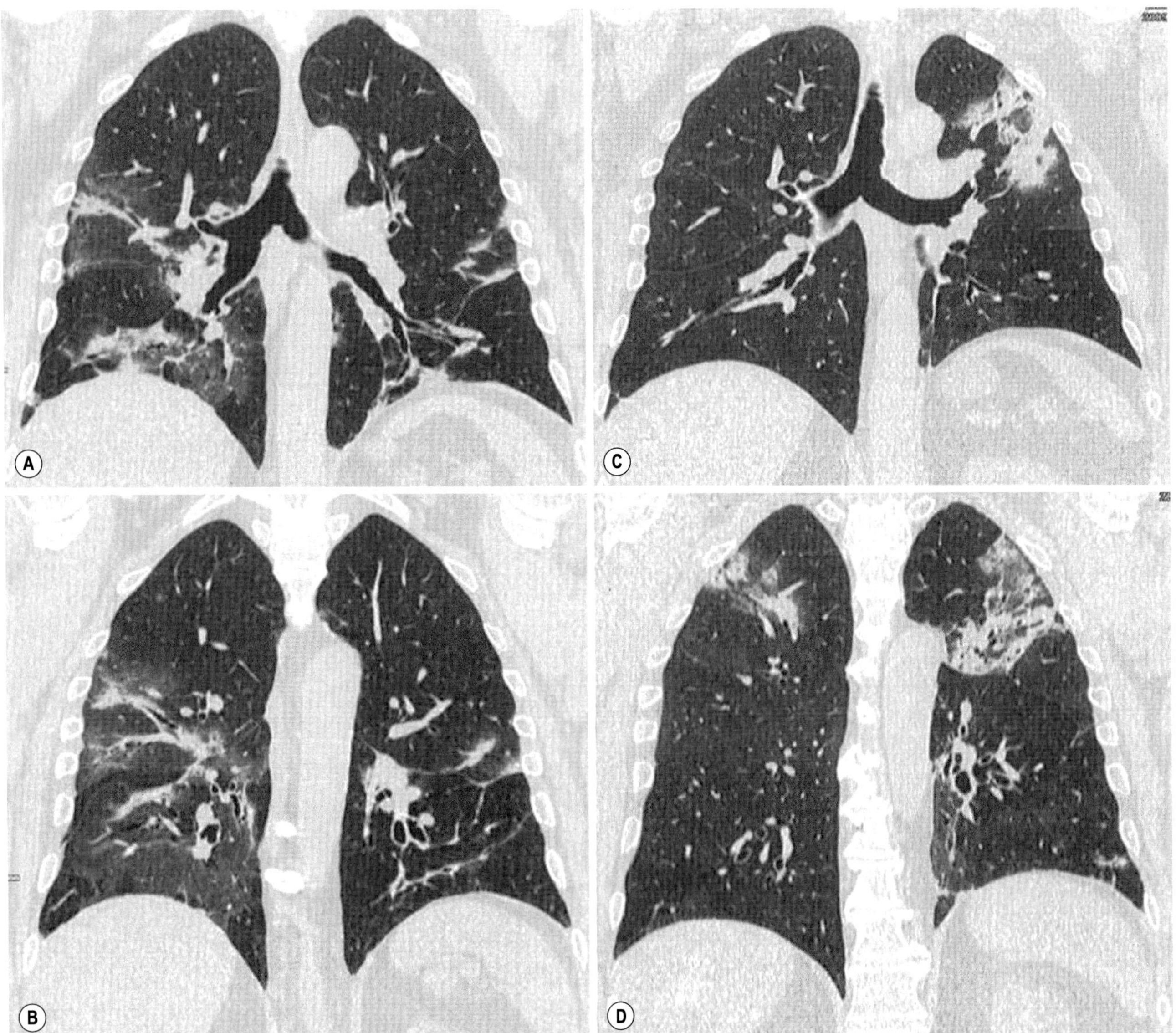

FIGURE 11-21 ■ **Cryptogenic organising pneumonia in a patient presenting with a cough, breathlessness and weight loss.** (A, B) Patchy multifocal consolidation and ground-glass opacities in the mid and lower zones. (C, D) Relapse caused by suboptimal treatment, 6 months later: there is patchy consolidation in the upper zones.

organising pneumonia (BOOP)' has also been used to describe this clinicopathological entity based on the findings of a paper published 2 years later.[64] However, because the airway changes are secondary to the dominant process in the air spaces and there is no evidence of a 'bronchiolitis obliterans', the term organising pneumonia is now preferred.[65]

The typical chest X-ray and CT signs of COP may be predicted from a knowledge of the histopathological changes.[66] Bilateral patchy areas of consolidation, which tend to be peripheral, are the characteristic findings on chest radiography (Fig. 11-21).[67] Although earlier series suggested a predilection for the mid and lower zones, data from CT indicate that all lung zones may be affected.[68] The changes of COP may be confined to one lung but this is uncommon (Fig. 11-22).[67] Consolidation in COP has a propensity for the subpleural and/or peribronchovascular regions in around two-thirds of patients. Cavitation is not a feature of COP but multifocal areas of ground-glass opacification with a surrounding rim of consolidation (termed the 'reverse halo' or 'Atoll' sign) has been described (Fig. 11-2).[69] Nodules, sometimes measuring up to 1 cm in diameter and representing focal areas of organising pneumonia, are seen in some patients and, occasionally, these may be the sole radiographic manifestation of COP;[67] as with areas of consolidation, there is no definite zonal predilection. In rare instances, a large solitary nodule or mass with irregular margins may be seen, prompting investigations for lung cancer.[70]

Murphy et al. reported linear opacities as the dominant HRCT abnormality in some patients with COP.[71] Two types of opacity (termed types I and II) were seen: type I opacities were intimately related to bronchi and extend radially towards the pleura. Type I opacities measured 2–4 cm in length and 1–2 mm in thickness. Areas of consolidation may coexist with type I linear opacities.

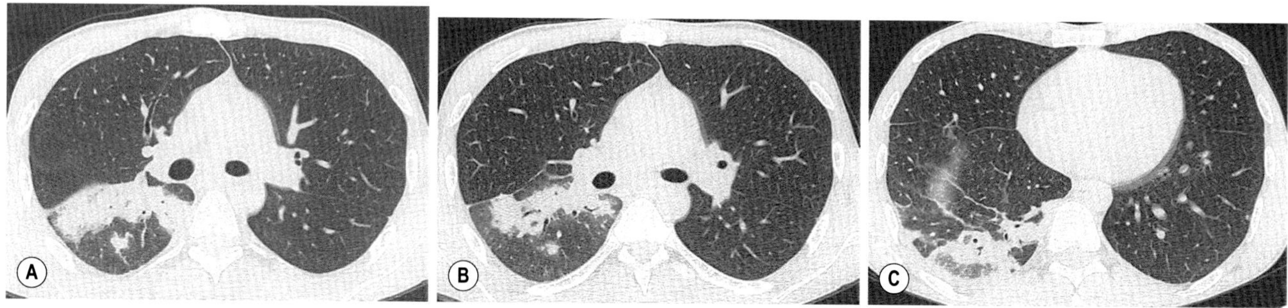

FIGURE 11-22 ■ A 37-year-old patient was treated with sulfasalazine for Crohn's disease and one month later developed dyspnoea and fever. HRCT shows right lower lobe consolidation (A, B) and the reversed halo sign (C), suggesting the diagnosis of organising pneumonia.

Type II linear opacities are subpleural and, unlike the type I pattern, are not related to airways. Type II linear opacities also tend to parallel the pleural surface but, like type I changes, they are frequently associated with multifocal airspace consolidation. More recently, a perilobular distribution of consolidation, giving rise to a distinctive CT appearance, has been also described[17,66] (Fig. 11-11).

Radiological distinction from pure infection (e.g. bacterial pneumonia) may be difficult, particularly when abnormalities are unilateral. Recognising the 'rhomboid' shape of the consolidation, traction features (bronchiectasis, fissures displacement), reversed halo sign and perilobular opacities may suggest the correct diagnosis of OP (Fig. 11-22).

EOSINOPHILIC LUNG DISEASE

Eosinophilic lung diseases are a diverse group of pulmonary disorders associated with peripheral or tissue eosinophilia. Indeed, many pulmonary diseases are known to be associated with a degree of blood eosinophilia (e.g. asthma, opportunistic infections), but these conditions are not usually considered to be eosinophilic lung diseases, in which a tissue eosinophilia is by definition pathogenically significant.[72] A simplified classification of the pulmonary eosinophilias is given in Table 11-5 and some of the entities encompassed within the broad category of eosinophilic pneumonia are discussed below.

Simple Pulmonary Eosinophilia (Löffler's Syndrome)

In 1932, Löffler reported a series of patients presenting with infiltrates on chest radiography, two of whom had a peripheral blood eosinophilia. The term Löffler's syndrome (synonymous with simple pulmonary eosinophilia) describes patients with transient radiographic infiltrates, minimal constitutional upset and an elevated eosinophil count in peripheral blood. The airspace opacification in Löffler's syndrome is fleeting and may be uni- or bilateral. Resolution of opacities within a period of days and, by definition, within a month is the rule. In many cases, no underlying aetiological factor is found but there is an association with parasitic infection, in particular infestation with *Ascaris lumbricoides*. CT findings include ground-glass opacities or consolidation principally in the periphery of the middle/upper lung zones, as well as single or multiple acinar nodules.[72]

TABLE 11-5 **Modified Classification of Eosinophilic Lung Disease**

Idiopathic
Simple pulmonary eosinophilia (Löffler's syndrome)
Acute eosinophilic pneumonia
Chronic eosinophilic pneumonia
Hypereosinophilic syndrome
Drug-Induced
Aminosalicylic acid
Para-aminosalicylic acid
Non-steroidal anti-inflammatory drugs
Captopril
Cocaine
Minocycline
Nitrofurantoin
Phenytoin
Infection
Parasitic (ascariasis, paragonimiasis, tropical eosinophilia)
Fungal (*Aspergillus*)
Bacterial (tuberculosis, atypical mycobacterial infection, *Brucella*)
Viral (respiratory syncytial virus)
Immunological Diseases
Wegener's granulomatosis
Churg–Strauss syndrome
Rheumatoid disease
Sarcoidosis
Neoplasms
Brochogenic carcinoma
Bronchial carcinoid
Lymphoma (Hodgkin's, non-Hodgkin's)

Acute Eosinophilic Pneumonia

In rare patients with pulmonary eosinophilia there is a more fulminant clinical illness beginning with a short febrile episode (< 1 month duration) but followed by significant respiratory distress.[73] Widespread airspace opacification on chest radiographs, more than 25% eosinophils in bronchoalveolar fluid and an eosinophilic pneumonia (in the absence of any known cause of eosinophil infiltration) are the principal findings: the term 'acute eosinophilic pneumonia' has been applied to this entity. A link with smoking is suspected and, in particular, there may be an association with a recent change in smoking habits.[74] The overwhelming majority of patients respond relatively quickly to corticosteroid treatment and relapses are rare.

On plain chest radiographs, there is bilateral airspace opacification and/or reticular infiltrates.[75] Pleural effusions are common. Areas of ground-glass opacification and consolidation are seen on CT and there may be smooth thickening of interlobular septa. The CT signs are similar to those seen in patients with pulmonary oedema or diffuse alveolar damage and the initial serum eosinophil count may be normal. Therefore, establishing a confident diagnosis of acute eosinophilic pneumonia can be difficult.[72]

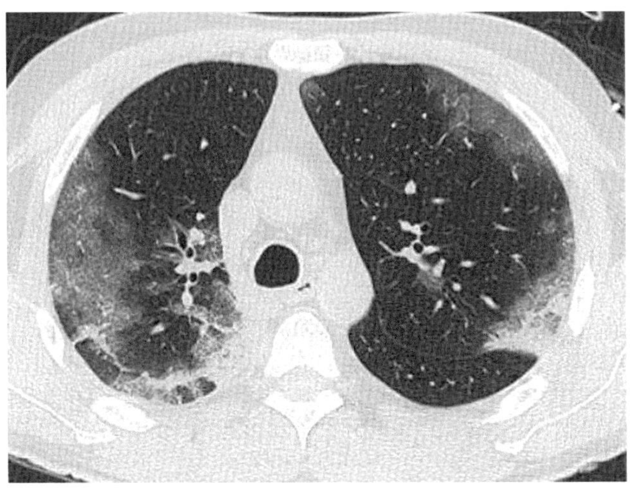

FIGURE 11-23 ■ Chronic eosinophilic pneumonia in a male patient complaining of a dry cough, weight loss and significant peripheral eosinophilia. HRCT through the upper lobes with bilateral patchy I areas of ground-glass opacification and consolidation in a peripheral distribution.

Chronic Eosinophilic Pneumonia

The clinical and radiological features of chronic eosinophilic pneumonia are strikingly different from the entities described above. As the term suggests, the clinical course of chronic eosinophilic pneumonia is generally more protracted and the symptoms are often more marked than in patients with simple pulmonary eosinophilia. There is frequently mild-to-moderate eosinophilia and increased serum IgE levels in the peripheral blood. The prognosis is good and most patients respond to steroid therapy.

The plain radiographic abnormalities in chronic eosinophilic pneumonia can be characteristic: patchy, non-segmental areas of consolidation are typical in the mid and upper zones.[2] A distinctive feature is that the opacities are peripheral and seem to parallel the chest wall, a finding that was considered to be the 'photographic negative of pulmonary oedema' by Gaensler and Carrington[2] (Fig. 11-23). Not surprisingly, the peripheral location of the consolidation and ground-glass opacity is more readily appreciated on CT. A number of other conditions may mimic chronic eosinophilic pneumonia at CT, including organising pneumonia. In one study, the most helpful distinguishing feature was the presence of nodules, seen in 32% of patients with COP but only 5% of patients with chronic eosinophilic pneumonia.[76]

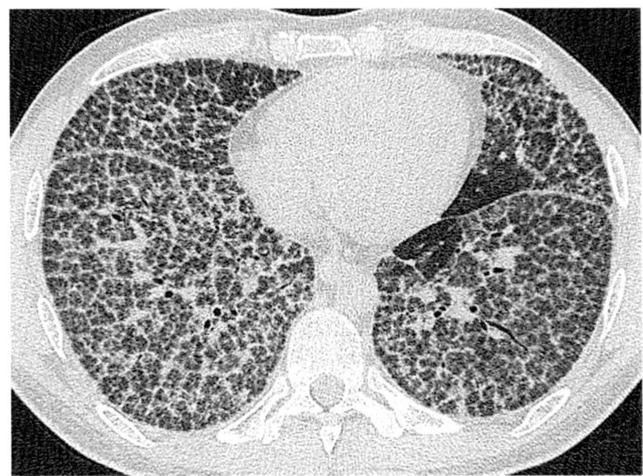

FIGURE 11-24 ■ 'Crazy-paving' pattern in alveolar proteinosis. Patchy but geographical ground-glass opacification is seen and there are numerous thickened interlobular septa in areas of ground-glass opacification.

PULMONARY ALVEOLAR PROTEINOSIS

Pulmonary alveolar proteinosis (PAP; also called alveolar lipoproteinosis and alveolar phospholipoproteinosis) is a rare disease characterised by the accumulation of a periodic acid-Schiff-positive lipoproteinaceous material in the alveoli.[77] Most cases are idiopathic but PAP is reported as a finding in patients with other conditions (notably lymphoma, chemotherapy, infections, dust inhalation) which alter phospholipid homeostasis.[77,78] PAP usually affects adults aged 20–50 years but has been described in children (in whom the outlook tends to be worse); there is a male predilection. The definitive diagnosis of PAP usually requires bronchoscopic lavage and/or biopsy, supported by imaging findings. Although spontaneous resolution is reported, the majority of patients require therapeutic (whole lung) bronchoalveolar lavage, a technique that has improved the outlook of patients with PAP.[79]

The chest radiographic changes of alveolar proteinosis are non-specific. In general, both lungs are affected and airspace opacification is most pronounced in the central lung, sometimes producing a 'bat's wing' appearance. The CT features are much more suggestive of alveolar proteinosis: a 'crazy-paving' pattern (comprising geographical areas of ground-glass opacification with thickened inter- and intralobular septa) is the characteristic feature which, in its classical form, is virtually diagnostic of PAP (Fig. 11-24).[4] However, it is worth remembering that, from time to time, a similar CT appearance is seen in some patients with adenocarcinoma, exogenous lipoid pneumonia and pulmonary oedema.[3]

ALVEOLAR MICROLITHIASIS

Pulmonary alveolar microlithiasis is a rare diffuse lung disease characterised by the deposition of tiny stones or calcipherites (measuring 250–750 μm in diameter and composed mainly of calcium phosphate) in alveoli. There is a high familial incidence and a genetic abnormality has been identified: mutations in the SLC34A2 gene (which codes for a sodium-dependent phosphate transporter in alveolar type II cells) leads to phosphate accumulation.[80] A wide age range (the peak incidence is between 30 and 50 years) has been reported but it seems likely that the disease begins in early life. Most patients are asymptomatic at the time of diagnosis and disease progression is variable. However, there is a tendency for pulmonary fibrosis and the development of cor pulmonale. The fibrosis of alveolar microlithiasis is associated with the formation of bullae, particularly at the apices.[80]

The classical finding on chest radiography is the widespread discrete high-density opacities (resembling grains of sand) seen in both lungs; when the infiltration is profuse there may be a 'white-out', with obscuration of the heart borders and diaphragm and the tiny stones may then only be seen on an overexposed radiograph.[81] A telltale line of black subpleural lung (caused by 5–10 mm diameter small cysts or paraseptal emphysema) may be seen and there may be thickening or beading of fissures.[81] Less commonly, apical blebs and thickened septal (Kerley B) lines may be seen. On CT, the characteristic finding is of widespread ground-glass opacification and/or a micronodular pattern. The changes are more pronounced in the lower zones and posteriorly. In about half of cases, calcification is uniform, producing a pattern of dense parenchymal opacification.[80] Thickening of fissures and interlobular septa may be present and in rare patients, a crazy-paving pattern has been reported.[82]

REFERENCES

1. Haddock JA, Hansell DM. The radiology and terminology of cryptogenic organizing pneumonia. Br J Radiol 1992;65(776):674–80.
2. Gaensler EA, Carrington CB. Peripheral opacities in chronic eosinophilic pneumonia: the photographic negative of pulmonary edema. Am J Roentgenol 1977;128(1):1–13.
3. Johkoh T, Itoh H, Muller NL, et al. Crazy-paving appearance at thin-section CT: spectrum of disease and pathologic findings. Radiology 1999;211(1):155–60.
4. Rossi SE, Erasmus JJ, Volpacchio M, et al. 'Crazy-paving' pattern at thin-section CT of the lungs: radiologic-pathologic overview. Radiographics 2003;23(6):1509–19.
5. Johkoh T, Ikezoe J, Kohno N, et al. Usefulness of high-resolution CT for differential diagnosis of multi-focal pulmonary consolidation. Radiat Med 1996;14(3):139–46.
6. Lui YM, Taylor JR, Zylak CJ. Roentgen—anatomical correlation of the individual human pulmonary acinus. Radiology 1973;109(1):1–5.
7. Van Allen CM, Lindskog GE, Richter HG. Collateral respiration. Transfer of air collaterally between pulmonary lobules. J Clin Invest 1931;10(3):559–90.
8. Miller WS. Historical sketch. In: Miller WS, editor. The Lung. Springfield: Charles C Thomas; 1947. pp. 162–202.
9. Itoh H, Murata K, Konishi J, et al. Diffuse lung disease: pathologic basis for the high-resolution computed tomography findings. J Thorac Imaging 1993;8(3):176–88.
10. Murata K, Itoh H, Todo G, et al. Centrilobular lesions of the lung: demonstration by high-resolution CT and pathologic correlation. Radiology 1986;161(3):641–5.
11. Webb WR. Thin-section CT of the secondary pulmonary lobule: anatomy and the image—the 2004 Fleischner lecture. Radiology 2006;239(2):322–38.
12. Gamsu G, Thurlbeck WM, Macklem PT, Fraser RG. Roentgenographic appearance of the human pulmonary acinus. Invest Radiol 1971;6(3):171–5.
13. Hansell DM, Bankier AA, MacMahon H, et al. Fleischner Society: glossary of terms for thoracic imaging. Radiology 2008;246(3):697–722.
14. Recavarren S, Benton C, Gall EA, et al. The pathology of acute alveolar diseases of the lung. Semin Roentgenol 1967;2:22–32.
15. Itoh H, Tokunaga S, Asamoto H, et al. Radiologic-pathologic correlations of small lung nodules with special reference to peribronchiolar nodules. Am J Roentgenol 1978;130(2):223–31.
16. Collins J, Stern EJ. Ground-glass opacity at CT: the ABCs. Am J Roentgenol 1997;169(2):355–67.
17. Ujita M, Renzoni EA, Veeraraghavan S, et al. Organizing pneumonia: perilobular pattern at thin-section CT. Radiology 2004;232(3):757–61.
18. Crapo JD. New concepts in the formation of pulmonary edema. Am Rev Respir Dis 1993;147(4):790–2.
19. Ketai LH, Godwin JD. A new view of pulmonary edema and acute respiratory distress syndrome. J Thorac Imaging 1998;13(3):147–71.
20. Harrison MO, Conte PJ, Heitzman ER. Radiological detection of clinically occult cardiac failure following myocardial infarctionl. Br J Radiol 1971;44(520):265–72.
21. Staub NC, Nagano H, Pearce ML. Pulmonary edema in dogs, especially the sequence of fluid accumulation in lungs. J Appl Physiol 1967;22(2):227–40.
22. Morgan PW, Goodman LR. Pulmonary edema and adult respiratory distress syndrome. Radiol Clin North Am 1991;29(5):943–63.
23. Woodring JH. Pulmonary artery-bronchus ratios in patients with normal lungs, pulmonary vascular plethora, and congestive heart failure. Radiology 1991;179(1):115–22.
24. Arai K, Takashima T, Matsui O, et al. Transient subpleural curvilinear shadow caused by pulmonary congestion. J Comput Assist Tomogr 1990;14(1):87–8.
25. Youngberg AS. Unilateral diffuse lung opacity; Differential diagnosis with emphasis on lymphangitic spread of cancer. Radiology 1977;123(2):277–81.
26. Fleischner FG. The butterfly pattern of acute pulmonary edema. Am J Cardiol 1967;20(1):39–46.
27. Gluecker T, Capasso P, Schnyder P, et al. Clinical and radiologic features of pulmonary edema. Radiographics 1999;19(6):1507–31; discussion 1532–3.
28. Zwikler MP, Peters TM, Michel RP. Effects of pulmonary fibrosis on the distribution of edema. Computed tomographic scanning and morphology. Am J Respir Crit Care Med 1994;149(5):1266–75.
29. Pistolesi M, Miniati M, Milne EN, Giuntini C. The chest roentgenogram in pulmonary edema. Clin Chest Med 1985;6(3):315–44.
30. Milne EN, Pistolesi M, Miniati M, Giuntini C. The radiologic distinction of cardiogenic and noncardiogenic edema. Am J Roentgenol 1985;144(5):879–94.
31. Aberle DR, Wiener-Kronish JP, Webb WR, Matthay MA. Hydrostatic versus increased permeability pulmonary edema: diagnosis based on radiographic criteria in critically ill patients. Radiology 1988;168(1):73–9.
32. Smith RC, Mann H, Greenspan RH, et al. Radiographic differentiation between different etiologies of pulmonary edema. Invest Radiol 1987;22(11):859–63.
33. Wiener-Kronish JP, Matthay MA. Pleural effusions associated with hydrostatic and increased permeability pulmonary edema. Chest 1988;93(4):852–8.
34. Goodman LR. Congestive heart failure and adult respiratory distress syndrome. New insights using computed tomography. Radiol Clin North Am 1996;34(1):33–46.

35. Herold CJ, Wetzel RC, Robotham JL, et al. Acute effects of increased intravascular volume and hypoxia on the pulmonary circulation: assessment with high-resolution CT. Radiology 1992;183(3):655–62.
36. Beigelman-Aubry C, Hill C, Guibal A, et al. Multi-detector row CT and postprocessing techniques in the assessment of diffuse lung disease. Radiographics 2005;25(6):1639–52.
37. Slanetz PJ, Truong M, Shepard JA, et al. Mediastinal lymphadenopathy and hazy mediastinal fat: new CT findings of congestive heart failure. Am J Roentgenol 1998;171(5):1307–9.
38. Storto ML, Kee ST, Golden JA, Webb WR. Hydrostatic pulmonary edema: high-resolution CT findings. Am J Roentgenol 1995;165(4):817–20.
39. Chabbert V, Canevet G, Baixas C, et al. Mediastinal lymphadenopathy in congestive heart failure: a sequential CT evaluation with clinical and echocardiographic correlations. Eur Radiol 2004;14(5):881–9.
40. Erly WK, Borders RJ, Outwater EK, et al. Location, size, and distribution of mediastinal lymph node enlargement in chronic congestive heart failure. J Comput Assist Tomogr 2003;27(4):485–9.
41. Lara AR, Schwarz MI. Diffuse alveolar hemorrhage. Chest 2010;137(5):1164–71.
42. Miller RR. Diffuse pulmonary hemorrhage. In: Thurlbeck WM, Churg AM, editors. Pathology of the Lung. New York: Thieme Medical Publisher; 1995. pp. 365–73.
43. Collard HR, Schwarz MI. Diffuse alveolar hemorrhage. Clin Chest Med 2004;25(3):583–92, vii.
44. Morgan PG, Turner-Warwick M. Pulmonary haemosiderosis and pulmonary haemorrhage. Br J Dis Chest 1981;75(3):225–42.
45. Buschman DL, Ballard R. Progressive massive fibrosis associated with idiopathic pulmonary hemosiderosis. Chest 1993;104(1):293–5.
46. Scadding JG. Clinical problems of diffuse pulmonary fibrosis. Br J Radiol 1956;29(348):633–41.
47. Ioachimescu OC, Sieber S, Kotch A. Idiopathic pulmonary haemosiderosis revisited. Eur Respir J 2004;24(1):162–70.
48. Goodpasture EW. The significance of certain pulmonary lesions in relation to the etiology of influenza. Am J Med Sci 1919;158:863–70.
49. Lee RW, D'Cruz DP. Pulmonary renal vasculitis syndromes. Autoimmun Rev 2010;9(10):657–60.
50. Brown KK. Pulmonary vasculitis. Proc Am Thorac Soc 2006;3(1):48–57.
51. Luqmani RA, Bacon PA, Beaman M, et al. Classical versus non-renal Wegener's granulomatosis. Q J Med 1994;87(3):161–7.
52. Cordier JF, Valeyre D, Guillevin L, et al. Pulmonary Wegener's granulomatosis. A clinical and imaging study of 77 cases. Chest 1990;97(4):906–12.
53. Weir IH, Muller NL, Chiles C, et al. Wegener's granulomatosis: findings from computed tomography of the chest in 10 patients. Can Assoc Radiol J 1992;43(1):31–4.
54. Maskell GF, Lockwood CM, Flower CD. Computed tomography of the lung in Wegener's granulomatosis. Clin Radiol 1993;48(6):377–80.
55. Kuhlman JE, Hruban RH, Fishman EK. Wegener granulomatosis: CT features of parenchymal lung disease. J Comput Assist Tomogr 1991;15(6):948–52.
56. Grotz W, Mundinger A, Wurtemberger G, et al. Radiographic course of pulmonary manifestations in Wegener's granulomatosis under immunosuppressive therapy. Chest 1994;105(2):509–13.
57. Attali P, Begum R, Ban Romdhane H, et al. Pulmonary Wegener's granulomatosis: changes at follow-up CT. Eur Radiol 1998;8(6):1009–113.
58. Wadsworth DT, Siegel MJ, Day DL. Wegener's granulomatosis in children: chest radiographic manifestations. Am J Roentgenol 1994;163(4):901–4.
59. Foo SS, Weisbrod GL, Herman SJ, Chamberlain DW. Wegener granulomatosis presenting on CT with atypical bronchovasocentric distribution. J Comput Assist Tomogr 1990;14(6):1004–6.
60. Agarwal R, Aggarwal AN, Gupta D. Another cause of reverse halo sign: Wegener's granulomatosis. Br J Radiol 2007;80(958):849–50.
61. Castaner E, Alguersuari A, Gallardo X, et al. When to suspect pulmonary vasculitis: radiologic and clinical clues. Radiographics 2010;30(1):33–53.
62. Davison AG, Heard BE, McAllister WA, Turner-Warwick ME. Cryptogenic organizing pneumonitis. Q J Med 1983;52(207):382–94.
63. Cordier JF. Cryptogenic organizing pneumonia. Clin Chest Med 2004;25(4):727–38, vi–vii.
64. Epler GR, Colby TV, McLoud TC, et al. Bronchiolitis obliterans organizing pneumonia. N Engl J Med 1985;312(3):152–8.
65. American Thoracic Society/European Respiratory Society International Multidisciplinary Consensus Classification of the Idiopathic Interstitial Pneumonias. This joint statement of the American Thoracic Society (ATS), and the European Respiratory Society (ERS) was adopted by the ATS board of directors, June 2001 and by the ERS Executive Committee, June 2001. Am J Respir Crit Care Med 2002;165(2):277–304.
66. Roberton BJ, Hansell DM. Organizing pneumonia: a kaleidoscope of concepts and morphologies. Eur Radiol 2011;21(11):2244–54.
67. Flowers JR, Clunie G, Burke M, Constant O. Bronchiolitis obliterans organizing pneumonia: the clinical and radiological features of seven cases and a review of the literature. Clin Radiol 1992;45(6):371–7.
68. Lee KS, Kullnig P, Hartman TE, Muller NL. Cryptogenic organizing pneumonia: CT findings in 43 patients. Am J Roentgenol 1994;162(3):543–6.
69. Kim SJ, Lee KS, Ryu YH, et al. Reversed halo sign on high-resolution CT of cryptogenic organizing pneumonia: diagnostic implications. Am J Roentgenol 2003;180(5):1251–4.
70. Akira M, Yamamoto S, Sakatani M. Bronchiolitis obliterans organizing pneumonia manifesting as multiple large nodules or masses. Am J Roentgenol 1998;170(2):291–5.
71. Murphy JM, Schnyder P, Verschakelen J, et al. Linear opacities on HRCT in bronchiolitis obliterans organising pneumonia. Eur Radiol 1999;9(9):1813–17.
72. Jeong YJ, Kim KI, Seo IJ, et al. Eosinophilic lung diseases: a clinical, radiologic, and pathologic overview. Radiographics 2007;27(3):617–37; discussion 637–9.
73. Allen JN, Pacht ER, Gadek JE, Davis WB. Acute eosinophilic pneumonia as a reversible cause of noninfectious respiratory failure. N Engl J Med 1989;321(9):569–74.
74. Rhee CK, Min KH, Yim NY, et al. Clinical characteristics and corticosteroid treatment of acute eosinophilic pneumonia. Eur Respir J 2013;41(2):402–9.
75. Cheon JE, Lee KS, Jung GS, et al. Acute eosinophilic pneumonia: radiographic and CT findings in six patients. Am J Roentgenol 1996;167(5):1195–9.
76. Arakawa H, Kurihara Y, Niimi H, et al. Bronchiolitis obliterans with organizing pneumonia versus chronic eosinophilic pneumonia: high-resolution CT findings in 81 patients. Am J Roentgenol 2001;176(4):1053–8.
77. Khan A, Agarwal R. Pulmonary alveolar proteinosis. Respir Care 2011;56(7):1016–28.
78. Prakash UB, Barham SS, Carpenter HA, et al. Pulmonary alveolar phospholipoproteinosis: experience with 34 cases and a review. Mayo Clin Proc 1987;62(6):499–518.
79. Ramirez J. Pulmonary alveolar proteinosis. Treatment by massive bronchopulmonary lavage. Arch Intern Med 1967;119(2):147–56.
80. Tachibana T, Hagiwara K, Johkoh T. Pulmonary alveolar microlithiasis: review and management. Curr Opin Pulm Med 2009;15(5):486–90.
81. Korn MA, Schurawitzki H, Klepetko W, Burghuber OC. Pulmonary alveolar microlithiasis: findings on high-resolution CT. Am J Roentgenol 1992;158(5):981–2.
82. Gasparetto EL, Tazoniero P, Escuissato DL, et al. Pulmonary alveolar microlithiasis presenting with crazy-paving pattern on high resolution CT. Br J Radiol 2004;77(923):974–6.

CHAPTER 12

Cardiac Anatomy and Imaging Techniques

Hans-Marc J. Siebelink • Jos J.M. Westenberg • Lucia J.M. Kroft • Albert de Roos

CHAPTER OUTLINE

Knowledge of the cardiac anatomy is essential for identifying and understanding cardiovascular disease in patients and is therefore important in clinical practice. To date, various imaging techniques such as conventional chest radiography, cardiac magnetic resonance (CMR) imaging, computed tomography (CT) and echocardiography are all used to assess aspects of cardiac and vascular anatomy. This chapter contains an overview of the techniques used and provides examples of the anatomy identified with these techniques.

NORMAL CHEST RADIOGRAPHY

Postero-anterior and lateral chest radiographs are commonly obtained in patients with cardiovascular disease. The chest radiograph provides an impression on the size of cardiovascular structures and the lung parenchyma. Specific cardiac chambers and large vessel anatomy can be recognised from chest radiography. Evaluation of the lung parenchyma and lung vasculature is helpful for assessing and grading heart failure. Valvular calcifications may be recognised as a clue for specific valvular disease. Figure 12-1 illustrates the normal chest radiograph, noting normal cardiovascular structures.

CARDIAC MAGNETIC RESONANCE

An advantage of choosing magnetic resonance for cardiac imaging is the free choice in obtaining imaging planes of cardiovascular anatomy in any arbitrary view, since this technique is not hampered by the limited availability of acoustic windows, as with ultrasound. This benefit is especially advantageous when imaging the morphology of the right ventricle (RV), which is excellently delineated by CMR, whereas in echocardiography, the assessment of RV geometry and function is challenging because of the particular crescent shape of the right ventricle wrapping around the left ventricle.[1] Furthermore, the unrestricted field of view of CMR allows superior visualisation of extracardiac and large vessel anatomy.

Single-plane two-dimensional (2-D) or multiple-plane 2-D or three-dimensional (3-D) imaging is possible with CMR. Dynamic functional information can be obtained by synchronising image acquisition to the RR interval of the electrocardiogram, using either prospective triggering or retrospective gating.[2] With prospective triggering, the operator needs to set the expected heart rate before the acquisition and triggering will be performed according to this defined heart rate. With retrospective gating, imaging is performed continuously and the electrocardiogram (ECG) signal is stored additionally. In retrospect, image reconstruction is synchronised to the stored ECG, providing time-resolved imaging in multiple phases of the cardiac cycle, which can be presented in cine mode.

Imaging planes in CMR are usually obtained in the orientation to the axes of the heart, or oriented to the major axes of the body. Therefore, the standard CMR planes of the heart are comparable to the standard cardiac views, well-known and established in other non-invasive imaging modalities such as echocardiography, cardiac CT, X-ray left ventricle angiography and nuclear medicine techniques.

The choice for a specific CMR protocol is mainly determined by the clinical questions that need to be answered. Standardised nomenclature for cross-sectional anatomy has been described,[3] facilitating comparison between different techniques and proper communication between imaging specialists.

Another important issue in clinical CMR imaging is the ability of the patient to collaborate during the examination and to perform breath-holding repeatedly and consistently. If a patient is capable of performing breath-holding, successive imaging planes are obtained with accelerated imaging, with the patient usually performing breath-holding in end expiration, as the anatomical level

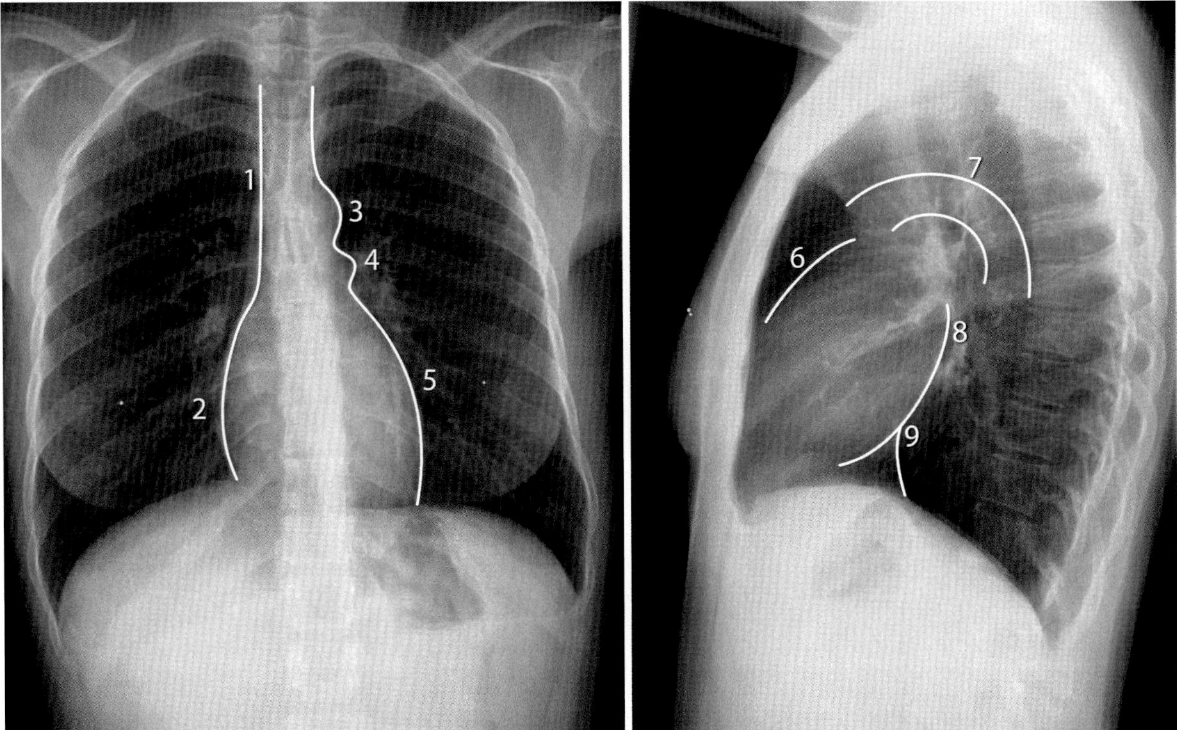

FIGURE 12-1 ■ Normal postero-anterior (left) and lateral (right) chest radiographs. Note normal cardiovascular structures: 1, contour of superior vena cava and other vessels; 2, contour of right atrium; 3, aortic knuckle; 4, left pulmonary artery at hilar level; 5, contour of left ventricle; 6, anterior contour of right ventricle and pulmonary outflow tract; 7, aortic arch; 8, upper posterior contour of left atrium; 9, lower posterior contour of left ventricle. Note relative bulging of left ventricular contour in relationship with inferior vena cava.

may be more reproducible than planes which are examined in inspiration.[4]

CMR techniques for anatomical evaluation include bright-blood and black-blood imaging, which essentially determines the contrast between myocardium and the intracardiac blood pool. For the assessment of left and right ventricular function, fast-gradient echo sequences are usually performed in combination with steady-state free-precession (SSFP) technique (balanced-TFE, True-FISP, Fiesta) for optimal contrast. On these bright-blood images, the blood pool is presented with bright signal, whereas the myocardium is represented dark with low signal. This results in an excellent definition of the left ventricular endocardial and epicardial borders, which is required for accurate image segmentation during cardiac volume and function quantification. Typically, SSFP images should be acquired with slice thickness of 6–8 mm and temporal resolution less than 45 ms to obtain optimal accuracy in ventricular function assessment.[5,6]

Additionally, cardiac morphology can be evaluated by double-inversion black-blood spin-echo sequences with fat suppression, providing gated, static images of the heart with high spatial resolution (optimally, in-plane acquired resolution of less than 2×2 mm^2 and slice thickness of 5–8 mm) in the orientation of the heart or the patient's body axes. Multiple other MRI techniques are available for tissue characterisation (e.g. T2-weighted sequences, delayed gadolinium-based contrast enhancement), extending the capabilities of CMR beyond anatomical and functional evaluation of the cardiovascular system.

Cardiac Axis Imaging Planes

To acquire imaging planes in the direction of the cardiac axes, SSFP scout views are used for planning. If available, free-breathing images obtained during real-time imaging can be used instead. Perpendicular to an anatomical transverse image, displaying the heart's four chambers, an acquisition plane is chosen through the middle of the atrioventricular junction at the level of the mitral valve and running through the apex (Figs. 12-2A, B). This plane is the so-called vertical long-axis (VLA) plane (Fig. 12-2C). On this VLA view, a plane is defined intersecting the apex and the middle of the mitral valve, resulting in the horizontal long-axis (HLA) view (Fig. 12-2D). This HLA view is almost comparable to the four-chamber view; however, often only a part of the left ventricular outflow tract is visualised in this HLA view. On the acquired HLA plane, the short-axis views (Figs. 12-2E, F) covering the entire left ventricle are planned parallel to the ring of the mitral valve and perpendicular to the line intersecting the apex.

For reproducibility and comparison purposes, the true two- and four-chamber views can still be obtained (Figs. 12-2G, H). The two-chamber view is planned perpendicular to the anterior and inferior wall of the left ventricle through the centre of the left ventricular cavity on a mid-ventricular short-axis (SA) image intersecting the apex. On the two-chamber view the apex, anterior and inferior wall of the left ventricle, the mitral valve and left atrium can be evaluated. The four-chamber view is planned also on a mid-ventricular SA image by a plane

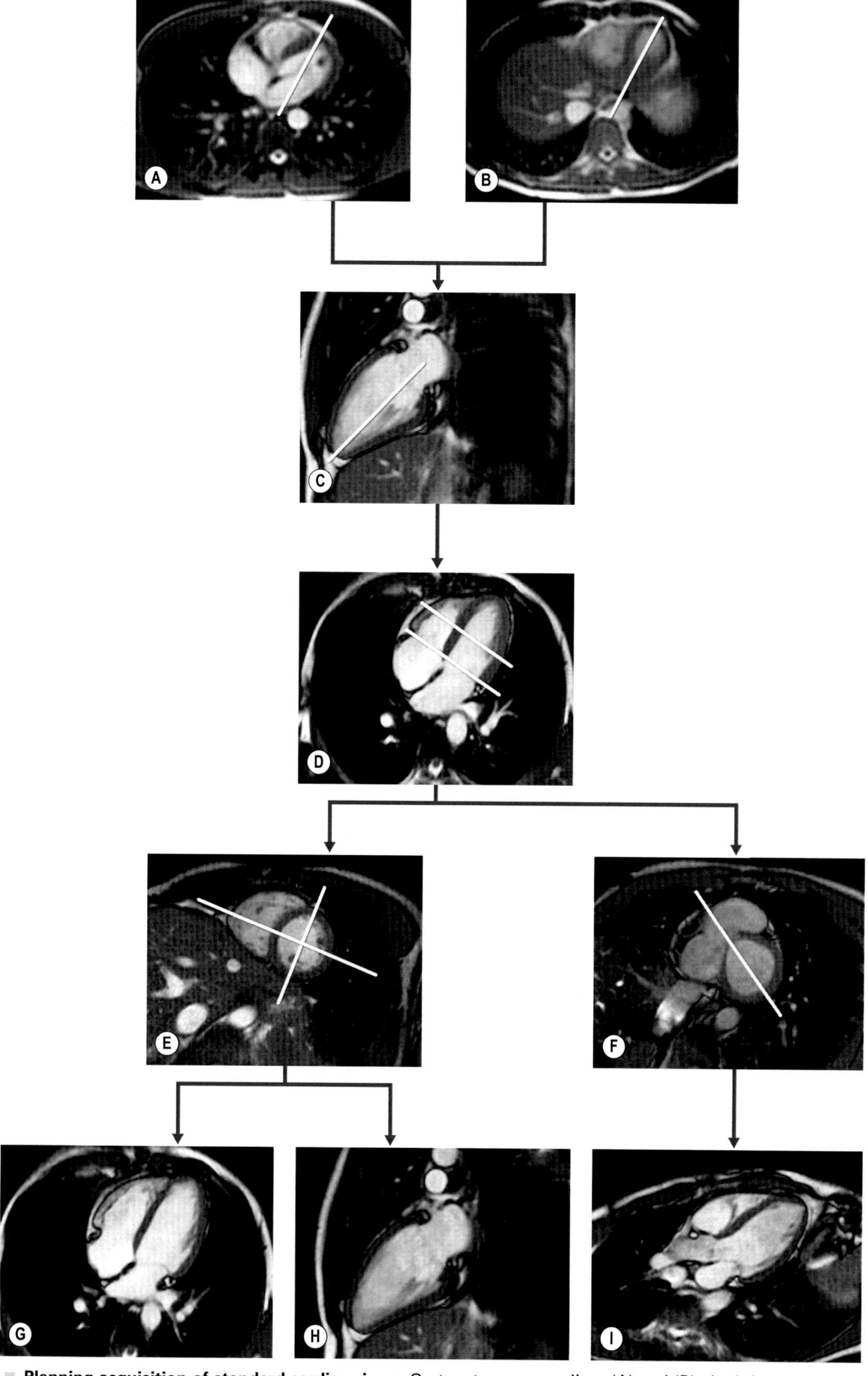

FIGURE 12-2 ■ **Planning acquisition of standard cardiac views.** On two transverse slices (A) and (B), the left ventricular vertical long-axis (VLA) (C) is planned by a plane transecting the mitral valve and the apex. The horizontal long-axis (HLA) (D) is obtained by acquiring a plane transecting the VLA through the mitral valve and apex. A short-axis image can be obtained perpendicular to HLA, at mid-ventricular (E) and basal level (F). The four-chamber (G) of the left ventricle (LV) is obtained as indicated from a plane transecting both LV and the right ventricle. The two-chamber (H) of the LV is acquired perpendicular to the four-chamber. The three-chamber LV (I) is obtained from a plane transecting the LV through the LV outflow tract.

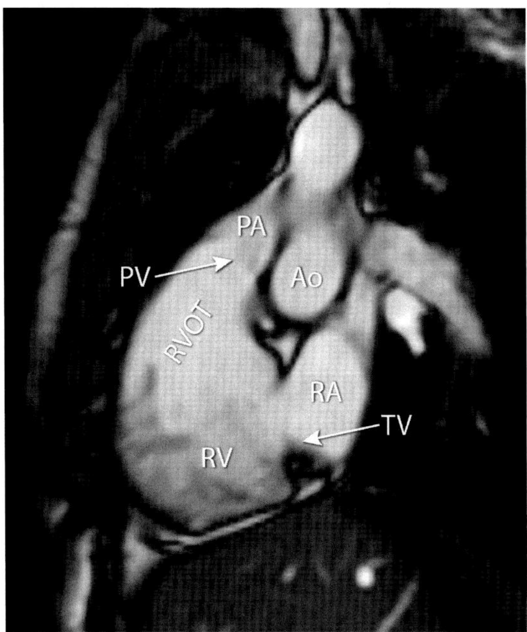

FIGURE 12-3 ■ Bright-blood acquisition of the right ventricle. Right ventricular outflow tract (RVOT), main pulmonary artery (PA) and pulmonary valve (PV). RA, right atrium; RV, right ventricle; TV, tricuspid valve; Ao, aorta.

through the centre of the left ventricular cavity and the acute margin of the right ventricle, also intersecting the apex (Fig. 12-2E). The four-chamber view depicts the interventricular septum, the lateral wall of the left ventricle, the free wall of the right ventricle, left and right atrium as well as the interatrial septum and both the mitral and tricuspid valves.

Routinely, the three-chamber or so-called left ventricular outflow tract (Fig. 12-2I) view is planned on a basal SA plane (Fig. 12-2F). This plane also intersects the apex. The left ventricular outflow tract view depicts the apex, the anteroseptal interventricular wall, the left ventricular outflow tract, the inferolateral wall, as the aortic and mitral valve, respectively.

The standard SSFP cine CMR protocol for assessing left ventricular function should include the two-, four- and three-chamber views in combination with SA images covering the entire left ventricle, resulting in images covering all described 17 left ventricular segments in two directions.[3]

Additionally, the right ventricular outflow tract can be obtained (Fig. 12-3). This view can be planned on a coronal image, depicting the outflow tract of the right ventricle. Alternatively, an optimised view of the right ventricular outflow tract view can be obtained from a plane outlining the tricuspid valve plane and the outflow tract. On this plane the outflow tract, pulmonary valve, tricuspid valve and the basal (diaphragmatic) part of the right ventricular wall are all visualised.

Body Axes Imaging Planes

For the evaluation of cardiac morphology, the pericardium, the great thoracic vessels and (para-) cardiac masses, imaging planes oriented to the main body axes are obtained. Also, the transverse (or axial), coronal (frontal) and sagittal planes are well known to clinicians, as these anatomical orientations are similar to clinical (cardiac) CT. Black- and bright-blood sequence approaches (Fig. 12-4) can be used in optimally adjusted planes to answer specific clinical questions. Black-blood images provide only static information in a single phase and are not suitable for quantification of left or right ventricular dimensions. For this analysis, SSFP multiphase images with appropriate temporal resolution are necessary.

Transversely oriented planes (Fig. 12-5) are especially useful for the evaluation of thoracic vascular structures as the ascending and descending thoracic aorta, the superior and inferior vena cava, the pulmonary trunk and right and left pulmonary artery. The right and left pulmonary veins entering the left atrium are also well depicted. Images in transverse orientation through the heart allow the evaluation of morphology of the ventricles and atria. Also the right ventricular free wall, the right ventricular outflow tract, the pericardium and mediastinum are well depicted. It has been suggested that right ventricular volume and function quantification by planimetry can be performed more accurately on transversely oriented images instead of SA images.[7]

Coronal or frontal anatomical views can be instructive for analysing the connection between the heart and the great vessels. An advantage of the frontal view is the similarity to the well-known anatomy from chest radiography. On sagittal images, the right ventricular outflow tract in relation to the pulmonary valve is well outlined and the connection of the right atrium with the superior and inferior vena cava can be studied.

Normal Anatomy on CMR Images

CMR images present distinct anatomical features of both atria and ventricles. For evaluating anatomy, either cardiac axes (Fig. 12-6) or body axes imaging planes (Figs. 12-4 and 12-5) can be chosen. The pericardial sac encloses the heart and the roots of the great vessels. The pericardial cavity is outlined by the parietal and visceral layer of the inner pericardium. Normal pericardium has a longer T1 than fat tissue, and therefore presents with low signal intensity on T1-weighted MR images, and can be well visualised due to the surrounding epicardial and pericardial fat. Normally, the thickness of the pericardium measures less than 4 mm on CMR images.

In normal cardiac anatomy, the right atrium can be recognised by identifying the corresponding broad-based triangular appendage. At the base, the tricuspid valve, positioned between the right atrium and the right ventricle, is located closer to the apex compared to the mitral valve.

The right atrium receives venous blood from the superior and inferior vena cava, and the coronary sinus. The coronary sinus enters the right atrium in the posterior atrioventricular groove. The appendage of the morphological left atrium has a narrow attachment to the atrium and is more tubular shaped. Characteristically, the left atrium receives in total four pulmonary veins, two on

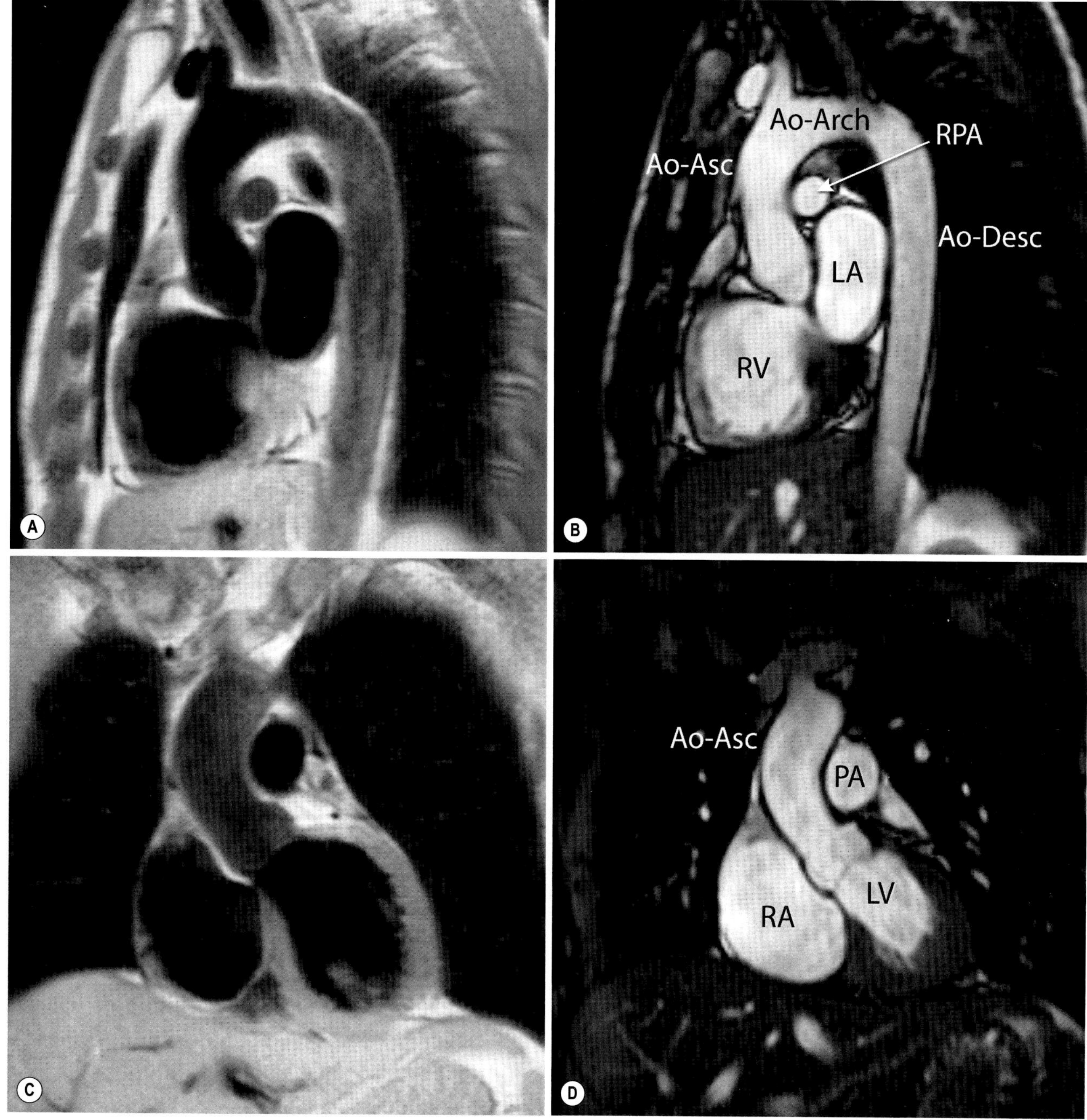

FIGURE 12-4 ■ **Normal cardiac anatomy on black-blood and bright-blood acquisitions, in sagittal (A, B) and coronal (C, D) views.** Ao-Asc, ascending aorta; Ao-Arch, aortic arch; Ao-Desc, descending aorta; RA, right atrium; LA, left atrium; RV, right ventricle; LV, left ventricle; PA, pulmonary artery; RPA, right pulmonary artery.

either side, although several variations of this occur. To date, imaging the venous anatomy of the heart is becoming more relevant. For example, during pre-ablation work-up for supraventricular arrhythmias the clinician needs to be informed about the exact anatomy of the left atrial morphology and number of the pulmonary ostia, as the left atrium and pulmonary veins are used to guide the interventional procedure.[8,9] The interatrial septum separates the two atria. As part of the interatrial septum, the fossa ovalis is very thin and can hardly be depicted on CMR images due to the limited spatial acquisition resolution.

The right ventricle is normally triangular in shape and anteriorly located relative to the left ventricle, directly behind the sternum. Morphologically, the right ventricle has typical features that can be depicted on CMR images. The right ventricle shows a muscular moderator band (Fig. 12-7), carrying branches of the conducting system. Furthermore, the right ventricle contains a muscular outflow tract (infundibulum or conus arteriosus) and

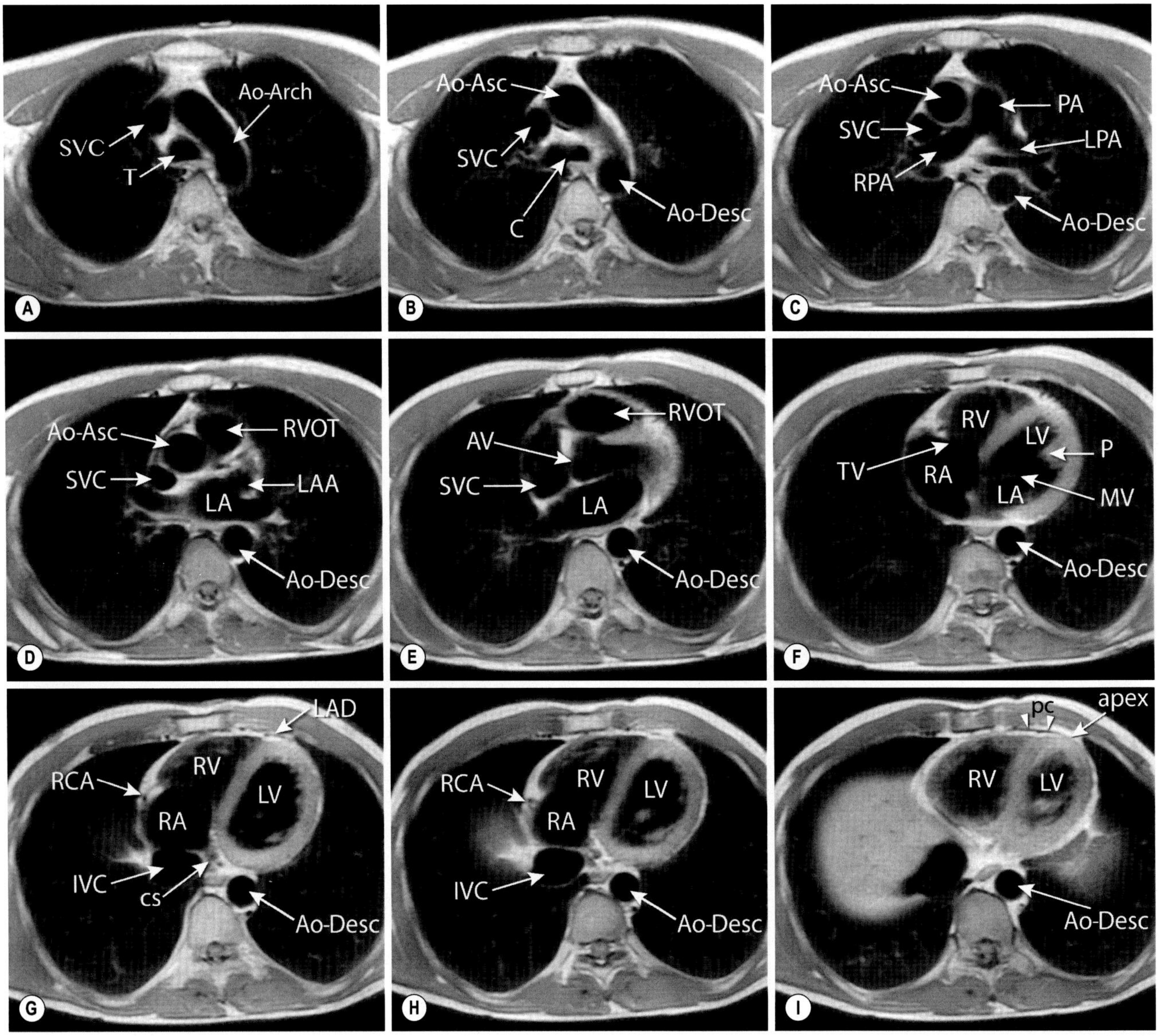

FIGURE 12-5 ■ **Normal cardiac anatomy on transverse black-blood acquisitions.** Ao-Asc, ascending aorta; Ao-Arch, aortic arch; Ao-Desc, descending aorta; RA, right atrium; LA, left atrium; RV, right ventricle; LV, left ventricle; RVOT, right ventricular outflow tract; ; PA, main pulmonary artery; RPA, right pulmonary artery; LPA, left pulmonary artery; LAA, left atrial appendage; TV, tricuspid valve; MV, mitral valve; P, papillary muscle; LAD, left anterior descending coronary artery; cs, coronary sinus; pc, pericardium; T, trachea; C, carina; IVC, inferior vena cava; SVC, superior vena cava.

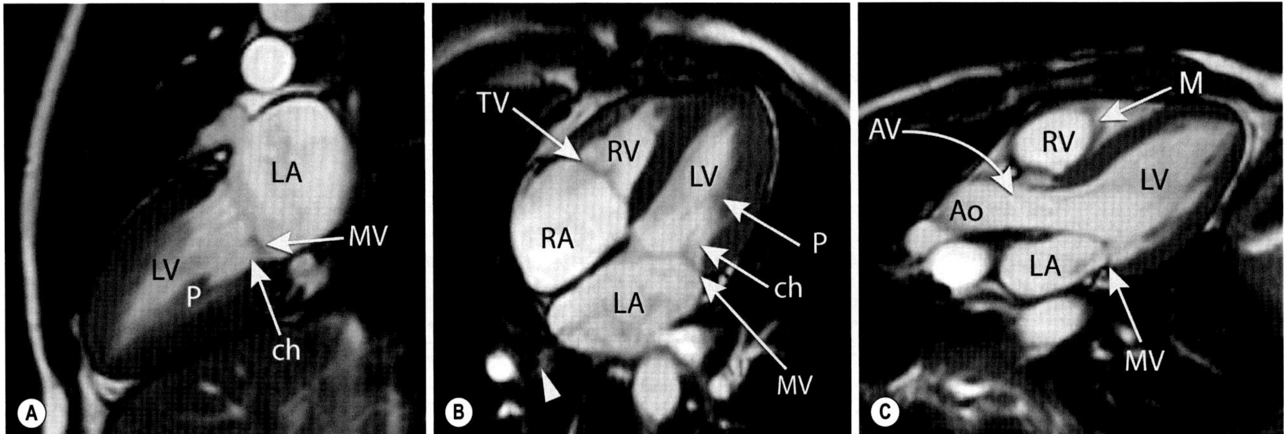

FIGURE 12-6 ■ **Normal cardiac anatomy on bright-blood two-, four- and three-chamber views.** RA, right atrium; LA, left atrium; RV, right ventricle; LV, left ventricle; P, papillary muscle; TV, tricuspid valve; MV, mitral valve; AV, aortic valve; Ao, aorta; M, moderator band; ch, chordae tendineae.

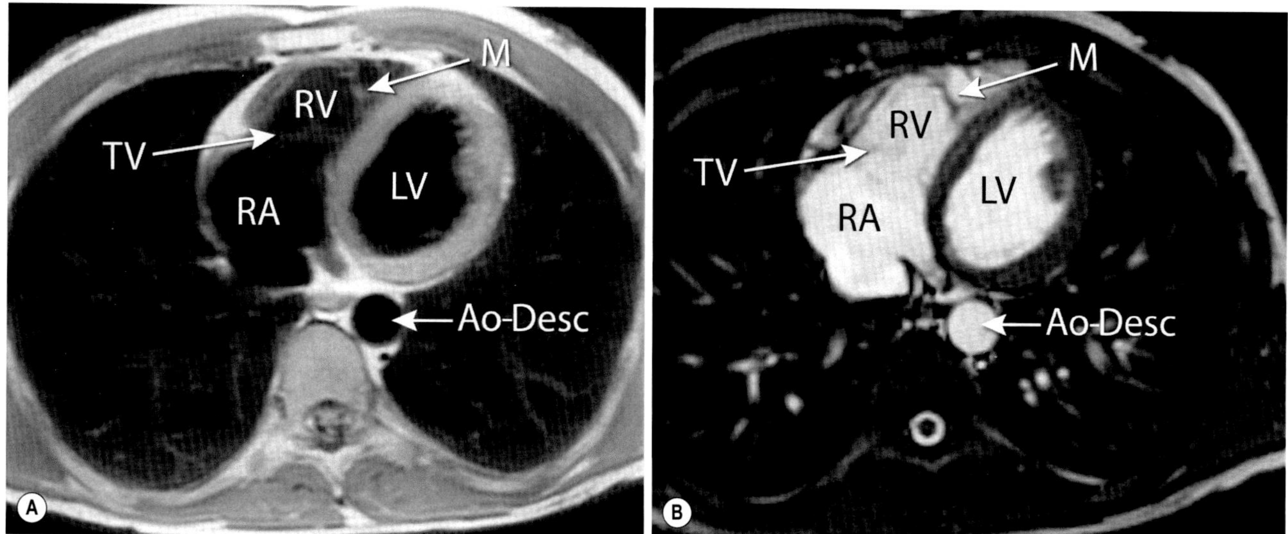

FIGURE 12-7 Transverse black-blood (A) and bright-blood (B) acquisition illustrating the moderator band in the right ventricle. RA, right atrium; RV, right ventricle; LV, left ventricle; TV, tricuspid valve; M, moderator band; Ao-Desc, descending aorta.

typically, the right ventricle wall is more trabeculated than the left. In normal anatomy, the left ventricle is positioned posteriorly and to the left. The septum is smooth with no trabeculae and the left ventricular outflow tract lacks a muscular part. The interventricular septum consists of a muscular and a membranous part. In particular, the membranous part is very thin and is therefore sometimes not depicted on CMR images. It is important to recognise these normal anatomical features of atrial and ventricular morphology, because the position of the atria and ventricles may be inversed in complex congenital heart disease.

At the outlet of each of the heart's four chambers, one-way valves that ensure blood flow in the proper direction are positioned. The blood flow through the atria into the ventricles is regulated by the atrioventricular valves (i.e. the tricuspid valve is related to the morphological right ventricle and the mitral valve is related to the morphological left ventricle). The pulmonary valve connects the outflow tract of the right ventricle to the pulmonary trunk, and the aortic valve connects the left ventricular outflow tract to the thoracic aorta. The normal tricuspid valve consists of three cusps, whereas the mitral valve consists of two cusps. Both the normal pulmonary and the aortic valve (Fig. 12-8) consist of three cusps. Opening of the atrioventricular valves is predominantly determined by pressure differences between the atria and ventricles. These differences are the result of the isovolumetric relaxation of the ventricles during diastole. Furthermore, the motion of the valves is regulated by papillary muscles, which originate from the inferolateral and anterolateral left ventricular myocardial wall and are connected to the valve leaflets by chordae tendineae. During contraction of the ventricle the papillary muscles also contract, pulling on the chordae tendineae, closing the valves and preventing blood flow from the ventricles into the atria (i.e. regurgitation). Normally, in the right ventricle three small papillary muscles can be depicted: the anterior, and posterior and septal papillary muscle. The left ventricle reveals two larger papillary muscles: the anterior and posterior papillary muscle.

Cine SSFP long-axis and SA images, as well as transverse images, are all well suited for depicting morphology and function of the valvular apparatus. The valve leaflets can be depicted if spatial resolution is adequate. Dedicated acquisitions of specific valvular planes are used to image the valve area, which is especially useful when studying aortic valve stenosis or incompetence. Both SSFP and fast gradient-echo sequences are used for valvular imaging. Papillary muscles are well visualised on both cine bright- and black-blood sequences. Chordae tendineae, on the other hand, are difficult to visualise on CMR due to the limited spatial resolution (Fig. 12-6).

COMPUTED TOMOGRAPHY IMAGING TECHNIQUES

With the introduction of 64- or more slice CT imaging devices, CT has been accepted as a diagnostic imaging tool for the evaluation of patients with suspected coronary artery disease and for several other cardiac indications. This includes evaluation of cardiac structures and function in adult congenital heart disease, evaluation of ventricular morphology, left and right systolic function, the pericardium and evaluation of intra- and extracardiac structures such as valves, masses and pulmonary veins.[10]

Cardiac CT requires intravenous injection of iodinated contrast agent, with the exception of CT calcium scoring that requires plain cardiac CT. Various cardiac CT imaging techniques are applied in clinical practice, depending on the CT device used, on the clinical question that must be answered and on patient-related parameters. Imaging can be performed with helical acquisition, with step-and-shoot 'sequential' acquisition or with wide-volume acquisition. With helical and with step-and-shoot acquisition, multiple heart beats are needed for cardiac imaging that requires a breath-hold of approximately

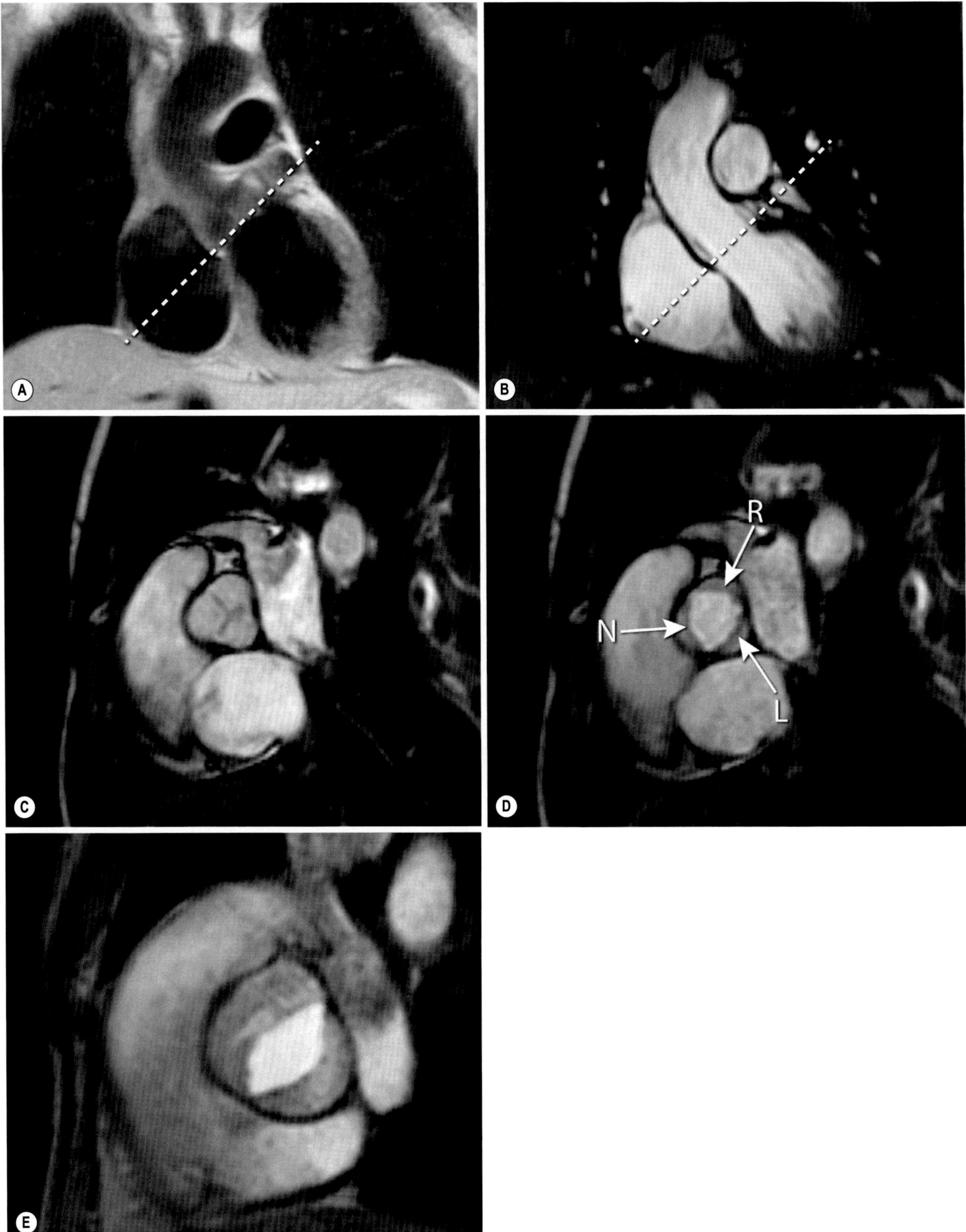

FIGURE 12-8 ■ **A segmented gradient-echo acquisition of the aortic valve.** In (A, B), the planning of the acquisition plane is presented in black-blood coronal view of the aorta during end diastole (A) and bright-blood at peak systole (B). In (C), a closed normal valve at end diastole and in (D), an opened normal valve with three cusps at peak systole is presented (L, left coronary cusp; R, right coronary cusp; N, non-coronary cusp). In (E), a bicuspid aortic valve is presented, with a fused non-coronary and right coronary cusp.

10 s. Images are reconstructed with a slice thickness down to 0.5 mm, with a temporal resolution down to 83 ms. Also, fast dual source helical techniques and wide-volume detectors that cover the whole heart allow for imaging of the heart within a single heart beat at radiation doses below 5 mSv.[11,12]

ECG recording is central in all cardiac CT techniques as to avoid motion artefacts. Patients are generally prepared with beta-blockers to slow down the heart rate below 65 beats per minute for optimal image quality. If only anatomical/morphological information is required, such as in coronary artery imaging, the acquisition can be prospectively triggered. This allows imaging during a predefined cardiac rest phase with least motion, which is at mid-diastole at approximately 75% of the cardiac -R cycle. In patients with high heart rates that are susceptible to motion artefacts, image acquisition may be performed with a wider acquisition interval during the cardiac cycle, allowing for selection and reconstruction of multiple cardiac phases for optimal motion-free imaging of each coronary artery.[13]

The current prospective triggering acquisition techniques have effectively reduced patient exposure to radiation.[14] With the older retrospective gating techniques, several consecutive cardiac cycles are continuously scanned with simultaneous recording of the ECG. This allows any cardiac phase to be reconstructed, but at the expense of a relatively high radiation dose in the range of 12–21 mSv. The technique may be used for combined imaging of the coronary arteries and ventricular function (ejection fraction). Radiation dose for functional analysis may be reduced by ECG-dose modulation techniques if coronary artery information is also needed, or by low-dose CT data acquisition throughout the cardiac cycle if only functional information is required.[13]

Cardiac CT imaging is a three-dimensional volume technique, which implies that any imaging plane can be reconstructed. Therefore, the use of 'standard views' is less critical than with projection invasive coronary angiography or echocardiography, or than with image-stack CMR. CT investigations are evaluated by reviewing the appropriate (multiplanar) image reconstructions that depend on the topic of interest and the clinical question that must be answered.

CT Imaging of Ventricles and Myocardial Tissue

The myocardial tissue can be visualised in any plane. The right ventricle can be best evaluated by scrolling through the transverse images (Fig. 12-9). Two-, three- and four-chamber and especially short-axis views are helpful for visualising the left ventricle and left ventricular myocardium (Fig. 12-10). The short-axis views can be used for 17-segment evaluation of the left ventricular myocardium,[3] and enable good correlation with echocardiography, CMR and nuclear medicine techniques.

Coronary Arteries by CT

Because of the good spatial and temporal resolution, the main coronary arteries and large side branches can be

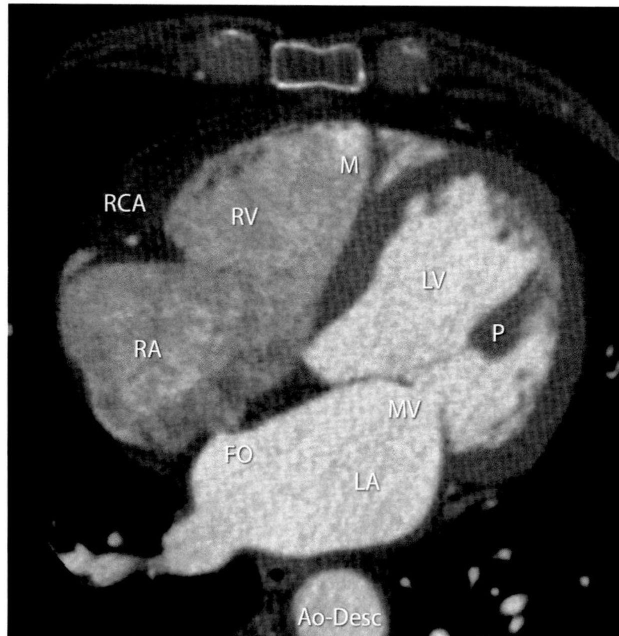

FIGURE 12-9 ■ **Right ventricle.** Transverse reconstruction showing the right ventricle (RV). Ao-Desc, descending aorta; FO, fossa ovalis; LA, left atrium; LV, left ventricle; M, moderator band; MV, mitral valve; RA, right atrium; RCA, right coronary artery; P, papillary muscle.

well visualised by coronary CT angiography. CT allows for evaluation of the dominance of coronary circulation. The location of origins and courses of the coronary arteries can be visualised for identifying coronary anatomical anomalies. CT allows evaluation of coronary lumen and vessel wall for assessing coronary artery stenoses.[10]

Dominance of the coronary arteries refers to the artery that gives rise to the posterior descending artery. The right coronary artery is dominant in approximately 80% of the population and the left circumflex artery in approximately 10%. The circulation is balanced (co-dominant) in the remaining population. Evaluating the dominancy of the coronary arteries prevents confusion with branch occlusion, as in right dominant circulation a relatively small circumflex artery can be expected and in left dominant circulation a small right coronary artery is expected (Fig. 12-11). Figure 12-12 shows normal coronary anatomy in transverse orientation with proximal, middle and distal segments of coronary arteries. Volume-rendered images show coronary anatomy in Fig. 12-13. The right coronary artery arises from the right sinus of Valsalva, and courses in the right atrioventricular groove (between the right atrium and right ventricle). Its side branches are usually visualised by scrolling through the transverse image stack: the conus branch coursing along the right ventricular outflow tract, the atrioventricular branch coursing posteriorly to the sinus node (at the junction of the superior vena cava and right atrium), the acute marginal/right ventricular branches along the right ventricular free wall (Fig. 12-11A), the posterior descending branch in the posterior interventricular groove and a posterolateral branch that continues in the left atrioventricular groove (Figs. 12-11, 12-12 and 12-13).

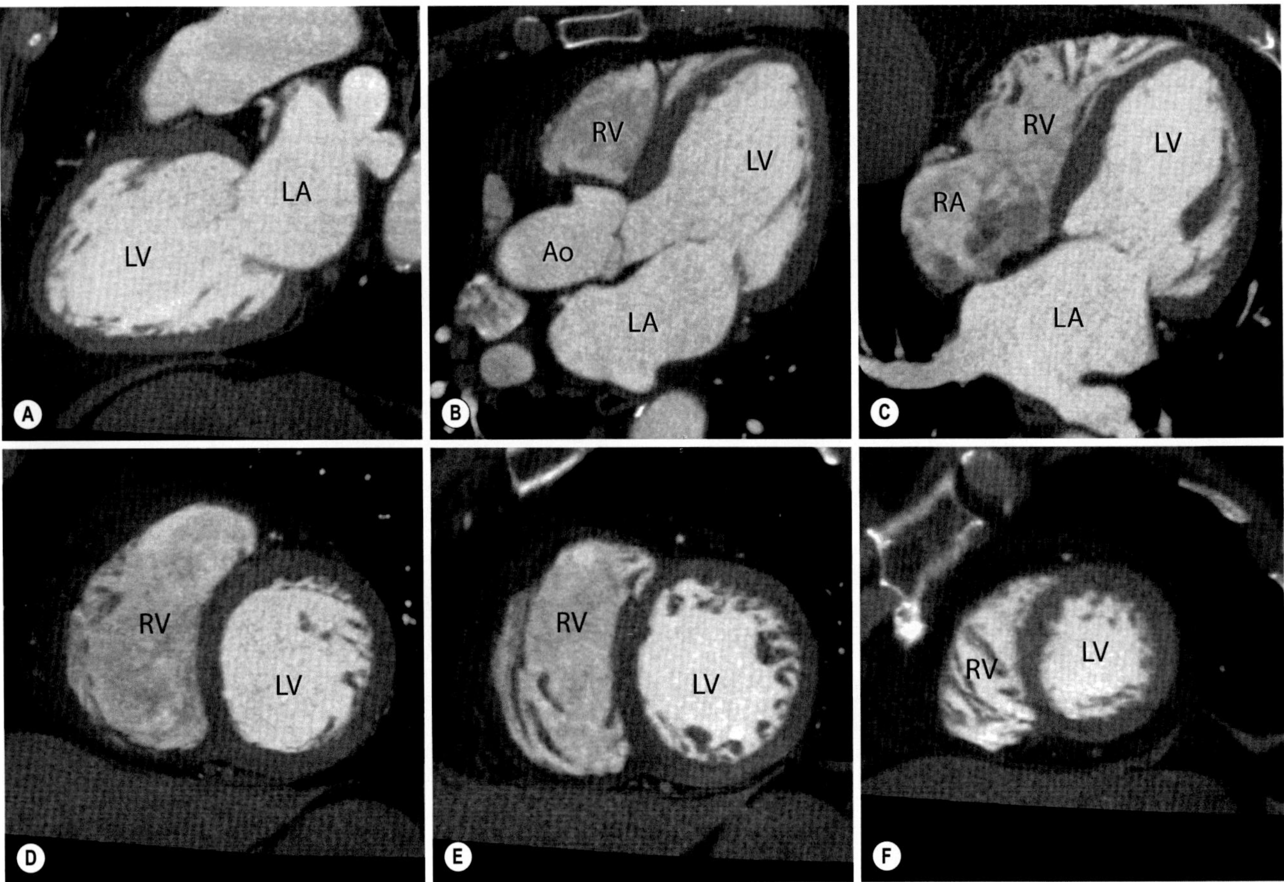

FIGURE 12-10 ■ **Left ventricular orientation.** Longitudinal two-chamber (A), three-chamber (B), and four-chamber (C) reconstructions. Left ventricular short-axis reconstructions at the base (D), mid ventricular (E) and apical level (F). Ao, aorta; LA, left atrium; RA, right atrium; LV, left ventricle; RV, right ventricle.

The left main coronary artery arises from the left sinus of Valsalva (Figs. 12-12 and 12-13). It divides into the left anterior descending artery that runs in the anterior interventricular groove (between the left and right ventricle) and in the circumflex artery that runs in the left atrioventricular groove (Fig. 12-12). In about one-third of the population, an intermediate artery that arises from the left main artery and that courses along the left ventricular wall between the left anterior descending and circumflex artery is present. The left main coronary artery may be absent in 1% of the population. In these cases, the left anterior descending and circumflex arteries arise from a common origin or separately from the left sinus of Valsalva (Fig. 12-14). The left anterior descending artery gives rise to septal branches that run straight down into the interventricular septum, and to (usually one to three) diagonal branches that course along the anterolateral left ventricular wall (Figs. 12-11 and 12-12). The circumflex artery gives rise to (usually one to three) obtuse marginal branches supplying the lateral free wall of the left ventricle (Figs. 12-11 and 12-12). In approximately one-third of the population, the sinus node branch arises from the left circumflex artery instead of the right coronary artery. Also, a left atrial circumflex branch that supplies part of the left atrium may be observed.

The coronary arteries and their major side branches can be classified by location by segment numbers or segment names, for locating coronary artery stenosis. Since several numeric classification systems are used in clinical and research practice, using numbers may be confusing. Therefore, it may be more practical to use the segment names (Fig. 12-12).[15]

Evaluation of the coronary arteries is done on original standard transverse views or orthogonal reconstructions as these images contain all the information without risk of reconstruction artefacts. (Curved) multiplanar and surface rendering reconstruction can be additionally helpful for overview and fast reading by projecting larger parts of the coronary arteries within single images (Fig. 12-15). For comparison with CT, Figs. 12-16 and 12-17 show views of the coronary anatomy obtained with invasive angiography. Invasive angiography is still considered the gold standard for evaluation of the coronary anatomy. It has a high temporal and spatial resolution and provides lumen evaluation that is not limited by the presence of calcium. The main disadvantage of invasive angiography is its invasive fashion, although at low risk of complications.

Valves

Echocardiography and CMR are the preferred imaging techniques for evaluating the cardiac valves, as these techniques allow for advanced functional imaging with

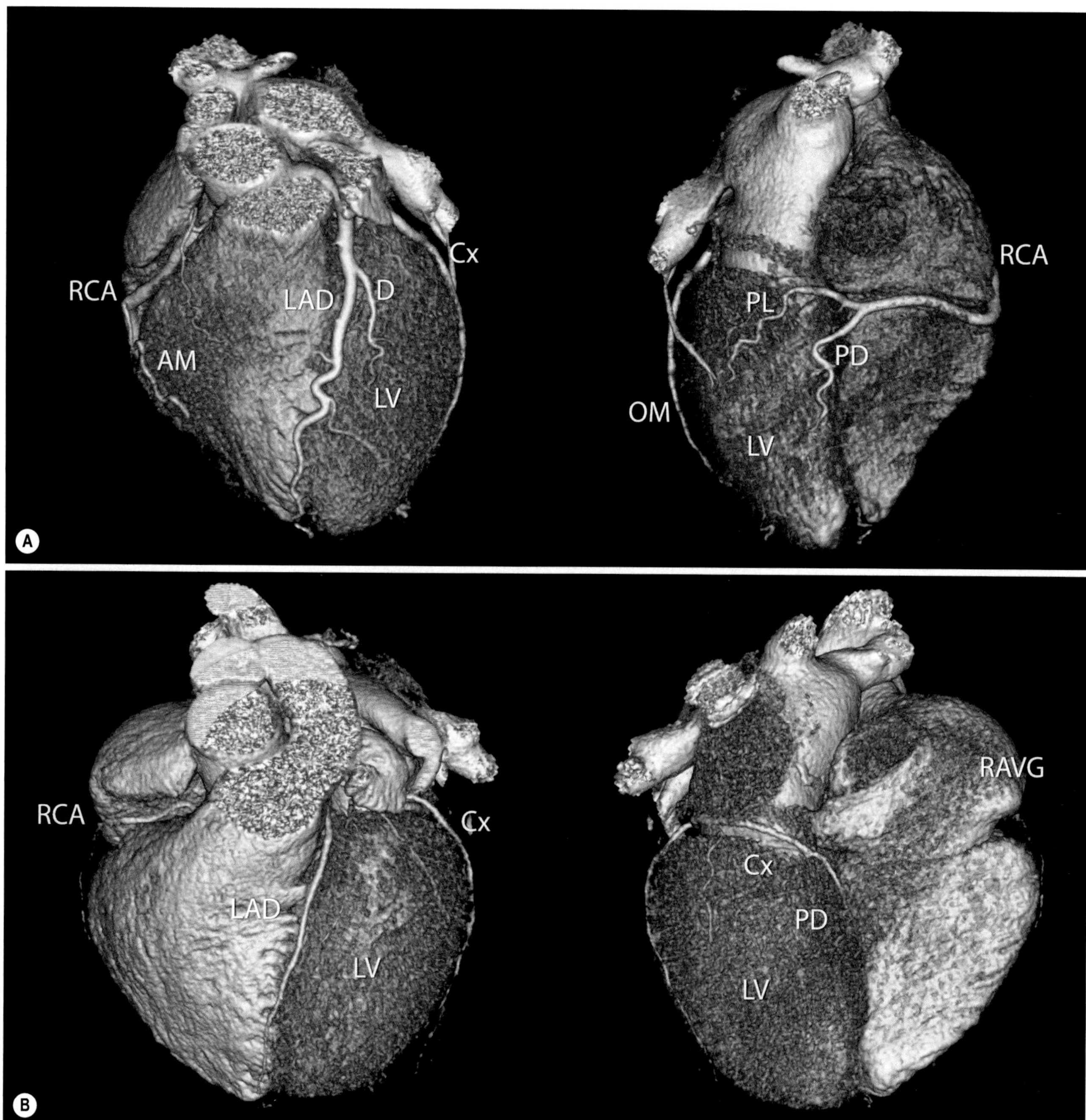

FIGURE 12-11 ■ **Coronary dominance.** Three-dimensional volume-rendered images with frontal view and view from below showing right dominant coronary artery circulation (A) and left dominant coronary artery circulation (B). In right dominant coronary artery circulation, the posterior descending artery (PD) arises from the right coronary artery (RCA). In left dominant coronary artery circulation, the PD arises from the circumflex artery (Cx) (B). Note the short RCA with empty right atrioventricular groove (RAVG) which is normal in left dominant coronary artery circulation, and should not be confused with RCA occlusion. Side branches visualised: AM, acute marginal branch; D, diagonal branch; OM, obtuse marginal branch; PL, posterolateral branch; LV, left ventricle.

superior temporal resolution, and without the use of ionising radiation. However, CT allows detailed information on aortic and mitral valve morphology and can provide functional information as well.[16] The pulmonary and tricuspid valve can also be visualised but have thinner cusps and are therefore more difficult to appreciate on CT.[17,18] For each valve, multiphase cine views may be helpful for evaluation.[17]

The normal aortic valve is composed of a fibrous annulus, three cusps (right coronary cusp, left coronary cusp, posterior or non-coronary cusp) and three commissures that separate the cusps. The dilatations in the aorta at each cusp are the sinuses of Valsalva. The aortic cusps open at systole and close at diastole with a small area of overlap. The normal aortic valve area at opening is 3.0–4.0 cm^2.[16] The aortic valve is well

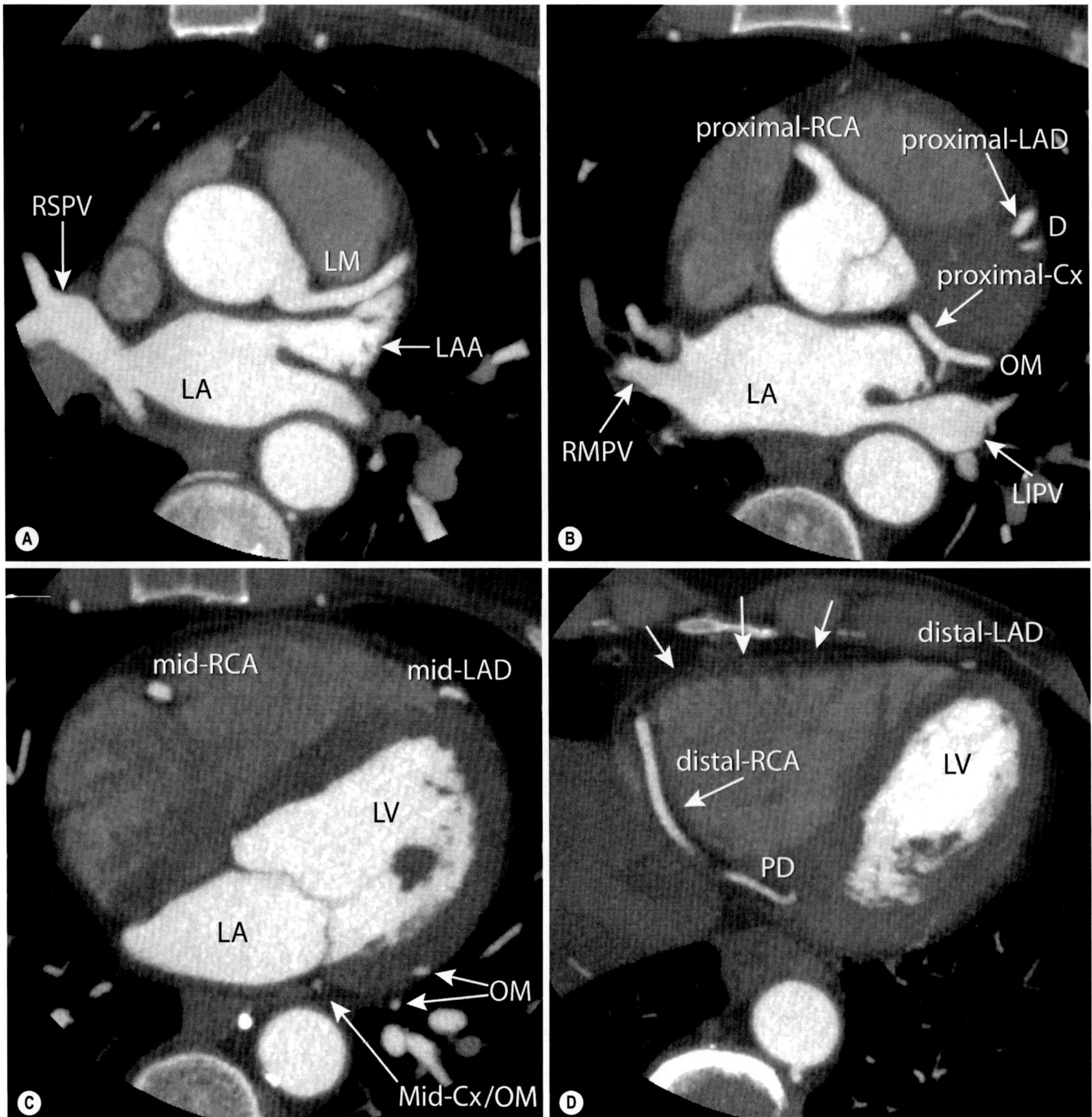

FIGURE 12-12 ■ **Coronary anatomy; segments.** Transverse reconstructions showing (A) the left main coronary artery (LM); (B) proximal right coronary artery (RCA), proximal left anterior descending artery (LAD) with diagonal side branch (D), and proximal circumflex artery (Cx) with obtuse marginal branch (OM); (C) mid-LAD, mid-RCA and mid-Cx/OM; (D) distal-RCA and posterior descending branch (PD), distal-LAD. Pericardium is visualised as a thin line (arrows in D). Visualised pulmonary veins: LIPV, left inferior pulmonary vein; RMPV, right middle pulmonary vein; RSPV, right superior pulmonary vein. LA, left atrium; LAA, left atrium appendage; LV, left ventricle.

visualised on coronal view and with MPR on coronal three-chamber view and parallel at the valvular plane itself (Fig. 12-18). A bicuspid aortic valve is present in 1–2% of the population (Fig. 12-19) and often results in complications such as aortic stenosis and/or regurgitation.[19]

The mitral valve is composed of a saddle-shaped fibrous annulus, two leaflets (a semicircular anterior leaflet and a rectangular posterior leaflet), two commissures, two papillary muscles (anterolateral and posteromedial) and chordae tendineae, which are fibrous tendons that arise from the papillary muscles and insert on the free edges of the leaflets.[16] The normal mitral valve area during opening in diastole is 4.0–5.0 cm^2. The mitral valve leaflets close with some overlap to prevent regurgitation.[16] The mitral valve can be visualised on

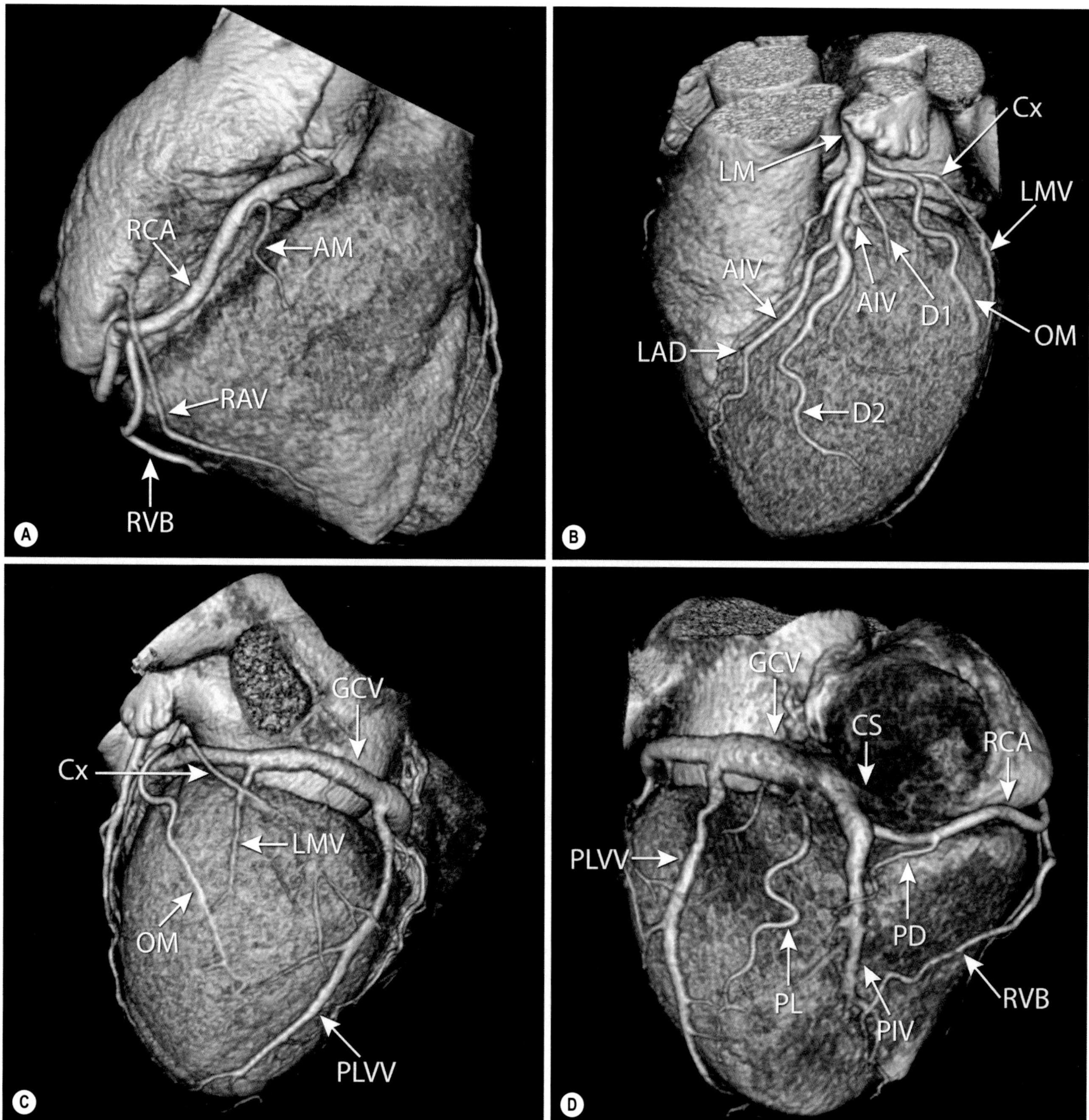

FIGURE 12-13 ■ **Coronary arteries and cardiac veins.** Volume-rendered reconstructions for coronary artery and cardiac venous anatomy. Coronary arteries and side branches: AM, acute marginal branch of RCA (A); Cx, circumflex artery (B, C); D1 and D2, first and second diagonal branch (B); LAD, left anterior descending artery (B); LM, left main coronary artery (B); OM, obtuse marginal branch (B, C); PD, posterior descending branch (D); PL, posterolateral branch from RCA (D); RCA, right coronary artery (A, D); RVB, right ventricle branch (running to distal part of posterior interventricular groove, A, D). Cardiac veins: AIV, anterior interventricular vein (B); CS, Coronary sinus (D); GCV, great cardiac vein (C, D); LMV, left marginal vein (C); PIV, posterior interventricular vein (D); PLVV, posterior left ventricular vein (C, D); RAV, right atrial vein draining directly into right atrium (A).

two-, three- and four-chamber and on short-axis MPR (Fig. 12-20).

The pulmonary valve contains a fibrous annulus, three cusps and three commissures separating the cusps. Optimum imaging views are the sagittal plane showing the right ventricular outflow tract and pulmonary valve, and with MPR at the valvular plane itself (Fig. 12-21). If the pulmonary cusps are easily visible, they are likely to be thickened.[17]

The tricuspid valve has three cusps (anterior, superior, inferior). The tricuspid valve is usually moderately visualised due to the thin cusps; its optimal views are transverse or four-chamber long- and short-axis views[17] (Fig. 12-22).

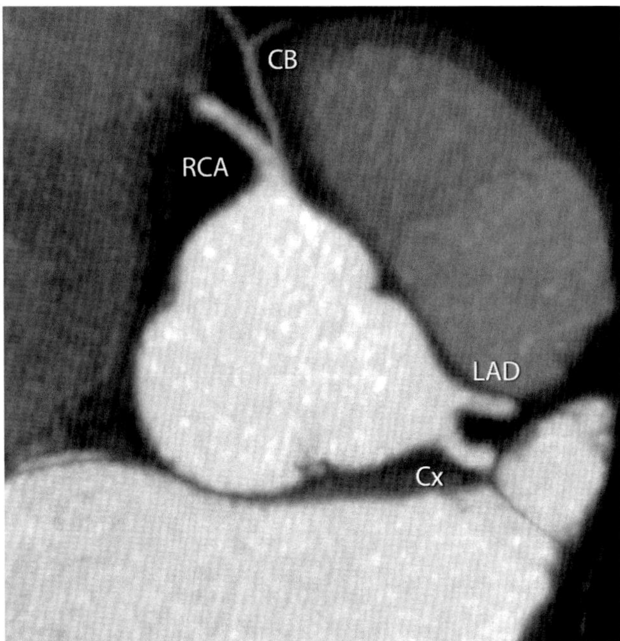

FIGURE 12-14 ■ **Absent left main.** Double oblique orientation parallel to the aortic root showing separate coronary ostia of left anterior descending artery (LAD) and circumflex artery (Cx). The left main artery is absent. Right coronary artery (RCA) with conus branch (CB).

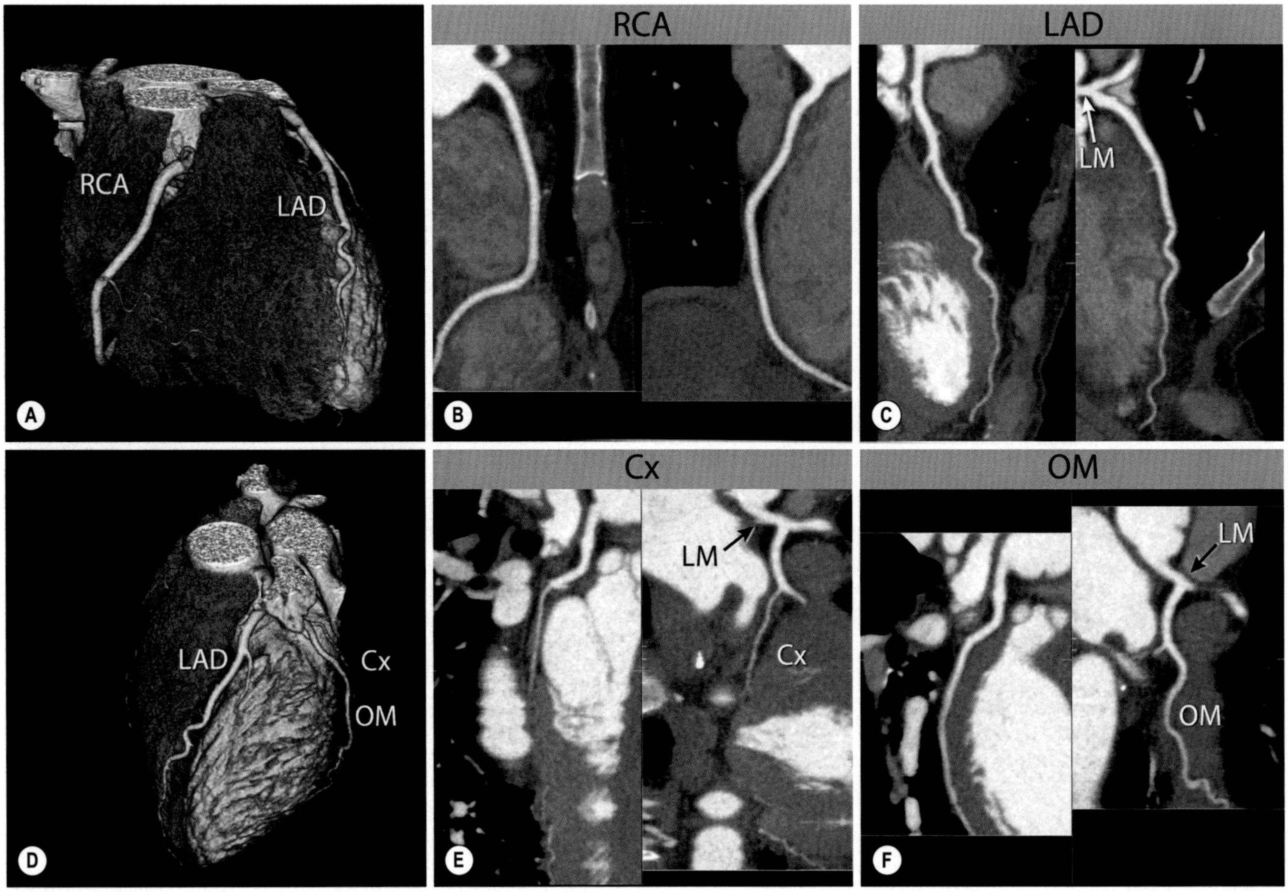

FIGURE 12-15 ■ **Full-length display of coronary arteries.** Three-dimensional volume-rendered reconstructions in right anterior oblique (A) and left anterior oblique (D) view and curved multiplanar reconstructions (B, C, E, F) showing each coronary artery in two longitudinal perpendicular directions: the right coronary artery (RCA, in B), left anterior descending coronary artery (LAD, in C), circumflex artery (Cx, in E) and obtuse marginal branch (OM, in F). Note that the OM is much larger than the Cx (E) itself, which is usually the case. LM, Left main.

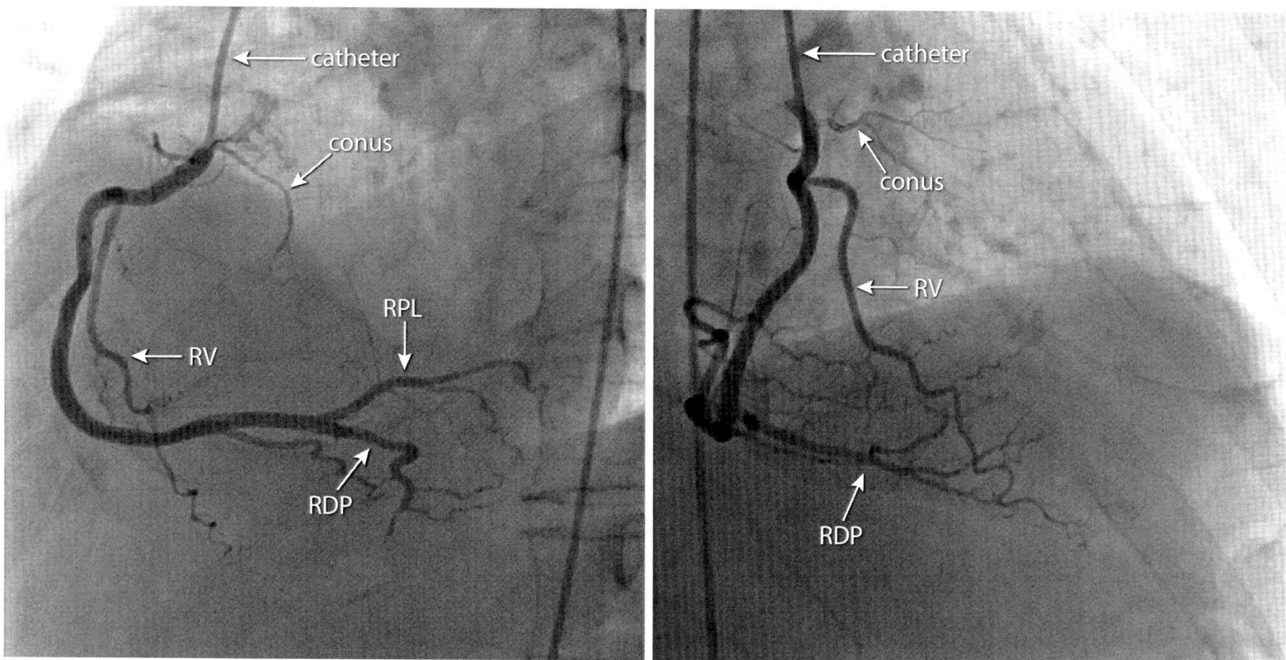

FIGURE 12-16 ■ **Invasive coronary angiography of the right coronary artery (RCA) in two different directions (left panel, left anterior oblique 45°; right panel, right anterior oblique 35°).** RV, right ventricular branch; RDP, right posterior descending branch; RPL, right posterolateral branch; conus, conus branch.

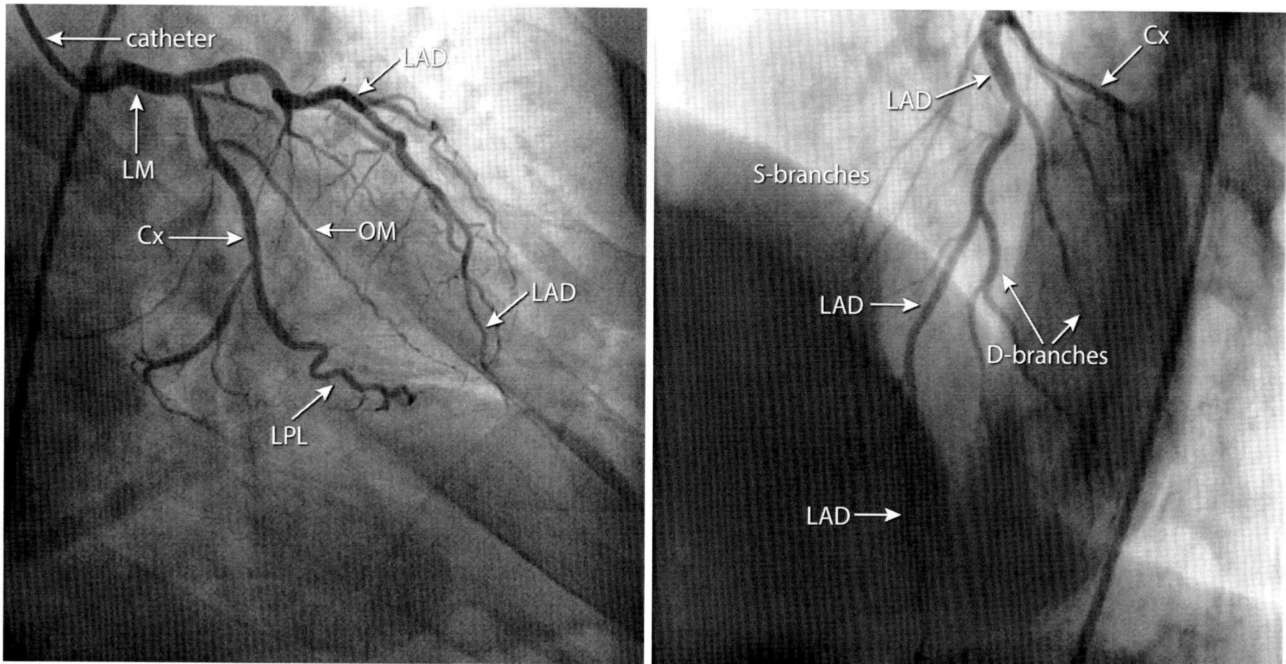

FIGURE 12-17 ■ **Invasive coronary angiography of the left coronary artery in two different directions (left panel, right anterior oblique 30°, 25° caudal angulation; right panel, left anterior oblique 50°, 25° cranial angulation).** LM, left main coronary artery; LAD, left anterior descending coronary artery; Cx, circumflex coronary artery; OM, obtuse marginal branch; LPL, left posterolateral branch, S-branches, septal branches; D-branches, diagonal branches.

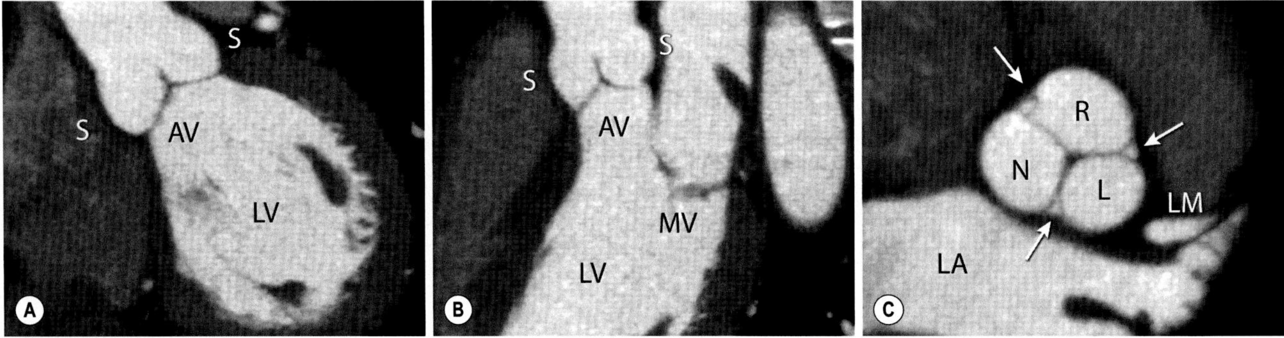

FIGURE 12-18 ■ **Aortic valve.** Multiplanar reconstructions at mid-diastole showing the closed aortic valve (AV) in coronal view (A), three-chamber view (B) and short-axis parallel to the aortic valve (C). S, sinus of Valsalva; MV, mitral valve; LV, left ventricle; LA, left atrium. Arrows in (C) point at the commissures.

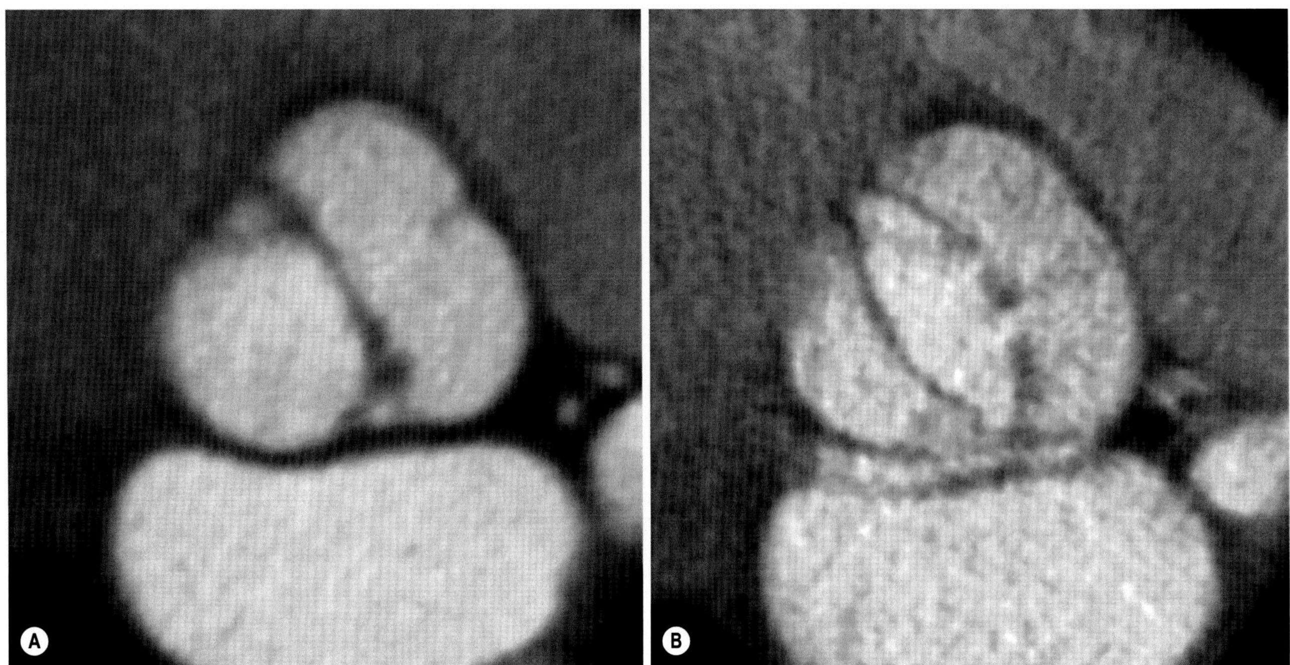

FIGURE 12-19 ■ **Bicuspid aortic valve.** 'Short-axis' double oblique transverse images parallel to the aortic valve, showing bicuspid aortic valve at diastole (A, closed) and at systole (B, slit-like opening due to fusion of left and right coronary cusp). Note the difference in noise level between the images, caused by ECG-dose modulation with full dose at diastole (during the cardiac rest phase for sharp imaging of the coronary arteries), and lower radiation dose at systole to save radiation dose.

Pulmonary Veins

CT provides an excellent view on the left atrium and pulmonary veins that can be used as road map for guiding radiofrequency catheter ablation therapy. Volume rendering (Fig. 12-23) and transverse views (Fig. 12-12) show the pulmonary vein and left atrium anatomy well. Orthogonal sagittal views may be used for pulmonary vein ostium evaluation.[20]

Other Structures

CT also visualises other (cardiovascular) structures in the same acquisition. Cardiac veins can be excellently visualised by CT.[21] The normal pericardium is visualised as a thin line (Fig. 12-12). Pulmonary CT angiography is the imaging test of first choice in patients suspected for pulmonary embolism,[22] and aortic CT angiography is the preferred imaging technique for evaluating patients with suspected acute aortic syndrome. Other thoracic structures beyond the heart and great vessels—the hilum, lungs, chest wall and bones—can be optimally visualised by viewing the images at the appropriate window-width and window-level settings.

ECHOCARDIOGRAPHY

Cardiac ultrasound is currently one of the most important imaging techniques in clinical cardiology because it is quickly performed, readily available (even at bedside) and bears low costs. Echocardiography has evolved from

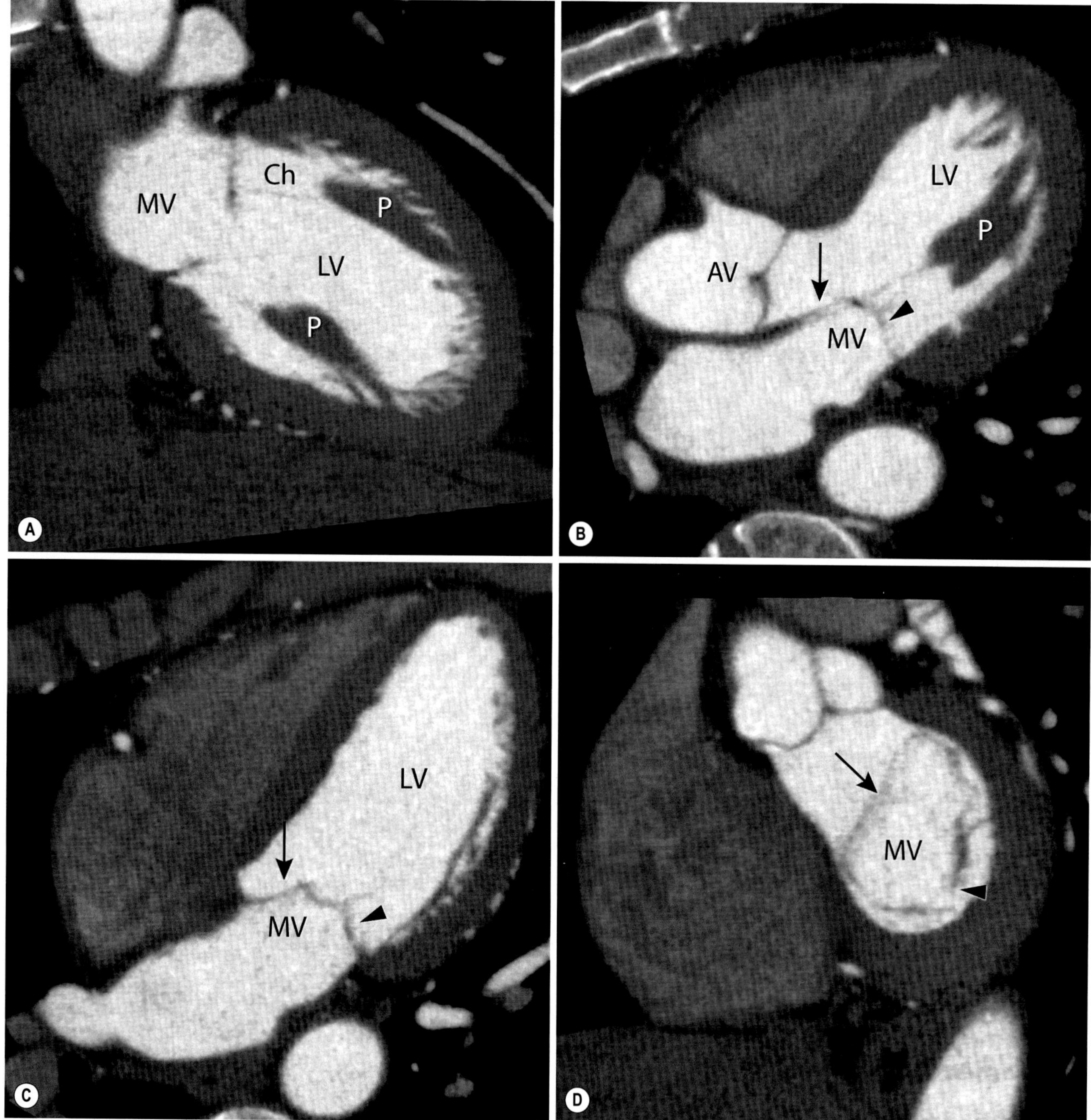

FIGURE 12-20 ■ **Mitral valve.** Multiplanar reconstructions at mid-diastole showing the mitral valve (MV) in longitudinal two-chamber view (A), three-chamber view (B), four-chamber view (C) and short-axis view (D). Anterior mitral leaflet (arrow), posterior mitral leaflet (arrowhead). P, papillary muscles; Ch, chordae tendineae; AV, aortic valve; LV, left ventricle.

M-mode ultrasound to 2-D and recently to 3-D image orientation. Echocardiography uses high-frequency ultrasound (2.0–7.5 MHz), and the nature of the ultrasound waves are such that the use of echocardiography is harmless and no X-rays are involved. The ultrasound waves show limited reflection on air and are attenuated by body fat. Therefore, in patients with chronic obstructive pulmonary disease and in obese patients, suboptimal windows with limited quality may be obtained.

Cardiac and vascular anatomy can be assessed with 2-D echocardiography, and cardiac and vascular function can be assessed by analysing the ECG traced cine images.[23] The temporal resolution of the cine images depends on the various settings and ranges typically from 30 to 100 frames per second (temporal resolution: 33–10 ms). With the use of Doppler technique, blood flow velocities can be measured to estimate pressure gradients in a non-invasive fashion and colour Doppler allows for non-invasive assessment of blood flow. The Doppler techniques are particularly important for the assessment of valvular function. Since the focus of this chapter is mainly on cardiac anatomy, functional and Doppler aspects are not addressed.

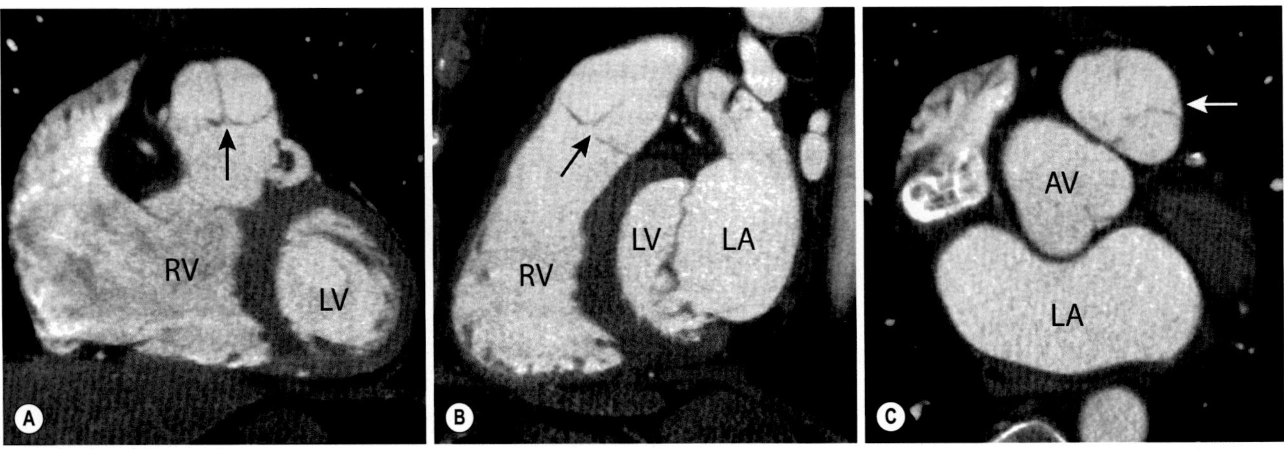

FIGURE 12-21 ■ **Pulmonary valve.** Coronal (A), sagittal (B) and multiplanar reconstruction parallel to the pulmonary valve (C) showing the pulmonary valve (arrows). AV, aortic valve; LA, left atrium; LV, left ventricle; RV, right ventricle.

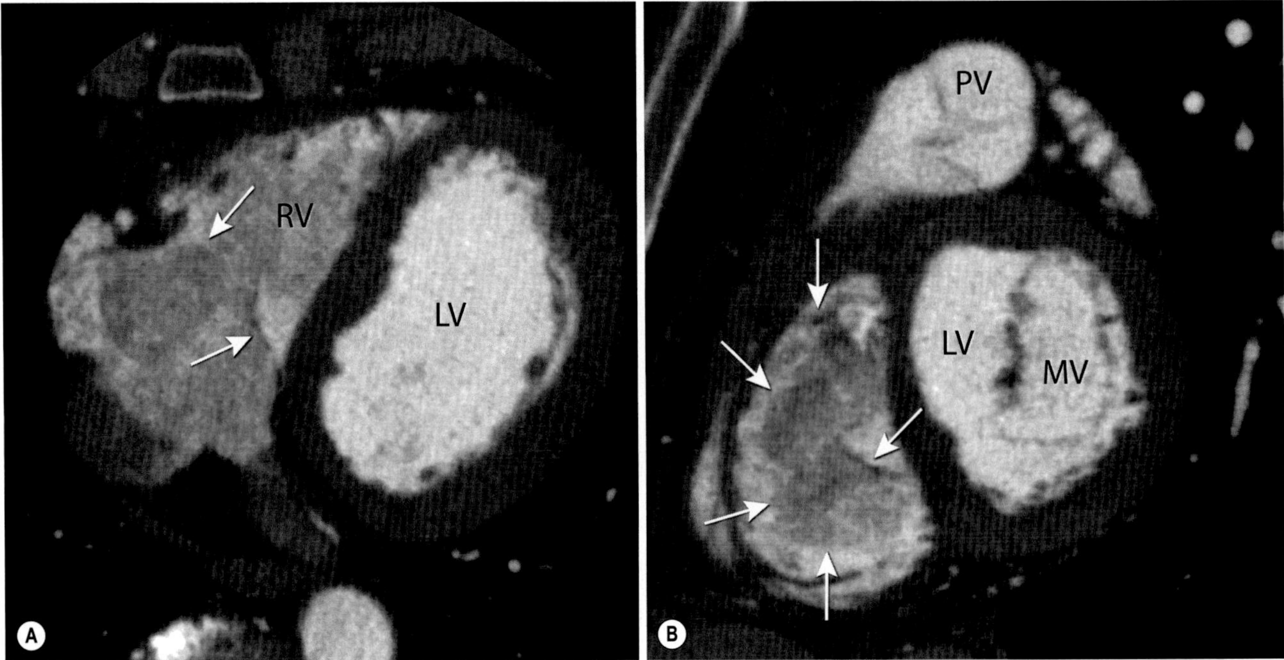

FIGURE 12-22 ■ **Tricuspid valve.** Transverse reconstruction (A) and short-axis reconstruction parallel to the tricuspid valve (B), showing the tricuspid valve (arrows). LV, left ventricle; RV, right ventricle; MV, mitral valve; PV, pulmonary valve. Note that the tricuspid valve is difficult to recognise as compared to the mitral valve (B).

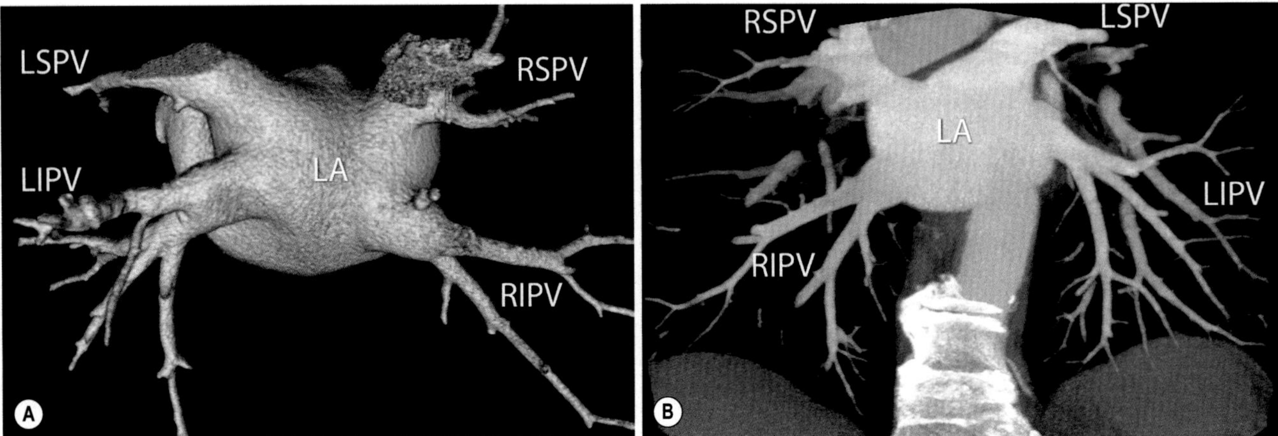

FIGURE 12-23 ■ **Pulmonary veins.** Volume-rendered (A) and maximum intensity projection (B) reconstructions, dorsal view (A) and frontal view (B). LA, left atrium; LIPV, left inferior pulmonary vein; LSPV, left superior pulmonary vein; RIPV, right inferior pulmonary vein; RSPV, right superior pulmonary vein.

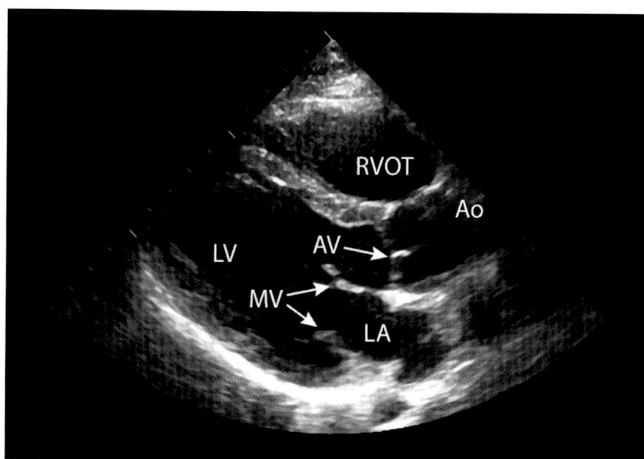

FIGURE 12-24 ■ **Parasternal long-axis view.** LV, left ventricle; LA, left atrium; RVOT, right ventricular outflow tract; Ao, aorta; AV, aortic valve; MV, mitral valve.

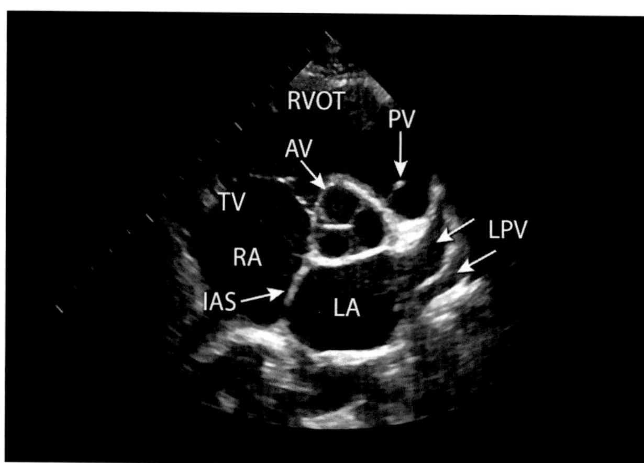

FIGURE 12-25 ■ **Parasternal short-axis aorta view.** RA, right atrium; LA, left atrium; IAS, interatrial septum; RVOT, right ventricular outflow tract; AV, aortic valve; TV, tricuspid valve; PV, pulmonary valve; LPV, left pulmonary veins.

Transthoracic echocardiography consists of several standard views and usually starts with the patient in the left lateral decubitus position at the left parasternal position at the third to fourth intercostal space. Then apical views are performed from the apex of the heart. In the supine position subcostal views and suprasternal views can be obtained. Additional custom-oriented views may be obtained depending on the clinical questions.

The parasternal position enables long- and short-axis views. The parasternal long-axis view (Fig. 12-24) shows the anteroseptal and the inferolateral/posterior wall of the left ventricle (LV). This view is used to assess end-diastolic and end-systolic LV dimensions and normal values are derived from this orientation.[24] Also dimensions of the left atrium, the aorta and the right and left ventricular outflow tract can be measured from this view.[24] Furthermore, identification of the aortic valve and mitral valve is possible. By rotating the transducer 90°, the parasternal short-axis view at the level of aortic valve (Fig. 12-25) allows assessment of the right atrium, left atrium, tricuspid valve, right ventricular outflow tract (in transverse orientation from the parasternal long-axis view), pulmonary veins, pulmonary valve and the interventricular septum. Of note, the view of the aortic valve is a transverse orientation from the parasternal long axis and provides clear identification of the aortic leaflets and also the pulmonary artery branches may be identified (Fig. 12-26). At the level of the basis of the left ventricle (Fig. 12-27) all six basal segments of the myocardium referring to the 17-segment model can be identified.[3] Also a part of the right ventricle, the mitral leaflets and occasionally the moderator band are shown. At the mid level of the left ventricle (Fig. 12-28) the six mid segments of the myocardium from the 17-segment model are identified, as well as a mid portion of the right ventricle and the papillary muscles. The last parasternal short-axis view is the apical view and shows the four apical segments (Fig. 12-29).

The apical views show the apex of the heart usually on top and the atria on the bottom of the image. The first apical view shows the left ventricle, right ventricle, left

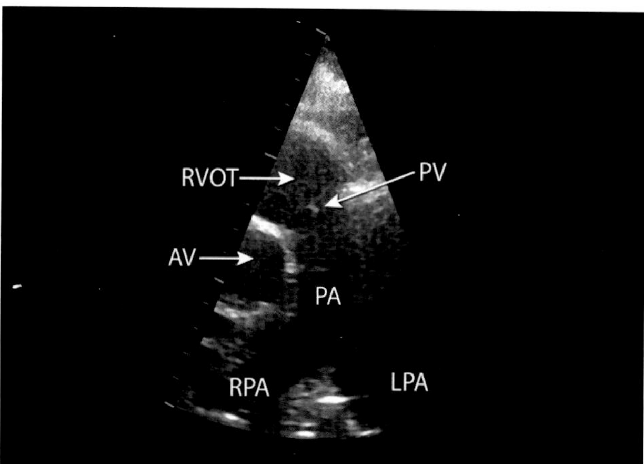

FIGURE 12-26 ■ **Parasternal short-axis pulmonary artery view.** RVOT, right ventricular outflow tract; AV, aortic valve; PV, pulmonary valve; PA, main pulmonary artery; RPA, right pulmonary artery; LPA, left pulmonary artery.

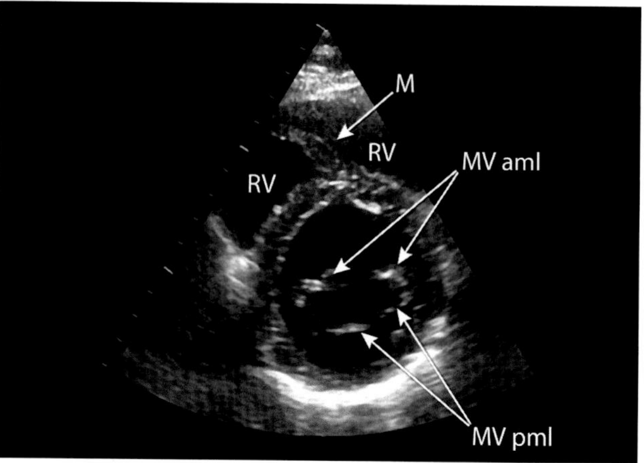

FIGURE 12-27 ■ **Parasternal short-axis basal left ventricle view.** LV, left ventricle; MV, mitral valve; MV aml, anterior leaflet mitral valve; MV pml, posterior leaflet mitral valve; RV, right ventricle; M, moderator band.

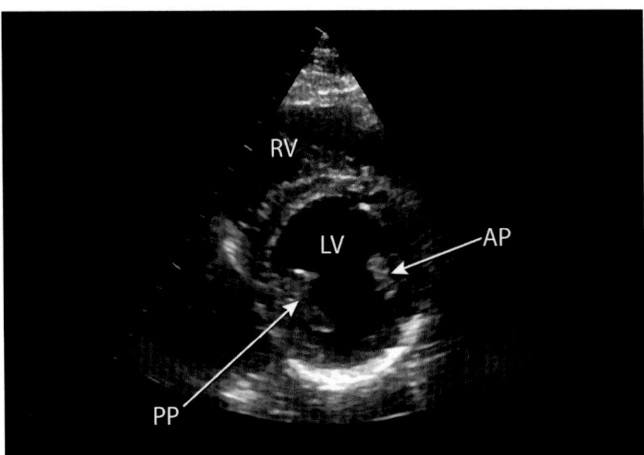

FIGURE 12-28 ■ **Parasternal short-axis mid left ventricle view.** LV, left ventricle; RV, right ventricle; AP, anterior papillary muscle; PP, posterior papillary muscle.

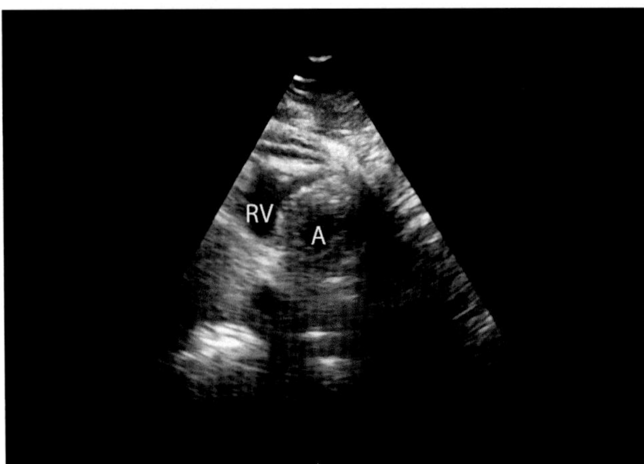

FIGURE 12-29 ■ **Parasternal short-axis apex left ventricle.** A, apex left ventricle; RV, right ventricle.

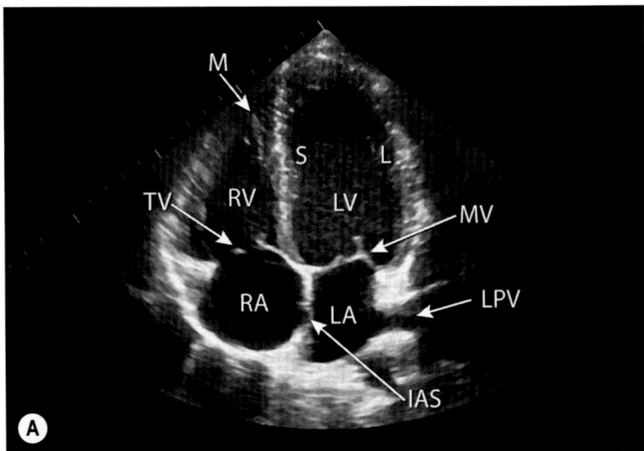

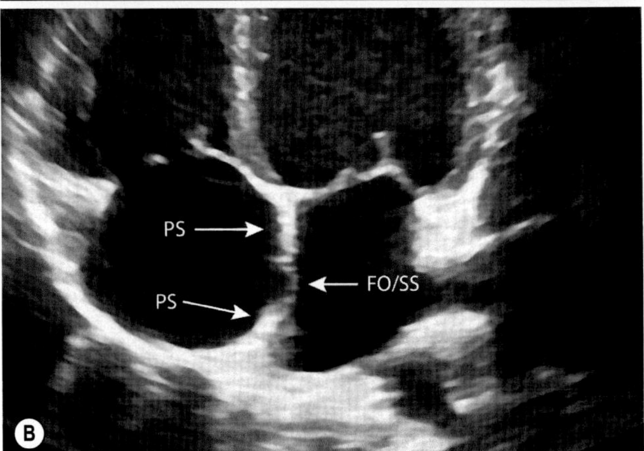

FIGURE 12-30 ■ (A) Apical four-chamber view. LV, left ventricle; S, septal myocardium; L, lateral myocardium; RV, right ventricle; LA, left atrium; RA, right atrium; MV, mitral valve; TV, tricuspid valve; M, moderator band; LPV, left pulmonary vein; IAS, inter-atrial septum; (B) detail of the inter-atrial septum. PS, primary septum; FO/SS, fossa ovalis/secondary septum.

atrium and right atrium and is therefore named the 'four-chamber' view, although the left atrium and right atrium are not real chambers (Fig. 12-30A). Furthermore, the interatrial septum (consisting of the primary and secondary parts; Fig. 12-30B), the pulmonary veins, mitral valve, tricuspid valve and the septal and lateral myocardium are identified. With a 90° rotation of the transducer from the four-chamber view, the two-chamber view is obtained (Fig. 12-31), showing the left ventricle with the anterior and inferior myocardium, and the left atrium as the second 'chamber'. From the four-chamber view also the five-chamber view (Fig. 12-32) is obtained, showing the four chambers and the aorta as the fifth chamber. This view identifies the anteroseptal- and inferolateral-posterior myocardium, the aortic valve and the left ventricular outflow tract. When the regular four-chamber view is angulated towards the right ventricle, the apical right ventricle view (Fig. 12-33) is obtained, showing a greater part of the right ventricle, and allows assessment of right ventricular function.

The subcostal views are performed via a subxiphoid approach with the transducer in the direction of the heart and show again a four-chamber view (Fig. 12-34), which

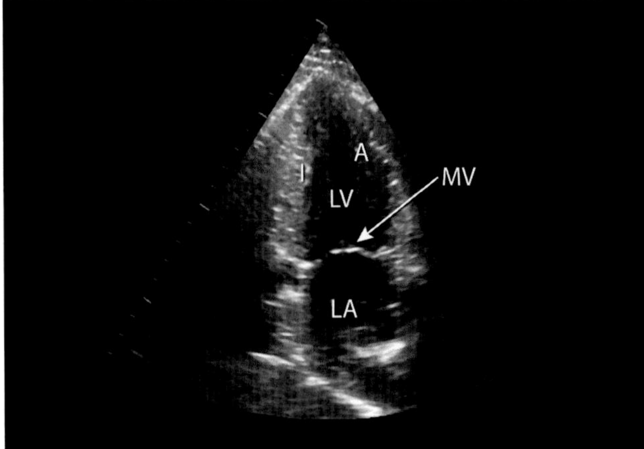

FIGURE 12-31 ■ **Apical two-chamber view.** LV, left ventricle; A, anterior myocardium; I, inferior myocardium; LA, left atrium; MV, mitral valve.

has the advantage of a detailed view on the pericardium and the pericardial space to assess pericardial effusion. This view is often used after thoracic operations in which the apical and parasternal windows are usually limited. Also the inferior vena cava is seen and the inferior vena

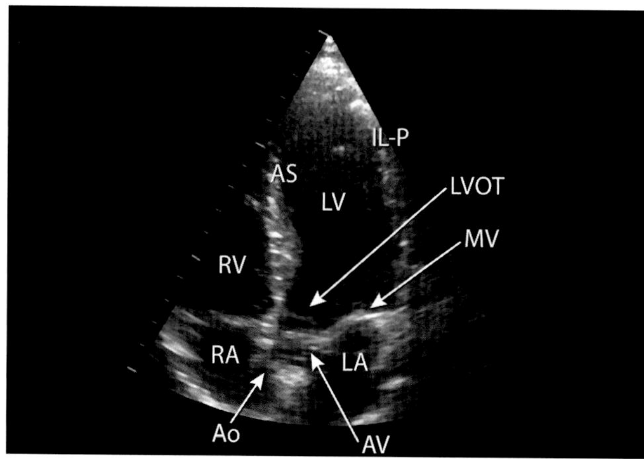

FIGURE 12-32 ■ **Apical five-chamber view.** LV, left ventricle; AS, anteroseptal myocardium; IL-P, inferolateral-posterior myocardium; LA, left atrium; MV, mitral valve; RV, right ventricle; RA, right atrium; AV, aortic valve; LVOT, left ventricular outflow tract; Ao, aorta-ascendens.

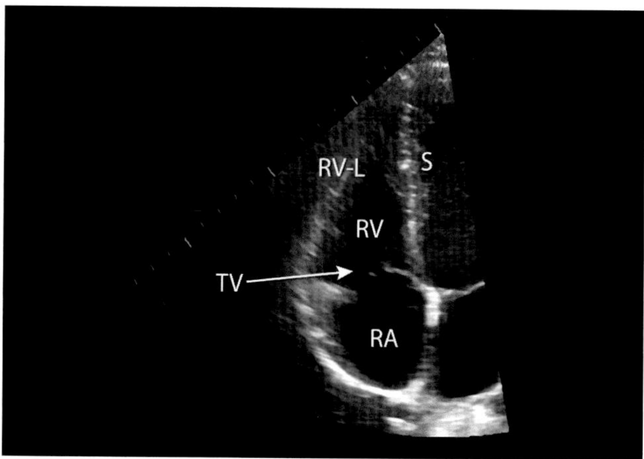

FIGURE 12-33 ■ **Apical right ventricle view.** RV, right ventricle; RA, right atrium; TV, tricuspid valve; S, septal myocardium; RV-L, right ventricle lateral myocardium.

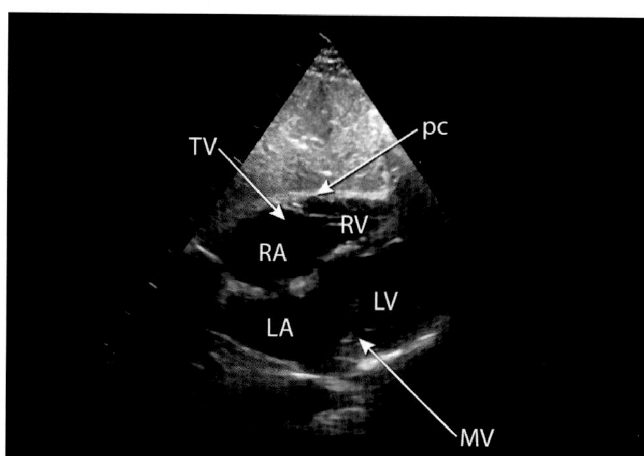

FIGURE 12-34 ■ **Subcostal four-chamber view.** LV, left ventricle; RV, right ventricle; LA, left atrium; RA, right atrium; MV, mitral valve; TV, tricuspid valve; pc, pericardium.

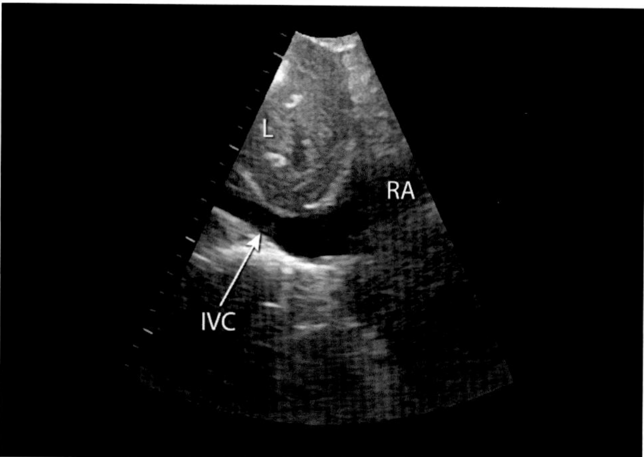

FIGURE 12-35 ■ **Subcostal inferior vena cava view.** L, liver; IVC, inferior vena cava; RA, right atrium.

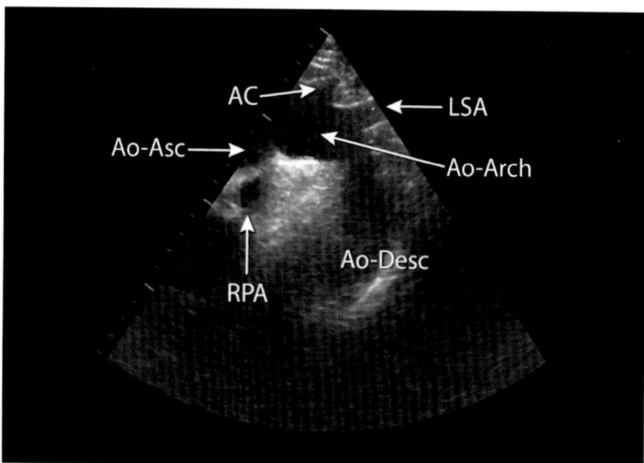

FIGURE 12-36 ■ **Suprasternal view.** Ao-Asc, ascending aorta; Ao-Arch, aortic arch; Ao-Desc, descending aorta; AC, common carotid artery; LSA, left subclavian artery; RPA, right pulmonary artery.

cava dimension, indicative for the right atrial pressure, can be measured (Fig. 12-35). The last standard view is the suprasternal view (Fig. 12-36) obtained from the suprasternal notch and this view enables assessment of the proximal ascending aorta, the aortic arch and its upper side branches and the descending aorta.

Valves

Apart from the above-mentioned structures, echocardiography is particularly suitable for assessing valvular anatomy and function with Doppler techniques. All four cardiac valves can be assessed with regular 2-D echocardiography, but in clinical practice most lesions affect the aortic valve and mitral valve. Echocardiographic example of a normal aortic valve (a detail from the parasternal short-axis aorta view; Fig. 12-25) allows identification of the three leaflets (Fig. 12-37). In case of a bicuspid aortic valve, echocardiography can distinguish the anatomy of a true bicuspid valve or a bicuspid valve with fused leaflets (Fig. 12-38). Also, the mitral valve anatomy can be looked

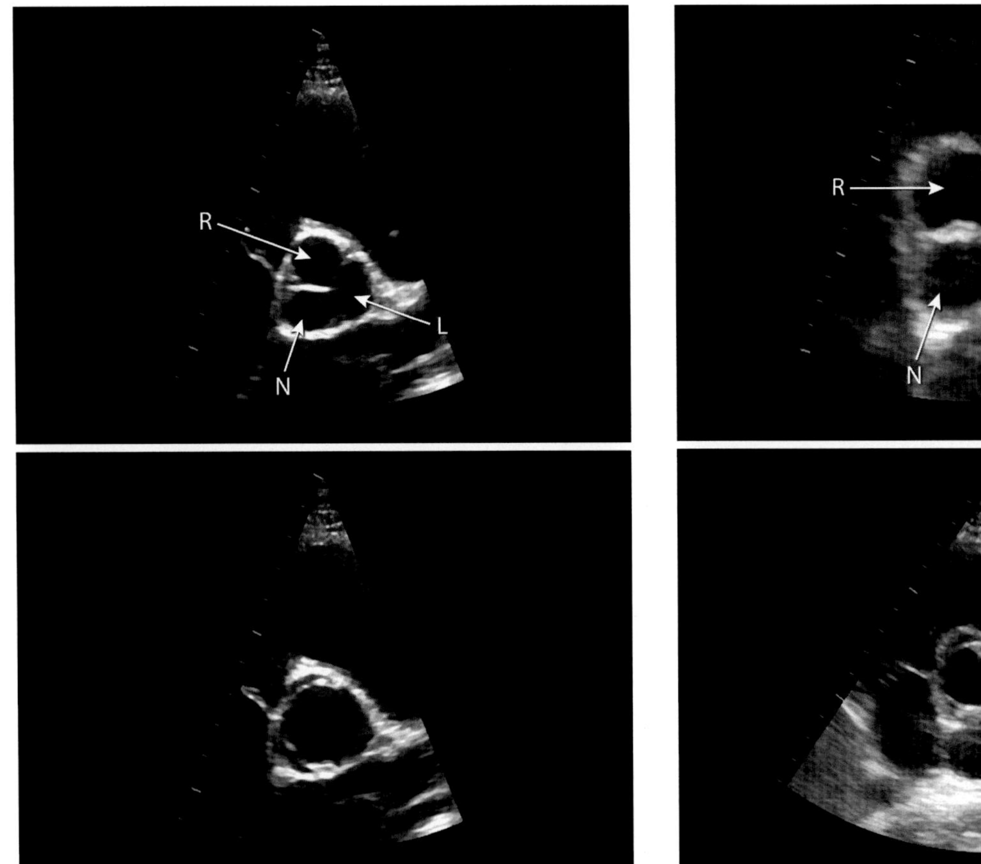

FIGURE 12-37 ■ **Aortic valve short-axis.** Normal aortic valve with right coronary cusp (R), left coronary cusp (L) and non-coronary cusp (N) in closed (upper panel) and open position (lower panel).

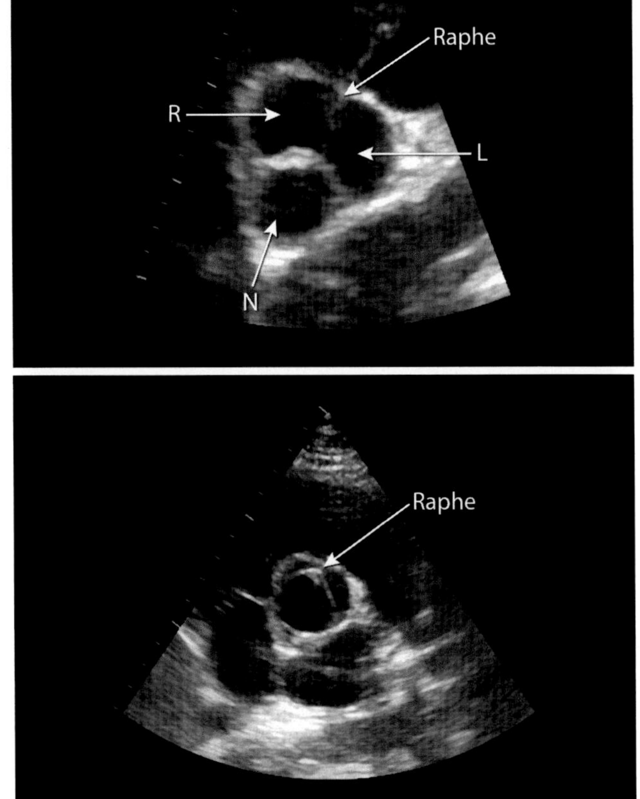

FIGURE 12-38 ■ **Bicuspid aortic valve.** Functionally bicuspid aortic valve with non-coronary cusp (N), and fusion (raphe) of the right coronary cusp (R) and left coronary cusp (L). Upper panel shows the aortic valve in closed and lower panel in open position.

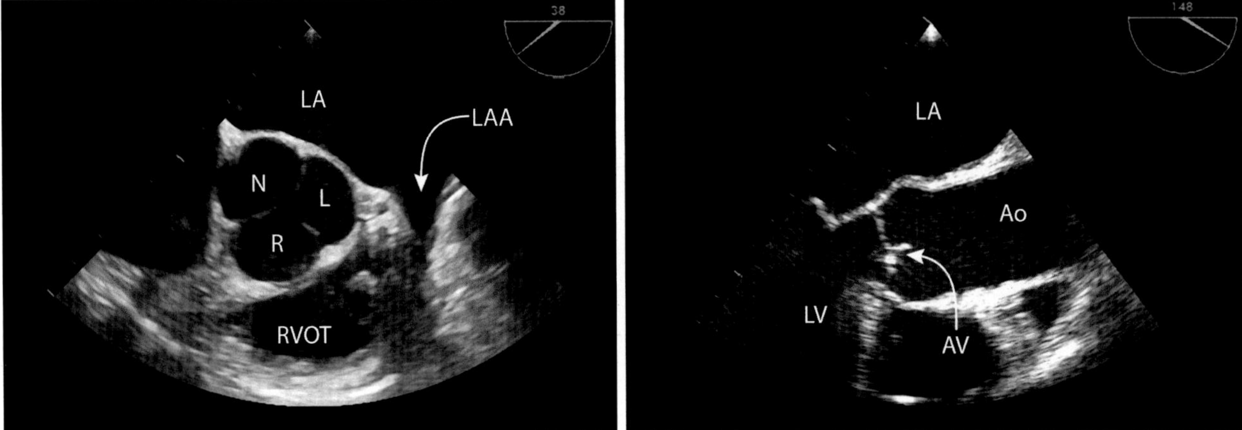

FIGURE 12-39 ■ **Transoesophageal echocardiographic view of the aortic valve in transverse/short-axis view (left panel) and longitudinal view (right panel).** N, non-coronary cusp; R, right coronary cusp; L, left coronary cusp; LA, left atrium; LAA, left atrial appendage; RVOT, right ventricular outflow tract; LV, left ventricle; AV, aortic valve; Ao, ascending aorta.

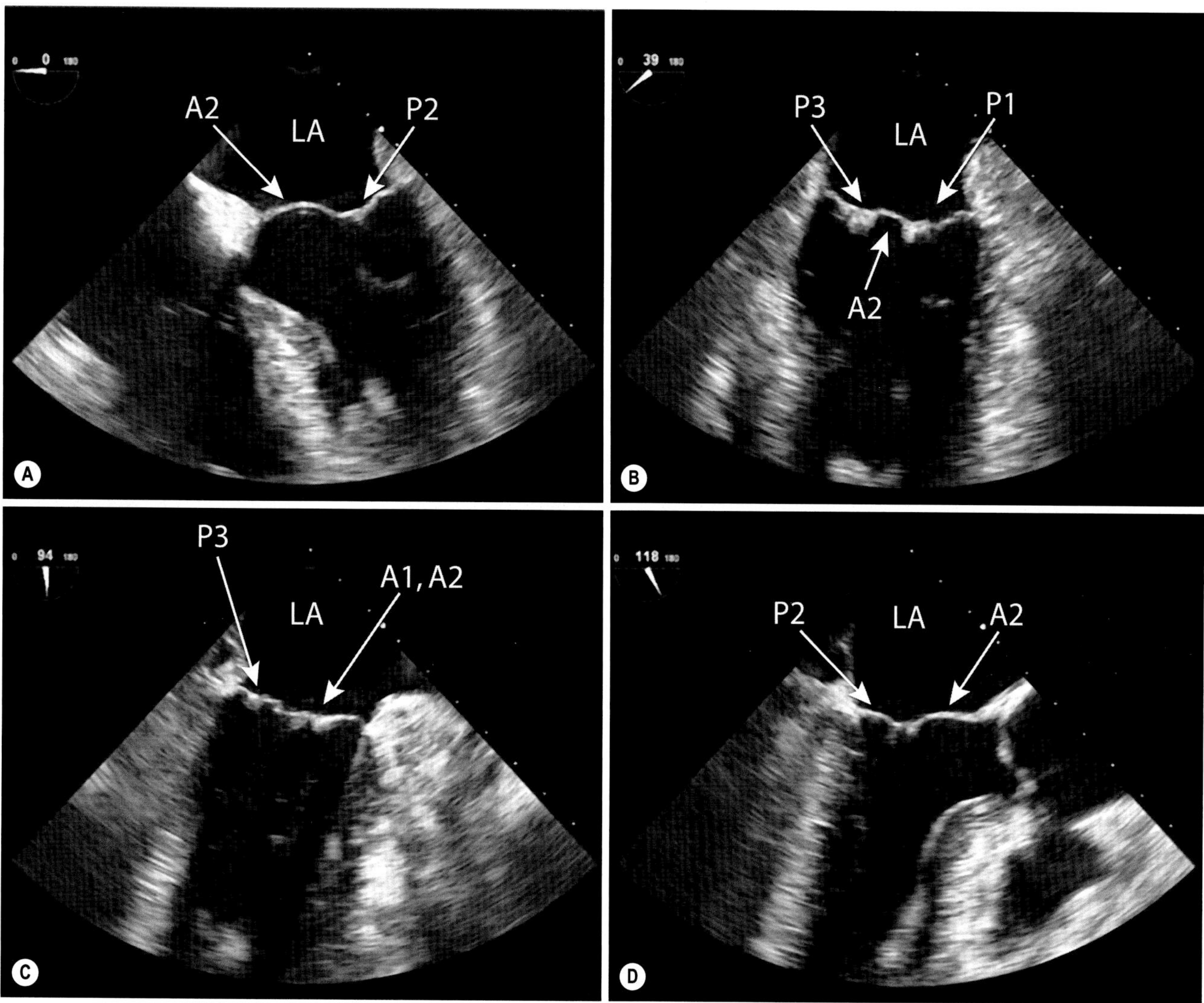

FIGURE 12-40 ■ **Transoesophageal echocardiographic views of the mitral valve.** With multiplanar views, the different parts of the anterior mitral valve leaflet (A1, A 2, A3) and the posterior leaflet (P1, P2, P3) can be visualised.

at with 2-D echocardiography in the parasternal long-axis view, the apical four-chamber view and the two-chamber view (Figs. 12-24, 12-30 and 12-31). For detailed assessment of the cardiac valves transoesophageal echocardiography can also be performed. Compared to transthoracic echocardiography, transoesophageal echocardiography provides closer views on the valves and atria with less attenuation since the oesophagus is situated posteriorly to the heart with almost no interposed tissue. The main disadvantage is discomfort for the patient, sometimes even requiring light anaesthesia. Figure 12-39 provides detailed anatomy of the aortic valve and other atrial structures such as left atrial appendage and pulmonary veins. Figure 12-40 shows anatomy of the mitral valve with identification of all the different parts of the anterior and posterior mitral valve leaflets. These detailed views provide better insight into the mechanism causing mitral valve regurgitation or stenosis, compared to transthoracic echocardiography.

For the mitral valve, an 'en face' view like in the aortic valve (Fig. 12-37) is usually not possible since the mitral valve is a saddle-shaped structure, and therefore the valve cannot be viewed in a single plane with a 2-D technique.

Also, recently, 3-D echocardiography was introduced for identifying valvular anatomy, and examples are shown in Figs. 12-41 and 12-42. Three-dimensional images provide a better orientation of the valve anatomy in relation to the surrounding structures. However, acquisition and spatial and temporal resolution of 3-D images are still to be improved.

Acknowledgement

G. Kracht, F. van der Kley and E. R. Holman are acknowledged for their assistance with the figures of this chapter.

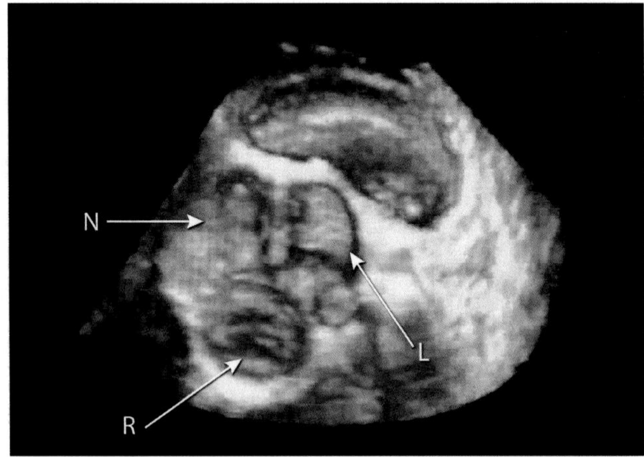

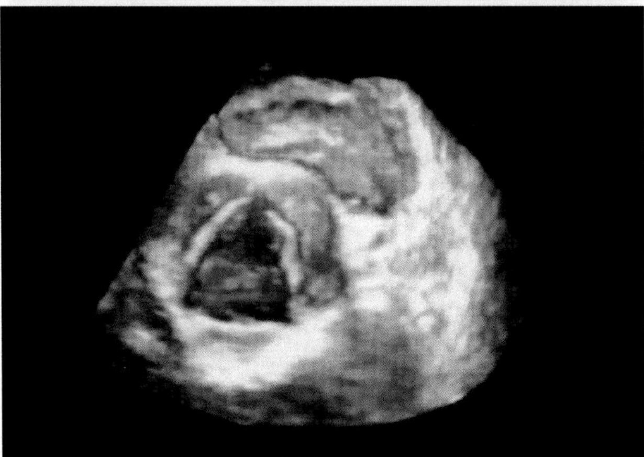

FIGURE 12-41 ■ **Three-dimensional view of the aortic valve in closed (upper panel) and in open position (lower panel).** The image is obtained with transoesophageal echocardiography. N, non-coronary cusp; R, right coronary cusp; L, left coronary cusp.

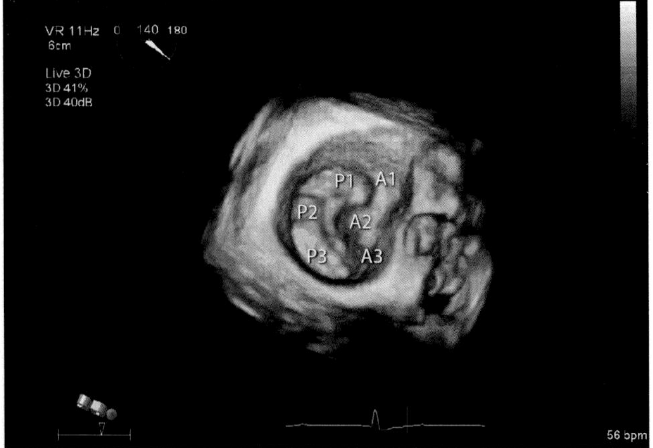

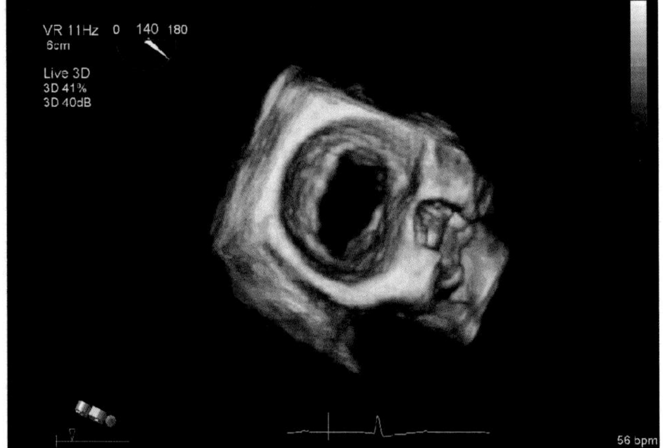

FIGURE 12-42 ■ **Three-dimensional view of the mitral valve with anterior leaflet and posterior leaflet in closed (upper panel) and in open position (lower panel).** The image is obtained with transoesophageal echocardiography and the valve is seen from the left atrium. The different parts of the anterior mitral valve leaflet (A1, A 2, A3) and the posterior leaflet (P1, P2, P3) can be determined.

REFERENCES

1. Ho SY, Nihoyannopoulos P. Anatomy, echocardiography, and normal right ventricular dimensions. Heart 2006;92:i2–13.
2. Lenz GW, Haacke EM, White RD. Retrospective cardiac gating: a review of technical aspects and future directions. Magn Reson Imaging 1989;7(5):445–55.
3. Cerqueira MD, Weismann NJ, Dilsizian V, et al. Standardized myocardial segmentation and nomenclature for tomographic imaging of the heart: a statement for healthcare professionals from the Cardiac Imaging Committee of the Council on Clinical Cardiology of the American Heart Association. Circulation 2002;105: 539–42.
4. Uribe S, Muthurangu V, Boubertakh R, et al. Whole-heart cine MRI using real-time respiratory self-gating. Magn Reson Med 2007;57:606–13.
5. Miller S, Simonetti OP, Carr J, et al. MR imaging of the heart with cine true fast imaging with steady-state precession: influence of spatial and temporal resolutions on left ventricular functional parameters. Radiology 2002;223:263–9.
6. Kramer CM, Barkhausen J, Flamm SD, et al. Standardized cardiovascular magnetic resonance imaging (CMR) protocols, society for cardiovascular magnetic resonance: board of trustees task force on standardized protocols. J Cardiovasc Magn Reson 2008;10: 10–35.
7. Alfakih K, Plein S, Bloomer T, et al. Comparison of right ventricular volume measurements between axial and short axis orientation using steady-state free precession magnetic resonance imaging. J Magn Reson Imaging 2003;18:25–32.
8. Mansour M, Holmvang G, Sosnovik D, et al. Assessment of pulmonary vein anatomic variability by magnetic resonance imaging: implications for catheter ablation techniques for atrial fibrillation. J Cardiovasc Electrophysiol 2004;15(4):387–93.
9. Van der Voort PH, van den Bosch HCM, Post JC, et al. Determination of the spatial orientation and shape of pulmonary vein ostia by contrast-enhanced magnetic resonance angiography. Europace 2006;8(1):1–6.
10. Taylor JA, Cerqueira M, Hodgson JM, et al. ACCF/SCCT/ACR/AHA/ASE/ASNC/NASCI/SCAI/SCMR 2010 appropriate use criteria for cardiac computed tomography: a report of the American College of Cardiology Foundation Appropriate Use Criteria Task Force, the Society of Cardiovascular Computed Tomography, the American College of Radiology, the American Heart Association, the American Society of Echocardiography, the American Society of Nuclear Cardiology, the Society for Cardiovascular Angiography and Interventions, and the Society for Cardiovascular Magnetic Resonance. J Am Coll Cardiol 2010;56:1864–94.
11. Einstein AJ, Elliston CD, Arai AE, et al. Radiation dose from single-heartbeat coronary CT angiography performed with a 320-detector row volume scanner. Radiology 2010;254:698–706.
12. Achenbach S, Marwan M, Ropers D, et al. Coronary computed tomography angiography with a consistent dose below 1 mSv using prospectively electrocardiogram-triggered high-pitch spiral acquisition. Eur Heart J 2010;31:340–6.
13. Van der Bijl N, Geleijns J, Joemai RM, et al. Recent developments in cardiac CT. Imaging Med 2011;3:167–92.
14. Earls JP, Berman EL, Urban BA, et al. Prospectively gated transverse coronary CT angiography versus retrospectively gated helical

technique: improved image quality and reduced radiation dose. Radiology 2008;246:742–53.
15. Meijer AB, OYL, Geleijns J, Kroft LJ. Meta-analysis of 40- and 64-MDCT angiography for assessing coronary artery stenosis. Am J Roentgenol 2008;191:1667–75.
16. Chhedda SV, Srichai MB, Donnino R, et al. Evaluation of the mitral and aortic valves with cardiac CT angiography. J Thorac Imaging 2010;25:76–85.
17. Manghat NE, Rachapalli V, van Lingen R, et al. Imaging the heart valves using ECG-gated 64-detector row cardiac CT. Br J Radiol 2008;81:275–90.
18. Chen JJ, Manning MA, Frazier AA, et al. CT angiography of the cardiac valves: Normal, diseased, and postoperative appearances. Radiographics 2009;29:1393–412.
19. Fedak PW, Verma S, David TE, et al. Clinical and pathophysiological implications of a bicuspid aortic valve. Circulation 2002;106: 900–4.
20. Jongbloed MR, Dirksen MS, Bax JJ, et al. Atrial fibrillation: Multidetector row CT of pulmonary vein anatomy prior to radiofrequency catheter ablation—initial experience. Radiology 2005;234: 702–9.
21. Jongbloed MR, Lamb HJ, Bax JJ, et al. Noninvasive visualization of the cardiac venous system using multislice computed tomography. J Am Coll Cardiol 2005;45:749–53.
22. Klok FA, Mos IC, Kroft LJ, et al. Computed tomography pulmonary angiography as a single imaging test to rule out pulmonary embolism. Curr Opin Pulm Med 2011;17:380–6.
23. Association Task Force on Practice Guidelines (ACC/AHA/ASE Committee to Update the 1997 Guidelines for the Clinical Application of Echocardiography). ACC/AHA/ASE. Guideline Update for the Clinical Application of Echocardiography: Summary Article. A Report of the American College of Cardiology/American Heart Association. Circulation 2003;108:1146–62.
24. Lang RM, Bierig M, Devereux RB, et al; Chamber Quantification Writing Group; American Society of Echocardiography's Guidelines and Standards Committee; European Association of Echocardiography. Recommendations for chamber quantification: a report from the American Society of Echocardiography's Guidelines and Standards Committee and the Chamber Quantification Writing Group, developed in conjunction with the European Association of Echocardiography, a branch of the European Society of Cardiology. J Am Soc Echocardiogr 2005;18:1440–63.

CHAPTER 13

Congenital Heart Disease: General Principles and Imaging

Andrew M. Taylor • Michael A. Quail

CHAPTER OUTLINE

INTRODUCTION

Congenital heart disease (CHD), although rare, with an incidence of 8 per 1000 births, has increased in prevalence due to the success of surgical and medical management in childhood. A significant proportion of patients with repaired CHD surviving to adulthood fall under the care of cardiologists outside tertiary centres for congenital cardiac care. Specialist cardiovascular and general radiologists require an understanding of the underlying morphological abnormalities and their physiology, methods of repair and how potential complications may be detected and assessed in their practice, using appropriate imaging techniques, such as ultrasound (US), cardiac magnetic resonance (CMR) and computed tomography (CT).

Congenital heart disease is *any* developmental malformation of the heart. The spectrum of disease falling into this classification ranges from simple lesions, for example bicuspid aortic valve, through to more complex diseases involving single ventricle lesions, such as hypoplastic left heart syndrome (HLHS). The developmental biology and genetic basis of CHD is under investigation, but apart from a few well-known associations—for example Di George syndrome (interrupted aortic arch, tetralogy of Fallot, truncus arteriosus), Down's syndrome (atrioventricular, ventricular and atrial septal defects), and Turner's syndrome (bicuspid aortic valve and coarctation)—the cause of the majority of clinical disease is unknown.

CLINICAL PRESENTATION

The clinical presentation of CHD in infancy may be dominated by a number of physiological states.

1. *Left-to-right shunts*: Redirection of blood from the systemic (left) to the pulmonary circulation (right) may occur at atrial, ventricular, or great vessel level. A proportion of already oxygenated blood is recirculated to the lungs with each heartbeat, resulting in inefficiency. The volume of the shunt and its location accounts for the observed signs. Chambers and vessels receiving the excessive volume enlarge and high pulmonary blood flow results in pulmonary plethora. Typical examples include atrial septal defects (ASDs), ventricular septal defects (VSDs) and patent ductus arteriosus (PDA). Patients are pink but increasingly breathless with larger shunts.
2. *Compromised systemic perfusion*: This may result from low stroke volume of a systemic ventricle (hypoplastic left heart syndrome), outflow tract obstruction (critical aortic stenosis) or aortic obstruction (interrupted aortic arch or coarctation). The clinical picture is one of poor peripheral perfusion, with low pulse volume; patients may be pink or blue (cyanotic). The ductus arteriosus may provide an effective temporary bypass for the obstruction, facilitating systemic perfusion with deoxygenated or mixed blood. However, as the duct closes (some days after birth), life-threatening systemic or lower body hypoperfusion ensues and often also pulmonary venous hypertension. Therapy is directed at maintaining the patency of the arterial duct using intravenous prostaglandins, intensive care for critically ill patients, and planning for surgical relief of the obstruction.
3. *Pulmonary venous congestion*: Obstruction to pulmonary venous return results in increased pulmonary venous pressure (elevated pulmonary capillary wedge pressure); at progressively higher transvascular gradients, colloid osmotic pressure is exceeded and extravasation of fluid into the interstitial and alveolar space occurs. Obstruction may occur in the pulmonary venous pathway (total anomalous pulmonary venous connection, TAPVD), in the atrium (cor triatriatum) or at the level of the left

ventricular inflow (supravalvular, valvular or subvalvular mitral stenosis or mitral regurgitation). Pulmonary venous congestion may also occur as a function of elevated left atrial pressure secondary to LV diastolic dysfunction: increased LV end diastolic pressure (valve disease, aortic coarctation, myocardial disease). The degree of pulmonary venous hypertension determines the clinical presentation. Patients with severe obstruction may present with hypoxia, cyanosis and dyspnoea due to pulmonary oedema, whilst patients with less severe obstruction may remain pink but may present later with failure to thrive.

The following three physiological states predominantly account for patients with cyanosis:

4. *Low pulmonary blood flow*: Reduction in pulmonary blood flow is commonly caused by obstruction to right ventricular outflow (tetralogy of Fallot or severe pulmonary stenosis). The increased resistance to RV outflow results in a redirection of systemic venous return to the left heart (right-to-left shunt) via an interatrial communication (patent foramen ovale or ASD) or a VSD. As lung function is normal, any pulmonary venous blood returns to the left atrium fully saturated, and mixes with the shunted systemic venous blood; however, because pulmonary flow is so low, there is insufficient oxygenated blood in the mix, resulting in cyanosis.
5. *Parallel circulations*: This occurs in transposition of the great arteries, where the aorta arises from the morphological right ventricle and the pulmonary artery from the left ventricle. In this condition, deoxygenated systemic venous return recirculates into the aorta and the oxygenated pulmonary venous return recirculates to the pulmonary artery, a situation clearly incompatible with life. Patients can only survive if there is sufficient mixing of the streams (shunt); this can occur best at atrial level through a large inter-atrial communication, less well at ventricular level (via a VSD) and even less well at great vessel level (via a PDA). Critical cyanosis may be managed medically by maintaining patency of the PDA by prostaglandins, but may require the creation of an artificial inter-atrial communication using cardiac catheterisation, until definitive treatment by surgically switching the great vessels.
6. *Intracardiac mixing*: Complete intracardiac mixing of blood may occur at atrial level (common atrium), ventricular level (all univentricular hearts), or great artery level (common arterial trunk). Patients are expected to be mildly cyanosed, depending on the relative amount of deoxygenated blood in the mix, and breathless, according to the amount of pulmonary blood flow.

Later Clinical Presentation

Most adult patients with CHD are survivors from childhood. This group may present with an interesting array of problems related to residual lesions or deteriorations of their initial repair or palliation (heart failure, valve regurgitation, conduit stenosis, baffle leaks). They require lifelong surveillance for anticipated problems arising from the 'unnatural history' of their underlying disorder.

New presentations of CHD continue beyond infancy into adulthood, usually because the underlying disorder has not yet produced symptoms. Common lesions include: left-to-right shunts, such as ASDs, VSDs or partial anomalous pulmonary venous drainage which only begin to be symptomatic in older patients; milder forms of LV or aortic obstruction such as coarctation of the aorta or valvular aortic stenosis which did not compromise systemic perfusion may progress and become symptomatic in later childhood or adulthood; and milder forms of RV obstruction such as pulmonary stenosis. Clearly, life-limiting conditions such as parallel circulation, significant shunts, severe intracardiac mixing or compromised systemic perfusion, would not normally be expected beyond childhood.

MORPHOLOGICAL DESCRIPTION AND SEQUENTIAL SEGMENTAL ANALYSIS

Numerous morphological abnormalities may be responsible for the physiological phenomena described above, and although initial management of an infant simply requires correct classification of the initial physiological pattern, subsequent surgical correction and medical management requires a precise anatomical diagnosis. The potential intrinsic complexity of CHD necessitates a systematic scheme of nomenclature that captures precisely the unique anatomy of each patient: this is called sequential segmental analysis. Using this approach, the clinician describes how the components of the heart and blood vessels are connected. This entails describing atrial situs (location of the atrial chambers and whether they are of left or right morphology), atrioventricular connections, ventriculo-arterial connections and other associated lesions in turn. Any cross-sectional imaging investigation may be used for this purpose, but transthoracic ultrasound is most commonly used for routine inpatient and outpatient assessment. In more complex lesions or when ultrasound provides an inadequate assessment (e.g. poor acoustic windows), CMR represents a powerful non-invasive technique giving morphological and haemodynamic information that ultrasound alone cannot provide.

Sequential Segmental Analysis

Step 1—Atrial Situs

Atrial situs is determined by an assessment of the morphology of each atrial appendage. Correct identification of the atrium allows the subsequent determination of the atrioventricular connection. The atrial appendages are the most consistent feature of the atrial mass; indeed, the venous attachments to each atrial chamber can form a variety of combinations. The right atrial appendage is a triangular shape, with a broad base and prominent pectinate muscles which extend around the right atrioventricular valve, whilst the left atrial appendage is a more elongated, tubular structure, and it has less extensive pectinate muscles which are confined within the appendage.

The most common lesions involve inversion of situs, or isomerism of the left or right atrial appendages. The non-cardiac thoracic and abdominal organs usually (but not always) demonstrate a similar 'sidedness' to that of the atrial chambers.

In the normal heart the morphological right atrium is located to the right of the morphological left atrium (situs solitus). The right lung is trilobed, with a shorter, early-branching bronchus, and the left lung is bilobed. In addition, the inferior caval vein (IVC) is to the right of the abdominal aorta, with a right-sided liver and left-sided spleen.

In situs inversus the mirror image of the normal anatomy is present.

Isomerism of the left atrial appendages is usually associated with bilateral bilobed lungs, polysplenia and IVC interruption. Isomerism of the right atrial appendages is usually associated with bilateral trilobed lungs, asplenia and a midline liver. In isomeric lesions there is often a common atrioventricular junction (instead of two separate and offset left and right junctions) with varying degrees of atrioventricular septal defect (AVSD). Gut malrotation is associated with both right- and left-sided isomerism. All of these abnormalities can be determined with CMR, particularly 3D balanced steady-state free precession (b-SSFP) technique.

Step 2—Ventricular Morphology

Determination of ventricular morphology allows analysis of atrioventricular (AV) and ventriculo-arterial connections. An AV connection is described as 'concordant' when the atria is connected to the expected ventricle (i.e. left atrium with left ventricle and right atrium with right ventricle); 'discordant' if the left atrium is connected to the right ventricle and right atrium to the left ventricle; 'ambiguous' if there is isomerism of the atrial appendages (e.g. two morphologically right atria connected to a left and right ventricle, respectively (one connection is concordant, the other discordant)); and finally 'univentricular' if both atria predominately connect to a single ventricle. Irrespective of atrioventricular concordance the AV valve is always concordant with the ventricle, i.e. the tricuspid valve connects to the morphological right ventricle and the mitral valve connects to the morphological left ventricle. The septal insertion of the tricuspid valve is more apical (apically 'offset') than that of the mitral valve, and allows determination of the ventricular morphology. The muscular structure of the ventricles also differs, the RV being more trabeculated than the LV, with a muscular infundibulum and mid-ventricular 'moderator band'. Although they are different in normal subjects, the size, shape and degree of trabeculation of the ventricles are not good indicators of ventricular origin, as all are dependent on load effects.

Step 3—Ventriculo-arterial Connection

Description of ventriculo-arterial connections represents the final element of sequential segmental analysis. This entails describing how each great vessel is connected to its respective ventricle. A ventriculo-arterial connection may be concordant (RV–PA, LV-aorta), discordant (RV–aorta, LV–PA), double outlet (e.g. RV–PA and aorta) or single outlet (e.g. LV and RV to common arterial trunk). The aorta and pulmonary arteries are defined by their typical branching patterns. Three-dimensional b-SSFP and contrast-enhanced MR angiography (MRA) techniques are particularly useful in determining the arrangement of the great vessels and the connections with their respective ventricles.

Step 4—Identification of Other Abnormalities

Other abnormalities to be considered include: abnormal venous connections, ASD, VSD, AVSD and valve abnormalities.

In general, most congenital cardiac lesions are single abnormalities that are easily described. However, almost any combination of abnormalities and connections can occur, and using the sequential segmental analysis method, the description of all conceivable combinations and diagnoses is possible. For more advanced reading, the reader is referred to the textbook *Paediatric Cardiology* by Anderson and colleagues.[1]

PHYSIOLOGICAL AND FUNCTIONAL ASSESSMENT

In addition to determining the morphology of underlying lesions, an assessment of their physiological impact on heart function is necessary. It is helpful to briefly consider a few parameters relating to normal cardiac function, which are commonly calculated by techniques such as CMR.

Stroke volume: This is the volume of blood (mL) pumped (displaced) by a ventricle with each heartbeat. The displaced volume is calculated by subtracting the volume of the ventricular cavity at end-diastole from the volume at end-systole. In the normal heart the stroke volume for each ventricle is the same and is also the same as the forward flow in the associated great artery. It may not be the same in the presence of a shunt or regurgitant valve. Here, discrepancies in interventricular volumes or great artery flows help locate and quantify the severity of shunts and valve regurgitation.

Cardiac output: This is how much blood each ventricular chamber pumps in one minute (L/min). It is calculated by multiplying the stroke volume (or great artery flow (mL)) by the heart rate (stroke (beat)/min). Cardiac output is increased by physiological stress (e.g. exercise, which increases both heart rate and stroke volume) and depressed in conditions that reduce either heart rate (bradyarrhythmias) or stroke volume (dilated cardiomyopathy, heart failure).

Ejection fraction: A useful assessment of gross systolic cardiac function is the percentage of blood ejected from the heart during each beat. This is calculated by dividing the stroke volume by the end-diastolic volume. Ejection fraction may be decreased if the systolic performance of the ventricle is impaired (cardiomyopathy).

NON-INVASIVE IMAGING TECHNIQUES

Imaging is fundamental to the diagnosis of CHD and is required at all stages of patient care. An ideal non-invasive investigation for imaging of CHD should be able to accurately and reproducibly delineate all aspects of the anatomy, including intracardiac abnormalities and abnormalities of extracardiac vessels, evaluate physiological consequences of CHD such as measurement of blood flow and pressure gradients across stenotic valves or blood vessels, be cost-effective and portable, provide data from fetal life to adulthood, not cause excessive discomfort and morbidity, and not expose patients to harmful effects of ionising radiation. No single investigation has fulfilled these entire requirements, and in the delivery of a CHD service, the imaging techniques discussed below play an important complementary role.

Ultrasound

Ultrasound is the initial imaging investigation used in the evaluation of patients with suspected CHD and should always be performed before other techniques are used. In most patients, ultrasound alone provides sufficient information to complete the diagnostic evaluation using a sequential segmental and functional analysis. In UK clinical practice, paediatric cardiologists have traditionally performed ultrasound. However, more recently neonatologists and radiologists have begun to use ultrasound in patients with suspected CHD where paediatric cardiology services are not immediately available. Cardiac anaesthetists also increasingly perform perioperative assessment using transoesophageal ultrasound. For a more comprehensive discussion of ultrasound in congenital heart disease, the reader is referred to Lai et al.[2]

Magnetic Resonance Imaging

As previously alluded, CMR probably provides the most comprehensive assessment available from a single non-invasive imaging investigation, but its immobility, cost, and limited availability constrain its general applicability. In our clinical practice it is used to define the morphology and physiology of the most complex CHD cases as well as providing routine surveillance for patients with repaired CHD such as tetralogy of Fallot and transposition of the great arteries. Extracardiac anatomy, including the great arteries and systemic veins, can be delineated with high spatial resolution. Vascular and valvular flow can be assessed, shunts can be quantified, and myocardial function can be measured accurately with high reproducibility, regardless of ventricular morphology. Finally, CMR provides high-resolution, isotropic, three-dimensional datasets. This allows for reconstruction of data in any imaging plane, facilitating visualisation of complex cardiac anomalies, without the use of ionising radiation.

The majority of CMR images are acquired using cardiac (ECG) gating during a single breath-hold to reduce the artefacts associated with cardiac and respiratory motion. For a complex case, CMR is performed over approximately 1 hour, though this time can be considerably reduced if a focused question is being addressed or by the incorporation of newer real-time sequences.

Imaging sequences can be broadly divided into:

- 'Black-blood' spin-echo images, where signal from blood is nulled and thus not seen—for accurate anatomical imaging.
- 'White-blood' gradient-echo or steady-state free precession images, where a positive signal from blood is returned—for anatomical, cine imaging and quantification of ventricular volumes, mass and function.
- Phase-contrast imaging, where velocity information is encoded for quantification of vascular flow.
- Contrast-enhanced MRA, where non-ECG-gated 3D data are acquired after gadolinium contrast medium has been administered for thoracic vasculature imaging.

All these sequences can be acquired in a single breath-hold, reducing the overall time in the CMR machine, and enabling the acquisition of accurate data in the majority of patients. Importantly, 'white-blood' cine images can be acquired in a continuous short-axis stack along the heart, enabling accurate quantification of right and left ventricular function.

Imaging should be performed in the presence of a cardiovascular MRI clinician in conjunction with an MRI technician to ensure that the appropriate clinical questions are answered. A comprehensive treatment of cardiovascular MRI is provided by the textbook by Bogaert and colleagues.[3]

Computed Tomography

CT is now well established for the assessment of the thoracic vasculature and large and small airways. Recent advances in multidetector CT (MDCT) have resulted in significant advances in spatial and temporal resolution. This has facilitated coronary artery imaging and gated cine imaging for ventricular function. The rapid acquisition times for MDCT have made it an attractive imaging investigation for CHD. Data can be acquired in a single breath-hold, which in younger patients may obviate the need for general anaesthesia. There are two main disadvantages of MDCT compared with CMR imaging. The first is the use of ionising radiation. This can be kept to a minimum, by using low kV, low mA acquisitions, with current modulation, and image acquisition over the minimal area of interest. Using such protocols, our mean dose for non-cardiac-gated cardiovascular MDCT in children is 1.2 ± 0.57 mSv. This equates to approximately 60 chest radiographs (standard PA chest radiograph = 0.02 mSv) or 6 months of background radiation exposure (UK average background radiation = 2.2 mSv per year). Furthermore, in critically ill patients the ability to perform a rapid examination without the need for general anaesthesia or even sedation may be more crucial, as the risk of prolonged sedation may be greater than that of radiation. The second disadvantage of current MDCT techniques is that easy quantification of cardiac function (at high heart rates) and arterial flow are not possible, especially when compared with cardiac-gated MR imaging. In our own practice, we currently use MDCT for the following indications in patients with CHD:

- Patients with vascular rings where airway information is very important.
- Patients undergoing assessment of pulmonary atresia with major aorta pulmonary collateral arteries (MAPCAs). CT before cardiac catheterisation will identify the number of large aorto-pulmonary collaterals and the presence of any central pulmonary arteries; this information is used to guide cardiac catheterisation. The main purpose of the cardiac catheterisation is to identify the temporal distribution of blood flow and define which areas of the lungs the pulmonary arteries, the MAPCAs, or both, supply. This significantly aids surgical planning for unifocalisation.
- Patients with abnormalities of pulmonary venous drainage—CMR of the pulmonary veins can be problematic.
- Patients with vascular stents, e.g. coarctation stents requiring postoperative assessment for pseudoaneurysms.
- Patients requiring investigation of coronary artery stenoses.
- Contraindication to MR imaging—permanent pacemaker, defibrillators, cerebral aneurysm clips, etc.

Conventional Radiology

Although CHD may be suspected on the basis of the chest X-ray (CXR), the technique precludes the detailed morphological assessment necessary for diagnosis and determination of specific underlying pathology should be de-emphasised.

The diagnostic accuracy of CXR in the assessment of infants with asymptomatic murmurs is poor; combined data from studies indicates the sensitivity and specificity are 0.29 (CI 0.24–0.35) and 0.86 (CI 0.83–0.88), respectively.[4,5] Even amongst experienced specialist paediatric radiologists the sensitivity is only 0.30 and amongst radiology trainees it is 0.16. Despite its poor performance as a screening tool, CHD may be suspected on the basis of a CXR due to higher specificity; but false-positive rates are significant.

The CXR, however, is not dispensable, and remains important in the subsequent management of patients with CHD, particularly in three situations:

1. Postoperatively, for identification of the position of intravascular catheters, chest drains and endotracheal tubes (Fig. 13-1A);
2. Identification of postoperative complications: consolidation, collapse, pleural effusion, pneumothorax, pneumomediastinum or pericardial collections (Fig. 13-1B); and
3. Perioperative, *physiological* assessment of the lungs and cardiomediastinal contour (see below).

Diagnostic Features

The ubiquity of the CXR in clinical practice warrants discussion of the diagnostic features that should prompt

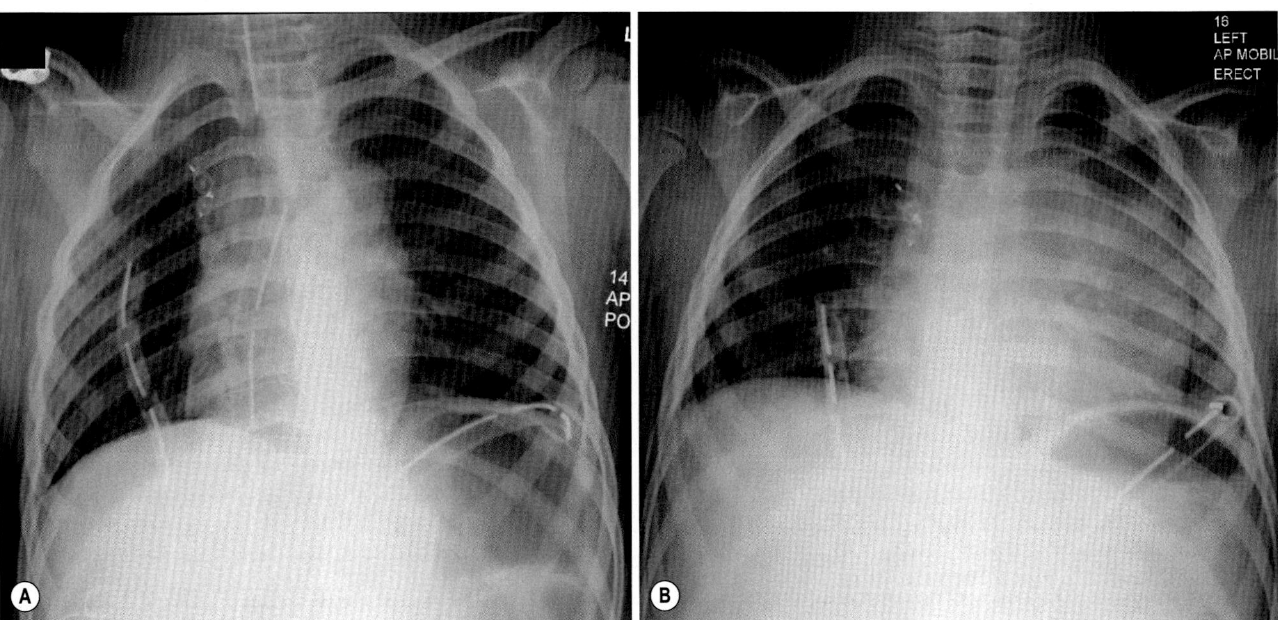

FIGURE 13-1 ■ **Perioperative CXR.** (A) A 3-year-old patient following total cavopulmonary connection surgery, postoperative CXR demonstrating tube positions in intensive care. Note two chest and one mediastinal drains, endotracheal tube and veno-venous collateral occluder device (right upper zone). (B) Third postoperative day following extubation and removal of mediastinal drain. Note change in cardiomediastinal contour caused by large pericardial clot, requiring evacuation.

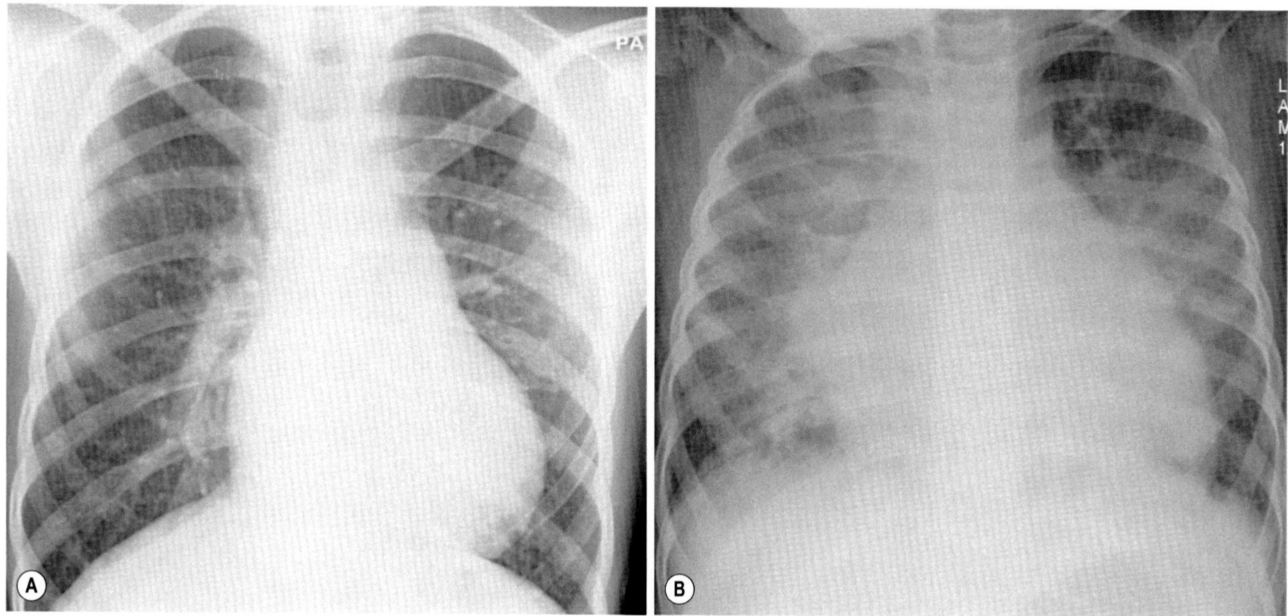

FIGURE 13-2 ■ **Physiological assessment using CXR.** (A) *Pulmonary plethora* in a patient with a VSD. Note the increased number and size of discrete vessels without haziness. (B) *Pulmonary oedema* in a supine patient with cor triatriatum (membranous obstruction to LA outflow) resulting in increased pulmonary venous pressure. Note cardiomegaly, perihilar alveolar haziness/consolidation and peribronchial cuffing.

suspicion of CHD. It is suggested that the reader avoid such terms as 'boot-shaped' or 'snowman' typically associated with specific lesions, when reporting images, as they can be misleading and often erroneous. More appropriate is a descriptive consideration of the cardiomediastinal contour and lungs, attempting to evaluate the predominant physiological profile discussed above. The reader may find it helpful to read this section in conjunction with the section on clinical presentation.

The Pulmonary Vasculature

Radiologically Normal Pulmonary Vascularity. Radiologically normal pulmonary vascularity is present in CHD if the patient is not in heart failure, if no large shunt is present, and if there is not a significant reduction in pulmonary blood flow, e.g. mild pulmonary stenosis. The pulmonary vasculature may, however, look normal on the conventional radiograph even in the presence of significant CHD.

Increased Pulmonary Perfusion (Pulmonary Plethora). Increased pulmonary perfusion (pulmonary plethora) is recognised by enlarged central and peripheral pulmonary arteries and veins in all zones (Fig. 13-2A), as occurs in situations with increased pulmonary blood flow: ASD, VSD and PDA with large left-to-right shunts (Table 13-1).

Decreased Pulmonary Perfusion (Oligaemia). Decreased pulmonary perfusion (oligaemia) (Fig. 13-3) is due to a reduction in pulmonary blood flow and is typically a phenomenon of cyanotic CHD. Dark lungs and sparse pulmonary vascular markings suggest the diagnosis. Image acquisition must be optimal, as overexposure will significantly confound correct interpretation. Pulmonary blood flow may be impaired by obstruction to normal flow through the right heart, e.g. tricuspid atresia, tetralogy of Fallot, pulmonary stenosis (Table 13-2).

TABLE 13-1 **Increased Pulmonary Perfusion (Plethora)**

Level of Shunt	Cardiac Lesion
Atria	Ostium secundum ASD[a]
	Ostium primum ASD (partial AVSD)[a]
	Sinus venosus defect
	Anomalous pulmonary venous drainage (partial;[a] total[b])
Atrioventricular valves	Complete AVSD
	Partial AVSD[a]
Ventricle	VSD[a]
	Double outlet ventricle[b]
	Single ventricle[b]
Great vessels	PDA[a]
	Aortopulmonary window
	Common arterial trunk[b]
	Coronary artery-RV fistula
	Transposition of great arteries[b]
	Systemic-to-pulmonary artery shunts (unrestrictive BT shunt)
Other	Vein of Galen malformation

[a]Common cause of plethora without cyanosis.
[b]Common cause of plethora with cyanosis.

Pulmonary Venous Congestion and Oedema. Pulmonary venous congestion and oedema (Fig. 13-2B) in CHD is due to functional or anatomical obstruction

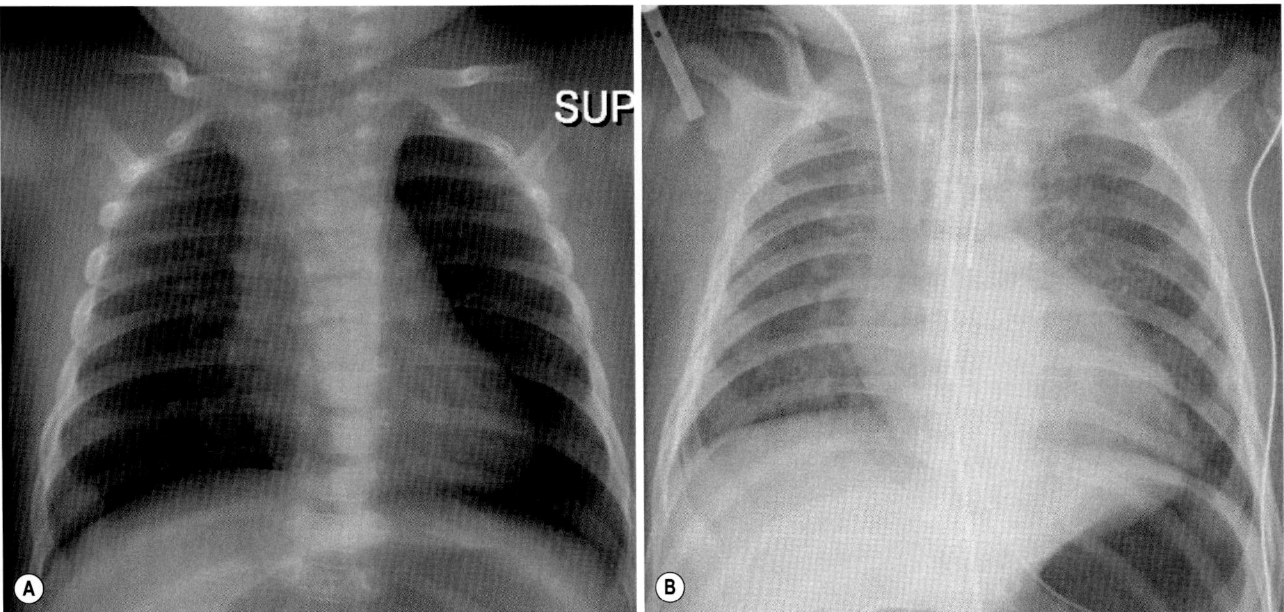

FIGURE 13-3 ■ **Pulmonary oligaemia.** (A) Supine AP CXR, in an 8-week-old patient with tetralogy of Fallot with severe pulmonary stenosis and cyanosis. Note black lungs with sparse, small-calibre vessels. (B) Supine AP CXR, in the same patient following construction of a right modified Blalock–Taussig (BT) shunt on the next day. Note the increased size of the left cardiac contour due to increased LV filling, increased pulmonary vascular markings, now plethoric, suggestive of high pulmonary blood flow arising from the shunt. Indeed, the patient had compromised systemic perfusion due to redistribution of cardiac output to the lungs, necessitating clipping the shunt to reduce its calibre.

TABLE 13-2 **Neonatal Pulmonary Oligaemia**

Level	Cardiac Lesion
Tricuspid valve	Tricuspid atresia Tricuspid stenosis Ebstein's anomaly
Right ventricular outflow	Pulmonary infundibular stenosis (severe) Pulmonary valvar stenosis (severe) Tetralogy of Fallot
Pulmonary artery	Pulmonary artery atresia Right or left pulmonary artery interruption (differential lung oligaemia) Peripheral pulmonary artery stenosis (regional oligaemia) Transposition of great arteries with pulmonary valve stenosis

TABLE 13-3 **Pulmonary Oedema and Venous Congestion**

Level	Cardiac Lesion
Pulmonary veins	Obstructed TAPVD Pulmonary vein stenosis
Left atrium	Cor triatriatum Mitral valve stenosis/atresia Left atrioventricular valve regurgitation
Left ventricle	Hypoplastic left ventricle LV endocardial fibro-elastosis Cardiomyopathy LV ischaemia—aberrant left coronary artery from pulmonary artery (ALCAPA)
Aorta	Aortic stenosis/atresia Coarctation/interruption of the aorta
Non-cardiac pulmonary oedema	Asphyxia Acute lung injury Intravenous overhydration

to pulmonary venous return. In addition to oedema formation due to increased transvascular pressure gradients, consideration should be given to other pathological processes such as increased vessel leakiness, for example due to acute lung injuries (Table 13-3). The usual adult pattern of basal oedema, resulting in alveolar hypoxia and constriction of lower pulmonary vasculature and redirection to the apices, does not apply to the supine infant. As pulmonary venous pressure increases, there is progressive accumulation of radiological signs, beginning with redistribution (in older children/adults), progressing to interstitial oedema (perivascular haziness, peribronchial cuffing, Kerley B lines, subpleural effusions) and finally migration of extravasated fluid centrally resulting in perihilar alveolar consolidation.

Systemic-to-Pulmonary Collateral Vessels. Abnormal systemic arterial connections to the pulmonary vasculature may occur as an adaptive mechanism to inadequate pulmonary blood flow. This usually occurs in the setting of pulmonary atresia associated with VSD, in which the RV and pulmonary arteries are not in continuity; instead, discrete MAPCAs and non-discrete networks of bronchial arteries are the source of pulmonary blood flow. It may also occur during staged management of the single ventricle. They may be recognisable by a nodular lung pattern in the central third of the lung parenchyma, with many small, rounded, opacities representing enlarged bronchial arteries seen end-on.

Pulmonary Arterial Hypertension. Pulmonary arterial hypertension may complicate unrepaired CHD. Increased pulmonary blood flow due to left-to-right shunting in unrepaired ASD, VSD or PDA gradually causes changes in the pulmonary vasculature, which over time leads to increased pulmonary vascular resistance and overt hypertension. The central pulmonary arteries enlarge and the peripheral pulmonary arteries become smaller than normal. In cases where pulmonary pressure exceeds systemic pressure, shunt reversal occurs, resulting in cyanosis, as occurs in Eisenmenger's syndrome.

Heart Size, Shape and Position

Abnormalities of the position of the cardiac apex, aortic arch, liver and stomach may be determined from examination of the CXR: the presence of situs inversus and left aortic arch may be discerned; however, this may or may not be associated with underlying CHD. Some assessment of global and regional heart size is possible (Fig. 13-3B), and should be described; however, the limitations of CXR in this regard should be considered. In a study comparing echocardiographical assessment of cardiac enlargement in 95 consecutive paediatric outpatients, the sensitivity of the CXR to identify cardiomegaly was only 58.8% (95% CI 32.9–81.6), specificity was 92.3% (95% CI 84.0–97.1).

SPECIFIC LESIONS

In the following discussion lesions have been classed as acyanotic and cyanotic for convenience. It is important to understand, however, that in various situations a lesion typically described in this way may present in the opposite manner, perhaps due to the presence or absence of a particular morphological feature, or the imposition of altered haemodynamics such as pulmonary hypertension. For example, tetralogy of Fallot with minimal outflow tract obstruction may have no cyanosis, or a VSD that is so large as to facilitate complete intracardiac mixing may produce cyanosis. Further, certain lesions do not fit easily into either category; for example, Ebstein's anomaly of the tricuspid valve when mild is acyanotic, but in its severe form is cyanotic. Similarly, congenitally corrected transposition of the great arteries, although acyanotic, is better understood when discussed alongside its cyanotic relative, simple transposition of the great arteries. For further illustrations and images, the reader is referred to the imaging atlas on congenital heart disease by Sridharan et al.[6]

ACYANOTIC LESIONS

Septal Defects

Atrial Septal Defects

Atrial septal defects are the most common congenital heart defect detected in adults. Irrespective of their type and location, they cause left-to-right shunting at the atrial level. This leads to atrial dilation, predisposing to tachyarrthymias, and right ventricular volume overload. The presence of an ASD is also an independent risk factor for thromboembolic stroke. This is due to the ability of thromboemboli, originating either in the right atrium or venous vasculature, to pass through the ASD into the systemic circulation.

Atrial septal defects are, anatomically and developmentally, a heterogeneous group of lesions (Fig. 13-4A). The specific nature of the ASD influences the natural history and management of this disease. Ostium secundum defects make up 80% of ASDs and are located in the fossa ovalis (Fig. 13-4B). These defects are due to failure of the septum secundum to form closure of the ostium secundum. Other forms of ASD are more properly termed inter-atrial communications, because they do not occur in the true morphological atrial septum. The ostium primum defect is actually a component of a common atrioventricular junction, also known as an atrioventricular septal defect. An AVSD usually occurs together with some degree of atrioventricular valve abnormality. The sinus venosus defect is found at the junction of the right atrium and either one of the caval veins (Fig. 13-4C). This type of ASD is less common, and is always associated with partial anomalous pulmonary venous drainage. The least common type of ASD occurs in the coronary sinus, and is termed an unroofed coronary sinus. In this case, there is deficiency of the coronary sinus wall in as it passes behind the left atrium, allowing shunting from left to right through the coronary sinus itself.

The management of atrial septal defects has changed in recent years, particularly with the increasing use of transcatheter ASD closure devices. Previously, surgical closure was only considered when a large left-to-right shunt led to RV volume overload, atrial dilation and symptoms. However, with the advent of transcatheter techniques, management has become more aggressive. Transcatheter techniques are only viable in patients with small to medium-sized ostium secundum defects that have adequate margins with which to anchor the device. Deficiency of the anterior or postero-inferior rim of the defect usually precludes transcatheter closure. Patients with large ostium secundum defects, or defects with deficiency of the anterior or postero-inferior rims, or with sinus venosus lesions, usually require operative repair. The clinical aim is to complete ASD closure before development of cardiac failure or atrial dilation, and timing of intervention depends on the haemodynamic status of the patient. Thus, evaluation of ASDs requires definition of type and location of the defect, quantification of the net shunt (pulmonary flow: systemic flow ($Q_p : Q_s$)), detection of any intra-atrial thrombus, assessment of RV volume and systolic function and visualisation of the pulmonary

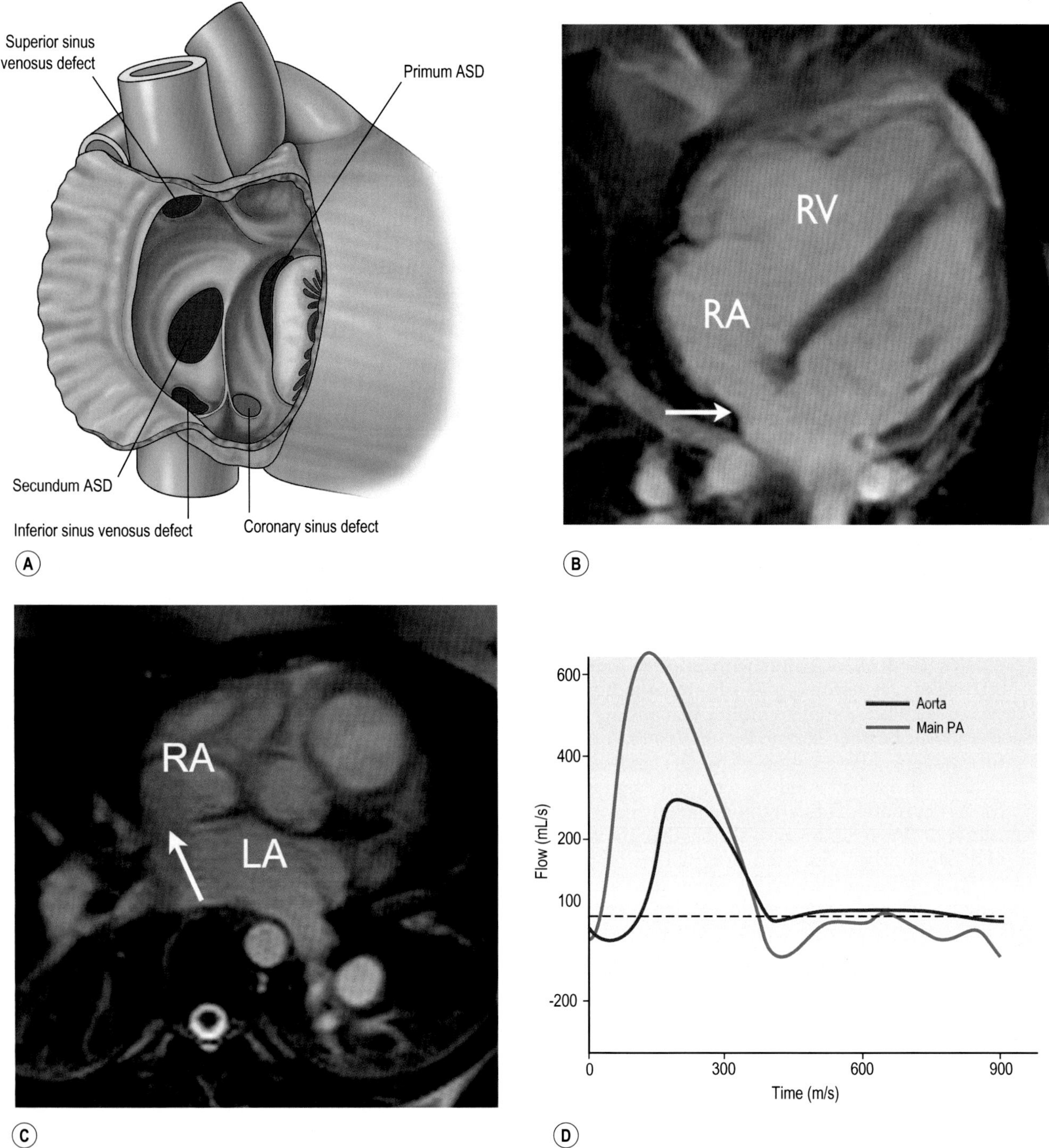

FIGURE 13-4 ■ **Atrial septal defects.** (A) Schematic drawing of ASD positions. (B) b-SSFP CMR image. Four-chamber view showing a large secundum ASD with posterior extension. The absence of a posterior rim (arrow) precludes insertion of an ASD closure device. Note the dilated right atrium (RA), and right ventricle (RV), and flattened interventricular septum. (C) b-SSFP CMR image. Axial view showing a large superior sinus venosus defect, with PAPVD of the right upper and right middle pulmonary veins, straddling the deficient atrial septum (arrow). (D) Plot of instantaneous flow (measured by velocity-encoded phase-contrast MRI) as a function of time showing a left-to-right shunt through an ASD; note increased pulmonary blood flow.

venous anatomy. Furthermore, in patients with ostium secundum defects, special attention must be given to delineating the anatomy of the margins of the defect as this influences planning invasive management.

Transthoracic ultrasound has a limited ability to visualise small ostium secundum and sinus venosus defects. In addition, detection of pulmonary venous abnormalities is technically difficult using the transthoracic approach. Transoesophageal ultrasound is the main imaging technique used to assess ASDs. However, transoesophageal ultrasound cannot be used to quantify the shunt ($Q_p:Q_s$) accurately and it can be difficult to delineate pulmonary venous anatomy. CMR has a significant role to play in the diagnosis and pre-interventional assessment of ASDs.

3D whole-heart techniques, with isotropic resolution, allow accurate multi-planar reformatting with no loss of resolution. These techniques allow 3D rendering of the atrial anatomy. Multi-slice 2D gradient echo techniques can be used to assess the dynamic 3D anatomy of the defect, and phase-contrast through-plane flow techniques can accurately size the cross-sectional dimensions of the defect, or diagnose multiple or fenestrated defects.

Haemodynamic assessment is also an important part of the evaluation of ASDs. Invasive catheterisation has previously been used to accurately quantify left-to-right shunts. Quantification of left-to-right shunts using velocity-encoded phase-contrast MR compares well to invasive catheterisation results (Fig. 13-4D). It has the benefit of being non-invasive and does not require exposure to ionising radiation. Ventricular overload can also be accurately assessed using multi-slice b-SSFP short-axis imaging and can give important information influencing the timing of intervention.

Key Imaging Goals

- Assess defect location, diameter and margin size—suitability for device anchorage
- Quantify right heart volume and function—assess volume overload
- Quantify shunt (Fig. 13-4D)
- Look for sinus venosus defect which has an associated partially anomalous pulmonary venous drainage.

Atrioventricular Septal Defects

An AVSD is a lesion caused by a deficiency of the tissues that normally interpose the atrial and ventricular chambers (Figs. 13-5A and C). The involved tissues include the atrial primum septum, the atrioventricular valves and the inlet portion of the ventricular septum. The feature shared by all AVSDs is a common AV junction guarded by a common AV valve, which may have either one or two orifices (Fig. 13-5A).

The common AV junction can be discerned by the loss of the usual 'offset' of the tricuspid and mitral valves in the normal heart. The valve, even when it has two orifices, is no longer referred to as a mitral and tricuspid valve; instead the valves are called left and right atrioventricular valves. The common valve typically has five leaflets, referred to as the superior bridging, right anterosuperior, right inferior/mural, inferior bridging and left mural leaflets (Figs. 13-5A and B).

The relative deficiency of the septal structures and the number of valve orifices gives rise to the classification as complete (both atrial and ventricular septal defects and single valve orifice), intermediate/incomplete (ventricular septal defect with two valve orifices) and partial (atrial septal defect with two valve orifaces, also called an ostium primum ASD). Another clinically useful description is the relative size of the ventricular chambers, allowing for classification as balanced (equal-sized ventricles) or unbalanced (disproportionate ventricles). AVSD can be associated with other cardiac abnormalities, including tetralogy of Fallot, subaortic stenosis, atrial isomerism and ventricular hypoplasia, which modify the presentation, prognosis and surgical management.

The diagnosis of AVSD is made in the neonatal period on the basis of transthoracic ultrasound. Other imaging investigations are usually not required. Surgical repair is carried out around 3–4 months of age and certainly before 6 months of age to prevent the development of pulmonary vascular disease. The repair involves closing the septal defects and creating competent left and right valves from the common atrioventricular valve tissue. The association of AVSD with trisomy 21 is well known; repair in this group is associated with *lower* mortality than non-trisomy 21.

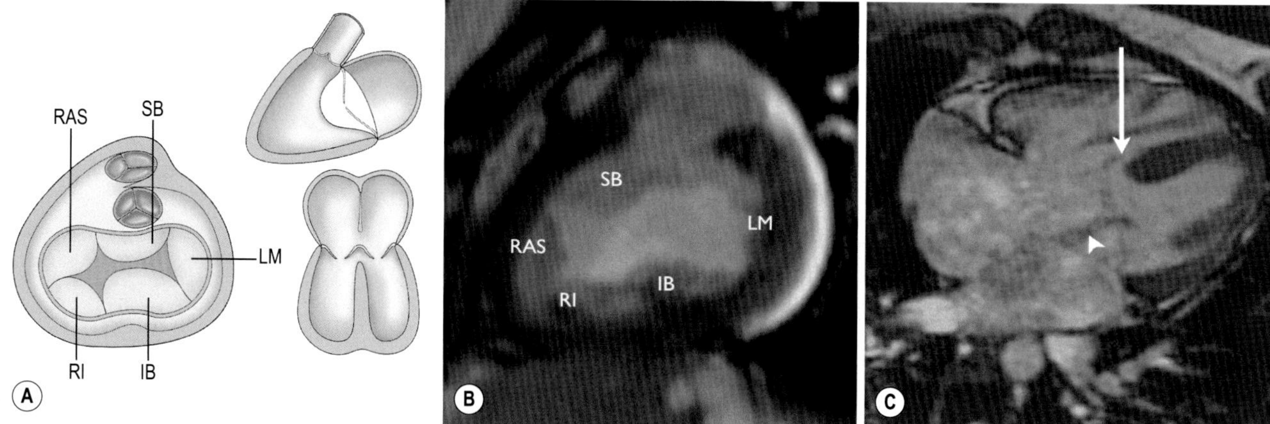

FIGURE 13-5 ■ **Atrioventricular septal defects.** (A) Schematic drawing of orthogonal views of a common atrioventricular valve: short-axis view from below (left), long-axis (top right), 4-chamber (bottom right). (B) Valve view showing a complete AVSD in a patient with right atrial isomerism and double outlet RV. Valve leaflets: SB = superior bridging leaflet, RAS = right anterosuperior leaflet, RI = right inferior (mural) leaflet, IB = inferior bridging leaflet, LM = left mural leaflet. (C) b-SSFP CMR image showing 4-chamber view of a balanced complete AVSD. There are large atrial and ventricular components. Note the VSD (arrow) and moderate left AV valve regurgitation (arrowhead).

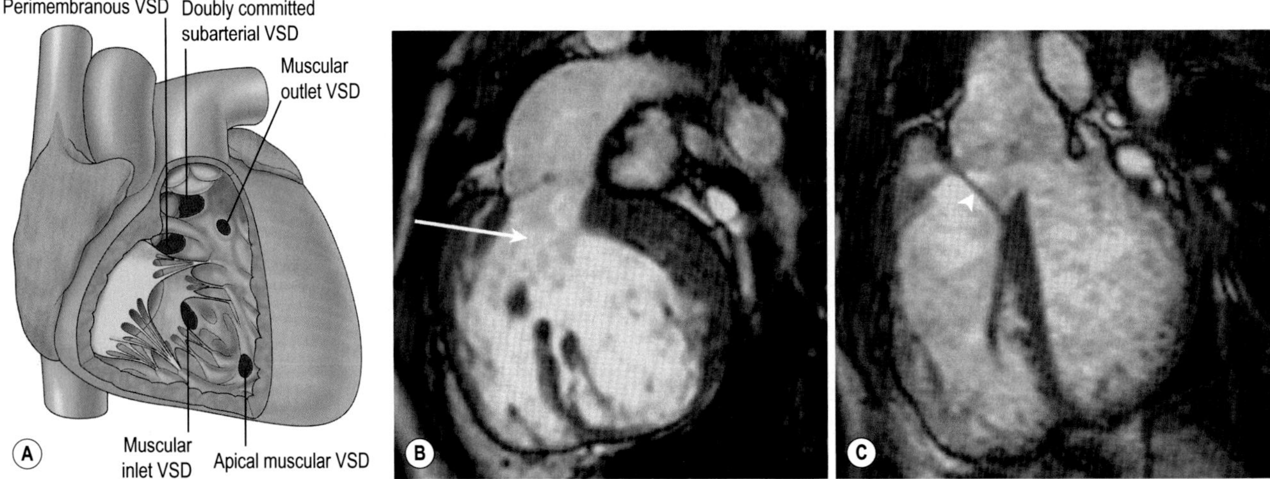

FIGURE 13-6 ■ **Ventricular septal defects.** (A) Schematic drawing of VSD positions viewed from the right ventricular aspect. (B) b-SSFP CMR image of a VSD (arrow) with overriding aorta in a patient with tetralogy of Fallot. (C) Coronal oblique view following correction with VSD patch (arrowhead).

Additional imaging techniques including CMR may be useful in the long-term management of patients with repaired AVSD, including surveillance for important late complications such as atrioventricular valve regurgitation (Fig. 13-5C).

Key Imaging Goals

- Assess ventricular proportion—unbalanced ventricle may not be suitable for biventricular repair
- Assess valve structure
- Identify associated abnormalities—isomerisim of the atrial appendages
- Quantify ventricular volume and function
- Quantify shunt
- Evaluate AV valve regurgitation.

Ventricular Septal Defects

The ventricular septum is a complex, almost helical 3D structure. Ventricular septal defects are the commonest form of CHD in childhood. Physiologically the defect causes left-to-right shunting, and the magnitude of the shunt determines the signs and symptoms. The volume of the shunt depends on the size of the defect and the relative resistances of the systemic and pulmonary circulations; at birth the pulmonary vascular resistance (PVR) is high, reducing the magnitude of the shunt (it also remains high for longer in patients with left-to-right shunts, explaining why infants may initially be asymptomatic). The degree of shunting is usually estimated by measuring the velocity of blood crossing the defect by ultrasound; if PVR is normal, higher-velocity jets indicate that the expected pressure difference between chambers is preserved, and are termed 'restrictive' defects; low-velocity jets suggest the LV and RV have similar pressures and that the defect is 'unrestrictive'. The exact volume of the shunt cannot be determined accurately by ultrasound, but, as described above for ASDs, it can be measured using velocity-encoded phase-contrast CMR (Fig. 13-4D).

The commonest location is the perimembranous region, accounting for 80% of VSDs; many small perimembranous VSDs close spontaneously. The rest of the ventricular septum is muscular and has three components: inlet, outlet (subarterial) and midmuscular regions (Fig. 13-6A). The appropriate management depends on the type and size of the defect.

Ultrasound is the mainstay of diagnosis; however, CMR can provide accurate 2D and 3D images that are particularly useful in complex defects. Multi-slice 2D gradient-echo techniques can be used to assess the dynamic 3D anatomy of the defect; however, multi-slice techniques suffer from poor through-plane resolution. Three-dimensional b-SSFP techniques with isotropic resolution allow accurate multi-planar reformatting, permitting 3D rendering of the ventricular anatomy. Image acquisition during the diastolic period is useful in assessing the anatomy of a VSD and its relationship to valvular structures (Fig. 13-6B).

Key Imaging Goals

- Assess position and size of defect(s)
- If outlet VSD, describe commitment to a particular vessel: subaortic, subpulmonary (Fig. 13-6B)
- Quantify shunt (note LV stroke volume contributes to the PA forward flow during systole)
- Quantify ventricular volume
- Assess aortic valve regurgitation and associated abnormalities
- Post repair, assess integrity of VSD patch (Fig. 13-6C).

Abnormalities of the Great Vessels

Patent Ductus Arteriosus

The arterial duct, in fetal life, connects the pulmonary artery to the aortic arch, allowing blood ejected from the

RV to bypass the high-resistance pulmonary circulation and enter the descending aorta. The ductal tissue constricts after birth, in response to changes in the blood gas composition. If the duct fails to close beyond the first few days of life, it is termed a PDA. The PDA permits a left-to-right shunt from the aorta into the pulmonary artery throughout the cardiac cycle. This leads to increased pulmonary blood flow, and dilation of the left heart. The length and diameter of the PDA, and the relative resistances of the pulmonary and systemic circulations, determine the volume of the shunt, which in turn determines the signs and symptoms of the lesion.

A common neonatal problem is the failure of the ductus arteriosus to close in the premature infant. In this situation, a PDA can confound the management of the lung disease associated with prematurity and can prolong ventilation. It can be comprehensively assessed by ultrasound in infancy, but in older patients the duct may not be easily demonstrated. CMR may be required to visualise and quantify the shunt in the same way as described for ASD and VSD.

Key Imaging Goals

- Assess position and size of defect(s)
- Quantify shunt
- Quantify volume overload
- Identify any associated intracardiac abnormalities.

Coarctation of the Aorta

Coarctation of the aorta is a luminal narrowing of a short section of the aorta (Fig. 13-7). It occurs most commonly at the site of insertion of the ductus arteriosus, and is thought to develop due to the presence of excessively integrated ductal tissue around the aortic isthmus, which contracts along with the ductus arteriosus at the time of birth. In severe coarctation, systemic perfusion will be compromised with ductal closure in infancy, due to increased luminal narrowing and the loss of the anatomical bypass provided by the duct itself. In less severe coarctation, the body maintains perfusion by renal mechanisms, resulting in systemic hypertension manifested proximal to the coarctation. Collateral arterial vessels develop over time to maintain lower body perfusion as the patient grows (Figs. 13-7A and C). Patients may present with unexplained hypertension as a teenager or adult and are at increased risk of the attendant micro- and macrovascular complications.

Treatment in infancy is usually by surgical excision of the narrowing, but in older subjects balloon angioplasty may be undertaken. Patients remain at increased risk of hypertension even if repaired in infancy.

Ultrasound is used in the initial diagnosis of infants, children and adults. Typical echocardiographic features include increased systolic and diastolic velocities across the stenosis (Fig. 13-7D). CMR or CT may be required postoperatively to establish if there is re-coarctation (up to 35% of patients in some series), aneurysmal dilatation, or LV hypertrophy secondary to hypertension. CMR is preferred to CT if there are no contraindications, as this reduces population radiation.

Imaging is crucial to establish the location and degree of stenosis, length of coarctation segment (Fig. 13-7B), associated aortic arch involvement (such as tubular hypoplasia), the collateral pathways (internal mammary and posterior mediastinal arteries), presence and relationship to an aberrant subclavian artery, post-stenotic dilatation and left ventricular hypertrophy.

Three-dimensional contrast-enhanced MRA can show the severity and extent of involvement (Fig. 13-7C). Assessment of collateral flow by measuring flows in the proximal and descending aorta can be performed. Reassessment of collateral flow following treatment can also be used to assess the success of the treatment. In patients with metal stents, high flip angle gradient-echo sequences can be used to overcome metal artefact and assess luminal narrowing.

CMR can also be used to assess secondary pathological features in patients with coarctation: e.g. aortic root dilatation associated with a bicuspid aortic valve (frequency in coarctation of 15%); aortic valve incompetence and stenosis; and ventricular function and left ventricular mass (an indirect indicator of increased left ventricular afterload).

Key Imaging Goals

- Describe location and degree of stenosis (MR flow mapping), length of coarctation segment
- Look for aortic root involvement and post–stenotic dilatation
- Assess aortic valve—often bicuspid
- Delineate collateral vessels
- Describe head and neck anatomy
- Assess ventricular function, volume and LV mass
- After repair, also look for re-coarctation or pseudoaneurysm
- Assess calibre of stented vessels (high flip angle gradient echo, or CT)
- Ultrasound—quantify Doppler-derived gradient across stenosis and identification of 'diastolic tail' on continuous-wave Doppler flow profile (Fig. 13-7D).

Interrupted Aortic Arch

Interrupted aortic arch results from a structural discontinuity between the ascending and descending aorta. The site of interruption relative to the brachiocephalic arteries forms the basis of classification. There is a high incidence of DiGeorge syndrome, which is also associated with variable thymic hypoplasia, the presence of which can be examined. Physiologically, systemic blood flow is provided distal to the interruption by deoxygenated blood via a patent arterial duct. The lower body will be cyanosed, and circulation may be comprised following duct closure. The site and length of interruption and any associated anomalies can be demonstrated well by CMR. Following repair, assessment is similar to that of coarctation. It is important to interrogate the repair site for residual narrowing, assess for the presence of LVOT obstruction due to posterior deviation of the outlet septum, and look for residual intracardiac shunts. Three-dimensional MRA and 3D whole-heart imaging are

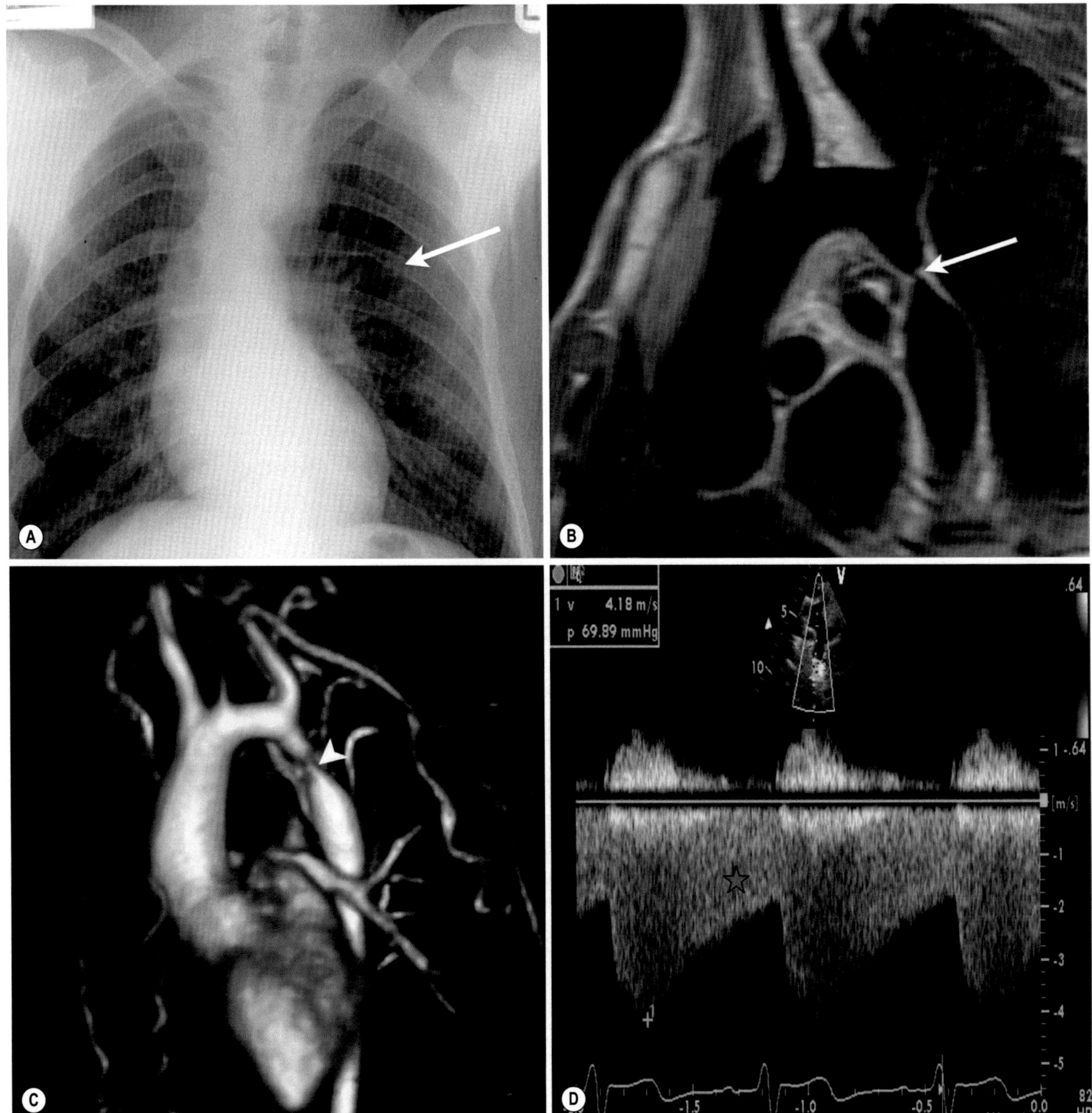

FIGURE 13-7 ■ Severe coarctation of the aorta. (A) PA CXR showing characteristic bilateral rib-notching (arrow), secondary to the development of collateral circulation. (B) Black-blood, spin-echo, oblique sagittal image through the aorta showing a tight discrete coarctation (arrow). (C) Volume-rendered 3D reconstruction of MR angiography showing a tight coarctation (arrowhead), and multiple enlarged collateral vessels. (D) Echocardiographic continuous-wave Doppler profile of the coarctation region, demonstrating increased velocity across the stenosis, 4.18 m/s (blue cross), corresponding to a pressure gradient of 70 mmHg from the simplified Bernoulli equation. There is also markedly increased diastolic velocity, characteristic in coarctation, termed 'diastolic tail' (red star).

particularly useful. Cine imaging will identify regions of flow acceleration.

Key Imaging Goals

- Describe the site of interruption and relationship of head and neck vessels
  - Type A—interruption distal to the left subclavian artery (29% of cases)
  - Type B—interruption between the left common carotid and the left common carotid (70% of cases)
  - Type C—interruption between the innominate artery and the left common carotid (1% of cases)
- Evaluate additional arch hypoplasia
- Measure aortic cross-sectional area proximal and distal to the interruption

- Measure the distance of the interruption gap
- Identify associated anomalies—VSD, LVOT obstruction, TGA, common arterial trunk
- Look for thymus—absence supports a diagnosis of DiGeorge syndrome.

Abnormalities of the Aortic Arch and Vascular Rings

The aortic arch connects the ascending aorta to the descending aorta. Abnormalities of this vascular section include disorders of sidedness. Arch sidedness refers to the side of the trachea that the aortic arch passes as it crosses a mainstem bronchus: there are three variations, left, right and double. In certain circumstances, the morphological pattern of the aortic arch and related structures (its branches or the ductus/ligamentum arteriosus) may produce a vascular ring, which can compress the trachea or oesophagus, producing symptoms of stridor or dysphagia. This usually involves the retro-oesophageal course of either the descending aorta or an aberrant subclavian artery combined with a ligamentum arteriosus on the opposite side of the arch, although non-ring structures such as anomalous origin of the left pulmonary artery from the right pulmonary artery or 'pulmonary artery sling' may also cause vascular compression.

Cross-sectional imaging (CMR or CT) can be regarded as the gold standard for the assessment of the aortic arch. For CMR, imaging begins with a simple transverse stack from the level of the larynx to the diaphragm. This information is augmented by 3D MRA. Using this information, patent vascular structures compressing the trachea/oesophagus can easily be identified. It is important to remember that some important components of a vascular ring may not be patent, and thus remain invisible on imaging—for example, the ligamentum arteriosus. However, clues to these structures often remain and include: dimples opposite the side of the aortic arch, a diverticulum opposite the side of the arch or if the proximal descending aorta descends on the opposite side of the arch.

Key Imaging Goals

- Describe side of aortic arch
- Delineate location and course of branches
- Identify presence of associated PDA, or dimple suggestive of ligamentum arteriosus
- Assess presence and level of compression of oesophageal/tracheal compression
- Identify associated abnormalities.

Valvular Heart Disease

Aortic Valve Disease

Congenital aortic valve disease is predominated by stenosis, which may occur at subvalvular, valvular or supravalvular levels. The haemodynamic consequence of aortic stenosis (AS) is pressure loading of the LV and the development of secondary concentric hypertrophy. Aortic regurgitation is usually a manifestation of treated aortic stenosis (e.g. balloon angioplasty) or secondary to pathological dilatation of the aortic root, which can occur in connective tissue disease (e.g. Marfan's syndrome). The haemodynamic consequence is volume loading of the LV and eccentric hypertrophy (dilatation).

Doppler ultrasound assessment of transvalvular pressure gradient is the commonest technique to assess severity of AS. However, transvalvular pressure gradients are flow dependent and measurement of valve area represents, from a theoretical point of view, the ideal way to quantify AS. However, inaccuracies in both gradients and valve area require consideration of a combination of flow rate, pressure gradient and ventricular function, as well as functional status; several investigations may be ended to elucidate. AS with a valve area < 1.0 cm^2 is considered severe; however, in patients with either unusually small or large body surface area, so-called 'indexed areas' with a cut-off value of 0.6 cm^2/m^2 are helpful. The presence of valvular stenosis can be identified by loss of signal on CMR cine images. Velocity mapping can be used to establish an accurate peak velocity across the stenosis and planimetry can assess the aortic valve area.

Ultrasound is also used routinely to assess AR, in particular using colour Doppler (to determine extension and width of regurgitant jet) and continuous-wave Doppler (to assess the rate of decline of aortic regurgitant flow and holodiastolic flow reversal in the descending aorta). However, these are semiquantitative measures; CMR permits precise assessment of the regurgitant volume and assessment of the volume and function of the eccentrically hypertrophied LV. It can also allow assessment of the effective regurgitant orifice area.

Subvalvular aortic stenosis is the least common form of AS and is more commonly caused by hypertrophic cardiomyopathy; however, it may occasionally be seen following repair of atrioventricular septal defects. Valvular aortic stenosis covers a broad spectrum of anomalies ranging from critical aortic stenosis presenting with compromised systemic perfusion in infancy sometimes associated with the hypoplastic left heart syndrome, to mild aortic stenosis due to a bicuspid aortic valve. Supravalvular aortic stenosis is a rare lesion that is typically associated with underlying Williams (Williams–Beuren) syndrome, a genetic disorder of the connective tissue protein elastin. Elastin is responsible for the normal distensibility of the aorta during systole and its subsequent recoil during diastole. In Williams–Beuren syndrome the reduced net deposition of arterial wall elastin leads to increased proliferation of arterial wall smooth muscle cells and multilayer thickening of the media of large arteries; this results in the development of obstructive hyperplastic intimal lesions. A characteristic hourglass narrowing of the aorta develops at the sinotubular junction, but in approximately 30% of cases there is a diffuse, tubular narrowing of the ascending aorta, often extending to the arch and the origin of the brachiocephalic vessels.

Key Imaging Goals

- Assess level and severity of stenosis, subvalvular, valvular, supravalvular—MR flow mapping
- Assess valve leaflet structure (bicuspid valve)
- Quantify aortic regurgitation

- Evaluate aortic root dilatation/hypoplasia
- Quantify LV volume and systolic function
- Measure effective orifice area
- Identify other arterial stenosis—head and neck vessels, renal arteries
- Ultrasound—quantify Doppler-derived gradient across stenosis or width and extent of regurgitant jet in AR.

Pulmonary Valve Disease

Obstructive lesions dominate congenital pulmonary valve disease, similar to the aortic valve, whereas significant pulmonary regurgitation (PR) is most often iatrogenic, following surgical or catheter-based interventions for obstructive lesions. Trivial pulmonary regurgitation is commonly discerned on ultrasound and can be considered physiological. Important congenital pulmonary regurgitation can occur in the absent pulmonary valve syndrome.

According to the site, PS is classified as valvular, subvalvular (infundibular) or supravalvular. They can occur as isolated findings, or in constellation with other lesions such as VSDs or more complex lesions (transposition of the great arteries, tetralogy of Fallot), which may significantly alter the clinical presentation.

Pulmonary stenosis (PS) and pulmonary regurgitation have physiological consequences analogous to aortic valve stenosis and regurgitation. In the former, RV ventricular pressure rises to overcome the obstruction, and maintain stroke volume. Compensatory mechanisms include RV hypertrophy. In PR, volume loading of the RV results in progressive dilatation and dysfunction, which is associated with adverse clinical outcomes.

In pulmonary valve stenosis, the pressure gradient across the valve is used to ascertain severity of the lesion more so than in left-sided valve conditions due in part to the difficulty in obtaining an accurate assessment of pulmonary valve area. The systolic pressure gradient is derived from the transpulmonary velocity flow curve using the simplified Bernoulli equation (pressure gradient = 4 × velocity^2). Mild stenosis is defined by a peak velocity under 3 m/s on continuous-wave Doppler, which corresponds to a peak gradient under 36 mmHg; moderate stenosis is defined by a peak velocity from 3 to 4 m/s, corresponding to a peak gradient between 36 and 64 mmHg; and severe stenosis is characterised by a peak velocity above 4 m/s, corresponding to a peak gradient above 64 mmHg. CMR assessment of PS can be performed in a similar fashion as outlined for AS, above.

CMR is the gold standard for the assessment of pulmonary regurgitation. As described for AS, quantification of the regurgitant volume, and its effect on the RV, can be precisely determined. RV volume and function cannot be accurately assessed by 2D ultrasound, but CMR measurements have been shown to be associated with adverse outcomes and can aid decision making for timing of interventions.

Key Imaging Goals

- Assess level and severity of stenosis, subvalvular, valvular, supravalvular—MR flow mapping
- Assess valve leaflet structure
- Quantify pulmonary regurgitation
- Evaluate main pulmonary artery dilatation/hypoplasia
- Quantify RV volume and systolic function
- Measure effective orifice area
- Ultrasound—quantify Doppler-derived gradient across stenosis.

Ebstein's Anomaly of the Tricupid Valve

Ebstein's anomaly is a congenital abnormality of the tricuspid valve. The septal and mural leaflets are more apically placed than normal, resulting in a malfunctioning, regurgitant tricuspid valve and atrialisation of the proximal right ventricle. The degree of displacement determines the clinical presentation. In severe cases there is gross right atrial enlargement and raised right atrial pressure. The anomaly is usually associated with an ASD and thus right-to-left shunting at the atrial level with subsequent cyanosis may occur. Ebstein's anomaly results in gross enlargement of the cardiac contour with a prominent curved right atrial border on the plain chest radiograph. Treatment is problematical, though expert surgical repair of the tricuspid valve is possible in some centres. Imaging should assess the valve morphology, quantify ventricular function and volume, and quantify right atrial enlargement.

Key Imaging Goals

- Describe apical displacement of the septal leaflet of the tricuspid valve
- Assess mobility of antero-superior and inferior tricuspid valve leaflets
- Note eccentric coaptation
- Quantify tricuspid regurgitation
- Quantify RA dilatation and size of atrialised RV
- Assess RV and LV volume, function and mass
- Quantify right-to-left shunt
- Exclude RVOT obstruction.

Coronary Artery Abnormalities

Anomalous Coronary Arteries

Coronary artery abnormalities are rare. They involve anomalous proximal and epicardial courses of the left coronary artery (LCA) and right coronary artery (RCA) (Fig. 13-8) or rarely anomalous *origin* of the left coronary artery from the pulmonary artery (ALCAPA). Anomalous course is increasingly important when interventions are carried out in close proximity to a coronary artery—for example, percutaneous pulmonary valve implantation into the pulmonary trunk and compression of the left coronary artery. Similarly the course of the coronary arteries is important during surgical repair of tetralogy of Fallot; a transannular patch repair may not be possible if the LCA arises from the RCA and passes anterior to the right ventricular outflow tract.

ALCAPA results in the left coronary artery territory being supplied with low-pressure deoxygenated blood; blood must therefore be supplied by collateralisation

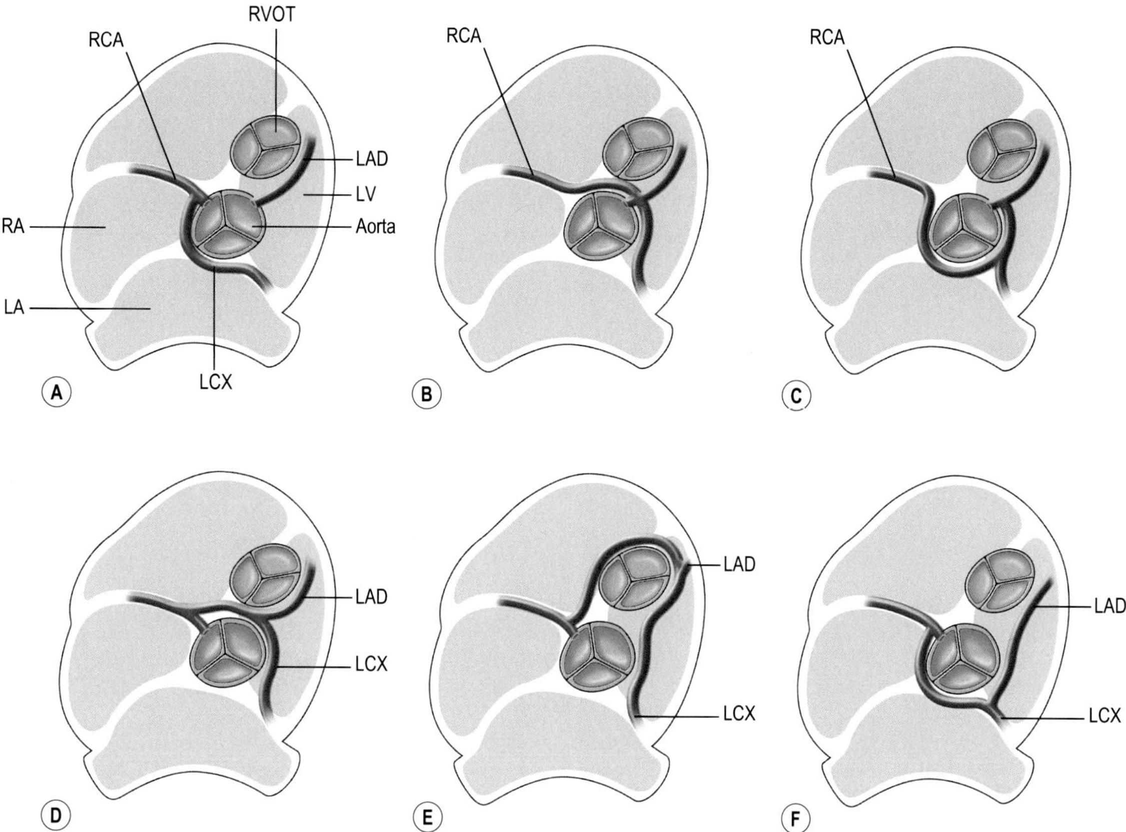

FIGURE 13-8 ■ **Coronary artery anomalies.** Schematic diagram of the coronary arteries viewed in the axial oblique plane on CMR. RA = right atrium, LA = left atrium, LV = left ventricle, RVOT = right ventricular outflow tract, LAD = left anterior descending artery, RCA = right coronary artery, LCX = left circumflex artery. (A) Anomalous LCX from RCA. (B) Anomalous RCA from left main stem (LMS), with interarterial course between pulmonary artery and aorta. (C) Anomalous RCA from LMS passing posteriorly between the aorta and atria. (D) Anomalous left coronary artery arising from RCA with interarterial course between the pulmonary trunk and aorta. (E) Anomalous left coronary artery arising from RCA passing anterior to pulmonary trunk. (F) Anomalous left coronary artery arising from RCA passing posteriorly between aorta and atria.

from RCA. Patients experience myocardial ischaemia and usually present at around 4–5months of age when pulmonary vascular resistance drops and LCA blood flow is reduced. Patients with sufficient collateralisation may survive to adulthood. Treatment usually involves surgical reimplantation of the coronary artery using a button transfer technique, or coronary artery bypass grafting.

From an anatomical point of view, coronary anomalies are classified according to the coronary artery involved, the origin of the anomalous coronary artery, and the anatomical course of the proximal segment (Fig. 13-8). From a clinical point of view, the anomalies are divided into 'benign' and 'malignant' lesions. The latter, especially those of ALCAPA and in cases where the LCA arises from the RCA and passes between the aortic root and right ventricular outflow tract or pulmonary artery, have an increased risk for developing myocardial ischaemia and sudden cardiac death.

Even with multiple projections, the precise location of the proximal course of the vessel in a patient with an abnormal origin of a coronary artery can be difficult to depict with conventional angiography and ultrasound. However, CMR and CT angiography provide reliable visualisation of the root of the arteries, and the coronary artery tree.

Key Imaging Goals

- Delineate coronary artery anatomy—CT may be better
- Look for myocardial perfusion defects—consider adenosine stress
- Identify areas of regional wall motion defects
- Assess ventricular function, volume and LV mass
- Identify mitral regurgitation—secondary to ischaemia
- Perform late gadolinium enhancement—to determine infarct size if present.

CYANOTIC CONGENITAL HEART DISEASE

Tetralogy of Fallot

Tetralogy of Fallot (TOF) is the most common cyanotic congenital heart defect, with an incidence of approximately 420 per million live births. It is caused by

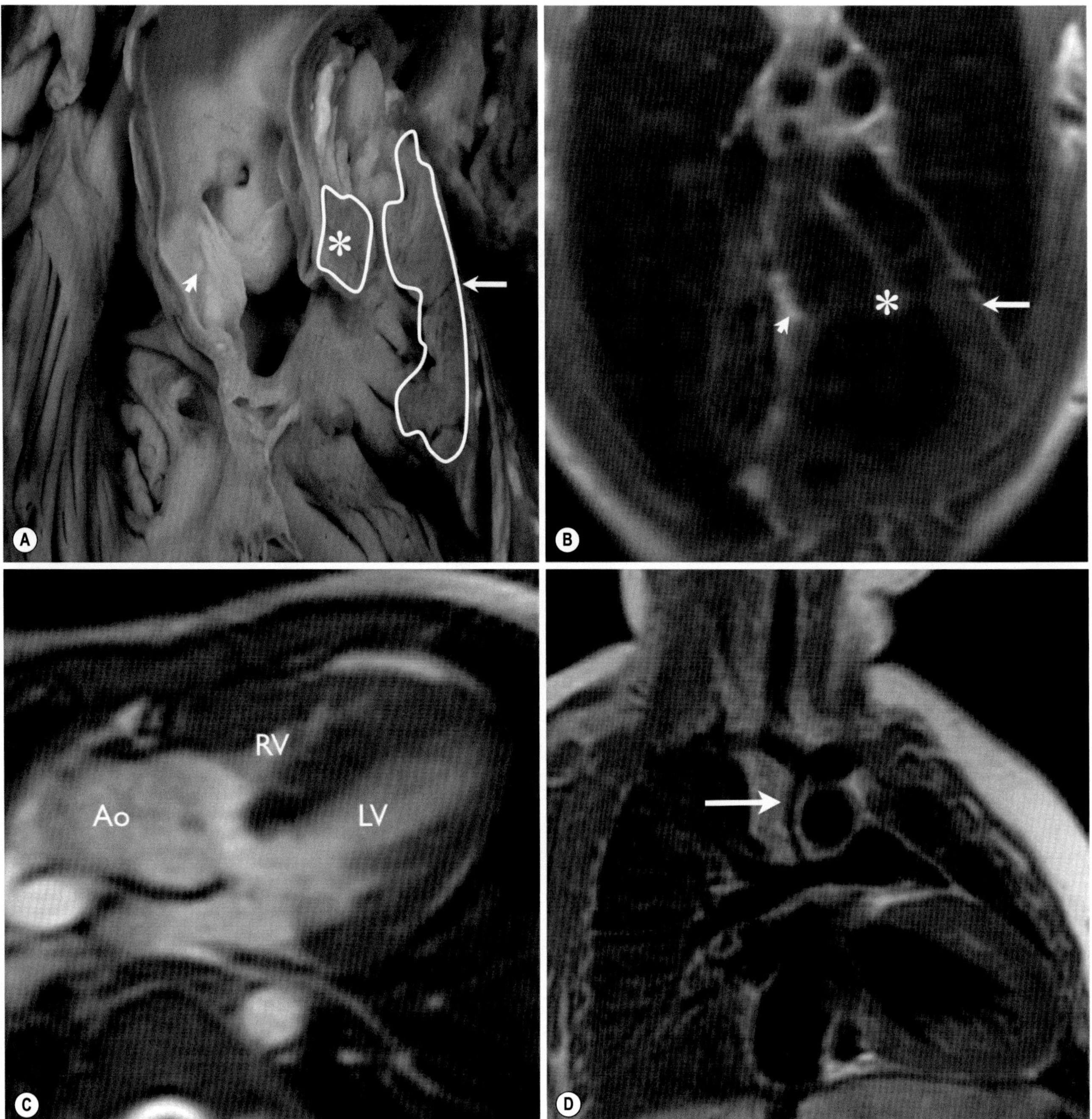

FIGURE 13-9 ■ **Tetralogy of Fallot.** (A, B) Right ventricular outflow tract, morphological specimen and corresponding black-blood spin-echo image in coronal view. The deviated outlet septum (asterisk), aortic root (arrowhead) and hypertrophied septoparietal trabeculations (arrow) are shown. (C) b-SSFP images of unrepaired tetralogy of Fallot: inflow/outflow view of the left ventricle (LV) shows a VSD with overriding aorta (Ao)—note the severe hypertrophy of the right ventricle (RV). (D) Black-blood, spin-echo image of right modified Blalock–Taussig shunt; 3.5-mm gortex tube from innominate artery to right pulmonary artery (arrow).

malalignment of the muscular outlet septum, which leads to right ventricular outflow (RVOT) obstruction, a subaortic VSD with aortic override and right ventricular hypertrophy (Figs. 13-9A–C). This produces the physiological pattern of low pulmonary blood flow and right-to-left shunt as described above. Current management consists of early single-stage reconstructive surgery, with closure of the VSD, and relief of the RVOT obstruction, usually by the placement of a transannular patch (across the pulmonary valve annulus) to enlarge the RVOT. Staged reconstruction is still required if there is severe cyanosis caused by a very narrow RVOT or significant hypoplasia of the central pulmonary arteries. In such cases a systemic-to-pulmonary anastomosis called a modified Blalock–Taussig (BT) shunt is placed (usually) between the innominate artery and the right pulmonary artery (Fig. 13-9D). This shunt is then taken down during subsequent definitive repair.

Transthoracic ultrasound is the optimal imaging investigation for the initial diagnosis and assessment of paediatric patients with possible tetralogy of Fallot. However, CMR has a role in untreated or shunt-palliated patients, in delineating pulmonary artery anatomy or excluding significant pulmonary artery distortion. While early surgical mortality from complete repair of tetralogy of Fallot is now very low, residual anatomical and haemodynamic abnormalities are common. These include right ventricle (RV) dilatation from pulmonary regurgitation, RV outflow tract aneurysm, RV outflow tract obstruction, pulmonary artery stenosis, residual atrial or ventricular septal defect, tricuspid valve regurgitation and aortic root dilatation.

CMR has emerged as the gold standard for the assessment of the right ventricle in patients with repaired TOF. Two-dimensional spin-echo black-blood and b-SSFP sequences can be used to define RVOT anatomy and quantitatively assess RVOT dilatation or stenosis. Velocity-encoded phase-contrast MR can accurately quantify the degree of pulmonary regurgitation and can be used to measure peak velocities at the level of RVOT obstruction, as well as differential regurgitation in the branch pulmonary arteries. MR assessment of right ventricular function/volumes with multi-slice short-axis b-SSFP imaging is particularly important when determining the timing and evaluating the impact of invasive therapeutic strategies.

Key Imaging Goals

- Describe the RVOT and pulmonary trunk anatomy
- Identify RVOT aneurysm
- Identify RVOT obstruction
- Quantify pulmonary regurgitation
- Assess branch PA anatomy and measure flow split
- Assess biventricular volume and function
- Exclude residual shunt ($Q_p:Q_s$)
- Measure aortic root for dilatation
- Delineate coronary artery anatomy (important for surgical or percutaneous pulmonary valve replacement).

Transposition of the Great Arteries

Transposition of the great arteries (TGA) is the second-commonest cyanotic CHD diagnosed in the first year of life, with an incidence of 315 per million live births. In this condition, the aorta arises from the right ventricle, and the pulmonary artery from the right ventricle (ventriculo-arterial discordance) (Fig. 13-10A). This produces the physiological pattern of parallel circulations described above which is incompatible with life. Treatment for TGA patients was revolutionised with the introduction of the Senning procedure, in which an intra-atrial baffle was used to divert blood from the right atrium to the left ventricle, and the left atrium to the right ventricle. A variation to the Senning procedure, the Mustard procedure uses a pericardial patch or prosthetic material to construct the intra-atrial baffle. However, although both these procedures produce a physiologically normal circulation, the patient is still left with a systemic RV. Patients surviving with these repairs may have unique complications such as pulmonary venous pathway or baffle obstruction, baffle leaks and failure of the systemic RV. Currently, the arterial switch operation has become the procedure of choice. In this operation, the great vessels are transected above the valve sinuses and sutured to their appropriate ventricle; the coronary arteries arising below this transection level must also be transferred separately (Fig. 13-10B). In cases of TGA associated with a VSD and subpulmonary stenosis, the Rastelli procedure (where blood from the LV is channelled through the VSD to the aorta) is preferred.

Key Imaging Goals

- Arterial switch repair
  - Identify any RVOT or LVOT obstruction
  - Assess branch pulmonary arteries, which may be narrowed as they straddle the aorta (Figs. 13-10C and D) (measure differential branch flow)
  - Identify aortic root dilatation
  - Assess coronary arteries for kinking, ostial stenosis
- Mustard/Senning
  - Assess patency of baffle and pulmonary venous pathway
  - Assess atrial baffles for leak (presence of shunt)
  - Quantify systemic RV volume and function
  - Perform late gadolinium enhancement for ventricular fibrosis/scar.

Congenitally Correct Transposition of the Great Arteries

Congenitally corrected transposition (CCTGA) is a rare disorder characterised by both atrioventricular discordance and ventriculo–arterial discordance (right atrium to left ventricle to pulmonary artery to lung (Fig. 13-11A); and left atrium to right ventricle to aorta). Thus, although the heart is anatomically abnormal, it is physiologically normal in terms of the pulmonary and systemic circuits. This lesion does not usually cause cyanosis; however, many of the problems are similar to those experienced by patients with TGA, particularly those treated by an atrial switch operation, and thus a systemic RV. CCTGA may be asymptomatic and in some patients is an incidental finding. However, the majority of patients with CCTGA have associated cardiac lesions (Fig. 13-11B), the most common being VSD. Pulmonary stenosis is present in approximately 50% of cases and tricuspid valve abnormalities (e.g. Ebstein's abnormality) are found in 20% of cases.

Even without associated abnormalities, the majority of patients with CCTGA eventually develop systemic ventricular failure. The main role of imaging is to evaluate associated lesions, quantification of ventricular function, and to assess postoperative complications.

Key Imaging Goals

- Describe A–V and V–A connections
- Identify associated VSD and tricuspid valve abnormalities
- Identify outflow tract obstruction
- Perform late gadolinium enhancement to assess for systemic RV fibrosis or scarring.

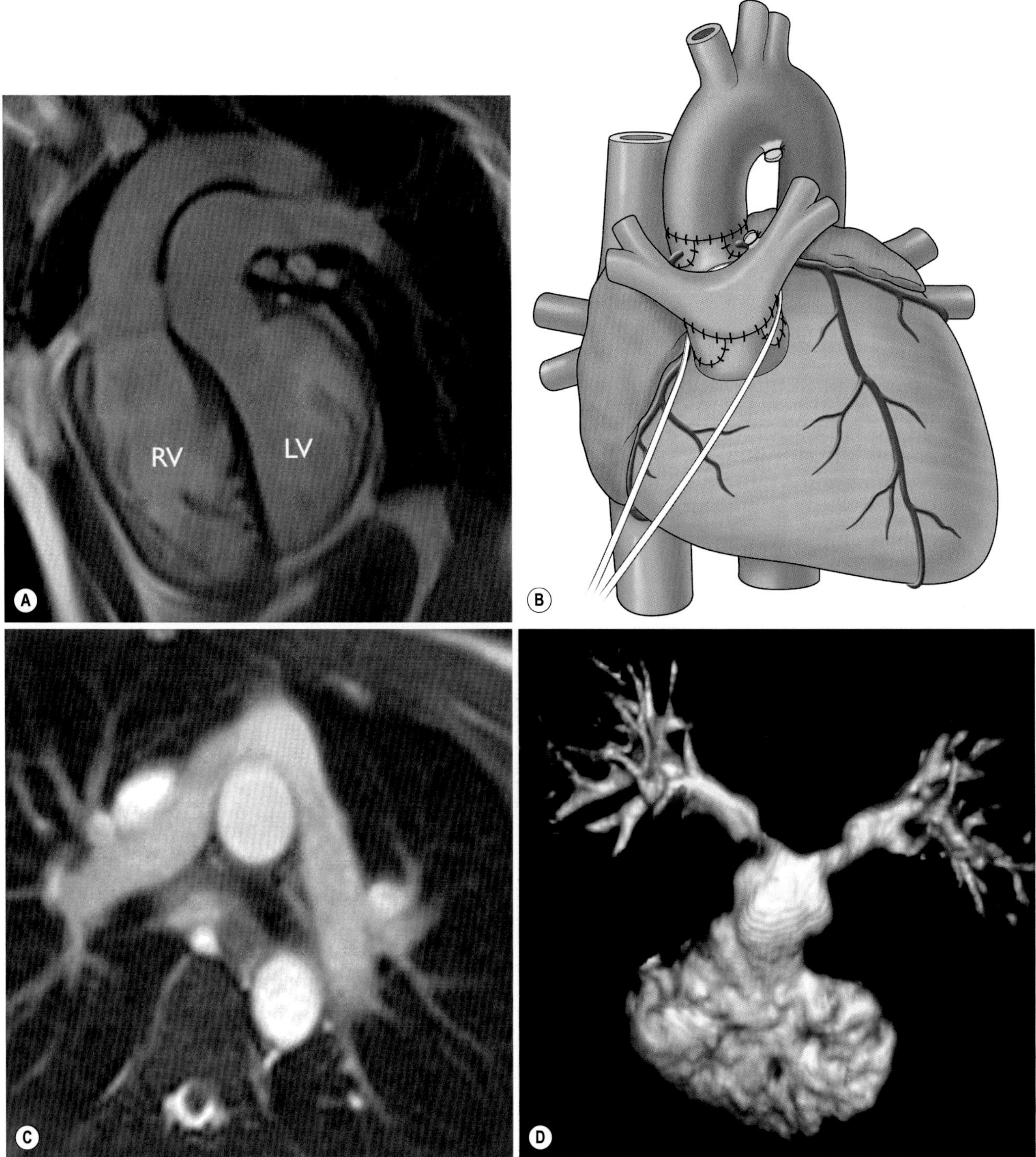

FIGURE 13-10 ■ **Transposition of the great arteries.** (A) b-SSFP CMR image showing an oblique sagittal outlet view of the aorta arising from the right ventricle (RV) and pulmonary artery arising posteriorly from the left ventricle (LV). (B) Schematic drawing of the arterial switch repair of TGA, showing the Le Compte manoeuvre with the translocation of the aorta and pulmonary artery. Note sites of coronary artery 'button' removal and subsequent reimplantation into the neo-aortic root. (C) b-SSFP CMR image showing the pulmonary arteries straddling the aorta following the arterial switch procedure with Le Compte manoeuvre. (D) Volume-rendered 3D reconstruction of a contrast-enhanced MRA showing bilateral proximal branch pulmonary artery narrowing.

Pulmonary Atresia

Pulmonary atresia is the lack of luminal continuity and absence of blood flow from the RV to the pulmonary artery. In its severe form, there is either partial or complete absence of the native pulmonary arteries. Pulmonary atresia can be separated into two groups depending on the presence of a VSD. As the diagnosis and subsequent management of these two groups are different, it is useful to consider them separately.

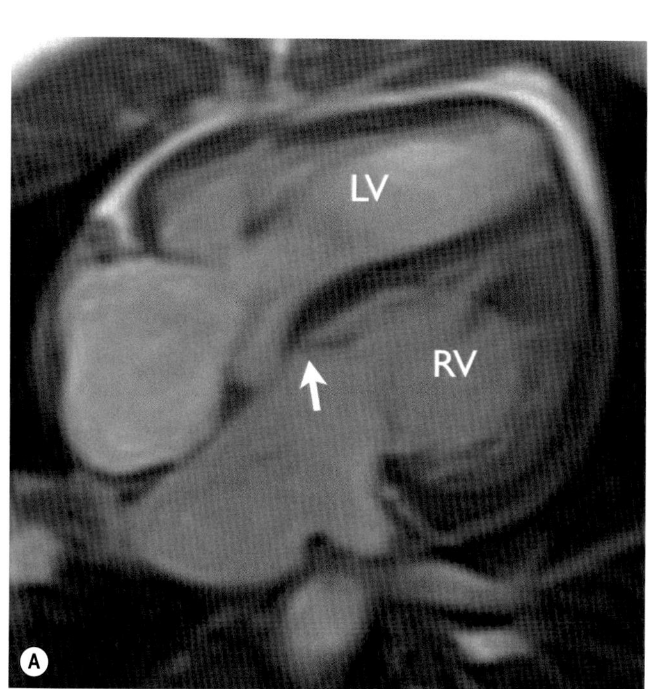

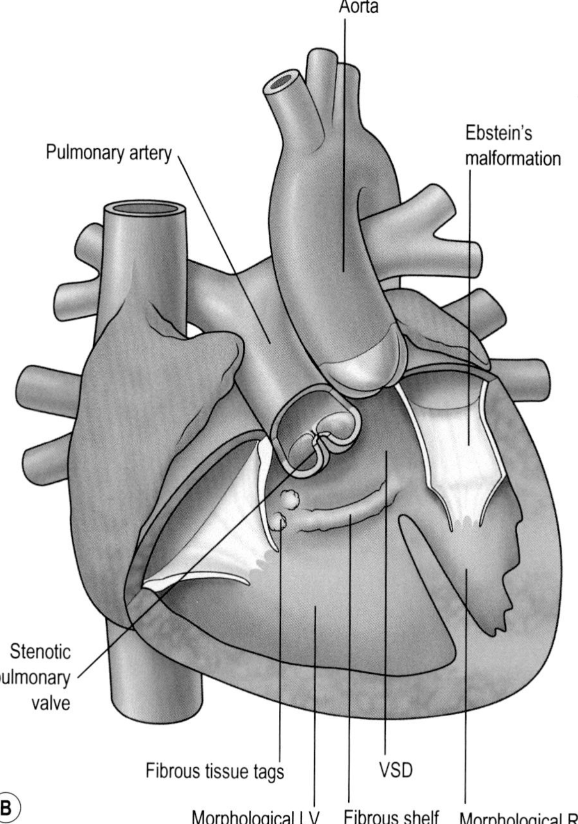

FIGURE 13-11 ■ **Congenitally corrected transposition of the great arteries.** (A) b-SSFP CMR image of CCTGA showing the discordant atrioventricular connection, with anterior LV. Note the apical offset of the left-sided tricuspid valve. (B) Schematic drawing of CCTGA and frequent associated lesions.

Pulmonary Atresia with a Ventricular Septal Defect. This is the more common variant and is considered by some to be a severe form of tetralogy of Fallot, with a subaortic VSD, overriding aorta. Pulmonary blood flow is supplied via major aortopulmonary collaterals (MAPCAs). Surgical repair aims to establish RVOT to the pulmonary artery continuity with a homograft (RV–PA conduit), repair the VSD and bring the aortopulmonary collaterals into the pulmonary circulation.

As with tetralogy of Fallot, the main role of imaging in patients with pulmonary atresia and a VSD is the assessment of postoperative complications. The most common long-term complication is homograft failure, usually mixed stenosis and regurgitation leading to right ventricular dysfunction. Conduit stenosis is often secondary to calcification of the non-viable homograft, and although calcified tissue is difficult to visualise using CMR, it is clearly seen on CT. Other long-term complications are similar to those found in tetralogy of Fallot.

Key Imaging Goals

- Characterise the presence or absence of the central PAs
- Characterise the source of pulmonary blood flow (PDA or multifocal MAPCAs)
- Quantify distance between RVOT and PA confluence
- Post-op (as for TOF): Assess RV–PA conduit function.

Pulmonary Atresia with an Intact Ventricular Septum. This is the less common variant of pulmonary atresia. The intact ventricular septum results in a variable degree of right ventricular hypoplasia. The type of surgical repair depends on the size and shape of the RV cavity. The presence of an RV infundibulum allows a biventricular repair. If the right ventricular cavity is small then single ventricular physiology is established and angiography demonstrates large venous sinusoids in the right ventricular wall. Imaging assessment is considered in the section below on the single ventricle.

Double Outlet Right Ventricle

The term double outlet right ventricle (DORV) refers to any cardiac anomaly in which both the aorta and the pulmonary artery originate, predominantly or entirely, from the right ventricle. In this situation the LV has no direct outlet to either great vessel and must eject blood into the RV through a ventricular septal defect. Rarely there may be no VSD and then the LV is very hypoplastic.

The physiological picture and type of surgical correction depend on the arrangement of the great vessels and the anatomy of the VSD. Cyanosis is not invariably present, and depends on the degree of pulmonary stenosis. The most common variant is a normal arrangement of the great vessels and a subaortic VSD. This variant is often referred to as the 'Fallot's type', as it is often associated with pulmonary stenosis and has a similar presentation. DORV may also be associated with an anterior aorta and a subpulmonary VSD known as the 'Taussig–Bing' anomaly.

Surgical correction for the 'Fallot type' variant consists of patch closure of the VSD, which redirects blood to the aorta, and correction of any pulmonary stenosis. For the Taussig–Bing anomaly the surgical approach depends on the presence of pulmonary obstruction. In the absence of pulmonary obstruction, correction consists of patch closure of the VSD and arterial switch. In the presence of obstruction, left ventricular flow is tunneled through the VSD to the aorta, and a RV–PA pathway is established—the Rastelli procedure.

Imaging plays an important role in preoperative assessment. The 3D anatomy of the VSD and the arrangement of the great vessels are well visualised by CMR and are particularly important when deciding the type of surgery. Spin-echo black-blood CMR of the VSD has been shown to compare well with surgical findings and is able to indicate the optimal type of repair.

Key Imaging Goals

- Describe arrangement of great vessels—normal with subaortic VSD (Fallot type), anterior Aorta with subpulmonary VSD (Taussig–Bing type)
- Describe VSD size, position and commitment
- Identify associated outflow tract obstruction
- Quantify shunt (may be left to right, or right to left)
- Quantify ventricular volume, function and mass
- Postoperatively evaluate as for TOF or TGA, described above, depending on type of DORV.

Common Arterial Trunk

Common arterial trunk (truncus arteriosus) is defined as a single arterial trunk arising from both ventricles, which overrides a large misaligned VSD. The pulmonary, systemic and coronary arteries all originate from the trunk. This produces the physiological pattern of cyanosis due to intracardiac mixing, as the simultaneous ejection of both ventricles into the common trunk merges streams. The classification of common arterial trunk relies on the branching pattern of the pulmonary artery. In type I, a short main pulmonary artery arises from the common trunk and subsequently divides. In type II, the right and left pulmonary arteries originate from the posterior wall of the common trunk and in type III, the right and left pulmonary arteries emerge from the lateral wall of the common trunk. The truncal valve is often abnormal with varying degrees of stenosis and insufficiency. About 40% of truncal arches are on the right side: most truncal arches rise higher in the mediastinum than the normal aortic arch.

Surgical repair consists of reconstruction of the common trunk to produce a systemic vessel from the left ventricle, patch closure of the VSD and establishment of a right ventricle-to-pulmonary artery conduit. The main role of CMR is in assessment of postoperative complications (homograft failure, truncal valve regurgitation, VSD patch leak). Imaging can be used to better delineate the vascular anatomy before surgery.

Key Imaging Goals

- Define morphological subtype:
  - Type I: RPA and LPA arise from a main PA segment
  - Type II: RPA and LPA arise from the posterior wall of the common trunk
  - Type III: RPA and LPA arise from lateral wall of the common trunk
- Describe truncal valve morphology (tricuspid, quadricuspid)
- Assess truncal valve function, stenosis or regurgitation
- Describe position of VSD
- Look for associated abnormalities, coarctation or interrupted aortic arch.

Anomalous Pulmonary Venous Drainage

Pulmonary veins may connect abnormally to a site other than the left atrium, usually the right atrium, systemic vein or coronary sinus. If all the veins connect abnormally, then it is described as total anomalous pulmonary venous connection/drainage (TAPVD), and if less than all the veins connect abnormally (usually only 1), then it is termed partial anomalous pulmonary venous connection/drainage (PAPVD). In TAPVD, a complete left-to-right shunt causes all of the pulmonary venous return to mix with systemic venous return. Survival is dependent on obligatory right-to-left shunting of the mixed pulmonary venous and systemic venous blood, usually at atrial level.

PAPVD is an acyanotic condition, which results in a physiology similar to an ASD. The number of veins involved determines the magnitude of the shunt and the clinical symptoms. It is associated with superior and inferior sinus venosus atrial septal defects (Fig. 13-4C).

In TAPVD the pulmonary veins coalesce posterior to the left atrium, but do not drain into it. Drainage from this venous confluence to the right atrium may be: (a) via an ascending vein to the innominate vein, and then to the SVC (supracardiac, 50% of patients, Fig. 13-12A); (b) the coronary sinus directly into the right atrium (cardiac, 15% of patients); (c) a descending vein, which passes through the diaphragm into either the IVC or portal venous system (infracardiac, 25% of patients, Fig. 13-12B); or (d) a mixture of these routes may coexist (mixed, 10% of patients).

The infracardiac type is usually associated with a degree of obstruction as the descending vein passes through the diaphragm (Fig. 13-12B). Thus, unlike the supracardiac and cardiac variants, which present with a left-to-right shunt, intracardiac mixing and cardiac failure, the clinical picture for infracardiac TAPVD is potentially more severe, with superimposed pulmonary venous hypertension, resulting in: tachypnoea,

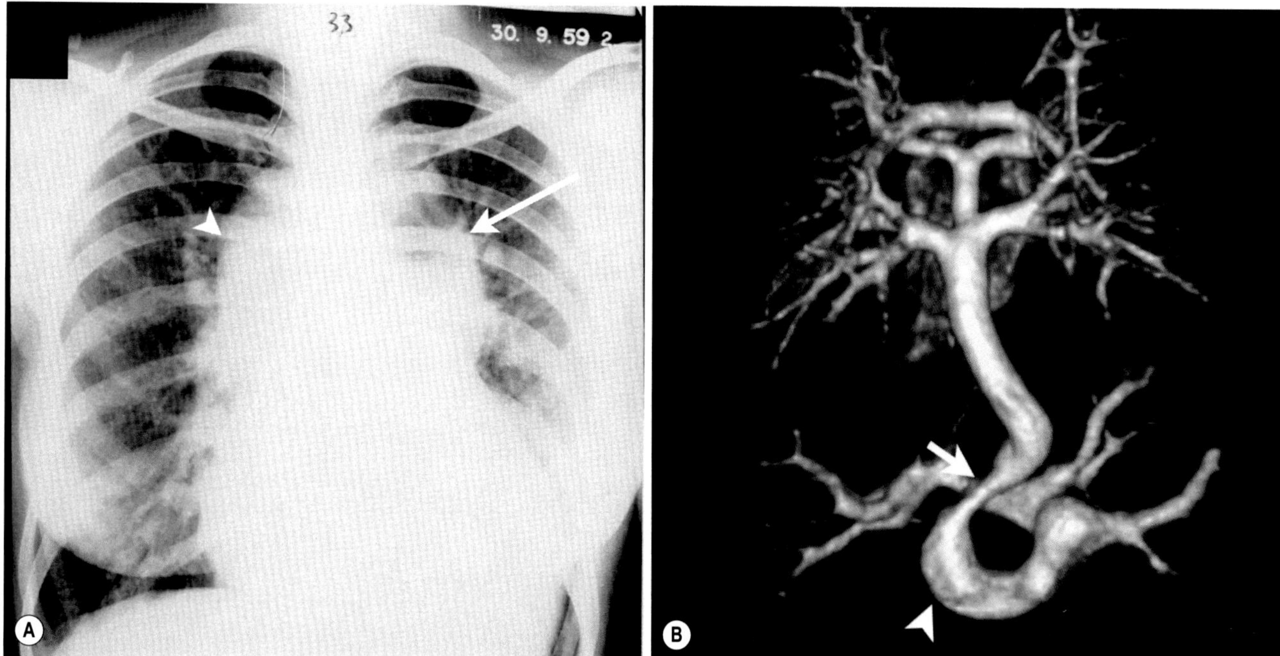

FIGURE 13-12 ■ **Total anomalous pulmonary venous drainage.** (A) PA CXR in a patient with unobstructed supracardiac TAPVD. Note dilated ascending vein (arrow) returning all pulmonary blood to the brachiocephalic vein. The arrowhead shows the dilated SVC. (B) Volume-rendered 3D reconstruction of MR angiography showing total anomalous infracardiac drainage of the pulmonary veins. Note the narrowing of the veins as they pass through the diaphragm (arrow) before draining into the portal vein (arrowhead).

tachycardia, liver enlargement, cyanosis, pulmonary oedema and respiratory distress. Symptoms usually appear within 24–36 h of birth. Importantly, the diagnosis of infracardiac TAPVD can be missed at ultrasound, and must always be considered in the differential diagnosis of pulmonary oedema on the neonatal chest radiograph (Fig. 13-2B).

Associations of TAPVD are complex cardiac anomalies such as isomerism of the atrial appendages, AVSD, pulmonary stenosis, DORV, HLHS, common arterial trunk, transposition of the great arteries and aortic coarctation. The anomalous pulmonary venous connection is easily visualised with ultrasound, but in patients with poor ultrasound acoustic windows, cross-sectional imaging with CMR and CT is very useful, often avoiding the need for a diagnostic X-ray catheterisation.

Key Imaging Goals

- Total anomalous pulmonary venous drainage
  - Describe pulmonary venous connection type: supracardiac, cardiac, infracardiac or mixed
  - Identify areas of pulmonary venous obstruction
  - Confirm obligatory right-to-left shunt
  - Identify associated abnormalities—Isomerism of the atrial appendages
- Partial anomalous pulmonary venous drainage
  - Describe pulmonary venous connection
  - Assess branch pulmonary arteries
  - Quantify ventricular volume, function and assess RA dilatation
  - Quantify shunt
  - Consider if shunt measured, but no ASD or VSD seen.

SINGLE VENTRICLES

The term single ventricle covers a wide range of different cardiac morphologies, e.g. hypoplastic left heart syndrome (Fig. 13-13A), tricuspid atresia or pulmonary atresia with intact ventricular septum. However, pragmatically, the term can be used to describe a group of patients, who, following surgical 'correction', have a circulation supported by one ventricle. Modern palliative management has resulted in long-term survival for many patients who would otherwise have died as infants.

This division extends the narrower morphological classification to include also functionally single ventricles: for example, where two ventricles are connected by a large VSD, which cannot be surgically septated due to atrioventricular valve apparatus straddling the ventricular septum (chordae tendinae attached to the septal crest or opposite ventricle) or when there is significant imbalance of the ventricular chambers, e.g. double inlet left ventricle.

The ultimate management goal is the creation of a single ventricle circuit with separation of the systemic and pulmonary circulations—a Fontan or total cavopulmonary circulation: such that the single ventricle pumps blood into the systemic circulation, and systemic venous return is directed to the pulmonary circulation without a ventricular pump. This is performed in a step-wise surgical fashion, involving two or three stages.

Systemic-to-Pulmonary Artery Shunt

In patients with inadequate pulmonary blood flow due to a hypoplastic RV (tricuspid atresia or pulmonary

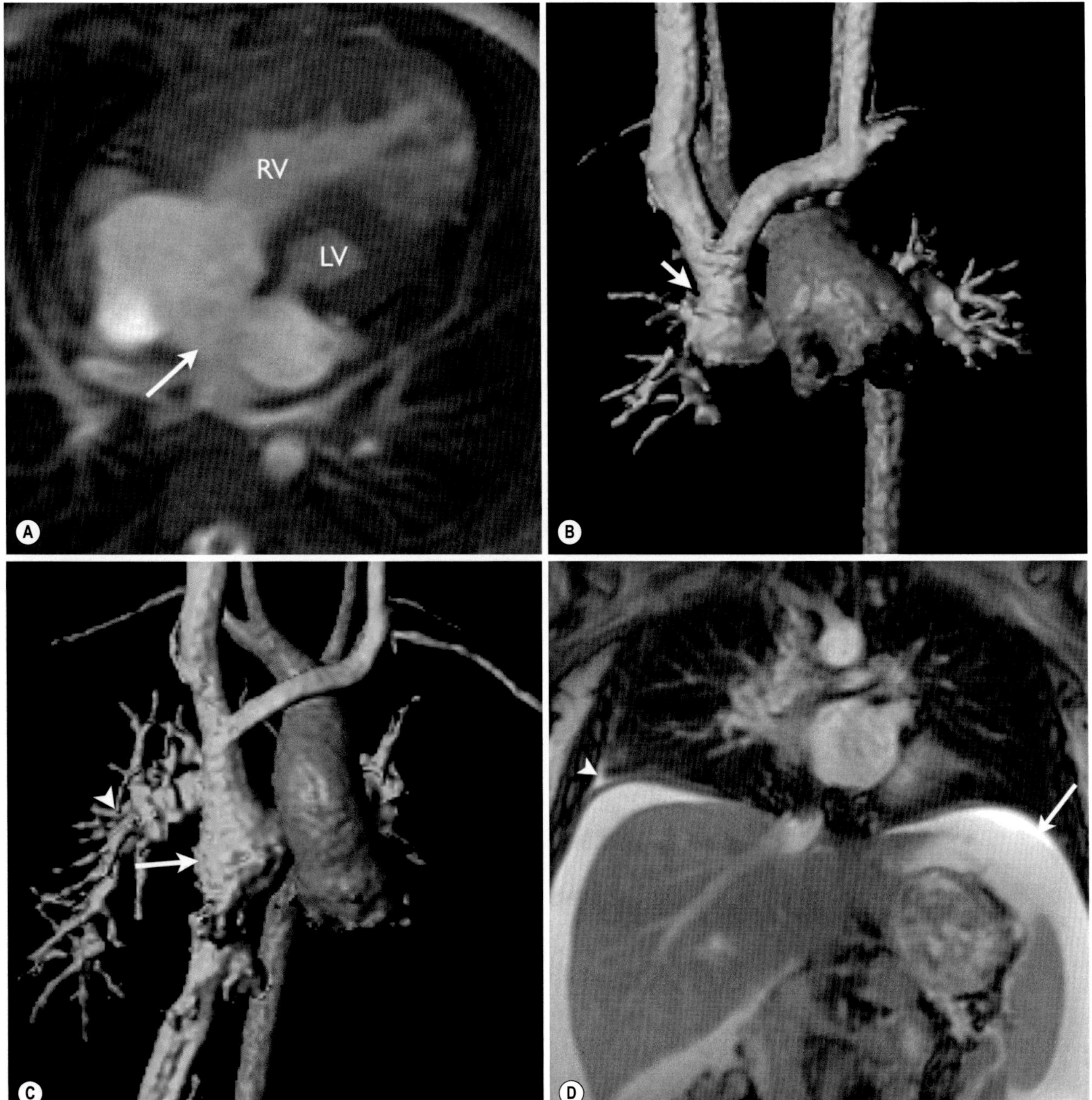

FIGURE 13-13 ■ **Single ventricle.** (A) b-SSFP CMR image showing hypoplastic left heart syndrome, with severe hypertrophy of the systemic RV. Note the large interatrial communication (arrowed), allowing mixing of systemic and pulmonary venous return. (B) Volume-rendered 3D reconstruction of an MR angiogram showing the Glenn, bidirectional cavopulmonary anastomosis (arrow) and (C) a lateral tunnel total cavopulmonary anastomosis (arrow) to the right pulmonary artery (arrowhead). (D) b-SSFP CMR image showing severe ascites (arrow), and right pleural effusion (arrowhead) in a patient with a failing TCPC circulation and protein-losing enteropathy.

atresia with intact ventricular septum) and in patients with hypoplastic left heart syndrome as part of the Norwood procedure, the first stage involves the creation of a systemic-to-pulmonary artery shunt such as a modified BT shunt (Fig. 13-9D). This is a temporising procedure in infants, in whom pulmonary vascular resistance is not low enough to proceed immediately with a Glenn procedure.

Key Imaging Goals Following Stage 1 (Pre-BCPC)

- Assess branch PA anatomy and exclude deformation at site of shunt insertion
- In hypoplastic left heart syndrome, assess aortic arch for residual obstruction or coarctation
- Assess systemic ventricular volume and function
- Identify any atrioventricular valve regurgitation
- Quantify aortic/neo-aortic valve regurgitation

- Evaluate adequacy of atrial communication
- Look for systemic-pulmonary or veno-venous collateral vessels
- Look for bilateral SVCs.

Bidirectional Glenn Circulation

The second stage in the creation of a single ventricular circulation is the bidirectional Glenn operation (superior cavopulmonary connection). It is usually performed around 3–9 months of age. In this procedure, an anastomosis is created between the SVC and the right pulmonary artery (such that the SVC blood flows into both arteries), and the SVC–RA junction oversewn (Fig. 13-13B). Any previous surgical systemic-to-pulmonary artery shunts are also taken down at this time. Imaging should be used to assess branch pulmonary artery narrowing and pulmonary venous obstruction; otherwise, the circulation may fail.

Key Imaging Goals Following Stage 2 (Pre-TCPC)

- Assess branch PA anatomy and SVC–PA connection
- Describe systemic venous return (SVC, IVC, hepatic veins)
- Quantify ventricular function and volume
- Identify atrioventricular valve regurgitation
- Describe outflow tracts and aortic arch
- Evaluate adequacy of atrial communication
- Look for veno-venous or systemic-to-pulmonary collateral vessels (common after BCPC) and quantify collateral flow
- At time of GA, assess pulmonary arterial pressure by transducing the pressure in the internal jugular vein
- Look for pulmonary vein stenosis.

Fontan Circulation

The Fontan circulation can be completed by a number of different surgical methodologies, but in the current era is performed by the creation of an intracardiac (lateral tunnel) (Fig. 13-13C) or extracardiac conduit between the IVC and the pulmonary arteries: total caval pulmonary connection (TCPC). It is usually performed between 18 months and 5 years. The classical Fontan operation involved connection of the SVC to the RPA (non-bidirectional Glenn procedure) and connection of the right atrium to the LPA. Right atrial dilatation is the major complication of the classical Fontan procedure and may cause arrhythmias, thrombosis or pulmonary vein compression, which can lead to failure of the Fontan circulation. CMR allows evaluation of the branch pulmonary arteries and their systemic venous connections, and can be used to accurately assess ventricular function. Despite optimal medical and surgical management, the intrinsic shortcomings of the TCPC invariably manifest as late attrition during follow-up. This situation, known as a 'failing Fontan', is particularly difficult to manage; systemic venous hypertension and low cardiac output may result in peripheral oedema, and unusual clinical syndromes of plastic bronchitis and protein-losing enteropathy (Fig. 13-13D). Ultimately this may result in death or necessitate high-risk cardiac transplantation.

Key Imaging Goals Following Stage 3 (Post-TCPC)

- Assess branch PA anatomy and SVC–PA, IVC–PA connections. Exclude stenosis.
- Quantify ventricular volume and function
- Identify atrioventricular valve regurgitation
- Evaluate flow in fenestration between conduit and RA if present
- Evaluate adequacy of atrial communication
- Look for veno-venous or systemic to pulmonary collateral vessels (common after BCPC) and quantify collateral flow
- At time of GA, assess pulmonary arterial pressure by transducing the pressure in the internal jugular vein
- Look for thrombus in RA if classical Fontan
- Identify any pulmonary vein stenosis.

CONCLUSION

Congenital heart disease is a complex area of medicine that requires a well-integrated understanding of anatomy and cardiovascular physiology. Using the principles illustrated in this chapter, cardiovascular imaging can be successfully utilised to guide medical and surgical management of patients with congenital heart disease. Ultrasound remains the first-line imaging investigation; however, when ultrasound cannot provide a complete diagnosis, cross-sectional imaging with CMR or CT is the next line of investigation. Catheter angiography is usually reserved for problem solving, coronary artery assessment, haemodynamics, and for catheter-guided therapeutic procedures.

It is hoped that the complementary nature of imaging investigations has been demonstrated, and that, when used in combination, ultrasound, CMR, CT and X-ray catheter angiography can provide a comprehensive assessment of patients with CHD.

REFERENCES

1. Anderson R, Baker J, Penny D, et al. Paediatric Cardiology. Edinburgh: Churchill Livingstone; 2010.
2. Lai WW, Mertens L, Cohen M, Geva T. Echocardiography in Pediatric and Congenital Heart Disease: From Fetus to Adult. Oxford: Wiley-Blackwell; 2009.
3. Bogaert J, Dymarkowski S, Taylor A, Muthurangu V. Clinical Cardiac MRI. New York: Springer; 2012.
4. Oeppen RS, Fairhurst JJ, Argent JD. Diagnostic value of the chest radiograph in asymptomatic neonates with a cardiac murmur. Clin Radiol 2002;57:736–40.
5. Birkebaek NH, Hansen LK, Elle B, et al. Chest roentgenogram in the evaluation of heart defects in asymptomatic infants and children with a cardiac murmur: Reproducibility and accuracy. Pediatrics 1999;103:E15.
6. Sridharan S, Price G, Tann O, et al. Cardiovascular MRI in Congenital Heart Disease: An Imaging Atlas. Berlin/London: Springer; 2010.

CHAPTER 14

Non-ischaemic Acquired Heart Disease

Luigi Natale • Agostino Meduri

CHAPTER OUTLINE

Non-ischaemic heart disease (NIHD) accounts for nearly half of the cardiac deaths. This group of diseases is extremely heterogeneous, including cardiomyopathies, valvular diseases, cardiac masses and pericardial diseases. Modern non-invasive imaging techniques have increased diagnostic accuracy for all these diseases, with a consequent decrease in the number of invasive procedures.

ROLE OF IMAGING

In the past, NIHD diagnosis was based on chest radiography and invasive angiography; the introduction of echocardiography has greatly modified the diagnostic approach, as both myocardium and heart chambers are visualised non-invasively, in real time and with the same examination. Furthermore, magnetic resonance has increased the role of non-invasive imaging, with a wider field of view, higher contrast resolution and tissue characterisation capabilities, coupled with extremely accurate, operator-independent functional assessment. Finally, multidetector ECG-gated CT has had a deep impact on non-invasive coronary artery imaging; recent technological improvements have also made CT effective in the assessment and therapeutic planning of NIHD, particularly in valve diseases and cardiac masses.

Chest Radiography

Chest radiography (CXR) still remains the first-line examination in both ischaemic and non-ischaemic heart disease. Its advantages are low cost, non-invasiveness, wide availability and unique information on pulmonary haemodynamics; of course, it is extremely non-specific and has a low sensitivity, particularly before disease is at an advanced stage.

CXR interpretation is based on a sequential procedure: the chest wall anatomy may explain modification in heart contours; pleural or parenchymal disease may cause non-specific symptoms such as chest pain. Analysis of vessel size and distribution which reflect the haemodynamic status, is fundamental in assessing heart disease: indeed, size and distribution are strictly related to capillary wedge pressure and pulmonary venous pressure, which equalises left atrial pressure and, consequently, end-diastolic left ventricular pressure (EDLVP). So, depending on the acute or chronic development of the disease, it is possible to obtain a non-invasive assessment of EDLVP.

Furthermore, a general assessment of the presence or absence of cardiomegaly will help to create a differential diagnostic list of possible diseases, with or without cardiomegaly. The next step is the analysis of modifications of cardiac contours in both frontal and lateral views which may be helpful in identifying specific chamber enlargement.

Echocardiography

Echocardiography is the most commonly performed imaging examination in the assessment of NIHD. It is a non-invasive, portable ultrasound technique that allows high-resolution, two- and three-dimensional (2D and 3D) views of the cardiac chambers, valves and pericardium. This technique, with either a transthoracic or transoesophageal approach, can assess cardiac anatomy and ventricular function. When combined with Doppler and colour-Doppler techniques, valvular regurgitation and stenosis and transvalvular pressure gradients can also be assessed.

Magnetic Resonance Imaging

Cardiac magnetic resonance imaging (CMR) is rapidly becoming very useful in the assessment of NIHD. Its role is most valuable in (1) serial measurement of ventricular function in patients with cardiomyopathy (considered superior to echocardiography in reproducibility); (2) evaluation and quantification of valve function, including stenosis and regurgitation; (3) morphology and extent of involvement in cardiac tumours; and (4) value of post-contrast delayed enhancement in assessing diagnosis and determining prognosis in many diseases, such as hypertrophic cardiomyopathy, dilated cardiomyopathy (DCM) and many types of infiltrative myocardial diseases including sarcoidosis and myocarditis.

Computed Tomography

Until recently, conventional computed tomography (CT) had a limited role in the evaluation of NIHD. The increasing use of ECG-gated subsecond multidetector CT techniques has the potential to make cardiac CT a viable alternative in assessing cardiac function. More recently cardiac CT has also been shown to be useful in the assessment of valvular function. However, as yet, CT has no demonstrable advantage over echocardiography or CMR in the evaluation of NIHD. Furthermore, despite recent reconstruction advances, radiation dose remains an issue. While imaging of the coronary arteries has become feasible with exposures below 1 mSv, even higher doses are necessary for functional assessment (full acquisition dose is needed over the complete heart cycle as opposed to prospective gating techniques for imaging of the coronaries).

CARDIOMYOPATHIES

According to the 2006 American Heart Association (AHA) definition,[1] cardiomyopathies (CMPs) are 'a heterogeneous group of diseases associated with mechanical and/or electrical dysfunction, usually exhibiting inappropriate hypertrophy or dilatation, due to a variety of causes, often genetic, confined to the heart or part of systemic disorder'. This classification divided CMPs into primary and secondary; primary CMPs are subdivided into genetic, mixed and predominantly non-genetic and acquired, while secondary CMPs are a variety of diseases that can affect the myocardium (Fig. 14-1).

In 2008, the European Society of Cardiology (ESC) proposed another classification,[2] based on different phenotypes (hypertrophic, dilated, etc.) that are subclassified into familial genetic and non-familial non-genetic (Tables 14-1 and 14-2). While the AHA classification is based more on pathology, the ESC classification is more clinical, as, for example, a hypertrophic phenotype can be due to many diseases that cause myocardial thickening—hypertrophic CMP, hypertensive CMP, Fabry disease, amyloidosis, etc. In this chapter the phenotype approach will be used, according to the ESC classification.

Hypertrophic Pattern

Increased myocardial thickness can be due to a variety of diseases, both familial and non-familial; among the familial, the classical hypertrophic cardiomyopathy (HCM) is the most common. It is autosomal dominant, and is defined as a sarcomere disease (with a number of different mutations), characterised by an excessive hypertrophy of the myocardium (not explained by other causes) in a non-dilated left ventricle.[1] Eleven mutations have been recognised with the most common affecting the β-myosin heavy chain. Pathologically there is disarray of myocytes with a variable amount of interstitial fibrosis, caused by

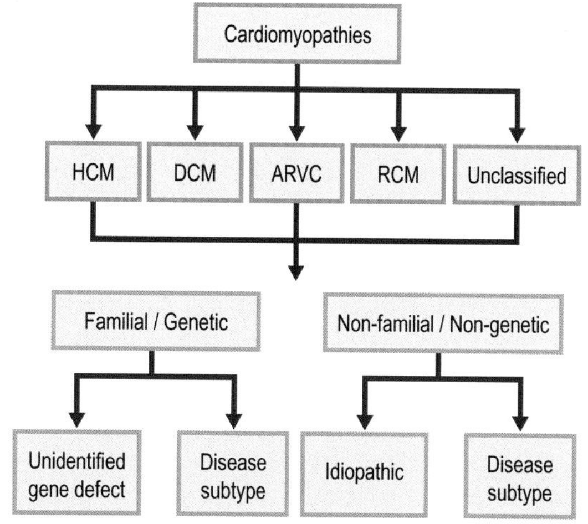

FIGURE 14-1 ■ Summary of classification system proposed by American Heart Association. (Modified from Maron et al.[1]).

TABLE 14-1 **Summary of Familial Diseases Causing Cardiomyopathies, by American Heart Association**

		Familial		
HCM	**DCM**	**ARVC**	**RCM**	**Unclassified**
• Familial (unknown gene) • Sarcomeric protein mutation • Glycogen storage disease • Lysosomal storage disease • Disorders of fatty acid metabolism • Carnitine deficiency • Phosphorylase B kinase deficiency • Mitochondrial cytopathies • Syndromic HCM • Other	• Familial (unknown gene) • Sarcomeric protein mutation • Cytoskeletal genes • Nuclear membrane • Mildly dilated CM • Intercalated disc protein mutations • Mitochondrial cytopathy	• Familial (unknown gene) • Intercalated disc protein mutations • Cardiac ryanodine receptor • Transforming growth factor-β_3	• Familial (unknown gene) • Sarcomeric protein mutation • Familial amyloidosis • Desminopathy • Pseudoxanthoma elasticum • Haemochromatosis • Anderson–Fabry disease • Glycogen storage disease	• Left ventricular non-compaction • Barth syndrome • LaminA/C • ZASP • α-Dystobrevin

Modified from Maron et al.[1]

TABLE 14-2 Summary of Non-familial Diseases Causing Cardiomyopathies, by American Heart Association

HCM	DCM	ARVC	RCM	Unclassified
• Obesity • Infants of diabetic mothers • Disorders of fatty acid metabolism • Athletic training • Amyloid	• Myocarditis • Kawasaki disease • Eosinophilic • Viral persistence • Drugs • Pregnancy • Endocrine • Nutritional • Alcoholic • Tachycardiomyopathy	• Inflammation?	• Amyloid • Scleroderma • Endomyocardial fibrosis • Carcinoid heart disease • Metastatic cancers • Radiation • Drugs	• Takotsubo cardiomyopathy

Modified from Maron et al.[1]

microvascular bed damage. Typically, increased septal thickness, exceeding 15 mm, is recognised at echocardiography; in the presence of ECG abnormalities and symptoms (such as chest pain, shortness of breath and dizziness, but also pre-syncope, syncope and arrhythmias), interventricular septum increased thickness is sufficient for diagnosis. Another echocardiographic criterion is a ratio between septal thickness and inferior wall of left ventricle at midventricular level higher than 1.3.[3]

CXR is often unhelpful: in concentric hypertrophy there may be a rounded third left cardiac contour, different from that due to aortic stenosis and systemic hypertension, which can both cause concentric hypertrophy of the left ventricle. Echocardiography can easily assess myocardial thickness (Fig. 14-2); however, there are many patterns of hypertrophy distribution, not all of them easily recognisable by ultrasound. Hypertrophy can be asymmetrical or septal, with or without left ventricle obstruction, symmetric, apical, midventricular, mass-like and non-contiguous.[4] In asymmetrical or septal forms, 25% of cases show a systolic obstruction of the left ventricle outflow tract (Fig. 14-3), due to the movement of the anterior leaflet of the mitral valve towards the hypertrophic interventricular septum, caused by the Venturi effect. This obstruction can be present at rest or only during/following physical exercise; it can be easily recognised at echocardiography and echo-Doppler.

Echocardiography has some limitations,[5] particularly in apical forms close to the low-frequency probe, and in mass-like forms where differential diagnosis with tumours can be difficult. In all these cases, and especially when the acoustic window is poor, MRI is extremely useful and accurate;[4] it provides precise measurement of wall thickness (Fig. 14-4), is more accurate in left ventricle mass quantification and can easily detect and quantify right ventricle involvement. Such morphological information can also be easily obtained by cardiac CT[6] (Fig. 14-5); modern CT equipment provides this information at a very low dose (1–3 mSv). However, the most relevant information is provided by MRI and refers to the presence of interstitial fibrosis; by means of the analysis of delayed enhancement after administration of contrast agent, fibrotic tissue can be easily detected as an area of 'bright' myocardium, due to the increased extravascular bed of collagen and its impaired washout, compared with normal 'dark' myocardium.[7] The distribution of delayed enhancement can be either diffuse, with elective localisation in the septum and relative sparing of subendocardial layer (different myocardial infarct scar) or at anterior and inferior septal insertion, or patchy, with large foci of intramural enhancement[8] (Fig. 14-5B).

Detection of fibrosis is extremely important, as it is strictly related to prognosis: a variety of published papers have reported the incidence of severe arrhythmias, due to re-entry mechanisms, and sudden cardiac death in young patients (<40 years) or progression to heart failure in older patients (>40 years) with HCM and severe fibrosis demonstrated at MRI.[9–11]

MRI can demonstrate that fibrotic tissue is probably due to impairment of intramural myocardial blood supply;[12] in fact, in the case of acute chest pain it is possible to see focal intramural areas of oedema (acute damage with non-ischaemic pattern) and vasodilator stress perfusion MRI can demonstrate a reduced myocardial flow reserve, corresponding to areas of fibrosis during late enhancement (Fig. 14-6). Finally, MRI permits recognition of associated findings, such as mitral regurgitation, and more sophisticated functional evaluation may reveal impairment of diastolic filling and radial or circumferential strain.

The hypertrophic phenotype that is increased myocardial thickness can be due to other cardiomyopathies; delayed enhanced MRI is particularly useful in the differential diagnosis,[8] particularly for storage disease such as Anderson–Fabry disease,[13] amyloidosis[14] and granulomatous non-infectious diseases, e.g. sarcoidosis.[15,16] In these cases, delayed enhancement patterns are different from those of HCM (Fig. 14-7); in Anderson–Fabry disease it is typically subepicardial in the lateral wall, with different presentations in amyloidosis. Due to the diffuse infiltration by amyloid and its link to gadolinium compounds, it is difficult to null myocardial signal, resulting in diffuse intermediate to bright signal intensity; alternatively, a patchy intramural pattern can be present, with small bright spots. Also sarcoidosis can present with the hypertrophic phenotype; again, a patchy pattern of distribution is more frequently present, with small foci, reflecting interstitial distribution of granulomas.

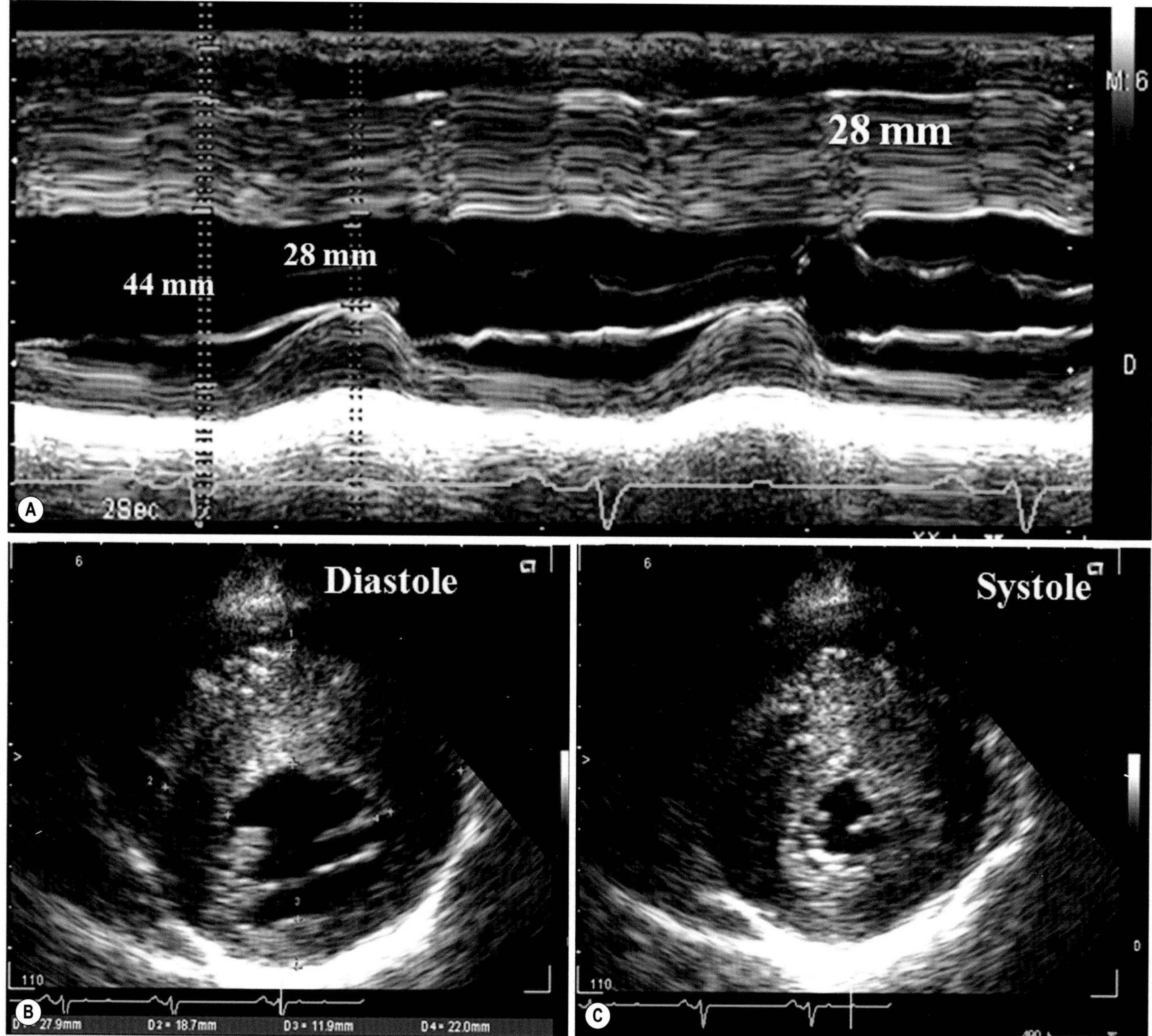

FIGURE 14-2 ■ M-mode (A) and B-mode (B, C) echocardiography in hypertrophic cardiomyopathy. M-mode allows measurements of left ventricle diastolic diameter (44 mm) and systolic diameter (28 mm), as well as thickened interventricular septum (28 mm). (B, C) Diastolic and systolic short-axis images, with clear evidence of hypertrophic septum.

Dilated Phenotype

Dilated cardiomyopathy (DCM) is defined as a left ventricular dilatation with systolic dysfunction not caused by abnormal loading (as in hypertension or valve disease) or coronary artery disease.[2] A dilated phenotype can have many different causes; among familial forms, autosomal dominant ones are more frequent, due to mutations of cytoskeletal, sarcomeric and other protein genes. Other forms are X-linked, such as muscular dystrophy. Non-familial DCMs include end-stage inflammatory diseases (infective and non-infective myocarditis), nutritional deficiencies, endocrine dysfunctions and drug toxicity.

Chest X-ray has limited sensitivity, as cardiac contour abnormalities can be observed only in advanced stages; typically, on frontal view the third left cardiac arch is enlarged, heart size is increased and, eventually, there are signs of left atrium enlargement (carina widening and double contour of second right cardiac arch) (Fig. 14-8). However, the most relevant role of CXR is the evaluation of pulmonary vasculature; due to increased left ventricular end-diastolic pressure (LVEDP), left atrium, pulmonary veins and capillary wedge pressures increase, with consequent balanced distribution or caudocranial redistribution of pulmonary vessels. In the case of high pressure values, further evolution can cause pulmonary oedema (interstitial to alveolar). Echocardiography is considered the first-line examination in clinically suspected DCM; echocardiographic criteria are increased left ventricle end-diastolic diameter (Fig. 14-9), exceeding normal values of 112% after age and body surface area correction, ejection fraction lower than 45% and

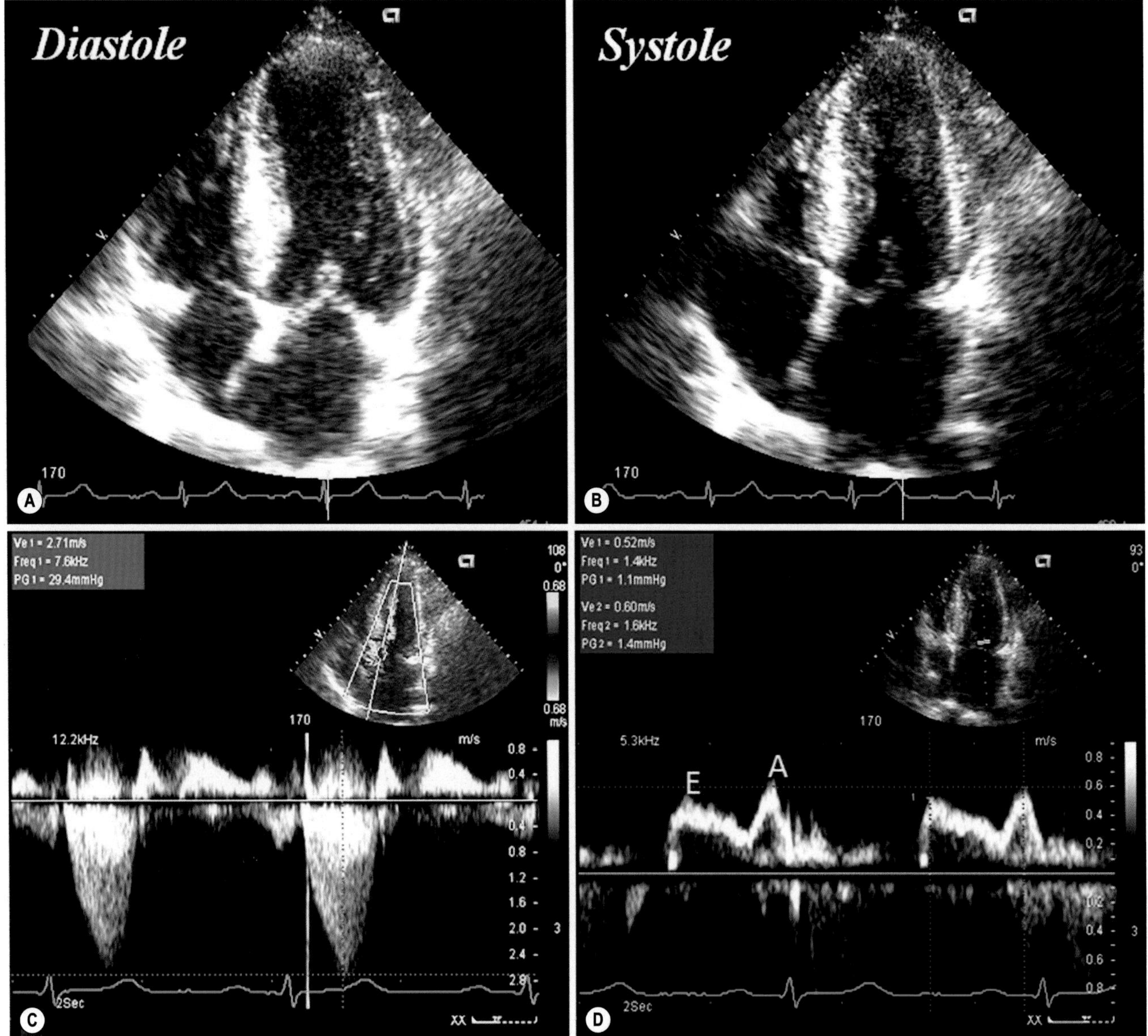

FIGURE 14-3 ■ **B-mode (A, B) and Doppler echocardiography (C, D) horizontal long-axis views, in hypertrophic cardiomyopathy.** (A, B) B-mode images show basal septal hypertrophy. (C) Doppler interrogation in outflow tract demonstrates a rest systolic gradient of 30 mmHg, while (D) transmitral flow evaluation shows an impairment of diastolic function, with reduced E wave equalised to A wave.

fractional shortening lower than 25%.[17] Another useful parameter is the spherical index that correlates the left ventricular end-diastolic volume with the long-axis diameter and which is increased in DCM.[18] Furthermore, echocardiography is able to demonstrate regional diffuse hypokinesis, sometimes restricted to apical segments, decreased forward flow velocities across all the valves and dominant E wave (early diastolic filling) at mitral flow interrogation, as well as complications such as mitral and/or tricuspid regurgitation and left ventricle thrombi.

In the case of poor acoustic window, CMR is extremely useful, because of the high intrinsic contrast resolution between blood and myocardium (Fig. 14-10); planimetric and volume measurements are extremely accurate and more reproducible than echocardiographic ones,[19] even if, in clinical settings, ultrasound measurements are commonly used. One of the major contributions of MRI is the differential diagnosis between ischaemic and non-ischaemic cardiomyopathy, which is crucial for decision making and treatment planning (revascularisation versus medical therapy and/or transplant); echocardiography, in fact, has a low specificity and thus differential diagnosis is not always easy. Using delayed enhancement technique, MRI is able to easily differentiate an ischaemic DCM (Fig. 14-11), demonstrating subendocardial or transmural scars, whereas non-ischaemic DCM late enhancement is absent or faint and limited to mesocardial layers, usually diffuse or septal (Fig. 14-12).[20] Another important indication for MRI is the evaluation of the left ventricle before therapeutic procedures. In general, ECG

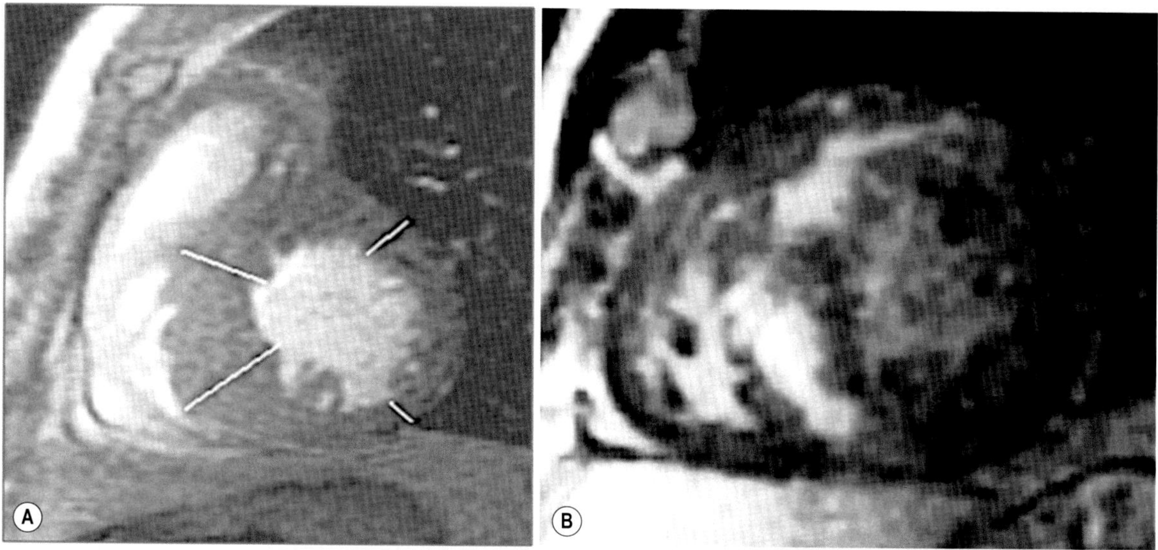

FIGURE 14-4 ■ **Hypertrophic cardiomyopathy.** (A) Cine-MRI frame showing typical localisation at basal septum. (B) Late gadolinium enhancement MRI short-axis image: thickened interventricular septum with large amount of fibrosis (hyperintense intramural foci).

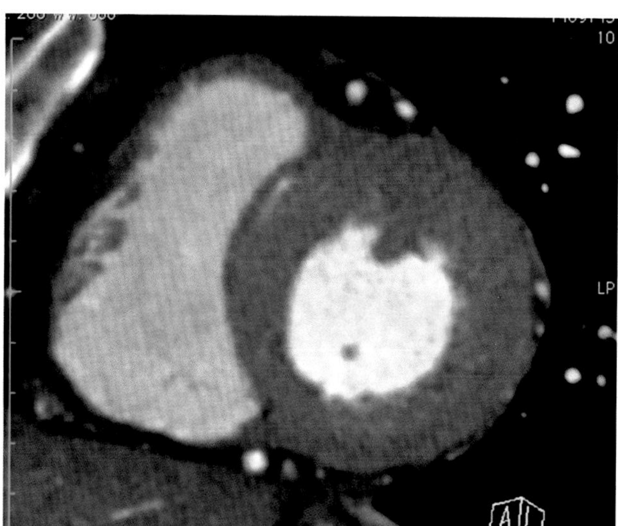

FIGURE 14-5 ■ **Cardiac CT in hypertrophic cardiomyopathy.** Short-axis midventricular image shows a diffuse left ventricle myocardial hypertrophy, with prevalent involvement of anterior wall.

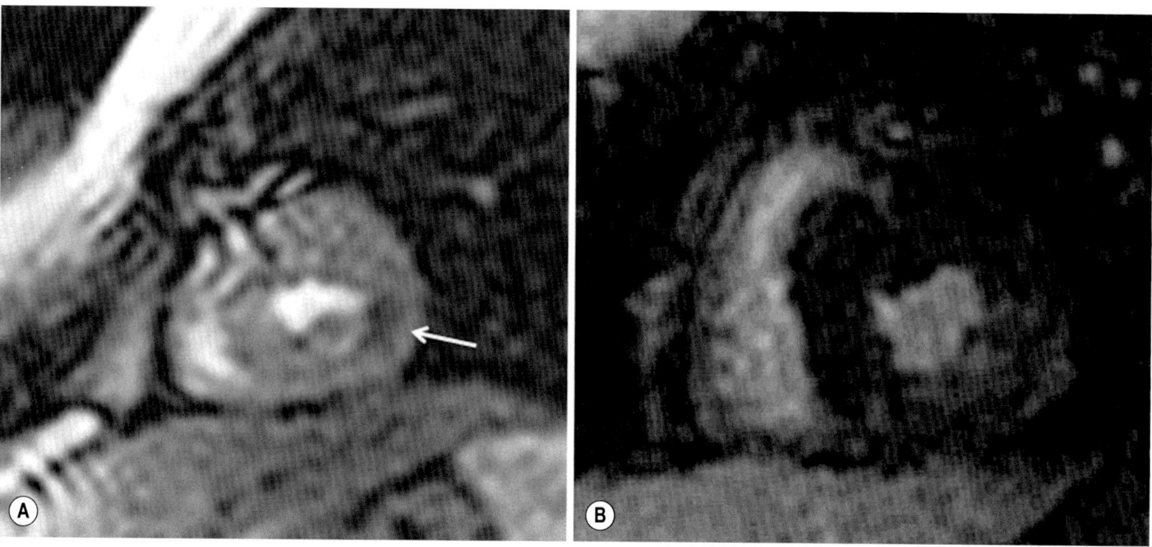

FIGURE 14-6 ■ **Gadolinium-enhanced MRI: short axis.** (A) First-pass frame showing intramural perfusion defect in lateral wall (arrow); (B) late enhancement due to fibrosis is evident in the same segment.

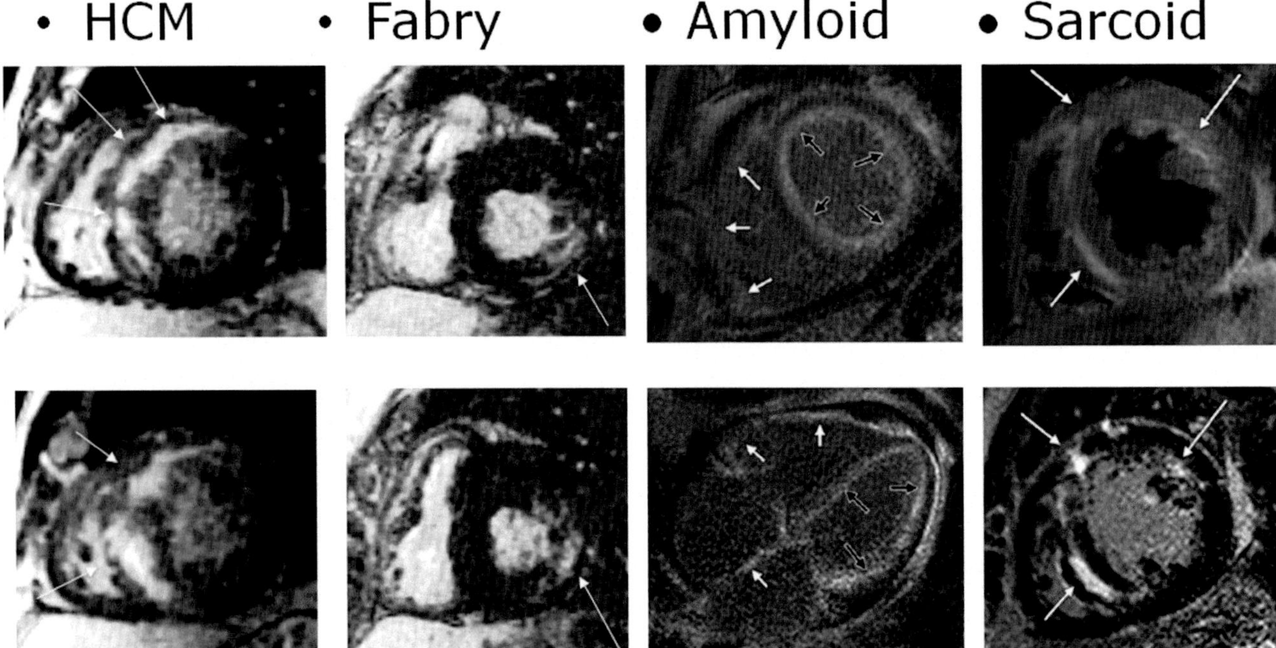

FIGURE 14-7 ■ **Different late gadolinium enhancement in hypertrophic phenotypes.** First column, large septal intramural late enhancement in hypertrophic cardiomyopathy (HCM) (arrows). Second column: intramural lateral wall late enhancement in Fabry disease (arrow). Third column: subendocardial diffuse late enhancement in amyloidosis (arrow in left ventricle, white arrows in right ventricle). Fourth column: T2w image (top) showing intramural hyperintense foci and striae due to oedema; lower image shows late enhancement in the same areas.

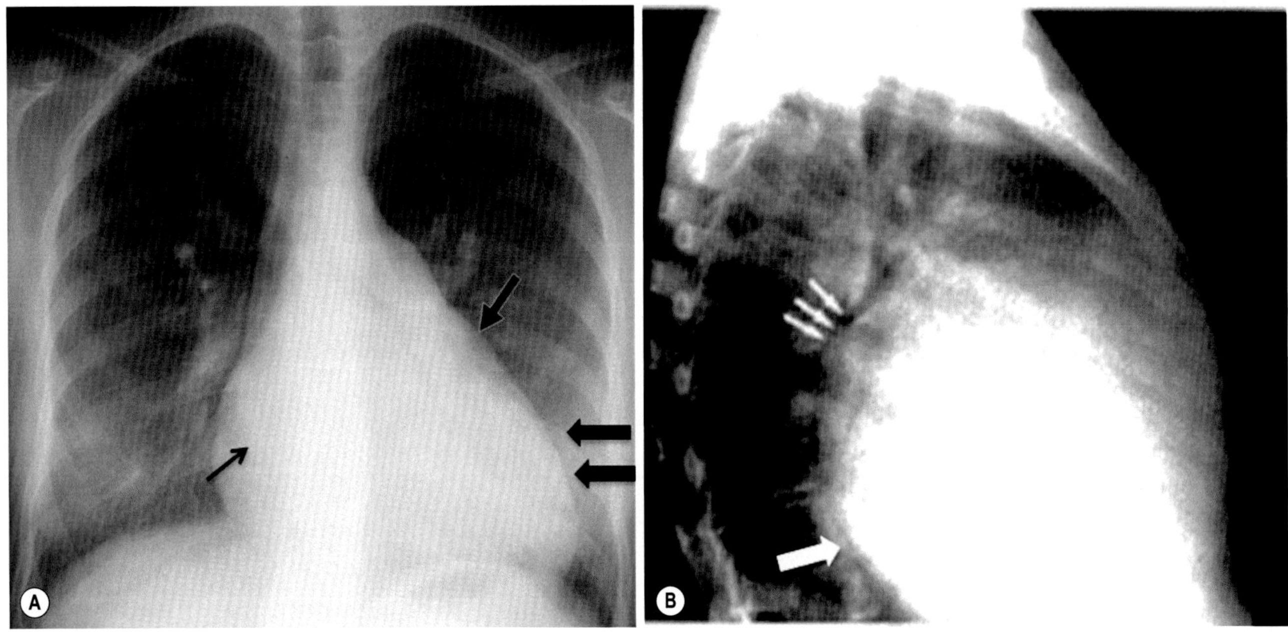

FIGURE 14-8 ■ **Primary dilative cardiomyopathy.** (A) Frontal view and (B) lateral view show overall increased cardiac size, with signs of left atrial enlargement (black arrows in A, thin white arrows in B), and left ventricle enlargement (thick black arrows in A, thick white arrow in B).

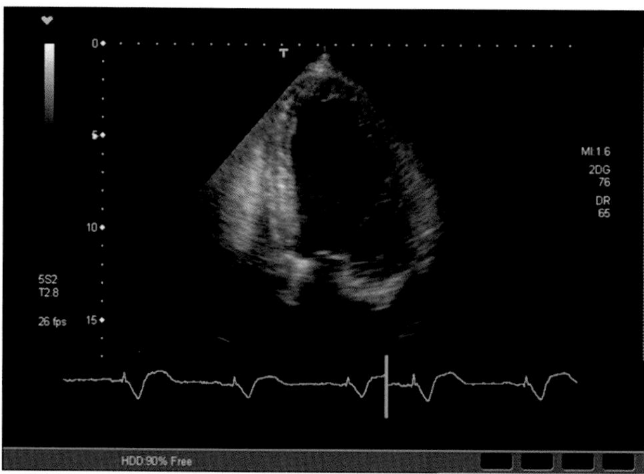

FIGURE 14-9 ■ Dilative cardiomyopathy. Echocardiography shows enlarged left ventricle.

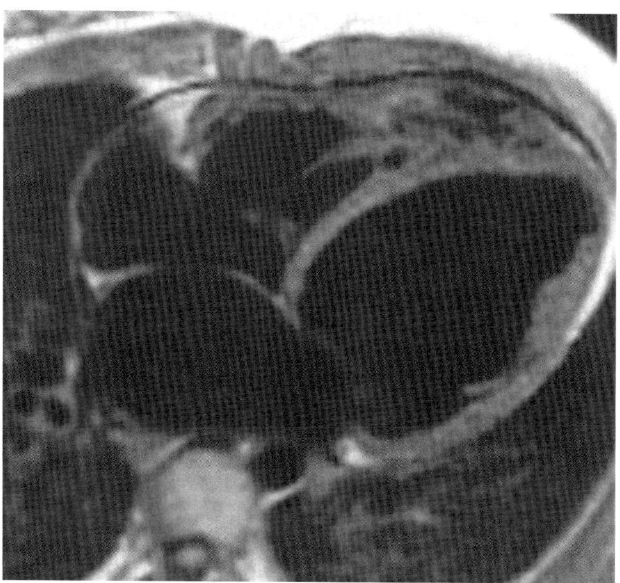

FIGURE 14-10 ■ Black-blood FSE T1w image of dilated cardiomyopathy. Left atrial and left ventricle enlargement is clearly evident.

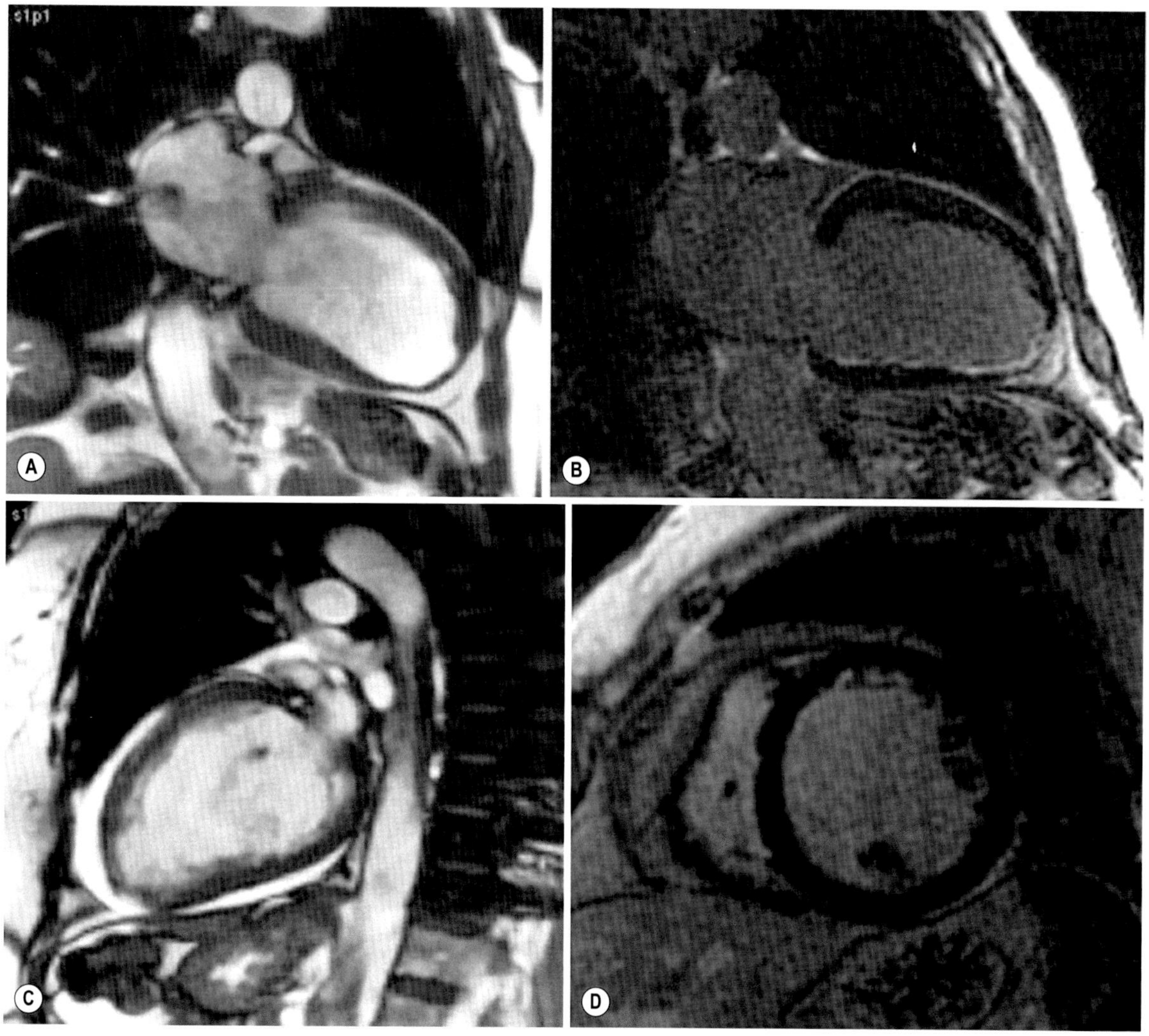

FIGURE 14-11 ■ Ischaemic versus non-ischaemic dilated cardiomyopathy. (A) Diastolic frame of two-chamber cine-MRI showing dilated left ventricle with inferoapical myocardial thinning. (B) Late enhancement in subendocardial layer of basal, mid and apical inferior segments, due to previous infarct in right coronary artery territory. (C) Diastolic frame of two-chamber cine-MRI showing dilated left Ventricle. (D) Short-axis late enhancement image, showing no gadolinium uptake.

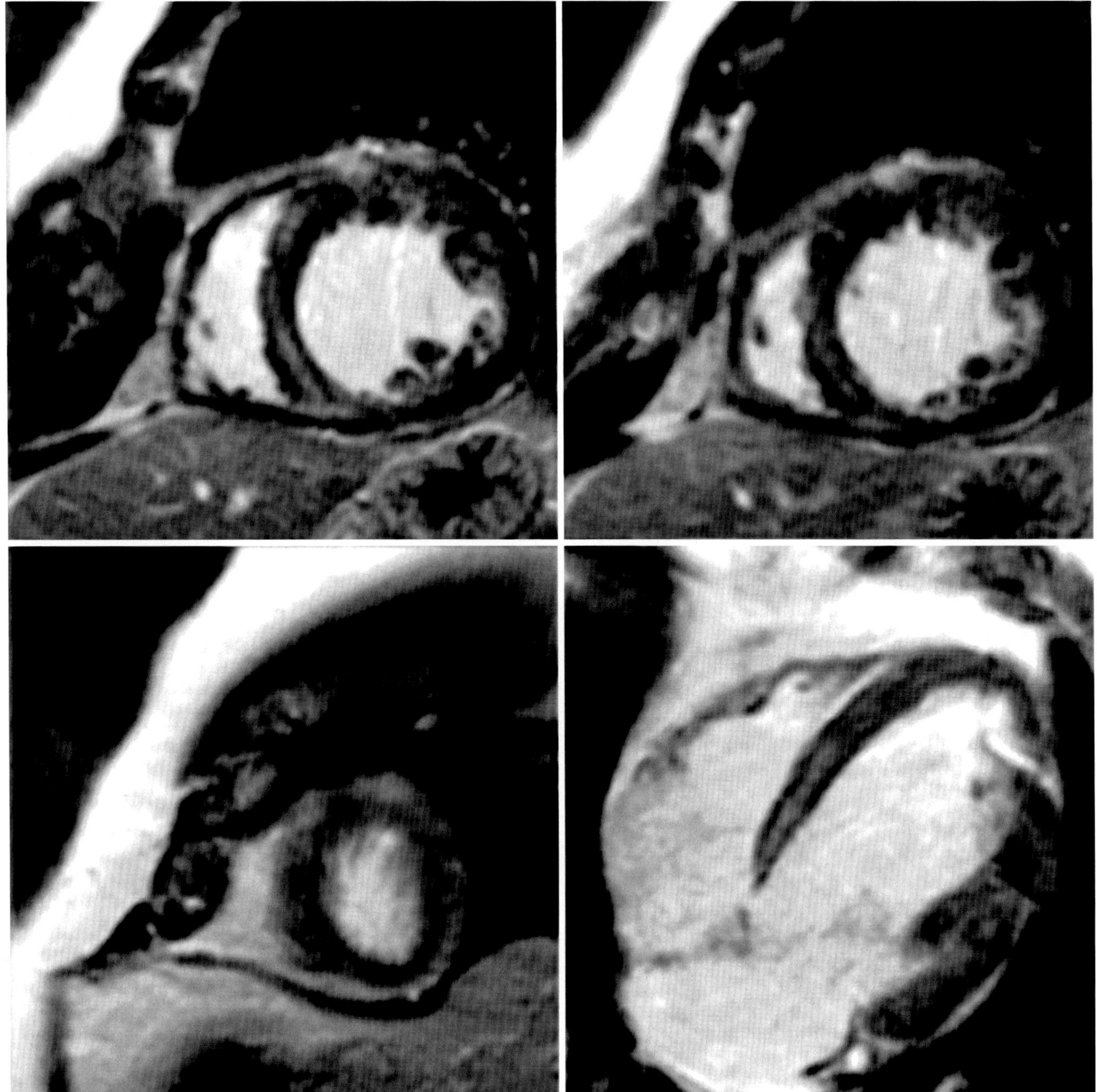

FIGURE 14-12 ■ Late gadolinium enhancement images in short-axis and four-chamber view, showing septal intramural contrast uptake in idiopathic dilated cardiomyopathy.

and echocardiography with Doppler interrogation are used in clinical practice,[21] but MRI is useful for assessing the presence of scar tissue in the inferior wall.[22] Finally, MRI is extremely accurate in thrombus detection (Fig. 14-13); contrast-enhanced images show the highest sensitivity, also in areas where echocardiography has false negatives, e.g. close to the apex.[23]

Differential diagnosis of non-ischaemic forms is only partially feasible with delayed enhancement technique: in general, intramural or mesocardial enhancement is more frequent in post-myocarditis DCM than in the idiopathic form, but this must be further investigated and confirmed.[8] Histology is still mandatory in these cases; in other secondary forms MRI is extremely useful, for example in dilated end stage HCM where the pattern and distribution of late enhancement help establish the correct diagnosis. The prognostic role of MRI in DCM is still under investigation; data are few and less robust than in HCM for risk assessment; left ventricular remodelling, ventricular tachycardia and sudden cardiac death seem to be related to the presence and amount of late enhancement.[24]

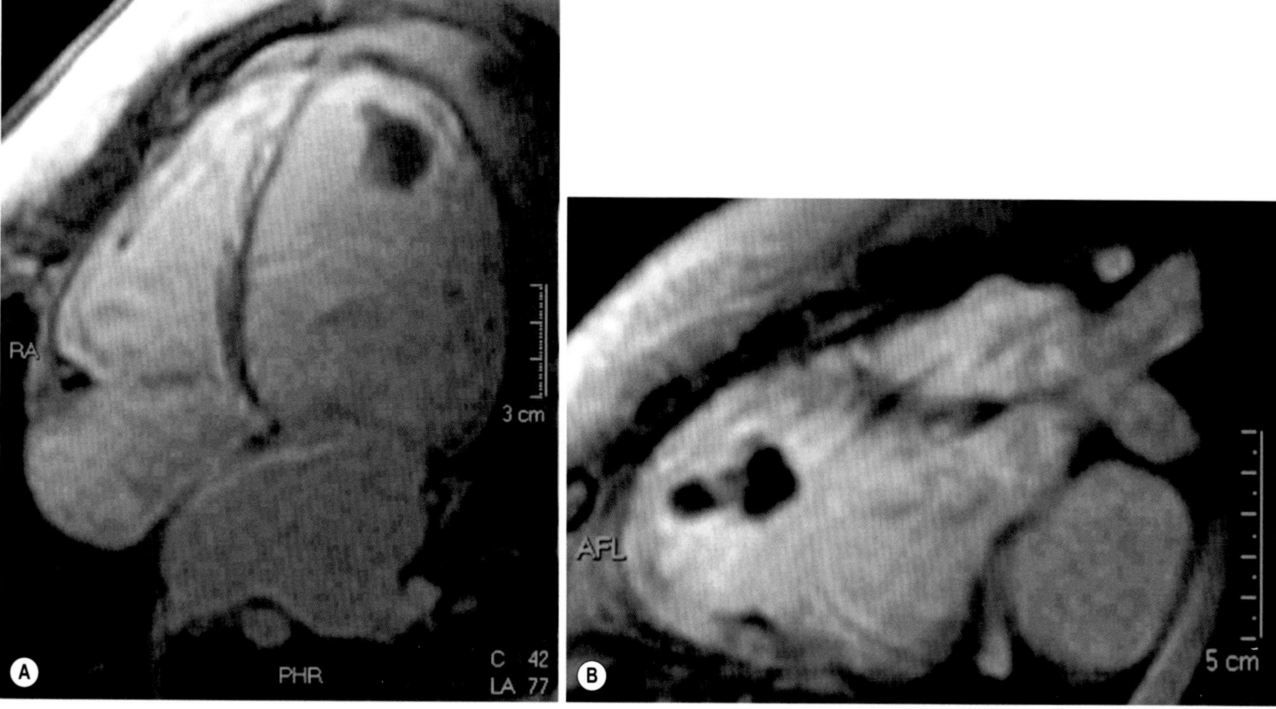

FIGURE 14-13 ■ **MRI of dilated cardiomyopathy complication.** Thrombi in left ventricle are evident in late enhancement four- (A) and two-chamber (B) views.

Cardiac CT can be used as an alternative to MRI in cases where echocardiography is difficult due to a poor acoustic window, to assess ventricular volumes and ejection fraction but, most importantly, it is useful in differential diagnosis between ischaemic and non-ischaemic forms, by means of its capability to exclude coronary artery disease (Fig. 14-14).[25] CT is also highly accurate in left ventricle thrombus detection, while late enhancement technique does not seem to be useful due to lower contrast resolution compared with MRI.

Restrictive Phenotype

In this phenotype, the increased wall stiffness causes a rapid pressure increase with only a small volume increase; this restrictive pattern can occur in a wide range of diseases. The wall thickness is normal.[2] Familial restrictive cardiomyopathy (RCM) is a very rare autosomal dominant disease; non-familial forms are caused by systemic disorders, such as amyloidosis, sarcoidosis, haemochromatosis, Anderson–Fabry disease, carcinoid heart disease, anthracycline toxicity, endomyocardial diseases, with or without hypereosinophilia (such as endomyocardial fibrosis) and endocardial fibroelastosis.

CXR is frequently negative; only at an advanced stage does left atrial enlargement become evident with signs of increased pulmonary venous pressure, as in mitral stenosis. Echocardiography often shows normal-sized ventricles, enlarged atria and normal or decreased contractile function; in some cases, such as in Loeffler's syndrome, or endomyocardial fibroelastosis or carcinoid syndrome, endocardial thickening is evident (Fig. 14-15). Doppler evaluation of mitral flow is particularly important, showing elevated early diastolic velocity, short deceleration time and low and shortened atrial velocity.[26] However, these abnormal parameters can be present also in the case of constrictive pericarditis, where pericardial stiffness does not allow ventricular filling; in this case, it is important to evaluate pericardial thickness, the interventricular septal kinetics and inferior vena cava flow during deep inspiration and expiration.[26,27]

The pericardium is not easily assessed by ultrasound, and here cardiac CT or MRI can play a major role; a cut-off value of 4 mm is highly predictive of pericardial constriction,[28] but it is important to remember that pericardial constriction without pericardial thickening can also occur. MRI can easily assess morphological and functional abnormalities of restriction (Fig. 14-16); T1- and T2-weighted (T1w, T2w) images can help in tissue characterisation (Fig. 14-17). As previously described, precontrast and delayed enhancement can be useful in differentiating some diseases, such as amyloidosis (Fig. 14-18), sarcoidosis and Anderson–Fabry disease (Fig. 14-7). Furthermore, cardiac MRI is extremely important in the assessment of iron overload of the myocardium (Fig. 14-19) as the measurement of T2* (transverse relaxation time in gradient-echo sequence) closely correlates with iron overload;[29,30] consequently, it is possible to modulate chelation therapy in these patients, which has made it possible to reduce the mortality for heart failure, the leading cause of death in this disease. Cardiac CT, as well as MRI, can be used in differentiating

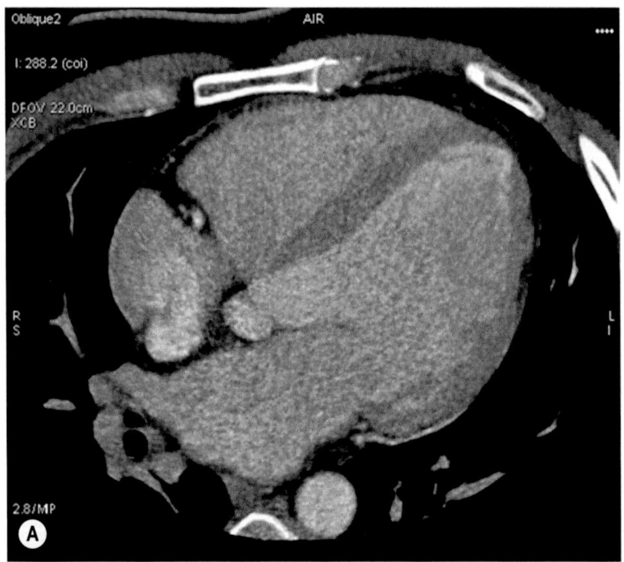

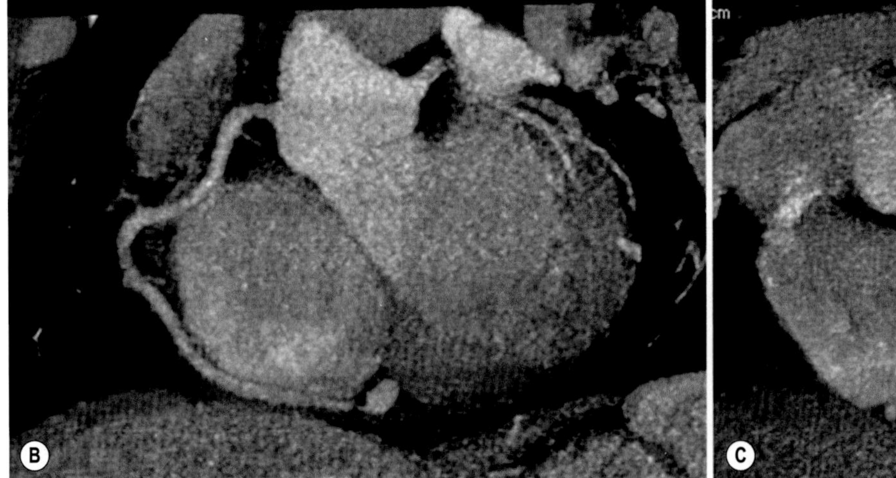

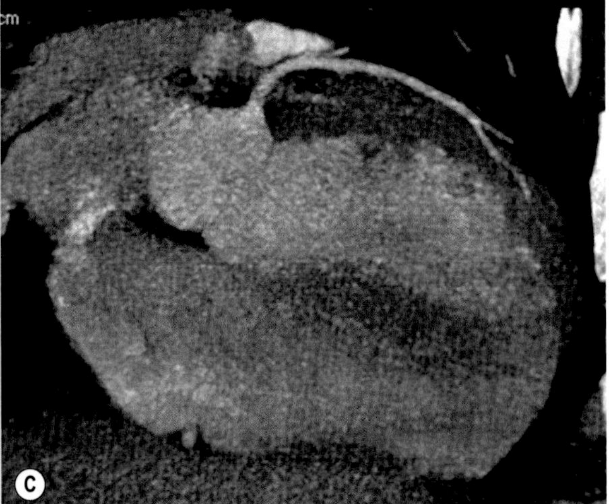

FIGURE 14-14 ■ **Cardiac CT in dilated cardiomyopathy.** (A) Left ventricle dilation in four-chamber view. (B, C) MIP reformatted images of right coronary artery, common trunk and left descending coronary artery showing no atherosclerotic lesions.

RCM from constrictive pericarditis, by means of pericardium thickness measurement (Fig. 14-20); a potential advantage over MRI is the assessment of pericardial calcification.[28]

Arrhythmogenic Right Ventricular Cardiomyopathy

Arrhythmogenic right ventricular cardiomyopathy (ARVC) is a relatively uncommon familial disease, usually autosomal dominant, characterised by various desmosome protein mutations. This results in right ventricle dysfunction, global or regional, with or without left ventricle involvement, in the presence of histopathological evidence of right ventricular myocardial replacement with fatty and fibrous tissue in various amounts. There is preferential localisation in the so-called triangle of dysplasia (outflow tract, inflow tract and apex). There are distinctive electrocardiographic abnormalities, according to previously published and recently revisited criteria.[31,32]

ARVC is a frequent cause of sudden cardiac death in young people, due to severe ventricular arrhythmias. For this reason, early diagnosis is crucial, based on the combination of many criteria proposed in 1994: familial history, ECG alterations, repolarisation abnormalities, arrhythmias (ventricular tachycardia with left bundle branch block, extrasystoles >1000/24 h), right ventricle systolic dysfunction, fibro-fatty replacement at endomyocardial biopsy. Based on the severity of the alterations, all these criteria are distinguished in major and minor; from their combination, a diagnosis of ARVC can be established, or excluded in their absence. In cases of doubt, it is important to regularly monitor the patient.

In 2010 these criteria were revisited and, particularly, quantitative parameters for right ventricle enlargement

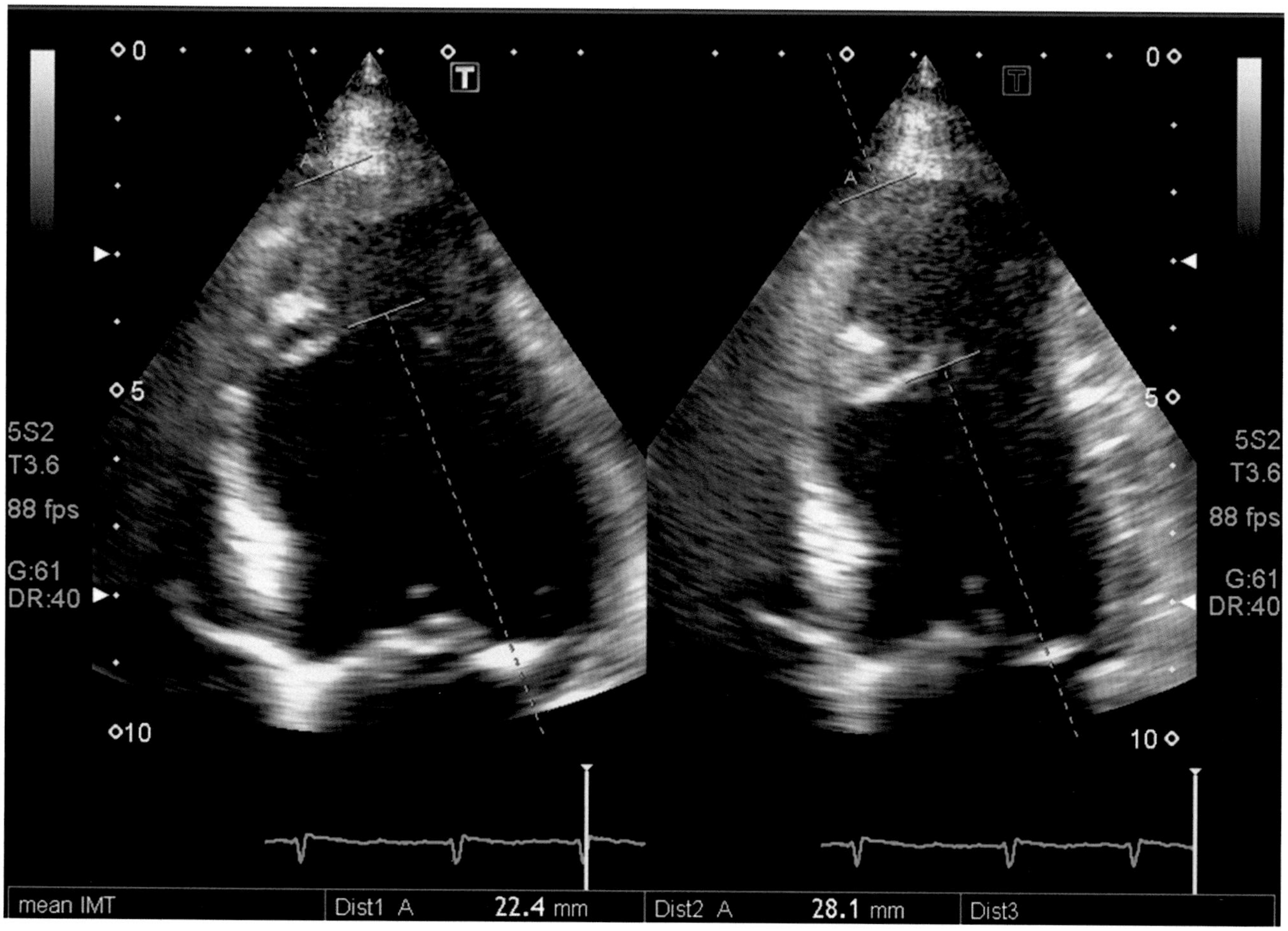

FIGURE 14-15 ■ **2D echocardiography in restrictive cardiomyopathy.** End-diastolic frame on left, end-systolic frame on right. In both images an endocardial thickening with thrombotic layer and calcifications are evident. Thickening of mitral valve is also present.

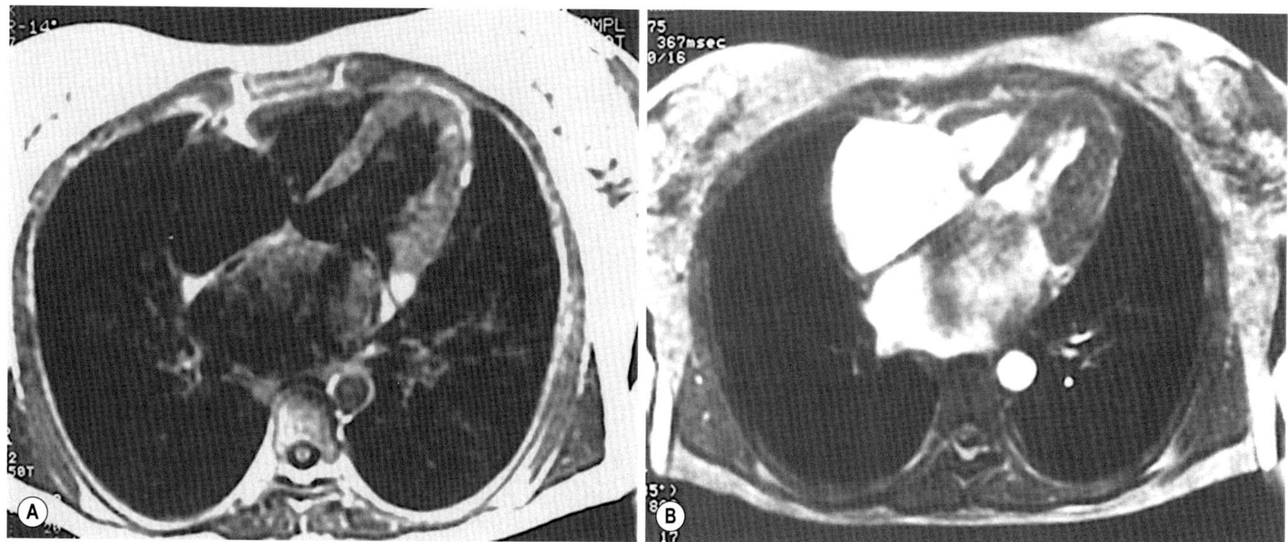

FIGURE 14-16 ■ **Restrictive cardiomyopathy.** (A) SE T1w image and (B) cine-MRI frame, both showing tubular shape of ventricles and enlarged atria. In (B) a flow void in the left atrium due to mitral regurgitation is evident.

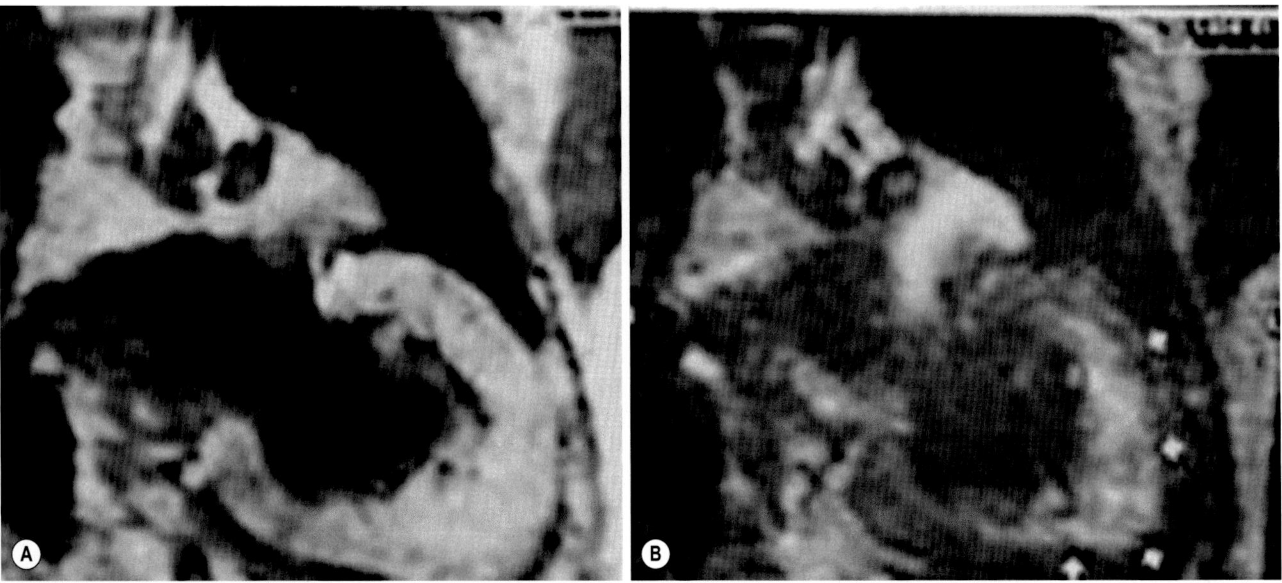

FIGURE 14-17 ■ Restrictive cardiomyopathy due to fibroelastosis. (A) SE T1w image shows an apparent thickened myocardium; (B) STIR image shows a thickened hyperintense endocardium (arrows) with normal myocardium.

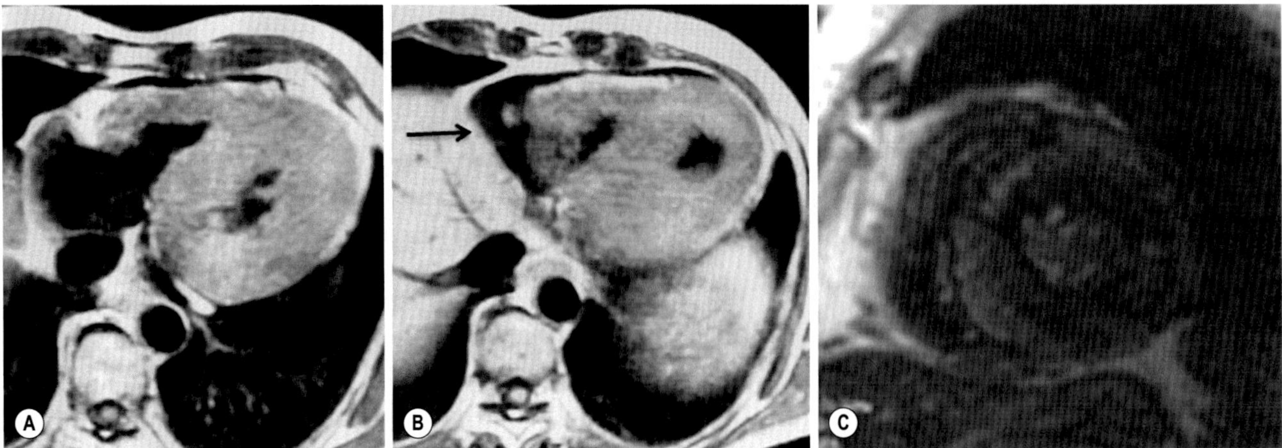

FIGURE 14-18 ■ Cardiac amyloidosis. (A, B) Contiguous T1w axial slices show marked myocardial thickening of both ventricles, with heterogeneous signal intensity; a small amount of pericardial effusion is present (arrows). (C) Late gadolinium enhancement short-axis image shows no myocardial suppression due to increased extracellular space and interstitial amyloid accumulation.

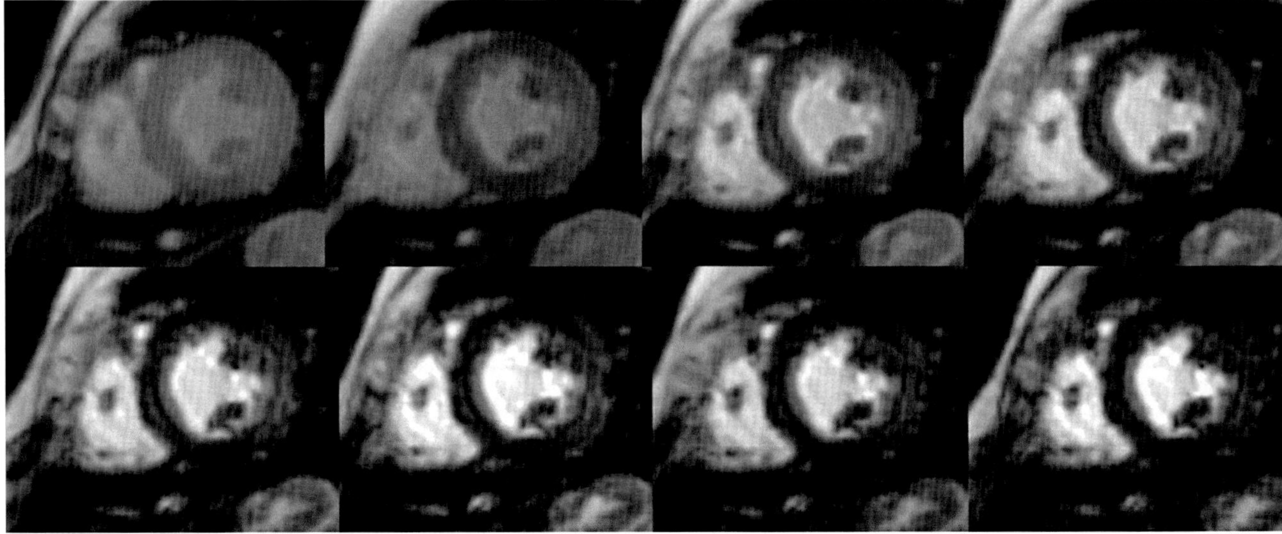

FIGURE 14-19 ■ Iron overload in major thalassaemia. Multi-echo fast gradient-echo sequence for T2* quantification; from a short TE (1.1 ms, top left) to a long TE (18 ms, bottom right), a rapid decay of myocardium signal intensity.

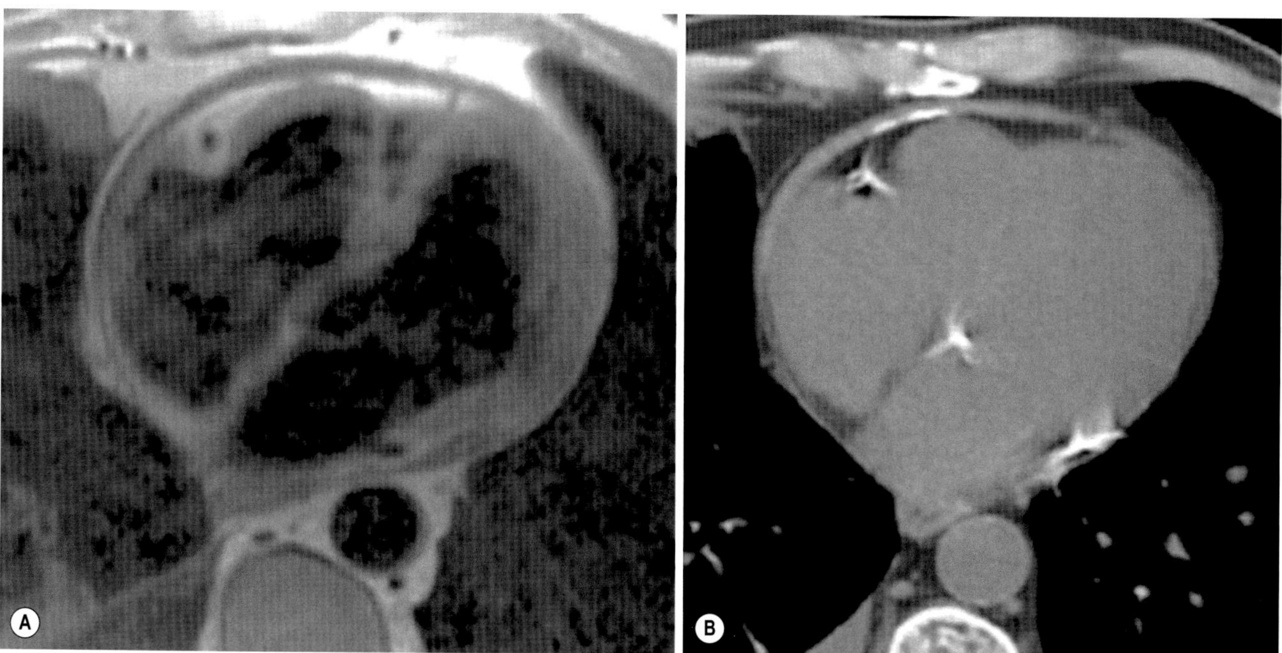

FIGURE 14-20 ■ Constrictive pericarditis. (A) This axial black-blood FSE image shows a diffuse pericardial thickening (5 mm), more evident anteriorly. Note also incomplete blood suppression in right atrium due to slow flow. (B) Axial unenhanced cardiac CT confirms pericardial thickening but also the presence of small calcifications.

TABLE 14-3 **European Society of Cardiology Classification of Secondary Cardiomyopathies**

Secondary Cardiomyopathies	
• Infiltrative • Storage • Toxicity • Endomyocardial • Inflammatory (granulomatous) • Endocrine	• Cardiofacial • Neuromuscular/neurological • Nutritional deficiency • Autoimmune/collagen • Electrolyte imbalance • Consequence of cancer therapy

Modified from Elliott et al.[2]

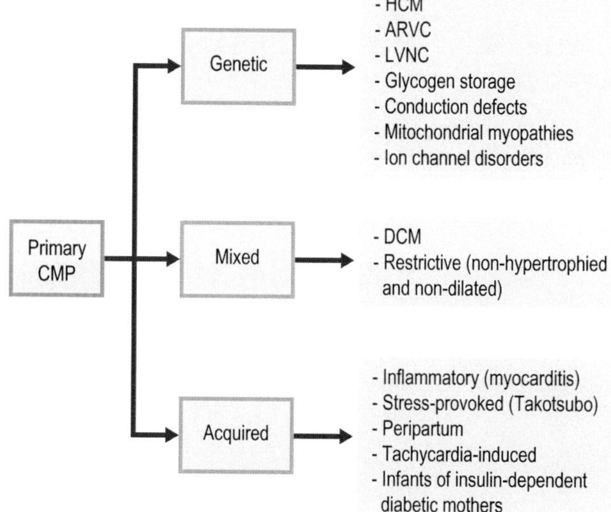

FIGURE 14-21 ■ European Society of Cardiology classification of primary cardiomyopathies. (Modified from Elliott et al.[2]).

and ejection fraction were introduced, by means of ultrasound or cardiac MRI measurements, aimed to increase sensitivity (Table 14-3 and Fig. 14-21).[2] MRI has been used in the past quite exclusively to demonstrate fatty infiltration of the right ventricle myocardium, particularly in the so-called triangle of dysplasia, the region contained between the subtricuspid area, the apex and the free wall of the outflow tract. However, the capability of assessing the presence of fat is strictly related to the amount of the fat, because of the limited spatial resolution: for this reason it is possible to recognise only cases with extensive replacement (Fig. 14-22). Another issue is the limitation of intramyocardial versus subepicardial differentiation of fat accumulation, partly because of limited spatial resolution but also because subepicardial fat accumulation can be recognised in other physiological and pathological conditions, such as obesity, steroid therapy and old age (Fig. 14-23).

In the revised criteria, MRI has been included only for the assessment of ventricular size and global/segmental functional assessment, as it has been demonstrated to be more sensitive than ultrasound for right ventricular systolic function evaluation; it is unique in volume measurements, as it uses a 3D approach (unlike ultrasound) that needs a geometrical assumption (not available for the right ventricle) for measuring volumes. Also, regional function is better evaluated by MRI: systolic bulging and aneurysms of the right ventricle anterior wall are easily detected (Fig. 14-24), also in the free wall, not always assessable by echocardiography.

Recent data have been published on the use of delayed enhancement technique to demonstrate the presence of fibrotic tissue[33] although this is not easy to visualise in the thin myocardium of the right ventricle. Cardiac CT is only relatively helpful, considering the wide role of MRI; however, in small series, CT has detected small foci of fat deposition/substitution even in the right ventricle, due to its high spatial resolution and good contrast resolution for fat.[34] However, CT is less suited to assessing regional wall motion abnormalities of the right ventricle.

Unclassified Cardiomyopathy

In this group two entities are included: left ventricular non-compaction and takotsubo cardiomyopathy. Left

FIGURE 14-22 ■ Arrhythmogenic right ventricular cardiomyopathy. Black-blood axial image shows a complete fatty substitution of right ventricle free wall (high signal intensity tissue); similar foci are evident in left ventricle apex and basal lateral wall (arrows).

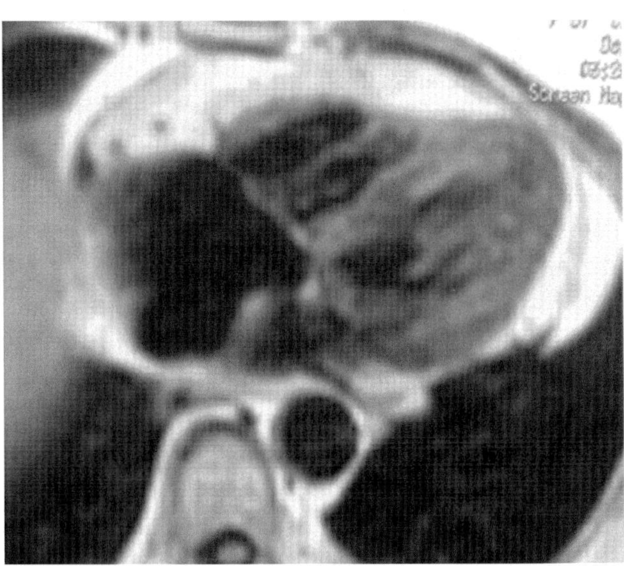

FIGURE 14-23 ■ T1w axial image in a patient receiving intensive steroid treatment. An increased amount of fat is evident in the mediastinum, prepericardial and subepicardial spaces, but normal right ventricle myocardium is visible.

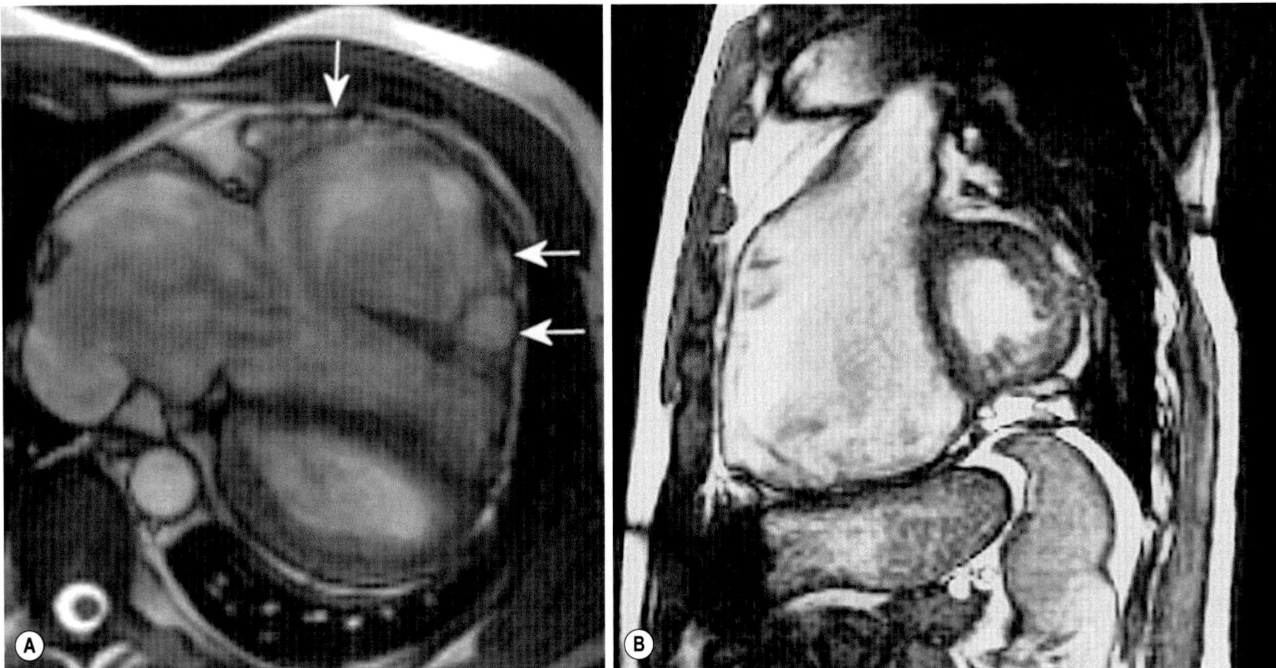

FIGURE 14-24 ■ Arrhythmogenic right ventricular cardiomyopathy. Cine-MRI axial (A) and short-axis (B) images show huge right ventricle dilation with small free-wall bulges (arrows in A).

ventricular non-compaction (LVNC) is characterised by prominent left ventricular trabeculae and deep intertrabeculae recesses;[35] this results in segments of thickened myocardium, composed of thin compacted epicardium with a thick endocardial layer. It is unclear whether LVNC is a separate CMP or a congenital or acquired trait shared by other phenotypes; it can be isolated or associated with congenital anomalies (complex cyanotic, Ebstein) or muscular dystrophies. It is frequently familial, with a wide range of abnormalities seen in about 25% of asymptomatic relatives.

Echocardiography is the first and often only diagnostic tool for assessing LVNC, especially in paediatric patients. Increased trabeculation is usually detected in mid-apical segments, on both lateral wall and septum (Fig. 14-25), with the latter normally being non-trabeculated. In difficult cases, MRI can be useful, using a cut-off value of 2.3 for the ratio between non-compacted and compacted myocardium (Fig. 14-26).[36] Furthermore, delayed enhancement is able to demonstrate the presence of fibrotic tissue in the compacted myocardium, more often in the forms associated with muscular dystrophies (Fig. 14-27).

Takotsubo CMP or transient left ventricular apical ballooning syndrome is characterised by a reversible regional systolic dysfunction, associated with chest pain and negative invasive coronary angiography; typical presentation is an acute coronary syndrome, more in post-menopausal women after a physical or emotional stress, with noradrenaline acting as a neuromediator.[37] Functional recovery usually occurs within days or a couple of weeks.

Echocardiography is usually able to detect the abnormal function and the ballooning,[38] but, because of the acute presentation, invasive coronary angiography is required to exclude obstructive coronary artery disease, according to guidelines. In these cases, after a negative coronary angiography, there is a strong indication for CMR, with the aim to differentiate a myocardial infarction with normal coronary arteries from an acute

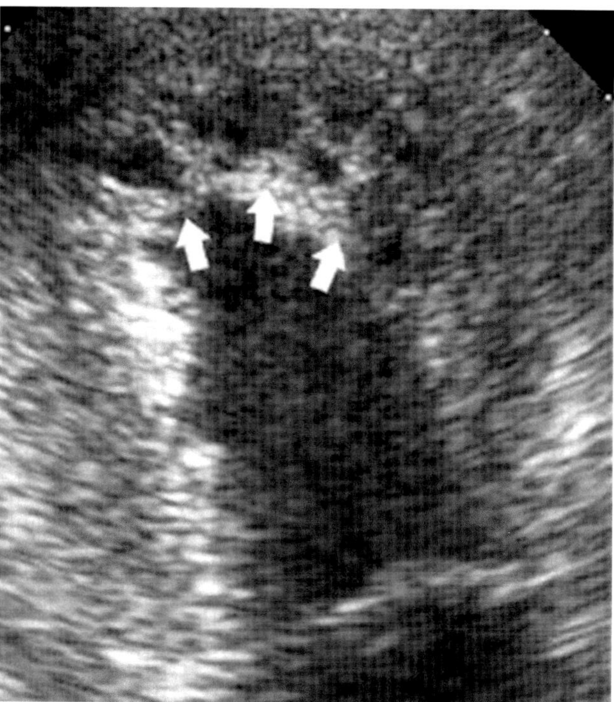

FIGURE 14-25 ■ **Echocardiography.** Two-chamber view shows thickened endocardium and increased trabeculation of left ventricle apex (arrows).

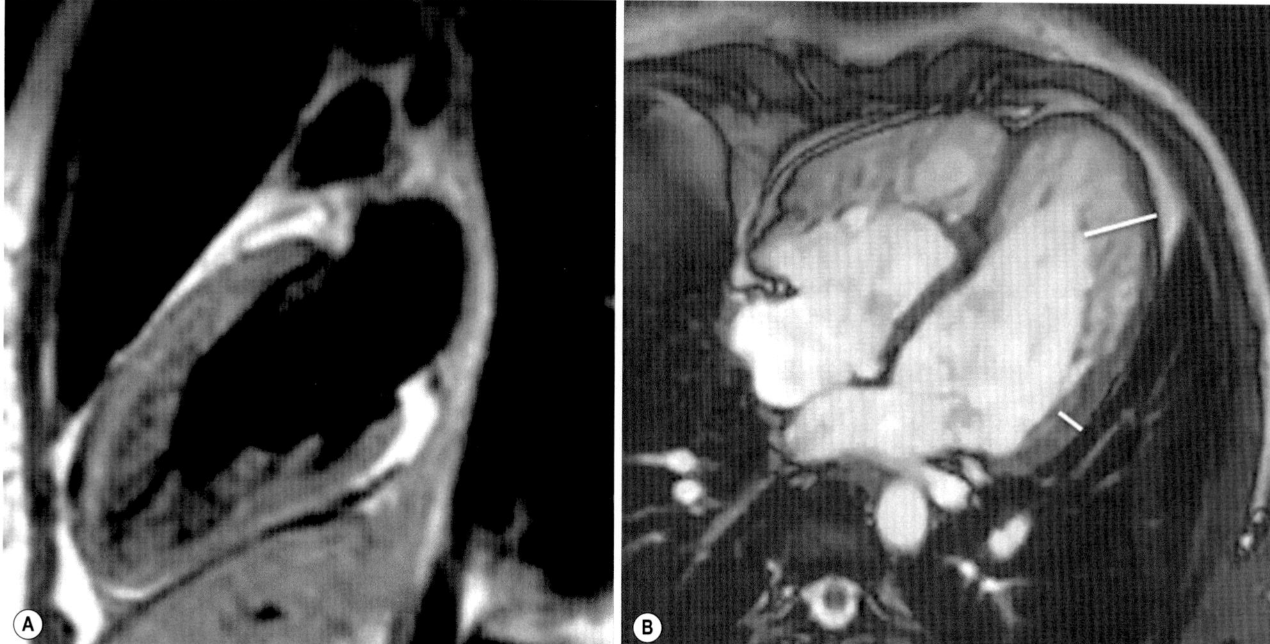

FIGURE 14-26 ■ **Left ventricular non-compaction.** (A) T1w black-blood vertical long-axis image shows increased number and thickness of myocardial trabeculae in mid and apical left ventricle regions. (B) Cine-MRI frame in horizontal long axis with measurement of non-compacted and compacted myocardium.

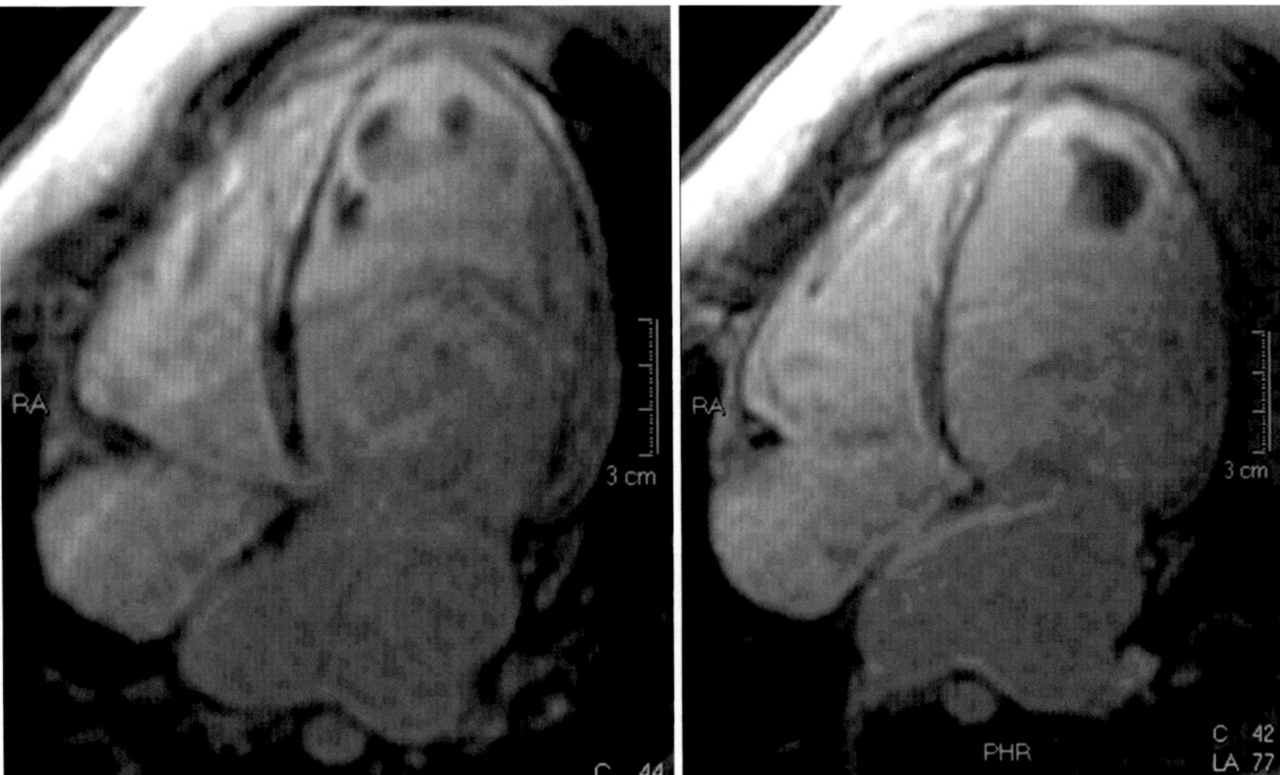

FIGURE 14-27 ■ **Left ventricular non-compaction.** Late enhancement images show contrast uptake in compacted myocardium (mostly at septal level), with subendocardial sparing, due to fibrotic changes. As an ancillary finding, multiple thrombi are visible.

myocarditis and a takotsubo CMP.[39] CMR is indeed able to detect the functional ballooning, but, more importantly, the oedema of the myocardium without any delayed enhancement, indicating the absence of necrosis and the reversibility of the damage (Fig. 14-28).[40]

Myocarditis

Myocarditis is not included in the ESC CMP classification as a single definite category, but is included in the acquired group as inflammatory CMP; in the AHA classification it is cited in the dilated phenotype for chronic myocarditis, while acute myocarditis does not show a precise phenotype. Consequently, myocarditis must be regarded separately from the classification, also when taking into consideration its increasing incidence and the recently increased possibilities to define the diagnosis.

Myocarditis is an acute or chronic inflammatory process affecting the myocardium, toxic or infective (viral, bacterial, rickettsial, fungal, parasitic), or due to hypersensitivity reactions.[1] It typically evolves through active healing and healed stages, with progression of inflammatory infiltrates, interstitial oedema, myocyte necrosis and finally scarring; in some cases, subclinical forms of viral myocarditis can trigger an autoimmune reaction causing immunological damage to the myocardium and/or cytoskeletal disruption, leading to a DCM phenotype with LV dysfunction. In these cases, viral persistence and chronic inflammatory infiltrates have been demonstrated.

Histology obtained through an endomyocardial biopsy is still considered the gold standard for the diagnosis,[41] based on the combination of leucocyte infiltration and necrosis defined by the so-called Dallas criteria,[42] though these criteria have been recently debated. Substantial refinement of the diagnosis can been reached by using molecular analysis of the specimens, such as DNA–RNA extraction and polymerase chain reaction.[43] Acute presentation can often mimic an acute coronary syndrome, with chest pain exertion dyspnoea, ECG abnormalities and mild enzyme elevation.[39,44] In this case there is an indication for invasive coronary angiography to exclude obstructive coronary artery disease, even if the presence of a recent viral infection or unexplained fever can indicate the correct diagnosis.

Echocardiography is usually performed to assess and quantify left ventricle systolic dysfunction; in the case of associated pericardial effusion, ultrasound can suggest the suspicion of an inflammatory process, but there is need for further examination. In the acute presentation, after negative coronary angiography, there is a strong indication to perform CMR, which can demonstrate oedema and delayed enhancement in the subepicardial layer, most frequently in the lateral and/or inferior wall (Fig. 14-29). This pattern easily allows differential diagnosis from acute myocardial infarction, where delayed enhancement is located in the subendocardial layer or is transmural, and from takotsubo CMP, where delayed enhancement is typically absent. However, a negative delayed enhancement study does not exclude an acute myocarditis, as

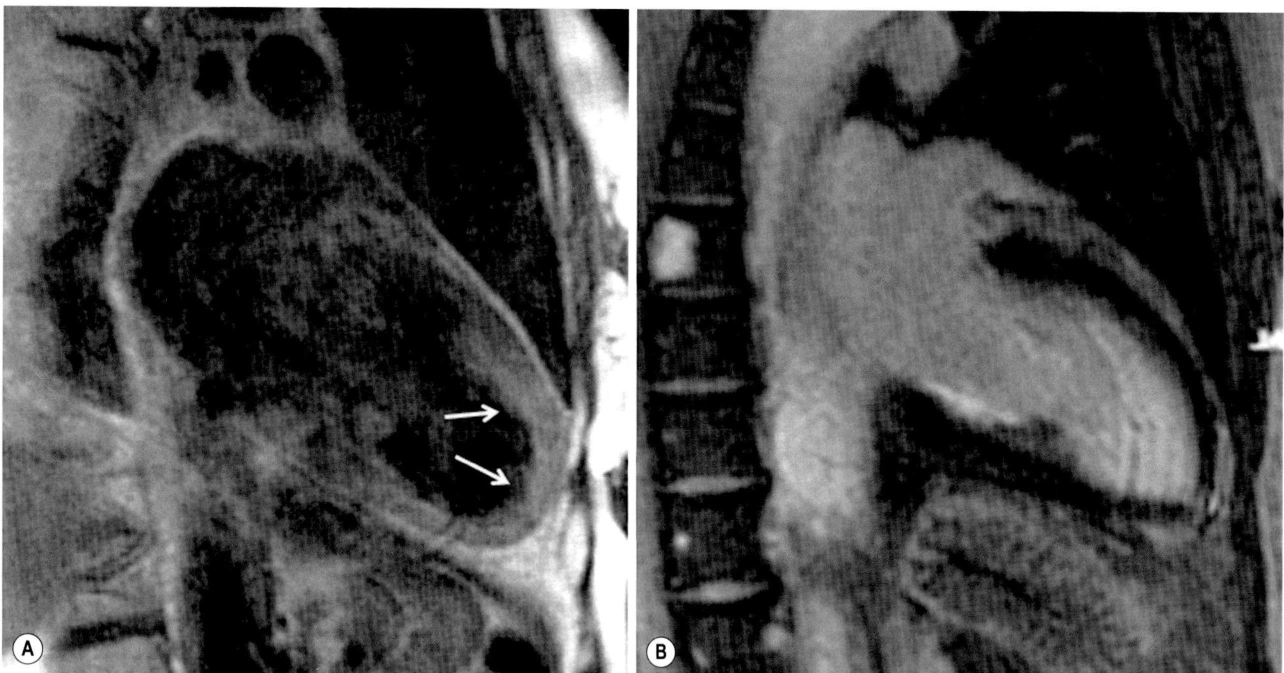

FIGURE 14-28 ■ **Takotsubo cardiomyopathy.** (A) T2w image in vertical long axis shows diffuse hyperintensity of the myocardium, due to oedema (arrows); (B) late enhancement image in the same plane shows no contrast uptake, demonstrating absence of any irreversible lesion.

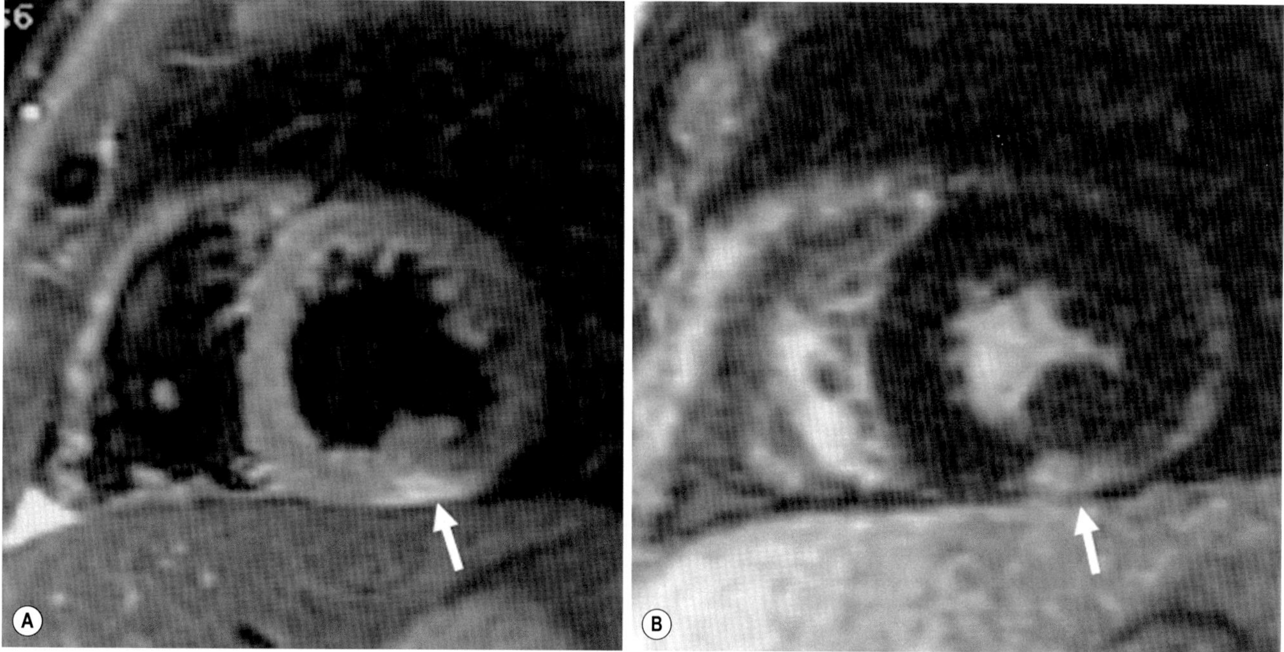

FIGURE 14-29 ■ **Acute myocarditis.** (A) T2w STIR short-axis image shows a subepicardial hyperintense area in inferior wall; (B) late enhancement image in corresponding plane shows contrast uptake with a non-ischaemic pattern. Patient presented 36 h before in emergency unit with chest pain and slight increase in cardiac enzymes; emergency coronary angiography was negative.

there is not always macroscopic detectable necrosis; in this case it is important to acquire MR images before and immediately after administration of contrast agent (early enhancement), in order to demonstrate inflammatory hyperaemia. The combination of oedema imaging (T2w sequences), basal, early and late enhancement imaging constitutes the cornerstone for the diagnosis, according to the so-called Lake-Louise criteria.[45] CMR is also useful and accurate for evaluating biventricular global and regional systolic function and eventually associated pericardial effusion, with or without pericardial enhancement, in the case of myopericarditis. Acute fulminant

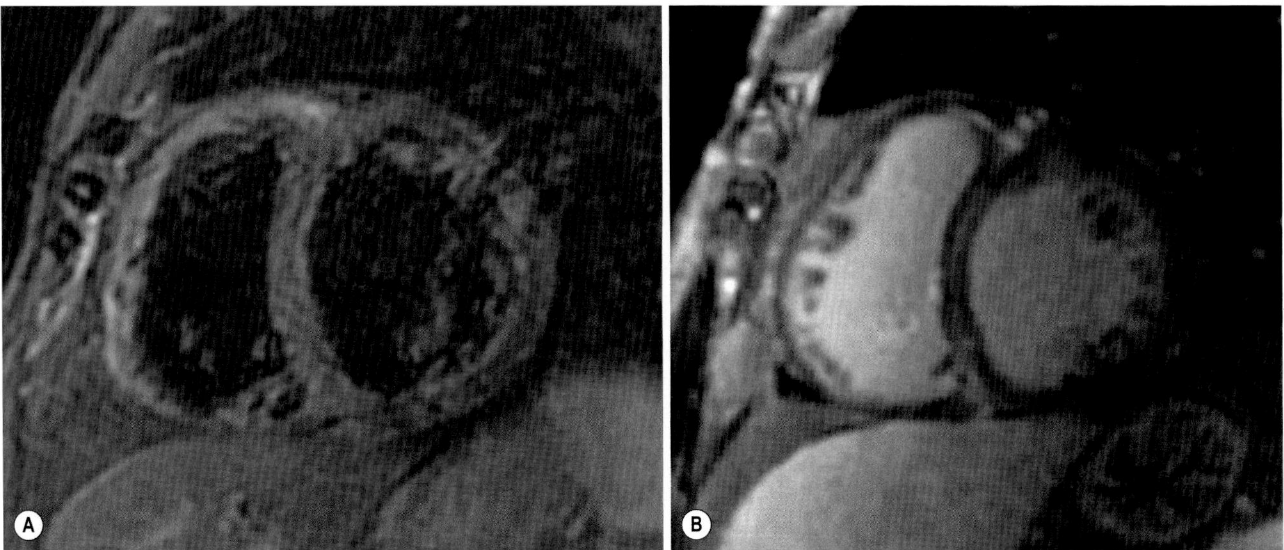

FIGURE 14-30 ■ Chronic myocarditis in patients presenting with new-onset severe tachyarrhythmia. (A) T2w STIR short-axis image shows no evidence of oedema; (B) late enhancement image in the same plane shows septal intramural contrast uptake. Septal endomyocardial biopsy demonstrated a lymphocytic infiltrate with interstitial fibrosis.

forms or cardiogenic shock can represent other rare but possible acute presentations.

Other clinical presentations can be more subtle, such as new-onset cardiac failure or tachyarrhythmias; these presentations are more often associated with chronic myocarditis. In these situations, echocardiography is useful for excluding other diseases: for example, a new onset of heart failure. In chronic myocarditis, MRI with late enhancement technique demonstrates fibrosis, typically located in the mesocardium.[46] Enhancement is generally less intense than in the acute forms, diffuse rather than patchy and located in the lateral wall or in the septum, the latter being more frequent in tachyarrhythmias (Fig. 14-30).

VALVULAR HEART DISEASE

Contrary to previous reports in the literature, the aetiology of acquired valve disease is now considered as being usually degenerative, rather than due to rheumatic or infective causes; the prevalence of mitral regurgitation and aortic stenosis is higher than that of mitral stenosis and aortic insufficiency. Also the age of onset is increasing. Radiographic findings are often minimal and non-specific, and the assessment is based on echocardiography.[47]

Mitral Valve Disease

In Western countries, non-rheumatic mitral valve disease is the most common manifestation of mitral disease; in non-Western countries, rheumatic heart disease is still quite prevalent. Among non-rheumatic diseases, mitral regurgitation is the most common, while non-rheumatic mitral stenosis is very rare. Many conditions can result in significant mitral regurgitation, affecting mitral leaflets (prolapse, endocarditis, mucopolysaccharidosis, lupus, rheumatoid arthritis) or subvalvular apparatus (annular dilatation, chordae tendineae rupture, annular calcification, myocardial infarction, hypertrophic cardiomyopathy). In mitral regurgitation, a portion of the left ventricular stroke volume is directed retrogradely into the atrium during systole, returning to the left ventricle during diastole, with consequent left ventricular volume loading. To maintain an adequate stroke volume both the left ventricular stroke volume and the ejection fraction increase.

Acute regurgitation may result from infective endocarditis or rupture of chordae tendineae/papillary muscles. Sudden volume loading into the non-compliant left atrium may result in markedly elevated atrial pressure, causing acute pulmonary oedema and symptoms of heart failure.[48] Rupture or elongation of chordae tendineae, ischaemic and non-ischaemic cardiomyopathy, hypertrophic obstructive cardiomyopathy and rheumatic heart disease are all causes of chronic mitral regurgitation.[48] In response to the chronic volume load both the left atrium and left ventricle dilate, thus serving as a reservoir for the regurgitant volume without necessarily increasing pulmonary vascular pressure. However, if the left ventricle decompensates and the forward stroke volume decreases, heart failure may arise.[48]

The appearances on CXR depend on the duration and severity of the mitral regurgitation and any other associated heart disease. Acute, severe mitral regurgitation may present with pulmonary oedema, but with a virtually normal heart size and shape (Fig. 14-31). After an interval, the heart usually decompensates by developing left ventricular dilatation, which may be marked (Fig. 14-32). Selective left atrial enlargement may be absent, slight or moderate, with or without left atrial appendage enlargement (Fig. 14-32). Pulmonary vascular changes reflect the haemodynamic derangement and the effects of treatment.

As previously described, mitral regurgitation can have many different causes such as mitral prolapse or chordae

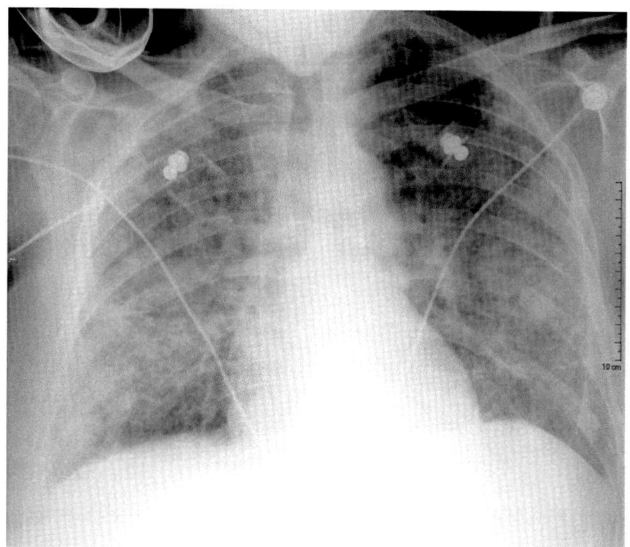

FIGURE 14-31 ■ Chest X-ray, frontal view, in intensive care unit shows signs of alveolar pulmonary oedema without cardiac enlargement.

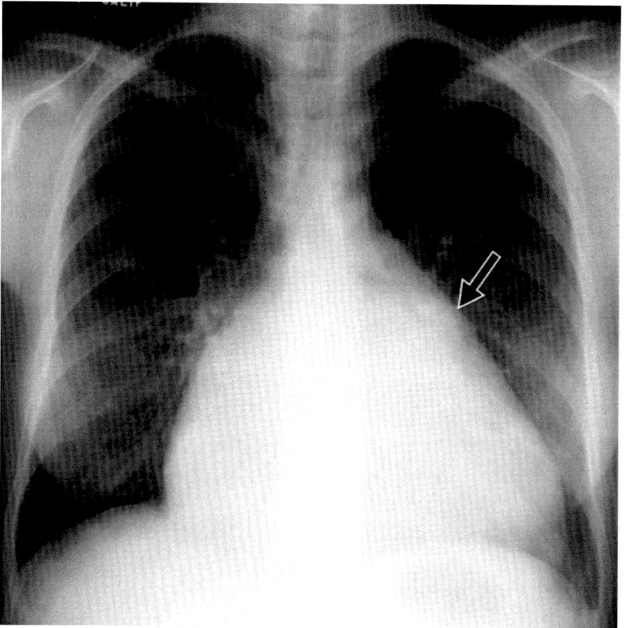

FIGURE 14-32 ■ **Chest X-ray shows left atrial appendage enlargement (arrow) in mitral regurgitation; subcarinal opacity with slight dislocation of upper left main bronchus is also evident due to left atrium enlargement.**

tendinee rupturae (during bacterial endocarditis, collagen diseases, acute myocardial infarction) or it may be functional (DCM, ischaemic).

Mitral Valve Prolapse

The most common cause of severe (non-ischaemic) mitral regurgitation is the mitral valve prolapse syndrome.[49] Mitral valve prolapse is defined as systolic bowing of the mitral leaflet more than 2 mm beyond the

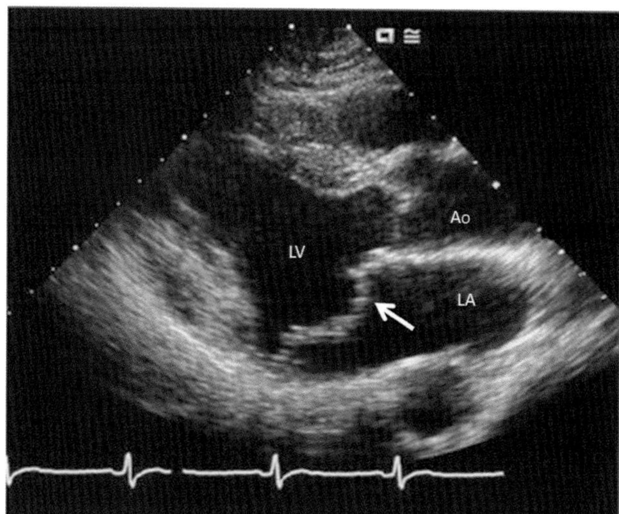

FIGURE 14-33 ■ **Mitral prolapse.** Echocardiography (parasternal long axis) shows wide anterior leaflet prolapse of the mitral valve.

annular plane into the atrium,[48] caused by rupture or elongation of the chordae tendineae. The middle scallop of the posterior leaflet is the most often affected.[48] Mitral valve prolapse is due to elongation of the chordae tendineae associated with myxomatous degeneration of the valve leaflets, occurring alone or in association with Marfan's syndrome and in patients with atrial septal defect. The diagnosis is typically made by echocardiography (Fig. 14-33), but it is also possible on CMR, with two- and three-chamber views preferred; associated imaging findings include leaflet thickening (thickness of >5 mm) and flail leaflet.[48] Cardiac CT also has good sensitivity for detecting mitral valve prolapse, small vegetations and ruptured chordae; furthermore, cardiac CT is useful for assessing valvular and subvalvular calcifications[50] and is increasingly used in valvular assessment. Prolapse of the mitral valve may be associated with chest pain and ECG changes, which may suggest ischaemic heart disease.

Chordal Rupture

Chordal rupture may complicate bacterial endocarditis, or less frequently myocardial infarction or connective tissue diseases, leading to flail of part of a leaflet; this is the eversion of the mitral leaflet tip into the atrium during systole,[48] preventing proper closure in systole and producing severe mitral regurgitation. In the case of an acute event, acute pulmonary oedema is seen on CXR, usually without cardiomegaly (Fig. 14-31).

Functional Mitral Regurgitation

Functional mitral regurgitation may occur in dilated cardiomyopathy or ischaemic cardiac failure. In this case the valve is normal, but regional wall motion abnormalities, left ventricular dilatation, tethering of chordae tendineae or annular dilatation, alone or in combination, lead to dysfunction of the mitral apparatus with 'functional' mitral regurgitation.[48] Mitral regurgitation in these

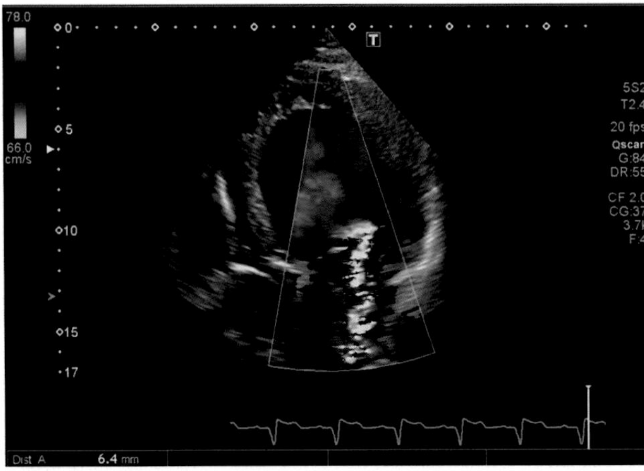

FIGURE 14-34 ■ **Mitral regurgitation.** Echo colour Doppler shows severe regurgitation in the left atrium and marked left ventricle enlargement (mitral annulus dilation).

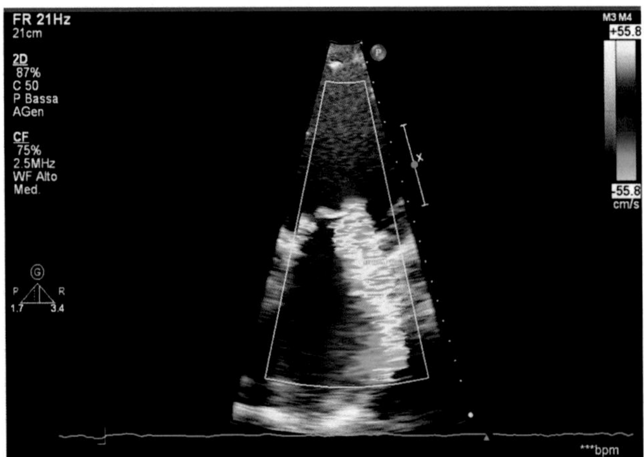

FIGURE 14-35 ■ **Mitral regurgitation.** Echo colour Doppler shows severe mitral regurgitation (apical 4C). Mosaic effect is evident with complete occupation of the left atrium.

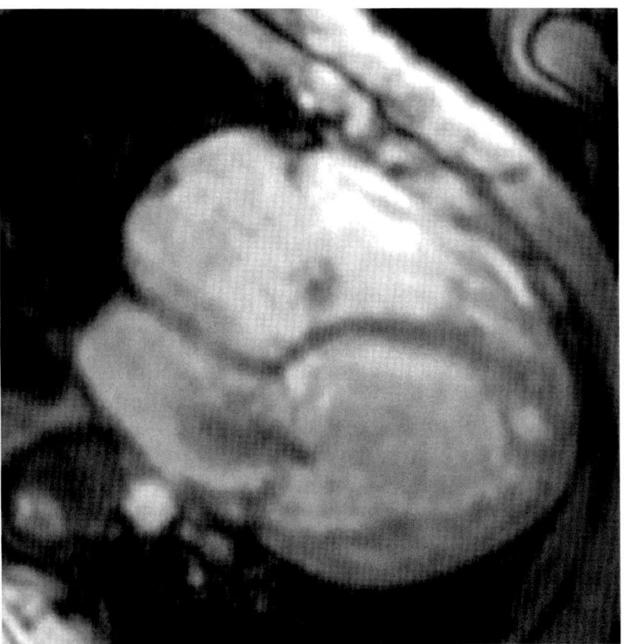

FIGURE 14-36 ■ Cine-MRI frame of functional mitral regurgitation (black jet directed from left ventricle to left atrium) in dilated cardiomyopathy.

situations is very common, but severe (Fig. 14-34). Mitral regurgitation detection and severity are usually assessed by 2D Doppler echocardiography, which can detect left atrial dilatation, increased atrial emptying volume and gradual closure of aortic valve during systole, coupled with visualisation of systolic regurgitant colour-coded flow within the left atrium. Pulsed Doppler interrogation is extremely sensitive also to small amounts of regurgitant flow; the extent of penetration and the area of the regurgitant jet within the left atrium allow for a semiquantitative estimation of the disease (mild, moderate, severe) (Fig. 14-35). However, in the case of asymmetrical jets (i.e. flail), this method underestimates the severity. Furthermore, continuous Doppler is very sensitive, giving a characteristic high-velocity, parabolic, systolic spectrum of the flow.

MRI identifies mitral regurgitation in cine as a retrograde jet through the mitral orifice from the left ventricle into the left atrium, due to turbulent flow and consequent spin dephasing (Fig. 14-36). Mitral valve regurgitation can be quantified as the difference between left and right ventricle stroke volumes (LVSV and RVSV). Every difference between the two measured stroke volumes indicates the amount of blood which comes back through the insufficient valve during diastole.[51] This estimation is valid only if the tricuspid valve is competent (tricuspid regurgitation is reported in up to 50% of patients with significant mitral regurgitation); moreover, the calculation of RVSV is less reproducible than LVSV due to the extensive trabeculation of the right ventricle.[51] In the case of combined aortic and mitral regurgitation, the difference represents the sum of regurgitant volumes.[51]

Phase contrast MRI can discriminate between antegrade and retrograde flow during the cardiac cycle; the mitral regurgitant volume (MRV) can be measured by MRI as the difference between the LVSV and the aortic forward flow. The regurgitant fraction (RF) is the ratio of the MRV divided by the LVSV.[51] It may also be possible to directly measure mitral flow by phase contrast velocity flow mapping at the tips of the mitral valve leaflets but this is better obtained with a specialised imaging sequence which tracks the motion of the mitral valve annulus during the cardiac cycle to adjust the plane of velocity encoding for diastolic mitral valve motion.[49,51,52] With cine-phase contrast MRI, mitral regurgitation can be calculated as left ventricular inflow through the mitral valve minus left ventricular outflow in the ascending aorta.[49] This approach is also applicable in patients with mitral and aortic regurgitation, since diastolic left ventricular inflow (= left ventricular mitral inflow and aortic regurgitation volume) is equal to the systolic left ventricular outflow (= aortic outflow and mitral regurgitant volume).[49]

The American Heart Association and the American College of Cardiology[53,54] have established echocardiographic criteria for grading the severity of mitral regurgitation. Even in the absence of inter-society established criteria for MRI, the measurements of regurgitant volume (RV) and fraction derived from LV volume and ascending aortic flow allow grading of regurgitation as:[48]

Mild: RV <30 mL/beat; RF <30%
Moderate: RV = 30–59 mL/beat; RF = 30–49%
Severe: RV >60 mL/beat; RF >50%.

For a comprehensive assessment of patients with mitral regurgitation, three components are mandatory: (1) quantification of regurgitation, (2) assessment of left ventricular adaptation to volume overload and (3) anatomy of mitral valve and subvalvular apparatus. Whereas MRI satisfies (1) and (2), the method of choice for assessing valve anatomy is echocardiography, although improvements in MR imaging strategies allow detection of morphological abnormalities such as flail mitral valve leaflets.[48]

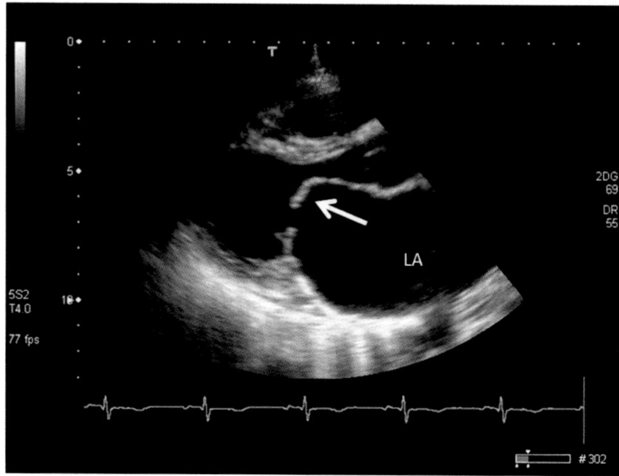

FIGURE 14-37 ■ **Mitral stenosis.** Echocardiography (parasternal long axis) shows marked thickening of mitral leaflets with restricted mitral valve orifice (doming anterior leaflet). Left atrial (LA) enlargement is evident.

Mitral Stenosis

Mitral stenosis is a structural abnormality of the mitral valve that prevents proper opening during diastolic filling of the left ventricle. Increased left atrial pressure is necessary to move blood across the stenotic mitral valve and into the left ventricle. Chronic elevation of left atrial pressure causes atrial dilatation and pulmonary venous hypertension. Atrial fibrillation (due to atrial dilatation) and dyspnoea (due to pulmonary venous hypertension) are common symptoms of mitral stenosis. Prolonged pulmonary venous hypertension may also lead to right ventricular dilatation and failure, as well as to tricuspid regurgitation.[48]

Mitral stenosis (MS) is highly prevalent in developing countries because of its association with rheumatic fever, but is also seen in developed countries.[55] The most common cause of MS is rheumatic fever. Isolated MS is twice as common in women as in men; it occurs in 40% of all patients presenting with rheumatic heart disease; a history of rheumatic fever can be elicited from approximately 60% of patients presenting with pure MS.[54]

Other causes of MS are very rare and include congenital anomalies, prior exposure to chest radiation, mucopolysaccharidosis, severe mitral annular calcification, ball valve thrombus and left atrial myxoma.[56] In cor triatriatum, the left atrium is divided by a membrane into two chambers; blood flow may be restricted before it reaches the mitral valve, mimicking mitral stenosis.[48] The main features of a stenotic mitral valve are leaflet thickening, nodularity, commissural fusion, with narrowing of the valve to the shape of a fish mouth. Leaflets might be calcified; chords may be fused and shortened.[55] The normal mitral valve cross-sectional area is 4–6 cm^2 and a gradient is rare unless the valve is less than 2 cm^2. Symptoms correlate with increasing mean left atrial pressure, when mitral valve area reduces to 1.5 cm^2.[55] The increase in left atrial pressure from obstruction across the mitral valve is reflected onto the pulmonary circulation, causing dyspnoea[57] and leading to pulmonary oedema. Haemoptysis may occur. In chronic severe mitral stenosis, secondary pulmonary hypertension may cause right ventricular failure and tricuspid regurgitation.[57] Occasional embolic episodes are related to the atrial fibrillation. Death is mainly due to heart failure or systemic embolism.

The standard for diagnosis and determination of the severity of mitral stenosis is 2D Doppler echocardiography.[57] Two-dimensional echocardiography evaluates the morphology of the mitral valve leaflets and the subvalvular apparatus. Leaflet thickening (Fig. 14-37) or calcification (hockey-stick deformity of the mitral valve leaflets is typical), leaflet mobility, and commissural or sub-valvular fusion can be seen. Narrowing of the mitral valve area can be appreciated.[57] Two-dimensional echocardiography also helps assess the suitability for mitral valve valvotomy: a pliable non-calcified valve could be suitable for balloon valvuloplasty or commissurotomy; a calcified fibrotic valve with subvalvular fusion may preclude valvotomy.[57]

Criteria for determining the severity of mitral valve obstruction are the mean mitral valve gradient and the mitral valve area: mild mitral stenosis is present when the area is >1.5 cm^2 and the mean gradient is <5 mmHg; moderate stenosis refers to an area of 1.0–1.5 cm^2 and a gradient of 5–10 mmHg; severe stenosis, when the area is <1.0 cm^2 and the gradient is >10 mmHg.[57]

Mitral valve area (MVA):

- is reliably calculated by planimetry from the short-axis view at the tip of the mitral valve leaflets; even higher accuracy might be achieved using 3D echocardiography.[55]
- is inversely related to diastolic half-time ($T_{1/2}$), which is the time it takes for the maximal mitral gradient to decrease by 50%. This can be obtained from the rate of velocity decrease during early and mid-diastole, as assessed on the transmitral velocity curve.

$$T_{1/2} = \mathrm{DT} \times 0.29; \mathrm{MVA} = 220/T_{1/2}$$

where $T_{1/2}$ = half-time and DT = deceleration time.

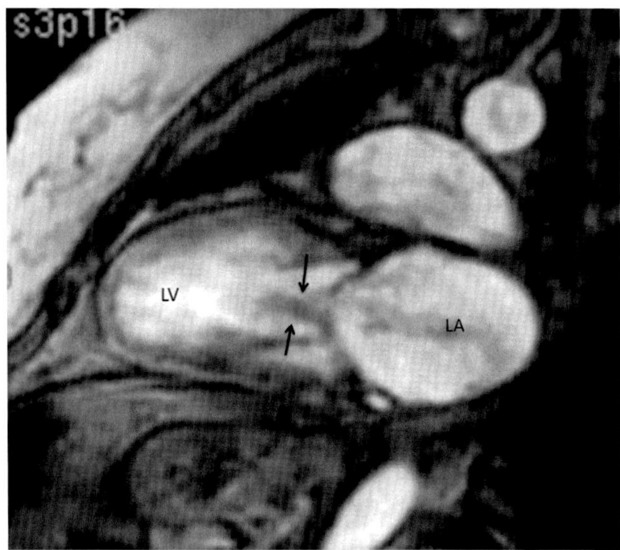

FIGURE 14-38 ■ **Cine-MRI frame of mitral stenosis.** A small flow void directed from left atrium (LA) to left ventricle (LV) is visible (arrows), due to mild mitral stenosis. Left atrium is enlarged.

- can be calculated with the continuity equation when the area derived from the half-time does not correlate with the mean transmitral gradient

  $$MVA = (LVOTTVI \times LVOTarea)/MVTVI$$

  where LVOT = left ventricular outflow tract, MV = mitral valve and TVI = time–velocity integral.[57]

Cine-MRI can be helpful in selected cases, however, with good visualisation of the restricted mitral leaflets and the anterograde jet due to turbulent flow across a stenotic valve orifice, best visible on the two chambers (Fig. 14-38) and LV outflow tract views.[58]

Mitral stenosis that is caused by rheumatic disease may have distinctive morphological features: restricted opening, thickened leaflets, commissural fusion, valve calcification and a 'fish-mouth' appearance on short-axis images. Bowing of a thickened and fibrotic anterior leaflet during diastole results in a 'hockey-stick' appearance best seen on two- or four-chamber images.[48]

Direct measurement of the orifice area can be performed in the same way as for aortic stenosis, by placing an imaging plane perpendicular to the direction of flow at the mitral valve tips during diastole[58] and drawing a contour around the smallest valve orifice.[48] The technique has good agreement with echocardiography, but care needs to be taken in positioning the plane at the tips in order to obtain an accurate valve area, and acquisition of multiple parallel thin slices may be helpful.[58] Diastolic flow and velocity can also be measured in this image plane; velocity-encoded CMR can be used as a robust tool to quantify MVA via mitral flow velocity analysis with the pressure half-time (PHT) method,[59] though the frequency of atrial fibrillation in severe mitral stenosis reduces the accuracy of the flow measurements.[58]

MVA planimetry can also be determined by MDCT although it frequently yields larger areas than calculated by Doppler transthoracic echocardiogram (TTE) or cardiac catheterisation; it may allow for reliable quantification of mitral valve stenosis and effectual discrimination among severity grades.[60] Mitral valve leaflet calcification on MDCT indicates mitral valve sclerosis or stenosis.[61] Cardiac catheterisation and angiocardiography are used in those rare situations where echocardiography has failed to elucidate the contribution of each valve lesion, or when coexistent coronary artery disease needs assessment.

Non-rheumatic causes of mitral stenosis usually produce non-specific imaging features such as valve thickening or leaflet fixation.[47] However, CT and MR imaging characteristics occasionally are suggestive of the cause of stenosis. Radiation-induced valve disease, for example, is associated with mitral premature calcification of the apparatus, lung fibrosis and focal vertebral abnormalities.[62] Calcification of the mitral leaflets, a cause of senescent mitral stenosis, may be depicted at CT. Non-valvular disease (e.g. ball-valve thrombus, left atrial myxoma) may also produce signs and symptoms of mitral stenosis (Figs. 14-20 and 14-22).

Rheumatic Mitral Valve Disease

Acute rheumatic disease can cause a pancarditis. During the acute phase, mitral regurgitation can be present; this is usually reversible. Chronic rheumatic mitral valve disease often leads to stenosis, due to fusion of the commissures, thickening and shortening of the chordae tendineae and fibrosis of the papillary muscles. Severe mitral regurgitation results from leaflet destruction. However, there is usually a combination of mitral stenosis and regurgitation, with the first counterbalancing the effects of the second, so both cannot be severe simultaneously.

Tricuspid Valve Disease

Tricuspid stenosis is generally rheumatic, more common in women than in men, and usually associated with tricuspid regurgitation and mitral stenosis. Most commonly, tricuspid regurgitation is functional and secondary to marked dilatation of the tricuspid annulus due to RV enlargement in the presence of pulmonary hypertension, mitral valve disease or mitral valve replacement, ischaemic heart disease or dilated cardiomyopathy. Tricuspid valve regurgitation may be directly caused by rheumatic disease. Severe tricuspid regurgitation can also occur in endomyocardial fibrosis and carcinoid heart syndrome (also responsible for stenosis). In Ebstein's anomaly, the insertion of the septal cusp of the tricuspid valve is displaced towards the apex of the right ventricle. Endocarditis can also cause tricuspid regurgitation

The clinical recognition of tricuspid valve disease can be difficult. On CXR, the main radiological sign is right atrial enlargement, which can be appreciated on frontal view as an increased prominence of the second right cardiac arch; in the lateral view, an enlarged right appendage is seen as increased retrosternal opacity between the aortic arch and the outflow tract of the right ventricle. Again, echocardiography is the most important diagnostic tool.

Colour Doppler can easily detect retrograde flow in the right atrium; by measuring the depth and area of the

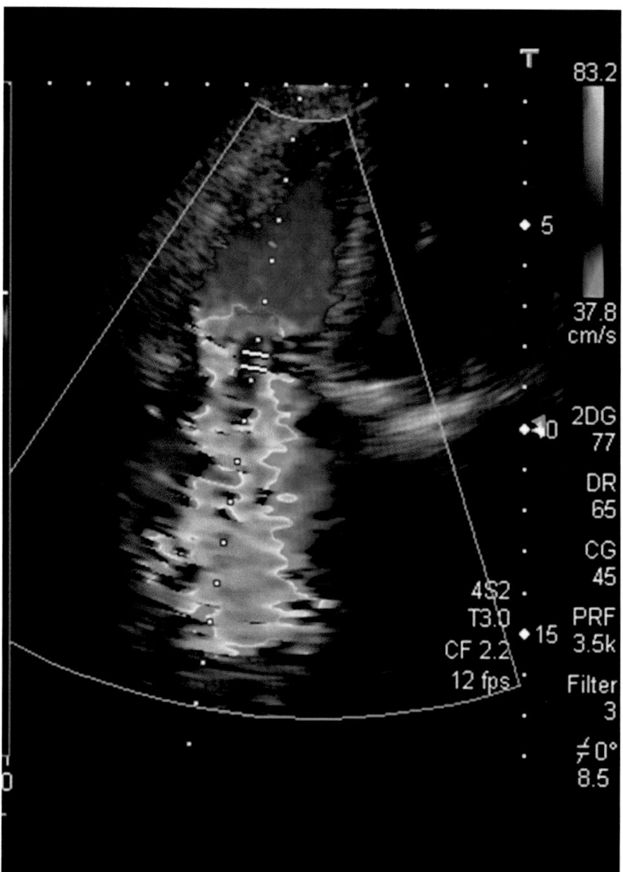

FIGURE 14-39 ■ **Tricuspid regurgitation.** Echo colour Doppler demonstrates severe tricuspid insufficiency with mosaic effect occupying entirely the right atrium.

jet's penetration, regurgitation can be semiquantitatively graded (Fig. 14-39).[63] At pulsed Doppler, regurgitation appears as a pansystolic turbulent signal in the right atrium; if retrograde flow is also appreciated in the inferior vena cava, regurgitation can be graded as severe. The estimation of the peak velocity of regurgitant flow through the valve at continuous Doppler is not useful for grading the regurgitation, but makes it possible to estimate the peak systolic pressure in the right ventricle and pulmonary artery, by applying the modified Bernoulli's formula. This parameter is extremely useful in evaluating the haemodynamic effect of all left chambers and myocardial diseases.

In tricuspid stenosis, echocardiography allows visualisation of the thickened valve leaflets and their limited motion, while Doppler allows visualisation and measurement of the jet. CMR, with steady-state free precession (SSFP) cine sequences, is used to delineate abnormal valvular morphology such as in Ebstein's anomaly or carcinoid heart disease.[64] Tricuspid regurgitation signal void seen in the right atrium is less evident than mitral regurgitation due to its lower velocity and turbulence (Fig. 14-40).[64] The regurgitant volume can be quantified by combining phase-contrast flow measurements at the pulmonary valve and RV stroke volume;[65] the regurgitant orifice can also be visualised with CMR,[64] which has shown some limitations in assessing the peak velocity of tricuspid regurgitation.

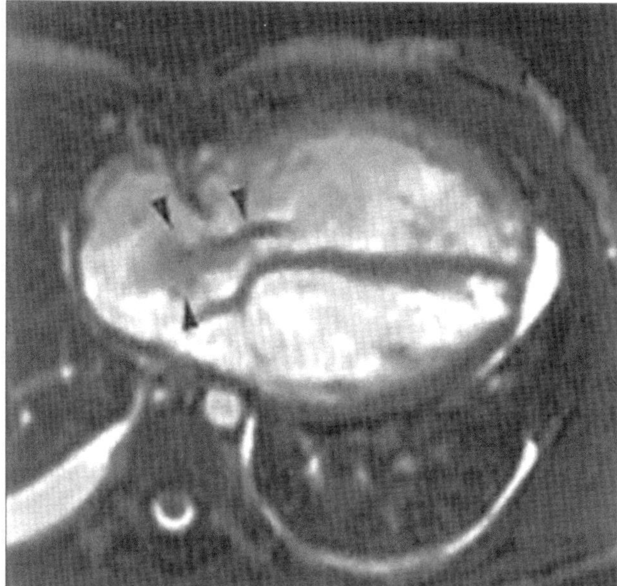

FIGURE 14-40 ■ **Cine-MRI frame of tricuspid regurgitation.** A retrograde black jet directed from right ventricle to right atrium is evident (arrowheads).

Aortic Valve Disease

Aortic Stenosis

The predominant cause of aortic stenosis in Western countries is degenerative calcific disease in middle-aged or elderly patients.[66] Compared with mitral stenosis, where calcium is deposited on an already stenosed valve, calcific aortic stenosis results from the calcification of the aortic cusps which causes obstruction. Rheumatic disease is a rare cause nowadays.

Clinical presentation may include breathlessness, chest pain, or syncope, with ECG signs of left ventricular hypertrophy. CXR can detect rounding of the cardiac apex, suggesting left ventricular hypertrophy (Fig. 14-41). Prominence of the ascending aorta (first right cardiac arch) may indicate post-stenotic dilatation (Fig. 14-41), but in older patients the whole thoracic aorta may be widened from atherosclerosis. In lateral view it is easier to demonstrate the presence of aortic valve calcification. Calcification in the aortic valve leaflets and adjacent aortic root is well shown by echocardiography (Fig. 14-42) and CT (Fig. 14-43). In younger patients it may be found in a congenitally bicuspid valve whereas 'degenerative' calcification is usually seen in patients over 65 years old. Calcified deposits are commonly distributed along the commissural edges of the leaflets. A valve calcium Agatston score of 150 has been shown to be 100% sensitive for discriminating between valve jet velocities under 2.5 m/s and those over 2.5 m/s;[67] however, 13.3% of patients with an increased gradient across the aortic valve at echocardiography had an Agatston score of less than 50.[68]

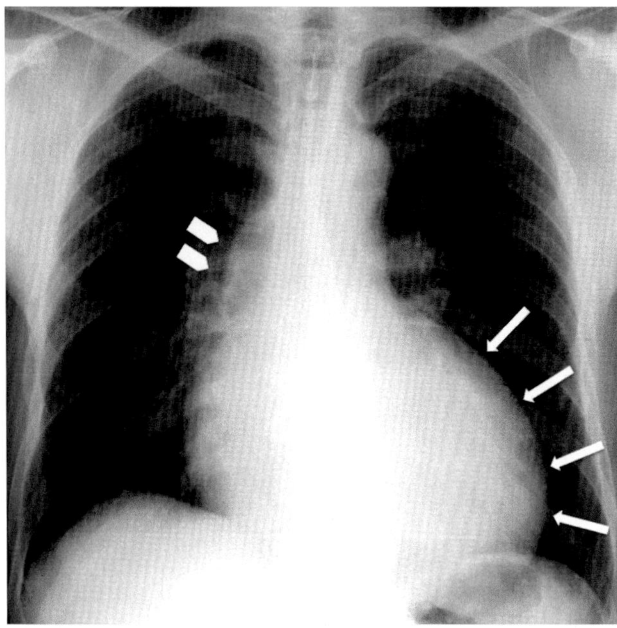

FIGURE 14-41 ■ Chest X-ray of aortic stenosis shows rounded profile of left ventricle (left third cardiac arch, white arrows), with slight enlargement of ascending aorta (right first cardiac arch, arrowheads).

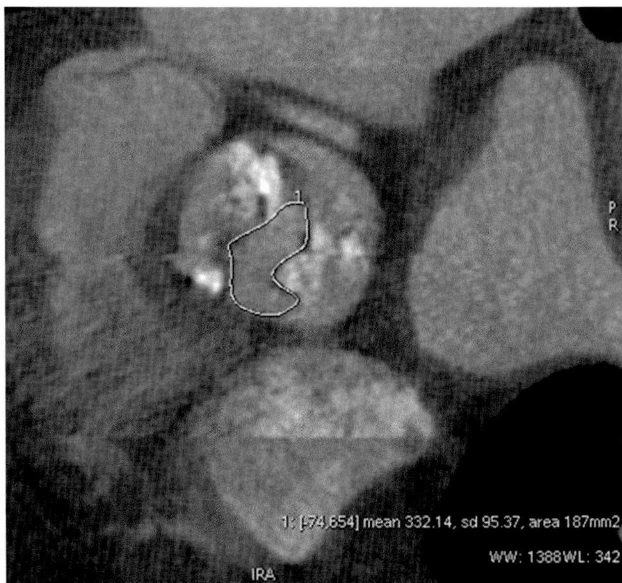

FIGURE 14-43 ■ **Cardiac CT.** Multiplanar short-axis reformation of aortic valve shows leaflet calcification with reduced systolic orifice. Manual contouring of the orifice allows stenosis quantification (moderate to severe: 187 mm^2).

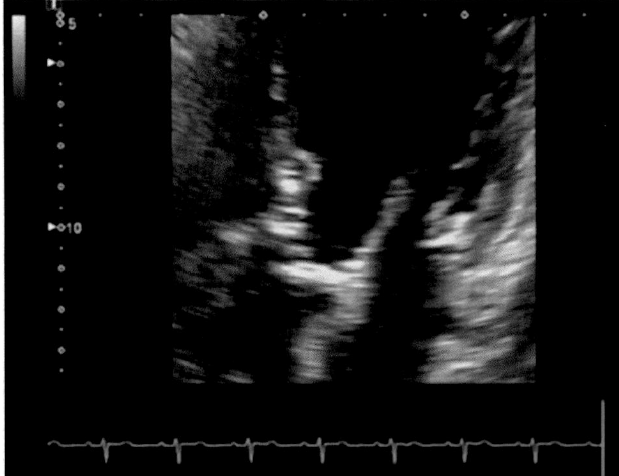

FIGURE 14-42 ■ **B-mode echocardiography, horizontal long axis, in aortic stenosis.** Hyperechoic calcified aortic leaflets; mitral annulus calcification is also evident.

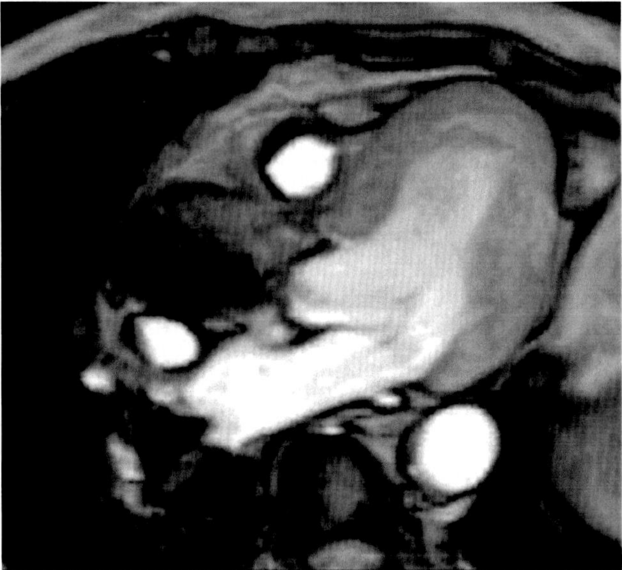

FIGURE 14-44 ■ **Cine-MRI frame in aortic stenosis.** In this three-chamber view, a large flow void due to blood flow acceleration is evident in ascending aorta.

Cardiac CT diagnosis of aortic stenosis is based on the demonstration of left ventricular hypertrophy, mild to moderate post-stenotic dilatation of the ascending aorta, calcification of the aortic valve, limited motion and reduced area of the aortic valve.[67] CMR can demonstrate impaired aortic valve opening and morphology of the valve (bicuspid or tricuspid), and can assess stenosis; however, it is less sensitive than CT for calcium detection. Coronal and oblique LV outflow tract views provide good qualitative assessment of the aortic valve.[58] In cine-MRI the area of systolic flow dephasing seen in the aortic root has a poor correlation with the severity of aortic stenosis (Fig. 14-44).

Direct planimetry of the aortic valve orifice, with both CT (Fig. 14-43) and MRI, is the most useful technique for quantifying stenosis severity, and is achieved by placing an imaging plane through the valve tips in systole.[58] Transvalvular velocity can be measured with cine phase contrast velocity mapping, though peak velocity may be less accurate (often underestimated) than continuous wave Doppler echo.[58] In-plane velocity mapping in the outflow tract is useful for identifying the location of maximal velocity, followed with through-plane velocity mapping in a plane perpendicular to the direction of flow, positioned at the identified location of maximal velocity.

The 'anatomical' orifice area (AOA) is not equivalent to the valve effective orifice area (EOA). The latter reflects the cross-sectional area of the transvalvular flow jet and is generally smaller than the valve area because there is a contraction of the flow downstream of the valve orifice. The EOA is given by the continuity equation

$$EOA = SV/VTI_{Ao}$$

where SV is the stroke volume and VTI is the velocity–time integral. There is a good agreement between CMR and Doppler–echocardiography for the estimation of valve EOA.[69]

CMR cine imaging differentiates subvalvular and supravalvular stenosis, accurately assesses the ascending aorta, which may be dilated, particularly with bicuspid aortic valves, and may influence surgical management.[58] Left ventricular function and hypertrophy are accurately measured by CMR, which is the most accurate method for determining ventricular volumes and mass. Late gadolinium enhancement imaging in patients with aortic stenosis has shown patchy mid-wall enhancement; this likely reflects focal areas of fibrosis and is associated with a worse prognosis.[58] In older adults with aortic stenosis, there is frequent association with coronary artery disease, and imaging of coronary arteries is indicated before surgery for valve replacement.

Rheumatic aortic stenosis is characterised by fusion of the commissures of the aortic valve cusps and is often associated with regurgitation and involvement of the mitral valve. At CXR the main signs are related to accompanying mitral valve disease, with left atrial enlargement. Post-stenotic dilatation of the aorta is rare in rheumatic aortic stenosis, but can be present in the case of associated aortic regurgitation. Gross aortic valve calcification is rare.

Aortic Regurgitation

Aortic regurgitation (AR) may result from disease of the cusps of the aortic valve (bicuspid, endocarditis, rheumatic disease), or from disease of the aortic walls (aortic dissection, Takayasu, Marfan, rheumatoid arthritis, Elhers–Danlos, trauma). Acute regurgitation can occur in bacterial endocarditis or, less frequently, be traumatic or related to aortic dissection. Chronic aortic regurgitation may be the result of congenital abnormality (e.g. bicuspid aortic valve, Fig. 14-45) or rheumatic heart disease. Aneurysms of the ascending aorta may cause dilatation of the valve ring, leading to aortic regurgitation. In a bicuspid valve the inadequately supported cusps allow progressive development of aortic regurgitation; a variable degree of stenosis can be present, because of inadequate development of the valve commissures or dystrophic calcification. In rheumatic aortic regurgitation, there is a slow destruction of the free edges of the cusps, often with commissural fusion. The slow onset of chronic aortic regurgitation allows the left ventricle to adapt and dilate to receive the regurgitant flow; due to compliance increase, end-diastolic pressure rises only when cardiac failure develops. Aortic regurgitation remains asymptomatic until the patient develops heart failure.

At CXR chronic aortic regurgitation appears as enlargement of the left ventricle on both views (Fig. 14-46), which correlates well with the severity of the condition and is one factor suggesting the need for surgical intervention. The enlargement can be reversible after treatment. The thoracic aorta may be moderately

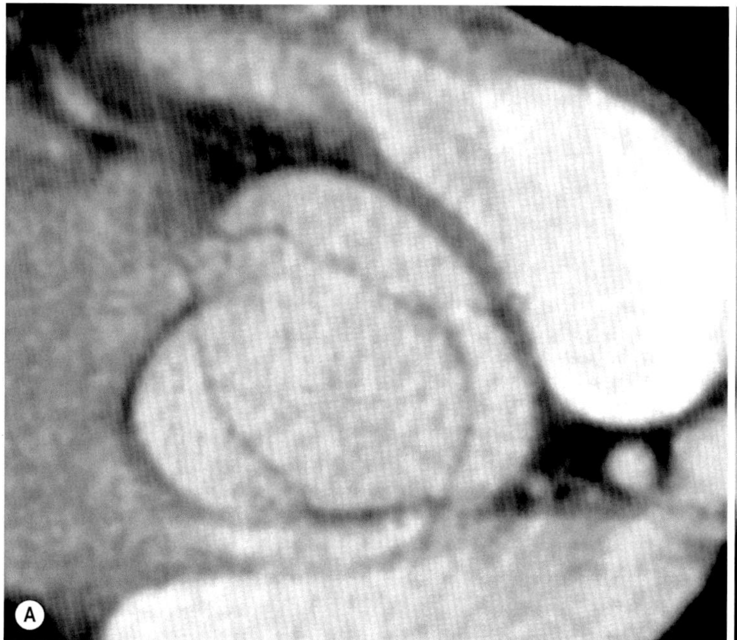

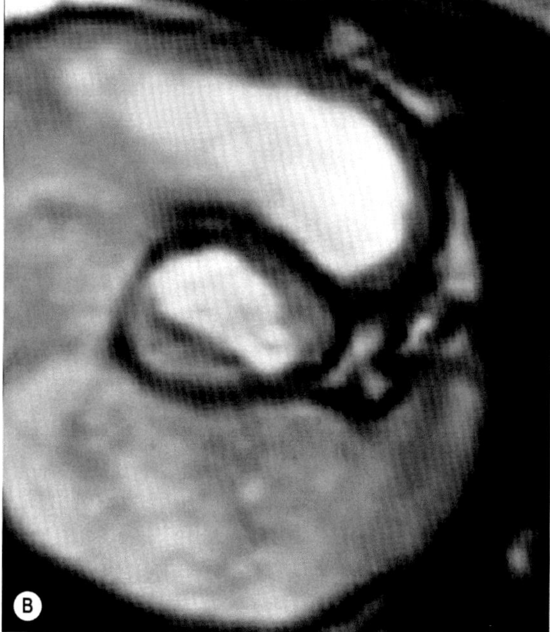

FIGURE 14-45 ■ **(A) Cardiac CT and (B) cine-MRI of a bicuspid aortic valve.** In both images only two semilunar leaflets are evident.

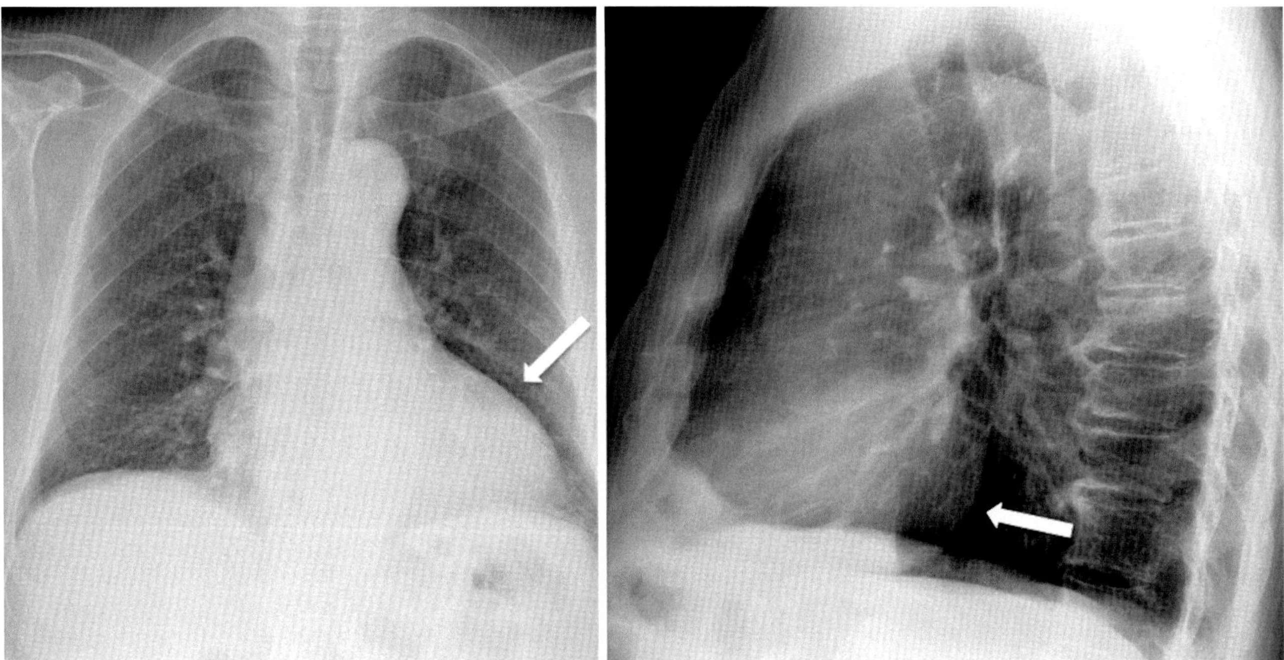

FIGURE 14-46 ■ **Chest X-rays of aortic regurgitation.** Frontal and lateral views demonstrate left ventricle enlargement, as left third cardiac arch widening in the frontal view, and second posterior arch in the lateral view (arrows).

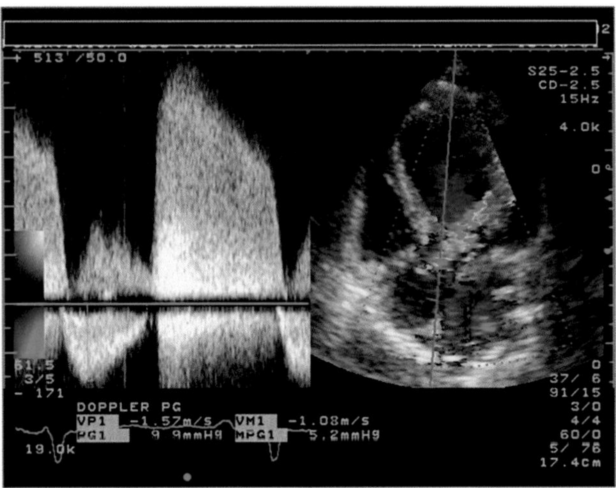

FIGURE 14-47 ■ **Aortic regurgitation.** Echo colour Doppler shows aortic insufficiency, with a wide jet, while continuous Doppler interrogation shows a steep decay of the curve indicating severity of regurgitation (rapid pressure drop during diastole). Pressure half-time is <250 ms.

enlarged. In acute regurgitation, the left ventricle is not dilated, while the rapid increase of ventricular pressure can cause pulmonary oedema.

Echocardiography is the main imaging technique for most patients with aortic valve disease. However, its most important role is in the assessment of timing for valve replacement; a progressive increase in regurgitation, together with deterioration of ventricular function, probably represents the best indicator for surgery.

Severity estimation is semiquantitatively obtained by means of Doppler; colour Doppler allows easy and immediate detection of regurgitation (Fig. 14-47). However, unlike the mitral regurgitant jet, the maximal length of the aortic jet does not correlate with severity;[70] the cross-sectional area of the jet performs better. Another good indicator is the width of the narrowest central part of the jet; a width ≥6 mm is related to a severe regurgitation with a sensitivity of 95% and specificity of 90%, while a width <3 mm represents a mild regurgitation.[71] Continuous Doppler makes it possible to estimate the transvalvular gradient, which drops rapidly in most severe cases. Pressure half-time is a good indicator of severity: 400 ms is a cut-off value separating mild from significant forms, while 200 ms indicates severe regurgitation.[72]

Finally, regurgitant volume and fraction can be measured by comparing the total stroke volume, measured at the aortic level, and the forward stroke volume, obtained at the mitral valve level, using pulsed Doppler;[73] however, this method shows some inaccuracies, particularly for mitral flow measurements.

CMR allows a good visualisation of the aortic valve and of the aortic root anatomy; the signal void jet of valvular insufficiency on cine sequences provides an approximate assessment of the severity of aortic regurgitation: a narrow jet width at the origin suggests a lower degree of regurgitation, while a wide jet suggests more severe regurgitation (Fig. 14-48).[74] Cine sequences may also help identify the cause of the regurgitation: for example, identifying annuloaortic ectasia (Fig. 14-48).

Velocity-encoded cine-MRI can quantify aortic regurgitation and regurgitant fraction with excellent accuracy (Fig. 14-49).[58] The imaging plane for flow mapping is an axial oblique one, perpendicular to the flow, and should be placed just above the aortic valve. Placing the plane closer to the valve minimises the underestimation of the regurgitation due to movement of the valve towards the LV apex during systole as blood between the imaging

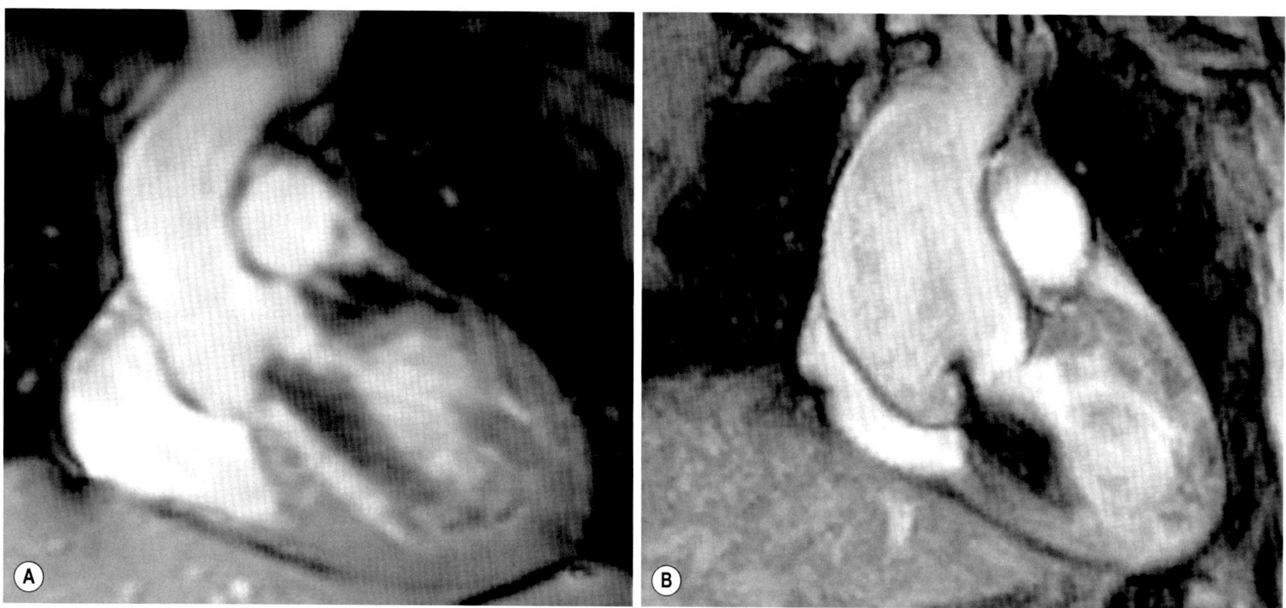

FIGURE 14-48 **Cine-MRI frames of aortic regurgitation.** Retrograde jets in left ventricle are evident as flow voids, in (A) with normal aortic bulb, in (B) with annuloaortic ectasia.

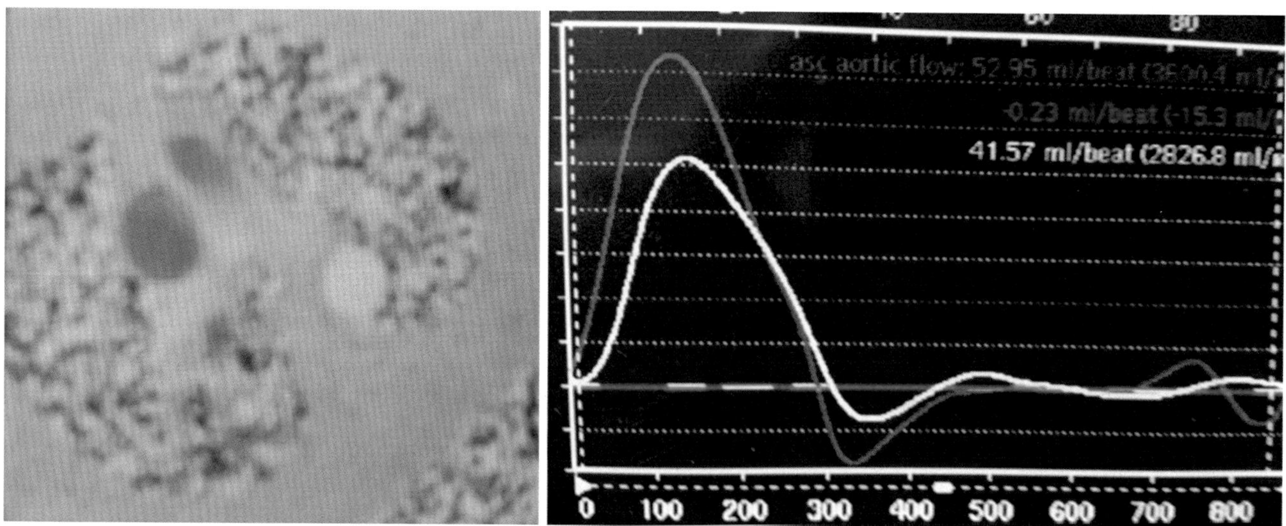

FIGURE 14-49 **MRI velocity map of mild aortic regurgitation.** Flow is measured in ascending (red line) and descending aorta (white line); area under the curve below zero (green line) represents regurgitant flow.

plane and the valve may return back to the ventricle during diastole, being lost to measurement. Non-breath-hold flow sequences are recommended.

In the absence of other valve regurgitation or shunts, aortic regurgitation can also be quantified from cine imaging by a comparison of the differences in LVSV and RVSV, obtained from a volume study or aortic and pulmonary trunk flow measurement. CMR reliably predicts the clinical course and outcome and is particularly useful for serial assessment. A regurgitant fraction >33% is an optimal threshold for identifying the need for valve surgery. A dilated aortic root can also suggest the need for replacement at the time of valve surgery.

Cardiac CT is currently not used in the primary diagnosis of AR, but the aortic valve should be reviewed in all patients undergoing CT angiography for possible concomitant underlying aortic regurgitation, particularly if echocardiography has not recently been performed.[75] Cardiac CT allows measurement of the aortic valve anatomical regurgitant orifice area by direct planimetry: by selecting end-diastolic CT data sets, the anatomical regurgitant orifice area (ROA) can be visualised as 'central valvular leakage area', reflecting an incomplete closure of the cusps (Fig. 14-50).[75] CT is thus able to detect the presence of AR and quantify the severity of AR with good correlation with the various echocardiographic parameters of AR.[76] However, a diagnosis of mild AR can be missed by CT in the presence of dense valvular calcification, or in bicuspid valves.[75] In the preoperative triage, CT can differentiate between bicuspid and tricuspid valve

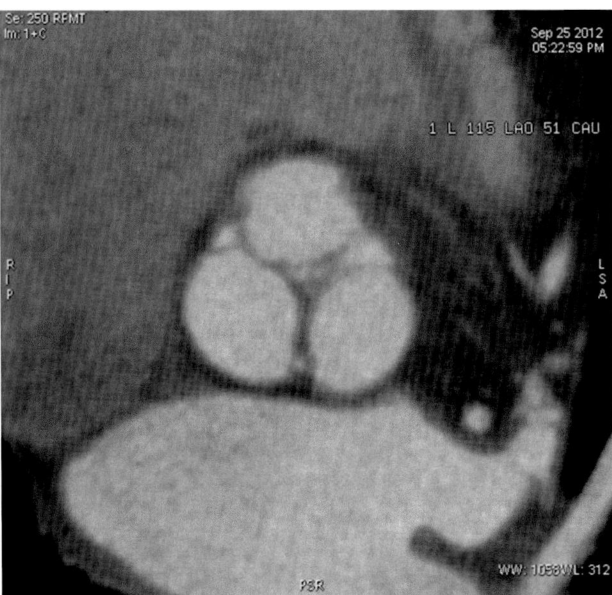

FIGURE 14-50 ■ Cardiac CT of aortic regurgitation. Multiplanar short-axis reformation of aortic valve demonstrates incomplete coaptation of leaflets, with central orifice.

morphology, and evaluates the aortic root, the ascending aorta and the coronary arteries within one imaging investigation.[77] Cardiac CT itself has recently shown promising results in depicting valvular abnormalities in infective endocarditis; in particular, evaluation of paravalvular involvement may be improved by CT.[75,76] CT may also provide a better morphological differentiation between valvular calcification and 'soft-tissue' lesions such as vegetations. The complications of endocarditis such as paravalvular abscess are well assessed by MRI and CT. Aortic root diseases such as annuloaortic ectasia or dissection are best investigated by CT angiography (CTA)[78] or MR angiography (MRA).

Prosthetic Cardiac Valves

There are two major types of artificial valves available for both aortic and atrioventricular placement, mechanical valves and bioprostheses (Fig. 14-51). Their specific characteristics should be structural durability, adaptation to the native valve annulus, chemically inert, free of thrombogenicity and without significant resistance to blood flow.[79] There are more than 40 types of cardiac valves, which differ in inlet and outlet diameters and flow patterns, action and complication rates, available for aortic, pulmonary, mitral and tricuspid replacement, as well as for vascular conduits. Complications are relatively frequent and depend on the specific models of prothesis; they include paravalvular leak, occluder variance or erosion, structural fracture, pseudoaneurysm, thrombosis, vegetations or tissue overgrowth. In bioprostheses, infective endocarditis and primary valve regurgitation can also occur. Finally, further complications to be considered are those of anticoagulation, embolism and post-pericardiotomy syndrome.

First-line examination of a prosthetic valve is echocardiography; radiology is mostly aimed at identifying the complications of prosthetic valves by means of chest radiography,[80] fluoroscopy, CT[81] and CMR. However, MRI diagnostic performances can be partially limited by the size of artefacts generated by the metallic components of the prosthesis. After valve replacement a baseline 2D and Doppler echocardiographic study should be obtained in order to compare follow-up studies performed on the suspicion of malfunction or complication.

There are a variety of different prosthetic valves: central ball occluder valve, central caged disc occluder valve, eccentric monocuspid disc valve, bileaflet disc valve and bioprosthesis. More recently, surgical techniques for valve reconstruction and annuloplasty have been introduced and developed. Practitioners should become familiar with the morphological differences and anatomical location of these types of valves in order to recognise them during the CXR examination (Figs. 14-52 to 14-54), at echocardiography (Fig. 14-55) or CT (Fig. 14-56). Morphology is difficult to assess using MRI due to the susceptibility artefact caused by metallic components of the prostheses (Fig. 14-57). Information about MR safety is available through the Magnetic Resonance Technology Information Portal, http://www.mr-tip.com.

Transcatheter aortic valve replacement implantation (TAVI) is an emerging technique developed for non-operable symptomatic patients with critical aortic stenosis; the device consists of an auto-expandable or a balloon-expandable stent with valve, which is delivered percutaneously by a transfemoral or a transapical approach. CT is an essential tool for TAVI planning, aimed to assess the size of the aortic root, the status of peripheral arteries (for the access) and the status of the coronary arteries.[82] As an alternative, CMR and MRA can be used.[83]

Complications of Prosthetic Valves

Structure Fracture

Structure fractures have been reported in some types of mechanical valves; CXR using microfocus, fluoroscopy and CT have been useful in identifying fractures of these radio-opaque components.

Porcine Bioprosthesis

The major problem with porcine bioprostheses is their poor durability. Cusp tears, degeneration, perforation, fibrosis and calcification appear on about the fifth post-operative year, and by the tenth year 20% have failed and require reimplantation.

Infective Endocarditis

Prosthetic valve endocarditis is an infrequent complication of cardiac valve replacement, with overall incidence ranging from 0.9 to 4.4%, and is most frequent within six months of valve replacement.

Organisms most frequently involved are coagulase-negative staphylococci, *Serratia marcescens*, streptococci,

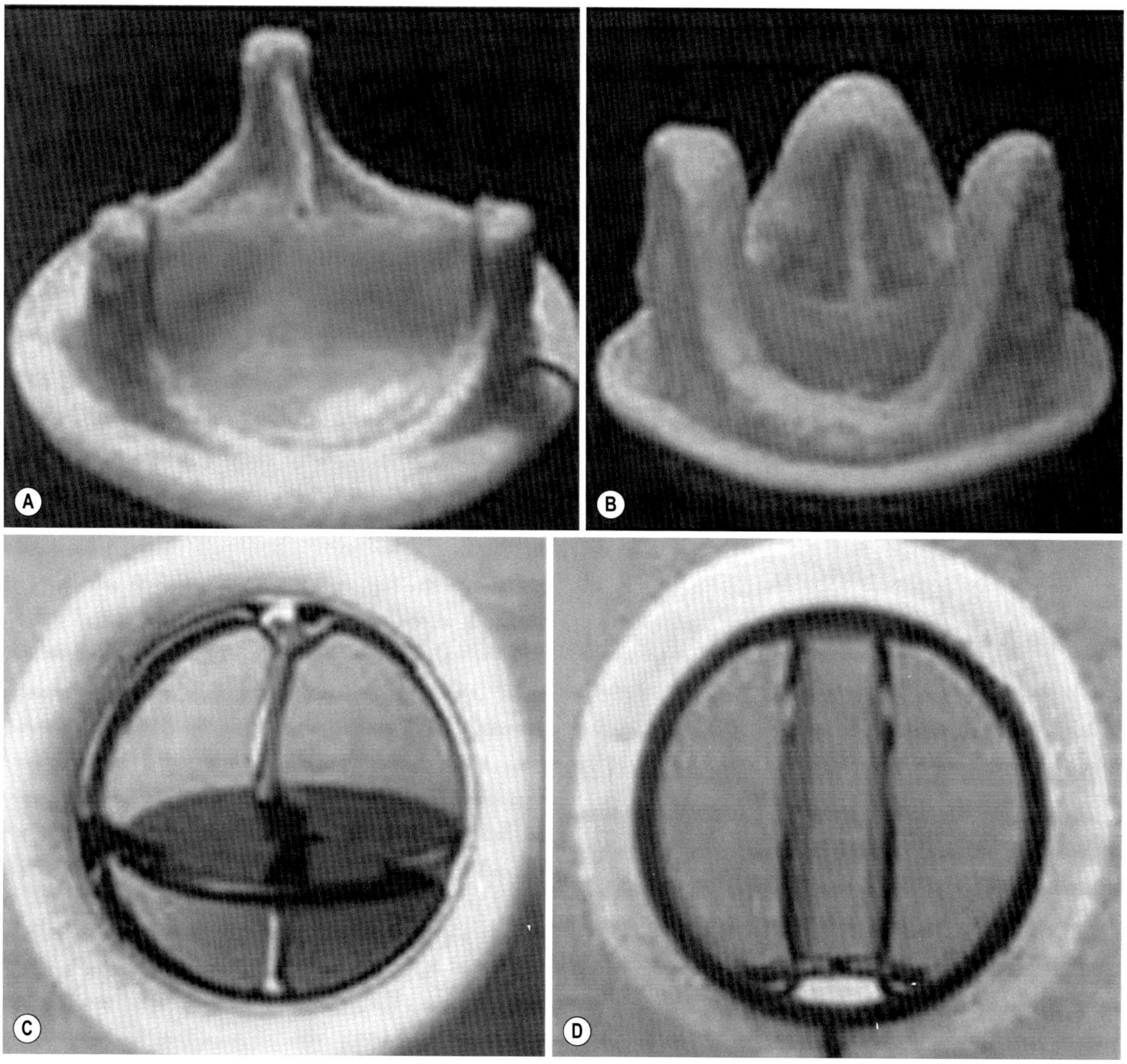

FIGURE 14-51 ■ Examples of biological (A, B) and mechanical (C, D) valvular prostheses.

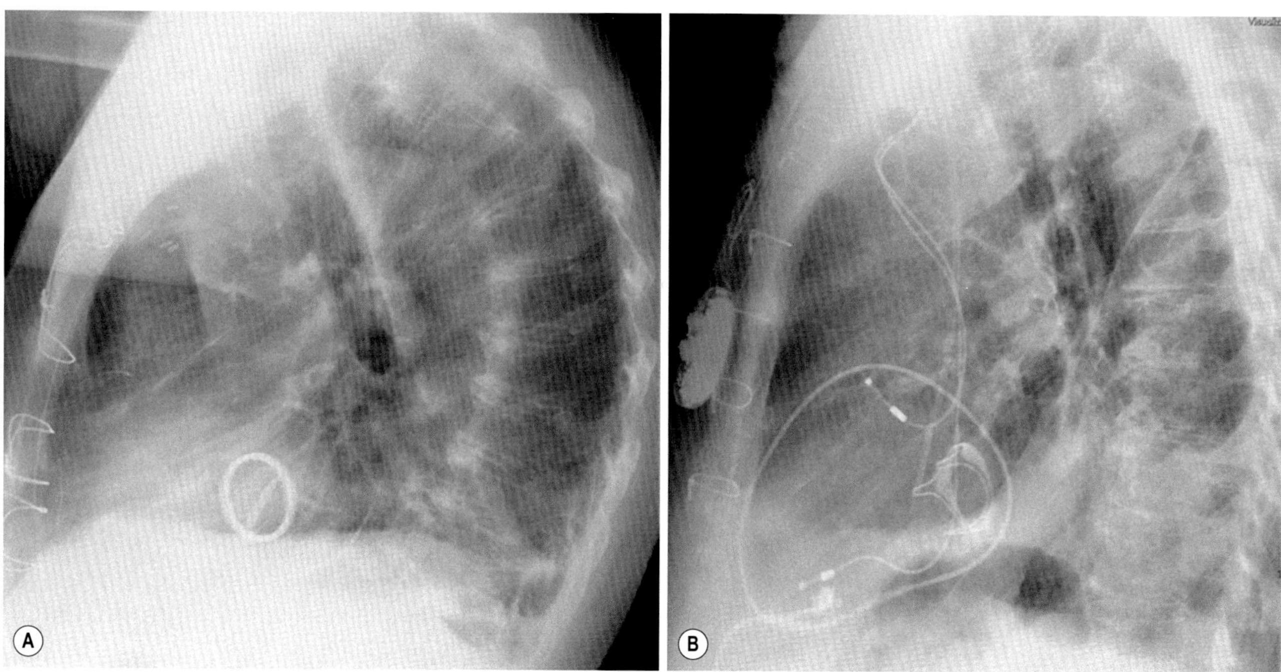

FIGURE 14-52 ■ Chest X-rays, lateral views, of mechanical (A) and biological (B) mitral valve prostheses.

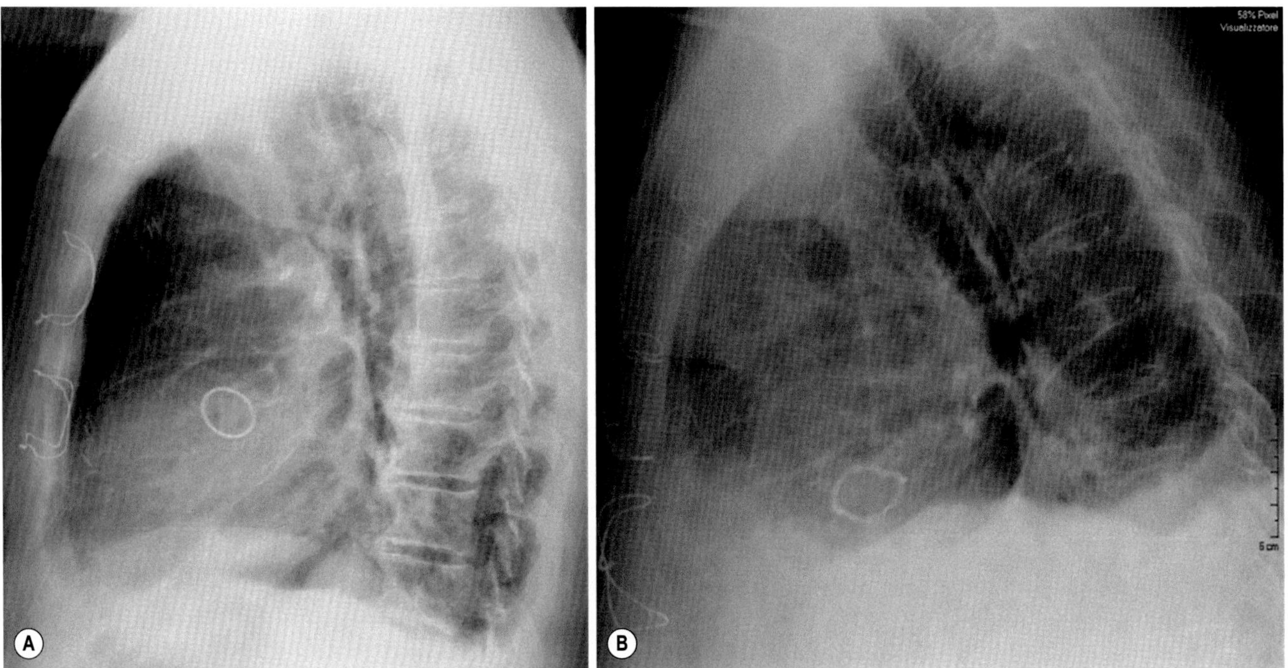

FIGURE 14-53 ■ **Chest X-rays, lateral views, of mechanical (A) and biological (B) aortic valve prostheses.**

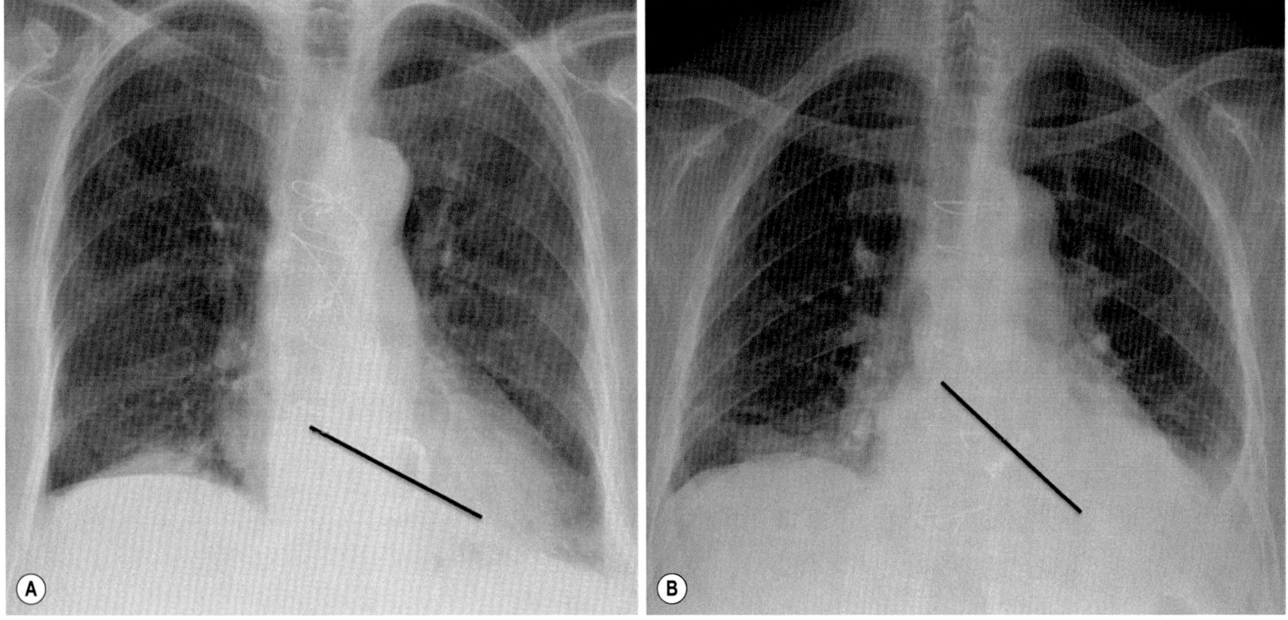

FIGURE 14-54 ■ Chest X-rays, frontal views, demonstrate the different orientation of the left atrioventricular vector and the left ventriculoaortic vector (black lines), respectively, in (A) mitral and (B) aortic valve replacements.

Candida albicans and *Staphylococcus aureus*. Diphtheroids are seen more frequently in early infective endocarditis, and there is a lower incidence of Gram-negative bacilli and fungal infections.[84] Infection typically develops in the coronary ostia, the ascending aorta and the aortic annulus, related to high-pressure regurgitant jets of blood which damage valve attachments and cause development of local abscesses. Pannus and vegetations obstruct flow through the valve orifice or limit occluder motion. Sinus of Valsalva and perivalvular pseudoaneurysms may develop;[85] they can be assessed by echocardiography (Fig. 14-58), CT (Fig. 14-59) or MRI (Fig. 14-60). Paravalvular insufficiency occurs as tissue fragments and sutures are destroyed by infection.

Two-dimensional echocardiography with transthoracic approach, or better, transoesophageal, can demonstrate site, form and size of vegetations or thrombi. However, cardiac CT has also been useful in identifying

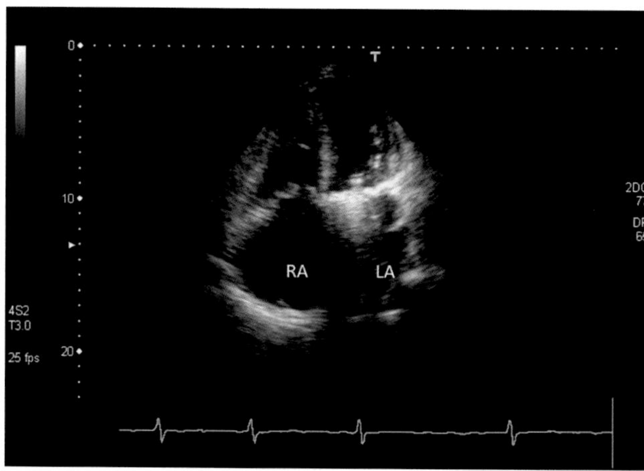

FIGURE 14-55 ■ **Echocardiography of a monoleaflet mitral valve, four-chamber view.** Right atrium (RA) enlargement with tricuspid leaflet thickening is also evident.

vegetations, and particularly pseudoaneurysms; MRI is limited in vegetation detection because of the artefacts generated by ferromagnetic components, while it is again useful for assessing pseudoaneurysms.

Valve Regurgitation

Minor regurgitation is relatively normal with many mechanical valves, but major regurgitation usually occurs as a result of ring dehiscence, thrombus, disc wear and sticking, cocking or vegetations of the valve leaflets. Dehiscence with valve detachment may occur in the case of infection or in a heavily calcified annulus or when there is underlying defective collagen, as in Marfan's syndrome. Perivalvular regurgitation or valve dysfunction should be suspected when sudden cardiac enlargement and pulmonary oedema occur. Echocardiography is the preferred tool for assessing dehiscence and regurgitation.

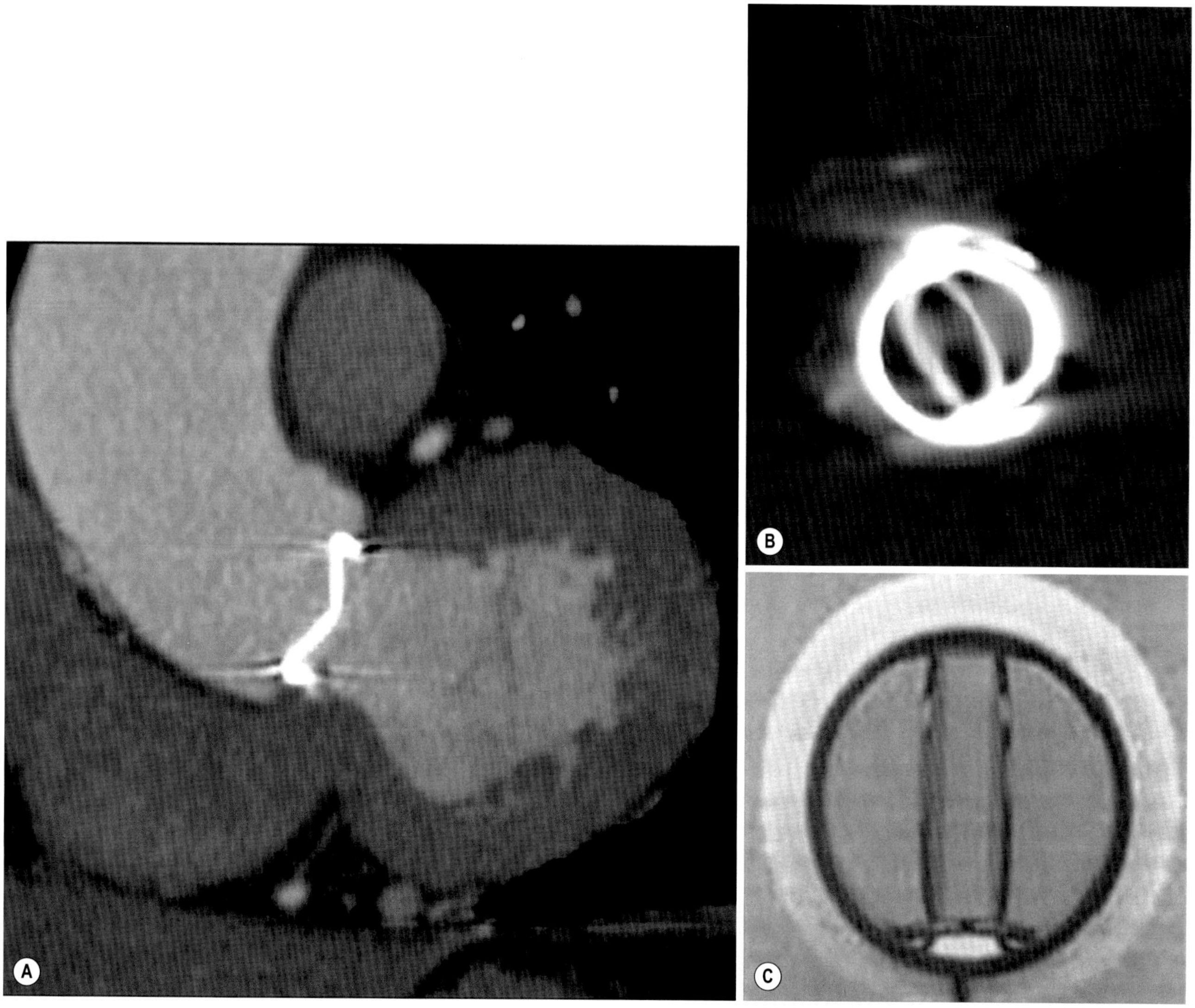

FIGURE 14-56 ■ **Cardiac CT of mechanical valvular prosthesis.** (A) Coronal reformatted image; (B) axial reformatted image of the valve; (C) corresponding image of the valve.

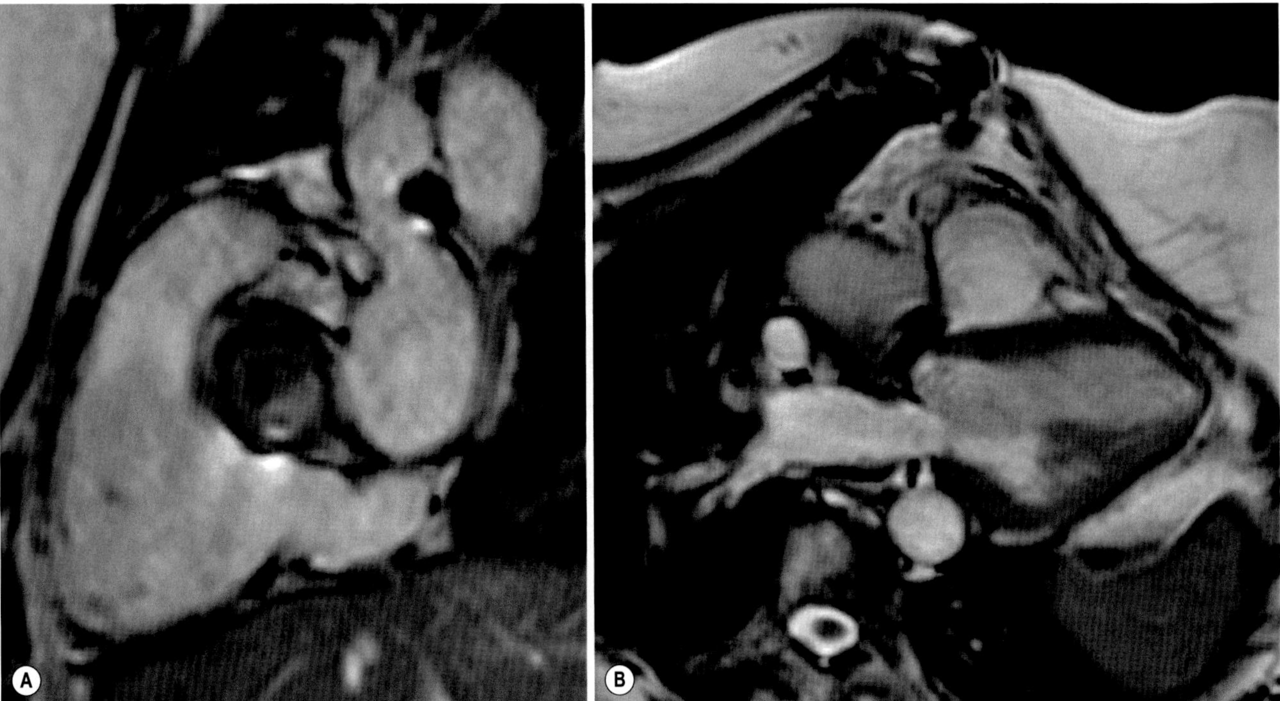

FIGURE 14-57 ■ Cine-MRI frames (A, short-axis view; B, three-chamber view) show the typical susceptibility artefact generated by the mechanical aortic valve prostheses.

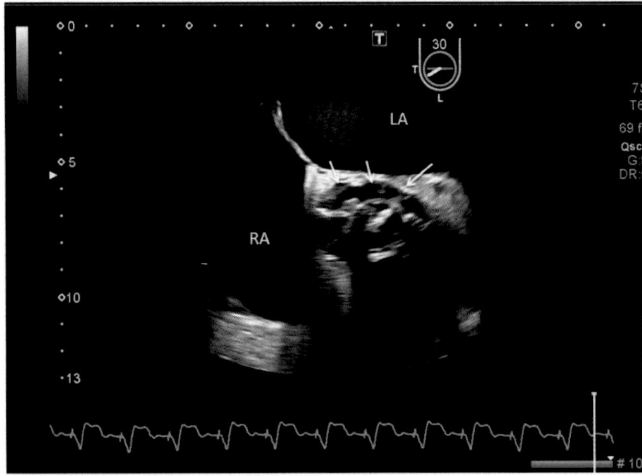

FIGURE 14-58 ■ **Transoesophageal echocardiography in paravalvular aortic abscess.** An anechoic rim anterior to a mechanical prosthesis is evident (arrows).

Thromboembolism

Thrombosis may occur spontaneously, despite adequate anticoagulation; the involvement of the valve orifice reduces the excursion of the occluding ball, disc or leaflet, and causes output reduction. Prosthetic mitral valve thrombosis is more common than aortic valve thrombosis. The frequency of thrombosis has decreased markedly during the past few years. With the early prostheses, the incidence of thromboembolism was 24–37%. Since the introduction of cloth-covered prostheses, the incidence has decreased to 3–5%.

Echocardiography is extremely useful in assessing the presence of the thrombus, as are CT and MRI, if the thrombus is large enough. As this complication represents a is a surgical emergency, immediate valve replacement or intervention by catheter remobilisation and intracardiac thrombolysis is required.

TUMOURS OF THE HEART

Cardiac tumours are rare. Metastases to the heart and pericardium are 40 times more frequent than primary tumours.[86,87] Approximately 75% of primary cardiac tumours are benign. Some cardiac tumours remain clinically silent, sometimes discovered incidentally; others present as heart failure, arrhythmia, chest pain or embolic disease.

The diagnosis is usually obvious when clinical evidence of cardiac involvement, arrhythmias or (haemorrhagic) pericardial effusion develops in a patient with a known primary malignant neoplasm. Intrathoracic, extracardiac tumours, benign or malignant, may produce cardiac symptoms and signs by compressing the heart and great vessels, and mimic obstructive lesions of these vessels. Obstructive murmurs developing in the course of the malignant disease are well recognised. Cardiac tumours and ventricular and aortic aneurysms may resemble each other radiographically. The guiding criteria in differentiating cardiac masses are age of the patient, chamber of origin, involvement of the interatrial septum, base of attachment, infiltrative growth, involvement of the valves and the pericardium and extension to extracardiac structures.[88]

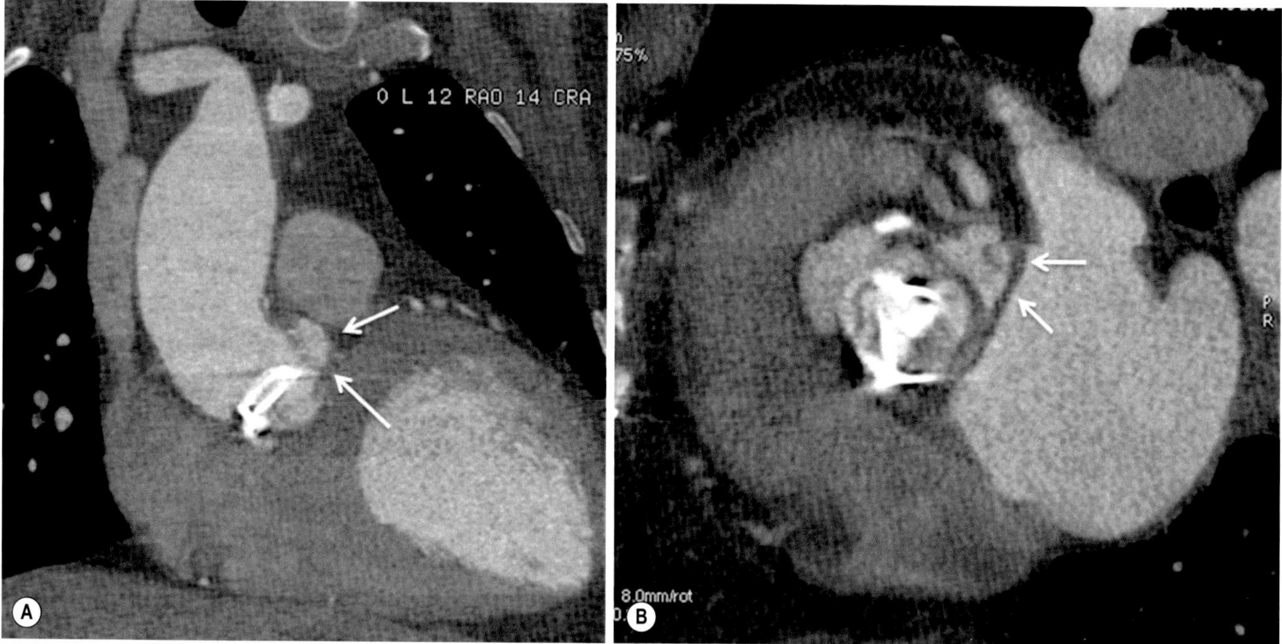

FIGURE 14-59 ■ **Cardiac CT of paravalvular aortic leak.** (A) Oblique coronal reformatted image of ascending aorta and (B) short-axis reformatted image of aortic valve demonstrate paravalvular extravasation of contrast medium around the prosthesis (arrows).

Echocardiography is the first-line imaging technique for the diagnosis of intracardiac tumours. Real-time imaging can show tumour mobility and distensibility features, which are typically seen in atrial myxomas and less likely in sarcomas and metastases. Because of MDCT's large field of view, the heart, paracardiac regions and lungs can be fully evaluated.[89] This allows a better diagnosis of the site and extension of the lesions; MDCT is also useful in tumour staging by identifying metastases.

With CT a densitometric evaluation of the lesion can also be performed, along with an assessment of the enhancement characteristics of the lesion. CT can depict calcifications and fat, and also helps in identifying the vascular supply of a cardiac mass.[89] ECG-gated CT may be useful when more precise evaluation of tumour extent and relationships is required.[86] MRI allows better soft-tissue characterisation than CT and can provide functional information such as flow direction and velocity, as well as a more reliable diagnosis of true invasion of cardiac structures by intrathoracic tumours.

Metastasis

Secondary cardiac tumours are 30–40 times more common than primary malignant neoplasms. The patterns of tumour spread are as follows:

1. Direct extension from intrathoracic tumours—lung and mediastinal tumours (Figs. 14-61 and 14-62) can invade the heart directly and generally cannot be excised. Lymphoma can extend to the pericardium and heart, changing its staging (Fig. 14-63).
2. Intralymphatic dissemination—this is possible in lung, oesophageal and breast carcinomas, with invasion of the pericardium generally causing haemorrhagic exudate. Due to the affinity for serous linings, adenocarcinomas frequently lead to pericardial metastases. Mesothelioma can involve the pericardium and less frequently the myocardium. Pericardial metastases are a sign of advanced disease and appear during tumour relapse.
3. Haematogenous metastasis from a systemic tumour such as malignant melanoma (Fig. 14-64), lymphoma, leukaemia, sarcoma or carcinoma (Fig. 14-65).
4. Intravascular dissemination—tumour thrombi from the kidneys, suprarenal glands as well as renal or hepatic tumours, which spread transvenously from the inferior vena cava (Fig. 14-66), whereas lung or thymic cancer can spread via the superior vena cava (SVC).

Lung carcinoma can invade the left atrium via the pulmonary veins or spread to the right atrium via the vena cava. In this case the formation of a mass in continuity with the systemic or pulmonary veins can be observed (Fig. 14-67). The evaluation of the atrial walls is important because if there is no invasion, tumour resection is not contraindicated.

CT is extremely useful in tumour localisation and staging for surgical resection. CT features that suggest a malignant nature of a cardiac neoplasm are wide attachment to the wall of the heart, destruction of the cardiac chamber wall, involvement of more than one cardiac chamber, invasion of the pericardium with diffuse or nodular thickening and pericardial effusion especially if haemorrhagic. Pericardial effusion can be loculated or can give rise to cardiac tamponade, especially if it forms rapidly. Nodular thickening is a much more specific sign of secondary localisation. CT is a relatively accurate technique for detecting direct invasion of the mediastinum and cardiovascular structures by lung cancer. The

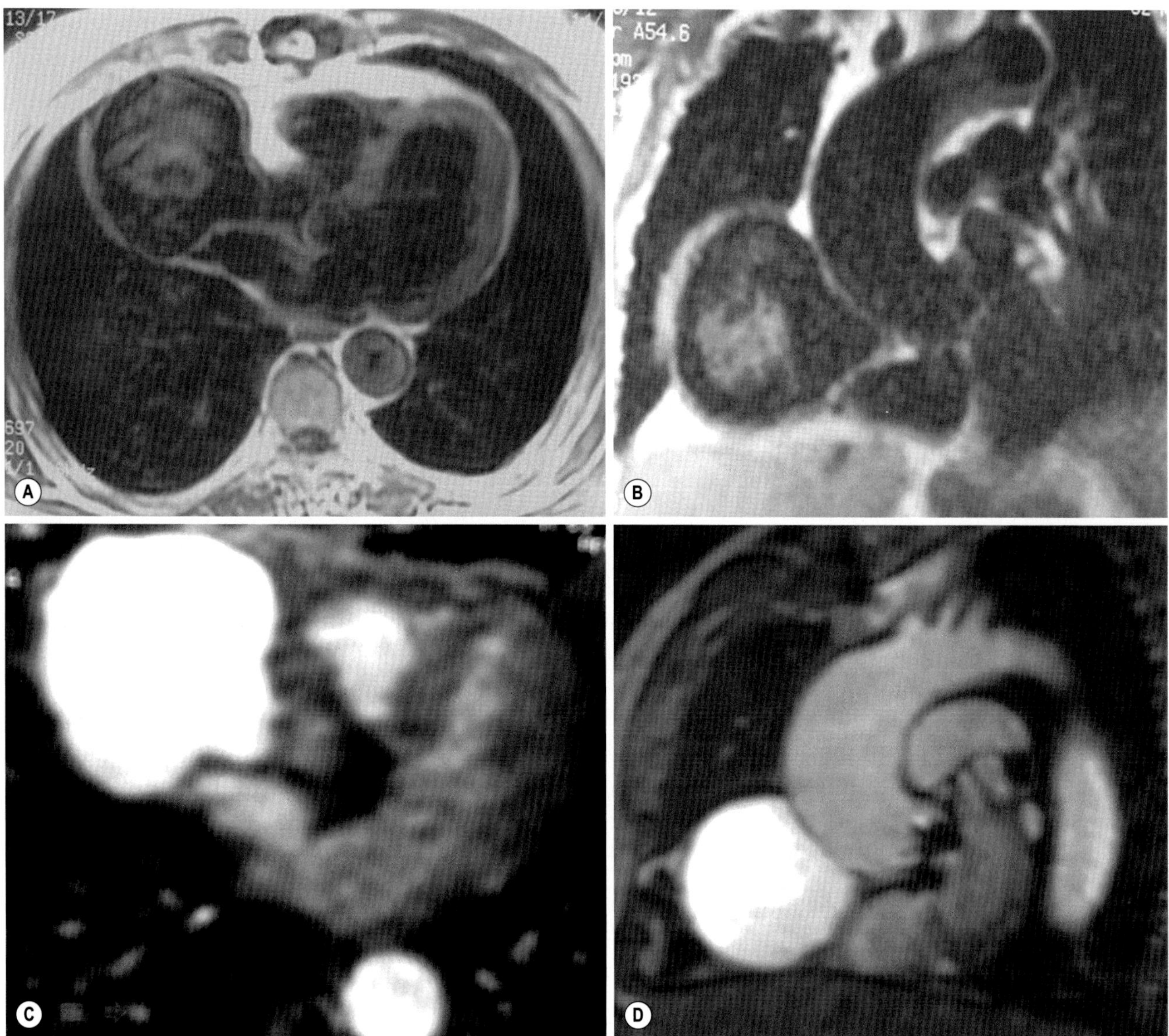

FIGURE 14-60 ■ **MRI of huge paravalvular leak after aortic valve replacement.** A large blood collection is evident, adjacent to aortic root, due to a paravalvular leak. (A, B) T1w axial and coronal oblique images show no signal in the collection because of flowing blood (the small amount of signal in the central part is due to slow turbulent flow). (C, D) Gadolinium enhanced gradient-echo images in the same planes demonstrate the passage of contrast medium in the collection; the susceptibility artefact of the mechanical valve is evident.

sensitivity for assessment of mediastinal invasion by CT ranges from 40 to 78% and specificity from 67 to 99%. The contact area between the thoracic mass and adjacent mediastinal structure, and the obliteration of intervening fat are the commonly seen CT features for local invasion, but neither is reliable. The normal sliding motion between two contacting areas can be helpful evidence of the absence of invasion and this feature can be demonstrated by MRI.

Primary Cardiac Tumours

Primary tumours of the heart are rare and the great majority are benign, the malignant tumours being sarcomas. Myxomas are by far the most common, followed by rhabdomyomas and fibromas. The clinical features of these tumours depend on their sites of origin. Intracavitary tumours are commonly pedunculated and may affect and/or occlude the valves, or fill cardiac chambers, leading to obstruction, arrhythmias and cardiac failure. Extension of tumours to the pericardium may produce haemorrhagic pericardial effusion that may lead to tamponade.

Cardiac Myxoma

Myxomas are the most common benign tumour, accounting for 25% of primary cardiac neoplasms; they occur more commonly in women. Patients may be asymptomatic or have the triad of peripheral embolic phenomena, symptoms and signs of mitral valve obstruction and constitutional symptoms of fever, anaemia, raised ESR and

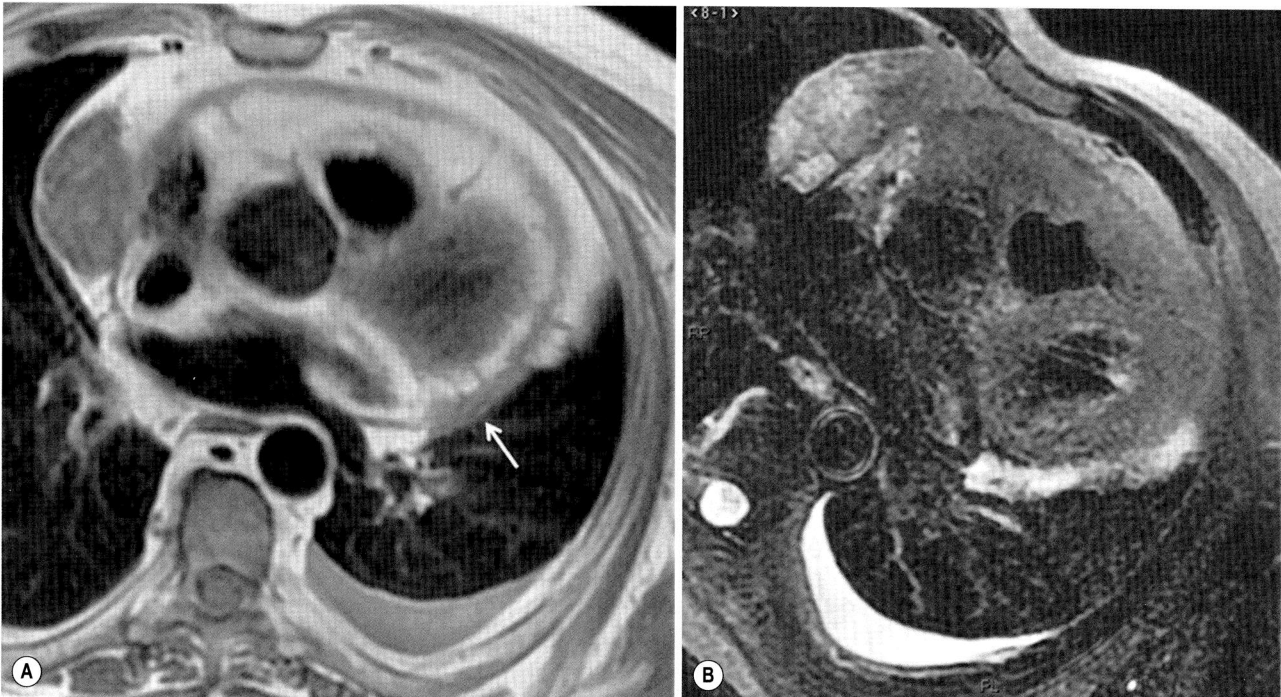

FIGURE 14-61 ■ Pericardial involvement in mediastinal malignant thymoma. (A) T1w axial image demonstrates an oval-shaped mediastinal lesion adjacent to thickened pericardium; lateral left pericardium shows a plaque-thickening due to tumour diffusion (white arrow). (B) T2w image shows high and heterogeneous signal intensity of the mass. A left pleural effusion is also present.

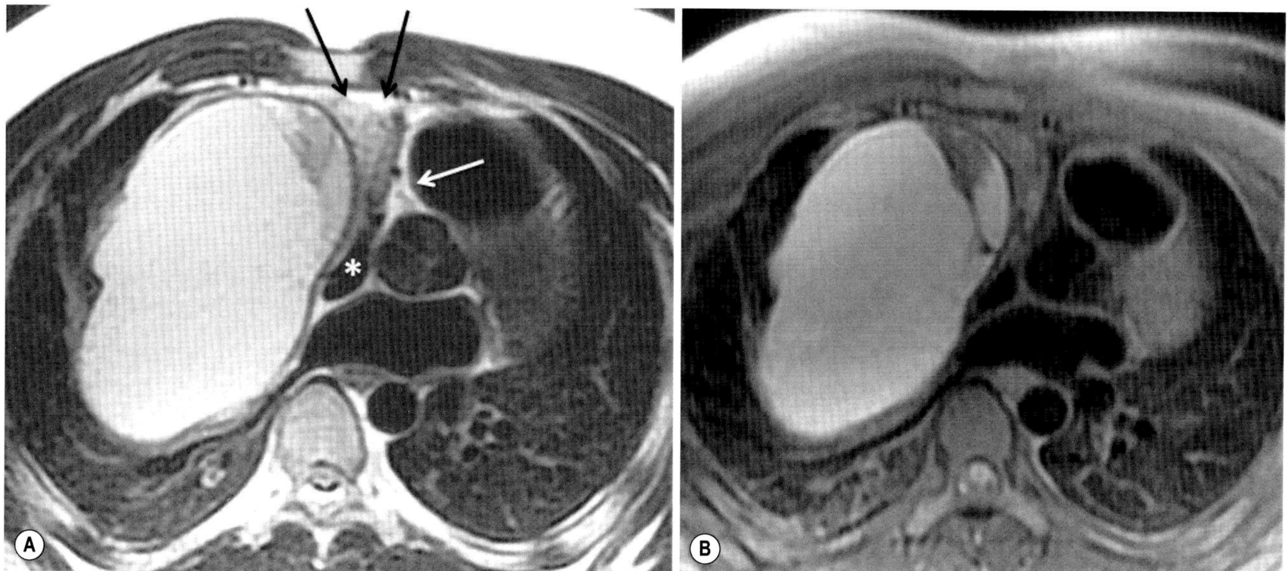

FIGURE 14-62 ■ Cystic teratoma of the pericardium, with right atrium involvement. (A) T2w axial image shows a large right paracardiac cystic tumour with eccentric solid component; extracapsular tissue (black arrows) also invades epicardial fat and abuts superior vena cava (*), contacting the right coronary artery (white arrow). (B) Post-contrast T1w corresponding axial image demonstrates enhancement of the solid components of the tumour.

sometimes finger clubbing mimicking infective endocarditis. Blood cultures, however, are sterile and splenomegaly does not occur. Familial myxomas constitute fewer than 10% of all myxomas, tend to present earlier (median age 20 years) and are more likely to have multiple myxomas at atypical locations and to develop recurrent tumours. Spotty skin pigmentation and endocrine abnormalities are associated with the autosomal dominant condition of Carney complex.[90] Symptoms related to peripheral embolisation are frequent, prompting the need for early resection.

Approximately 90% are solitary lesions; they commonly arise in the left (75%) or right atrium (20%). In 85% of cases they are characteristically attached to the

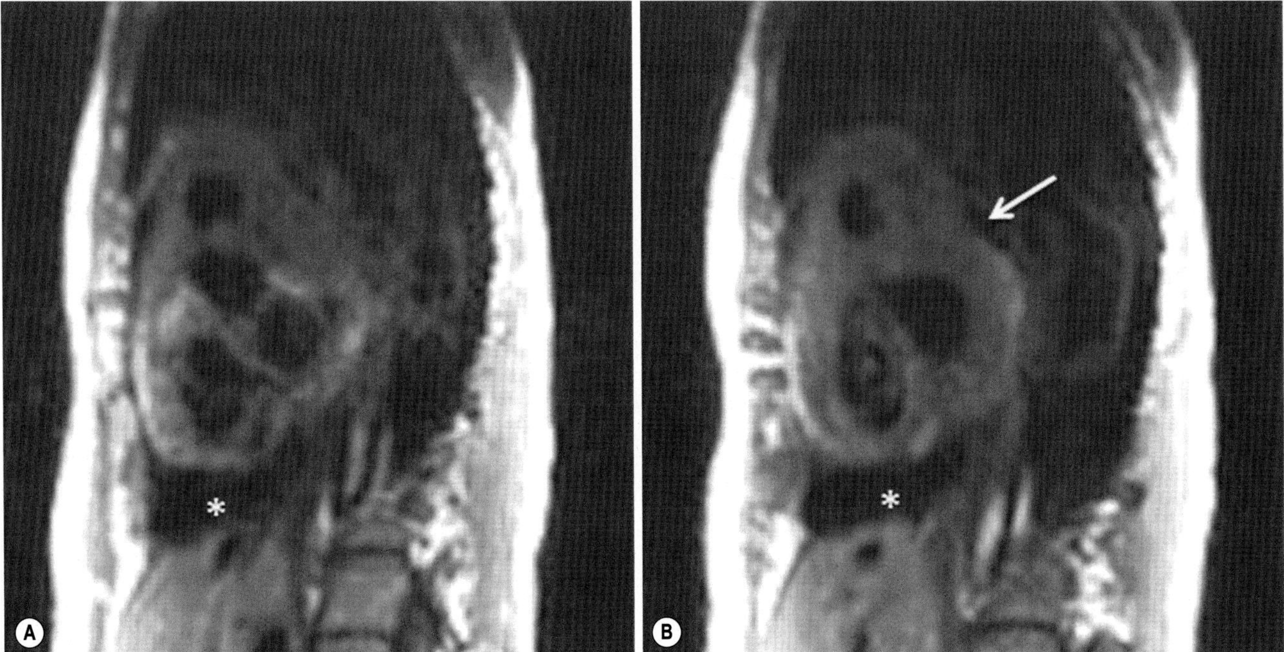

FIGURE 14-63 ■ **Two black-blood short-axis T1w MRI images of mediastinal NHL, with great vessel encasement, pericardial and myocardial infiltration (arrow) and inferior pericardial effusion (*).**

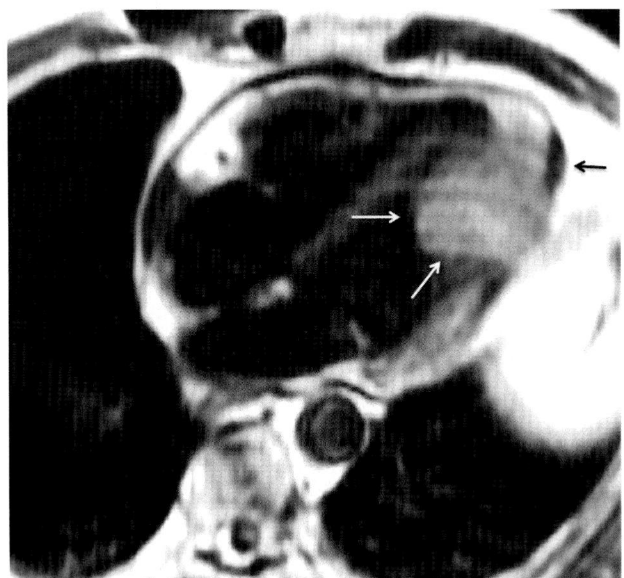

FIGURE 14-64 ■ **T1w axial image shows a rounded slightly hyperintense lesion in the left ventricle, arising from left lateral wall (white arrows).** A small amount of pericardial effusion is evident (black arrow).

interatrial septum near the fossa ovalis.[91] Growth through the fossa ovalis with tumour in both atria is recognised.[92] Myxoma tends to be pedunculated or polypoid with a lobulated surface; the less common villous type has gelatinous, fragile surface extensions that are prone to fragmentation and embolisation.[92] Owing to a pedunculated attachment, myxomas are often mobile but they can sometimes be broad based and relatively fixed. Most are solitary and range in size from 1 to 15 cm.

On CXR, the heart can be enlarged and there is often evidence of selective left atrial enlargement, though rarely is there a large appendage, which would suggest rheumatic heart disease. Pulmonary venous hypertension, pulmonary oedema or even pulmonary arterial hypertension may be present. Appearances on the chest radiograph may, however, be normal. The rare calcified myxoma may be identified on chest radiograph or CT.

The first-line examination, which usually sufficient for diagnosis, is echocardiography. It can assess the presence of a hyperechoic mass, usually attached to the interatrial septum, with a heterogeneous texture in large lesions; the pedicle, as well as the lesion crossing the mitral orifice, can be easily detected (Fig. 14-68). Both MRI and MDCT[86] are capable of demonstrating myxomas. ECG-gated MDCT depicts an intracavitary mass with well-defined margins and lobulated surface; given their gelatinous nature, in baseline conditions they are heterogeneously hypodense. Calcification is present in about 14% of lesions, more frequently in right-sided lesions. Arterial phase contrast enhancement is usually not apparent[93] but heterogeneous enhancement due to the presence of cystic or necrotic areas is recognised on studies performed with a longer delay time.[92] The main differential diagnosis is intracavitary thrombi, which usually have no pedicle and appear hypodense and non-enhancing. On MDCT, prolapse through the mitral valve orifice is the only reliable discriminatory finding indicating myxoma.

MRI can also be useful; myxomas demonstrate an intermediate but variable signal intensity on spin-echo images similar to that of myocardium. A heterogeneous appearance is typical because of their complex architecture and varying components of myxoid, haemorrhagic, cystic, calcified, ossified and fibrous tissue.[94] They are predominantly hypointense to myocardium on T1w

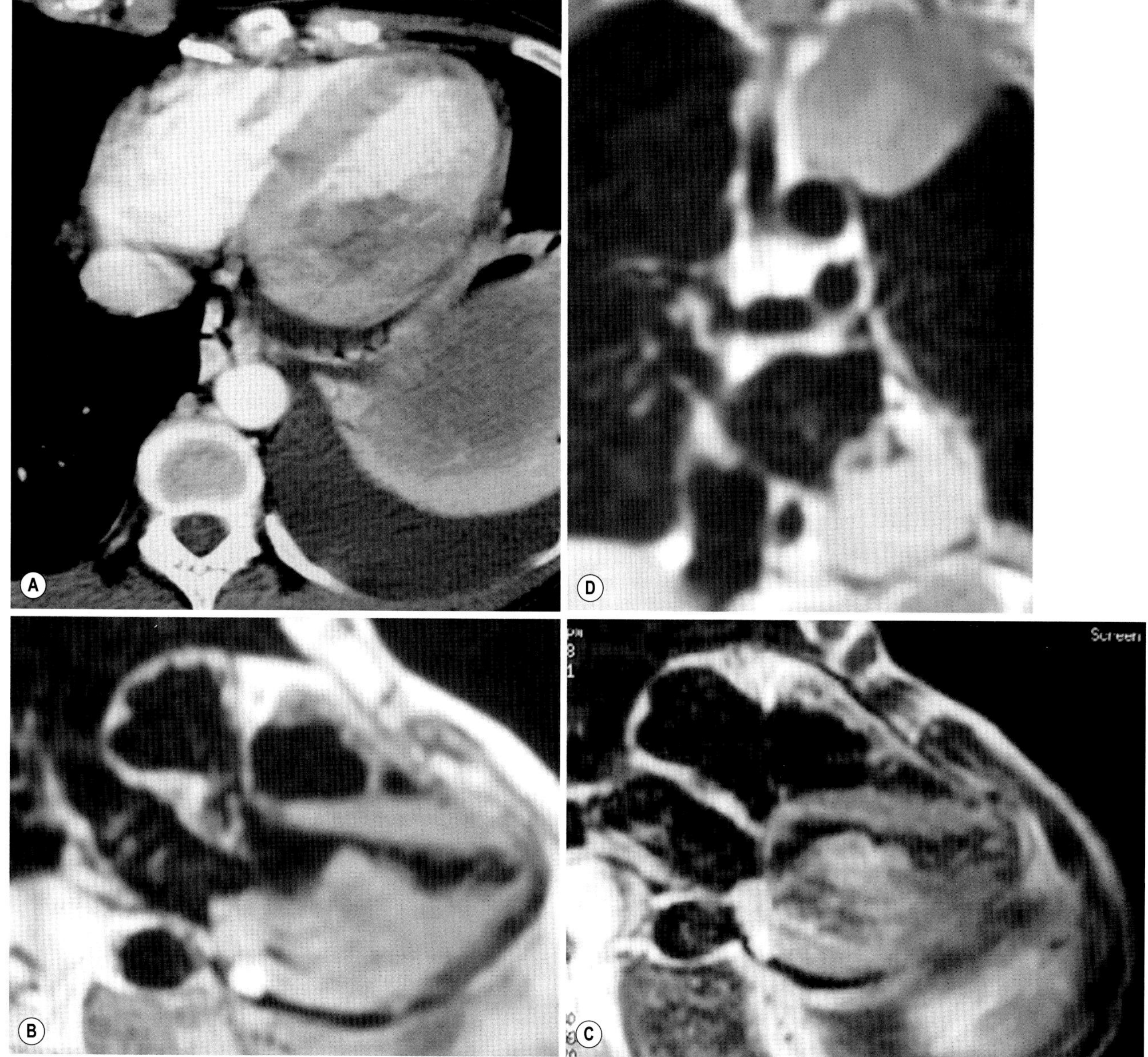

FIGURE 14-65 ■ **Left ventricle lung cancer metastasis.** (A) Contrast-enhanced CT image shows a heterogeneous mass in the left ventricle. (B, C) T1w and T2w horizontal long-axis MRI demonstrate the large implant of the lesion, involving the lateral wall of the left ventricle, with T2 high signal heterogeneity. (D) The left superior sulcus tumour is evident on the coronal T1w image.

images and hyperintense on T2w images (Fig. 14-69). On gradient-echo images, myxomas often have a low signal intensity caused by partial calcification. Myxomas are usually hypointense relative to the blood pool and hyperintense to myocardium on SSFP sequences (Fig. 14-70).[95] Intratumoural subacute or chronic haemorrhage appears as high or heterogeneous signal intensity on both T1w and T2w sequences. Moderate enhancement after intravenous Gd-DTPA is caused by increased vascularisation but this can be heterogeneous due to admixed cystic or necrotic areas. Cine-MRI display may show the mobility of the tumour, including prolapse through the mitral or tricuspid valve orifice in diastole (Fig. 14-71). The attachment point for pedunculated lesions can be suggested on cine review. First-pass enhancement is usually mild or not apparent; most lesions demonstrate at least some delayed enhancement, which is usually patchy (Fig. 14-70), although some myxomas will have a homogeneous enhancement pattern.[96] Differential diagnosis with an atrial thrombus can be obtained by MRI.

Thrombus usually occurs in an enlarged chamber, atrial appendage is commonly involved and atrial fibrillation is likely to be present. Myxomas can be sessile or pedunculated and are commonly attached to the interatrial septum. Thrombi are usually sessile and readily distinguished by complete absence of both first-pass and delayed enhancement, which are seen to a variable degree in myxomas. Mitral valve prolapse has also been reported as having high sensitivity for myxoma over left atrial thrombus.[93] However, surgical resection is

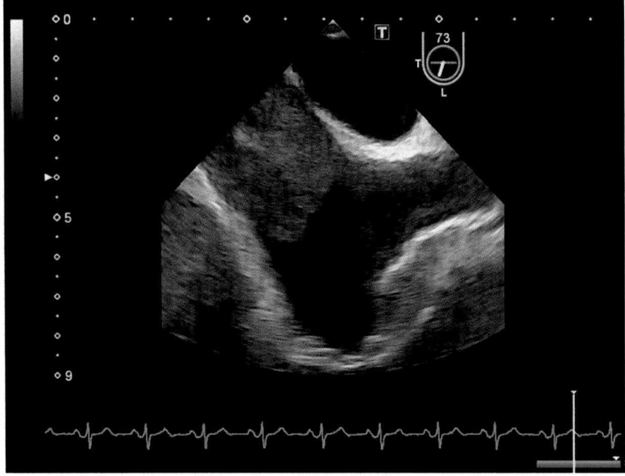

FIGURE 14-66 ■ 2D echocardiography of neoplastic thrombus from renal cell carcinoma in inferior vena cava and right atrium.

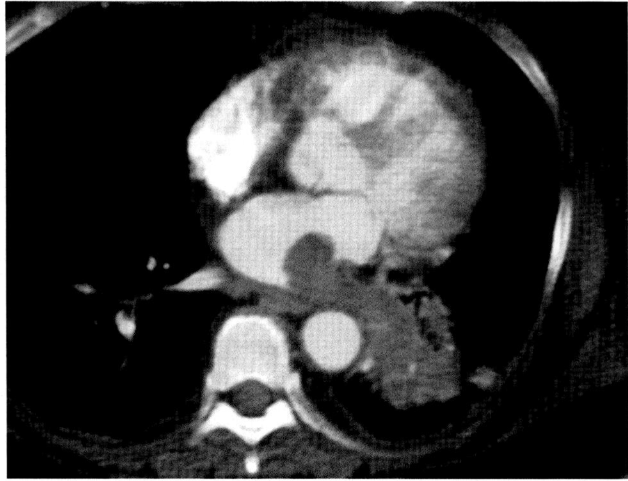

FIGURE 14-67 ■ Enhanced CT image shows direct invasion of left atrium from a left lower lobe bronchogenic carcinoma.

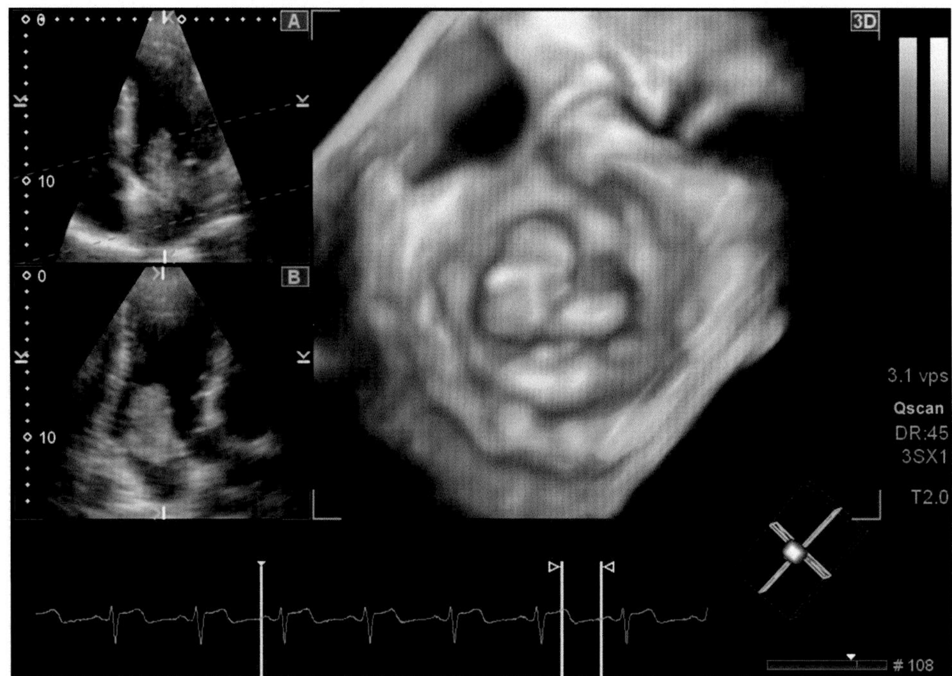

FIGURE 14-68 ■ **Echocardiography (2D and 3D) of atrial myxoma.** On the left, systolic and diastolic frames show a large hyperechoic tumour of the left atrium passing through the mitral valve; on the right, a 3D short-axis image shows the tumour across the mitral valve.

required for definitive diagnosis and to prevent major complications.

Lipomas

Lipomas are slow-growing neoplasms composed of mature adipose tissue. They may arise from the epicardium, myocardium or endocardial surfaces, including the interatrial septum. They occur commonly in the right atrium at the level of the interatrial septum. An epicardial location, a narrow attachment point and growth into the pericardial space are typical.[97] Cardiac lipomas can have highly variable appearances on echocardiography.[96] On CT, lipomas appear well circumscribed and show homogeneous fat attenuation (–50 to –150 HU) (Fig. 14-72).[86] Occasionally they may display internal soft-tissue septa. Lipomatous hypertrophy of the interatrial septum consists of an accumulation of brown fat with a diameter greater than 2 cm; it characteristically spares the mid septum (the fossa ovalis), which gives a dumbbell-like appearance.[98] Lipomatous hypertrophy of the interatrial septum is often found incidentally on routine chest CT (Fig. 14-72). Lipomas have high signal intensity on MRI due to their short T1 and long T2 relaxation, consistent with fat (Fig. 14-72). There should be no soft-tissue component and no contrast enhancement (Fig. 14-72) and both of these features are considered suspicious for the presence of sarcomatous elements.[98]

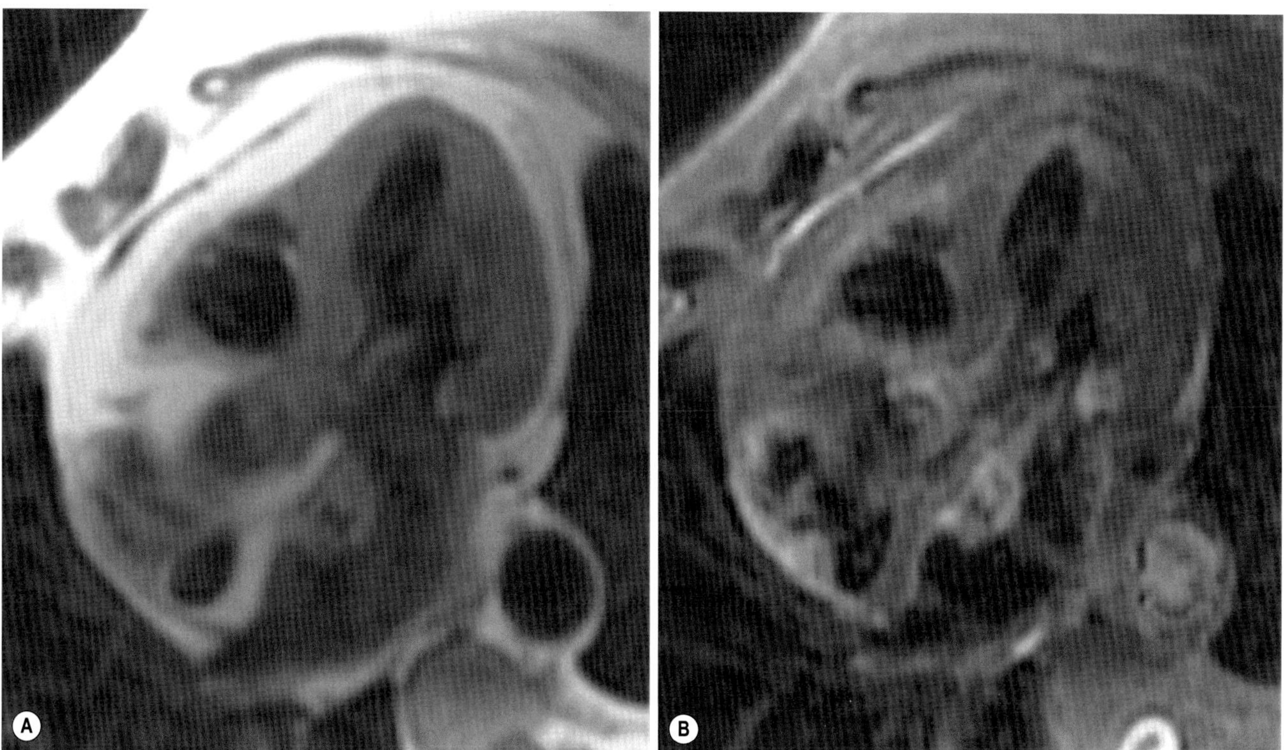

FIGURE 14-69 ■ (A) FSE T1w horizontal long-axis view of left atrial myxoma: typical localisation in the area of fossa ovalis, with heterogeneous signal intensity; central hypointense area is due to calcifications. (B) FSE T2w fat-suppressed image, same plane: lesion shows heterogeneous hyperintensity with central dark area.

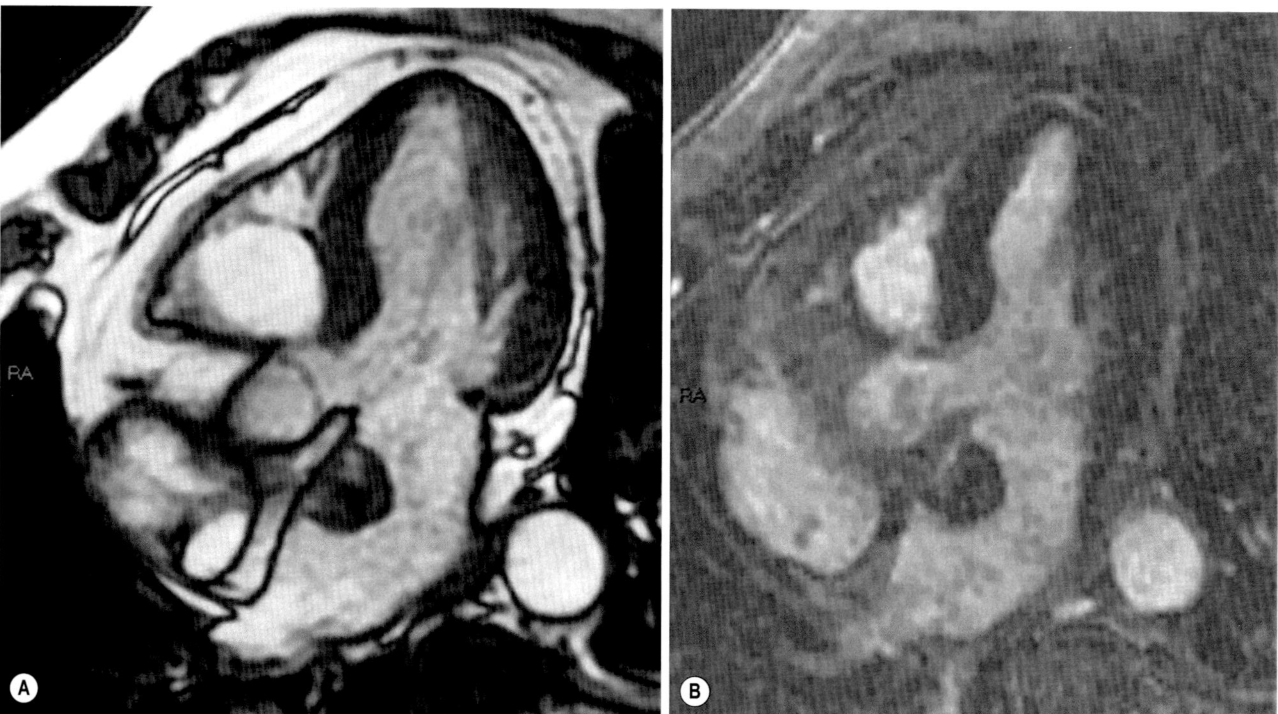

FIGURE 14-70 ■ **Same case as described in the caption to Fig. 14-45.** (A) On SSFP image slight heterogeneous hyperintensity of the lesion compared with myocardium is evident; (B) late gadolinium enhancement image shows tiny foci of contrast uptake caused by fibrotic changes.

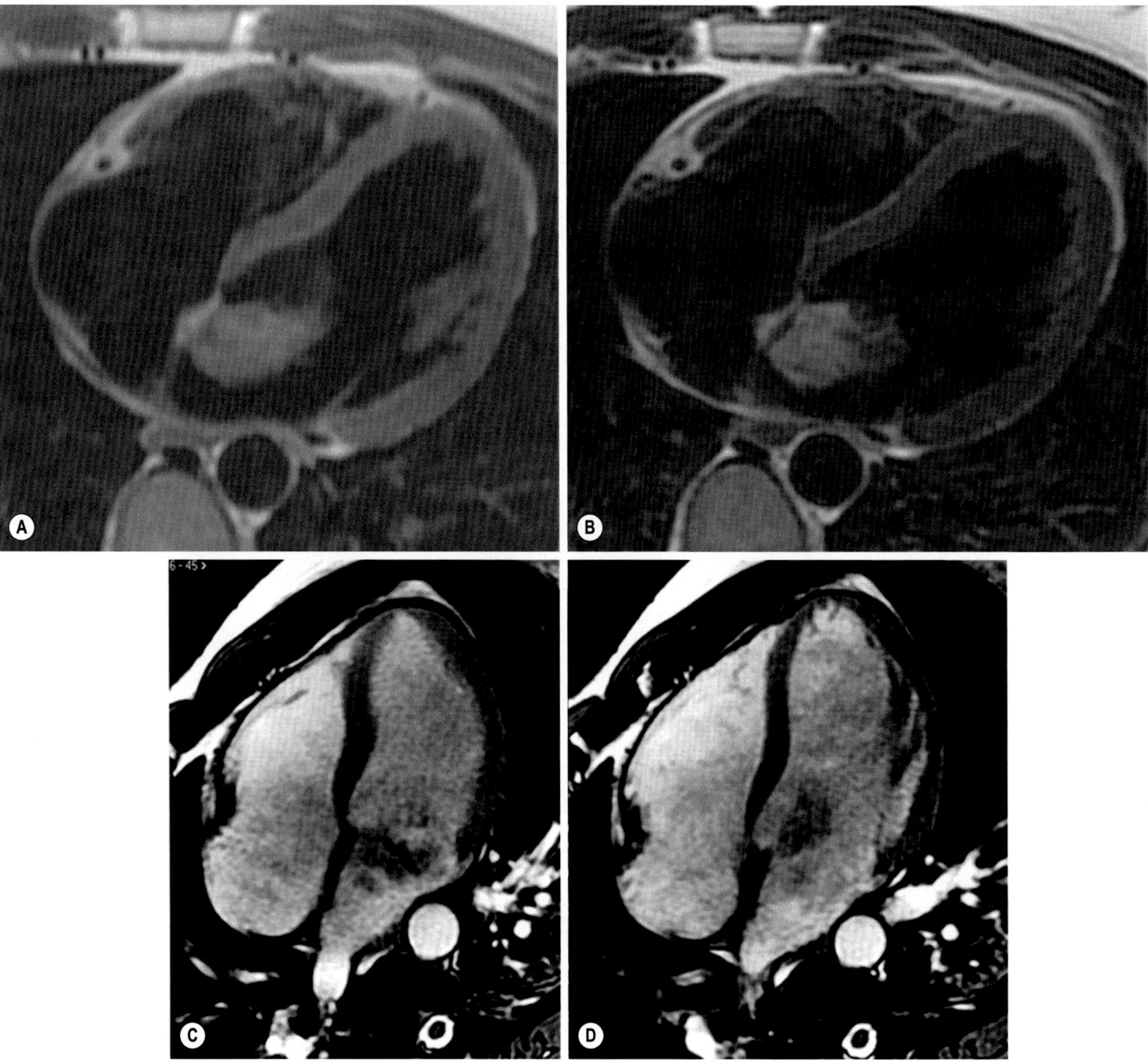

FIGURE 14-71 ■ **Atrial myxoma of fossa ovalis.** (A, B) Axial T1 and T2 images show heterogeneity in signal intensity of the lesion. (C) and (D) are systolic and diastolic frames of cine-MRI: prolapse of the pedunculated myxoma through the mitral orifice is evident.

Rhabdomyomas

These are the most frequent (40%) cardiac neoplasm in infants and children and are mostly found in patients less than one year of age. They occur in association with tuberous sclerosis in up to 50% of cases, where they may be congenital and manifest in the neonatal period. Arrhythmias, which may be fatal, are their main presenting feature. They are usually intramural, may occur in any location in the heart but are more common in the ventricles. They may be small and multiple, and measure around 3–4 cm in diameter, rarely up to 10 cm. These tumours are often inoperable because they are commonly deep-seated, poorly demarcated and multiple; however, the majority of cardiac rhabdomyomas regress spontaneously.[98] Echocardiographic appearance is variable, from isoechoic (not easily differentiated from normal myocardium) to hyperechoic (more often in neonates and children) (Fig. 14-73). On CT, the lesions are enhancing, and when multiple may display diffuse thickening of the myocardium. On MRI, rhabdomyomas have signal intensity similar to that of the adjacent myocardium on T1w images and relatively increased signal intensity on T2w images.[98]

Fibroma

A fibroma is usually a single tumour of the ventricular wall, generally on the left, and may be resectable. The presentation is with arrhythmia or congestive cardiac failure, and plain radiographs can show an enlarged heart. Though the tumour is rare, it is of radiological interest in that it may calcify and show characterising whorls of calcium, which may suggest the specific diagnosis. On

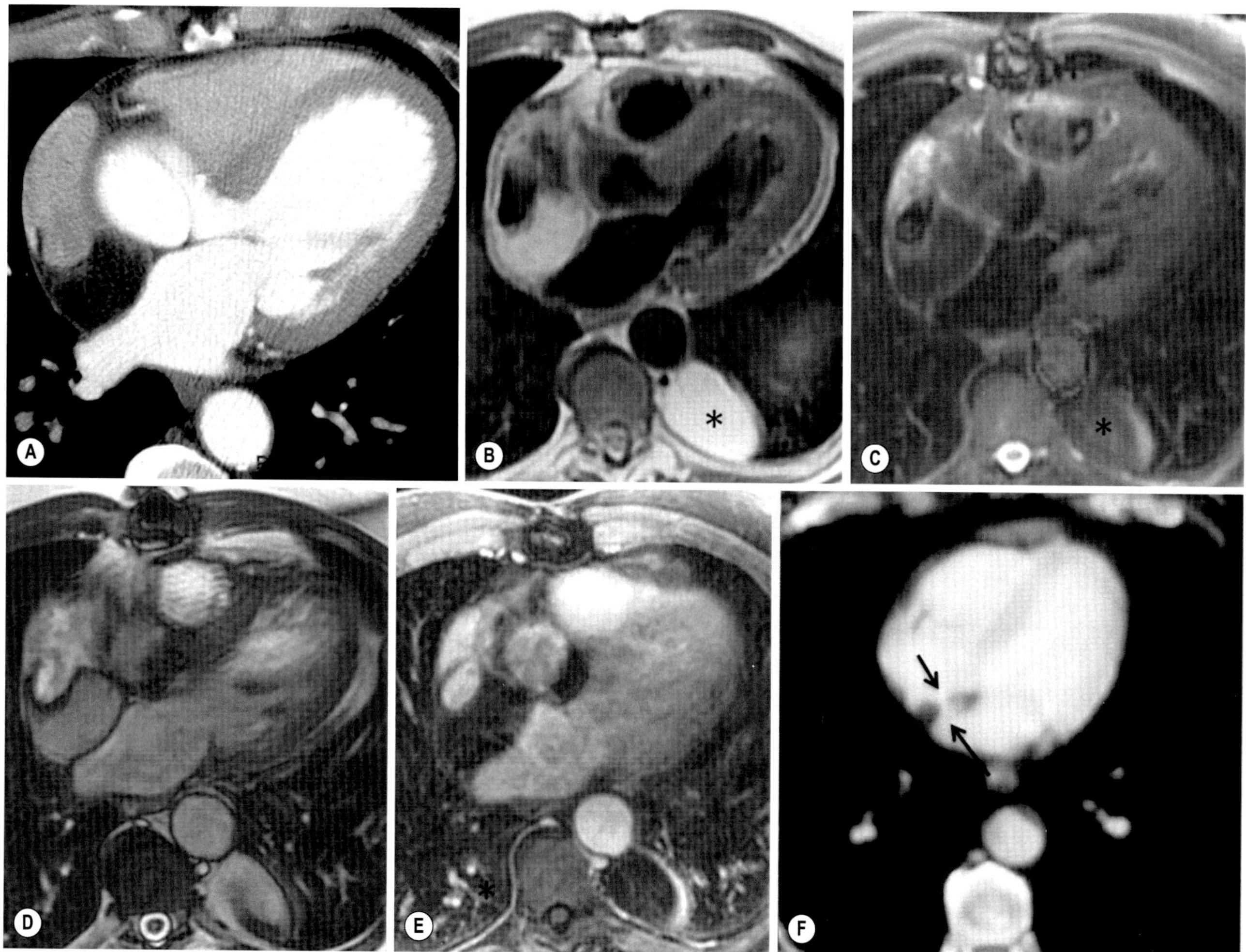

FIGURE 14-72 ■ Atrial septum lipoma. (A) Cardiac CT shows a marked hypodense well-defined lesion; (B) T1w image demonstrates marked hyperintensity of the lesion, completely suppressed in STIR image (C). In (D) a frame from cine-SSFP shows high to intermediate signal intensity of the tumour, while post-contrast T1 GRE image does not demonstrate enhancement (E). Furthermore, in all the MR images, a subpleural lipoma is evident (*). (F) A different case of lipomatous infiltration of the interatrial septum is reported, just to show the classical sparing of the fossa ovalis (arrows).

MDCT, fibroma appears as a well-defined or infiltrative mass, usually large (5 cm) with dystrophic calcifications and minimal enhancement. On MRI, fibromas are usually poorly vascularised, intramurally located with well-circumscribed margins and a surrounding rim of compressed myocardium. On both T1w and T2w images they yield low signal compared with normal myocardium because of their dense fibrous composition. They have variable signal intensity on SSFP, and do not deform on tagged sequences. Delayed enhancement may be homogeneous, peripheral or heterogeneous. Fibromas that demonstrate little or no delayed enhancement may resemble a focal hypertrophic cardiomyopathy.[98]

Papillary Fibroelastoma

Papillary fibroelastoma is the second most common benign cardiac tumour.[96] A fibroelastoma is nearly always solitary; it can arise from any endocardial surface but the majority originate on the atrial surface of the mitral valve and aortic side of the aortic valve. Most are small (<1 cm) and remain clinically silent, and may cause systemic embolisation or sudden cardiac death secondary to coronary artery embolisation. Echocardiography usually establishes the correct diagnosis, showing a small hyperechoic lesion attached to valve leaflets (Fig. 14-74). They are occasional findings on ECG-gated CT where they appear as a focal low-attenuation mass arising from a valve surface.[86,99] Detection with MRI can be difficult because of their small size; fibroelastomas are well circumscribed with intermediate signal intensity on T1w and T2w images.[100] Usually there is no delayed enhancement; however, a uniform enhancement may reflect gadolinium accumulation within fibroelastic tissue.[101] In SSFP cine sequences they appear mobile, well circumscribed and of low signal, with peritumoural turbulent flow.[102]

Haemangioma

Usually found in the ventricles, haemangiomas may occur in multiple locations.[103] These lesions are hyperintense on T2w images and iso- or hyperintense on T1w images.

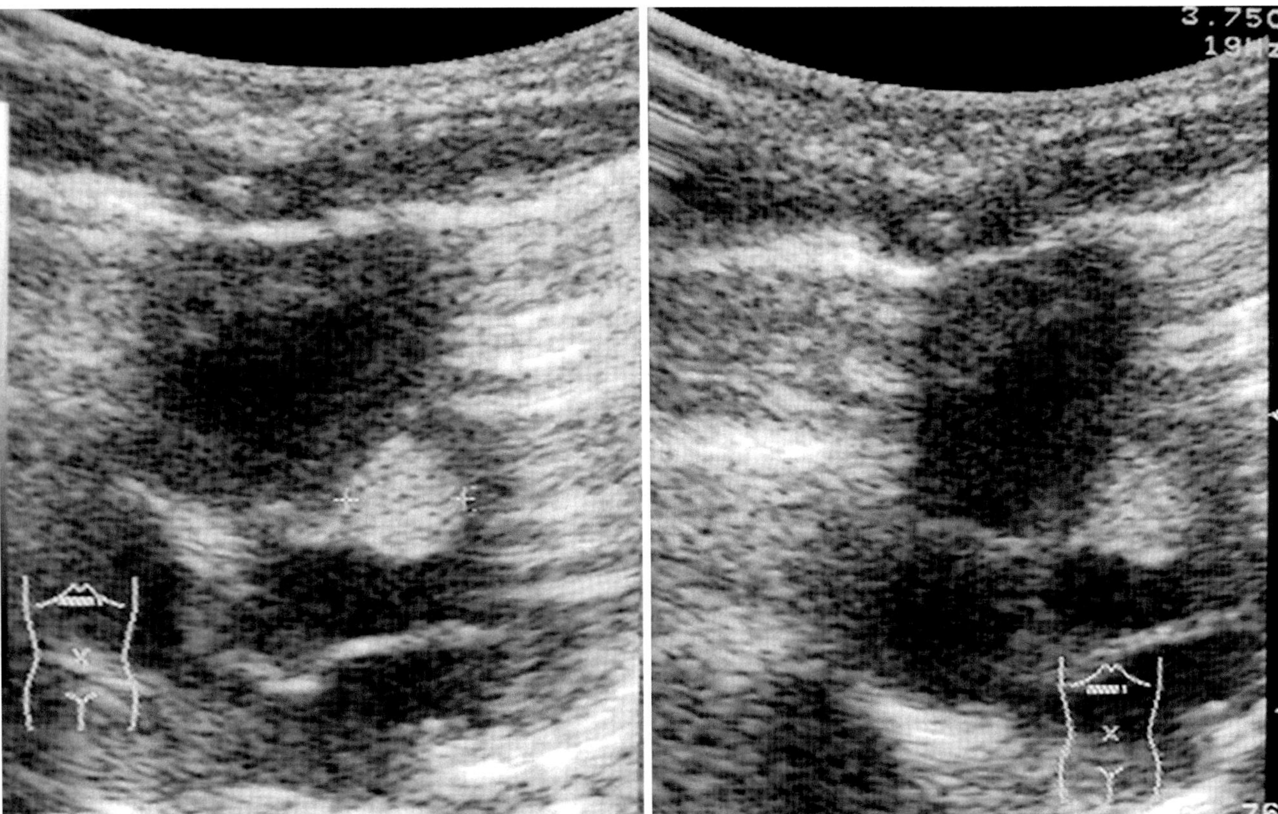

FIGURE 14-73 ■ 2D echocardiographic subcostal view shows a typical rhabdomyoma (hyperechoic rounded lesion) attached to the basal interventricular septum (calipers).

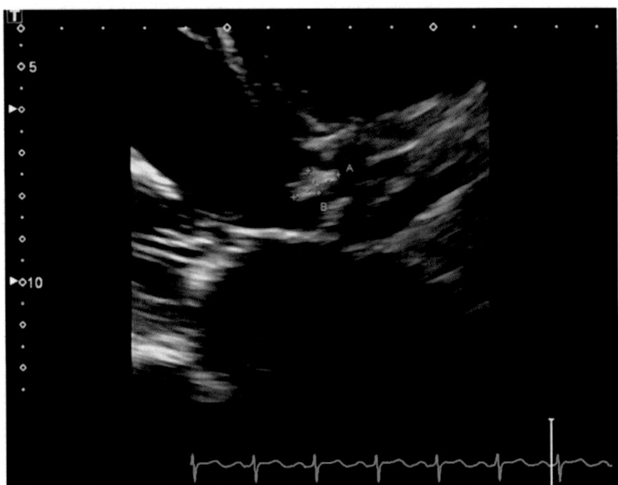

FIGURE 14-74 ■ B-mode echocardiography shows a small hyperechoic lesion (calipers) attached to valve leaflets. At surgery a fibroelastoma was found and resected.

Contrast enhancement is strong, sometimes heterogeneous due to calcifications and internal septations.[96] On CT, they appear as heterogeneous foci of calcification; enhancement is intense.[98]

Hydatid Disease

Hydatid disease may involve the heart. The cysts behave as a benign myocardial tumour—well-circumscribed, loculated lesions; they may calcify. Echocardiography can usually assess the correct diagnosis, but MDCT and eventually MRI can be useful.

Primary Malignant Tumours of the Heart

Malignant primary cardiac tumours can be broadly divided into sarcomas, lymphomas and primary pericardial malignancy.[95] Imaging findings suggestive of a malignant cardiac tumour include a right atrial location, involvement of more than one cardiac chamber, size >5 cm, a haemorrhagic pericardial effusion, a broad base of attachment, extension into the mediastinum or great vessels and a moderate to strong or heterogeneous delayed enhancement pattern.[104,105]

Sarcomas

Sarcomas account for nearly all primary malignant cardiac neoplasms and are the second commonest primary tumour after myxoma.[105] Angiosarcoma is the most common malignant tumour of the heart. Peak incidence is in the fourth decade and there is a strong male predominance.[105] They usually present with arrhythmias, symptoms of right heart failure, pericardial effusion, often haemorrhagic, cardiac tamponade and features of valvular or vena cava obstruction.[96] Diagnosis is usually late and metastases are present in most cases (lungs, liver, bones, lymph nodes and brain). Most angiosarcomas arise in the right atrium, are mainly intramural and

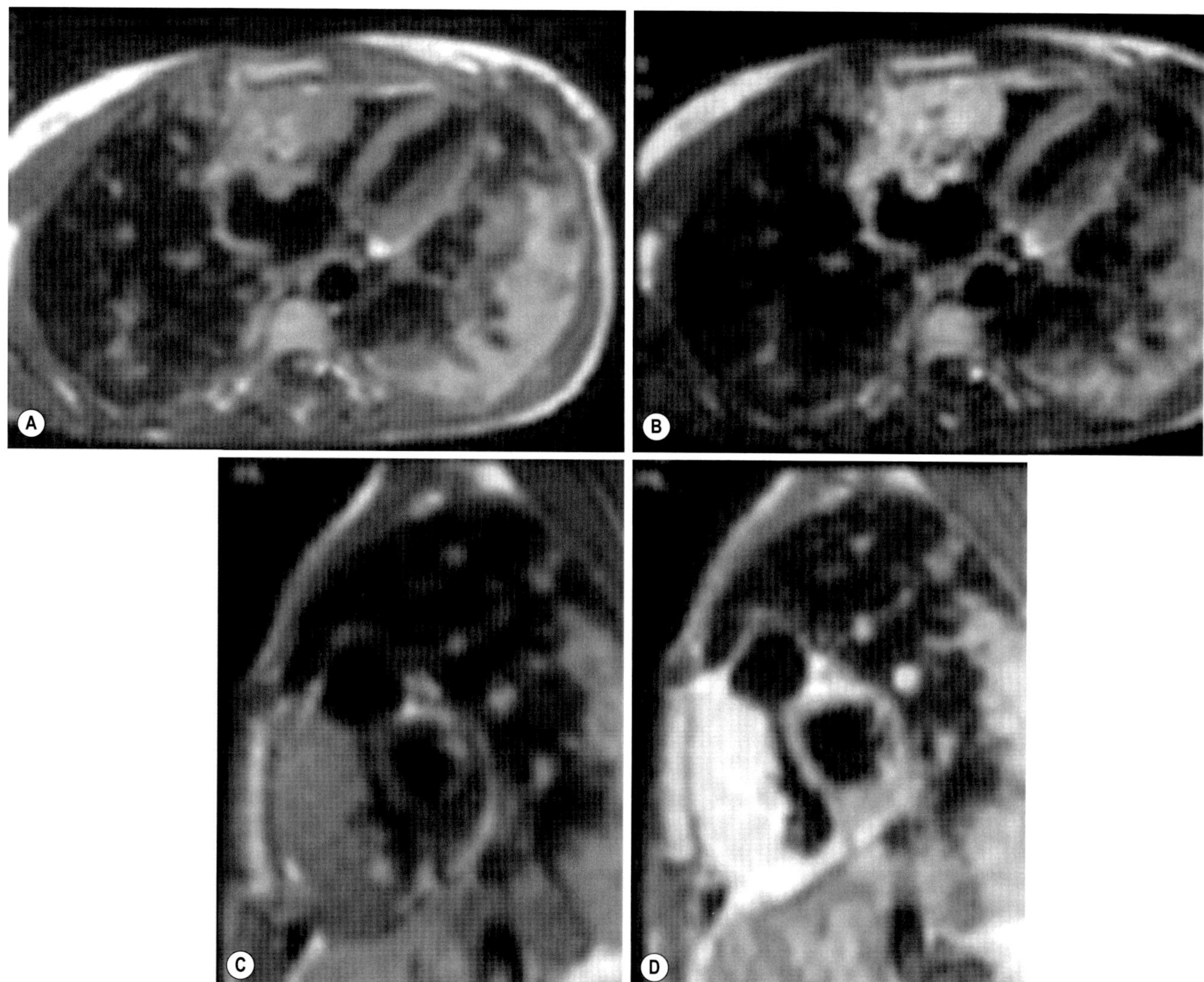

FIGURE 14-75 ■ **Angiosarcoma of right ventricle.** (A) Axial T1w image shows a large tumour with irregular margins, involving free wall of right ventricle, right atrioventricular groove, tricuspid annulus and right atrium wall; furthermore, multiple nodules are visible in both lungs, with large consolidation in left inferior lobe; (B) T2w image demonstrates high signal intensity of the tumour. (C, D) Pre- and post-contrast T1w short-axis images show strong enhancement of the tumour and the lung metastasis. Biopsy confirmed the suspected angiosarcoma.

infiltrating, though they may fill the chamber, and may extend to the pericardium, vena cavae, tricuspid valve, right coronary artery and right ventricular free wall. As many as 25% originate in other cardiac chambers or the pericardium. Involvement of the pericardium may lead to tamponade.

The heart is usually enlarged on the plain radiograph, and echocardiography will show a mass which is atypical of myxoma, with or without an effusion. Some particular characteristics may help in recognising an angiosarcoma on MRI (Fig. 14-75):[106] a large infiltrating, broad-based mass with a cauliflower appearance; heterogeneous signal intensity (T1 isointense, T2 hyperintense) originating from necrosis and intratumoural haemorrhage; and intralesional flow voids which may reflect large vascular channels.[107] Homogeneous or heterogeneous strong enhancement, the latter with a sunray appearance, is common on enhanced MRI.[96] On MDCT, they appear as a heterogeneously enhancing mass. A high attenuation pericardial effusion is frequent and caused by haemorrhage and/or tumour debris.[86,108] A left atrial location, even if rare, is possible (Fig. 14-76).

Sarcomas with Myofibroblastic Differentiation. These tumours include undifferentiated sarcoma, leiomyosarcoma, fibrosarcoma, liposarcoma and osteosarcoma; they predominate in adulthood (fourth or fifth decade) and have slow infiltrative growth patterns. Most patients die of local effects. Survival depends on effective surgical resection. They originate most often from the posterior wall of the left atrial wall (fibrosarcoma in 30% of the cases from either ventricle and 20% from pericardium; liposarcoma from any chamber or pericardium). MRI findings are relatively non-specific. Liposarcoma rarely contains significant fat but necrosis and haemorrhage predominate; osteosarcoma may present calcifications that appear as signal void in all sequences. MDCT is better suited for the detection of calcific components.

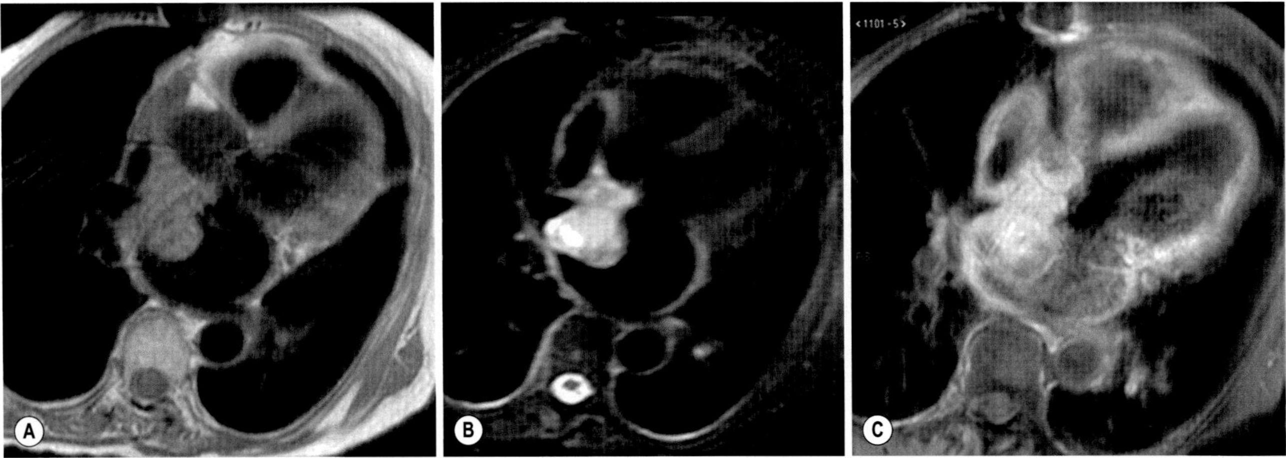

FIGURE 14-76 ■ **Interatrial mass, involving both atria.** (A) T1w axial image shows an isointense lesion, while (B) the T2w image demonstrates a marked hyperintensity. (C) In post-contrast T1w image a strong and homogeneous enhancement of the mass is visible. Biopsy revealed an angiosarcoma; compared with the case shown and described in Fig. 14-49, this localisation is uncommon.

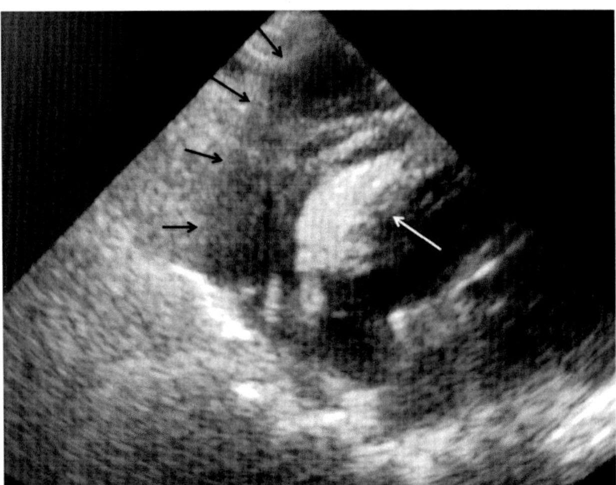

FIGURE 14-77 ■ 2D echocardiographic subcostal image in a case of rhabdomyosarcoma shows a hyperechoic mass infiltrating the right atrioventricular groove (white arrow). Pericardial effusion is also evident (black arrows).

Rhabdomyosarcoma. It predominates in childhood; the much less frequent pleomorphic sub-type occurs in adults.[105] This tumour appears as a large, bulky, infiltrative mass with central necrosis, has no chamber predilection and may involve the valves.[109] At echocardiography, texture is variable, from hyperechoic to heterogeneous in larger lesions, and, often associated with pericardial effusion (Fig. 14-77). On MRI, signal intensity is heterogeneous on T1w and T2w images.[95] On MDCT, attenuation is low, with peripheral enhancement.[109]

Lymphoma

Primary cardiac lymphoma is an aggressive B-cell lymphoma, usually occurring in immune-compromised patients. It is rare, confined to the heart or pericardium with no evidence of extracardiac disease and involves the right atrium, less frequently more than one chamber and the pericardium. On MRI, cardiac lymphoma may appear as multiple myocardial nodules iso- or slightly hyperintense relative to normal myocardium with heterogeneous enhancement or as diffuse pericardial infiltration with a haemorrhagic pericardial effusion.[105,110] On MDCT, it appears isoattenuating relative to myocardium.[111]

PERICARDIAL DISEASES

Anatomy

The pericardium is a fibroserous, relatively inelastic sac that surrounds the heart and extends cranially to cover the pulmonary trunk, SVC and ascending aorta.[112] It is made up of an inner visceral and outer parietal layer with a serosal lining; these layers surround a virtual cavity which under normal circumstances contains a small quantity of fluid (15–30 mL).

Its functions are:[113]

- Mechanical: protecting the heart, acting as a barrier against local inflammation, limiting its movement within the mediastinum and maintaining ventricular compliance.
- Membranous: forming the serous pericardial fluid and producing surfactant and prostacyclins.
- Ligamentous: limiting cardiac displacement.

On CT, the pericardium appears as a thin line of fibrous tissue enveloping the heart, well contrasted with the surrounding low attenuation of the outer mediastinal fat and inner epicardial fat.[114] Visualisation of the pericardium on CT strongly correlates with the amount of fat present.[115] Although the pericardium is visible over the right atrium and right ventricle in most individuals, it is often not visible over the lateral and posterior walls of the left ventricle.

On MR, the pericardium is well demonstrated by the high natural contrast between the two layers, fluid in the cavity, and the pericardial and epicardial fat. On

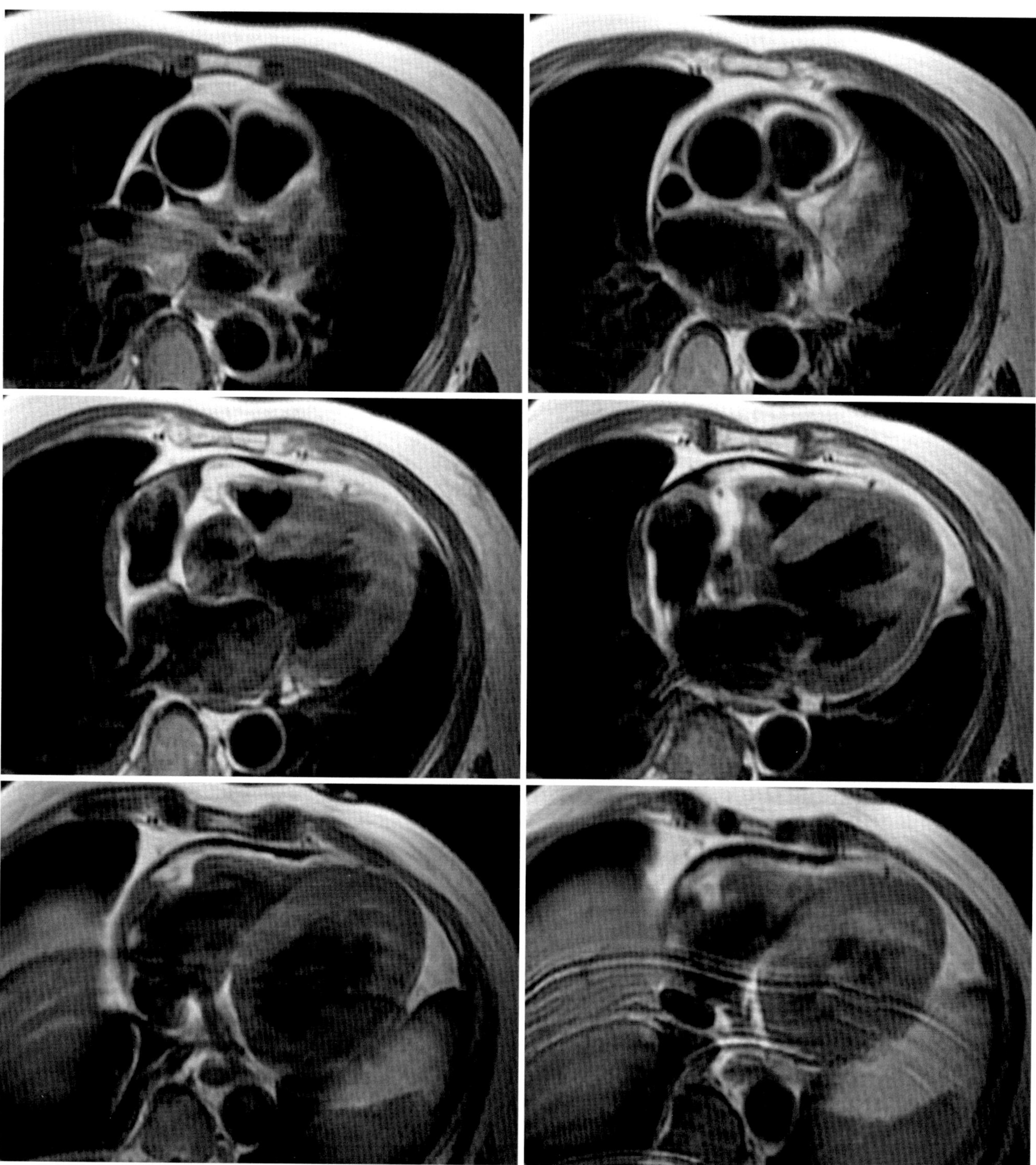

FIGURE 14-78 ■ **T1w axial images show the dark line of the pericardium (with a small amount of fluid within) between the high signal intensity of the prepericardial and subepicardial fat.**

black-blood sequences it appears as a thin low-intensity line surrounded by the high signal of pericardial and subepicardial fat (Fig. 14-78). Its hypointensity is related to the fibrous structure of the layers, to the non-linear movement of the fluid, and also to chemical-shift phenomena at the interface with the adipose tissue. In these sequences the layers appear hypointense, in contrast with the marked hyperintensity of the pericardial fluid. On MR angiographic sequences the pericardium may have intermediate signal.

Several studies have examined the thickness of the normal pericardium: 1.2 mm in diastole and 1.7 mm in systole, with a maximum of 4 mm.[113] The pericardium is best appreciated where it is well delineated from the surrounding fat, e.g. over the right ventricular surface, while it is more difficult to visualise near the lung, particularly

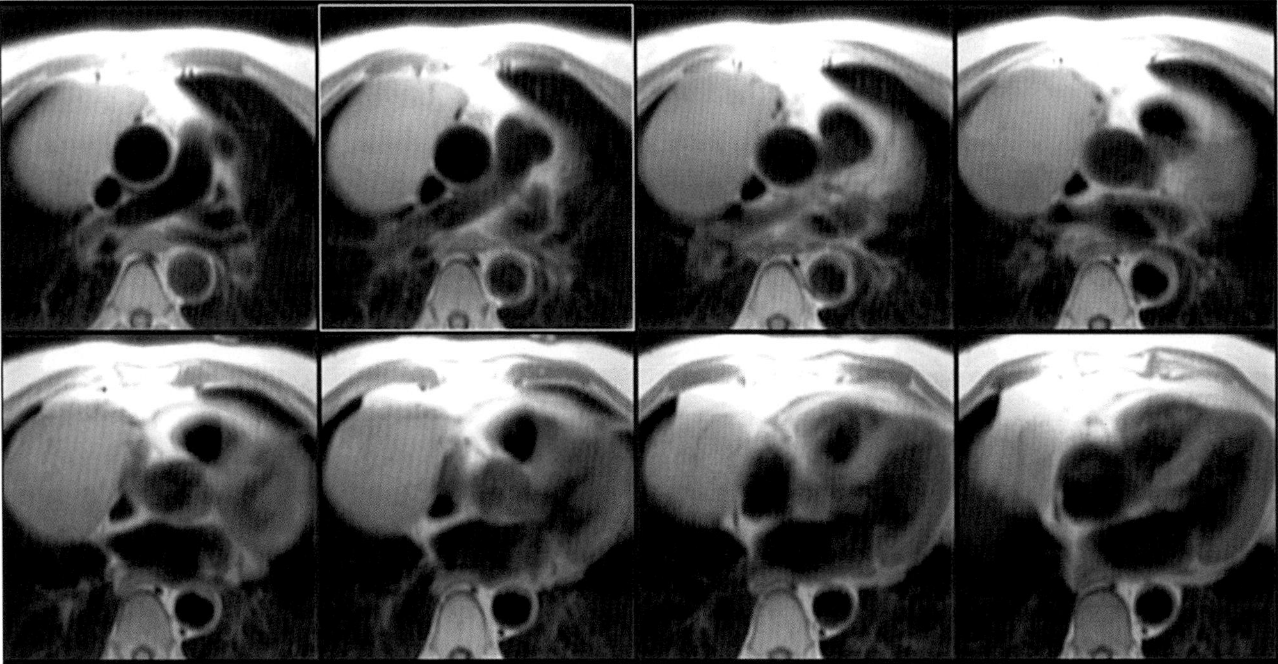

FIGURE 14-79 ■ **Pericardial cyst.** Contiguous black-blood T1w axial images show a well-defined lesion close to superior vena cava and right atrium, with intermediate signal intensity due to proteinaceous fluid content.

along the posterolateral surface of the left ventricle, where it can be seen in only 61% of cases.

The pericardium forms several recesses: these are cavities between the outer fibrous and inner serous layers of the pericardium, where small amounts of fluid may be present. Knowledge of their anatomy can help differentiate them from pathological findings. The superior pericardial recess forms from the transverse sinus and is wrapped around the right wall of the ascending aorta. Its anterior extension can be seen between the ascending aorta and pulmonary trunk with a characteristic triangular shape; its posterior extension, directly behind the ascending aorta, has a crescentic shape; its right lateral part insinuates between the ascending aorta and SVC. The superior pericardial recess may be mistaken for an aortic dissection, mediastinal mass, lymph node or thymus. The oblique pericardial sinus is the most posterior pericardial space: it is situated behind the left atrium and may be misinterpreted as an oesophageal lesion or bronchogenic cyst. On MDCT, the pericardial recesses are visible as defined anatomical structures in up to 44% of the cases.[116] Cine-MRI may help differentiate the normal pericardial recesses from abnormal lesions.

Pericardial Cysts

Pericardial cysts are usually round or oval in shape; they occur most frequently at the cardiophrenic angles, especially on the right. Pericardial cysts are rare congenital abnormalities; they are, however, the most common benign pericardial mass. Most often they are asymptomatic, representing an incidental finding on the CXR, and in some cases may cause compression on the cardiac chambers and right ventricular outflow tract obstruction.[117] Pericardial cysts usually have thin, smooth walls without internal septations and attach to the pericardium directly or by a pedicle. On CXR, pericardial cysts appear as a sharply demarcated mass causing a well-circumscribed, abnormal prominence of the cardiac border in the region of the right cardiophrenic angle.[118]

CT correctly demonstrates the position and extent of these lesions which appear as well-defined masses with fluid density and no enhancement after intravenous contrast agent.[114] Usually, their size and shape alters with respiration or body position. On MRI, pericardial cysts have low signal on T1w images, but they can appear hyperintense when the cystic fluid has high protein content (Fig. 14-79); signal intensity is homogeneously high on T2w images; no enhancement is evident after intravenous gadolinium. Pericardial cysts must be differentiated from other mediastinal cysts (e.g. bronchogenic or thymic) and from circumscribed fluid collections. Hydatid pericardial cysts may be trabeculated with the presence of daughter cysts.

Pericardial Defects

Complete or partial pericardial defects are extremely rare;[119] they result from an incomplete embryonic pericardial development, secondary to an insufficient intra-uterine vascularisation. Partial defects are more frequent than complete absence and may be associated with other complex anomalies, either cardiac (Fallot, interatrial septal defects, patent duct arteriosus) or extra-cardiac (bronchogenic cyst, hiatal hernia). The absence of the pericardium may cause cardiac or left lung herniation

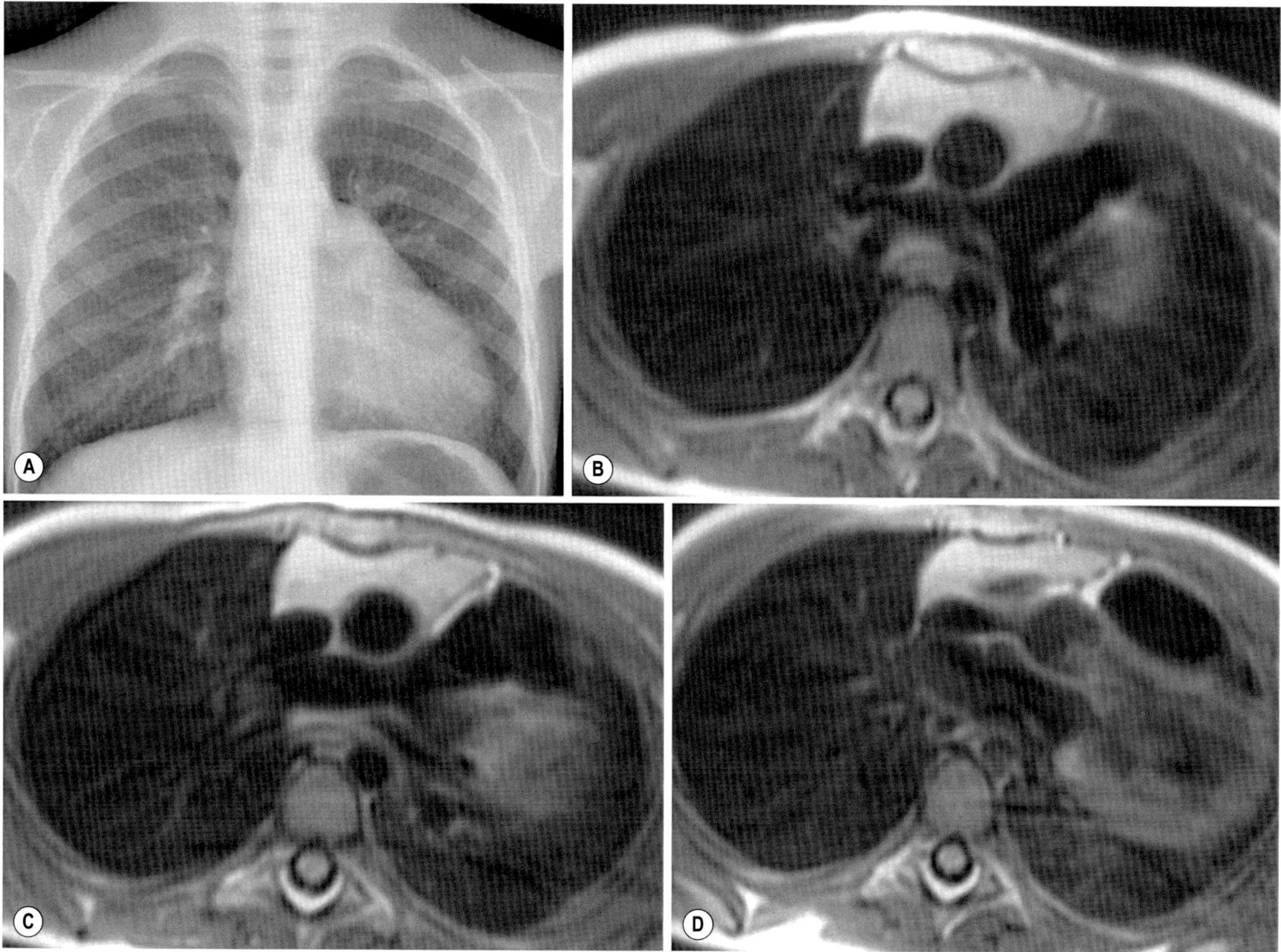

FIGURE 14-80 ■ **Partial pericardial agenesis.** (A) Chest X-ray, frontal view, shows prominent left second cardiac arch, with deep incisure between first and second left cardiac arch; main pulmonary trunk is deeply located in the lung. (B-D) Serial T1w axial MR images show pulmonary trunk (B, C) out of mediastinal margins (acute angle with anterior mediastinal fat) while the heart (D) is completely rotated towards the left, occupying the left hemithorax.

through the defect. Pulmonary tissue can be seen interposed between the aorta and the pulmonary artery. The clinical presentation is related to the site and extent of the defect: it may be asymptomatic or become symptomatic when herniation or strangulation through the defect leads to infarction of the left appendage or to coronary compression.

In the case of complete pericardial absence, CXR may show leftward displacement of the cardiac silhouette, a focal bulge in the region of the main pulmonary artery, lung interposition between the aorta and the pulmonary artery and between the left hemidiaphragm and the inferior cardiac border (Fig. 14-80). On CT or MRI, the pericardial defects can be more clearly defined: in the complete absence of the left side of the pericardium, lung tissue is interposed between the main pulmonary artery and aorta; bulging of the left atrial appendage can occur through the defect. The heart is usually rotated to the left (Fig. 14-80). This abnormal location can change and become more evident in left lateral decubitus. Pericardial defects may be difficult to directly diagnose, even with CT and MRI, as the left pericardium is not always well represented.

Pericardial Diverticulum

A pericardial diverticulum is very rare; it can be congenital or acquired.[120] It is an evagination of the parietal serous layer through small gaps in the fibrous external layer and it should be suspected when a complete wall cannot be identified in all parts of the lesion.[121] It is usually located at the right cardiophrenic angle; it tends to grow with time, eventually requiring surgery. The chest radiograph shows an abnormal shadow at the right side of the heart; CT demonstrates a well-circumscribed water attenuation lesion.

Pericardial Effusion

Under normal conditions the pericardium contains 15–30 mL of fluid; a quantity greater than 50 mL is considered abnormal. The causes include cardiac failure, renal or hepatic insufficiency, infection (bacterial, viral or fungal) and neoplastic lesions (pulmonary, mammary or lymphoma).[122]

The CXR can be positive when the pericardium contains at least 200 mL of fluid: the cardiac silhouette

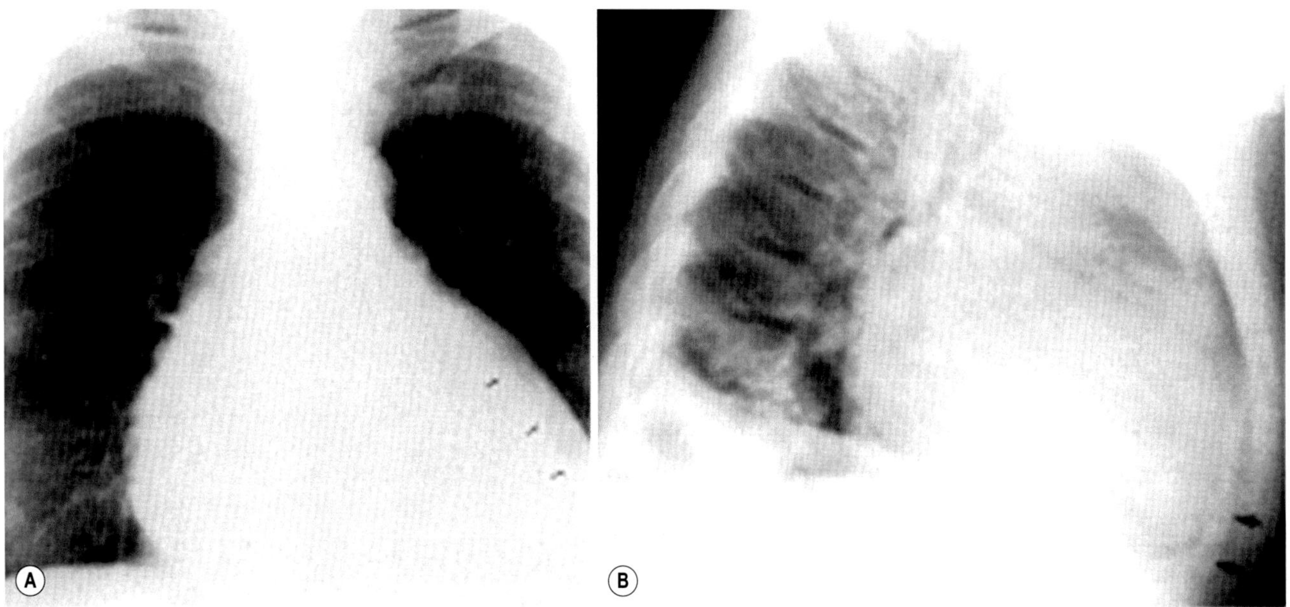

FIGURE 14-81 ■ Pericardial effusion, chest X-rays. (A) Frontal view shows double contouring of left third cardiac arch (small arrows); (B) lateral view demonstrates a retrosternal opacity (arrows), contoured by fat radiolucency (prepericardial and epicardial).

enlarges symmetrically, resulting in a flask configuration. The cardiophrenic angles are acute. On the lateral view, there is loss of the retrosternal clear space and a water density separates substernal from epicardial fat; on the frontal view, a curvilinear lucency can be seen along the left cardiac border (Fig. 14-81). Change in size can be rapid, with no changes in pulmonary vascular pattern.

Echocardiography is considered the primary imaging investigation for the evaluation of pericardial effusion.[115] The normal small amount of fluid is not detectable with echocardiography or is seen in systole as a thin posterior echo-free space. A small pericardial effusion is usually only seen behind the LV free wall; moderate and large effusions surround the heart. The character of the effusion cannot be reliably diagnosed by its echocardiographic appearance.[123] Pericardial fluid collections are usually well documented by ultrasound; however, the accuracy of echocardiography can be significantly limited. Anterior epicardial fat, pulmonary atelectasis or pleural effusion can all mimic a pericardial effusion; false negatives occur instead with small loculated collections. In obese or emphysematous patients the heart may be difficult to examine and it becomes difficult to differentiate between thickened pericardium, fat and fluid.[124]

The distribution of pericardial fluid is not uniform, due to gravity (Fig. 14-82); it is commonly localised along the posterolateral wall of the left ventricle, inferolateral to the right ventricle and in the superior pericardial recess. The size, severity and extent of the pericardial effusion may be better assessed using CT or MRI than with transthoracic echocardiography. Loculated effusions, especially those in anterior locations, can be difficult to detect at echocardiography but are readily demonstrated at CT or MR imaging.[125] Generally a distance greater than 4 mm between the pericardial leaflets is considered abnormal; in moderate effusions (100–500 mL), pericardial space anterior to the right ventricle is greater than 5 mm. A more precise evaluation of the fluid volume can be achieved by tracing the contours of the cavity.

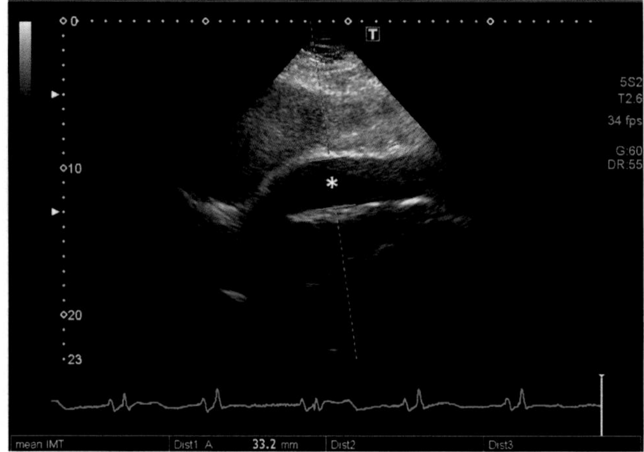

FIGURE 14-82 ■ B-mode echocardiography shows anterior anechoic fluid collection (*).

A severe acute effusion can compress the cardiac chambers, altering ventricular filling while decreasing cardiac output. This phenomenon is called cardiac tamponade. Symptoms depend on its severity and on the time course of its development; it can be rapidly lethal. The diagnosis of tamponade is clinical and confirmed with echocardiography that shows right atrial compression, diastolic collapse of the RV free wall, increased respiratory variation of mitral and tricuspid diastolic blood flow velocities, abnormal right-sided venous flows with decreased inferior vena cava collapsibility with inspiration.

MRI can help assess the functional effects on diastolic filling and cardiac function. CT or MRI is indicated

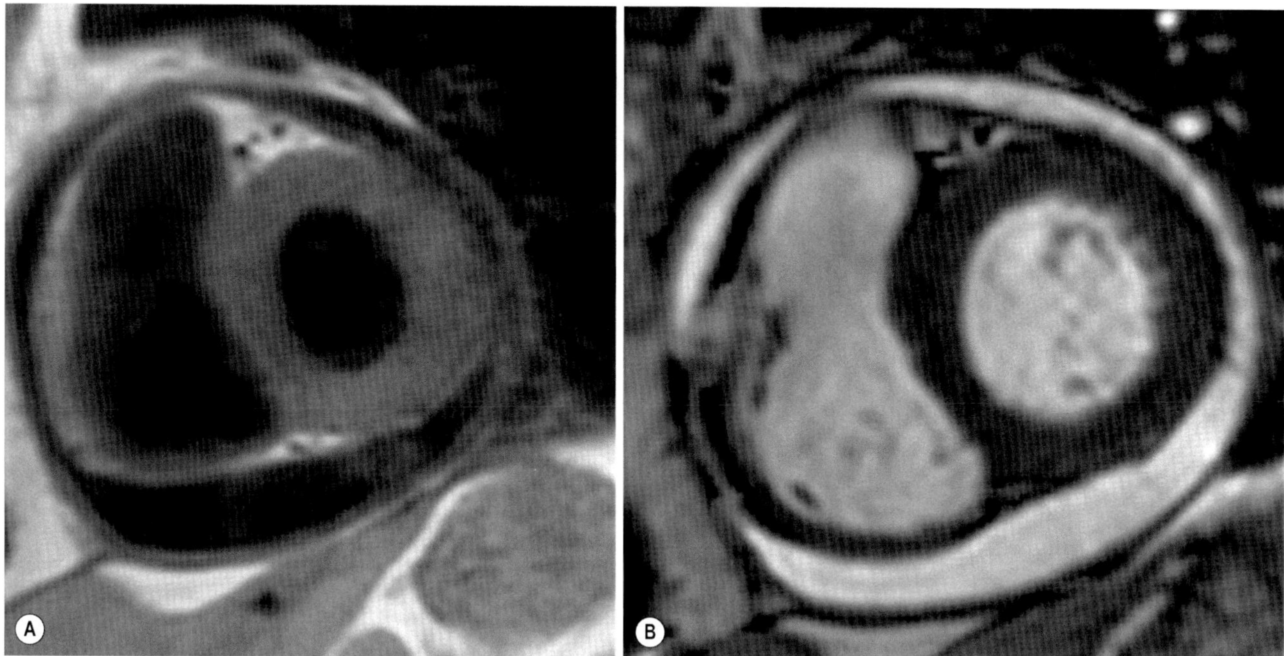

FIGURE 14-83 ■ **Pericardial effusion in pericarditis.** (A) T1w short-axis image shows no signal in the effusion, with mild thickening of the pericardium. (B) Cine-MRI frame shows hyperintense signal of the effusion, due to its prolonged T2 (SSFP signal is T2/T1-dependent).

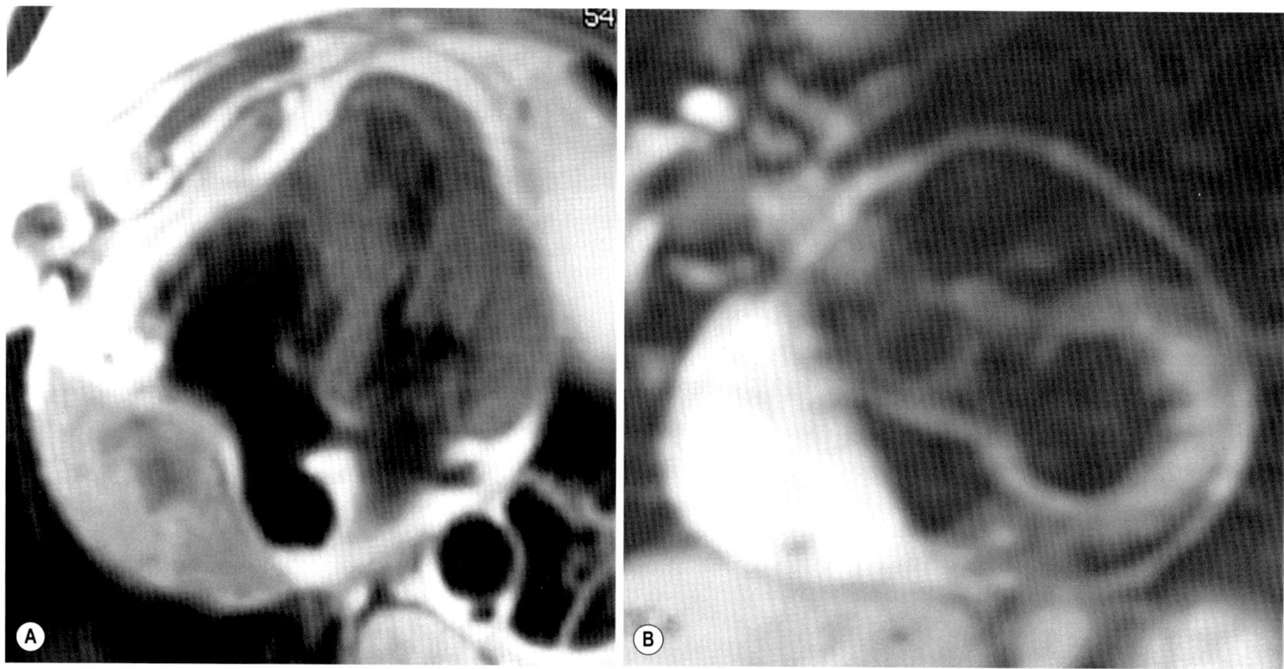

FIGURE 14-84 ■ **Pericardial haematoma (post-endomyocardial biopsy).** (A) T1w horizontal long-axis image shows well-circumscribed high signal pericardial collection, abutting right atrium. (B) T2w fat-saturated short-axis image demonstrates the high signal of the collection due to acute bleeding.

if the effusion is suspected to be complicated by haemorrhage, loculations, pericardial inflammation, thickening or constriction. A transudate typically has a low density (0–20 HU), whereas a higher CT attenuation value (up to 50 HU or more) indicates the effusion is more likely to be a purulent exudate or a haemopericardium associated with malignancy or with hypothyroidism.[115]

Pericardial effusions are in general hyperintense on T2w, gradient-recalled echo (GRE) and SSFP images (Fig. 14-83). Transudative or exudative effusions without debris are usually hypointense on T1w images (Fig. 14-83); proteinaceous or haemorrhagic effusions are T1-hyperintense (Figs. 14-83 and 14-84) but can be hypointense due to flow-void effects. GRE and SSFP

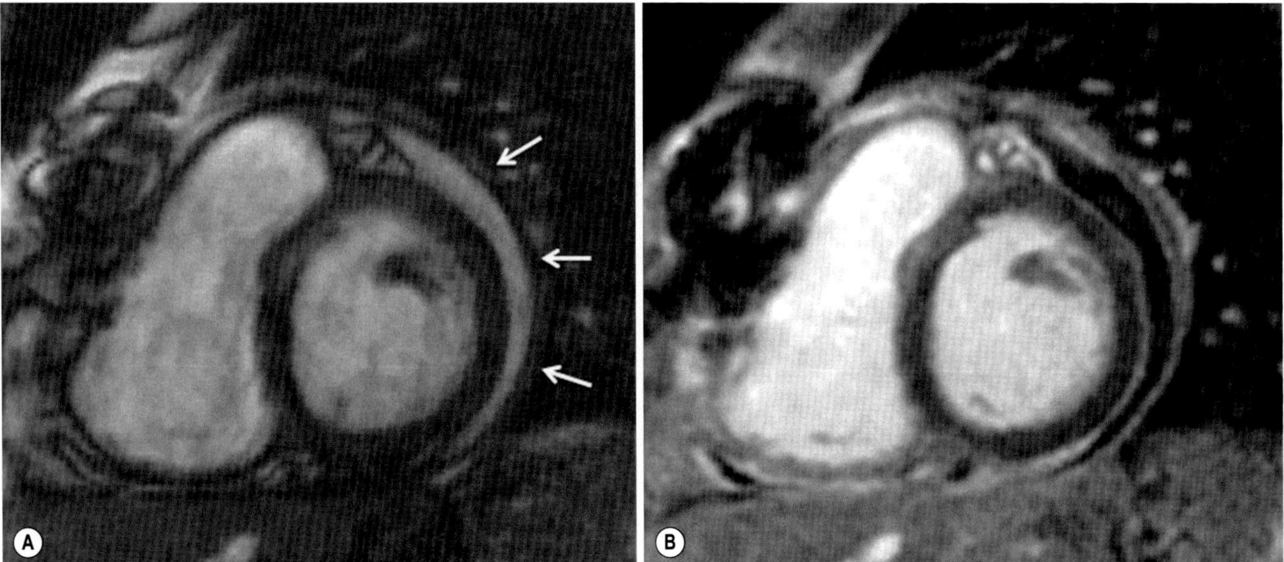

FIGURE 14-85 ■ **Pericarditis.** (A) Cine-MRI frame, short-axis image demonstrates mild pericardial effusion (arrows). (B) Delayed post-gadolinium enhancement, same plane, shows contrast uptake of pericardial layers, due to inflammation.

images can show fibrinous strands of coagulated blood. Accessory findings, such as pericardial thickening or leaflet enhancement, can suggest the inflammatory or neoplastic nature of the effusion. When a pericardial effusion is secondary to a malignancy there may also be associated irregularity and nodularity. Because most or all of the chest is evaluated during CT or MR imaging of the pericardium, associated abnormalities in the mediastinum and lungs may also be detected during the examination.[115]

Pericardial Inflammation

Pericardial inflammation can be idiopathic (in 30% of cases it is not possible to identify a cause). In most cases, its origin is infectious (viral, bacterial, mycobacterial or fungal); tuberculosis must be suspected in immunocompromised patients. Pericarditis may be caused by systemic diseases (rheumatoid arthritis, lupus erythematosus, scleroderma) or secondary to uraemia.[125] It can follow an acute transmural myocardial infarction (epistenocardiac pericarditis) while Dressler's syndrome or post-infarctual pericarditis arises later and has an autoimmune aetiology. Direct or indirect thoracic trauma can result in pericarditis. Radiotherapy for the treatment of lung, breast or mediastinal cancer has caused an increase of pericarditis and constrictive pericarditis. Symptoms vary according to the severity of the inflammation. In the acute phase there is usually chest pain but a subclinical course is possible.

The acute inflammation of the pericardial leaflets is characterised by the presence of highly vascularised granulation tissue, pericardial fluid and initial fibrin deposits that can determine with time the adhesion of the leaflets. The chronic phase is instead characterised by a progressive sclerosis of the pericardial leaflets because, with the deposition of fibrin, fibroblasts and collagen fibres, the pericardium becomes thickened and inelastic, characteristics of constrictive pericarditis. A thickened pericardium may not, however, determine constrictive pericarditis.[115]

CT shows increased thickness and enhancement of pericardial layers, unsharp pericardial borders and surrounding fat increased density. It may not easily differentiate a small effusion from pericardial thickening.[115] In cases where a pericardial effusion is absent, CT abnormalities may not be impressive, yielding a mild, diffusely thickened pericardium enhancing after intravenous administration of contrast material. Calcification is better detected with CT; on MR, calcification appears as a focal hypointense area, difficult to distinguish from fibrous tissue. MR signal intensity of the thickened pericardium can be highly variable, depending on the activity and nature of the inflammation. In the chronic fibrous forms, on T1w and T2w sequences, the pericardium appears as a low-intensity signal band;[126] in subacute forms, signal intensity can be intermediate or high and indistinguishable from high signal effusion (Fig. 14-84).[115] Late enhancement sequences are helpful for detecting the acute inflammatory conditions and for better defining the different components of the thickened pericardium and delineating pericardial leaflets from the effusion. Saturation of the adipose tissue signal is particularly useful in cases of myocardial pericarditis as it separates the myocardial enhancement from the hyperintense contrasted pericardium (Fig. 14-85).

Constrictive Pericarditis

Constrictive pericarditis is a chronic disease characterised by the fusion of the visceral and parietal leaflets: the pericardial sac becomes a fibrous or fibrocalcific inextensible rind that envelops the heart and determines a serious impairment of the diastolic filling. Patients with constrictive pericarditis have elevated systemic pressures and symptoms related to the low cardiac output, in particular with right cardiac failure, such as dyspnoea,

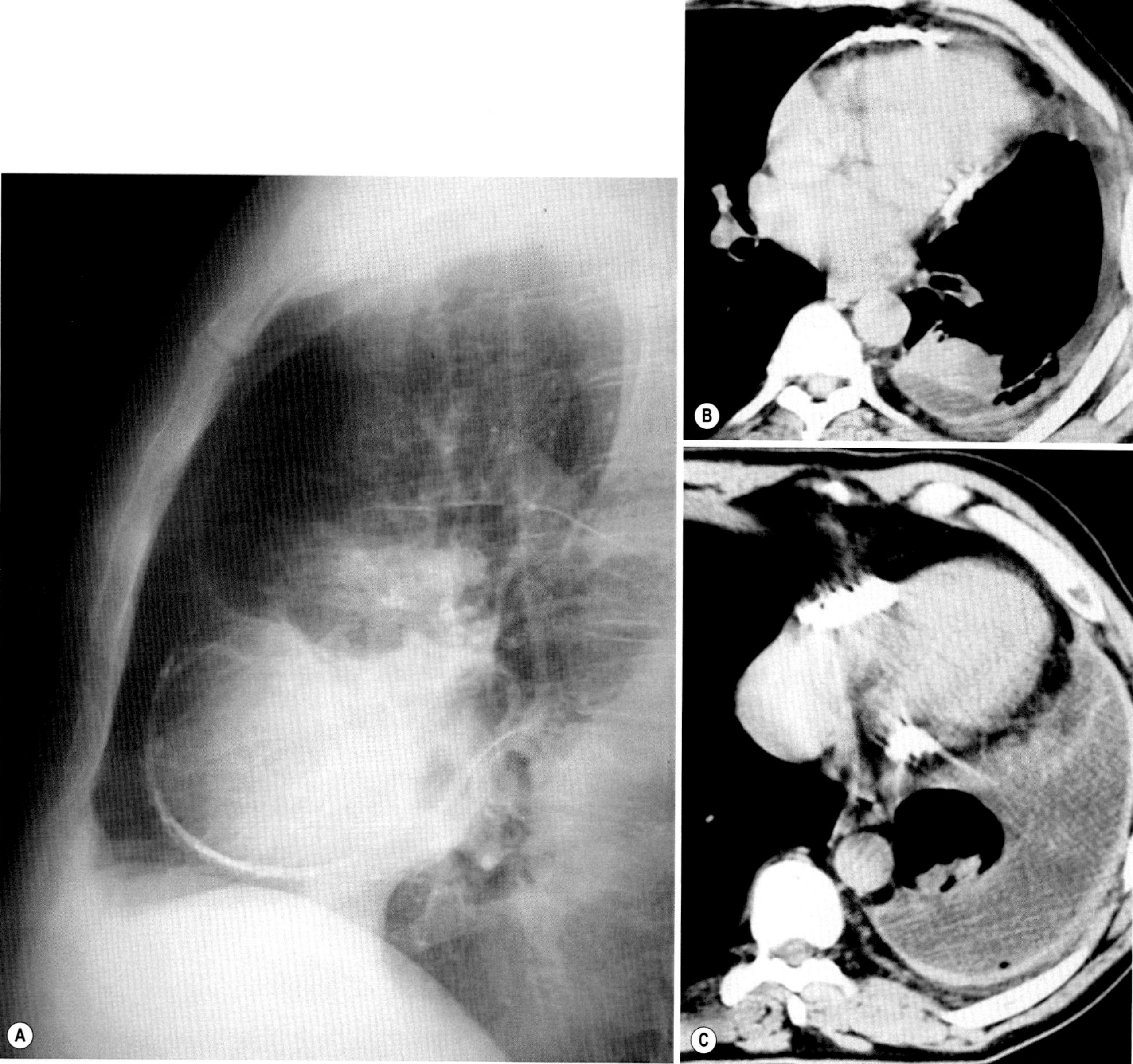

FIGURE 14-86 ■ **Constrictive pericarditis.** (A) Chest X-ray, lateral view, shows thick pericardial calcifications. (B, C) CT images demonstrate the presence, site and thickness of pericardial calcifications in a patient with pleuro-pulmonary tuberculosis.

orthopnoea and fatigue, and occasionally may present with liver enlargement and ascites. The inextensible pericardium determines the equalisation of the telediastolic pressure in the cardiac chambers with inversion of the interventricular septum convexity highly dependent on the respiratory acts. Constrictive pericarditis can be idiopathic; more frequently it is a consequence of cardiac surgery and radiation therapy. Other causes include subclinical acute viral infections, connective tissue disease, uraemia and neoplasm.[115] A tubercular aetiology is rare nowadays. As symptoms are non-specific, it is necessary to exclude the other causes of impaired ventricular filling (pulmonary hypertension, myocardial infarction, restrictive cardiomyopathy). It is important to identify pericardial constriction as the cause of the impaired ventricular filling as these patients may benefit from pericardectomy, while medical therapy is more appropriate in the restrictive forms. This differentiation is particularly important in radiotherapy patients.

On CXR, the heart, in particular the left atrium, may be enlarged with dilatation of the SVC and of the azygos vein, so that the right and left cardiac borders appear straightened.[118] Pericardial calcification is seen in 40–50% of the patients as plaque-like or linear calcified densities along the cardiac surface and in the atrioventricular grooves (Fig. 14-86). The main echocardiographic findings in constrictive pericarditis are pericardial thickening, abnormal motion of the interventricular septum, diastolic flattening of the LV posterior wall, dilated inferior vena cava with reduced inspiratory collapse, and increased

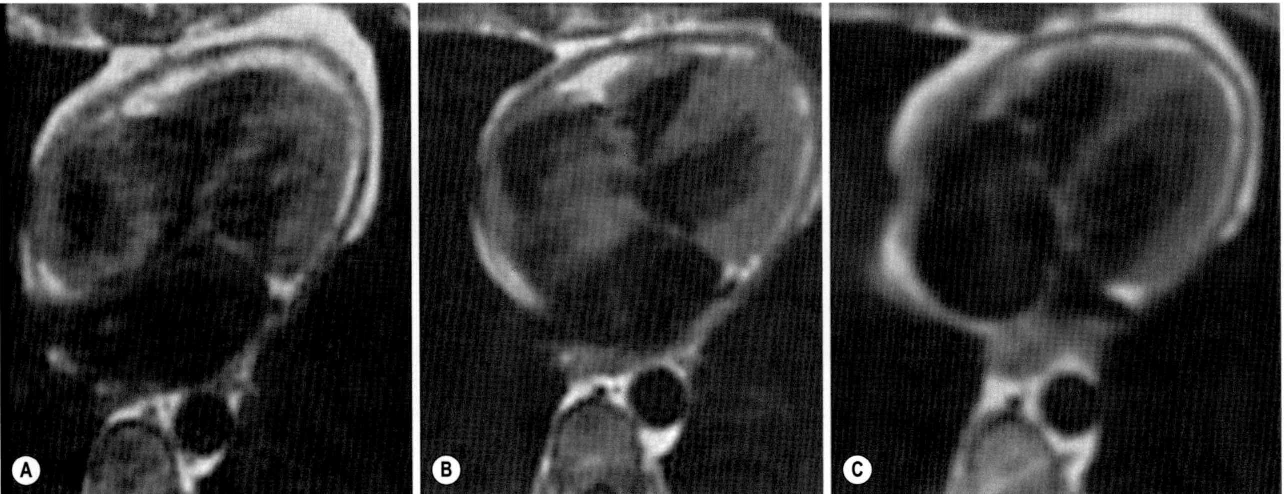

FIGURE 14-87 ■ **Constrictive pericarditis.** Axial craniocaudal T1w images show a marked and diffuse pericardial thickening in patient with previous tuberculosis. Right atrial enlargement is evident in the images B and C.

respiratory variation of mitral and tricuspid blood flow. Constriction allows early diastolic filling, but with abrupt termination in mid-diastole. Echocardiography may erroneously estimate pericardial thickness; moreover, some regions of the pericardium may not be easily accessible. A transoesophageal approach, although limited by a narrow field of view and being relatively invasive, allows better visualisation of the pericardium. Respiration-correlated Doppler techniques are particularly useful.[115]

CT and MRI can aid the diagnosis of constrictive pericarditis. Pericardial constriction appears as a more or less diffuse thickening of the pericardium that may present irregular margins; it is more often localised along the free right ventricular wall and the atrioventricular junction. A pericardial thickening >4 mm is suggestive of pericardial constriction in those patients with corresponding clinical findings, whereas a thickness >5–6 mm is highly specific for constrictive pericarditis. However, pericardial constriction can be present even in patients with normal pericardial thickness. MRI has been shown to be better than CT at differentiating between pericardial fluid and thickened pericardium, although CT shows any calcification better. MR imaging has a reported accuracy of 93% for differentiating between constrictive pericarditis and restrictive cardiomyopathy on the basis of depiction of thickened pericardium (≥4 mm).[115]

Cardiac constriction symptoms depend mainly on the site of the lesions. Focal lesions of the pericardial leaflets at the level of the atrioventricular junction or at the basal level of both ventricles can impair significantly ventricular filling. The haemodynamic impact is therefore related not only to the morphological characteristics of the increased thickness but also mainly to the reduced compliance and the site of the lesion. Pericardial constriction may be occult under normal conditions, as some patients develop symptoms only after a sudden water imbalance. In other cases myocardial constriction is related to the presence of pericardial effusion.

CT, unlike MRI, is very sensitive in demonstrating calcification of the pericardium (Fig. 14-86). At MRI, fibrous or calcific pericardium is hypointense on T1w, T2w (Fig. 14-87) and cine sequences. During the advanced phases of the disease pericardial leaflets don't usually show enhancement. Enhancement of the pericardium on post-contrast CT and MRI should eventually be related to a residual inflammation. The altered filling pattern causes a particular tubular morphology of the ventricles (more often of the right ventricle) and consequent atrial dilatation that can be seen at both CT and MR imaging. They can show at the same time the dilatation of the inferior vena cava and of the hepatic veins as well as the presence of pleural effusion and ascites. Cine-MRI can help to assess pericardial rigidity during the cardiac cycle and to document the reduced expansibility of the ventricles during the diastolic filling.[127] MR dynamic studies may allow differentiation of a normal pericardium from a rigid, sclerotic one: normal pericardium moves in synchrony with myocardium during a cardiac cycle; this characteristic is lost when the pericardium is thickened.

In pericardial constriction the heart is isolated from the normal respiratory changes in intrathoracic pressure. Reduced pericardial compliance accentuates coupling between the ventricles; that is, each ventricle directly influences the volume and pressure in the other ventricle. Cardiac filling pressures are increased with pressure equalisation in all four cardiac chambers. In constrictive pericarditis, septal flattening or inversion is evident on early diastolic ventricular filling, and serpentine septal motion can be seen on cardiac long-axis view. Because of the respiratory-related variation in cardiac filling (enhanced RV filling on inspiration, enhanced LV filling on expiration), this paradoxical movement is most pronounced at onset of inspiration. Assessment of these effects is usually performed by echocardiography and cardiac catheterisation.

CMR, with the exception of intracardiac pressure measurements, may provide valuable information too, and has the intrinsic advantage that findings may be directly linked to morphological abnormalities.

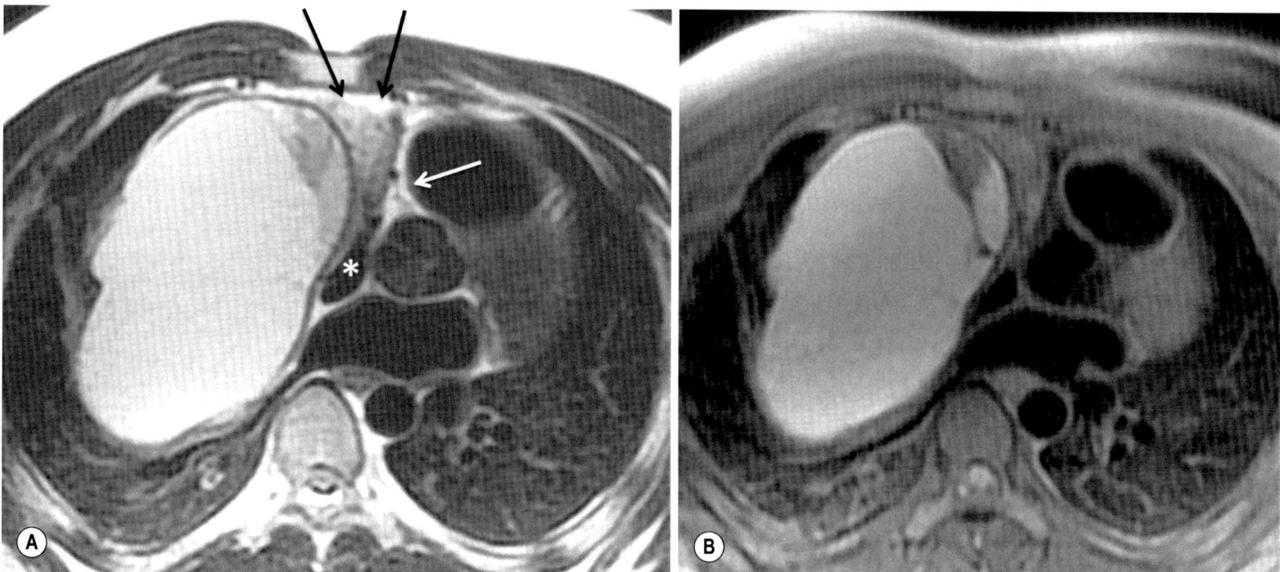

FIGURE 14-88 ■ **Cystic teratoma of the pericardium, with right atrium involvement.** (A) T2w axial image shows a large right paracardiac cystic tumour with eccentric solid component; extracapsular tissue (black arrows) invades also epicardial fat and abuts superior vena cava (*), contacting the right coronary artery (white arrow). (B) Post-contrast T1w corresponding axial image demonstrates enhancement of the solid components of the tumour.

Ventricular dimensions and the systolic dynamics can be used to differentiate constrictive pericarditis from restrictive myocarditis: in particular, in restrictive cardiomyopathy patients, septal paradoxical movement is absent and ventricular dimensions may be normal.

Pericardial Masses

Primary tumours of the pericardium are rare while pericardial metastases can be found in 22% of the postmortems of patients who died from metastatic disease. The most common primary malignant tumours of the pericardium are mesothelioma, sarcomas (fibrosarcoma, angiosarcoma, liposarcoma) and malignant teratoma (Fig. 14-88). Benign tumours are lipoma[128] and teratoma.[129] Tumours that more frequently give pericardial metastases are lung or breast carcinoma, leukaemia and lymphoma. Metastatic pericardial implants are often small and difficult to identify; they cause a large effusion that is often haemorrhagic and disproportionate in size to the tumour itself. The appearance of pericardial haematoma depends on the age of the collection.

Invasion by contiguity from mediastinal masses can be identified by a focal disruption of the pericardial line and the presence of pericardial effusion; MRI and CT can define the tumour implantation site and margins, as it is surrounded by the contiguous adipose tissue and effusion (Fig. 14-61). Tissue characterisation of pericardial tumours is not always possible and biopsy is necessary for a definitive diagnosis. Because of its adipose nature, lipoma has low CT density and high MR T1 and T2 signal intensity; metastatic melanoma may have high signal intensity on T1w images because of the paramagnetic effect of melanin. Calcium or fat in a pericardial mass suggests teratoma. Fibroma has low signal intensity on T2w images re-phrase needed. Mesothelioma of the pericardium may manifest as pericardial effusion, occasionally accompanied by pericardial nodules or plaques. Pleural mesothelioma may also invade the pericardium directly. Lymphoma, sarcoma and liposarcoma typically appear as large heterogeneous masses frequently associated with serohaematic pericardial effusion.[115]

REFERENCES

1. Maron BJ, Towbin JA, Thiene G, et al. Contemporary definitions and classification of the cardiomyopathies: an American Heart Association scientific statement from the Council on Clinical Cardiology, Heart Failure and Transplantation Committee; Quality of Care and Outcomes Research and Functional Genomics and Translational Biology Interdisciplinary Working Groups; and Council on Epidemiology and Prevention. Circulation 2006; 113:1807–16.
2. Elliott P, Andersson B, Arbustini E, et al. Classification of the cardiomyopathies: a position statement from the European Society of Cardiology Working Group on Myocardial and Pericardial Diseases. Eur Heart J 2008;29:270–6.
3. Maron BJ. Asymmetry in hypertrophic cardiomyopathy: the septal to free wall ratio revisited. Am J Cardiol 1985;55:835.
4. Chun EJ, Choi SI, Jin KN, et al. Hypertrophic cardiomyopathy: assessment with MR imaging and multidetector CT. Radiographics 2010;30:1309–28.
5. Prasad K, Atherton J, Smiyh CG, et al. Echocardiographic pitfalls in the diagnosis of hypertrophic cardiomyopathy. Heart 1999; 82(suppl.3):III8–15.
6. Williams TJ, Manghat NE, McKay-Ferguson A, et al. Cardiomyopathy: appearances on ECG-gated 64-detector row computed tomography. Clin Cardiol 2008;63:464–74.
7. Moon JC, Reed E, Sheppard MN, et al. The histological basis of late gadolinium enhancement cardiovascular magnetic resonance in hypertrophic cardiomyopathy. J Am Coll Cardiol 2004;43: 2260–4.
8. Mahrholdt H, Wagner A, Judd RM, et al. Delayed enhancement cardiovascular magnetic resonance assessment of non-ischemic cardiomyopathies. Eur Heart J 2005;26:1461–74.
9. Moon JC, McKenna WJ, McCrohon JA, et al. Toward clinical risk assessment in hypertrophic cardiomyopathy with gadolinium cardiovascular assessment. J Am Coll Cardiol 2003;41: 1561–7.

10. Kwon DH, Smedira NG, Rodriguez ER, et al. Cardiac magnetic resonance detection of myocardial scarring in hypertrophic cardiomyopathy: correlation with histopathology and prevalence of ventricular tachycardia. J Am Coll Cardiol 2009;54:242–9.
11. Spirito P, Bellone P, Harris KM, et al. Magnitude of left ventricular hypertrophy and risk of sudden death in hypertrophic cardiomyopathy. N Engl J Med 2000;342:1778–85.
12. Sipola P, Lauerna K, Husso-Saastamoinen M, et al. First-pass MR imaging in the assessment of perfusion impairment in patients with hypertrophic cardiomyopathy and the Asp175Asn mutation of the alpha-tropomyosin gene. Radiology 2003;226: 129–37.
13. Moon JC, Sachdev B, Elkington AG. Gadolinium enhanced cardiovascular magnetic resonance in Anderson-Fabry disease. Evidence for a disease specific abnormality of the myocardial interstitium. Eur Heart J 2003;24:2151–5.
14. Maceira AM, Joshi J, Prasad SK. CMR in amyloidosis. Circulation 2005;111:186–93.
15. Vignaux O, Dhote R, Duboc D. Detection of myocardial involvement in patients with sarcoidosis applying T2-weighted, contrast enhanced, and cine magnetic resonance imaging: initial results of a prospective study. J Comput Assist Tomogr 2002;26:762–7.
16. Patel MR, Cawely PJ, Heitner JF. Improved diagnostic sensitivity of contrast enhanced cardiac MRI for cardiac sarcoidosis. (Abstract). Circulation 2004;108(Suppl.):645.
17. Thomas DE, Wheeler R, Yousef ZR, et al. The role of echocardiography in guiding management in dilated cardiomyopathy. Eur J Echocardiogr 2009;10:iii15–21.
18. Harjai KJ, Edupuganti R, Nunez E. Does left ventricular shape influence clinical outcome in heart failure? Clin Cardiol 2000; 23:813–19.
19. Hundley WG, Bluemke DA, Finn JP, et al. ACCF/ACR/AHA/NASCI/SCMR 2010 Expert Consensus Document on Cardiovascular Magnetic Resonance. A Report of the American College of Cardiology Foundation Task Force on Expert Consensus Documents. Circulation 2010;121:2462–508.
20. McCrohon JA, Moon JC, Prasad SK, et al. Differentiation of heart failure related to dilated cardiomyopathy and coronary artery disease using gadolinium-enhanced cardiovascular magnetic resonance. Circulation 2003;108(1):54–9.
21. Verdas PE, Auricchio A, Blanc JJ, et al. Guidelines for cardiac pacing and cardiac resynchronization therapy. The Task Force for Cardiac Pacing and Cardiac Resynchronization Therapy of the European Society of Cardiology. Developed in collaboration with the European Heart Rhythm Association. Europace 2007;9: 959–98.
22. Bleeker GB, Kaandorp TA, Lamb HJ, et al. Effect of posterolateral scar tissue on clinical and echocardiographic improvement after cardiac resynchronization therapy. Circulation 2006;113: 969–76.
23. Srichai MB, Junor C, Rodriguez LL, et al. Clinical, imaging, and pathological characteristics of left ventricular thrombus: a comparison of contrast-enhanced magnetic resonance imaging, transthoracic echocardiography, and transesophageal echocardiography with surgical or pathological validation. Am Heart J 2006;152: 75–84.
24. Assomull RG, Prasad SK, Lyne J, et al. Cardiovascular magnetic resonance, fibrosis and prognosis in dilated cardiomyopathy. J Am Coll Cardiol 2006;48(10):1977–85.
25. Taylor AJ, Cerqueira M, Hodgson JM, et al. ACCF/SCCT/ACR/AHA/ASE/ASNC/NASCI/SCAI/SCMR 2010 Appropriate Use Criteria for Cardiac Computed Tomography. A Report of the American College of Cardiology Foundation Appropriate Use Criteria Task Force, the Society of Cardiovascular Computed Tomography, the American College of Radiology, the American Heart Association, the American Society of Echocardiography, the American Society of Nuclear Cardiology, the North American Society for Cardiovascular Imaging, the Society for Cardiovascular Angiography and Interventions, and the Society for Cardiovascular Magnetic Resonance. J Cardiovasc Comput Tomogr 2010;4:407.
26. Appleton CP, Hatle LK, Popp RL. Demonstration of restrictive ventricular physiology by Doppler echocardiography. J Am Coll Cardiol 1988;11:757.
27. Nihoyannopoulos P, Dawson D. Restrictive cardiomyopathies. Eur J Echocardiogr 2009;10:iii23–33.
28. Wang ZJ, Reddy GP, Gotway MP, et al. CT and MR imaging of the pericardium. Radiographics 2003;23:S167–180.
29. Anderson LJ, Holden S, Davies B, et al. Cardiovascular T2-star (T2*) magnetic resonance for the early diagnosis of myocardial iron overload. Eur Heart J 2001;22:2171–9.
30. Ramazzotti A, Pepe A, Positano V, et al. Multicenter validation of the magnetic resonance T2* technique for segmental and global quantification of myocardial iron overload. J Magn Reson Imag 2009;30:62–8.
31. McKenna WJ, Thiene G, Nava A, et al. Diagnosis of arrhythmogenic right ventricular dysplasia/cardiomyopathy. Task Force of the Myocardial and Pericardial Disease Working Group of the European Society of Cardiology and the Scientific Council on Cardiomyopathies of the International Society and Federation of Cardiology. Br Heart J 1994;71:215–18.
32. Marcus FI, McKenna WJ, Sherrill D, et al. Diagnosis of arrhythmogenic right ventricular cardiomyopathy/dysplasia: proposed modification of the Task Force Criteria. Circulation 2010;121: 1533–41.
33. Tandri H, Saranathan M, Rofriguez ER, et al. Non-invasive detection of myocardial fibrosis in arrhythmogenic right ventricular cardiomyopathy wing delayed enhancement magnetic resonance imaging. J Am Coll Cardiol 2005;48:2277–84.
34. Kimura F, Matsuo Y, Nakajima T, et al. Myocardial fat at cardiac imaging: how can we differentiate pathologic from physiologic fatty infiltration? Radiographics 2010;30:1587–602.
35. Jenni R, Oechslin EN, van del Loo B. Isolated ventricular non-compaction of the myocardium in adults. Heart 2007;93: 11–15.
36. Petersen SE, Selvanayagam JB, Wiessmann F, et al. Left ventricular non-compaction. Insights from cardiovascular magnetic resonance imaging. J Am Coll Cardiol 2005;46:101–5.
37. Gianni M, Dentali F, Grandi AM, et al. Apical ballooning syndrome or takotsubo cardiomiopathy: a systematic review. Eur Heart J 2006;27:1523–9.
38. Pilgrim TM, Wyss TR. Takotsubo cardiomyopathy or transient left ventricular apical ballooning syndrome: A systematic review. Int J Cardiol 2008;124:283–92.
39. Lockie T, Nagel E, Redwood S, et al. Use of cardiovascular magnetic resonance imaging in acute coronary syndromes. Circulation 2009;119:1671–81.
40. Eitel I, Behrendt F, Schindler K, et al. Differential diagnosis of suspected apical ballooning syndrome using contrast-enhanced magnetic resonance imaging. Eur Heart J 2008;29:2651–9.
41. Cooper LT, Baughman KL, Feldman AM, et al. The role of endomyocardial biopsy in the management of cardiovascular disease: a scientific statement from the American Heart Association, the American College of Cardiology, and the European Society of Cardiology. Endorsed by the Heart Failure Society of America and the Heart Failure Association of the European Society of Cardiology. J Am Coll Cardiol 2007;50:1914–31.
42. Aretz HT. Myocarditis: the Dallas criteria. Hum Pathol 1987; 18:619–24.
43. Basso C, Calabrese F, Angelini A, et al. Classification and histological, immunohistochemical, and molecular diagnosis of inflammatory myocardial disease. Heart Fail Rev 2012;Oct 25. [Epub ahead of print].
44. Natale L, De Vita A, Baldari C, et al. Correlation between clinical presentation and delayed-enhancement MRI pattern in myocarditis. Radiol Med 2012;117(8):1309–19.
45. Friedrich MG, Sechtem U, Schulz-Menger J, et al. Cardiovascular magnetic resonance in myocarditis: A JACC White Paper. J Am Coll Cardiol 2009;53:1475–87.
46. De Cobelli F, Pieroni M, Esposito A, et al. Delayed gadolinium-enhanced cardiac magnetic resonance in patients with chronic myocarditis presenting with heart failure or recurrent arrhythmias. J Am Coll Cardiol 2006;47:1649–54.
47. Chen I, Otto CM. Longitudinal assessment of valvular heart disease by echocardiography. Curr Opin Cardiol 1998;13: 397–403.
48. Morris MF, Maleszewski JJ, Suri RM, et al. CT and MR imaging of the mitral valve. Radiographics 2010;30:1603–20.
49. Schwitter J. Valvular heart disease: assessment of valve morphology and quantification using MR. Herz 2000;25:342–55.
50. Ghosh N, Al-Shehri H, Chan K, et al. Characterization of mitral valve prolapse with cardiac computed tomography: comparison to

echocardiographic and intraoperative findings. Int J Cardiovasc Imag 2012;28:855–63.
51. Apostolakis EE, Baikoussis NG. Methods of estimation of mitral valve regurgitation for the cardiac surgeon. J Cardiothor Surg 2009;4:34.
52. Kilner PJ, Gatehouse PD, Firmin DN. Flow measurement by magnetic resonance: a unique asset worth optimising. J Cardiovasc Magn Reson 2007;9:723–8.
53. Bonow RO, Carabello BA, Kanu C, et al. ACC/AHA 2006 guidelines for the management of patients with valvular heart disease: a report of the American College of Cardiology/American Heart Association Task Force on Practice Guidelines (writing committee to revise the 1998 Guidelines for the Management of Patients With Valvular Heart Disease): developed in collaboration with the Society of Cardiovascular Anesthesiologists: endorsed by the Society for Cardiovascular Angiography and Interventions and the Society of Thoracic Surgeons. Circulation 2006;114:e84–231.
54. Bonow RO, Carabello BA, Chatterjee K, et al. Focused update incorporated into the ACC/AHA 2006 guidelines for the management of patients with valvular heart disease: a report of the American College of Cardiology/American Heart Association Task Force on Practice Guidelines. Circulation 2008;118:e523–661.
55. Chandrashekhar Y, Westaby S, Narula J. Mitral stenosis. Lancet 2009;374:1271–83.
56. Maganti K, Rigolin VH, Sarano ME, et al. Valvular heart disease: diagnosis and management. Mayo Clinic Proc 2010;85: 483–500.
57. Nishimura RA. Valvular stenosis. In: Murphy JG, Lloyd MA, editors. Mayo Clinic Cardiology Concise Textbook. Mayo Clinic Scientific Press—Informa Healthcare; 2007. pp. 523–34.
58. Myerson SG. Heart valve disease: investigation by cardiovascular magnetic resonance. J Cardiovasc Magn Reson 2012;14:7–23.
59. Lin SJ, Brown PA, Watkins MP, et al. Quantification of stenotic mitral valve area with magnetic resonance imaging and comparison with Doppler ultrasound. J Am Coll Cardiol 2004;44:133–7.
60. Lembcke A, Durmus T, Westermann Y, et al. Assessment of mitral valve stenosis by helical MDCT: comparison with transthoracic Doppler echocardiography and cardiac catheterization. Am J Roentgenol 2011;197:614–22.
61. Mahnken AH, Mühlenbruch G, Das M, et al. MDCT detection of mitral valve calcification: prevalence and clinical relevance compared with echocardiography. Am J Roentgenol 2007;188: 1264–9.
62. Rozenshtein A, Boxt LM. Computed tomography and magnetic resonance imaging of patients with valvular heart disease. J Thorac Imag 2000;15:252–64.
63. Fisher EA, Goldman ME. Simple, rapid method for quantification of tricuspid regurgitationby two-dimensional echocardiography. Am J Cardiol 1989;63:1375–8.
64. Christiansen JP, Karamitsos TD, Myerson SG. Assessment of valvular heart disease by cardiovascular magnetic resonance imaging: a review. Heart Lung Circ 2011;20:73–82.
65. Sommer G, Bremerich J, Lund G. Magnetic resonance imaging in valvular heart disease: Clinical application and current role for patient management. J Magn Reson Imag 2012;35:1241–52.
66. Passik CS, Ackermann DM, Pluth JR, et al. Temporal changes in the causes of aortic stenosis. A pathological study of 646 cases. Mayo Clin Proc 1987;52:119–23.
67. Vogel-Claussen J, Pannu H, Spevak PJ, et al. Cardiac valve assessment with MR imaging and 64-section multi-detector row CT. Radiographics 2006;26:1769–84.
68. Liu F, Coursey CA, Grahame-Clarke C, et al. Aortic valve calcification as an incidental finding at CT of the elderly: severity and location as predictors of aortic stenosis. Am J Roentgenol 2006;186:342–9.
69. Garcia J, Marrufo OR, Rodriguez AO, et al. Cardiovascular magnetic resonance evaluation of aortic stenosis severity using single plane measurement of effective orifice area. J Cardiovasc Magn Reson 2012;14:23.
70. Louie EK, et al. Early diastolic interaction between the aortic regurgitant jet and mitral inflow. A pulsed Doppler study (abstract). J Am Coll Cardiol 1987;9:83A.
71. Tribouilloy CM, Enriquez-Sarano M, Bailey KR, et al. Assessment of severity of aortic regurgitation using the width of the vena contracta: a clinical color Doppler imaging study. Circulation 2000;102:558–64.
72. Teague SM, Sublett KL, Anderson J, et al. Doppler half-time index correlates with the severity of aortic regurgitation. Circulation 1984;70(suppl):394.
73. Zoghbi WA, Enriquez-Sarano M, Foster E, et al. Recommendations for evaluation of the severity of native valvular regurgitation with two-dimensional and Doppler echocardiography. J Am Soc Echocardiogr 2003;16:777–802.
74. Aurigemma G, Reichek N, Schiebler M, et al. Evaluation of aortic regurgitation by cardiac cine magnetic resonance imaging: plane analysis and comparison by Doppler echocardiography. Cardiology 1991;78:340–7.
75. Feuchtner GM. The utility of computed tomography in the context of aortic valve disease. Int J Cardiovasc Imag 2009; 25:611–14.
76. Jassal DS, Shapiro MD, Neilan TG, et al. 64-slice multidetector computed tomography (MDCT) for detection of aortic regurgitation and quantification of severity. Invest Radiol 2007;42: 507–12.
77. Gahide G, Bommart S, Demaria R, et al. Preoperative evaluation in aortic endocarditis: findings on cardiac CT. Am J Roentgenol 2010;194:574–8.
78. Takahashi K, Stanford W. Multidetector CT of the thoracic aorta. Int J Cardiovasc Imag 2005;21:141–53.
79. Kotler MN, Goldman A, Parry WR. Non-invasive evaluation of cardiac valve prosthesis. In: Kotler MN, Steiner RM, editors. Cardiac Imaging: New Technologies and Clinical Applications. Philadelphia: Davis; 1986. pp. 201–41.
80. Steiner RM, Mintz GS, Morse D, et al. The radiology of cardiac valve prostheses. Radiographics 1988;8:277–98.
81. Boxt LM. CT of valvular heart disease. Int J Cardiovasc Imag 2005;21:105–13.
82. Bennett CJ, Maleszewski JJ, Araoz PA. CT and MR imaging of the aortic valve: radiologic-pathologic correlation. Radiographics 2012;32:1399–420.
83. La Manna A, Sanfilippo A, Capodanno D, et al. Cardiovascular magnetic resonance for the assessment of patients undergoing transcatheter aortic valve implantation: a pilot study. J Cardiovasc Magn Reson 2011;13:82.
84. Heimberger TS, Duma RJ. Infections of prosthetic heart valves and cardiac pacemakers. Infect Dis Clin North Am 1989;3: 221–45.
85. Winkler ML, Higgins CB. MRI of perivalvular infections pseudoaneurysms. Am J Roentgenol 1986;7:253–6.
86. Hoey ETD, Mankad K, Puppala S, et al. MRI and CT appearances of cardiac tumours in adults. Clin Radiol 2009;64: 1214–30.
87. Chiles C, Woodard PK, Gutierrez FR, et al. Metastatic involvement of the heart and pericardium: CT and MR imaging. Radiographics 2001;21:439–49.
88. Meduri A, Natale L. Cardiac and mediastinal masses. In: Cademartiri F, Casolo G, Midiri M, editors. Clinical Applications of Cardiac CT. Milan: Springer-Verlag; 2008. pp. 313–24.
89. Rajiah P, Kanne JP, Kalahasti V, et al. Computed tomography of cardiac and pericardial tumors. J Cardiovasc Comp Tomogr 2011;41:16–29.
90. Carney JA, Gordon H, Carpenter PC, et al. The complex of myxomas, spotty pigmentation, and endocrine overactivity. Am J Cardiol 1987;147:527–34.
91. Schvartzman PR, White RD. Imaging of cardiac and paracardiac masses. J Thorac Imag 2000;15:265–73.
92. Grebenc M, Rosado-de-Christenson M, Green C, et al. Cardiac myxoma: imaging features in 83 patients. Radiographics 2002; 22:673–89.
93. Scheffel H, Baumueller S, Stolzmann P, et al. Atrial myxomas and thrombi: comparison of imaging features on CT. Am J Roentgenol 2009;192:639–45.
94. Luna A, Ribes R, Caro P, et al. Evaluation of cardiac tumors with magnetic resonance imaging. Eur Radiol 2005;15:1446–55.
95. Sparrow PJ, Kurian JB, Jones TR, et al. MR imaging of cardiac tumors. Radiographics 2005;25:1255–76.
96. Randhawa K, Ganeshan A, Hoey ETD. Magnetic resonance imaging of cardiac tumors: part 1, sequences, protocols, and benign tumors. Curr Probl Diagn Radiol 2011;40:158–68.
97. Salanitri JC, Pereles FS. Cardiac lipoma and lipomatous hypertrophy of the interatrial septum: cardiac magnetic resonance imaging findings. J Comp Assist Tomogr 2004;28:852–6.

98. Grebenc ML, Rosado de Christenson ML, Burke AP, et al. Primary cardiac and pericardial neoplasms: radiologic-pathologic correlation. Radiographics 2000;20:1073–103.
99. Kondruweit M, Schmid M, Strecker T. Papillary fibroelastoma of the mitral valve: appearance in 64-slice spiral computed tomography, magnetic resonance imaging, and echocardiography. Eur Heart J 2008;115:831.
100. Wintersperger BJ, Becker CR, Gulbins H, et al. Tumors of the cardiac valves: imaging findings in magnetic resonance imaging, electron beam computed tomography, and echocardiography. Eur Radiol 2000;10:443–9.
101. Kelle S, Chiribiri A, Meyer R, et al. Images in cardiovascular medicine. Papillary fibroelastoma of the tricuspid valve seen on magnetic resonance imaging. Circulation 2006;117:e190–1.
102. Syed IS, Feng D, Harris SR, et al. MR imaging of cardiac masses. Magn Reson Imag Clin North Am 2008;16:137–64.
103. O'Sullivan PJ, Gladish GW. Cardiac tumors. Semin Roentgenol 2008;43:223–33.
104. Hoffmann U, Globits S, Schima W, et al. Usefulness of magnetic resonance imaging of cardiac and paracardiac masses. Am J Cardiol 2003;92:890–5.
105. Randhawa K, Ganeshan A, Hoey ETD. Magnetic resonance imaging of cardiac tumors: part 2, malignant tumors and tumor-like conditions. Curr Probl Diagn Radiol 2011;40:169–79.
106. Di Bella G, Gaeta M, Patanè L, et al. Tissue characterization of a primary cardiac angiosarcoma using magnetic resonance imaging. Rev Esp Cardiol 2010;63:1382–3.
107. Deetjen AG, Conradi G, Möllmann S, et al. Cardiac angiosarcoma diagnosed and characterized by cardiac magnetic resonance imaging. Cardiol Rev 2012;14:101–3.
108. Shin MS, Kirklin JK, Cain JB, et al. Primary angiosarcoma of the heart: CT characteristics. Am J Roentgenol 1987;148:267–8.
109. Araoz PA, Mulvagh SL, Tazelaar HD, et al. CT and MR imaging of benign primary cardiac neoplasms with echocardiographic correlation. Radiographics 2000;20:1303–19.
110. Kubo S, Tadamura E, Yamamuro M, et al. Primary cardiac lymphoma demonstrated by delayed contrast-enhanced magnetic resonance imaging. J Comput Assist Tomogr 2004;28:849–51.
111. de Lucas EM, Pagola MA, Fernández F, et al. Primary cardiac lymphoma: helical CT findings and radiopathologic correlation. Cardiovasc Interv Radiol 2004;27:190–1.
112. Rajiah P, Kanne JP. Computed tomography of the pericardium and pericardial disease. J Cardiovasc Comput Tomogr 2010;4(1): 3–18.
113. Francone M, Calabrese FA, Iacucci I, Mangia M. Malattie del pericardio. In: De Cobelli F, Natale L, editors. Risonanza magnetica cardiaca. Milan: Springer Verlag Italia; 2010. pp. 165–76.
114. Bogaert J, Centonze M, Vanneste R, Francone M. Cardiac and pericardial abnormalities on chest computed tomography: what can we see? Radiol Med 2010;115:175–90.
115. Rienmüller R, Gröll R, Lipton MJ. CT and MR imaging of pericardial disease. Radiographics 2004;42:587–601.
116. O'Leary SM, Williams PL, Williams MP, et al. Imaging the pericardium: appearances on ECG-gated 64-detector row cardiac computed tomography. Br J Radiol 2010;83:194–205.
117. Schweigert M, Dubecz A, Beron M. The tale of spring water cysts. Texas Heart Inst J 2012;39(3):330–4.
118. Rozenshtein A, Boxt LM. Plain-film diagnosis of pericardial disease. Semin Roentgenol 1999;34:195–204.
119. Ratib O, Perloff JK, Williams WG. Congenital complete absence of the pericardium. Circulation 2001;103:3154–5.
120. Guler A, Sahin MA, Kadan M, et al. Incidental diagnosis of asymptomatic pericardial diverticulum. Texas Heart Inst J 2011; 38:206–7.
121. Peebles CR, Shambrook JS, Harden SP. Pericardial disease—anatomy and function. Br J Radiol 2011;84:S324–337.
122. Bogaert J, Francone M. Cardiovascular magnetic resonance in pericardial diseases. J Cardiovasc Magn Reson 2009;11:14.
123. Adelmann G, Goldstein SA, Weissman NJ. Pericardial disease. In: Weissman N J, Adelmann G A, editors. Cardiac Imaging Secrets. Philadelphia: Hanley & Belfus; 2004. pp. 260–7.
124. Francone M, Dymarkowsky S, Kalantzi M, Bogaert J. Magnetic resonance imaging in the evaluation of the pericardium. A pictorial essay. Radiol Med 2005;109:64–76.
125. Oh KY, Shimizu M, Edwards WD, et al. Surgical pathology of the parietal pericardium: a study of 344 cases (1993–1999). Cardiovascular Pathol 2001;10:157–68.
126. Kovanlikaya A, Burke LP, Nelson MD, Wood J. Characterizing chronic pericarditis using steady-state free-precession cine MR imaging. Am J Roentgenol 2002;179:475–6.
127. Smith W, Beacock D, Goddard A, et al. Magnetic resonance evaluation of the pericardium. Br J Radiol 2001;74:384–92.
128. Puvaneswary M, Edwards JR, Bastian BC, Khatri SK. Pericardial lipoma: ultrasound, computed tomography and magnetic resonance imaging findings. Australas Radiol 2000;44:321–4.
129. Choi YW, Jang IIS, Jeon SC, et al. Pericardium: anatomy and spectrum of disease on computed tomography. Curr Probl Diagn Radiol 2002;31:198–209.

CHAPTER 15

Ischaemic Heart Disease

Jan Bogaert

CHAPTER OUTLINE

INTRODUCTION

Ischaemic heart disease (IHD), the leading cause of morbidity and mortality in developed countries, poses an enormous financial burden on our society. Although the mortality associated with IHD has declined, due to therapeutic improvements and to prevention campaigns reducing the incidence of fatal and non-fatal myocardial infarction, the prevalence of IHD will continue to increase. Worldwide, it is estimated IHD will become the number one cause of death at the end of this decade. Survivors of a first myocardial infarction are thought to be at increased risk of death from IHD at later ages due to heart failure and late cardiac complications. Other contributing factors are an increasing prevalence of type II diabetes, physical inactivity and obesity. In times of constrained financial budgets, the increasing prevalence of IHD will urge for rational use of diagnostic and therapeutic means. Thus rational, evidence-based use of diagnostic and therapeutic means is needed to provide affordable medicine in the coming years. Cardiac computed tomography (CCT) and cardiovascular magnetic resonance (CMR) have emerged in the past decade as important players in imaging of IHD and in preclinical detection of coronary artery disease (CAD), and are appealing to practioners in the assessment of patient prognosis.[1–3] The aim of this chapter is to discuss how imaging techniques, with an emphasis on CCT and CMR, can be used to study the highly complex and heterogeneous disease entity of IHD (Table 15-1).

PATHOPHYSIOLOGY OF ISCHAEMIC HEART DISEASE

Coronary artery disease (CAD), i.e. the process of atherosclerotic plaque formation, is the usual cause of IHD. Symptoms of myocardial ischaemia occur when the coronary blood flow is significantly impaired. This may happen when the coronary artery lumen is slowly and progressively impinged by an evolving atherosclerotic plaque (*chronic stable plaque*), or when a coronary artery plaque ruptures (or less frequently plaque erosion) and a thrombus is formed with a sudden occlusion of the lumen causing an *acute coronary syndrome* (Fig. 15-1).

An acute coronary occlusion triggers in the myocardial perfusion territory distal to the occlusion, i.e. *the jeopardised myocardium* or *myocardium at risk*, an ischaemic cascade starting with metabolic disturbances followed by regional dysfunction, ECG changes and finally onset of anginal symptoms (Fig. 15-2). Systolic contraction typically ceases within seconds after coronary occlusion. After approximately 20–30 min of sustained ischaemia, irreversible myocardial damage (i.e. *myocardial infarction*) occurs with myocardial cell swelling, apoptosis, ultimately leading to myocyte necrosis. Cellular necrosis always initiates at the endocardial side of the myocardium with the lateral boundaries of infarction closely corresponding to the myocardium at risk, and follows a transmural wave front progression, taking 3 to 6 hours to reach the subepicardium[4] (Fig. 15-3). The amount of necrosis is mainly determined by extent of myocardium

TABLE 15-1 **Contribution of Imaging Techniques for Studying IHD Patients**

	CMR	Cardiac Ultrasound	CCT	Nuclear Medicine	Cardiac Catheterisation
Coronary Arteries					
Anatomy	++	+	++(+)	0	++(+)
Patency	+	–	+(+)	0	+++
Calcifications	–	–	+++	0	+
Wall imaging and characterisation	+	0 (+++)[a]	+(+)	0	0
Flow and flow reserve	–	–	–	0	++(+)
Microvascular dysfunction	++	0	?	+(+)	0
Cardiac Function					
Systolic function					
Global	+++	++	++	++(+)	++
Regional	+++	++	+(+)	++	++
Stress imaging	+++	++	?	++	?
Diastolic function	++	+++	0	?	–
Myocardial strain	++	++[b]	0	0	0
Myocardial Perfusion	++(+)	+(+)	+	++(+)	–
Ischaemic Myocardial Damage					
Myocardial ischaemia	++(+)	++	0	++(+)	+
Myocardial edema	+++	–	–	–	–
Myocardial stunning	++	++	0	++	+
Myocardial infarction	+++	+	+	++	+
Myocardial viability	++(+)	++	0	++(+)	+
Myocardial Metabolism	0 (++)[c]	0	0	++	0
IHD-Related Complications					
Valve regurgitation	++(+)	++(+)	–	0	++
Thrombus formation	+++	++	+++	0	+
Aneurysm formation	+++	++	+++	–	+++
Pericardial effusion	+++	++	+++	–	+
Pericardial inflammation	+++	+	++	–	0

+++, Excellent; ++, good; +, average; –, poor; 0, not possible; ?, unknown.
[a]Intravascular ultrasound.
[b]Tissue Doppler imaging.
[c]MR spectroscopy.

at risk and degree of transmural progression. Current therapeutic strategies aim to timely restore coronary flow by percutaneous coronary intervention (PCI) or thrombolysis. This will stop the transmural progression of necrosis, and salvages the ischaemic, but still viable, myocardium. However, despite the beneficial effects of reperfusion, the process of cell death may continue during the first hours of reperfusion, a phenomenon called *myocardial reperfusion injury*.[5] This occurs in the infarct core and is characterised by a lack of reperfusion at myocardial capillary level (i.e. *microvascular obstruction* or *no-reflow phenomenon*) despite an effective recanalisation of the infarct-related artery.

Myocardial infarctions are usually classified by (a) location (anterior, inferior, lateral), (b) size (focal necrosis, small (<10%), moderate (10–30%) and large (>30% of LV myocardium) and (c) temporally as evolving (<6 h), acute (6 h–7 days), healing (7–28 days) and healed (>28 days).[6] Though myocardial infarctions usually affect the left ventricle, extension toward the right ventricle may occur. Isolated right ventricular infarctions, conversely, are seldom. In the days, weeks and months following the acute event, the heart undergoes a remodelling with changes in ventricular size, shape and function with changes not limited to the infarcted myocardium but involving the remote myocardium as well. In an early phase, tissue oedema, haemorrhage and acute inflammation lead to an expansion of the infarct size.[4] Eventually this may result in an early ventricular rupture or may rapidly evolve toward an aneurysm. During infarct healing an opposite phenomenon occurs, with a progressive replacement of the necrotic myocardium by a collagen-rich fibrous scar causing a thinning of the affected myocardial wall.[4] Depending on the extent of the infarct, part of the ventricle loses contractile force, and as compensatory mechanism usually the ventricle dilates to maintain stroke volume. This, however, is a potentially adverse event, because it may trigger the evolution towards a dilated ischaemic cardiomyopathy and ultimately ischaemic heart failure.

If the duration of coronary occlusion is brief (<15 min), no myocardial infarction occurs but recovery of the myocardial dysfunction is typically delayed and is closely related to the length of ischaemia, a condition known as *stunned myocardium*.[7] This is typically encountered in patients with stable or unstable angina, and coronary vasospasm. When a milder degree of ischaemia persists for a longer time, myocytes become chronically dysfunctional by downregulation of energy consumption through a lower level of aerobic and/or anaerobic metabolism. If perfusion is restored to these dysfunctional areas, function may return to normal, although the recovery

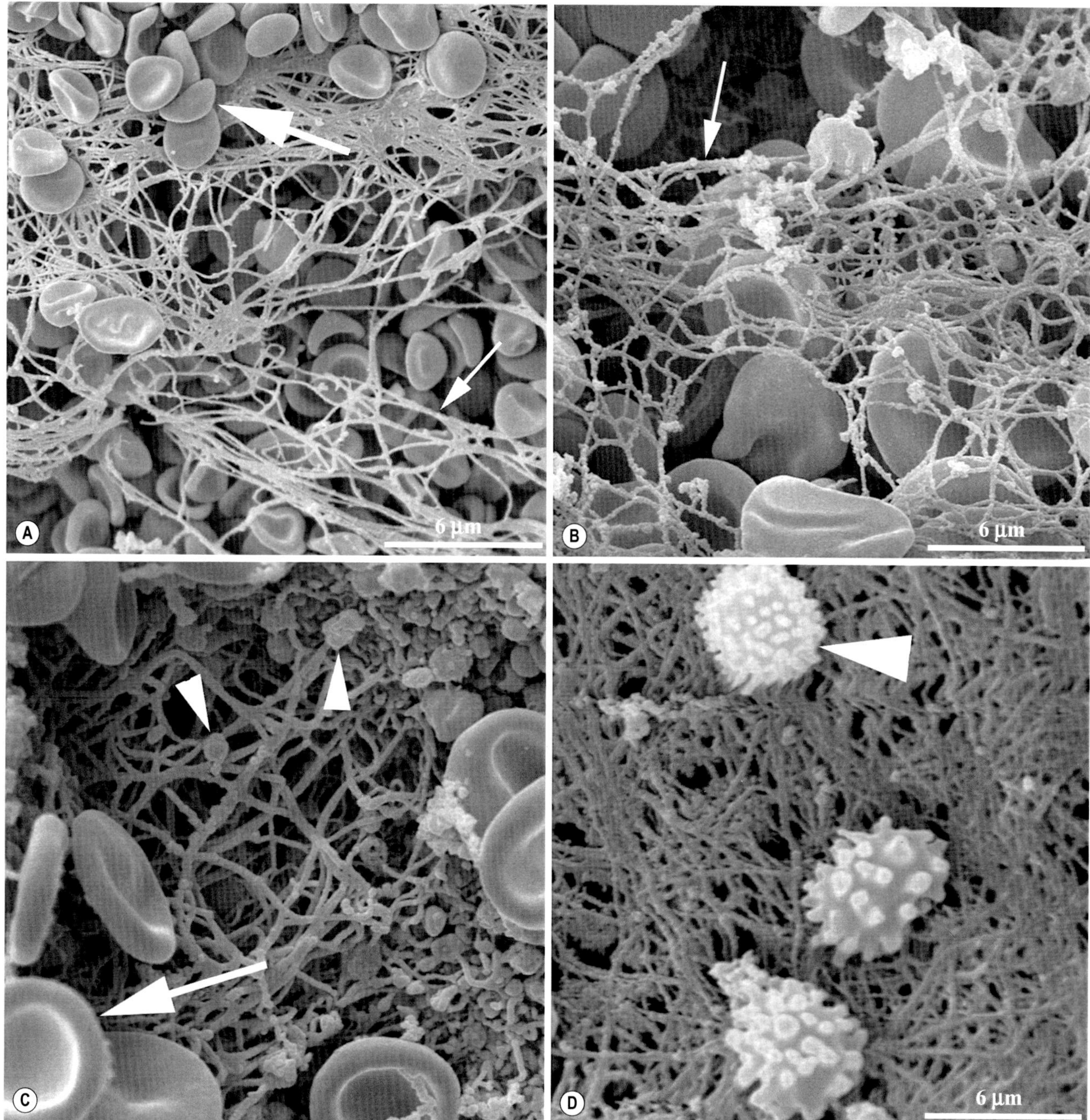

FIGURE 15-1 ■ **Electron microscopy of a fresh thrombus extracted from four different patients with an acute myocardial infarction (3000× magnification).** Presence of red blood cells (big arrow) and platelets (small arrowhead) entrapped in the fibrin clot (small arrow) and a variable amount of white bloods (big arrowhead). (Courtesy Dr J Zalewski, Cracow, Poland.)

is typically slow, taking up to more than one year in severe forms.[8,9] This condition, known as *hibernating myocardium*,[10] should be differentiated from chronic myocardial dysfunction caused by irreversibly damaged myocardium. Patients typically present with moderate to severely reduced ventricular function, presence of several stenotic lesions on their coronary angiogram and symptoms of heart failure. Because of the cost of revascularisation procedure and the inherent risk related to these interventions, in particular when performed in patients with poor cardiac function, it is crucial to determine preoperatively the benefit of a revascularisation procedure.[11] It should be emphasised IHD patients may present with a mixture of different ischaemic substrates (ischaemic, stunned, hibernating, necrotic/scarred myocardium) urging for accurate myocardial tissue characterisation in order to choose the best therapeutic option.

CORONARY ARTERY IMAGING

The process of atherosclerotic plaque formation usually involves the epicardial part of the coronary artery system. The diagnosis of CAD is made on conventional coronary

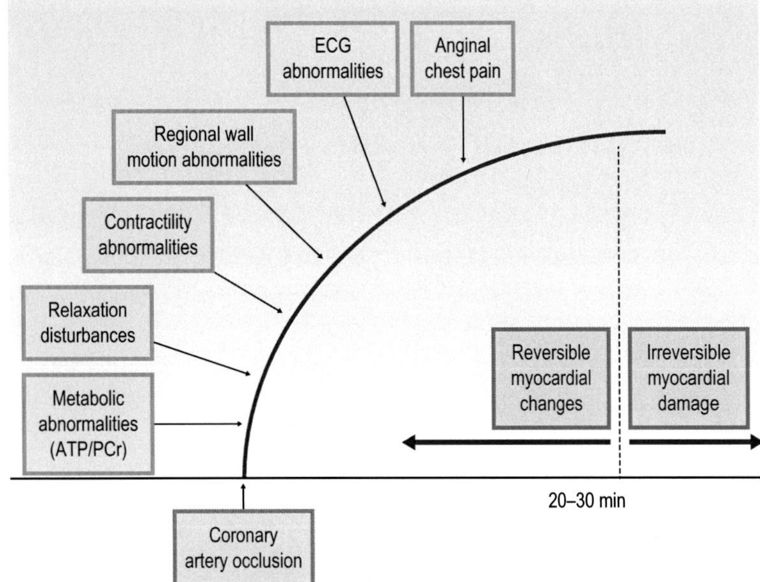

FIGURE 15-2 The ischaemic cascade. Series of events occurring in the ischaemic myocardium following a coronary artery occlusion. While changes are initially reversible, after 20–30 min irreversible myocardial damage occurs.

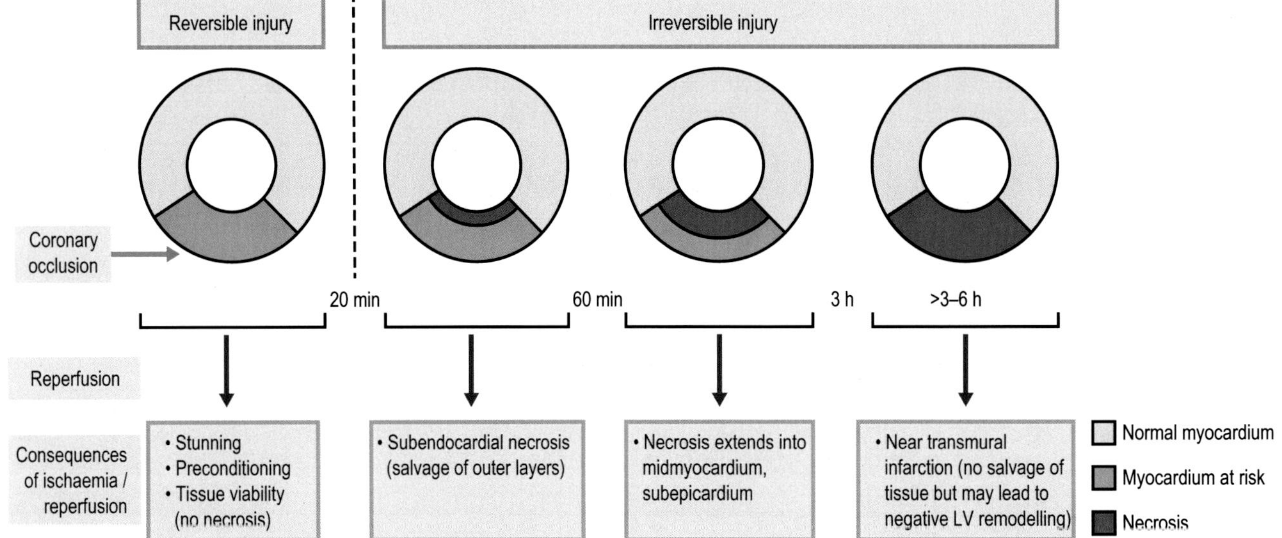

FIGURE 15-3 Effects of ischaemia and reperfusion on myocardial tissue viability and necrosis. Studies in anesthetised canine model of proximal coronary artery occlusion. (Based on Kloner RA, Jennings RB 2001 Consequences of brief ischemia: stunning, preconditioning and their clinical implications. Circulation 104: 2981–2989.)

angiography by impingement and narrowing of the coronary artery. Significant CAD is considered in the presence of a diameter stenosis of ≥ 70% in a major vessel or ≥ 50% in the left main, and usually results in referral for intervention. Though coronary angiography provides valuable information regarding the severity and length of stenosis, CA occlusions, number of vessels affected, stenosis configuration (smooth, ulcerated), presence of thrombus, collateral vessels, CA anatomy and variants, this technique faces several limitations. Mild or non-stenotic CAD is not visualised and no information is provided regarding the plaque composition, or degree of vascular remodelling. Thus, a normal coronary angiogram does not exclude CAD, and a stenotic plaque may be just the tip of the iceberg in some CAD patients. It should be emphasised that in the majority of patients presenting with an acute myocardial infarction the event is caused by rupture of a non- or minimally stenotic plaque. Because of its invasive nature, the need to administrate iodinated contrast agent and radiation issues, use of conventional coronary angiography should be limited to symptomatic patients with high pre-test likelihood of obstructive CAD. Finally, the relationship between myocardial ischaemia and CAD is complex, and many patients fulfilling the criteria of significant CAD turn out not to have a flow-limiting stenosis when measuring the fractional flow reserve (FFR, the ratio of maximum blood flow distal to a stenotic lesion to normal maximal flow in the same vessel). While treatment should be reserved for patients with myocardial ischaemia, the oculostenotic reflex yields the risk of overuse of revascularisation.[12] Oculostenotic reflex refers to the tendency to overestimate the functional importance of intermediate coronary artery lesions. Other issues such as collateral vessels and number and length of plaques should be considered in the decision-making. In a minority of patients presenting with typical anginal chest pain and ST-segment depression on exercise testing, no abnormalities are found on conventional coronary angiography. In these patients diffuse subendocardial perfusion defects have been reported on stress perfusion imaging, suggesting that microvascular dysfunction ('syndrome X') is the cause of myocardial ischaemia and anginal chest pain.

Thanks to technological advances in the field of CCT and CMR, non-invasive coronary angiography has become a reality and these novel techniques get integrated into daily clinical care.[13] Current state-of-the-art multidetector CT (at least 64 or more slices) affords coronary artery imaging with sufficient spatial and temporal resolution for clinical use. A typical clinical examination consists of an unenhanced CCT for detection and quantification of coronary calcium, and a contrast-enhanced CCT for coronary artery imaging, detection of coronary artery plaques and, to some extent, characterisation of the non-calcified plaques (Figs. 15-4 and 15-5). Patients are optimally suited if they have a regular heart

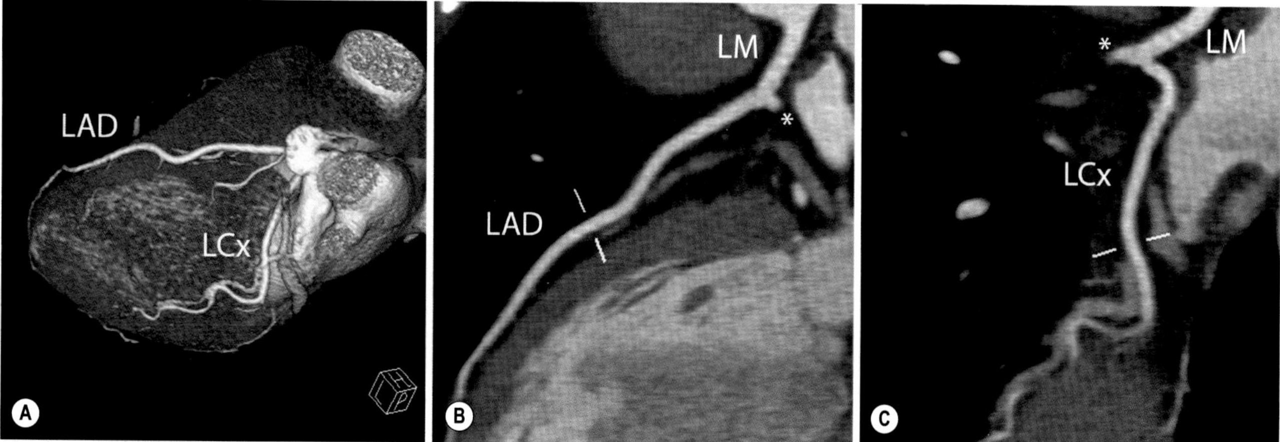

FIGURE 15-4 ■ **Cardiac computed tomography of the left coronary artery: normal findings.** Volume-rendered view (A), curved reformatted view (B, C). Abbreviations: LAD, left anterior descending coronary artery; LCx, left circumflex coronary artery; LM, left main coronary artery.

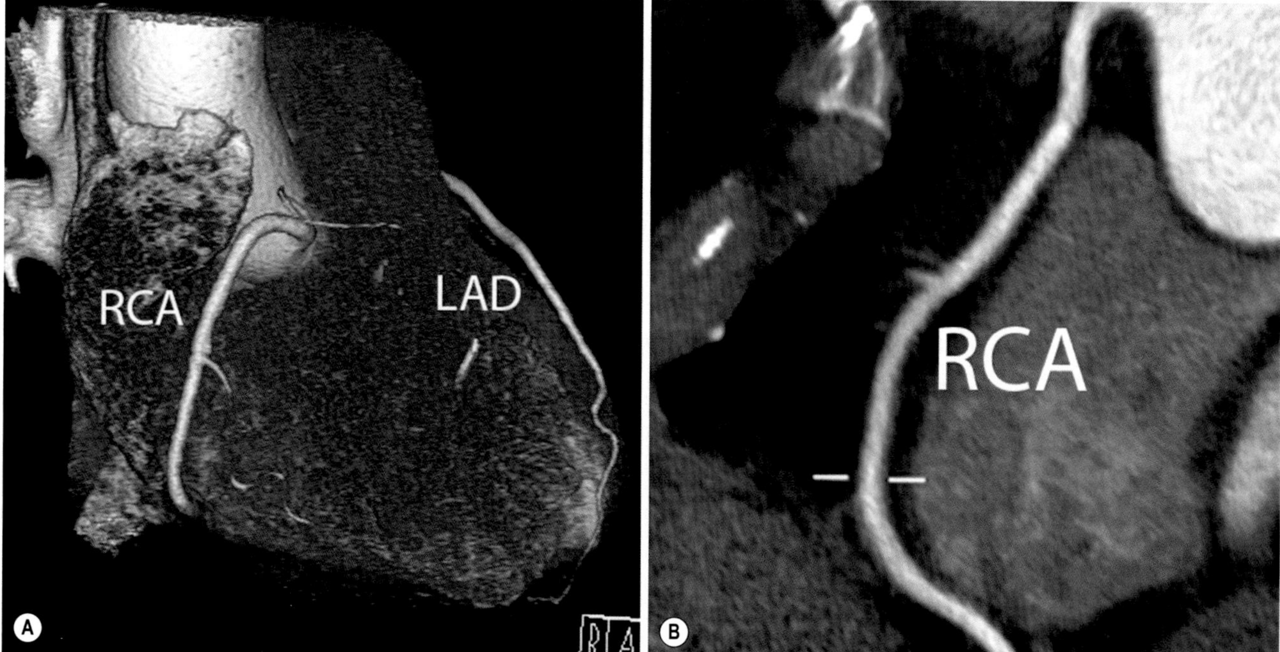

FIGURE 15-5 ■ **Cardiac computed tomography of the right coronary artery: normal findings.** Volume-rendered view (A), curved reformatted view (B). Abbreviations: LAD, left anterior descending coronary artery; RCA, right coronary artery.

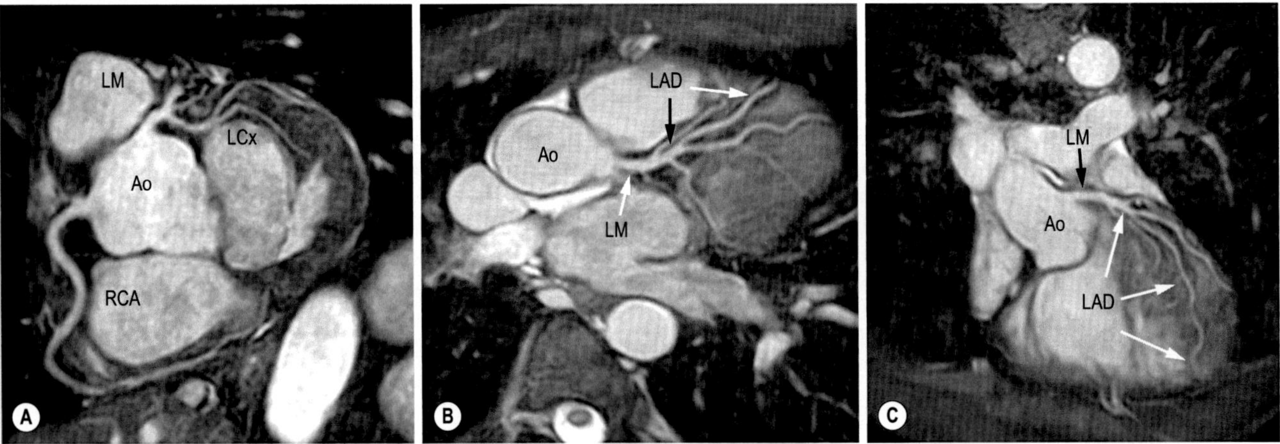

FIGURE 15-6 ■ Coronary MR angiography in a healthy volunteer. (A–C) Three different curved reformatted views using Soap-Bubble Tool (Philips, Best, The Netherlands). Abbreviations: Ao, aorta; LAD, left anterior descending coronary artery; LCx, left circumflex coronary artery; LM, left main coronary artery; RCA, right coronary artery.

rate and rhythm, a body mass index below 40 kg/m^2 and a normal renal function. The examination is performed following intravenous injection of contrast agent. Image quality can be substantially improved by lowering the patient's heart rate to < 65 bpm, which is usually achieved by administering β-blockers.[13–15] Coronary vasodilatation can be achieved using sublingual nitroglycerin administration. With the newest-generation imaging, not only can the heart be imaged in less than one heartbeat but also the radiation can be substantially reduced (~0.7–3 mSv). Further reduction in radiation dose can be achieved with iterative reconstruction algorithms.[16] Coronary MR angiography is achieved using high-resolution imaging targeted to each coronary artery separately, or using a whole-heart approach. Images are acquired during repeated breath-holds or during free breathing using a respiratory trigger algorithm (Fig. 15-6). Sequences are available for luminal and for wall imaging. Despite enormous efforts of CMR experts worldwide, coronary MR angiography is at present still not incorporated in daily clinical care, mainly because of long acquisition times, unreliable image quality and the availability and ease of use of CCT. However, clinically interesting indications for coronary MR angiography are imaging of congenital anomalies of the coronary arteries, coronary artery imaging in (postoperative) patients with congenital heart disease and diagnosis (and follow-up) of patients with coronary aneurysms in Kawasaki's disease (Figs. 15-7–15-9).

Calcification in the coronary arteries occurs, with exception of patients with advanced chronic kidney disease, almost exclusively in patients with coronary atherosclerosis (Fig. 15-10). Since the amount of coronary calcium roughly correlates to the atherosclerotic plaque extent, detection and quantification of coronary calcium is of interest for patient risk stratification.[13] Most patients with an acute coronary syndrome (ACS) show coronary calcium, and the amount of calcium in these patients is substantially greater than in age- and gender-matched subjects without CAD. It should be emphasised that coronary calcification is not related to plaque (in)stability and only weakly related to the severity of luminal stenosis (Fig. 15-11). In young symptomatic patients, a negative coronary calcium image does not exclude coronary artery stenoses. The Agatston score, less frequently volume or mass scores, is used to quantify the amount of calcium. Reference data sets stratified by age and gender are available for interpreting coronary calcium shown by CT. In the 2010 Appropriate Use Criteria for CCT, coronary calcium scoring was considered appropriate in asymptomatic low-risk patients without known CAD and with a family history of premature IHD, and for stratifying intermediate-risk patients for future cardiac events.[14] Moreover, coronary calcium scoring is of value on the decision to perform the use of contrast CT angiography in symptomatic patients. Above a CCS > 400, a contrast CT angiography is considered uncertain or inappropriate.[1]

Coronary CT angiography offers high accuracy for detection and especially for ruling out significant CAD (Fig. 15-12). Two recent multicentre trials reported a sensitivity of 95–99%, specificity of 64–83%, negative predictive value of 97–99% and a positive predictive value of 64–86% to identify patients with at least one coronary artery stenosis among individuals at low to intermediate risk for CAD.[13] The lower positive predictive value is explained by the tendency to overestimate the degree of stenosis by coronary CT angiography. In particular, calcified plaques tend to be overestimated by the so-called blooming artefact. Coronary CT angiography performs best in symptomatic patients with a low to intermediate likelihood of CAD. In these patient groups, according to the 2010 Appropriate Use Criteria for CCT, coronary CT angiography was deemed appropriate for detecting CAD in symptomatic patients without known heart disease, and also in those presenting with a clinical suspicion of ACS but having normal ECG and cardiac biomarkers, uninterpretable/non-diagnostic ECG or equivocal biomarkers. Coronary CT angiography yields promise to determine and to quantify the coronary plaque burden, and to a certain extent to characterise the plaque composition. Using intravascular ultrasound (IVUS) as reference technique, lipid-rich plaques yielded mean

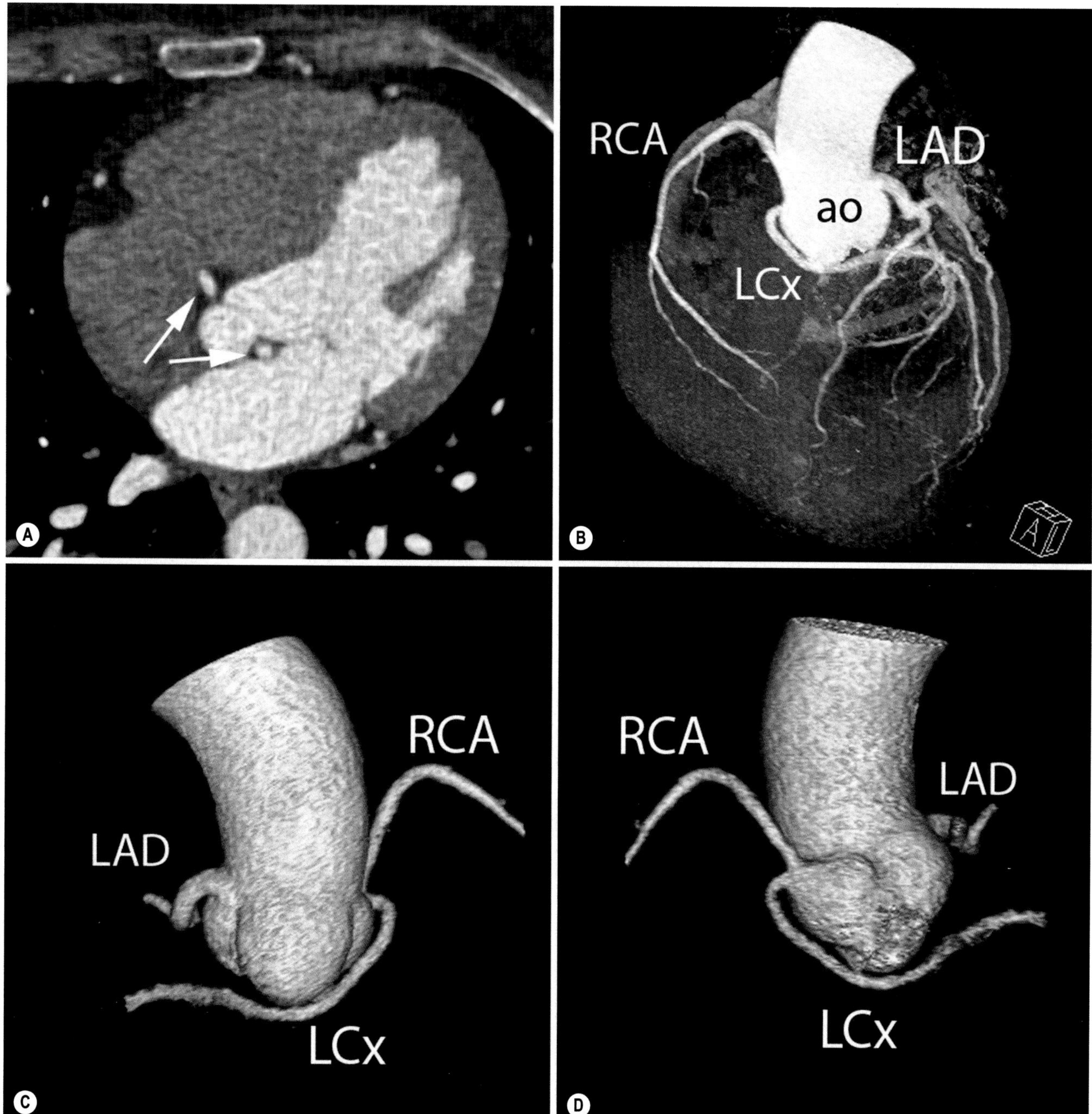

FIGURE 15-7 ■ Benign form of congenital anomaly of the left circumflex coronary artery. Common origin of RCA and LCx coronary artery with retro-aortic course of LCx. The abnormal retro-aortic course of the LCx can be diagnosed on the axial CCT images (arrows, A). The origin and course can be well appreciated on the volume-rendered views (B–D). Abbreviations: ao, aorta; LAD, left anterior descending coronary artery; LCx, left circumflex coronary artery; RCA, right coronary artery.

attenuation values between 11 and 99 HU versus 77–121 HU for fibrous plaques.[13] Finally, CCT is excellent for depicting anomalous coronary arteries and myocardial bridging.[17,18]

FUNCTIONAL IMAGING

Assessment of cardiac function is essential in the diagnostic work-up of IHD patients. For instance, in patients admitted with an acute myocardial infarction, the dead myocardium ceases to contribute to the expulsion of blood, shifting the workload to the non-affected ('remote') myocardium. Though a compensatory increase in contractility may occur in these areas, the net result is usually a decrease in (global) ventricular functional performance. Several imaging techniques can be applied for functional cardiac imaging, e.g. echocardiography, CMR, nuclear medicine (planar radionuclide ventriculography, gated blood pool single photon emission computed

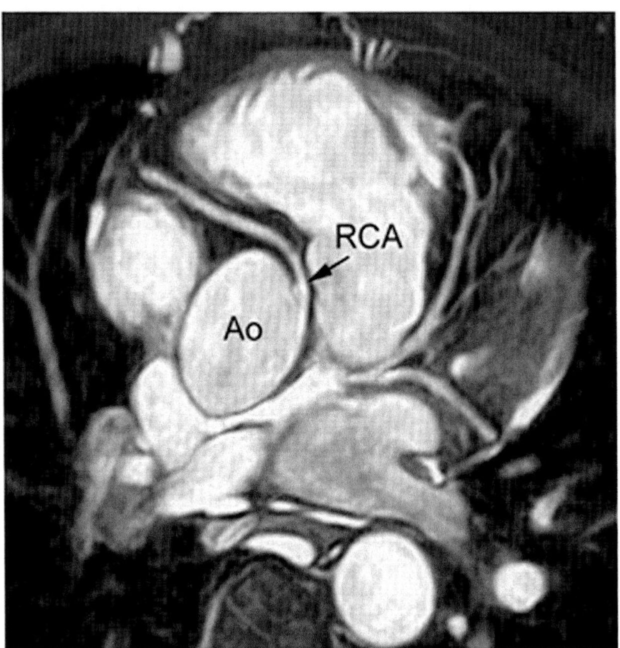

FIGURE 15-8 ■ Malignant form of congenital anomaly of the right coronary artery. Coronary MR angiography. The right coronary artery arises from the left aortic cusp and has a proximal interarterial course (between aortic root and pulmonary trunk). Abbreviations: Ao, aorta; RCA, right coronary artery.

tomography (SPECT)), catheter angiography and CCT. Requirements are that techniques are accurate, reproducible and preferably non-invasive. Global ventricular function is usually assessed by measuring the volume at end diastole (maximal filling) and at end systole (maximal emptying) (Fig. 15-13). Subtracting both volumes yields the amount of blood expulsed by the ventricle (i.e. stroke volume). Dividing the stroke volume by the end-diastolic volume yields the ejection fraction, while multiplying the stroke volume with the heart rate yields the cardiac output. Moreover, these values can be indexed to body surface area or body weight. Two approaches can be used for this purpose: (a) assumption techniques comparing the ventricle to a geometrical model, and (b) volumetric techniques. Since ventricles have a complex anatomy, their volumes can be quantified using the slice-summation technique; i.e. the ventricle is cut in a set of continuous slices, and the volume (and volume changes during the cardiac cycle) of each slice is (are) quantified. Summing the volumes of these slices yields the ventricular volume. Volumetric quantification is more accurate and reproducible than assumption techniques, at the expense of a more time-consuming analysis. Regional ventricular function is assessed either visually or (semi-)-quantitatively. Ventricular wall motion during systole is usually visually graded as normokinetic, hypokinetic (decreased but still present), akinetic (completely absent), dyskinetic (wall moving outward during contraction) and hyperkinetic (increased). Systolic wall thickening can be visually graded as normal, diminished, absent, wall thinning or increased. Moreover, it is often expressed as percentage systolic wall thickening (normal values are typically in the range of 40%).[19] The American Heart Association has recommended the use of a 17-segment model to express regional functional and morphologic parameters.[20] The left ventricle is divided longitudinally in a basal level (segments 1–6), a mid-level (segments 7–12), an apical level (segments 13–16) and an apical segment (segment 17) (Fig. 15-14). Segments 1, 7 and 13 represent the anterior LV wall, and a numbering in anticlockwise direction is followed (viewing the LV from apically). Moreover, segments can be attributed to a coronary artery perfusion territory; e.g. segments 1, 2, 7, 8, 13, 14, 17 typically belong to the left anterior descending coronary artery perfusion territory. Segments 3, 4, 9, 10, 15 belong to the right coronary artery, while segments 5, 6, 11, 12, 16 belong to the left circumflex coronary artery. This relation, however, may vary, depending on the coronary anatomy. The strength of this model is that the segmentation is technique-independent. It should be emphasised that functional abnormalities in IHD are not limited to the left ventricle but may affect the right ventricle as well. As discussed in the paragraph on stress imaging, it can be necessary to evaluate the functional cardiac response during stress conditions. Indications are detection of haemodynamic significant coronary artery stenosis, viability assessment in chronic dysfunctional myocardium and depiction of the presence and extent of stunned myocardium in patients with acute myocardial infarction.

Cardiac ultrasound is a first-line technique for assessing cardiac function in IHD patients. It can be performed bedside, provides valuable information regarding cardiac structure and function and allows the visualisation of complications such as aneurysm or thrombus formation post-infarction. Novel techniques such as velocity vector imaging or strain imaging are promising tools for studying myocardial motion and deformation with good feasibility in the clinical setting.[21] However, in many patients image quality is suboptimal, and geometric assumptions are used in clinical routine to assess ventricular volume and function. Bright-blood CMR, using the balanced steady-state free-precession sequence, has become one of the preferred techniques for assessing cardiac function. Whereas competing techniques need to administer iodinated contrast material (CCT) or radioactive tracer (isotope ventriculography) for volumetric/functional ventricular imaging, these CMR sequences yield a high intrinsic contrast between blood and surrounding myocardium. To obtain dynamic information, images are acquired at multiple time points during the cardiac cycle. Loading these images in a cine mode enables the appreciation of dynamic phenomena such as myocardial wall motion/thickening or motion of valve leaflets (i.e. cine imaging). Though normally acquired within a series of repeated breath-holds, in uncooperative patients or in patients with atrial fibrillation, non-gated real-time cine imaging is a valuable alternative for estimating the degree of ventricular dilatation and dysfunction, for visualising focal aneurysm formation or for image concomitant valve pathology. Cine imaging is performed along the cardiac axes, using a combination of short- and long-axis planes. If needed, images along other planes such as the three-chamber view can also be obtained. This approach allows a full appreciation of regional ventricular function (Fig. 15-15). Ventricular volumes, mass and function are

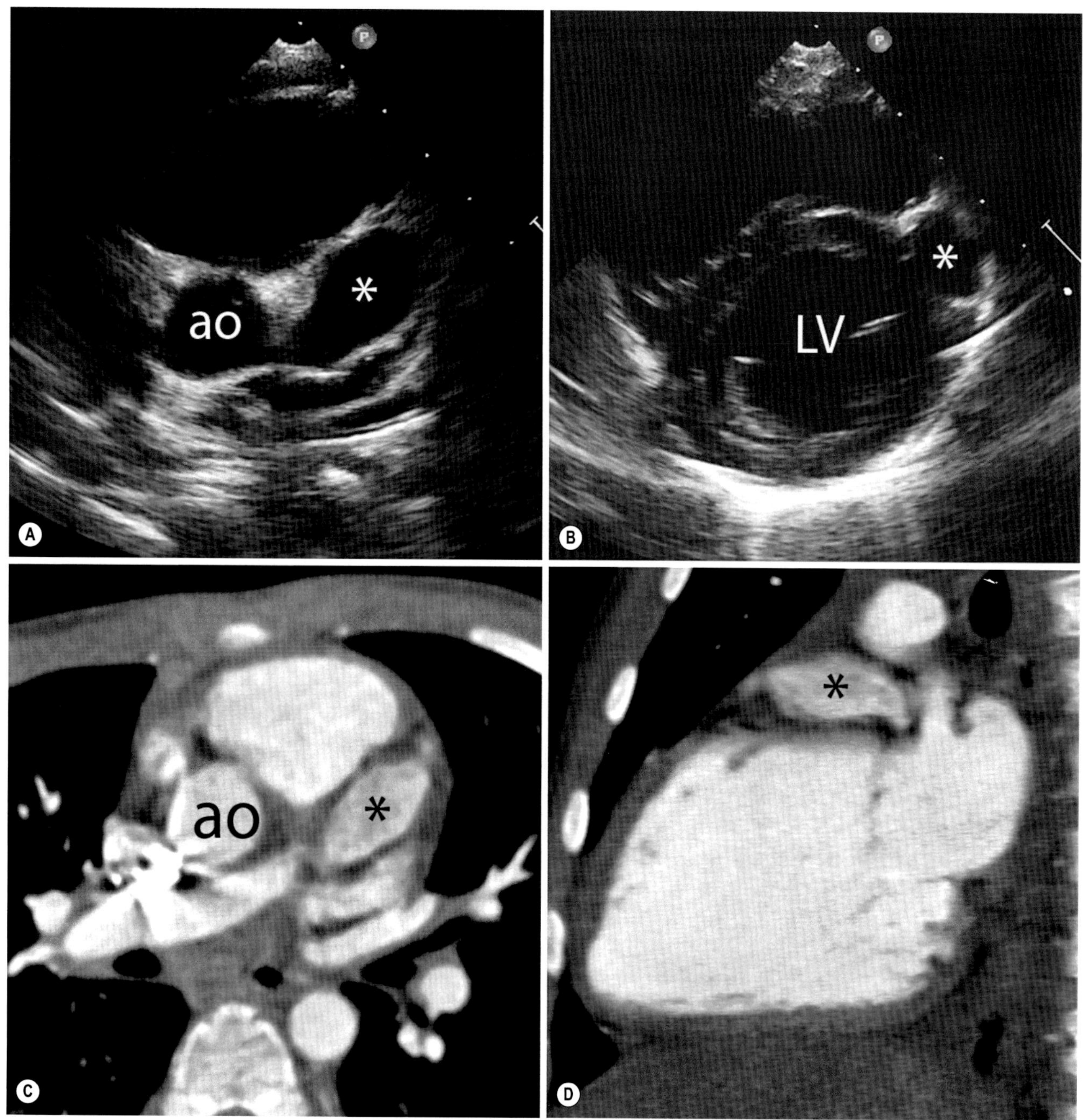

FIGURE 15-9 ■ Aneurysm of the left anterior descending coronary artery in a young patient with Kawasaki's disease. Echocardiography (A, B) and CCT (C, D). Presence of a fusiform aneurysm (*) (36 × 15 mm) in the proximal part of the left anterior descending coronary artery. The ultrasound and CCT findings match well. No evidence of thrombus formation in the aneurysm. Abbreviations: ao, aorta; LV, left ventricle.

usually quantified using a stack of short-axis slices encompassing the ventricles. To elucidate the complex mechanisms of myocardial deformation in normal and pathologic conditions, tag lines or grids can be non-invasively imprinted on the myocardium.[22] Clinical use has been impeded by the elaborative post-processing, but novel techniques such as fast direct colour-coded strain visualisation using strain-encoded (SENC)-CMR are appealing for stress imaging.[23] Merging functional imaging with morphological (infarct/oedema imaging) or perfusion imaging is an interesting pathway for assessing the functional performance in the diseased and normal parts of the heart.[23]

Cardiac CT is an interesting alternative to CMR for left and right ventricle assessment in patients unable to undergo a CMR study.[14,24] The administration of contrast agent should be adapted to obtain enhancement of the right ventricular cavity. It is imperative to mention that techniques for reducing radiation dose such as prospective triggering do not allow for functional imaging since

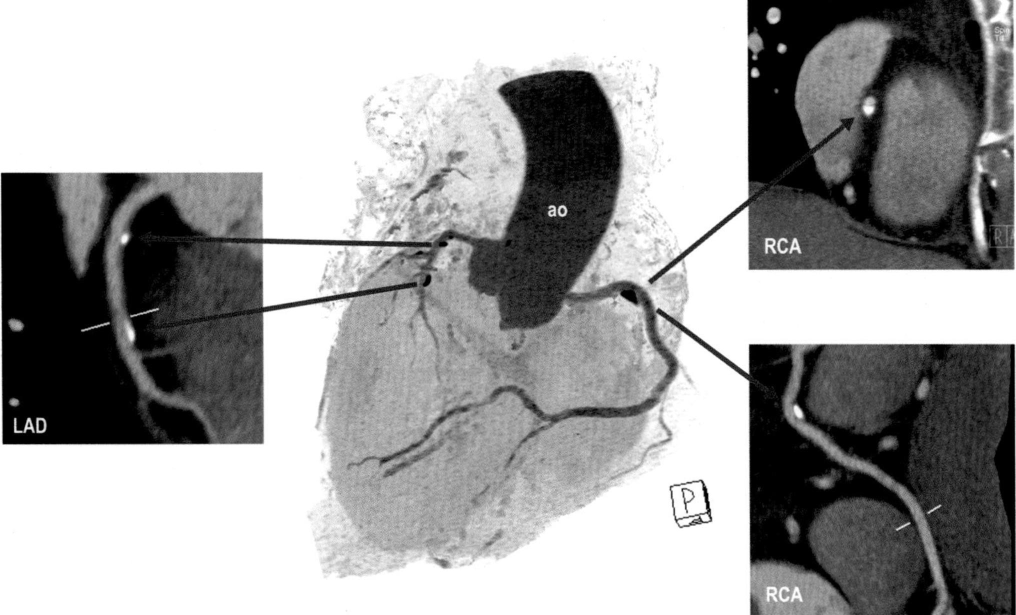

FIGURE 15-10 ■ **Visualisation of calcified non-stenotic plaques by CCT.** Presence of three calcified plaques in right coronary artery and left anterior descending coronary artery. The calcified plaques do not impinge on the coronary artery lumen but cause an enlargement of the external border, a phenomenon called positive remodelling. Abbreviations: ao, aorta; LAD, left anterior descending coronary artery; RCA, right coronary artery.

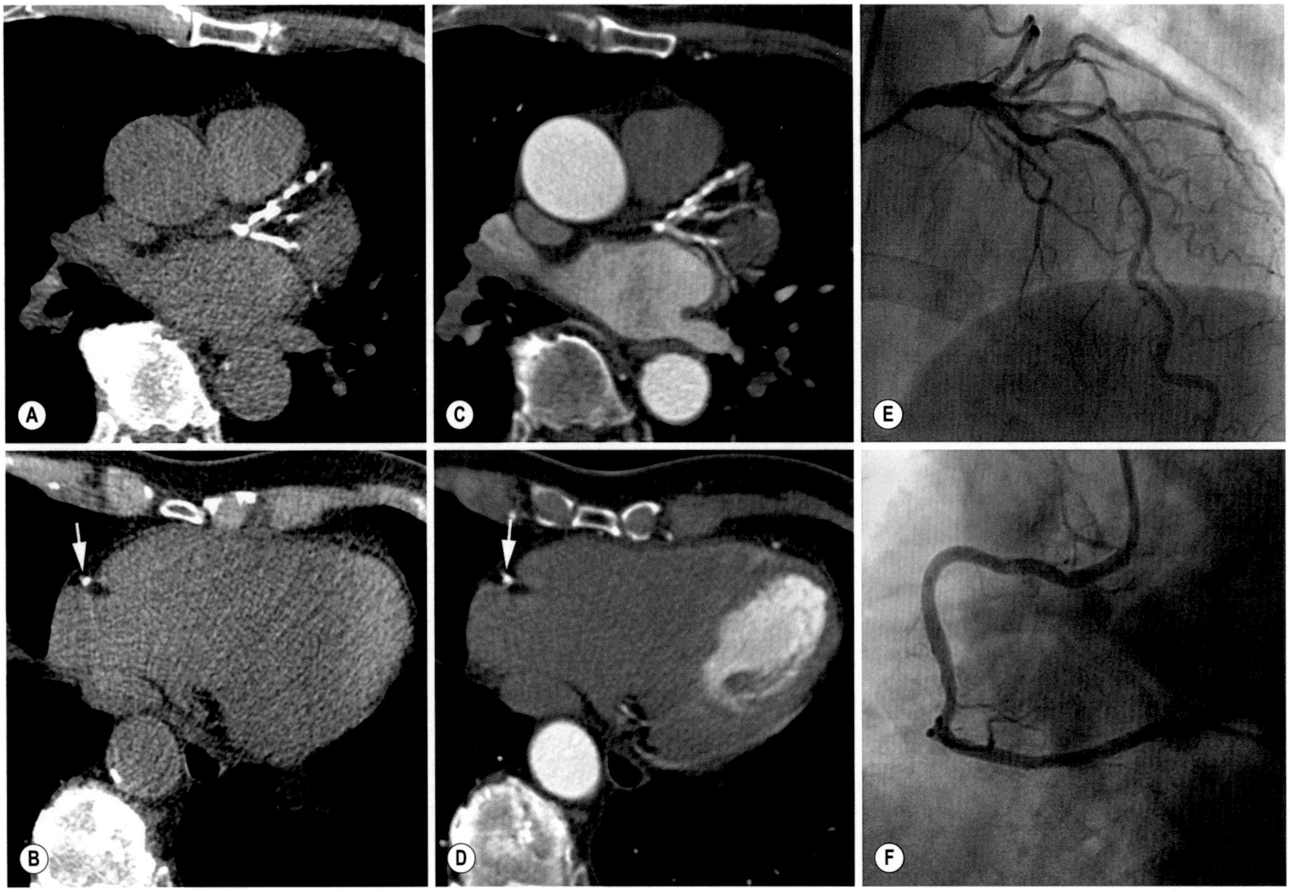

FIGURE 15-11 ■ **The calcium paradox.** Unenhanced CCT (A, B), contrast-enhanced CCT (C, D) and coronary angiography of left (E) and right (F) coronary artery. Presence of diffuse calcified coronary atherosclerosis (total calcium score: 1251) and suspicion of several coronary artery stenoses on contrast-enhanced CCT (C, D). However, as clearly shown by coronary angiography, except for a mild (40%) stenosis in proximal LAD, no flow-limiting stenoses are found.

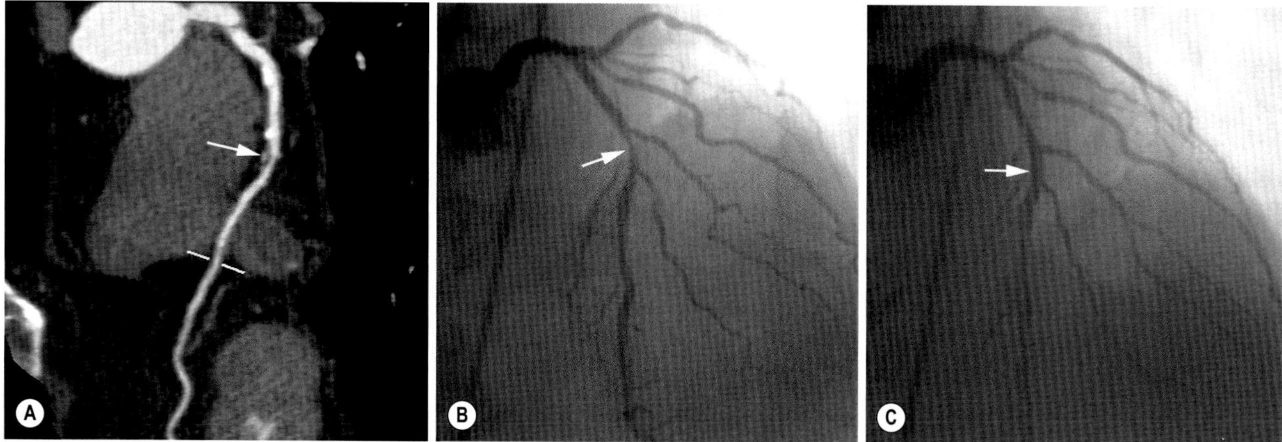

FIGURE 15-12 ■ **Flow-limiting stenosis in mid left anterior descending (LAD) coronary artery.** Contrast-enhanced CCT (A), coronary angiography before (B) and after PCI (C). Presence of an atherosclerotic plaque with mixed density in mid LAD impinging on coronary artery lumen (arrow, A) and several non- or minimally stenotic calcified plaques. At coronary angiography, a 70% excentric stenosis is found in mid LAD (arrow, B). The patient was treated with a 3-mm bare metal stent. No residual stenosis was present post-PCI (arrow, C).

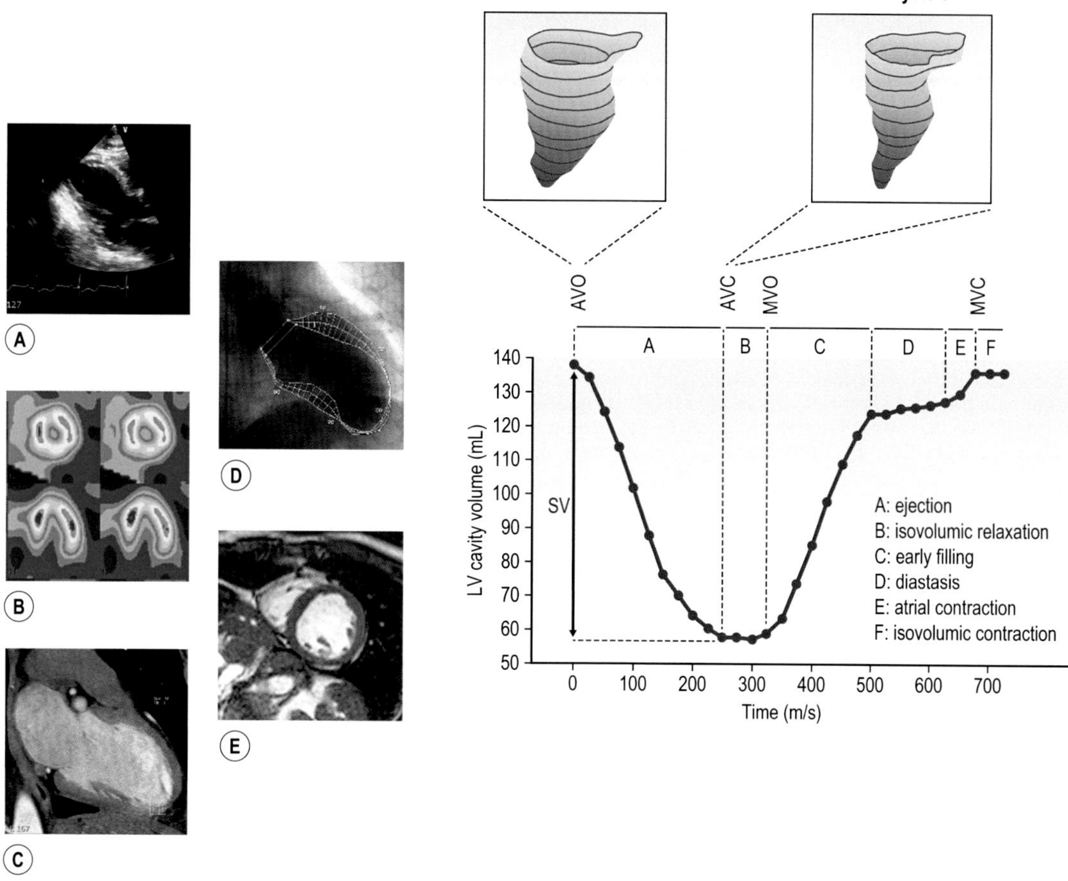

FIGURE 15-13 ■ **Imaging techniques used for assessment of cardiac function.** On the left, five different imaging techniques are shown: echocardiography (A), nuclear medicine (B), CCT (C), cardiac catheterisation (D) and CMR (E), which are used daily to assess ventricular volumes and function. The graph shows the time–volume changes of the left ventricular (LV) cavity during a cardiac cycle. At time 0 corresponding to end diastole, the LV has its largest volume. After aortic valve opening (AVO) part of this volume (stroke volume (SV)) is ejected into the thoracic aorta during ventricular contraction ('ejection'). Between aortic valve closure (AVC) and mitral valve opening (MVO), the LV volume remains constant (isovolumic relaxation phase). At the moment of mitral valve opening (MVO) LV filling occurs, and is characterised by three phases, i.e. early filling, diastasis and atrial contraction. The last phase of the cardiac cycle is the isovolumic contraction between mitral valve closure (MVC) and AVO. Most techniques measure the changes in LV volume at end diastole (maximal filling) and end systole (maximal emptying) to express LV volumes and ejection fraction.

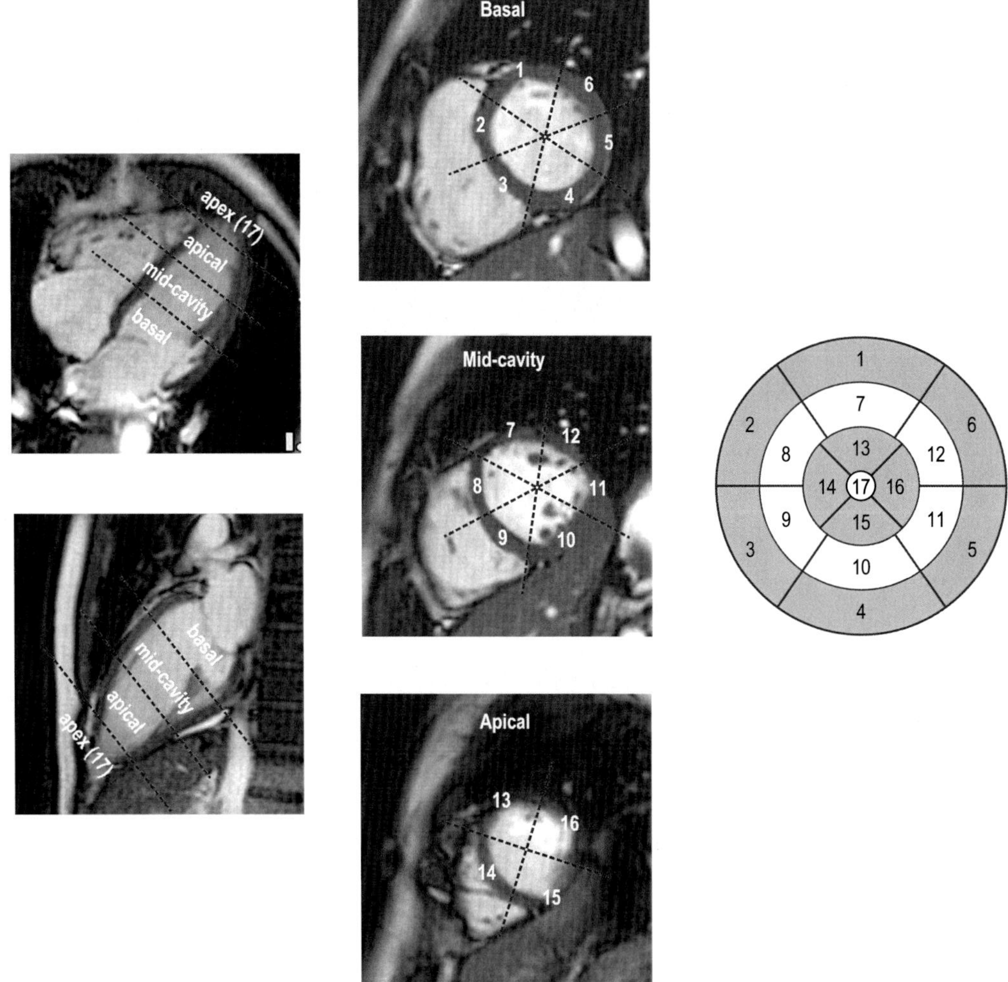

FIGURE 15-14 ■ Seventeen-segment approach to LV segmentation as proposed by the American Heart Association. The left ventricle is divided in longitudinal direction (left) into a basal, mid-cavity, and an apical short-axis ring (middle). Subsequently these short-axis rings are divided into six basal, six mid-cavity and four apical segments, with segment 17 being the apex seen on the long-axis views (left images). Basal: 1, anterior; 2, anteroseptal; 3, inferoseptal; 4, inferior; 5, inferolateral; 6, anterolateral. Mid-cavity: 7, anterior; 8, anteroseptal; 9, inferoseptal; 10, inferior; 11, inferolateral; 12, anterolateral. Apical: 13, anterior; 14, septal; 15, inferior; and 16, lateral. Bull's eye plot (right) representation of all segments of the left ventricle. The segment numbers refer to the same segments.

data are acquired during a brief period of the cardiac cycle, usually at mid-diastole.

In many hospitals, planar radionuclide ventriculography is an established technique for assessing left ventricular volumes and function. Alternatively, gated blood pool SPECT can be used to assess wall motion and regional ejection fraction.[25]

STRESS IMAGING

In patients with chronic stable CAD, treatment goals are threefold: relief of symptoms and ischaemia; prevention of premature cardiovascular death; and prevention of progression of CAD leading to myocardial infarction, left ventricular dysfunction and congestive heart failure. Management of CAD, however, remains highly challenging as several studies have shown that revascularisation fails to improve mortality over medical treatment in randomised trials.[26,27] The explanation of this paradox lies most likely in the poor relation between stenosis severity in diffuse CAD and coronary flow physiology.[28,29] Whereas anatomical techniques (conventional coronary angiography, CCT) provide limited information regarding the impact of a stenosis on the coronary flow, stress testing can be recommended to assess the extent of myocardial ischaemia before coronary angiography. Though prospective trials are still lacking, there is substantial evidence that a moderate to severe ischaemic burden greater than 5–10%, with or without angina, is an indication for revascularisation, whereas those patients without clear evidence of myocardial ischaemia likely benefit from an optimum medical treatment (e.g. high-dose statins, risk factor modification) to alter the natural history of CAD.[12,30] During cardiac catheterisation the functional severity of a stenosis can be determined by the FFR

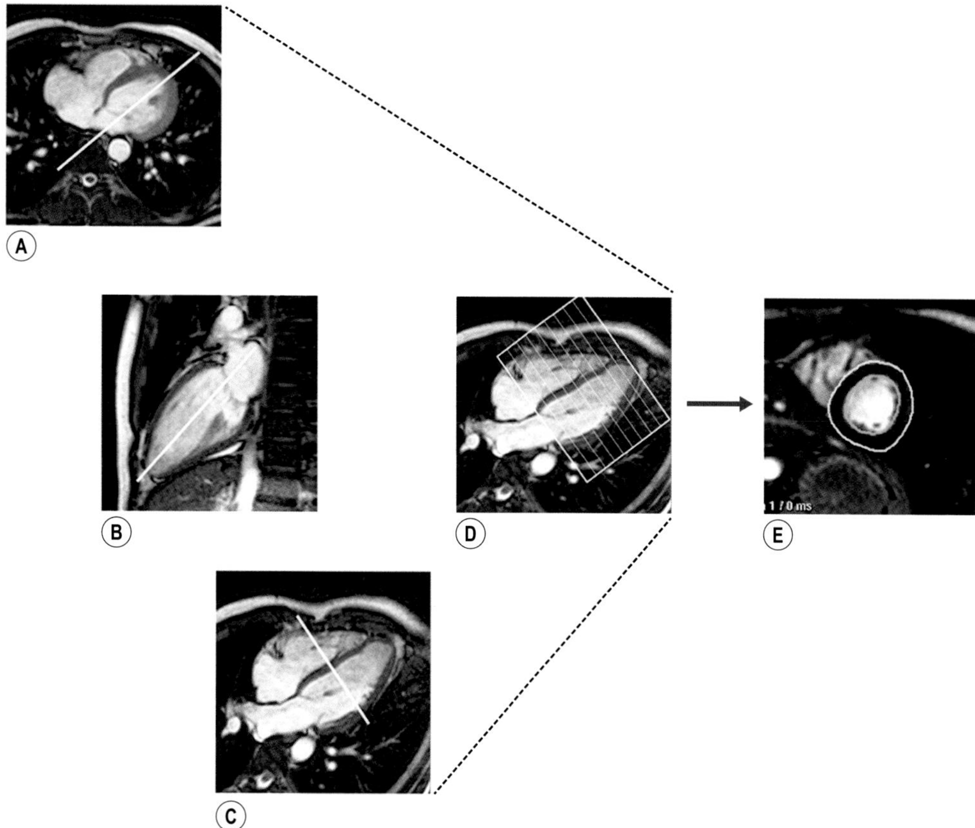

FIGURE 15-15 ■ CMR approach for quantification of LV function. A standardised approach is used to assess LV volumes, function and mass. CMR imaging is started with axial images (A). The vertical long-axis plane (B) is aligned from the axial plane through the mitral valve and LV apex, which may be on a separate more inferior slice. The horizontal long-axis plane (C) is aligned from the vertical long-axis plane through the mitral valve and LV apex. The short axis (E) is aligned from the vertical long-axis and horizontal long-axis planes—perpendicular to both. For quantification of LV volumes, function and mass, the set of short-axis images is positioned completely encompassing the left ventricle (D). Contouring the endocardial (green line, E) and epicardial border (yellow, E) of the short-axis images at end diastole and end systole makes it possible to calculate LV end-diastolic and end-systolic volume, stroke volume, ejection fraction and LV myocardial mass.

expressing the maximum achievable blood flow to the myocardium supplied by a stenotic artery as a fraction of normal maximum flow. A normal value is 1.0 and a value of 0.75 reliably identifies stenoses associated with inducible ischaemia. The diagnostic accuracy of FFR is >90%.[31] Though FFR may be helpful with patients presenting with diffuse CAD at cardiac catheterisation, in which stenoses may benefit from angioplastic interventions, non-invasive testing for reversible (or inducible) ischaemia is warranted to optimally stratify patients with stable CAD.

Non-invasive testing for reversible ischaemia is achieved by stressing the heart and evaluating whether during stress, symptoms of angina, ECG signs of myocardial ischaemia, ischaemia-induced myocardial wall motion abnormalities or myocardial perfusion disturbances occur. Exercise ECG test (EET), although widely used in daily practice, has a low sensitivity (0.44 to 0.92, median 0.63) and moderate specificity (0.41 to 0.8, median 0.77),[33] and a normal test does not exclude CAD. In particular, EET is a poor diagnostic test in low-risk populations (such as women) owing to its low positive value in a population with a low prevalence of the disease. The limited accuracy of EET in diagnosing CAD is also due in part to its position near the bottom of the ischaemic cascade. Therefore, diagnosis of CAD may be improved by use of non-invasive tests higher up in the ischaemic cascade than EET, assessing abnormalities in myocardial function or in myocardial perfusion during stress conditions. While we are most familiar with myocardial perfusion scintigraphy and stress echocardiography for these purposes, several other single or hybrid techniques have emerged in the field of stress imaging such as stress perfusion CMR, stress function CMR, stress perfusion CT, combined coronary and stress myocardial perfusion imaging by CCT and hybrid cardiac SPECT/CT or cardiac positron emission tomography (PET)/CT.[32–36]

Nuclear medicine is currently the cornerstone in the assessment of myocardial perfusion in CAD patients, and it has an established role in risk stratification for major adverse cardiac events.[37] Most often SPECT is used to diagnose and evaluate the severity of CAD, while PET is more accurate but also more expensive and less available.[36] SPECT measures the relative myocardial distribution of radionuclides, such as thallium-201 (^{201}Tl), technetium-99m (^{99m}Tc) and sestamibi (MIBI). Study protocols are specific for the different tracers; for instance,

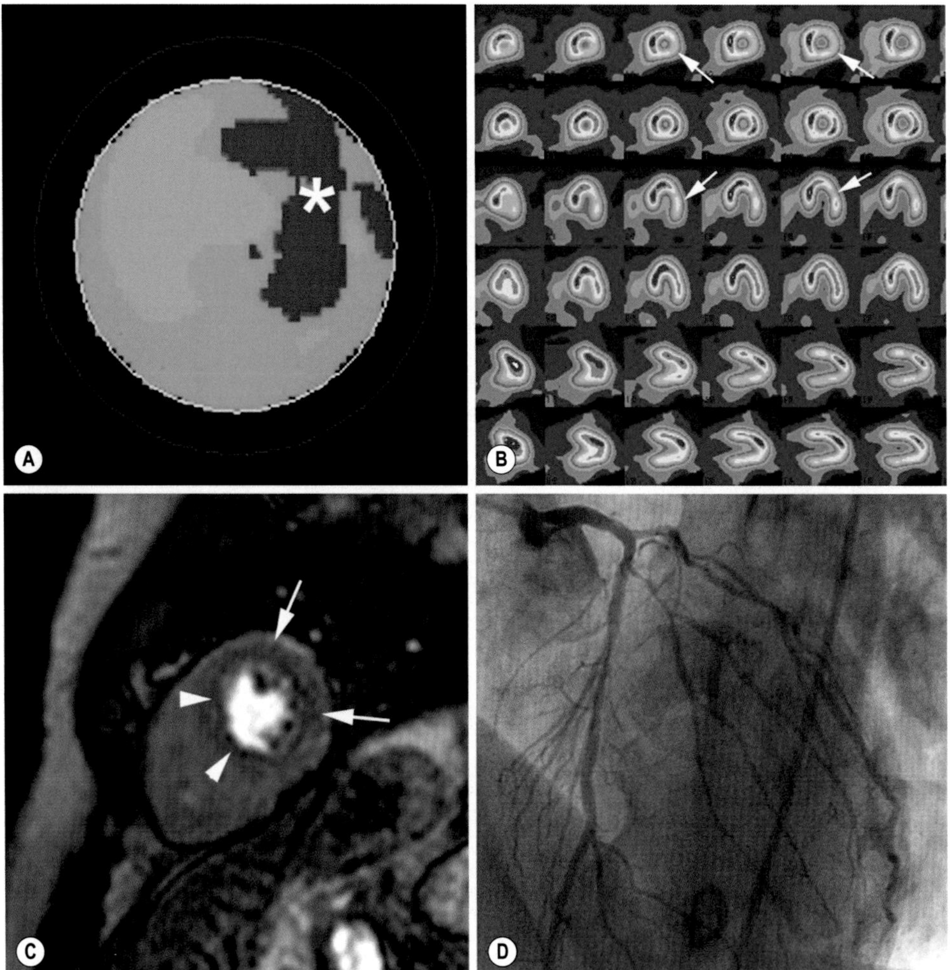

FIGURE 15-16 ■ **Myocardial ischaemia testing, MIBI SPECT versus CMR.** A 49-year-old man with type I diabetes, no symptoms, no anginal pain. MIBI SPECT shows reversible perfusion defect in lateral LV wall with an estimated ischaemia of 19% of LV myocardium) (*, A) (arrows, B). Stress perfusion CMR shows extensive stress-induced perfusion defect in lateral LV wall (arrows, C) and subendocardial perfusion in anterior LV wall and septum (arrowheads, C). LGE CMR shows moreover partial infarcisation of both papillary muscles (images not shown). At coronary angiography (D) severe two-vessel CAD is shown with distal LCx 80% stenosis, 1st lateral 80% stenosis, and mid anterior LAD 70% stenosis and distal LAD 80% stenosis. Coronary artery bypass graft surgery was performed with LIMA to LAD and free LIMA from LIMA to LCx. (MIBI SPECT courtesy of O. Gheysens, Department of Nuclear Medicine, UZ Leuven, Leuven, Belgium.)

MIBI SPECT is performed using an injection of tracer during stress and a second injection at rest (or vice versa), while ^{201}Tl is injected during stress, and the redistribution of tracer is measured at rest after a delay (e.g. 4 h). In regions with impaired myocardial perfusion the number of counts is lower than in the normally perfused myocardium, resulting in a 'defect'. *Reversible* defects (i.e. present on stress but absent at rest) are caused by flow-limiting stenoses and should be differentiated from *fixed* defects (i.e. present at rest/redistribution at rest) reflecting myocardial scarring (Fig. 15-16). The severity of the defect (i.e. reduction in counts) is related to stenosis severity while the extent of the defect is related to the myocardium supplied by the stenotic artery. Although SPECT is widely used in clinical practice, yielding good sensitivity, i.e. 89% (95% CI, 84–93%) and moderate specificity, i.e. 65% (95% CI, 54–74%), certain pitfalls need to be mentioned. Radiation exposure of the injected isotopes ranges between 8 and 20 mSv, depending on the protocol used. Subendocardial and small infarcts may be missed by SPECT because of the lack in spatial resolution (Fig. 15-17). To avoid false-positive readings and to improve the test specificity, use of attenuation correction methods and gated analysis of wall motion is recommended. Finally, in patients with multivessel CAD, hypoperfusion of the entire myocardium may mask regional abnormalities. PET is very useful for assessing myocardial perfusion and metabolism. Assessment of myocardial perfusion can be performed with nitrogen-13 ammonia, oxygen-15 H_2O, rubidium-82 or carbon-11 acetate. PET has several advantages over SPECT, such as a higher spatial resolution and the possibility of measuring absolute myocardial blood flow.[36] This is advantageous in patients with balanced ischaemia caused by left main or three-vessel CAD in which maximal myocardial blood flow is reduced in all regions of the left ventricle, or in patients in whom the myocardial ischaemia is caused by microvascular dysfunction. The reported sensitivity of

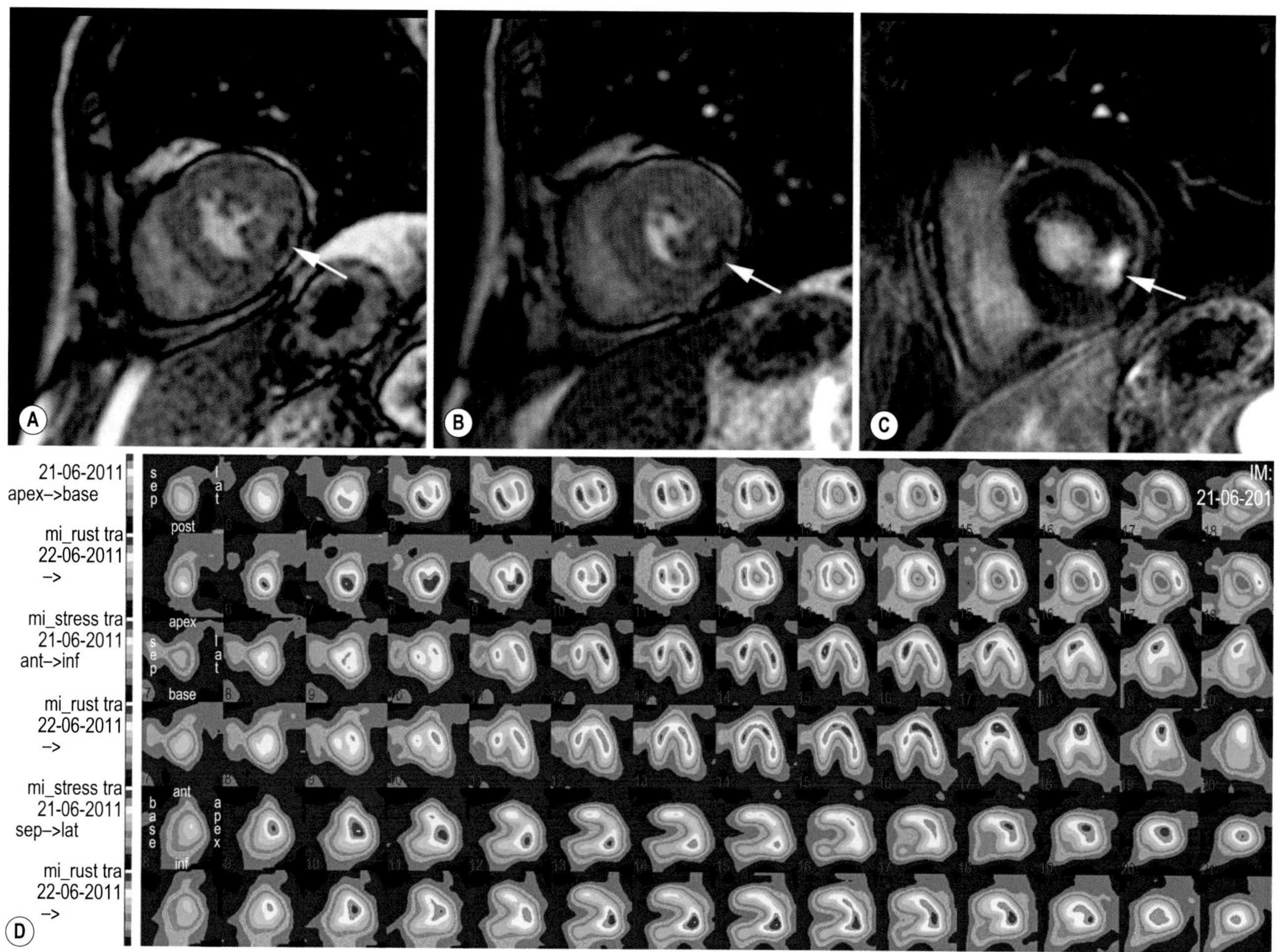

FIGURE 15-17 ■ Small inferolateral myocardial infarct, MIBI SPECT versus CMR. History of PCI with stent placement in LAD coronary artery in 45-year-old man. MIBI SPECT shows reversible defect in mid/apical LV anterior wall (±10% of LV myocardium) and decreased tracer activity in mid/basal inferolateral wall. Rest perfusion (A) and stress perfusion (B) CMR show focal hypointense appearance of the mid/basal LV inferolateral wall during first pass of contrast (arrow, A, B). On LGE CMR, this area shows a focal, almost completely transmural enhancement (arrow, C), compatible with healed myocardial infarction. No evidence of myocardial ischaemia in LAD territory in stress perfusion CMR (D). (MIBI SPECT courtesy of O. Gheysens, Department of Nuclear Medicine, UZ Leuven, Leuven, Belgium.)

PET for detecting angiographic stenosis ≥ 50% is 91% (range 83–100%) and the specificity is 89% (range 73–100%).[38] Drawbacks of PET are patient exposure to radiation (although less than SPECT), availability and limited half-life of PET tracers, cost and availability of PET, false-positive myocardial perfusion defects due to misregistration and the limited spatial resolution when compared to CMR.

CMR uses the changes in myocardial signal intensity during the first pass of a bolus of contrast through the heart to assess myocardial perfusion. This necessitates fast imaging sequences with saturation pre-pulses to suppress myocardial signal and to obtain T1-weighting. Use of three short-axis slices assures sufficient coverage of the left ventricle, enabling a regional 16-segment perfusion assessment[20] (Fig. 15-14). Similar to nuclear imaging, myocardial hyperaemia (induced by an infusion of vasodilator such as dipyridamole or adenosine) makes it possible to depict haemodynamic significant stenoses. Hypoperfused myocardium appears on CMR as a non- or slow-enhancing part of the myocardium ('perfusion defect') (Fig. 15-18). The defect, typically, obeys anatomical borders as well as the boundaries of the coronary artery perfusion territories, and the extent is determined by the position of the stenosis along the coronary artery. Semi-quantitative measures show a decline in the upslope during first pass of contrast agent, and when related to the upslope during resting conditions, the myocardial perfusion reserve (MPR) ratio is typically decreased. Several studies, including a recent prospective trial in 752 patients, showed the superiority of stress perfusion CMR over SPECT with a sensitivity of 86.5 versus 66.5%, specificity of 83.4 versus 82.6%, positive predictive value of 77.2 versus 71.4% and negative predictive of value 90.5 versus 79.1%, for CMR and SPECT respectively.[39–41] These favourable results can be largely explained by the superior spatial resolution of CMR (e.g. an in-plane pixel resolution up to 1.1×1.1 mm^2 is achievable with the newest high-resolution CMR perfusion sequences) compared to SPECT, enabling visualisation of smaller,

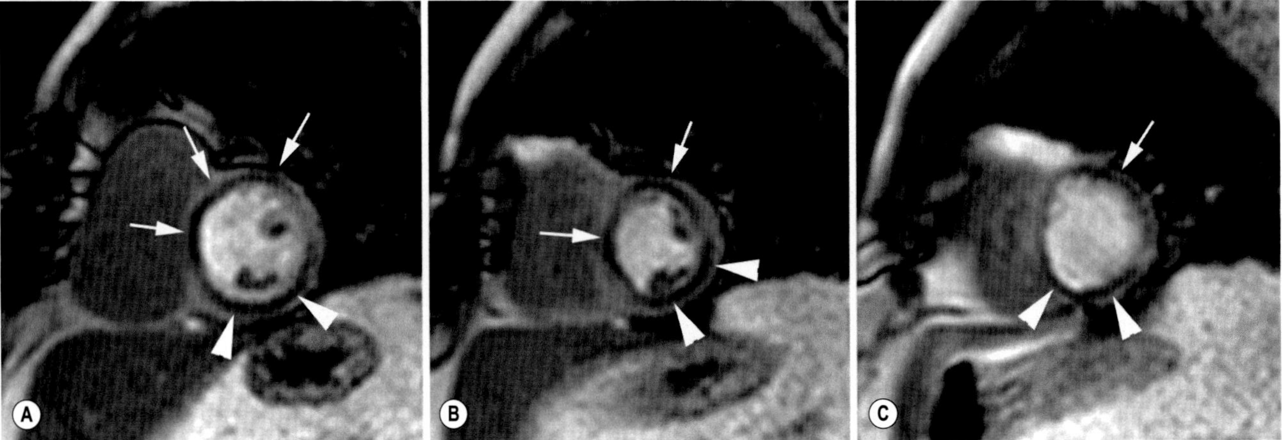

FIGURE 15-18 ■ Stress perfusion CMR in patient with severe three-vessel CAD. (A–C) A 62-year-old man with history of CABG presenting with increasing complaints of angina chest pain post-surgery. Medical treatment yielded unsatisfactory relief of symptoms. Stress perfusion CMR shows extensive perfusion defect in the anteroseptal LV wall (arrows) and inferolateral wall (arrowheads). Surgical re-intervention is planned.

subendocardially located, perfusion defects not infrequently. Moreover, CMR is not hampered by soft-tissue and attenuation artefacts. Similar to PET, absolute myocardial blood flow can be quantified with myocardial perfusion CMR.[42] Currently, the value of CCT to study myocardial perfusion under stress conditions is under investigation. In particular, because perfusion imaging can be combined with coronary artery imaging, this combined approach is highly appealing for studying the haemodynamic effects of a coronary artery plaque, and its consequences on myocardial perfusion. Although early reports are appealing, it should be mentioned that at present radiation issues are still substantial (approximately 10 mSv) and that only a limited part of the heart can be studied.[43]

In analogy to stress echocardiography, stress function studies can be performed safely in an MR environment. Dobutamine, a β-agonist, increases oxygen consumption by increasing myocardial contractility and heart rate. A stepwise dose increment of dobutamine allows for the evaluation of the myocardial response at each stress level. Whereas normally supplied myocardium shows a progressive increase in myocardial contractility, myocardium supplied by a flow-limiting coronary stenosis becomes ischaemic when the compensatory increase in coronary blood supply is insufficient to match the increased demand in oxygen (thus when the coronary flow reserve is superseded). This, in turn, will cause a decrease in regional contractility and lead to wall motion abnormalities (WMAs). Using a combination of long- and short-axis cine CMR sequences, regional contractility can be assessed in all segments of the left ventricle. Imaging is started in resting conditions, and the same set of sequences is repeated for each stress level. Dobutamine infusion is started at low dose (5 μg/kg body weight per minute). Cine images are analysed for new (or worsening) WMAs. If normal, the dose of dobutamine is increased using steps of 5–10 μg/kg, and the above approach is repeated. The test is considered positive for obstructive CAD when WMAs develop or worsen, or when the patient develops chest pain at a certain stress level. If the target heart rate of the patient, defined as (220 – age) × 0.85, is not reached at 40 μg/kg dobutamine, intravenous atropine can be additionally administered up to 1–2 mg using fractionate doses of 0.25 mg every minute (Fig. 15-19). Dobutamine administration needs to be stopped on patient request, and is also discontinued if the systolic blood pressure decreases >20 mmHg below the baseline systolic blood pressure, the systolic blood pressure decreases >40 mmHg from a previous level, the blood pressure increases to above 240/120 mmHg or when severe arrhythmias occur. Since this is a potentially harmful examination, haemodynamic parameters such as heart rate and blood pressure should be closely monitored, cardiac resuscitation material should be available and teams should be trained in case of cardiac complications for fast patient evacuation from the magnet. Wahl et al. showed that in experienced hands, high-dose dobutamine–atropine stress MRI is safe, with minimal side effects.[44] Besides detection of flow-limiting coronary stenoses in patients suspected of obstructive CAD, low-dose stress function imaging (≤20 μg/kg dobutamine) enables differentiation between viable and non-viable dysfunctional myocardium in patients with chronic CAD. Also in patients with a recent myocardial infarction, low-dose stress imaging can differentiate between stunned and irreversibly damaged myocardium. High-dose dobutamine–atropine stress CMR yields good sensitivity (83–96%) and specificity (80–100%) for detection of significant CAD. In particular, patients with poor echocardiogeneity benefit from CMR stress testing. Novel CMR techniques such as SENC-CMR, allowing strain visualisation, provide incremental value for the detection of CAD as compared to conventional wall motion readings, and have the strength to detect CAD at lower stress levels.[23]

MYOCARDIAL INFARCT IMAGING

Assessment of the electrical cardiac activity using 12-lead electrocardiography and analysis of cardiac biomarkers are central diagnostic techniques in patients presenting

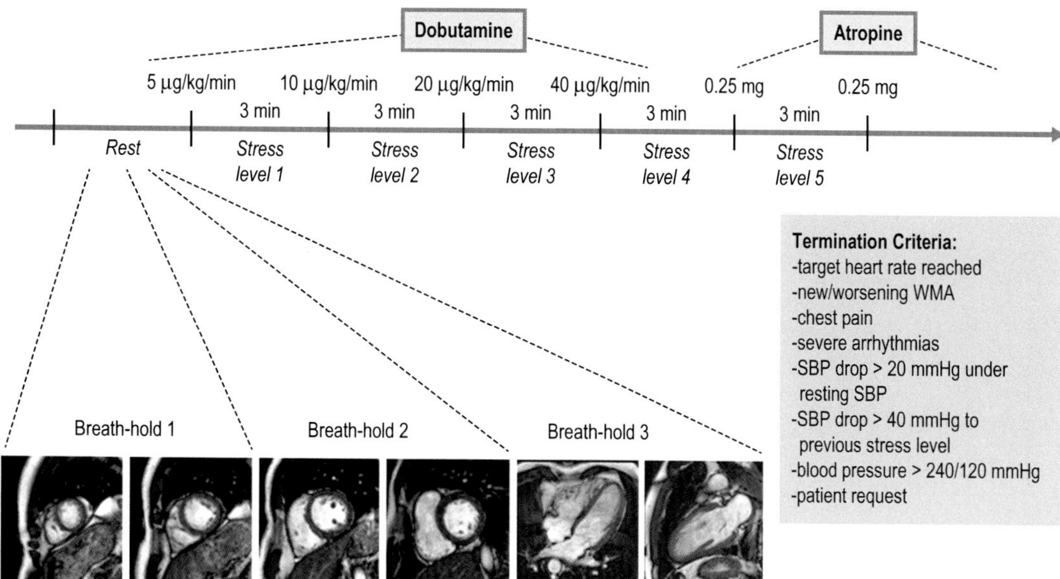

FIGURE 15-19 ■ **Practical scheme for dobutamine stress CMR.** Per stress level, four short-axis and two long-axis cine studies are obtained in three consecutive breath-holds, making it possible to evaluate the left ventricle for new wall motion abnormalities (WMAs). If termination criteria are not met at the highest dobutamine dose, atropine can be additionally administered.

with an ACS. Firstly, a patient's triage and treatment are to a large extent based on ECG changes indicative of new ischaemia (new ST-T changes or new left bundle branch block), and development of new pathological Q waves (Fig. 15-20). The ECG allows the clinician to suggest the infarct-related artery, to estimate the amount of myocardium at risk and to detect prior (healed) myocardial infarction. In infarcts presenting an ST-segment elevation, the degree of ST-resolution post-reperfusion reflects the success of reperfusion.[6] Secondly, as myocardial cell death is characterised by a release of different proteins into the circulation from the damaged myocytes, increased cardiac blood biomarkers are indicative of recent myocardial necrosis. The preferred biomarker at present is cardiac troponin (I or T), which has a nearly absolute myocardial tissue specificity as well as high clinical sensitivity.[6] If troponin assays are not available, the best alternative is creatine kinase-MB. Because of the complex release characteristics of these cardiac proteins, it is still unclear whether the peak value or a single point measurement of cardiac biomarkers provides the best estimate of myocardial infarct size. Moreover, neither blood biomarkers nor ECG provides a good insight in the evolving processes in the jeopardised myocardium. Imaging techniques such as cardiac ultrasound and cardiac catheterisation visualise an acute myocardial infarction indirectly by the impact of the infarction on wall motion or wall strain but do not visualise the necrotic myocardium. Gated SPECT shows a myocardial infarction as a fixed defect with loss in regional function. However, small (subendocardial) infarcts are not infrequently missed because of the lack in spatial resolution (Fig. 15-19).[45] In the past decade, CMR has emerged as the in vivo reference technique for myocardial infarction imaging, and it has the advantage of being multiparametric, thus offering substantial complementary information to the standard diagnostic and imaging tools (Fig. 15-21). Though in recent years several papers have reported on the use of CCT for myocardial infarct imaging, it is currently unclear what is the clinical value, though this technique may be valuable, for example, in patients unable to undergo CMR, or for infarct imaging as part of a more comprehensive CCT including coronary artery and myocardial perfusion imaging.[46]

Tissue characterisation of the jeopardised myocardium by CMR is basically twofold. Firstly, increased free water in the ischaemic myocardium prolongs T2 relaxation, and the prolongation is related to the duration of ischaemia. Using T2-weighted imaging techniques such as the short inversion time inversion recovery (STIR) fast spin-echo sequences ('T2W-imaging'), myocardial oedema is shown as bright, while normal myocardium appears dark (Fig. 15-22). Abnormalities occur rapidly after onset of coronary artery occlusion (i.e. in the first 30 min after onset of ischaemia) and are considered to reflect the area at risk to become necrotic.[47,48] Myocardial oedema is most evident the first days post-infarction, and then slowly fades away due to processes of infarct healing. Healed infarcts, conversely, present similar or decreased signal intensity to normal myocardium. Myocardial oedema, however, is not specific for myocardial infarction but may occur in other conditions such as acute myocarditis or stress cardiomyopathy (tako-tsubo cardiomyopathy) as well. Secondly, administration of extracellular gadolinium-based contrast agents results in a time-varying enhancement of infarcted myocardial tissue, which is different from normal myocardium. Since wash-in and wash-out of contrast are dynamic processes, timing of imaging is important; the optimal time is somewhere between 10 and 25 min after administration of contrast agent. Because imaging is late or delayed, this sequence is often called late (or delayed) gadolinium enhancement ('LGE') imaging. The contrast between

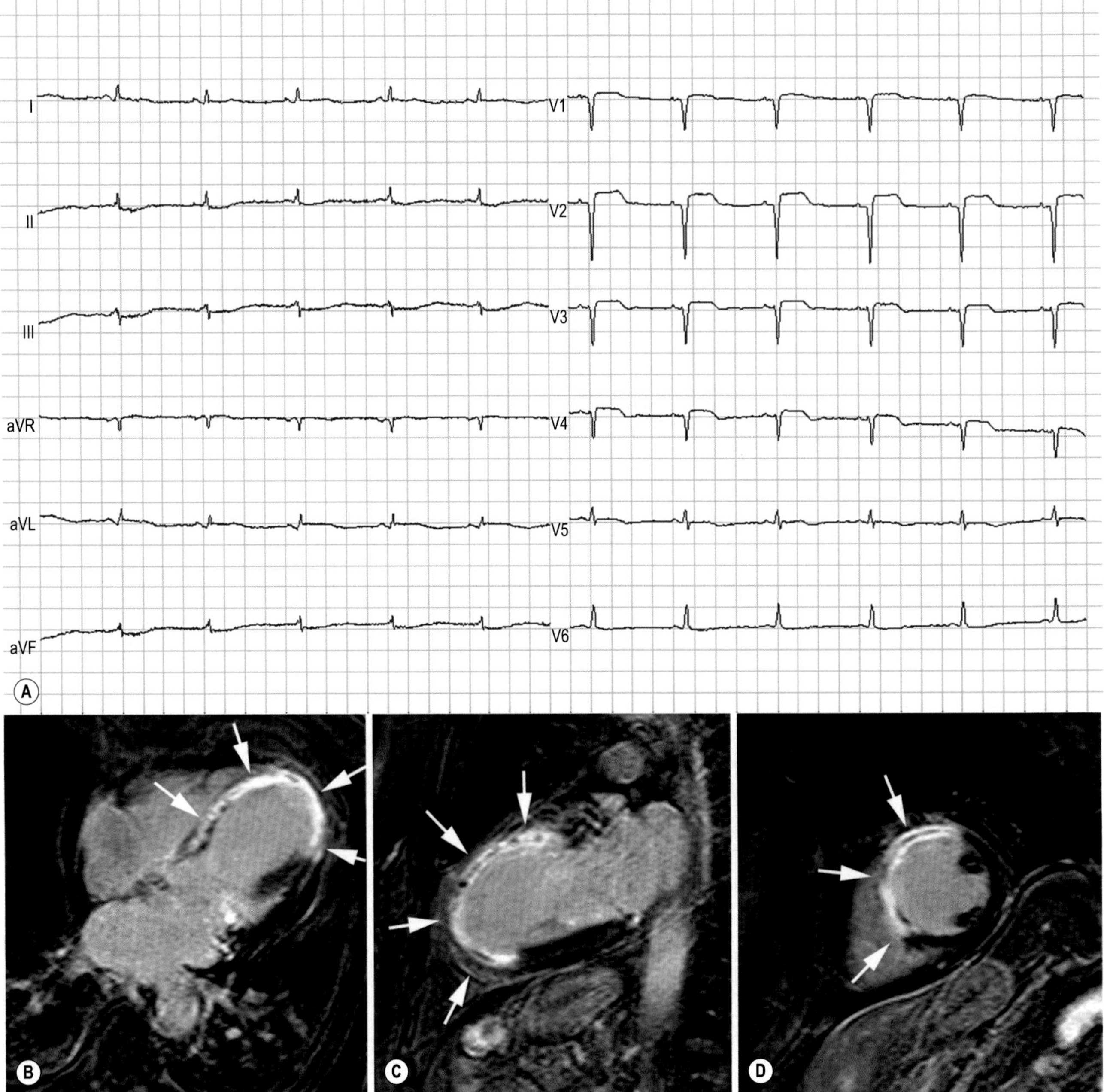

FIGURE 15-20 ■ Extensive acute anteroseptoapical myocardial infarction. ECG-CMR correlate. (A) Successful PCI of occluded proximal left anterior descending (LAD) coronary artery. Both CMR and ECG were obtained 3 days after the acute event. The ECG shows anterior necrosis with QS complex in V1–V4 and persistent ST segment elevation with positive T-waves in the same leads. These findings suggest lack of myocardial tissue perfusion (i.e. microvascular obstruction). LGE-CMR in horizontal long axis (B), vertical long axis (C) and midventricular short axis (D) show transmural enhancement in segments 1, 2, 7, 8, 13–15 and 17, reflecting extensive necrosis in the LAD perfusion territory. Presence of microvascular obstruction inside the infarct area as suggested on ECG. The extent of microvascular obstruction was more prominent on CMR images obtained early after contrast administration.

normal and abnormal myocardium can be significantly increased, adding an inversion prepulse to the 2D or 3D segmented gradient-echo sequence. By correctly choosing the length of inversion time, the signal of normal myocardium is nullified, thus resulting in an improved visualisation of the infarcted myocardium. For a contrast dose of 0.2 mmol/kg, inversion times typically range between 200 and 300 ms. Use of a Look–Locker sequence may be of help in determining the optimal inversion time. The phase-sensitive image reconstruction (PSIR) technique allows infarct imaging without the need to adjust inversion times.[49] The LGE CMR combining high spatial with high contrast resolution allows depiction of subtle myocardial damage as small as 1 g (e.g. papillary muscle necrosis or peri-procedural myocardial damage), which is of prognostic significance (Fig. 15-23). Though LGE CMR is a robust, well-validated and accurate tool for depicting myocardial necrosis in the acute setting of MI

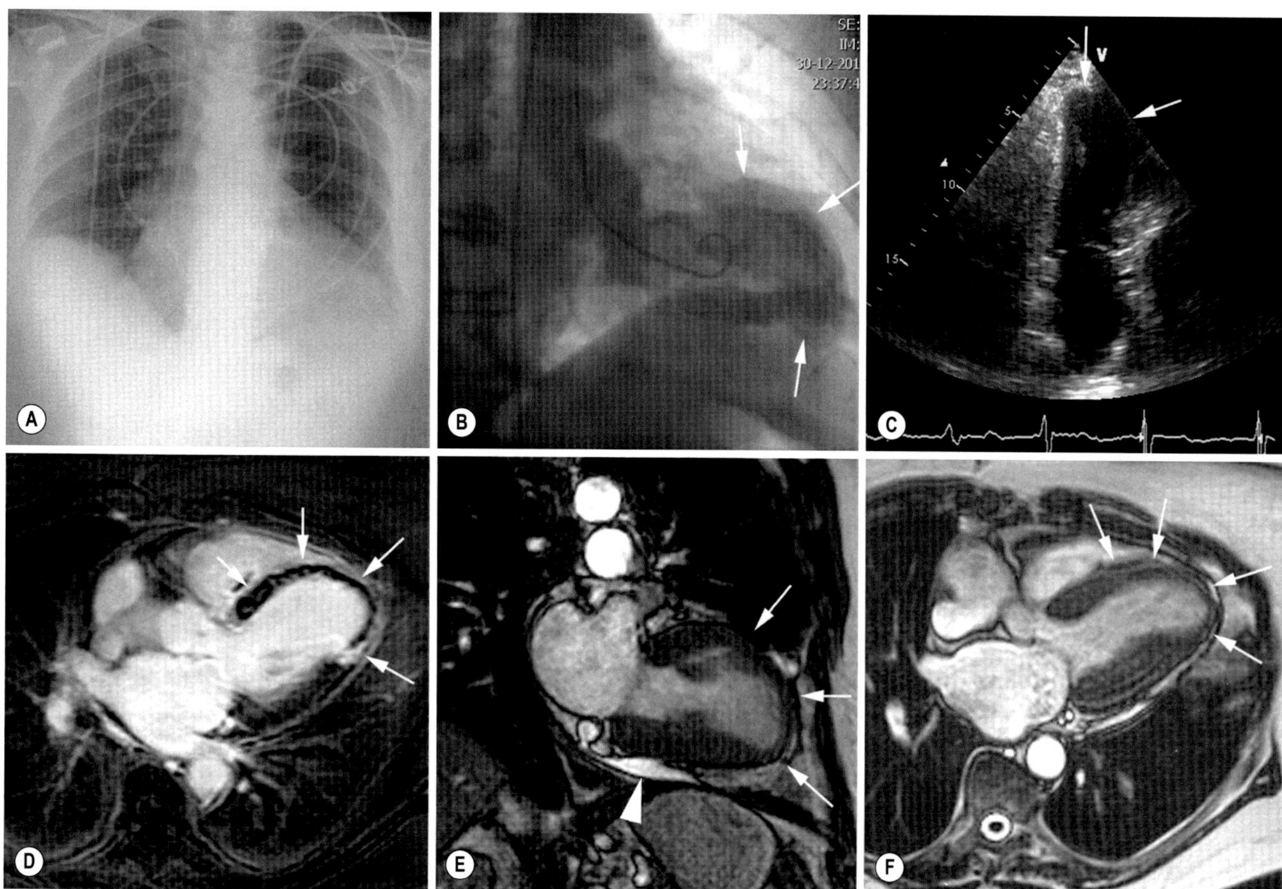

FIGURE 15-21 ■ Comparison of imaging techniques in assessing patients with an acute myocardial infarction. Conventional chest film (A), cardiac catheterisation (B), cardiac ultrasound (C) and CMR using LGE CMR (D), and cine CMR in vertical long-axis (E) and horizontal long-axis (F). Conventional CXR (bedside radiograph) shows moderate cardiomegaly without evidence of pulmonary oedema. LV contrast ventriculography (RAO position, end-systolic time frame) shows extensive area of decreased contractility involving the anterior wall, apex and the apicoinferior LV wall (arrows, B). Cardiac ultrasound (longitudinal parasternal view) reveals similar information (arrows, C). LGE CMR shows extensive myocardial infarction involving the majority of the ventricular septum, apical two-thirds of the anterior wall, apex, and apical inferolateral wall (arrows, D). While the periphery of the infarct is strongly enhanced, centrally an extensive zone of microvascular obstruction remains on LGE CMR, reflecting severe microvascular damage. The functional consequences of the infarction can be well appreciated on cine CMR (arrows, E, F). Small amount of pericardial fluid (arrowhead, E).

(Fig. 15-24), some incompletely resolved issues remain regarding the specificity of enhancement,[50] and myocardial enhancement may be seen in several non-ischaemic myocardial diseases as well.[51] Finally, a free bonus of LGE CMR is its excellent ability to demonstrate infarct-related complications such as thrombus formation, or inflammatory pericarditis (Fig. 15-25).[52,53]

Thus, a combination of T2-imaging and LGE CMR can be used to determine areas at risk and extent of infarction. The difference between both reflects the degree of salvaged myocardium ('myocardial salvage'). With increasing ischaemia time, salvageable myocardium decreases at the expense of increasing infarct size, while the myocardium at risk remains constant.[54] Thus, early reperfusion may result in complete myocardial salvage (i.e. aborted infarction). Myocardial salvage is independently associated with early ST-segment resolution and is an independent predictor of adverse ventricular remodelling and major cardiac events.[55,56]

Estimation of the *infarct size* is imperative for assessing infarct severity. Moreover, it is an important prognosticator for determining adverse ventricular remodelling and patient outcome,[57] and therefore this parameter is often used as surrogate end point to assess efficacy of novel treatments.[58] However, several parameters other than infarct size should be taken into consideration when assessing infarct severity. Amongst them is the transmural extent of necrosis. Increasing *infarct transmurality* is related to lack of inotropic reserve and impaired recovery of contractile function, and is associated with more pronounced post-infarct wall thinning, aneurysm formation and adverse ventricular remodelling.[59] Another important parameter is microvascular obstruction or no-reflow, which is present in up to 50% of patients. It can be defined as lack of restoration of blood flow at myocardial level despite a successful recanalisation of the coronary artery.[60] No reflow is related to myocardial damage and ischaemia time, and it is independently associated with

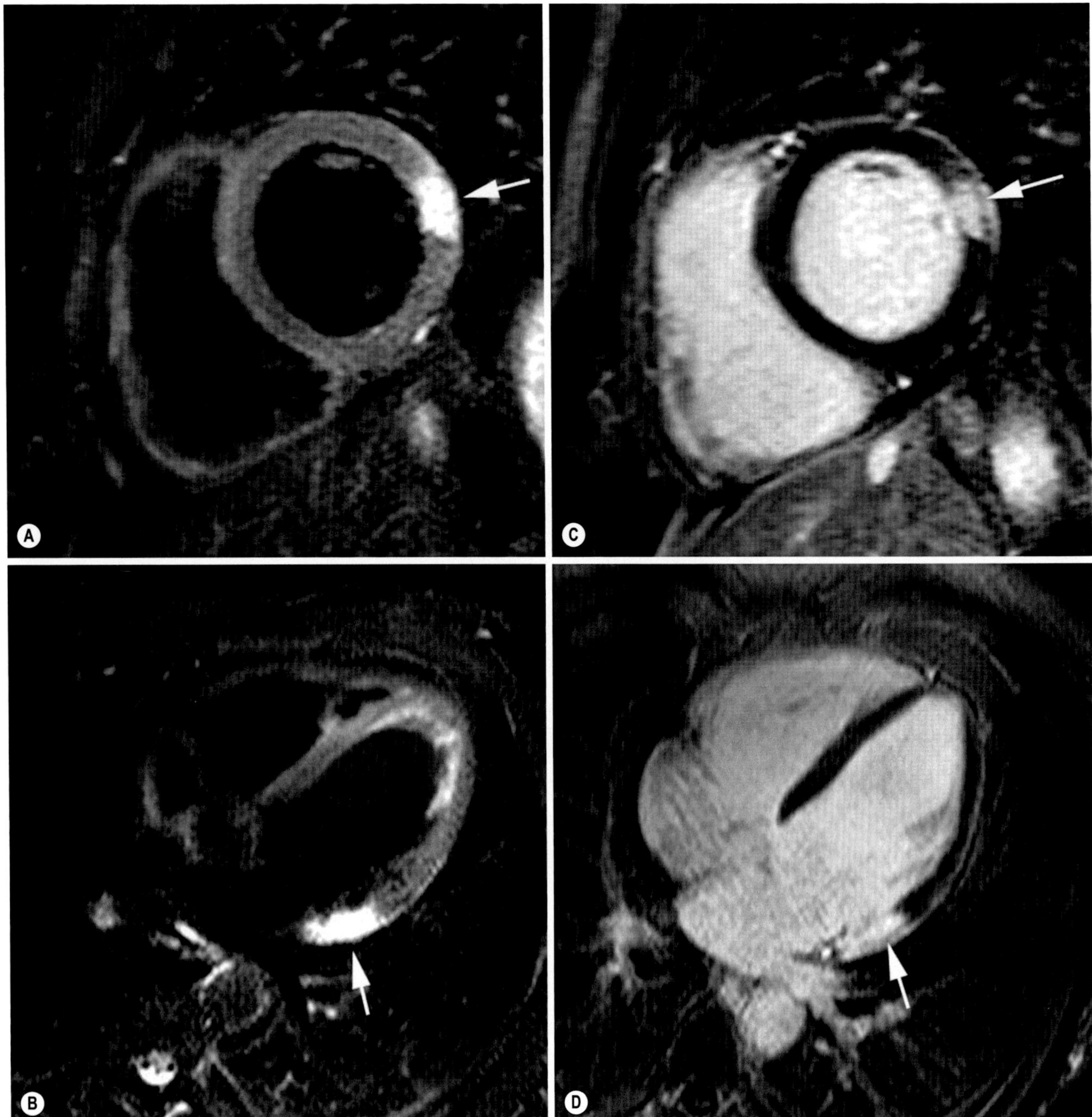

FIGURE 15-22 ■ **Acute laterobasal myocardial infarction.** A 37-year-old man admitted with retrosternal chest pain irradiating to the mandibula. Positive cardiac enzymes and ST-segment elevation in anterior and lateral ECG leads. Coronary angiography shows proximal occlusion of the first lateral branch of the left circumflex coronary artery. T2-weighted imaging in short axis (A) and horizontal long axis (B). LGE CMR in short axis (C), and horizontal long axis (D). Sharply defined zone of myocardial oedema in anterior and lateral wall (segments 1, 6) (arrows, A, B). LGE CMR shows strong enhancement in anterior and lateral wall (segments 1, 6) (arrows, C, D). The extent of enhancement coincides very well with the extent of myocardial oedema, which means that the major part of the jeopardised myocardium has been irreversibly damaged. In other words, myocardial salvage is very low.

lack of functional recovery, adverse remodeling and worse patient outcome.[54,61] Contrast-enhanced CMR is a preferred technique for depiction of microvascular obstruction (Fig. 15-26). Early imaging is recommended for appreciating the maximal extent of microvascular obstruction because its size decreases over time due to gadolinium molecules diffusing into the no-reflow zone. Visualisation of no-reflow zones can be improved by using longer inversion times on the order of 500 ms. Another parameter reflecting infarct severity is post-reperfusion myocardial haemorrhage. Restoration of myocardial perfusion is often associated with interstitial extravasation of red blood cells caused by severe microvascular damage. Thus, intramyocardial haemorrhage reflects microvascular injury and serves as marker for reperfusion injury. T2-weighted imaging has the

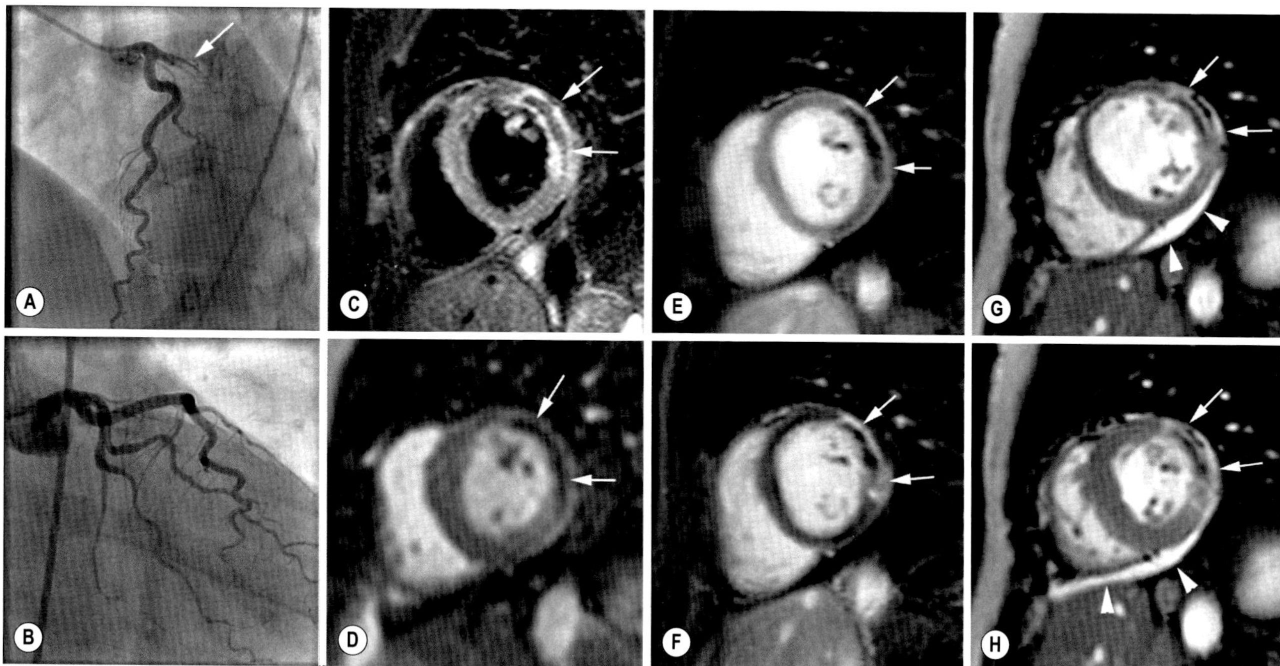

FIGURE 15-26 **Acute transmural lateral myocardial infarction with microvascular obstruction and haemorrhagic component.** Coronary angiography before (A) and after (B) PCI. CMR using T2-weighted imaging (C), first-pass perfusion imaging (D), early (E) and late (F) post-contrast CMR and cine imaging after contrast administration at end diastole (G) and end systole (H). All CMR images are acquired in midventricular short axis. Before PCI, the proximal left circumflex artery is completely occluded (arrow, A). Successful recanalisation of the occluded coronary artery (B). T2-weighted imaging shows bright signal in the lateral wall with presence of a 'dark' core (arrows, C). Presence of microvascular obstruction which can be well appreciated during first-pass perfusion (arrows, D) and early post-contrast administration (arrows, E). At LGE transmural enhancement of the lateral wall has occurred, reflecting a transmural myocardial infarction (arrows, F), while the extent of microvascular obstruction is decreased. Cine imaging shows severely impaired function in the lateral wall (arrowheads, G, H) while the remainder of the LV wall still contracts appropriately. Presence of a moderate amount of pericardial fluid mainly located inferiorly (arrowheads, G, H). The post-reperfusion myocardial haemorrhage can be recognised by the dark core in the jeopardised myocardium on T2-weighted imaging.

ventricle can contain a mixture of different ischaemic substrates. Thus, the goal is to determine those patients that might benefit from a revascularisation procedure and those in whom medical therapy should be considered, bringing us to the issue of 'myocardial viability' assessment. Different techniques using different approaches are currently available for myocardial viability assessment. Best-known techniques are PET and stress echocardiography. PET uses a combination of a flow (e.g. NH_3) and metabolism (e.g. fluorodeoxyglucose (FDG)) tracer to determine whether dysfunctional myocardium is viable (mismatch pattern) or non-viable (match pattern) (Fig. 15-28), while echocardiography assesses the improvement in myocardial contractility using a low dose of dobutamine (i.e. 5–10 μg/kg body weight). Viable myocardium, having a contractile reserve, shows a functional improvement. Non-viable myocardium, in contrast, shows no functional improvement or even a worsening in wall motion. Compared to normal myocardium, the contractile reserve in dysfunctional but viable myocardium is limited, explaining why at higher doses of dobutamine (i.e. 20 μg/kg body weight) the wall motion worsens, i.e. the so-called 'biphasic effect' of viable myocardium.

In recent years, CMR has emerged as an interesting alternative to PET and stress echocardiography. The approaches used by CMR to assess myocardial viability are largely emulated from those used by other techniques, but this technique takes advantage of a superb spatial and contrast resolution and a multiparametric approach, allowing the clinician a much broader picture of the diseased heart compared to that of its closed competitors. In analogy to PET, MR spectroscopy can be used to measure metabolic spectra (e.g. ATP and phosphocreatine) in heart failure patients.[66] A first approach consists of assessing end-diastolic wall thickness. A normal (or preserved) wall thickness is considered viable while a thinned wall is deemed to reflect non-viability. The rationale is that scar formation in a myocardial infarction leads to a wall thinning. The higher the infarct transmurality, the more pronounced the degree of wall thinning.[67] This approach yields a high sensitivity (95%, range 94–100%), but a low specificity (41%, range 19–53%) to predict functional recovery after revascularisation (Fig. 15-27).[65] Thus, a thin dysfunctional wall (<6 mm) has a low likelihood of recovering function, though infrequently reversed remodelling has been described. The weakness of this approach is its poor performance to predict recovery in dysfunctional segments with preserved wall thickness. A second approach is low-dose dobutamine stress function CMR, yielding specificities (83%, range 70–95%) and sensitivities (74%, range 50–89%) similar to those of dobutamine echocardiography.[65] The third and clinically most used approach for

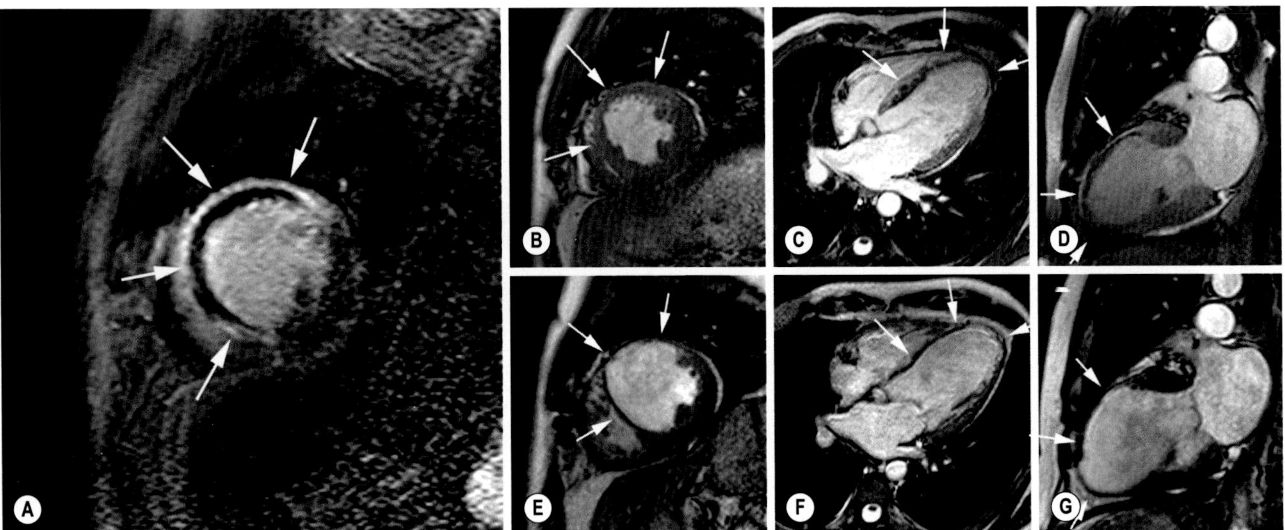

FIGURE 15-27 ■ Adverse ventricular remodelling post acute myocardial infarction. Patient with extensive anterior myocardial infarction. Short-axis LGE CMR (A) early post-infarction shows extensive transmural enhancement (arrows; segments 1, 2, 7, 8, 13–15, 17) with large zone of microvascular obstruction. Cine CMR early (B–D) and 6 months (E–G) post-infarction. Note the important wall thinning of the involved segments with aneurysm formation at 6-month follow-up (arrows, E–G). The end-diastolic volume increased from 257 mL at baseline to 432 mL at follow-up while the ejection fraction decreased from 36 to 18%.

viability imaging is LGE CMR. It is highly accurate and reproducible for sizing healed infarcts,[68] and is therefore routinely used to depict infarct-related myocardial scarring. Moreover LGE CMR is helpful for differentiating dilated cardiomyopathy from LV dysfunction related to CAD[69] and it has prognostic significance.[70] Myocardial LGE in dysfunctional segments in patients with stable CAD is associated with non-viability obtained by SPECT imaging and dobutamine echocardiography, while absence of LGE correlates with measures of viability, regardless of resting contractile function. In particular the transmural extent of LGE[11] determines the likelihood of improvement in contractility after revascularisation. In dysfunctional segments without LGE, 78% of segments improved contractility post-revascularisation, versus 2% of segments with a scar involving >75% of wall thickness. Though this technique yields an excellent sensitivity (95%, range 91–99%), specificity is low (45%, range 37–54%). Because none of the above approaches are perfect in predicting or excluding functional recovery after revascularisation, diagnostic accuracy can be improved using a combined approach. For example, viability imaging can be started with LGE CMR to determine presence and transmural extent of myocardial scarring. In patients presenting dysfunctional segments with intermediate grades of scar transmurality (i.e. 25–50%), the likelihood of recovery is uncertain. Additional low-dose dobutamine stress imaging makes it possible to determine whether these segments have contractility reserve. Moreover, use of the thickness of non-enhanced rim as determined by LGE imaging may provide additional value regarding viability.[71] A cut-off value of 3 mm for the non-enhanced rim was superior to end-diastolic wall thickness with a cut-off of 5.4 mm for viability assessment.

Cardiac resynchronisation therapy (CRT) has emerged as an effective therapy for heart failure.[72] Imaging has an increasingly important role in determining those patients that might benefit from CRT. The goals of imaging are threefold: (a) assessment of the degree of mechanical dyssynchrony, (b) myocardial scar imaging and (c) coronary venous imaging. Ventricular performance can be improved if the contraction of the different parts of the ventricle is synchronised. The degree of mechanical dyssynchrony can be quantified using conventional cine techniques as well as more advanced techniques such as myocardial tagging, displacement encoding with stimulated echoes (DENSE) and tissue velocity mapping, and can be considered valuable alternatives to other techniques such as tissue Doppler imaging (TDI). Secondly, correct placement of the CRT leads is crucial for improving mechanical dyssynchrony. Ventricular scar mapping can be achieved using LGE CMR, making it possible to determine the presence, location and extent of myocardial scarring. Finally, information regarding the coronary vein anatomy is important since this pathway is often used for CRT lead placement. Coronary vein anatomy is not only highly variable but also the veins may be affected by previous myocardial infarction. Cardiac CT is currently the preferred technique for imaging the coronary veins.[72] Finally, imaging is important in patients with cardiac or circulatory assist devices. These devices are increasingly used to support patients in cardiogenic shock (intra-aortic counterpulsation balloon pump) or to temporarily replace the function of the left ventricle awaiting a cardiac transplantation (ventricular assist devices) (Fig. 15-29).[73] Complications related to intra-aortic balloon pump include occlusion of the aortic branches causing ischaemia, aortic dissection and balloon rupture with gas embolisation. Complications related to ventricular assist devices include pneumothorax, haemothorax, postoperative haemorrhage in the pericardium of mediastinum, infection, obstruction or dislocation of the cannula, and mechanical failure.

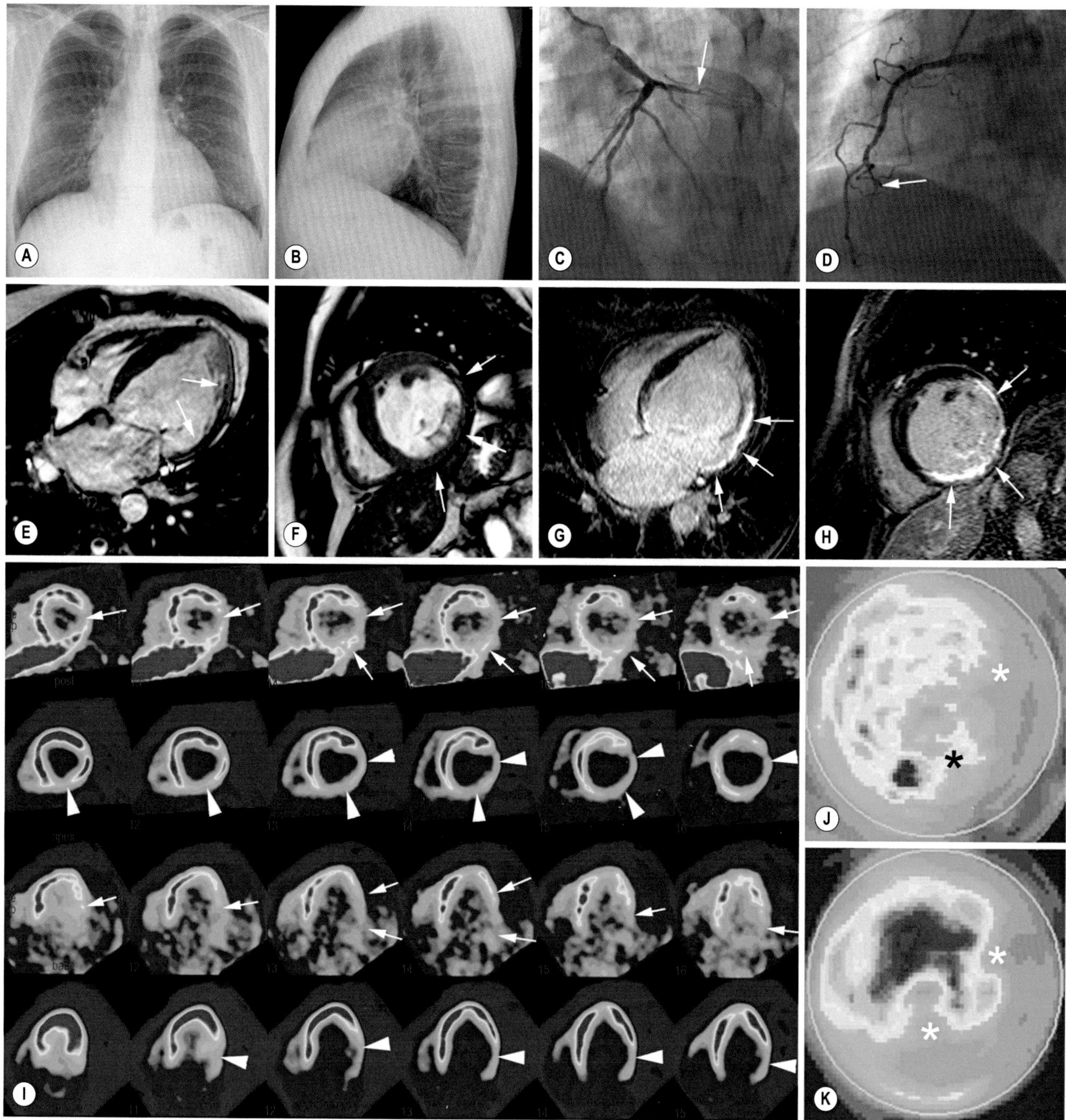

FIGURE 15-28 ■ **Viability imaging.** Viability imaging in 57-year-old patient presenting ischaemic cardiomyopathy and increasing dyspnoea (NYHA III). Chest film (A, B) shows moderate cardiomegaly with redistribution of the pulmonary vascularisation to the upper lung fields, reflecting increased pulmonary venous pressures. Coronary angiography shows complete occlusion of the proximal left circumflex coronary artery (arrow, C), and mid right coronary artery (arrow, D). Cine CMR in horizontal long axis (E) and short axis (F) shows severely dilated left ventricle (end-diastolic volume 453 mL, ejection fraction 36%) with severe thinning of the entire inferolateral wall (arrows, E, F). Presence of a severe mitral regurgitation due to mitral valve enlargement secondary to LV dilatation (regurgitant fraction 37%). LGE CMR shows presence of transmural enhancement in the inferolateral wall reflecting a healed extensive inferolateral myocardial infarction (arrows, G, H). PET imaging with perfusion imaging (NH_3 as tracer) and myocardial metabolism imaging (fluorodeoxyglucose (FDG) as metabolic tracer). Reconstructed slices in short axis and horizontal long axis (I), NH_3 (J) and FDG (K) polar maps. Presence of an extensive perfusion defect in the entire inferolateral wall (*, J) that matches perfectly with the lack of metabolism on FDG-PET (*, K). This match pattern reflects irreversibly damaged myocardium. The PET and CMR abnormalities correlate perfectly. (FDG/NH_3 PET courtesy of O. Gheysens, Department of Nuclear Medicine, UZ Leuven, Leuven, Belgium.)

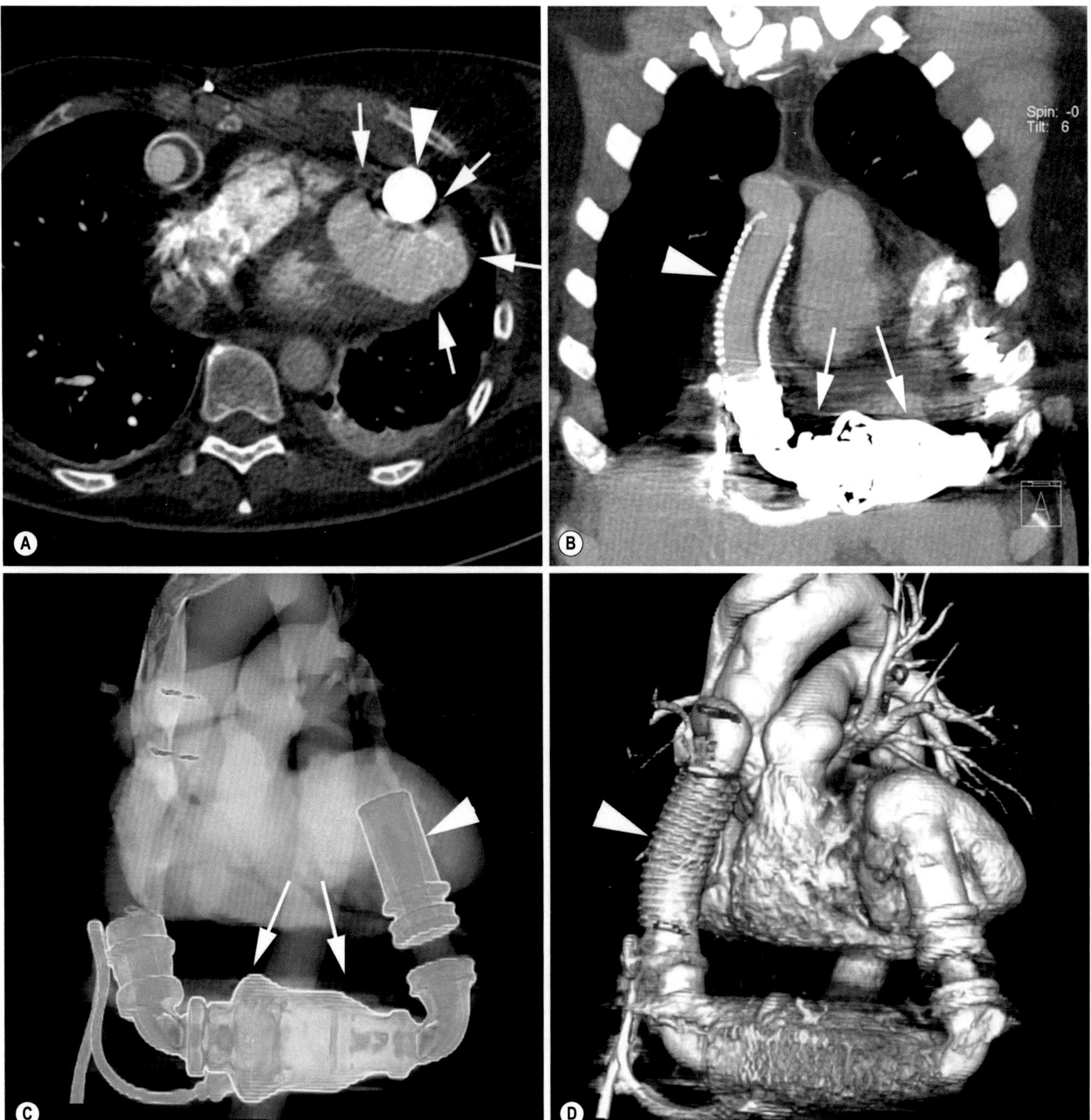

FIGURE 15-29 ■ **Left ventricular assist device.** A 45-year-old woman with history of extensive anterior myocardial infarction presenting with symptoms of heart failure. The patient received a left ventricular assist device (Heartmate II, Thoratec) awaiting cardiac transplantation. CCT with axial (A) and coronal (B) images, angiographic view (C) and volume-rendered view (D). Presence of wall thinning with extensive aneurysm formation in the LV apex (arrows, A). The inflow cannula is inserted into the LV apex (arrowhead, A, C). The pump is positioned beneath the heart (arrows, B, C). The outflow cannula with a graft conduit connects to the ascending aorta (arrowhead, B, D).

IMAGING OF COMPLICATIONS RELATED TO ISCHAEMIC HEART DISEASE

An acute myocardial infarction can cause a series of potentially lethal complications. Early detection is mandatory. In daily practice, echocardiography is readily available and can be performed bedside, while MRI and CT can provide complementary information in selected cases. Acute myocardial rupture in patients with extensive transmural myocardial necrosis is often lethal. The patient may survive if the rupture of the myocardium is contained by pericardial adhesions, forming a false aneurysm. A true aneurysm is formed if some myocardial elements are contained in the aneurysmal wall. False aneurysms can be differentiated from true aneurysms because they usually present a orifice smaller than the maximal internal diameter, whereas in true aneurysms

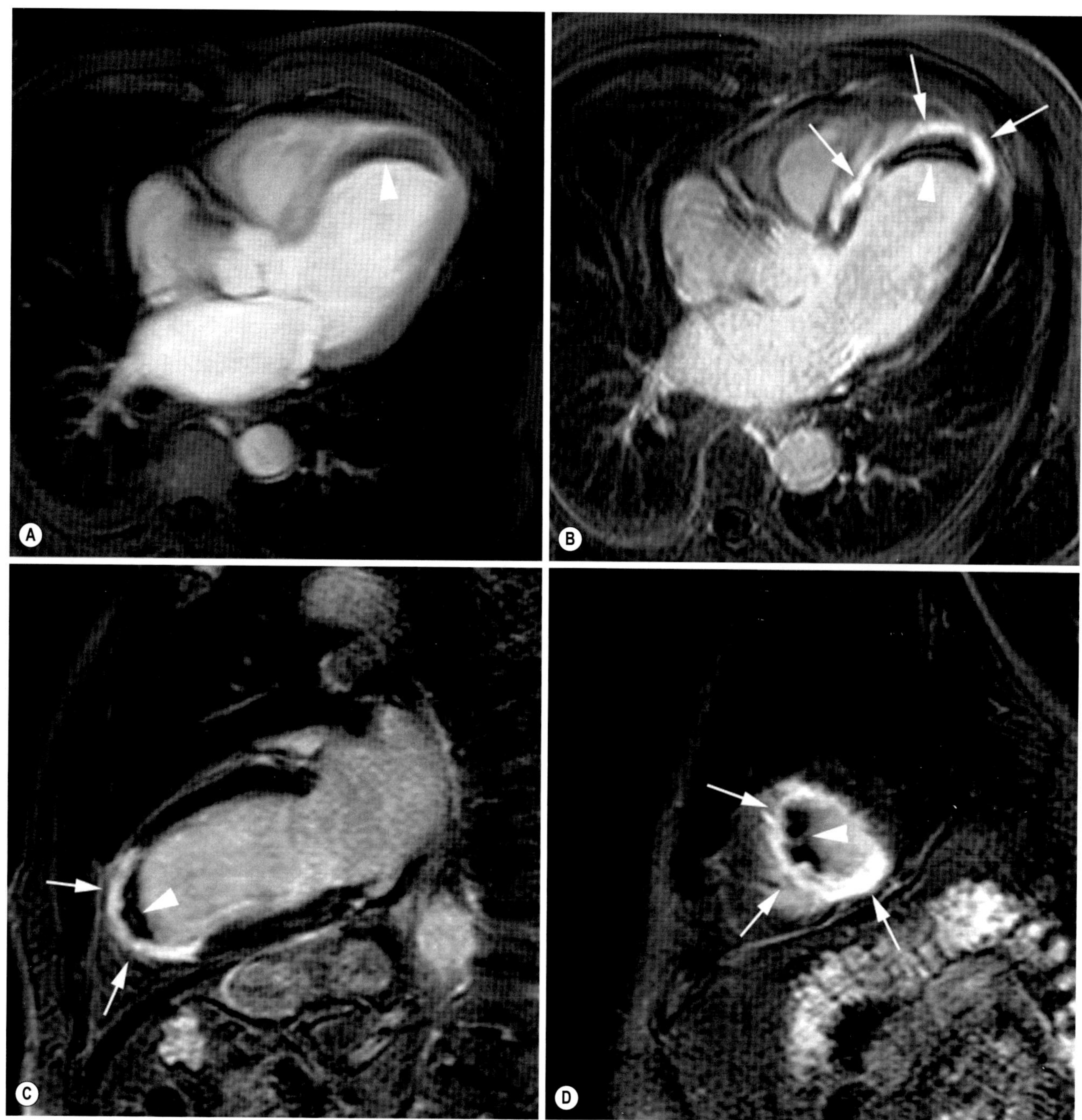

FIGURE 15-30 ■ **Thrombus formation post-infarction.** Contrast-enhanced inversion-recovery CMR early following contrast administration using a long inversion time (i.e. 500 ms) (A). LGE CMR in horizontal long axis (B), vertical long axis (C) and apical short axis (D). On early imaging, the myocardium is brightly hyperintense, and the blood pool is strongly enhanced. An intracavitary structure as a thrombus is visible as a hypointense structure (arrowhead, A). On LGE CMR the irreversibly damaged myocardium in the LAD perfusion territory (segments 7, 8, 13, 14, 17) is strongly enhanced (arrows, B–D) and the adjacent mural thrombus is well visible (arrowhead, B–D).

dimensions are similar. Moreover, pericardial enhancement is frequently found in false aneurysms while it rarely occurs in true aneurysms.[74]

Ventricular thrombus formation is a frequent complication following a myocardial infarction, and is not infrequently found in patients with ischaemic dilated cardiomyopathy. A thrombus is found in approximately 10% of patients with an anterior myocardial infarction (Fig. 15-30). The presence of an aneurysm predisposes to thrombus formation. Early thrombus detection is of paramount importance to avoid neurologic and peripheral embolic events, and to initiate anticoagulation therapy. Small-sized thrombi are easily missed by transthoracic echocardiography, in particular when located in the apex or when trapped in the endocardial trabeculations. CCT and CMR facilitates the diagnosis of thrombi, since the blood pool is enhanced by the injection of contrast material, thus improving the detection of

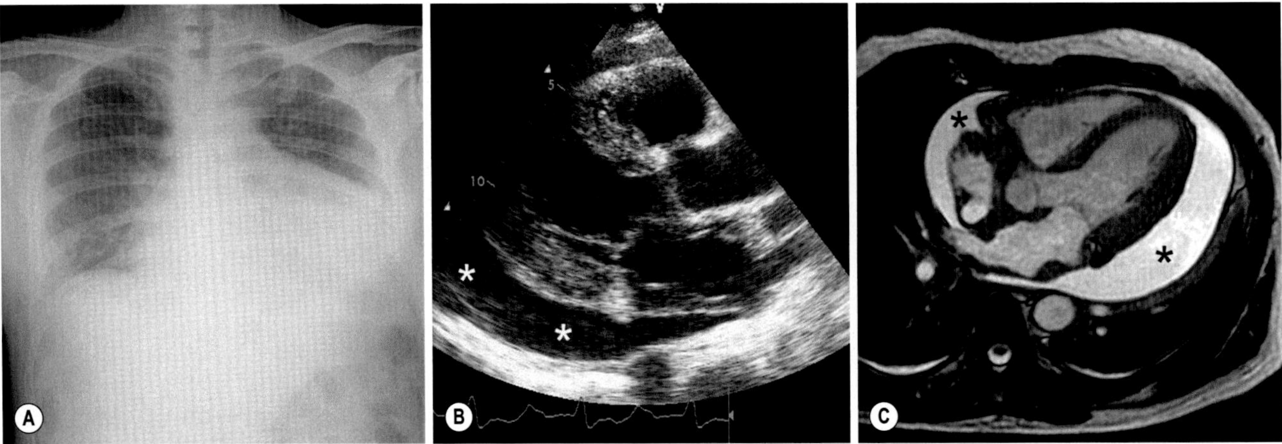

FIGURE 15-31 ■ Severe pericardial effusion. Chest radiograph (A), transthoracic echocardiography (B) and CMR (cine imaging)(C). Presence of severe cardiomegaly caused by lateral displacement of the left heart border. The abnormalities are caused by a moderate to severe pericardial effusion as clearly visible on cardiac ultrasound (*, B). CMR confirms the cardiac ultrasound findings (*, C). The majority of the pericardial effusion is left-sided located (maximal width 38 mm), explaining the chest film findings.

intraluminal masses such as thrombi. It could be said that thrombus detection by contrast-enhanced CMR is a free bonus since contrast agent administration is obligatory for infarct detection. It is advisable to always carefully inspect the cardiac cavities for possible thrombi.[52] Since thrombi appear hypointense on LGE CMR, differentiation with no-reflow zones in patients with an acute myocardial infarction may be challenging, especially for less experienced people. Besides a difference in location (intramyocardial versus intraluminal), no-reflow zones become smaller over time, whereas thrombi remain usually constant. Use of a longer inversion time (e.g. 500 ms) facilitates depiction of thrombi in the vicinity of normal myocardium.

Pericardial inflammation can occur early post-infarction and is typically found in transmural infarctions. This condition should be differentiated from late post-infarction pericarditis (Dressler's syndrome). Amongst the different cardiac imaging techniques, CMR has become one of the preferential techniques for demonstrating associated pericardial pathology in infarct patients.[75] The presence, location and severity of pericardial effusion can be well demonstrated by cine imaging (Fig. 15-31). In the presence of pericardial inflammation, the pericardial layers strongly enhance following contrast administration. The LGE CMR technique is very well fitted for this purpose (Fig. 15-25). Recent studies have shown that residual/persistent inflammation in patients suspected of constrictive pericarditis is characterised by pericardial enhancement, whereas in fibrotic end stages the pericardium does not enhance any longer. Real-time cine imaging is useful for evaluating the impact of the thickened pericardial layers on ventricular filling. In the case of pericardial constriction, the ventricular interdependence (or coupling) is increased. The hallmark is an inspiratory septal flattening/inversion of the ventricular septum during early ventricular filling, and the presence/absence can be easily evaluated by real-time cine imaging. Mitral valve leakage can be caused by valve ring dilatation secondary to adverse ventricular remodelling post-infarction and/or infarction of the papillary muscle(s). High spatial resolution 3D LGE CMR improves detection of papillary infarction.[76] This and other studies have shown that presence of necrosis of both papillary muscles is related to mitral regurgitation.[77]

PROGNOSIS ASSESSMENT IN ISCHAEMIC HEART DISEASE

In asymptomatic patients, as well as in patients with suspected or known CAD, risk assessment and prediction of future cardiac events are important. Traditional risk assessment classifies patients as high risk, intermediate risk or low risk. Although this classification is of great help in adapting or intensifying lifestyle (primary prevention) or medication (e.g. statins), most high-risk patients will never experience a cardiac event, while patients belonging to the intermediate- or low-risk group are not event-free, emphasising the need to improve prognosis assessment. Well known, well validated and widely used is coronary calcium score, reflecting the atherosclerotic burden in a patient. In asymptomatic patients without evidence of CAD, coronary calcium scoring adds prognostic information beyond clinical risk factors.[78] In particular, asymptomatic adults belonging to the intermediate-risk group (i.e. 10 to 20% 10-year risk of events) can be 'up'- or 'down'-graded, depending upon their Agatston calcium score.

In symptomatic patients suspected of CAD, the severity of CAD and/or presence of myocardial ischaemia are important prognosticators for future events.[37,79] It should be emphasised that a negative coronary calcium score in symptomatic patients does not exclude obstructive CAD and is associated with increased cardiovascular events.[80] Moreover, the severity of CAD assessed by CCT predicts, together with LV ejection fraction, all-cause mortality.[37] In the absence of myocardial ischaemia on SPECT, future cardiac events are highly unlikely.[79] There is also cumulating evidence that CMR is important in the management of cardiovascular disease.[3,81–84] The risk of future events is increased when resting LV ejection fraction is impaired (EF < 40%), LV hypertrophy is present (defined as LV wall thickness ≥12 mm or LV mass >96 g/m^2 in men and >77 g/m^2 in women), when the patient exhibits a positive stress perfusion or stress dobutamine test or when myocardial (hyper)-enhancement is found on LGE CMR. In a recent study by Bingham and Hachamovitch 908 consecutive patients with suspicion of CAD and/or myocardial ischaemia underwent a multiparametric CMR exam including assessment of LV volume/mass/function, stress perfusion, myocardial enhancement and aortic flow.[3] A normal study yielded a low risk of cardiac events, whereas all CMR parameters had incremental values over pre-CMR data for prediction of adverse events.

In patients without a history of myocardial infarction but a clinical suspicion of CAD, evidence of ischaemia-related myocardial scarring carries an increased risk for future major adverse cardiac events (MACE) independent of the extent of LGE.[85–87] In patients presenting an ACS in whom myocardial infarction is excluded by cardiac biomarkers and ECG, stress perfusion MRI is an accurate and independent predictor of future cardiac events.[88] Moreover, a large number of MRI studies have shown that several parameters other than infarct size are important in predicting adverse remodelling and patient outcome following an acute myocardial infarct.[89] These include microvascular obstruction, post-infarction myocardial haemorrhage and myocardial salvage.[56,57,61,62,89]

In ischaemic cardiomyopathy patients, the extent of myocardial enhancement is a strong and independent predictor of all-cause mortality/cardiac transplantation, even in the presence of traditional well-known prognosticators such as ejection fraction, congestive heart failure and age.[70] Gerber and colleagues recently showed improved outcome in patients with complete revascularisation of viable myocardium compared to those with no or incomplete revascularisation, stressing the importance of correct characterisation of the dysfunctional myocardium.[90]

ROLE OF CONVENTIONAL CHEST RADIOGRAPHY IN ISCHAEMIC HEART DISEASE

Even though 'advanced' imaging techniques are nowadays central in the diagnosis of heart diseases, the contribution of conventional chest radiography in evaluating IHD patients should not be neglected. Valuable information can be provided regarding the cardiac size, enlargement of a specific cardiac chamber or pulmonary filling status, and the chest X-ray is of great help to exclude pulmonary, pleural or aortic disease such as aortic aneurysm. In cardiac-ill patients, bedside radiographs are easily obtainable. Left-sided cardiac decompensation in patients with recent myocardial infarction or ischaemic cardiomyopathy leads to an apical redistribution of pulmonary vascularisation, onset of pulmonary interstitial and alveolar oedema and pleural effusion. Chest radiographs makes it possible to closely monitor the effects of the installed heart failure therapy, and to demonstrate concomitant pulmonary disease such as infection or ARDS. It also serves to check the correct positioning of devices such as endotracheal tube, central venous catheters, pulmonary artery catheters, and pacing leads.[73] Infarct-related complications, such as pericardial effusion/haematoma or aneurysm formation, can be detected on chest CXRs, though echocardiography, CMR and CCT are definitely superior (Fig. 15-31).

DIFFERENTIAL DIAGNOSIS IN ISCHAEMIC HEART DISEASE

In patients suspected of having an ACS, the current ACC/AHA/UA/STEMI guidelines recommend a classification into (1) 'definite' ACS, (2) 'possible' ACS, (3) chronic stable CAD or (4) non-cardiac cause of chest pain.[91] This classification is based on the patient's history, physical examination, 12-lead ECG and initial cardiac biomarkers. In patients with normal/non-diagnostic ECG or normal initial biomarkers, however, the question arises as to whether the symptoms arise from unstable angina pectoris, which is characterised by ischaemia without myocardial damage to release detectable quantities of markers of myocardial injury. Those patients with 'possible' ACS are usually admitted for observation 12 h or more from symptom onset and usually stress testing is performed to provide evidence of myocardial ischaemia. As an alternative in these patients, CCT is recommended to demonstrate or exclude significant CAD in those with low or intermediate pretest probability of CAD, while the role of CCT for patients with a high pretest likelihood is uncertain.[14] A negative CCT, defined as no CAD or stenosis < 50%, yields an excellent negative predictive value for ACS or MACE,[92,93] while in those patients having a positive CCT, ischaemia testing can be subsequently performed. CCT is also of interest for ruling out other causes of chest pain related to pathology of the pulmonary arteries (i.e. pulmonary embolism) and thoracic aorta (i.e. aortic dissection). This so-called *triple rule-out* approach needs an adaptation of contrast medium administration to assure sufficient enhancement of pulmonary arteries, coronary arteries and thoracic aorta during imaging.[94] Though promising, the value of triple rule-out CCT in the emergency department is still uncertain.[15]

In a small but important group of patients presenting with chest pain and elevated cardiac biomarkers, subsequent coronary angiography reveals normal or non-flow limiting CAD, questioning what is the underlying cause of the clinical presentation, with a number of possible causes such a non-cardiac aetiologies, myocardial infarction with a recanalised coronary artery and acute myocarditis.[95,96] In these patients CMR can be recommended. If patients have experienced an ischaemic event, T2-weighted imaging will show myocardial oedema while myocardial enhancement on LGE CMR is suggestive of myocardial necrosis and the functional consequences can be evaluated with cine imaging. Not infrequently, smaller coronary artery branches that were initially not recognised on coronary angiography are

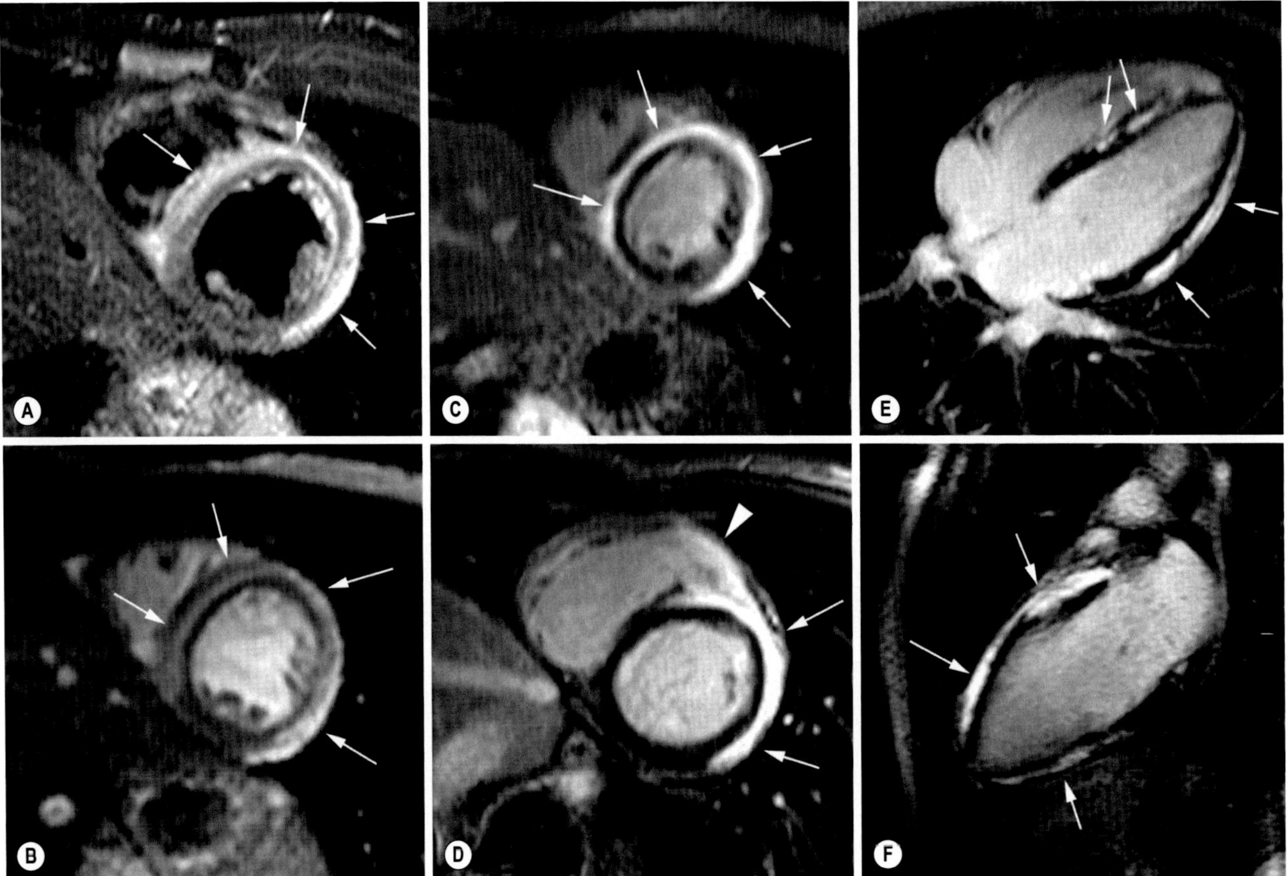

FIGURE 15-32 ■ **Fulminant myocarditis.** A 17-year-old man admitted with severe respiratory-related retrosternal chest pain. Increased serum biomarkers (troponin I: 83 μg/L). Coronary angiography shows normal coronary arteries. Short-axis T2-weighted CMR (A). Short-axis cine imaging post-contrast administration (B). LGE CMR in cardiac short axis (C, D), horizontal long axis (E) and vertical long axis (F). Presence of diffuse subepicardially located myocardial oedema (arrows, A). LGE CMR shows strong subepicardial enhancement in LV (arrows, C, D, F, G), and focal strong enhancement in RV (arrowhead, D). The subepicardial enhancement is nicely visible on cine imaging post-contrast administration (arrows, B). CMR findings of severe form of acute myocarditis. Myocardial biopsy shows lymphohistiocytic infilrate.

affected. The same CMR approach is of great help in depicting patients with acute myocarditis. These patients show a different pattern of myocardial enhancement on LGE CMR than acute myocardial infarction patients, i.e. midwall/subepicardial enhancement instead of subendocardial enhancement with variable transmural spread (Fig. 15-32). Also in patients with tako-tsubo cardiomyopathy (also called stress cardiomyopathy), CMR is helpful in depicting the reversible nature of cardiac abnormalities consisting of functional abnormalities, myocardial oedema on T2-weighted imaging and lack of myocardial enhancement on LGE CMR.[97] It typically occurs in elderly women and is initiated or related to emotional stress. Most commonly, the apical half of the left ventricle is affected, not respecting a coronary artery perfusion territory. Though patients may need cardiac support during the acute phase, abnormalities are usually rapidly and completely reversible. In patients with heart failure related to dilated cardiomyopathy, the pattern of myocardial enhancement on LGE CMR makes it possible to differentiate between CAD and non-CAD causes of ventricular dilatation and dysfunction.[98]

REFERENCES

1. Lockie T, Nagel E, Redwood S, Plein S. The use of cardiovascular magnetic resonance imaging in acute coronary syndromes. Circulation 2009;119:1671–81.
2. Kim HW, Farzaneh A, Kim RJ. Cardiovascular magnetic resonance in patients with myocardial infarction. Current and emerging applications. J Am Coll Cardiol 2010;55:1–16.
3. Bingham SE, Hachamovitch R. Incremental prognostic significance of combined cardiac magnetic resonance imaging, adenosine stress perfusion, delayed enhancement, and left ventricular function over pre-imaging information for the prediction of adverse events. Circulation 2011;123:1509–18.
4. Reimer KA, Jennings RB. The wavefront progression of myocardial ischemic cell death. II. Transmural progression of necrosis within the framework of ischemic bed size (myocardium at risk) and collateral flow. Lab Invest 1970;40:633–44.
5. Yellon DM, Hausenloy DJ. Myocardial reperfusion injury. N Engl J Med 2007;357:1121–35.
6. Thygesen K, Alpert JS, White HD; on behalf of the Joint ESC/ACCF/AHA/WHF Task Force for the Redefinition of Myocardial Infarction. Universal definition of myocardial infarction. Circulation 2007;116:2634–53.
7. Braunwald E, Kloner RA. The stunned myocardium: prolonged, postischaemic ventricular dysfunction. Circulation 1982;66:1146–9.
8. Bax JJ, Visser FC, Poldermans D, et al. Time course of functional recovery of stunned and hibernating segments after surgical revascularization. Circulation 2001;104:I314–18.

9. Bondarenko O, Beek AM, Twisk JW, et al. Time course of functional recovery after revascularization of hibernating myocardium: a contrast-enhanced cardiovascular magnetic resonance study. Eur Heart J 2008;29:2000–5.
10. Rahimtoola SH. The hibernating myocardium. Am Heart J 1989;117:211–20.
11. Kim RJ, Wu E, Rafael A, et al. The use of contrast-enhanced magnetic resonance imaging to identify reversible myocardial dysfunction. N Engl J Med 2000;343:1445–53.
12. Pfisterer ME, Zellweger MJ, Gersh BJ. Management of stable coronary artery disease. Lancet 2010;375:763–72.
13. Achenbach S, Raggi P. Imaging of coronary atherosclerosis by computed tomography. Eur Heart J 2010;31:1442–8.
14. Taylor AJ, Cerqueira M, Hodgson J, et al. ACCF/SCCT/ACR/AHA /ASE/ASNC/SCAI/SCMR 2010 Appropriate Use Criteria for Cardiac Computed Tomography. A Report of the American College of Cardiovascular Foundation Appropriate Use Criteria Task Force, the Society of Cardiovascular Computed Tomography, the American College of Radiology, the American Heart Association, the American Society of Echocardiography, the American Society of Nuclear Cardiology, the Society for Cardiovascular Angiography and Interventions, and the Society for Cardiovascular Magnetic Resonance. Circulation 2010;122:e525–55.
15. Mark DB, Berman DS, Budoff MJ, et al. ACCF/ACR/AHA/NASCI/SAIP/SCAI/SCCT 2010 expert consensus document on coronary computed tomographic angiography. A report of the American College of Cardiology Foundation Task Force on Expert Consensus Documents. Circulation 2010;121:2509–43.
16. Singh S, Kalra MK, Gilman MD, et al. Adaptive statistical iterative reconstruction technique for radiation dose reduction in chest CT: a pilot study. Radiology 2011;259:565–73.
17. Datta J, White CS, Gilkeson RC, et al. Anomalous coronary arteries in adults: depiction at multi-detector row CT angiography. Radiology 2005;235:812–18.
18. Leschka S, Koepfli P, Husmann L, et al. Myocardial bridging: depiction rate and morphology at CT coronary angiography—comparison with conventional coronary angiography. Radiology 2008;246:754–62.
19. Bogaert J, Rademakers FE. Regional nonuniformity of the normal adult human left ventricle. A 3D MR myocardial tagging study. Am J Physiol 2001;280:H610–20.
20. Cerqueira MD, Weissman NJ, Dilsizian V, et al. Standardized myocardial segmentation and nomenclature for tomographic imaging of the heart: a statement for healthcare professionals from the Cardiac Imaging Committee of the Council on Clinical Cardiology of the American Heart Association. Circulation 2002;105:539–42.
21. Jurcut R, Pappas CJ, Masci PG, et al. Detection of regional myocardial dysfunction in patients with acute myocardial infarction using velocity vector imaging. J Am Soc Echocardiogr 2008; 21:879–86.
22. Bogaert J, Bosmans H, Maes A, et al. Remote myocardial dysfunction after acute anterior myocardial infarction: impact of left ventricular shape on regional function. A magnetic resonance myocardial tagging study. J Am Coll Cardiol 2000;35:1525–34.
23. Korosoglou G, Futterer S, Humpert PM, et al. Strain-encoded cardiac MR during high-dose dobutamine stress testing: comparison to cine imaging and to myocardial tagging. J Magn Reson Imaging 2009;29:1053–61.
24. Maffei E, Messalli G, Martini C, et al. Left and right ventricle assessment with cardiac CT: validation study vs. cardiac MR. Eur Radiol 2012;22(5):1041–9.
25. Kim S-J, Kim I-J, Kim Y-S, Kim Y-K. Gated blood pool SPECT for measurement of left ventricular volumes and left ventricular ejection fraction: comparison of 8 and 16 frame gated blood pool SPECT. Int J Cardiovasc Imaging 2005;21:261–6.
26. Boden WE, O'Rourke RA, Teo KK, et al. for the COURAGE Trial Research Group. Optimal medical therapy with or without PCI for stable coronary disease. N Engl J Med 2007;356:1503–16.
27. BARI 2D Study Group, Frye RL, August P, Brooks MM, et al. A randomized trial of therapies for type 2 diabetes and coronary artery disease. N Engl J Med 2009;360:2503–15.
28. Tonino PA, De Bruyne B, Pijls NH, et al. Fractional flow reserve versus angiography for guiding percutaneous coronary intervention. N Engl J Med 2009;360:213–24.
29. Gould KL. Does coronary flow trump coronary anatomy? J Am Coll Cardiol Img 2009;2:1009–23.
30. Hachamovitch R, Hayes SW, Friedman JD, et al. Comparison of the short-term survival benefit associated with revascularization compared with medical therapy in patients with no prior coronary artery disease undergoing stress myocardial perfusion single photon emission computed tomography. Circulation 2003;107:2900–7.
31. Blech GJW, De Bruyne B, Pijls NJ, et al. Fractional flow reserve to determine the appropriateness of angioplasty in moderate coronary stenosis. A randomized trial. Circulation 2001;103: 2928–34.
32. Greenwood JP, Maredia N, Younger JF, et al. Cardiovascular magnetic resonance and single-photon emission computed tomography for diagnosis of coronary heart disease (CE-MARC): a prospective trial. Lancet 2012;379:453–60.
33. Rocha-Filho JA, Blankstein R, Shturman LD, et al. Incremental value of adenosine-induced stress myocardial perfusion imaging with dual-source CT at cardiac CT angiography. Radiology 2010;254:410–19.
34. George RT, Arbab-Zadeh A, Cerci RJ, et al. Diagnostic performance of combined noninvasive coronary angiography and myocardial perfusion imaging using 320-MDCT: the CT angiography and perfusion methods of the CORE320 multicenter multinational diagnostic study. AJR Am J Roentgenol 2011;197:829–37.
35. Dvorak RA, Brown RKJ, Corbett JR. Interpretation of SPECT/CT myocardial perfusion images: common artifacts and quality control techniques. Radiographics 2011;31:2041–57.
36. Di Carli MF, Murthy VL. Cardiac PET/CT for the evaluation of known or suspected coronary artery disease. Radiographics 2011;31:1239–54.
37. Iskandrian S, Iskandrian AE. Risk assessment using single-photon emission computed tomographic technetium-99m sestamibi imaging. J Am Coll Cardiol 1999;32:57–62.
38. Blankstein R, Di Carli MF. Integration of coronary anatomy and myocardial perfusion imaging. Nat Rev Cardiol 2010;7:226–36.
39. Nandalur KR, Dwamena BA, Choudhri AF, et al. Diagnostic performance of stress cardiac magnetic resonance imaging in the detection of coronary artery disease. A meta-analysis. J Am Coll Cardiol 2007;50:1343–53.
40. Schwitter J, Wacker CM, Van Rossum AC, et al. MR-IMPACT: comparison of perfusion-cardiac magnetic resonance with single-photon emission computed tomography for the detection of coronary artery disease in a multicentre, multivendor, randomized trial. Eur Heart J 2008;29:480–9.
41. Greenwood JP, Maredia N, Younger JF, et al. Cardiovascular magnetic resonance and single-photon emission computed tomography for diagnosis of coronary heart disease (CE-MARC): a prospective trial. Lancet 2012;379:453–60.
42. Hsu LY, Ingkanisorn WP, Kellman P, et al. Quantitative myocardial infarction on delayed enhancement MRI. Part II: clinical application of an automated feature analysis and combined thresholding infarct sizing algorithm. J Magn Reson Imaging 2006;23:309–14.
43. Wang Y, Qin L, Shi X, et al. Adenosine-stress dynamic myocardial perfusion imaging with second-generation dual-source CT: comparison with conventional catheter coronary angiography and SPECT nuclear myocardial perfusion imaging. AJR Am J Roentgenol 2012;198:521–9.
44. Wahl A, Paetsch I, Gollesch A, et al. Safety and feasibility of high-dose dobutamine-atropine stress cardiovascular magnetic resonance for diagnosis of myocardial ischaemia: experience in 1000 consecutive patients. Eur Heart J 2004;25:1230–6.
45. Wagner A, Mahrholdt H, Holly TA, et al. Contrast-enhanced MRI and routine single photon emission computed tomography (SPECT) perfusion imaging for detection of subendocardial myocardial infarcts: an imaging study. Lancet 2003;361:374–9.
46. Vliegenthart R, Henzler T, Moscariello A, et al. CT of coronary heart disease: part I, CT of myocardial infarction, ischemia, and viability. AJR Am J Roentgenol 2012;198:531–47.
47. Aletras AH, Tilak GS, Natanzon A, et al. Retrospective determination of the area at risk for reperfused acute myocardial infarction with T2-weighted cardiac magnetic resonance imaging. Histopathological and displacement encoding with stimulated echoes (DENSE) functional validations. Circulation 2006;113:1865–70.
48. Friedrich MG. Myocardial edema—a new clinical entity? Nat Rev Cardiol 2010;7:292–6.

49. Kellman P, Dyke CK, Aletras AH, et al. Artifact suppression in imaging of myocardial infarction using B1-weighted phased-array combined phase-sensitive inversion recovery dagger. Magn Reson Med 2004;51:408–12.
50. Ibrahim T, Hackl T, Nekolla SG, et al. Acute myocardial infarction: serial cardiac MR imaging shows a decrease in delayed enhancement of the myocardium during the 1st week after reperfusion. Radiology 2010;254:88–97.
51. Mahrholdt H, Wagner A, Judd RM, et al. Delayed enhancement cardiovascular magnetic resonance assessment of non-ischaemic cardiomyopathies. Eur Heart J 2005;26:1461–74.
52. Mollet NR, Dymarkowski S, Volders W, et al. Visualization of ventricular thrombi with contrast-enhanced magnetic resonance imaging in patients with ischaemic heart disease. Circulation 2002;106:2873–6.
53. Taylor AM, Dymarkowski S, Verbeken E, Bogaert J. Detection of pericardial inflammation with late-enhancement cardiac magnetic resonance imaging: initial results. Eur Radiol 2006;16:569–74.
54. Francone M, Bucciarelli-Ducci C, Carbone I, et al. Impact of primary coronary angioplasty delay on myocardial salvage, infarct size, and microvascular damage in patients with ST-segment elevation myocardial infarction. Insight from cardiovascular magnetic resonance. J Am Coll Cardiol 2009;54:2145–53.
55. Eitel I, Desch S, Fuernau G, et al. Prognostic significance and determinants of myocardial salvage assessed by cardiovascular magnetic resonance in acute reperfused myocardial infarction. J Am Coll Cardiol 2010;55:2470–9.
56. Masci PG, Ganame J, Strata E, et al. Myocardial salvage by CMR correlates with LV remodeling and early ST-segment resolution in acute myocardial infarction. J Am Coll Cardiol Img 2010;3: 45–51.
57. Wu E, Ortiz JT, Tejedor P, et al. Infarct size by contrast enhanced cardiac magnetic resonance is a stronger predictor of outcomes than left ventricular ejection fraction or end-systolic volume index: prospective cohort study. Heart 2008;94:730–6.
58. Fuster V, Sanz J, Viles-Gonzalez JF, Rajagopalan S. The utility of magnetic resonance imaging in cardiac tissue regeneration trials. Nat Clin Pract Cardiovasc Med 2006;3(Suppl 1):S2–7.
59. Tarantini G, Cacciavillani L, Corbetti F, et al. Duration of ischemia is a major determinant of transmurality and severe microvascular obstruction after primary angioplasty. A study performed with contrast-enhanced magnetic resonance. J Am Coll Cardiol 2006; 46:1229–35.
60. Niccoli G, Burzotta F, Galiuto L, Crea F. Myocardial no-reflow in humans. J Am Coll Cardiol 2009;54:281–92.
61. Hombach V, Grebe O, Merkle N, et al. Sequelae of acute myocardial infarction regarding cardiac structure and function and their prognostic significance as assessed by magnetic resonance imaging. Eur Heart J 2005;26:549–57.
62. Ganame J, Messalli G, Dymarkowski S, et al. Impact of myocardial hemorrhage on left ventricular function and remodelling in patients with reperfused acute myocardial infarction. Eur Heart J 2009; 30:662–70.
63. Masci PG, Francone M, Desmet W, et al. Right ventricular ischemic injury in patients with acute ST-segment elevation myocardial infarction. Characterization with cardiovascular magnetic resonance. Circulation 2010;122:1405–12.
64. Gheorghiade M, Sopko G, De Luca L, et al. Navigating the crossroads of coronary artery disease and heart failure. Circulation 2006;114:1202–13.
65. Schinkel AF, Bax JJ, Poldermans D, et al. Hibernating myocardium: diagnosis and patient outcomes. Curr Probl Cardiol 2007;32: 375–410.
66. Bottomley PA, Wu KC, Gerstenblith G, et al. Reduced myocardial creatine kinase flux in human myocardial infarction. An in vivo phosphorus magnetic spectroscopy study. Circulation 2009;119: 1918–24.
67. Baer FM, Voth E, Schneider C, et al. Comparison of low-dose dobutamine-gradient-echo magnetic resonance imaging and positron emission tomography with [18F]fluorodeoxyglucose in patients with chronic coronary artery disease. A functional and morphological approach to the detection of residual myocardial viability. Circulation 1995;91:1006–15.
68. Mahrholdt H, Wagner A, Holly TA, et al. Reproducibility of chronic infarct size measurement by contrast-enhanced magnetic resonance imaging. Circulation 2002;106:2322–7.
69. McCrohon JA, Moon JCC, Prasad SK, et al. Differentiation of heart failure related to dilated cardiomyopathy and coronary artery disease using gadolinium-enhanced cardiovascular magnetic resonance. Circulation 2003;108:54–9.
70. Cheong BYC, Muthupillai R, Wilson JM, et al. Prognostic significance of delayed-enhancement magnetic resonance imaging. Survival of 857 patients with and without left ventricular dysfunction. Circulation 2009;120:2069–76.
71. Kühl HP, van der Weerdt A, Beek A, et al. Relation of end-diastolic wall thickness and the residual rim of viable myocardium by magnetic resonance imaging to myocardial viability assessed by fluorine-18 deoxyglucose positron emission tomography. Am J Cardiol 2006;97:452–7.
72. Al Jaroudi W, Chen J, Jaber WA, et al. Nonechocardiographic imaging in evaluation for cardiac resynchronization therapy. Circ Cardiovasc Imaging 2011;4:334–43.
73. Godoy MCB, Leitman BS, de Groot PM, et al. Chest radiography in the ICU: part 2, evaluation of cardiovascular lines and other devices. AJR Am J Roentgenol 2012;198:572–81.
74. Konen E, Merchant N, Gutierrez C, et al. True versus false left ventricular aneurysm: differentiation with MR imaging—initial experience. Radiology 2005;236:65–70.
75. Bogaert J, Francone M. Cardiovascular magnetic resonance in pericardial diseases. J Cardiovasc Magn Reson 2009;11:14.
76. Peters DC, Appelbaum EA, Nezafat R, et al. Left ventricular infarct size, peri-infarct zone, and papillary scar measurements: a comparison of high-resolution 3D and conventional 2D late gadolinium enhancement cardiac MRI. J Magn Reson Imaging 2009; 30:794–800.
77. Okayama S, Uemara S, Soeda T, et al. Clinical significance of papillary muscle late enhancement detected via cardiac magnetic resonance imaging in patients with single old myocardial infarction. Int J Cardiol 2011;146:73–9.
78. Detrano R, Guerci AD, Carr JJ, et al. Coronary calcium as a predictor of coronary events in four racial or ethnic groups. N Engl J Med 2008;358:1336–45.
79. Chow BJW, Small G, Yam Y, et al. Incremental prognostic value of cardiac computed tomography in coronary artery disease using CONFORM. COroNary computed tomography angiography evaluation for clinical outcomes: an inteRnational multicenter registry. Circ Cardiovasc Imaging 2011;4:463–72.
80. Villines TC, Hulten EA, Shaw LJ, et al. Prevalence and severity of coronary artery disease and adverse events among symptomatic patients with coronary artery calcification scores of zero undergoing coronary computed tomography angiography. J Am Coll Cardiol 2011;58:2533–40.
81. Flett AS, Westwood MA, Davies LC, et al. The prognostic implications of cardiovascular magnetic resonance. Circ Cardiovasc Imaging 2009;2:243–50.
82. Walsh TF, Dall'Armellina E, Chughtai H, et al. Adverse effect of increased left ventricular wall thickness on five year outcomes of patients with negative dobutamine stress. J Cardiovasc Magn Reson 2009;11:25.
83. Bodi V, Sanchis J, Lopez-Lereu MP, et al. Prognostic value of dipyridamole stress cardiovascular magnetic resonance imaging in patients with known or suspected coronary artery disease. J Am Coll Cardiol 2007;50:1174–9.
84. Bodi V, Husser O, Sanchi J, et al. Prognostic implications of dipyridamole cardiac MR imaging: a prospective multicenter registry. Radiology 2012;262:91–100.
85. Kwong RY, Chan AK, Brown KA, et al. Impact of unrecognized myocardial scar detected by cardiac magnetic resonance imaging on event-free survival in patients presenting with signs or symptoms or coronary artery disease. Circulation 2006;113:2733–43.
86. Kwong RY, Sattar H, Wu H, et al. Incidence and prognositic implication of unrecognized myocardial scar characterized by cardiac magnetic resonance in diabetic patients without clinical evidence of myocardial infarction. Circulation 2008;118: 1011–20.
87. Steel K, Broderick R, Gandla V, et al. Complementary prognostic values of stress myocardial perfusion and late gadolinium enhancement imaging by cardiac magnetic resonance in patients with known or suspected coronary artery disease. Circulation 2009;120: 1390–400.
88. Ingkanisorn WP, Kwong RY, Bohme NS, et al. Prognosis of negative adenosine stress magnetic resonance in patients presenting to

an emergency department with chest pain. J Am Coll Cardiol 2006;47:1427–32.
89. Dall'Armellina E, Karamitsos TD, Neubauer S, Choudbury RP. CMR for characterization of the myocardium in acute coronary syndromes. Nat Rev Cardiol 2010;7:624–36.
90. Gerber BL, Rousseau MF, Ahn SA, et al. Prognostic value of myocardial viability by delayed enhancement magnetic resonance in patients with coronary artery disease and low ejection fraction: impact of revascularization therapy. J Am Coll Cardiol 2012;59: 825–35.
91. Anderson JL, Adams CD, Antman EM, et al. ACC/AHA 2007 guidelines for the management of patients with unstable angina/ non ST-elevation myocardial infarction: a report of the American College of Cardiology/American Heart Association Task Force on Practice Guidelines for the Management of Patients with Unstable Angina/Non ST-Elevation Myocardial Infarction): developed in collaboration with the American College of Emergency Physicians, the Society for Cardiovascular Angiography and Interventions, and the Society of Thoracic Surgeons: endorsed by the American Association of Cardiovascular and Pulmonary Rehabilitation and the Society for Academic Emergency Medicine. Circulation 2007;116: e148–304.
92. Hoffmann U, Nagurney JT, Moselewski F, et al. Coronary multidetector computed tomography in the assessment of patients with acute chest pain. Circulation 2006;114:2251–60.
93. Rubinshtein R, Halon DA, Gaspar T, et al. Usefulness of 64-slice cardiac computed tomographic angiography for diagnosing acute coronary syndromes and predicting clinical outcome in emergency department patients with chest pain of uncertain origin. Circulation 2007;115:1762–8.
94. Vrachliotis TG, Bis KG, Haidary A, et al. Atypical chest pain: coronary, aortic, and pulmonary vasculature enhancement at biphasic single-injection 64-section CT angiography. Radiology 2007; 243:368–76.
95. Arai AE. Using magnetic resonance imaging to characterize recent myocardial injury: utility in acute coronary syndrome and other clinical scenarios. Circulation 2008;118:795–6.
96. Assomull RG, Lyne JC, Keenan N, et al. The role of cardiovascular magnetic resonance in patients presenting with chest pain, raised troponins, and unobstructed coronary arteries. Eur Heart J 2007; 28:1242–9.
97. Eitel I, von Knobelsdorff-Brenkenhoff F, Bernhardt P, et al. Clinical characteristics and cardiovascular magnetic resonance findings in stress (takotsubo) cardiomyopathy. JAMA 2011;306:277–86.
98. McCrohon JA, Moon JC, Prasad SK, et al. Differentiation of heart failure related to dilated cardiomyopathy and coronary artery disease using gadolinium-enhanced cardiovascular magnetic resonance. Circulation 2003;108:54–9.

CHAPTER 16

Pulmonary Circulation and Pulmonary Thromboembolism

Ieneke J.C. Hartmann • Cornelia M. Schaefer-Prokop

CHAPTER OUTLINE

PULMONARY CIRCULATION

The pulmonary circulation is unique in many ways as its appearance reflects the patho-physiological unit of ventilation and perfusion, e.g. its response to hypoxia is arterial constriction as opposed to arterial dilatation in the systemic circulation. Secondly, the pulmonary vasculature is directly influenced by cardiac function and vice versa, as illustrated most prominently by venous congestion due to left heart failure or pulmonary hypertension causing right ventricular dysfunction or even failure. In addition it follows a dual flow model (both pulmonary and bronchial circulations supply the lung).

Appreciation of pulmonary anatomy and normal physiology enables a better understanding of abnormal conditions (and their relevant radiographic features).

Acute pulmonary embolism can be life threatening and has a high mortality if undiagnosed; chronic pulmonary embolism leads to pulmonary hypertension and right heart failure. Imaging plays a major role for diagnosing acute and chronic PE since clinical symptoms are frequently non-specific. The second half of this chapter is therefore devoted to demography, pathophysiology and imaging features of pulmonary thromboembolism.

PULMONARY CIRCULATION ANATOMY

Pulmonary Arteries

The *pulmonary trunk* originates from the right ventricle. In adults the main pulmonary artery measures approximately 5 cm in length and is entirely enveloped within the pericardium. At its base there is the pulmonary valve consisting of three cusps and preventing the blood flowing back at diastole. The pulmonary sinuses are situated between the cusps of the pulmonary valves and the dilation of the pulmonary arterial wall. These sinuses prevent the valves from sticking to the wall when they open.

At about the level of the fifth thoracic vertebra, it divides into the longer right and the shorter left pulmonary artery.

The *left pulmonary artery* runs superiorly over the left main bronchus to enter the left hilum. Within the hilum it may either continue directly into the left interlobar artery from which the segmental branches to the upper and lower lobe come off directly, or it may bifurcate into an ascending and descending branch. The ascending branch then divides almost immediately into the apico-posterior and anterior segmental branches which supply the left upper lobe. The descending branch gives a branch to the lingula which itself divides into two segmental arteries (superior and inferior lingular segmental artery). The next branch from the descending branch is the superior segmental artery, supplying the superior segment of the left lower lobe (segment 6). Subsequent branches supply the remaining 4 segments of the left lower lobe.

The *right pulmonary artery* runs under the aortic arch, posterior to the superior vena cava and anterior to the right main bronchus, and just before entering the hilum it divides into the ascending (truncus anterior) and the descending (interlobar) branch. The ascending branch divides into apical, anterior and posterior segmental branches. The posterior segmental branch may however also originate at the bifurcation of the right main pulmonary artery or the right descending trunk. The interlobar artery gives rise to the middle lobe artery (which further divides into the lateral and medial segmental branches) and the right lower lobe artery, which immediately gives off the artery to the superior segment of the right lower lobe. As on the left side, subsequent branches supply the remaining 4 segments of the right lower lobe.

The arterial branching follows and runs parallel to the divisions of the bronchial tree (and having the same name), supplying each bronchopulmonary segment. The branching pattern of the lobar and especially the segmental arteries shows a high variation, whereas for the more proximal arteries it is fairly constant. In addition, supernumerary (accessory) branches exist that are not accompanied by bronchial branches and give additional arterial supply to the lung parenchyma. These arteries are usually located in the periphery of the lung.

Normal sizes of the pulmonary arteries have been assessed with CT. There are some contradicting data on the correlation between pulmonary artery diameter and height, weight, BSI and age; in general, diameters tend to be slightly higher in men. According to the literature, in adults, the upper limit of normal for the diameter of the pulmonary trunk is 29–33 mm[1–3] (for women 27 mm is suggested[1]), and for the right and left pulmonary artery 23 and 22 mm, respectively.[3]

The pulmonary artery-to-aorta ratio is used for the screening and evaluation of pulmonary hypertension: A PA-to-Ao ratio of >1 or 1.1 has been proposed as being suggestive of pulmonary hypertension, although data on the diagnostic accuracy of this ratio to PA pressures are contradicting.[4] The PA-to-Ao ratio decreases with age because the ascending aortic diameter increases with age and body size, whereas the PA increases with body size only. In addition, the PA may enlarge in some diseases (e.g., pulmonary fibrosis) without a correlating increase in PA pressure.[5] The pulmonary artery-to-bronchus ratio, which can be assessed on both plain chest film and CT, is especially helpful in the assessment of congestive heart failure and volume overload.[6] It has been also suggested to be used for the assessment of pulmonary hypertension.

Pulmonary Veins

The pulmonary veins, classically two on each side, transport the oxygenated blood from the lung back to the left atrium of the heart. The veins run independently from the pulmonary arteries and bronchi towards the heart. The superior pulmonary veins drain the blood from the upper lobes, including the middle lobe on the right side; the inferior pulmonary veins drain the lower lobes. In addition, the veins from the visceral pleura drain into the pulmonary veins, whereas the veins of the parietal pleura drain into the systemic circulation via the veins of the thoracic wall. There is great interest in variations in pulmonary venous anatomy with regards to ablation of pacemaker centres,

Bronchial Arteries

Bronchial arteries supply various parts of the intrathoracic structures: they are responsible for the majority of oxygen supply to the bronchial tree from the central main bronchi to the respiratory bronchioles and lung parenchyma, the upper oesophagus, part of the pericardium, and the visceral pleura. The smallest, most peripheral branches anastomose with branches from the pulmonary arteries in the walls of the bronchioles and the visceral pleura. Systemic branches supplying the thoracic wall also supply the parietal pleura.

The place of origin as well as the number of the bronchial arteries is subject to considerable variation. In more than 70%, the bronchial arteries arise from the descending thoracic aorta, most commonly between the levels of T5 and T6. In most individuals there are 2 to 4 bronchial arteries present, arising either independently or from a common trunk.

The *right* bronchial artery usually (78%) arises within a common stem, with the first aortic intercostal (intercostobronchial artery) from the posteromedial aspect of the descending aorta. On the *left* side, there is generally a superior and an inferior branch, both arising from the anterior aspect of the descending thoracic aorta. The bronchial arteries run into the hilum, where they branch parallel and close to the bronchus to the peripheral airways. The diameter of these arteries is small, usually 1–1.5 mm at its origin within the mediastinum.

Anomalous bronchial arteries, defined as bronchial arteries that originate outside the levels of T5 and T6, are found in up to 21% of patients with haemoptysis.[7] These anomalous arteries arise in the majority of cases from the aortic arch, less frequently from the lower part of the descending aorta or from major aortic branches such as the subclavian arteries, the thyrocervical trunk, brachiocephalic artery, or the internal mammary artery. Bronchial arteries can be distinguished from non-bronchial systemic arteries in that the first ones run into the pulmonary parenchyma parallel to the bronchi in contrast to the non-bronchial systemic collateral arteries. In the periphery, bronchial arteries arise form anastomoses with the pulmonary arteries.

Venous return occurs either via bronchial veins into the azygos vein (right side), accessory hemiazygos vein or left superior intercostal vein (left side), or via the bronchopulmonary arterial anastomoses into the pulmonary veins.

PULMONARY CIRCULATION PHYSIOLOGY

The pulmonary circulation is, unlike the systemic circulation, a low-pressure system. There is only a relatively small pressure difference between the pulmonary arteries (mean pressure 12–20 mmHg) and the left atrium (7–12 mmHg). The pressure in the capillaries and the veins approximates the pressure in the left atrium. That is the reason why elevated pressure in the left ventricle / left atrium (e.g. mitral valve disease) leads via the capillary bed to an increased pulmonary artery pressure.

As with the airways, the cross-sectional area of the pulmonary vasculature increases towards the periphery of the lung. The resistance in the capillaries contributes considerably to the whole vascular resistance. At rest, only one-third of the capillaries are perfused; with increasing cardiac output under stress, the remaining capillaries will be recruited by increasing pressure in order to contribute to gas exchange.

The hydrostatic pressure within the pulmonary capillaries tends to force fluid into the interstitium of the lung. This is partly counteracted by the plasma oncotic (colloid osmotic) pressure, which attracts fluid back into the capillaries. Imbalance of these pressure ratios can lead to abnormal fluid shift and thus overflow of fluid into the lung parenchyma. The pulmonary interstitial space is usually kept dry by pulmonary lymphatic channels. They drain any excess fluid which enters the interstitium from the alveoli, and their capacity can increase by a factor of ten if needed (e.g. chronic cardiac insufficiency).[8] However, if the rate of accumulation of fluid exceeds the capacity of lymphatic clearance, fluid will begin to accumulatewithin the interstitium. If this process continues, it leads to alveolar fluid accumulation when gas exchange may become compromised (gas exchange is not usually compromised by the presence of interstitial oedema alone).

An important difference between the pulmonary and systemic vasculature is the response to hypoxia. In the pulmonary system hypoxia results in local vasoconstriction, causing diversion of blood to regions of better ventilation.[9]

Although contrary to the vascular response in the rest of the body, this mechanism serves to protect the alveolar–arteriolar pO_2 balance and thus to minimise ventilation–perfusion differences in cases of diffuse and regional disease; i.e. it supplies blood to regions of the lung that will most efficiently oxygenate it. This homeostatic mechanism (Euler–Liljestrand reflex) is responsible for 'matched defects' seen in cases of pneumonic consolidation on ventilation–perfusion imaging. This mechanism is also responsible for different vascular calibres in patients with lobular air trapping, as seen in 'mosaic perfusion' caused by pulmonary embolism.

The bronchial arteries primarily perfuse airways, pulmonary vessel walls, interstitium and pleura. While the more centrally localised bronchial veins drain into the right atrium, the peripherally located smaller bronchial veins drain into the left atrium. This explains why increased left atrial pressure during left heart failure causes bronchial wall thickening (cuffing).

The blood circulation is influenced by gravity and body position. In the upright position, most blood perfusion volume is in the basal part of the lung as illustrated by increased lung parenchyma density and larger vessel calibres. In the apical part of the lung (zone I) the intra-alveolar pressure is larger than the intravenous and intra-arterial pressure independent of ventilation and blood volume. In the basal part of the lung (zone III) intravenous and intra-arterial pressure exceed the intra-alveolar pressure. In the middle part (zone II) the intra-arterial pressure is higher than the intra-alveolar pressure followed by the intravenous pressure. In a lying position zone I is ventrally localised and zone III dorsally accompanied by an apico-basal gradient. In case of acute volume overload or left cardiac failure, especially the vessels in zone III are affected.[10]

PULMONARY VASCULAR PATTERNS

Pulmonary Venous Hypertension

Pulmonary venous hypertension (PVH) is caused by increased resistance in the pulmonary veins and is defined by an elevation of the mean pressure > 12 mmHg. An increased venous pressure automatically leads to an increased capillary pressure. Increase of the mean PVH to 12–20 mmHg results in a redistribution of blood volume (grade 1), a PVH of 20–25 mmHg to an interstitial oedema (grade 2) and a PVH of > 25–30 mmHg to an alveolar oedema (grade 3).

The most common reason, by far, is left-sided heart disease (Table 16-1) due to left ventricular failure, mitral valve disease, or aortic valve disease. The severity of mitral valve stenosis can be non-invasively gauged by assessing the degree of PVH. In cases of aortic valve disease, however, the degree of PVH is more indicative of myocardial failure than severity of stenosis. It has to be noted that an increased left ventricular pressure load does not immediately result in PVH. Only an elevated end-diastolic left ventricular pressure leads to elevation of the left atrial pressure and subsequently to PVH. The pulmonary venous pressure can be estimated from the pulmonary artery wedge pressure (PAWP) using a Swan-Ganz catheter and is usually < 12 mmHg.

The radiological findings can be thought of as a progressive series of changes that occur in response to the underlying changes in physiology.[11,12]

Three grades of severity of pulmonary congestion are differentiated (Table 16-2).

TABLE 16-1 Causes of Pulmonary Venous Hypertension and Pulmonary Oedema

- Left ventricular outflow obstruction (aortic stenosis, aortic coarctation, hypoplastic left heart)
- Left ventricular failure
- Mitral valve disease
- Left atrial myxoma
- Fibrosing mediastinitis
- Pulmonary veno-occlusive disease

TABLE 16-2 Patterns of Oedema and Corresponding Pulmonary Venous Hypertension

	Vascular Redistribution Grade 1 (mmHg)	Interstitial Oedema Grade 2 (mmHg)	Alveolar Oedema Grade 3 (mmHg)
Acute	12–19	20–25	> 25
Chronic	15–25	25–50	> 30

Vascular Redistribution (Grade 1)

As pulmonary venous pressure rises, the upper lobe veins distend. They initially reach the size of, and eventually become larger than, the lower lobe vessels (thus reversing the normal 'gravity-dependent' pattern). This is described as 'upper lobe venous diversion' and is often the first recognised radiological sign of pulmonary venous hypertension (Fig. 16-1). The same vascular calibres of upper and lower lobe veins do not indicate increased PVH if seen in a bedside radiograph.

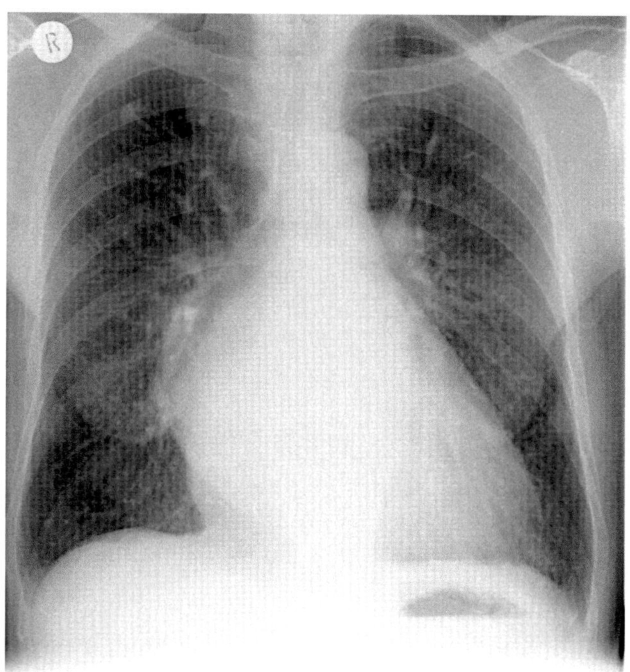

FIGURE 16-1 ■ Upper lobe venous distension.

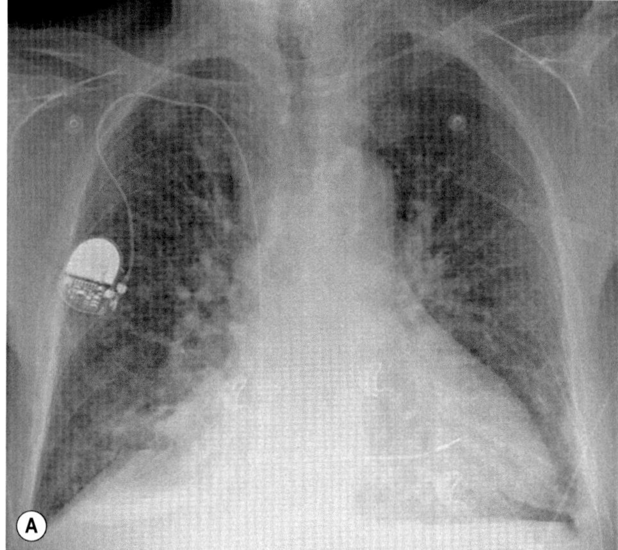

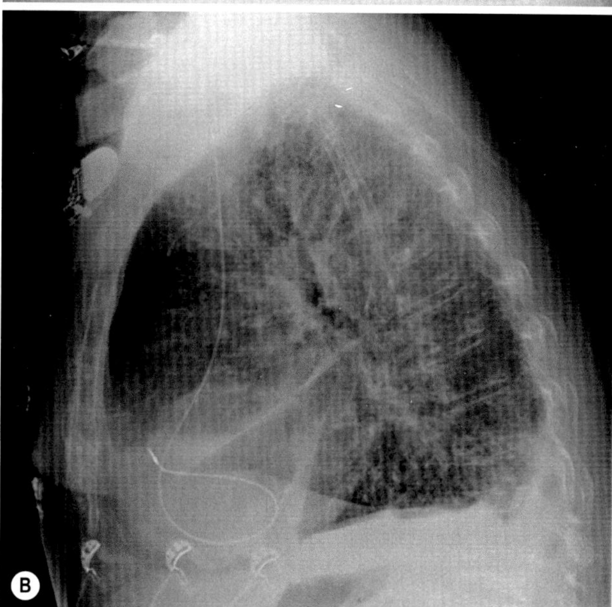

FIGURE 16-2 ■ **Interstitial oedema.** Thickened interlobular septa (Kerley B) at the base of the right lower lobe, bronchial wall thickening (cuffing), overall distended veins and a small pleural effusion with fluid in the interlobar fissures.

Patients suffering from their first episode of acute PVH elevation tend to immediately develop an interstitial or alveolar oedema. Only recurrent periods or chronically increased PVH result in distended veins.

Interstitial Oedema (Grade 2)

If the pulmonary venous pressure continues to rise and exceeds the plasma oncotic pressure, fluid will begin to accumulate in the lung interstitium. This is known as *interstitial pulmonary oedema*. Typical radiological signs of an interstitial oedema are interstitial (Kerley) lines (Fig. 16-2) caused by thickening of the interlobular septa as a result of fluid accumulation within the lung.

Kerley B lines are the most obvious ones and are short (1 cm or less) interlobular septal lines, found predominantly in the lower zones peripherally, and parallel to each other but at right angles to the pleural surface. *Kerley A* lines are deep septal lines (lymphatic channels), radiating from the periphery (not reaching the pleura) into the central portions of the lung and approximately 4 cm long. Their presence normally indicates a more acute or severe degree of oedema.

Septal lines can be differentiated from blood vessels as the latter are not visible in the outer 1 cm of the lung. In addition, deep septal lines do not branch uniformly (as is the case for blood vessels) and are seen with a greater clarity (as they represent a sheet of tissue) than a blood vessel of similar calibre (Fig. 16-3A).

Under normal circumstances septal lines caused by interstitial fluid overload would be expected to disappear after suitable reduction in pulmonary venous pressure. Exceptionally, however, they may persist, e.g. in longstanding PVH, where haemosiderin deposition or fibrosis has occurred. Other causes of persistent septal lines include idiopathic interstitial fibrosis, lymphangitis carcinomatosa and pneumoconiosis.

Other signs of interstitial fluid overload include perihilar haze (loss of visible clarity of the lower lobe and hilar vessels), peribronchial cuffing (apparent thickening of proximal bronchial walls as a result of interstitial fluid accumulating around their walls) and thickening of the interlobar fissure due to thickened subpleural interstitium (to differentiate from interlobar pleural effusion).

Alveolar Oedema (Grade 3)

As the pulmonary venous pressure continues to increase fluid begins to accumulate in the alveolar spaces. This is termed alveolar oedema. Kerley B lines, airspace nodules,

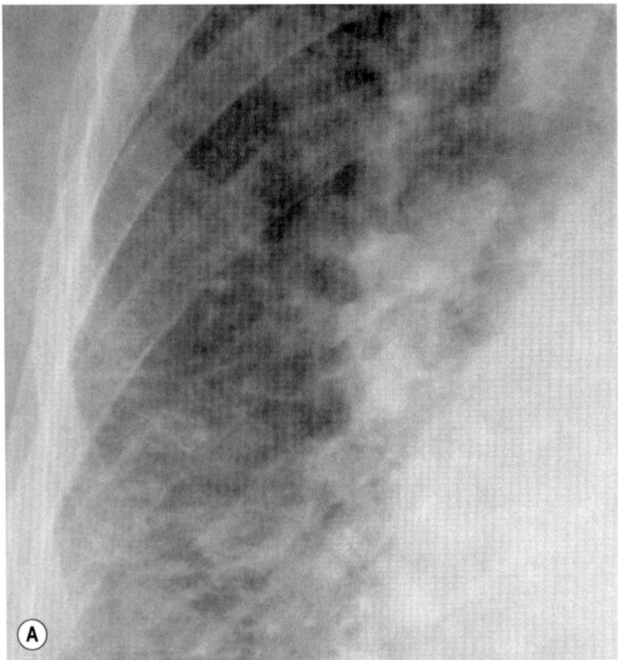

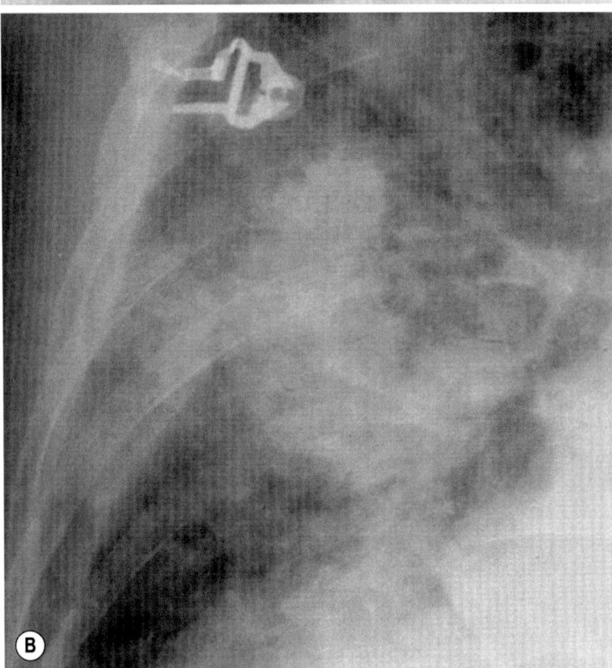

FIGURE 16-3 ■ **Magnified view of interstitial (A) and alveolar oedema (B).** Note the sharp thickened interlobular septa in (A) versus the opacification ranging from ground glass to dense consolidation in (B).

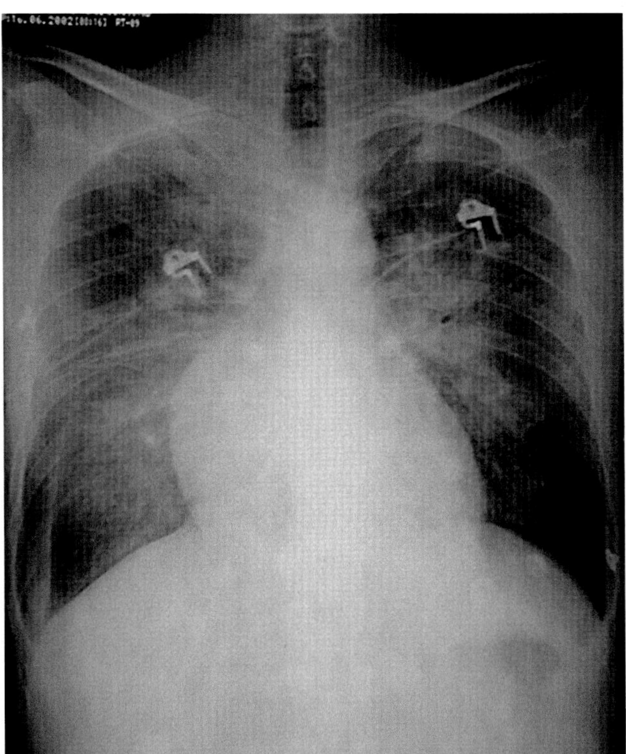

FIGURE 16-4 ■ **Alveolar pulmonary oedema.** Bilateral hilar consolidation due to alveolar fluid accumulation (bat's wing oedema).

bilateral symmetric consolidation in the mid and lower lung zones and pleural effusions may be seen.

Depending on the amount of alveolar fluid overload, there are many variations of increased lung density, ranging from subtle haziness to dense consolidations with air bronchograms (Fig. 16-3B).

Certain patterns of opacification may suggest particular diagnoses.[13] The often-cited 'perihilar bat's wing' pattern of airspace consolidation is seen most commonly in left ventricular and renal failure, whereas alveolar oedema localised to the right upper zone is suggestive of severe mitral regurgitation (Fig. 16-4). The latter is thought to be a result of predominant regurgitant blood flow in the right upper lobe pulmonary vein, from the superiorly and posteriorly positioned mitral valve. A predominantly upper lobe oedema is seen in patients with a severe head trauma (neurogenic oedema). Alveolar fluid accumulation changes with patient position and gravity: asymmetric consolidations mimicking a pneumonia may be the result of left- or right-sided position of the patient.

Computed tomography (CT) findings of oedema are similar as the radiographic findings, although very atypical patterns are possible, causing differential diagnostic difficulties.[14,15]

An interstitial oedema is characterised by (smoothly) thickened interlobular septa that do not follow the hydrostatic gradient (Fig. 16-5A). Also the peribronchovascular interstitium is thickened to be seen best in the perihilar area. Mostly, there is also at least subtle increased parenchymal density due to alveolar fluid overload.

Alveolar oedema may initially be recognised as peribronchovascular airspace nodules progressing to diffuse ground-glass or dense airspace consolidation (Fig. 16-5B). Increased density may follow a ventrodorsal gradient but can also be localised predominantly perhilar or in a patchy distribution, the latter causing sometimes quite atypical patterns (Fig. 16-6).

In *chronic pulmonary venous hypertension* signs of pulmonary arterial hypertension may also develop. In addition, a fine nodular 'interstitial' pattern may appear throughout both lungs. These nodules represent haemosiderin

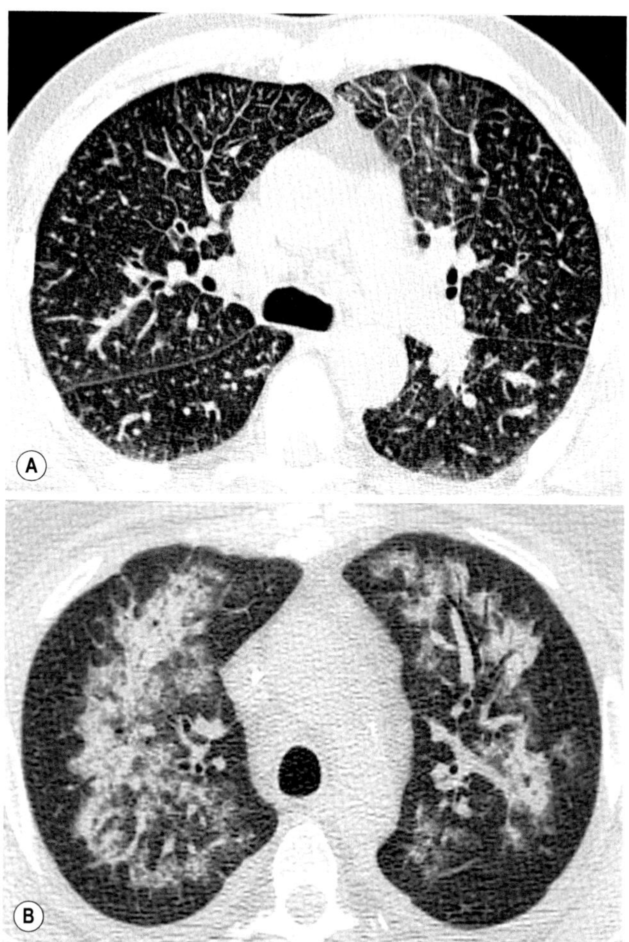

FIGURE 16-5 ■ Interstitial oedema (A) is characterised by thickened interlobular septa and focal areas of increased density. Alveolar oedema (B) causes dense consolidations which can be diffuse or more patchy in distribution. The subpleural area may be spared.

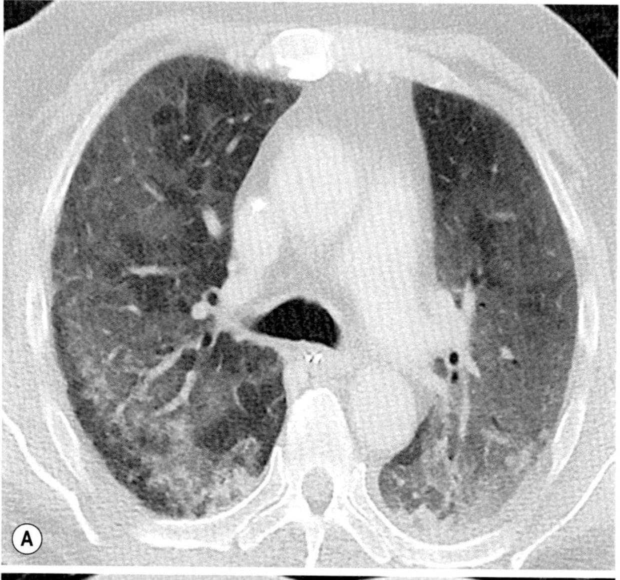

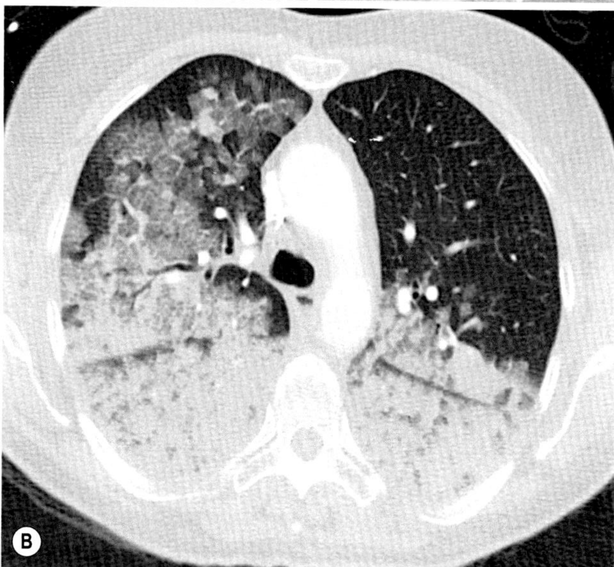

FIGURE 16-6 ■ **Two patients with alveolar oedema.** The distribution of fluid is very variable, causing different patterns of opacifications, ranging from ground glass to consolidation. Note the subpleural sparing on the right side and the ventrodorsal gradient on the left side in (A), both relatively typical features of oedema. The distribution, however, can be also very asymmetric and sharply demarcated, as in (B).

deposition. This pattern was previously most commonly seen in patients with long-standing severe mitral stenosis.

Pre-existing underlying lung disease influences the pattern and distribution of oedema, Patients with extensive emphysema do not develop homogeneous consolidation; even though degree of pulmonary venous pressure or fluid overload would otherwise lead to an alveolar oedema, the fluid remains within the interstitium, leading to thickened septa and a rather 'interstitial' fluid distribution, meaning that the radiographic appearance may lead to underestimation of the severity of oedema in these patients (Figs. 16-7 and 16-8).

Although most cases of PVH are associated with valvular and/or myocardial dysfunction leading to cardiomegaly, this is not always the case. An important example of this is in the early post-myocardial first 24–48 h post-infarction. This is due to an acute decrease in myocardial compliance, which essentially resolves in the first week post-infarction. Other situations where signs of pulmonary oedema may be seen associated with a normal heart size is in patients with non-cardiogenic pulmonary oedema, in patients with acute overhydration or drug-induced lung oedema (e.g. heroin, aspirin, nitrofurantoin).

Cardiogenic oedema has to be differentiated from other underlying diseases resulting in an imbalance of hydrostatic pressure, colloid osmotic pressure or capillary permeability, all of them resulting in pulmonary oedema (Table 16-3).

Pulmonary Arterial Hypertension

Pulmonary hypertension (PH) is a progressive disease leading to substantial morbidity and mortality. PH results from a number of diseases with different

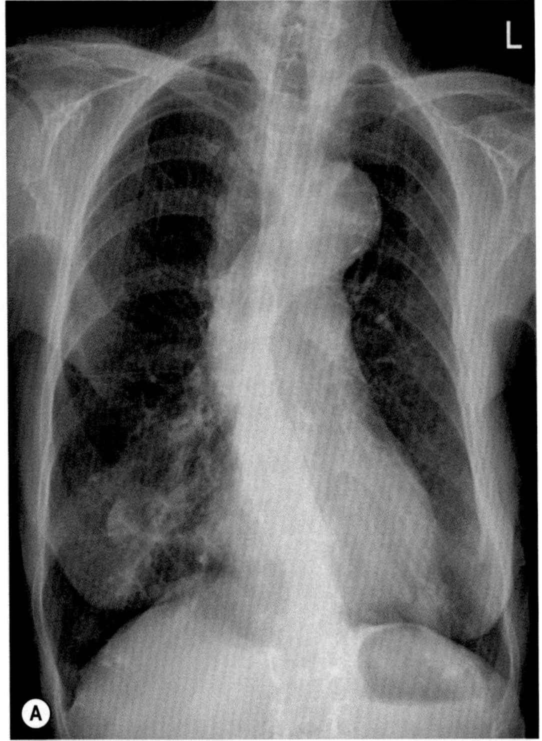

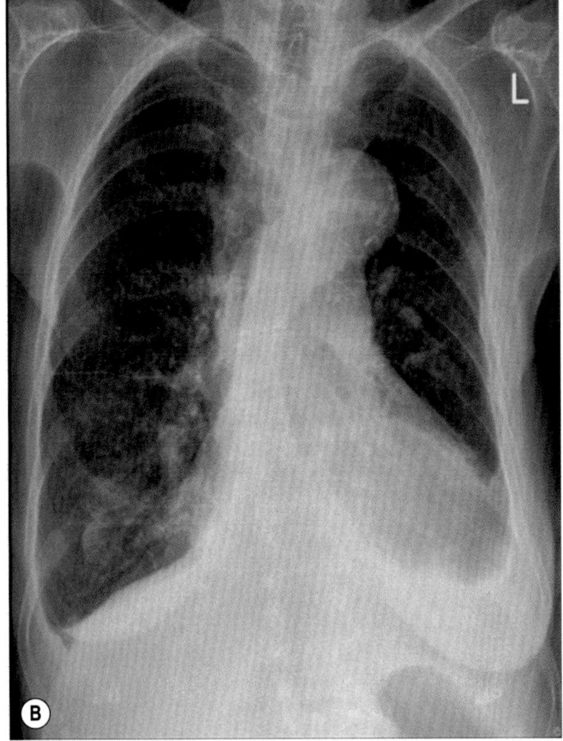

FIGURE 16-7 ■ Patient with severe COPD without (A) and with (B) signs of pulmonary fluid overload and cardiac decompensation. Note the only discrete increase of vascular markings in (B) while the pleural effusion and the enlarged heart indicate the severity of disease.

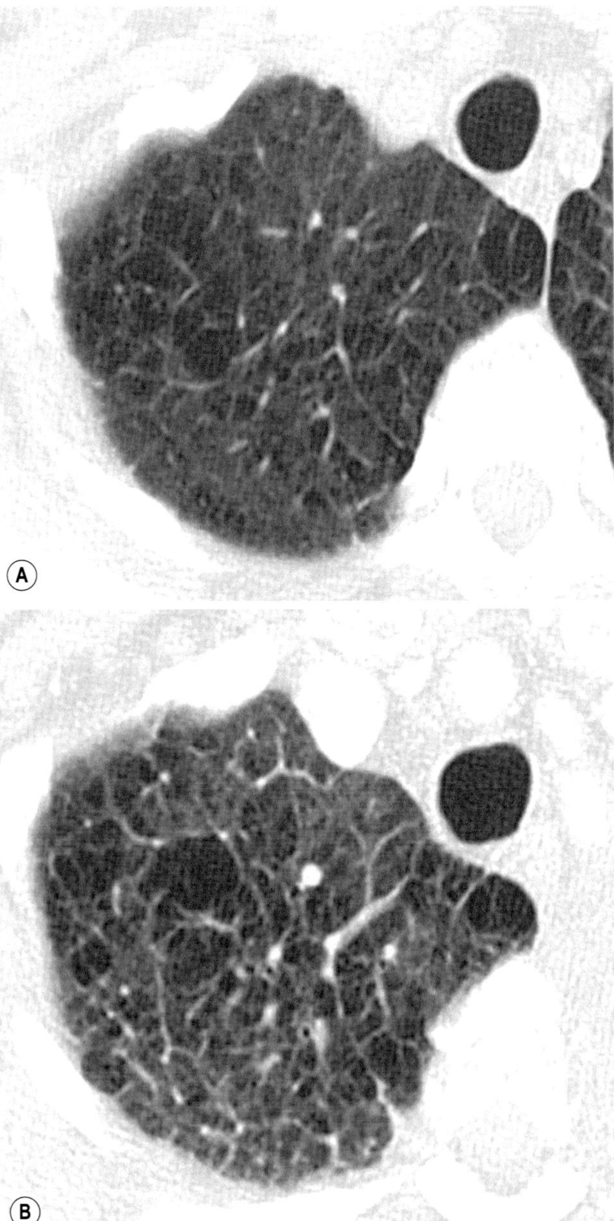

FIGURE 16-8 ■ **Corresponding CT images in the same patient show severe centrilobular emphysema without (A) and with (B) increased septal thickening due to fluid overload but no consolidations.**

pathophysiologies, treatments and prognosis. Diagnosis is often delayed because of the non-specificity of clinical symptoms. Imaging (HRCT, CTPA and MRI) play a crucial role in the diagnostic work-up of pulmonary hypertension and are particularly important for identifying patients with recurrent or chronic pulmonary thromboembolism and for assessing the feasibility of pulmonary thrombendarterectomy.[16]

PH is a clinical and haemodynamic syndrome that results in increased vascular resistance in the pulmonary circulation, usually involving a combination of vasoconstriction and remodelling of the small vessels. Haemodynamically it is defined as a systolic pulmonary artery pressure of > 35 mmHg or a mean pulmonary artery pressure of > 25 mmHg at rest or > 30 mmHg with exertion. An increase in pulmonary vascular resistance and subsequent compensatory right ventricular (RV) hypertrophy lead to elevated pulmonary pressure, which often

TABLE 16-3 Differential Diagnosis of Pulmonary Oedema

1. Increased hydrostatic pressure
   A. Cardiogenic
      - Heart disease (left ventricular failure, mitral valve disease, left atrial myxoma)
      - Pulmonary venous disease (veno-occlusive disease, mediastinal fibrosis)
      - Pericardial disease (constrictive pericardititis, pericardial effusion)
      - Drugs (anti-arrhythmic drugs, beta-blockers)
   B. Non-cardiogenic
      - Renal failure
      - IV fluid overload
   C. Neurogenic
2. Decreased colloid osmotic pressure
   - Hypoproteinaemia
   - Rapid re-expansion of lung
   - Transfusion of crystalloid fluid
3. Increased capillary permeability
   - Aspiration (near drowning, Mendelson's syndrome)
   - Inhalational injury
   - Trauma (contusion, radiation injury)
   - Injury via bloodstream (shock, sepsis, fat embolism, drugs, anaphylaxis, high altitude, acute large airway obstruction)

results in increased RV afterload and failure. The disorder is progressive, leading to right heart failure and death within a medium of 2.8 years after diagnosis.[17,18]

PH can be found in multiple clinical conditions. The current classification of PH (Table 16-4) was developed at the 4th World Symposium on Pulmonary Hypertension in Dana Point, CA, in 2008 and represents a modification of the previous Venice classification. The goal of the new classification is to group together different manifestations of disease sharing similarities in pathophysiological mechanisms, clinical presentation and therapeutic approaches.[19]

Group 1 describes the group of patients with pulmonary arterial hypertension (PAH) characterised by the presence of pre-capillary PH in the absence of other causes of PH due to lung diseases (groups 3 and 5), chronic PE (group 4) or other rare diseases (group 5). Group 1 PAH have a mean pulmonary artery pressure > 25 mmHg and a pulmonary capillary wedge pressure < 15 mmHg, and comprises idiopathic and heritable PH, PH in association with connective tissue diseases, HIV infection, portal hypertension or rare diseases such as pulmonary veno-occlusive disease and/or pulmonary capillary haemangiomatosis.

Group 2 comprises patients with PH due to left heart disease, causing an increased pulmonary artery pressure and an elevated pulmonary capillary wedge pressure > 15 mmHg (Table 16-5).[20]

The diagnostic work-up of patients with PH includes a medical history, physical examination, echocardiogram, cardiac catheterisation and advanced imaging such as CT, MR and scintigraphy.

Radiographically, cardiac enlargement (right atrial and ventricular enlargement), enlargement of the central pulmonary arteries (main pulmonary artery and its branches down to the segmental level) (Fig. 16-9) and tapering of peripheral arterial branches (vessels beyond segmental level)—termed 'peripheral pruning'—are seen. In long-standing cases the central pulmonary arteries may develop calcification due to atheroma, which is a feature not seen in non-hypertensive pulmonary arteries. Central arterial

TABLE 16-4 Classification of Pulmonary Hypertension According to the 4th World Symposium in Dana Point, CA in 2008

1. Pulmonary arterial hypertension (PAH)
   - Idiopathic
   - Heritable
   - Drug and toxin induced
   - Associated with connective tissue diseases, HIV, portal hypertension, congenital heart disease, schistosomiasis, chronic haemolytic anaemia
   - Persist neonatal pulmonary hypertension
   - Pulmonary veno-occlusive disease/capillary haemangiomatosis
2. PH due to left heart disease
   - Systolic dysfunction
   - Diastolic dysfunction
   - Valvular disease
3. PH due to lung disorder and/or hypoxemia
   - COPD
   - Interstitial lung diseases
   - Pulmonary diseases with mixed restrictive/obstructive pattern
   - Sleep disordering breathing
   - Alveolar hypoventilation disorder
   - Chronic exposure to high altitude
   - Developmental abnormalities
4. Chronic thromboembolic pulmonary hypertension
5. Pulmonary hypertension with unclear multifactorial mechanisms
   - Haematological disorders
   - Systemic disorders (sarcoidosis, LCH, LAM, vasculitis
   - Metabolic disorders (Gaucher, thyroid disorders, glycogen storage disease)
   - Others (tumoural obstruction, fibrosing mediastinitis, chronic renal failure)

TABLE 16-5 Haemodynmic Definitions of Pulmonary Hypertension (PH)

Definition	Haemodynamic Characteristics	Clinical Groups (see Table 16-3)
PH	P – PA > 25 mmHg	All
Pre-capillary PH	P – PA > 25 mmHg P – PCW < 15 mmHg CO: normal or reduced	1—PAH 3—PH due to lung diseases 4—CTEPH 5—PH with unclear/ multifactorial mechanisms
Post-capillary PH	P – PA > 25 mm HG P – PCW > 15 mmHg CO: normal or reduced	2—PH due to left heart disease

P – PA = mean pulmonary artery pressure; P – PCW = pulmonary capillary wedge pressure; CO = cardiac output.

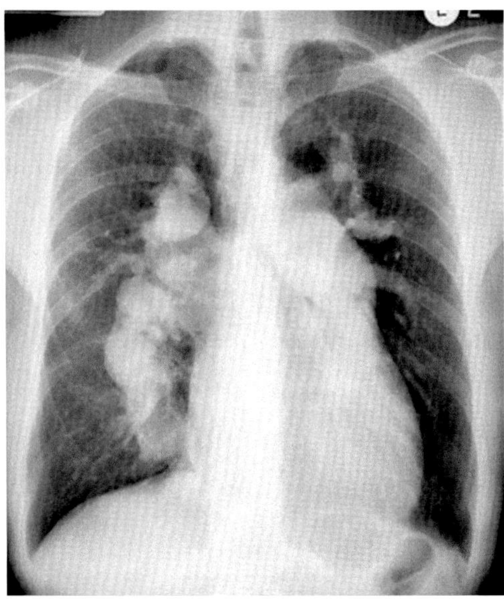

FIGURE 16-9 ■ **Pulmonary arterial hypertension with massively enlarged pulmonary arteries.**

enlargement may mimic enlarged hilar lymph nodes. However, careful scrutiny usually allows differentiation, as lymphadenopathy characteristically has a lobulated border whereas arterial enlargement has a smoother outline. A recognised method of assessing pulmonary arterial size is by measuring the size of the right descending pulmonary artery. Enlargement may be diagnosed if the transverse diameter of the artery at its midpoint is greater than 17 mm. Although it is not known at what exact stage PH causes visible changes on a CXR, it is likely that they become apparent only in severe stages of PH. Overall, although relatively specific, the sensitivity of chest radiography for the diagnosis of (mild) PAH is therefore low.

Transthoracic ultrasound (*TTE; transthoracic echocardiography*) is often used as screening tool and in fact is recommended to be performed in all patients with suspected PH.[21] By measuring the tricuspid regurgitant jet, the systolic PA pressure is estimated. When peak tricuspid regurgitation velocity is difficult to measure (trivial/mild tricuspid regurgitation), use of contrast enhanced ultrasound significantly increases the Doppler signal, allowing for more precise measurement of the peak tricuspid regurgitation velocity. However the literature is not uniform with respect to diagnostic accuracy of TTE; bedside measurements show considerable user dependency and examinations may suffer from variable quality, especially in patients with chronic lung disease.

The *ventilation–perfusion lung scintigram* is a nuclear medicine test performed in patients with PH to look for potentially treatable chronic thromboembolic pulmonary hypertension (CTEPH). According to the ESC/ERS guidelines published in 2009 it is recommended in all patients as the screening method of choice to diagnose or rule out CTEPH. A normal or low probability VQ result effectively excludes CTEPH with a sensitivity of 90–100% and a specificity of 94–100%. Unmatched perfusion defects are also seen in PVOD and sometimes in patients with PAH, and CTA is used in those as a complementary investigation.

Traditional pulmonary angiography is still required in many patients for the work-up of CTEPH to identify patients who may benefit from thrombendarterectomy. Angiography may also be helpful in the evaluation of possible vasculitis or pulmonary arteriovenous malformations.

Right heart catheterisation is indicated in all patients with PAH to confirm the diagnosis, to evaluate the severity and when PAH-specific drug therapy is considered. *Vasoreactivity testing* is indicated in patients with IPAH, heritable PAH and other types of PAH; however, it should only be performed in specific centres and under controlled conditions. It is not recommended for other PH groups.

MRI plays an important role in diagnosis of PH because of its ability to assess right ventricular dysfunction causes by increased afterload. MR angiography for the assessment of pulmonary vasculature and parenchyma perfusion can be combined with dynamic quantitative assessment of ventricular volumes and function (Fig. 16-10). Phase-contrast imaging allows for the assessment of PA blood flow.[22] Cardiac MR provides direct evaluation of the RV size, morphology and function, and allows non-invasive assessment of blood flow including stroke volume, cardiac output (CO), distensibility of the PA and RV mass. CMR data may be used to assess right heart haemodynamics, particularly for follow-up purposes. A decreased stroke volume, increased RV end-diastolic volume and decreased LV end-diastolic volume are indicative of a poor prognosis.[23] With MR perfusion techniques it is possible to distinguish between patients with CTEPH and patients with PAH. Vascular obstruction leads to wedge-shaped perfusion defects while in PAH the perfusion is overall reduced and inhomogeneous. Quantitative evaluation of perfusion found a significantly reduced pulmonary blood flow (PBF) and prolonged mean transit time (MTT) in patients with PAH compared to healthy volunteers; no correlation, however, was found between these quantitative measures and the mean PAP.[24]

Computed tomography plays a major role in assessing patients with PH. In addition to its indisputable role in diagnosing acute and chronic pulmonary embolism (see below), it allows assessment of the central as well as peripheral vascular structures, including the lung parenchyma, which plays an important role for the differential diagnosis. Signs to assess or indicate pulmonary hypertension refer to the vasculature, the right ventricle itself and the lung parenchyma.[25–27]

Vascular Signs

- A diameter of the main pulmonary artery at the level of its bifurcation > 29 mm was found to have a sensitivity of 87% at a specificity of 89% for diagnosis of PH. If this finding is combined with an arterial-bronchial ratio > 1 on the segmental level in at least three lobes, the specificity increased to 100%. A PA:AA ratio > 1 was highly specific (92% for a PH > 20 mmHg) (Fig. 16-11).

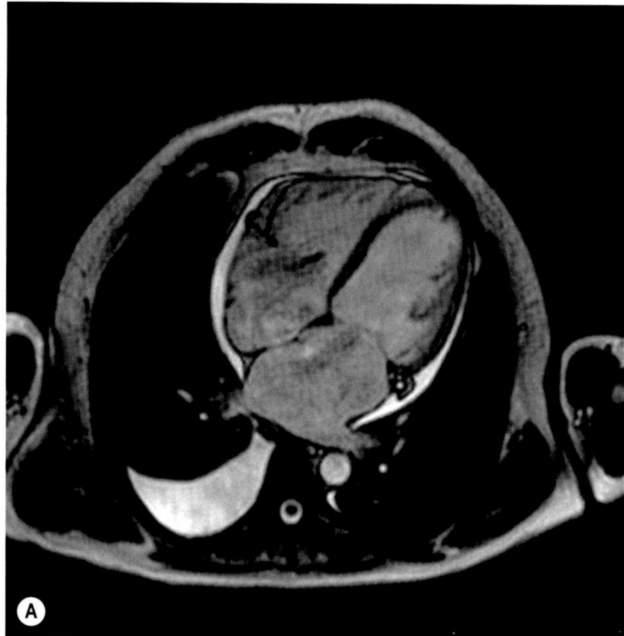

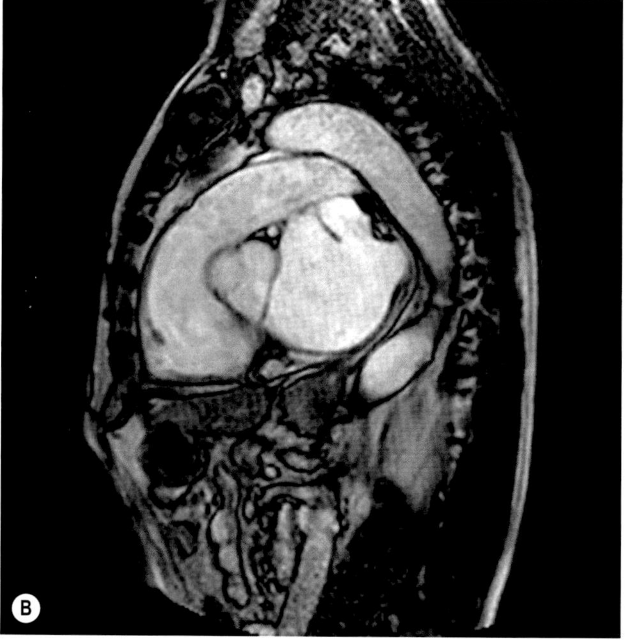

FIGURE 16-10 ■ MR of the heart showing the regurgitation jet (arrows) in both atria due to tricuspid and mitral valve insufficiency. Note the enlargement of all chambers, the pericardiac and pleural effusion in (A) and the enlarged pulmonary trunk (> 3 cm) compared to the aorta in (B). (Courtesy of N. Prakken, MMC, Amersfoort, NL.)

A wide variation of the upper limit of the PA diameter is reported in the literature. Although it is likely that the PA diameter is correlated to patent size or stage in cardiac cycle, neither the ratio of PA:AA nor normalisation of the PA to the BMI increased the correlation with the mean PAP. The PA diameter can be considerably increased in patients with interstitial lung disease (e.g. up to 4 cm), which is not necessarily associated with PH.

From a practical point of view, the PA:AA ratio has become the most widely accepted sign for many radiologists.

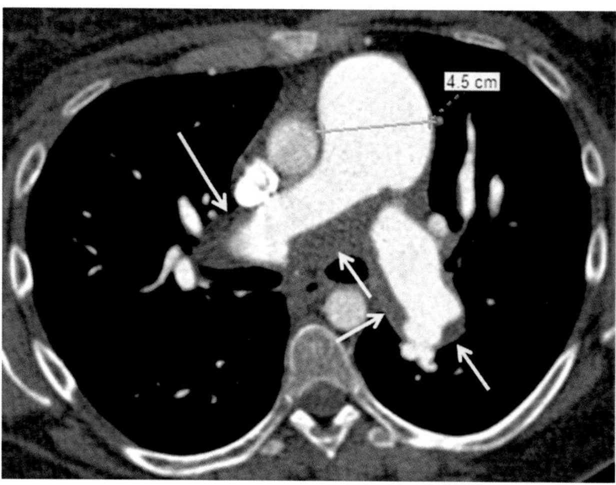

FIGURE 16-11 ■ CT in a patient with CTEPH demonstrating an enlarged pulmonary trunk and enlarged main pulmonary arteries when compared to the ascending aorta. There is eccentric thrombus with irregular margins and obtuse angles to the vessel wall (arrows).

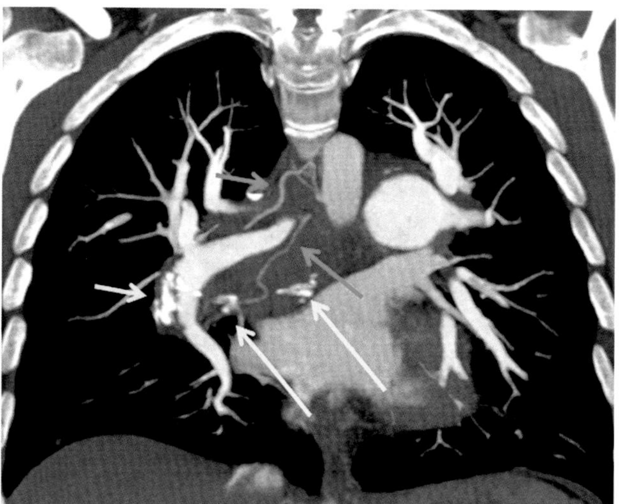

FIGURE 16-12 ■ Coronal maximum intensity projection showing dilatation of bronchial arteries (blue arrows) and a thrombus with calcifications (yellow arrows) in the central pulmonary arteries.

- Dilatation of bronchial arteries (> 1.5 mm) is an indicator that they participate in blood oxygenation due to (major) occlusion of pulmonary arteries (Fig. 16-12). They are most frequently seen in patients with CTEPH but are present also in patients with Eisenmenger or IPAH, making it a not 100% discriminating finding between PH, IPAH or CTEPH. The presence of dilated bronchial arteries in CTEPH predicted a better postsurgical outcome after thromboendarterectomy.

Cardiac Signs

- Flattening and later bowing of the cardiac septum and dilatation of the short-axis diameter of RV as compared to the LV (RV:LV >1) are indicative of

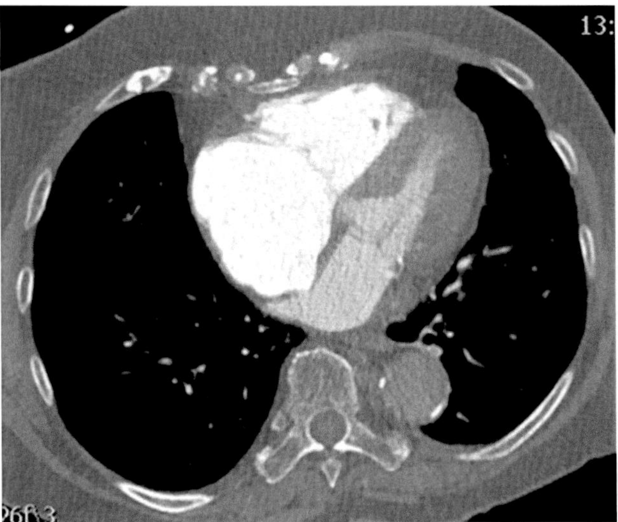

FIGURE 16-13 ■ Enlargement of the right atrium and right ventricle in a patient with severe pulmonary hypertension.

increased pulmonary pressure, though most of experience with respect to the usefulness of this sign refers to acute pulmonary embolism (Fig. 16-13).

- Reflux of contrast medium into the inferior cava and hepatic veins is seen in association with tricuspid regurgitation secondary to PH. Reflux into the inferior vena cava is also seen in normal pressure patients with injection rates exceeding 3mL/s; however, reflux into the peripheral hepatic veins is considered abnormal (Fig. 16-14).
- Fluid collection in the anterior pericardiac recess (> 10–15 mm in depth) has been reported in association with increased ventricular strain in association with PH.

Parenchymal Signs

- Mosaic perfusion is a hallmark of CTEPH, reflecting peripheral vascular obstruction.
- In patients with Eisenmenger and IPAH, tiny serpiginous intrapulmonary vessels may be seen (so-called neovascularity) arising from centrolobular arterioles not conforming to the usual pulmonary artery anatomy.
- Diffuse centrilobular acinar opacities, sometimes confluent to areas of patchy ground glass indicate the rare disease of capillary hemangiomatosis if associated with signs of pulmonary hypertension (Fig. 16-15A). Alternatively, there might be thickened interlobular septa described as being suggestive for pulmonary veno-occlusive disease (Fig. 16-15B). Today both diseases are considered as two spectra of the same entity. It is important that radiologists recognise this pattern and suggest the presence of this disease (group 1 according to the Dana classification), as patients indeed suffering from pulmonary haemangiomatosis/PVOD will develop life-threatening oedema if treated with the usual pulmonary hypertension medication. Lymphadenopathy and pleural effusion are frequent additional findings.[28]

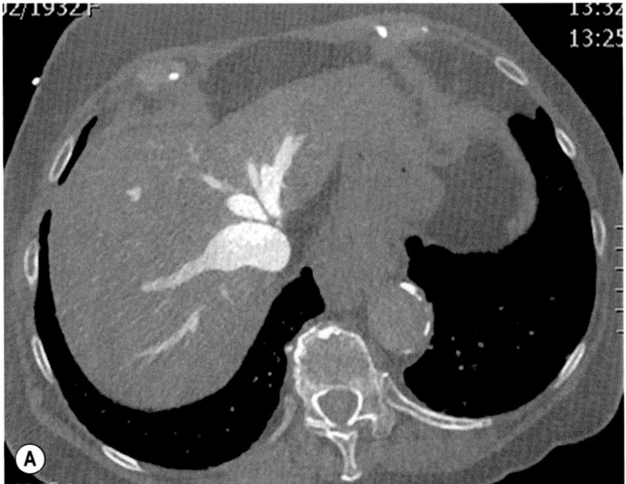

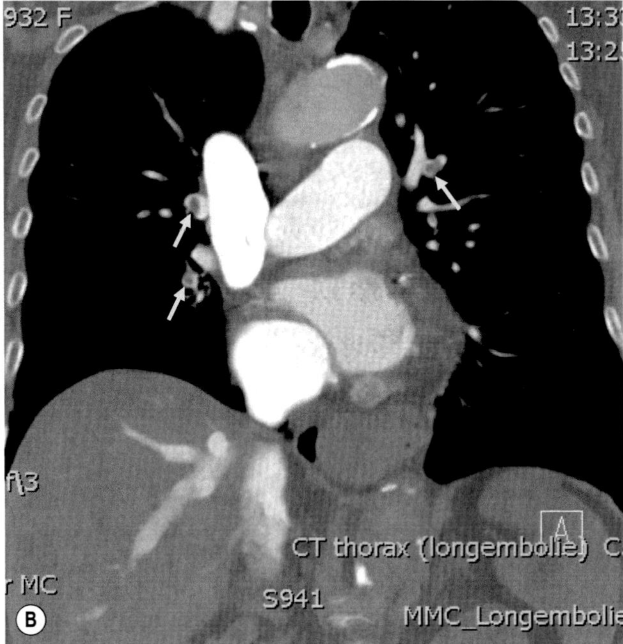

FIGURE 16-14 ■ Retrograde flow of contrast medium in the hepatic veins (A) in a patient with acute pulmonary embolism (yellow arrows) (B).

Pulmonary Arteriovenous Malformations

Pulmonary arteriovenous malformations (PAVMs) may be diagnosed on clinical grounds and/or by familial screening in patients with hereditary haemorrhagic telangiectasia (HHT). When acquired, they may be seen in conjunction with liver cirrhosis, schistosomiasis and metastatic thyroid carcinoma.

Clinically they may produce systemic arterial desaturation and give rise to signs of dyspnoea, hypoxia, cyanosis and heart failure. When they rupture, massive haemoptysis and haemothorax occur. Direct communication between a pulmonary artery and vein causes paradoxical embolism, which is responsible for two-thirds of neurological symptoms in patients with HHT. Although 10% of cases present in the first decade, most do not

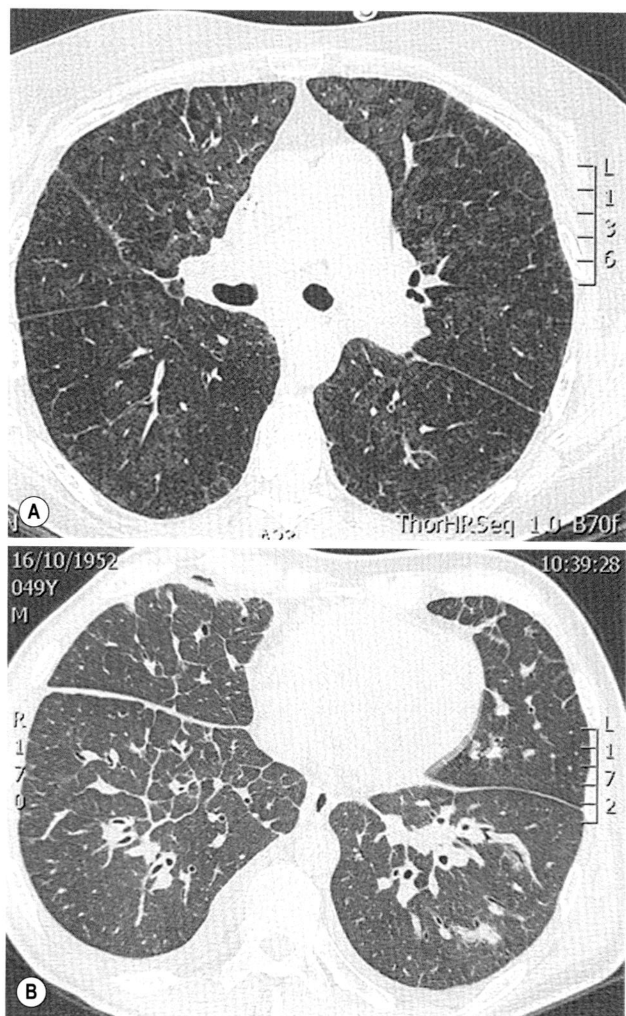

FIGURE 16-15 ■ Two patients with severe pulmonary hypertension and parenchymal findings typical for capillary hemangiomatosis (A) and pulmonary veno-occlusive disease (PVOD) (B). Both patterns are considered to represent twp spectra of the same disease. (Courtesy of Esther Nossent, VU, Amsterdam.)

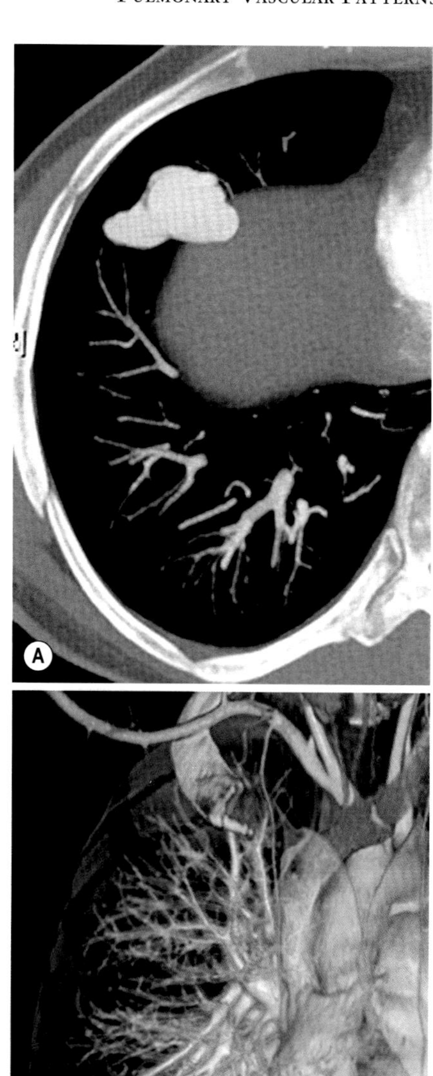

FIGURE 16-16 ■ Arteriovenous malformation (simple type) with one feeding artery and draining vein. Axial MIP (A) and coronal VRT (B) demonstrating the angioarchitecture. (Courtesy of M. Prokop, RUMC Nijmegen, NL.)

manifest clinically until the third or fourth decade. Multiple lesions are seen in up to 50% of cases.

PAVMs can be treated non-invasively by embolotherapy or by surgery; the preference goes for the first in the majority of cases. Exact knowledge of the angioarchitecture is necessary before interventional procedures and can be achieved using modern CTA techniques and 3D reconstructions.

Two types of PAVMs can be differentiated:

1. The simple type, consisting of a single feeding artery and one or several draining veins (80%).
2. A complex PAVM, consisting of more than one feeding arteries and one or more draining veins (20%).

Radiographically they may appear as round, oval, or lobulated opacities with an associated prominent vascular shadow, but if small and discrete they may not be detected on plain chest radiography.[15] They occur most frequently in the lower lobes.

Although pulmonary angiography has been considered the 'gold standard' for the diagnosis of PAVMs, CT angiography using thin slices for acquisition and 3D reconstructions with VRT and MIP for visualisation has largely taken over the diagnostic task because of its excellent capacity to three-dimensionally illustrate the angioarchitecture (Fig. 16-16). Remy and colleagues found that CT was more sensitive than pulmonary angiography (98% versus 60%).[29] MR can also be used; however, it suffers from lower spatial resolution compared with the MDCT technique.

PULMONARY THOMBOEMBOLIC DISEASE

ACUTE PULMONARY THROMBOEMBOLISM

Pulmonary thromboembolism (PE) is a frequently occurring disease caused by obstruction of a pulmonary artery by a thrombus. The annual incidence of clinically detected pulmonary embolus (PE) is estimated to be 23–69 patients per 100,000 per year.[30,31] PE may not only cause morbidity but also is a potentially lethal disease: of all patients who develop PE, it directly causes or contributes to the patient's death in one-third of the cases. If the patient is treated with anticoagulants, mortality due to PE is reduced to 8%.[32] The causes of undetected PE are twofold: PE may remain clinically silent, or the non-specific clinical signs and symptoms did not arouse suspicion of PE.

Most patients present with pleuritic chest pain, tachypnoea, and/or dyspnoea.[33] The classic clinical triad of sudden chest pain, dyspnoea and haemoptysis is present in only the minority of the cases. Other symptoms and signs may be: cough, syncope, tachycardia, fever, signs of DVT, but patients may also present with cardiac arrest.

Obstruction of the pulmonary artery may have several physiological effects. The severity of effects are in general directly related to the extent of obstruction, such as arterial hypoxia, alveolar dead space, pulmonary dead space due to surfactant depletion, reduced lung volume and pulmonary arterial hypertension. In order to raise the pulmonary arterial pressure significantly, it is estimated that at least 50% of the vascular bed needs to be obstructed. Other factors resulting in vasoconstriction such as humoral agents and reflex mechanisms are considered to play an additional role.

Several factors may predispose to the development of PE such as increasing age, previous venous thromboembolic disease (VTE), instrumentation (e.g. indwelling intravenous catheters), neoplastic disease, immobilisation, (orthopaedic) surgery, hypercoagulable state and hormonal treatment including oral contraceptives, and pregnancy.[34] In some cases, the underlying cause remains unknown.

In more than 90% of the cases the thrombus originates from the deep veins of the legs or pelvis (deep vein thrombosis; DVT). Consequently, PE and DVT are considered part of the same disease entity, VTE. From this thrombus a part (embolus) breaks off and is transported by the blood flow through the right side of the heart into the pulmonary arteries. Emboli normally lodge either at the bifurcation of branching pulmonary arteries (a few are situated at the bifurcation of the main pulmonary artery, so-called 'saddle emboli') or in the peripheral small pulmonary branches. Once an embolus is lodged in a pulmonary artery, it is normally either lysed by the patient's fibrinolytic system or becomes organised with recanalisation. The degree to which each of these processes occurs depends to some extent on the patient's fibrinolytic system, the amount of thrombus deposited on the embolus and the degree of organisation of the embolic material itself. In cases of repeated thromboembolism without lysis of the embolic material, arterial hypertension is likely to develop.

The embolus results in either a reduction or a cessation of the distal perfusion. Because of the collateral circulation offered by the bronchial arteries, which increases in case of PE, lung viability is preserved in the majority of cases and pulmonary infarction usually does not occur in patients who do not suffer from pre-existing cardiovascular disease. However, if an impaired circulation exists, e.g. due to chronic congestion, the presence of PE may result in local hypoxia, capillary damage, exudation, haemorrhage and coagulation necrosis. Pulmonary infarction eventually develops only in up to 15% of the thromboembolic events[35] and is seen most commonly in the lower lobes. When a part of the visceral pleura is involved in this process, ischaemia may result in inflammation, which may irritate or fuse with the sensitive parietal pleura, eventually causing pain. Pulmonary infarcts become revascularised from the periphery, leading to either complete resolution or the development of small scars. Occasionally, pulmonary infarcts become secondarily infected, resulting in abscess formation.

Diagnosing Acute Pulmonary Embolism

Since PE is frequent, resulting in high morbidity and mortality, clinical signs and symptoms are usually non-specific, and the standard treatment with anticoagulants may also result in morbidity and mortality due to the increased bleeding risk, a good clinical work-up of patients is of utmost importance. However, of all the patients with clinically suspected PE, only up to one-third of them have thromboembolic disease.

Clinical (Pre-Test) Probability Estimate and D-Dimer Testing

There are no reliable bedside tests available to diagnose PE. ECG and measurement of arterial pO_2 are not diagnostic for PE, and are more useful in suggesting other causes for the patient's symptoms, e.g. myocardial infarction.

A D-dimer blood test (a degradation product of fibrin in the process of fibrinolysis; an increased D-dimer suggests activation of the coagulation and fibrinolytic systems) has a very high negative predictive value (NPV). However, the NPV is not 100%, meaning that a negative test cannot exclude PE. The D-dimer test generally is performed in combination with a clinical probability estimate, usually a clinical prediction rule. Several clinical prediction rules, such as the Wells and Geneva rules, have been developed, of which the original and the simplified Wells rule are the best evaluated and most frequently used (Table 16-6). However, the performance of these clinical prediction rules vary between different patient groups and in different clinical settings.[36,37] The combination of a negative D-dimer test and a low or intermediate clinical probability estimate reliably rules out PE and no further testing is indicated.[34] This combination is

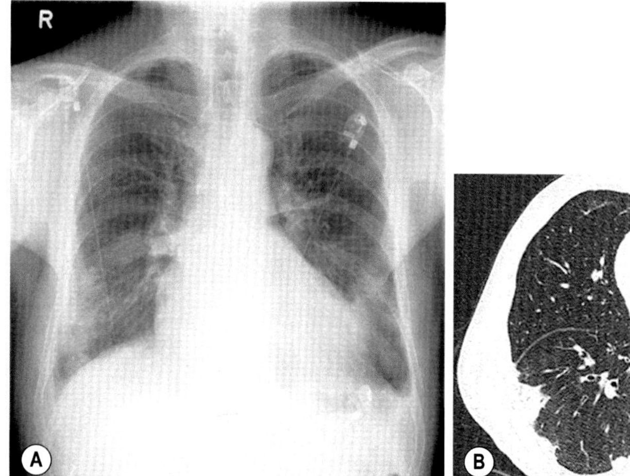

FIGURE 16-17 ■ CXR (A) and CT (B) demonstrating pleurally based wedge-shaped opacities (Hampton's hump). (Courtesy of W. van Lankeren, Erasmus MC, Rotterdam, NL.)

TABLE 16-6 **Wells Clinical Prediction Rule**

	Original Version (points)	Simplified Version (points)
Previous PE or DVT	1.5	1
Heart rate > 100 beats/min	1.5	1
Surgery or immobilisation < 4 weeks	1.5	1
Haemoptysis	1	1
Active cancer	1	1
Clinical signs of DVT	1	1
Alternative diagnosis less likely than PE	3	1
Clinical probability		
PE unlikely	≤ 4	≤ 1
PE likely	> 4	> 1

found in up to 51% of outpatients or those seen via the emergency ward.[38] In all other circumstances (high clinical suspicion and/or positive D-dimer testing) further diagnostic work-up using imaging is warranted. The D-dimer test is non-specific as there are many causes of activation of the thrombolytic system such as inflammation, pregnancy, recent operation, neoplastic disease and increasing age. Consequently, this test is of limited value in hospitalised patients.

Imaging Findings

Plain Chest Radiography

The chest X-ray may be normal (up to 40% of patients with PE) or show non-specific findings, even in extensive PE. The chest X-ray is performed not to diagnose PE but to exclude other causes of the symptoms, such as pneumonia, pleuritis, or pneumothorax. Although they are infrequently present, yet non-specific, there are several signs related to PE and therefore suggestive but still they do not confirm the diagnosis of PE. The most important ones being:

- *Hampton's hump.* This is a pleural-based, wedge-shaped opacity with the apex of the triangle pointing towards the occluding vessel/hilum. It is typically not seen in the first 24 h after the PE and represents a parenchymal infarction (Fig. 16-17). It may take 3–5 weeks up to months to resolve, and a band-like opacity due to scarring or focal pleural thickening may remain. The opacity may not always be triangular as the infarction may be surrounded by haemorrhage. If the infarcted area becomes secondarily infected, cavitation may occur. The latter may also be caused by septic emboli. These opacities may not only be seen in case of infarction but can also be the result of only oedema and haemorrhage. The latter are usually found in the lower lobes, from 12 h to several days after the thromboembolic event and show relatively rapid resolution (up to 7–10 days).
- *Westermark sign*, defined by a hyperlucent area with decreased vascularity due to oligaemia of the involved part of the lung. Although this finding is not specific for PE, PE should be considered, especially if newly found.
- *'Knuckle' or 'sausage' sign*, describing a dilatation of a central pulmonary artery due to occlusion by the embolus with collapse or constriction of the distal arteries resulting in an abrupt tapering of these arteries.

Other secondary findings that may be present are: plate-like atelectasis, (haemorrhagic) pleural effusion, and an elevation of the diaphragm, either due to pleuritic pain or as a result of decreased pulmonary compliance. If PE is severe, signs of right ventricular failure may be encountered, such as dilatation of the right heart, the superior vena cava and the azygos vein.

Transthoracic or Transoesophageal Ultrasound (Echocardiography)

This examination is the first imaging method of choice in cardiorespiratory unstable patients in whom massive PE is suspected. The right ventricular function can be assessed and central pulmonary emboli be detected. As this technique has a low sensitivity for peripheral emboli, its use is not recommended in stable patients. The advantage of this technique is the assessment of other cardiovascular diseases that may explain the patient's symptoms, such as cardiac tamponade or acute myocardial infarction.

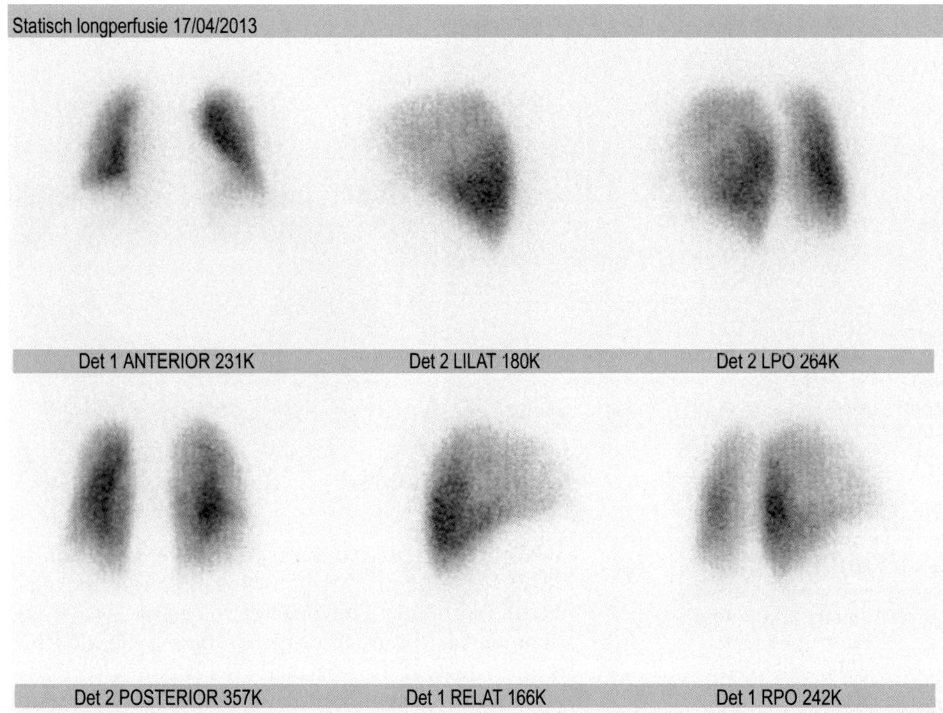

FIGURE 16-18 ■ **Static perfusion scan in 6 standard views (anterior, posterior and left/right posterior oblique) performed 6 months after acute PE reveals normal distribution of the activity. No perfusion defects are demonstrated.**

Conventional Pulmonary Angiography

Until recently, pulmonary angiography was considered the gold standard for the diagnosis of PE. For several reasons, e.g. costs, limited availability and invasiveness of the procedure, it has not gained general acceptance. In experienced hands it remains a valuable examination with a low complication rate (mortality 1% and non-fatal complications < 5%[39,40]); however, for diagnostic purposes it may only have a role if CT is not available or a definite diagnosis cannot be obtained otherwise. Thrombectomy or selective thrombolysis by conventional pulmonary angiography is performed in some centres as a treatment option in a subgroup of patients with PE.

Compression Ultrasound of the Legs

The majority of the PE originates from the deep venous system of the lower extremities and pelvis. If DVT is diagnosed in a patient with clinically suspected PE, no further evaluation is needed and the patient can be treated for PE. In skilled hands compression ultrasound (CUS) achieves a 92–95% sensitivity and 98% specificity for the diagnosis of acute DVT.[41] However, the presence of DVT can be confirmed in only a minority of patients with proven PE. A negative CUS of the legs, the best investigation to evaluate DVT, does not exclude the presence of PE and further imaging is warranted.

Ventilation–Perfusion Scintigraphy

This is a nuclear investigation starting with the assessment of the pulmonary blood flow (perfusion (Q) scintigraphy) by intravenously injection of technetium (Tc)-99m labelled macro-aggregated albumin (MAA) particles. These particles are transported to the pulmonary circulation where they get trapped in a minor proportion of the small pulmonary capillary bed. Traditionally, images are then obtained in 6 or 8 views by counting the radiation emitted by the particles in the lung with a gamma camera (Fig. 16-18). Alternatively, with a single photon emission computed tomography (SPECT) camera (either with or without low-dose CT) a volumetric data set is obtained, but the latter increases the investigation time and often higher doses of technetium are used.[42] Data on this topic are limited but there may be a higher diagnostic accuracy with SPECT as compared to planar imaging (Figs. 16-19A, B).

When thrombus is present, the particles cannot get into the small vessels, resulting in a perfusion defect. A normal perfusion study rules out PE with almost 100% certainty and further investigation is not indicated. If a perfusion defect is present, further imaging is warranted. Depending on the number and size of the perfusion defects, additional ventilation imaging can be performed to increase the specificity. Ventilation (V) scintigraphy is performed by inhalation of a radioactive gas. Krypton-81m (81mKr) is the optimal imaging agent for this purpose as it emits high-energy photons (190 keV) and owing to its short half-life can be continuously administered to the patient, including during perfusion imaging.

Once ventilation and perfusion images are obtained, they are then compared to observe for V/Q 'mismatches'. When segmental perfusion defects are present and ventilation is normal, there is a high probability for PE (>95%) and the patient can be treated for PE without further investigation. All other V/Q results, i.e. subsegmental perfusion defects or ventilation defects matching the segmental perfusion defects (occurring in 60–70% of the V/Q-scans)[43] are called non-diagnostic or indeterminate as other diseases such as asthma and chronic

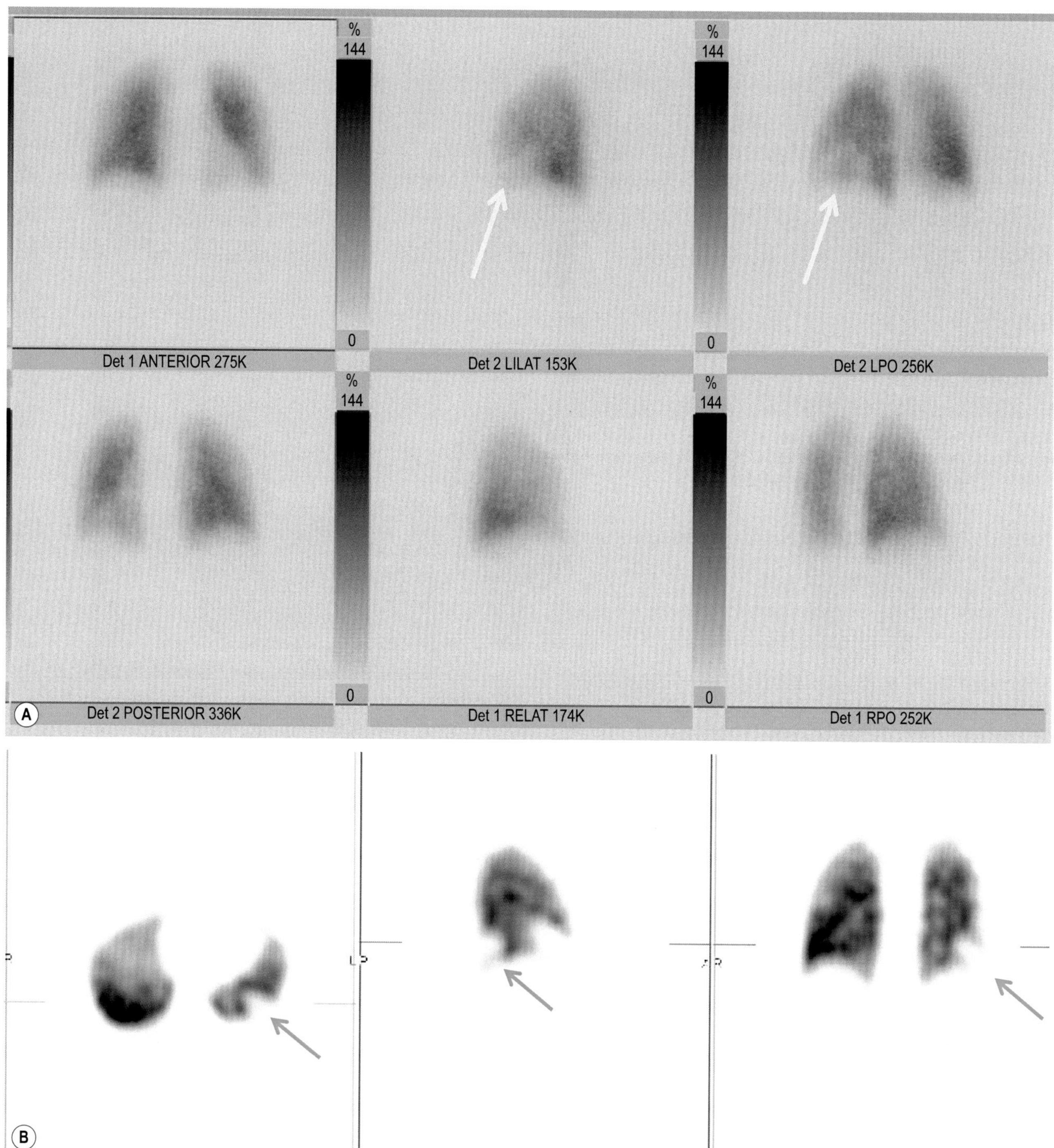

FIGURE 16-19 ■ **Additional SPECT reveals a wedge-shaped perfusion defect.**

obstructive pulmonary disease may also cause these defects. Further investigation therefore is indicated as only up to 30–40% of the patients with an indeterminate result eventually have PE.[43,44]

Perfusion scintigraphy is a good initial imaging investigation in patients with a normal chest X-ray and no history of pulmonary disease; in this setting a normal result or a segmental perfusion defect is a reliable finding which leads to few non-diagnostic results. Perfusion scintigraphy should also be considered when a relative contraindication for CT (see below) exists, such as severe renal impairment.

CT Pulmonary Angiography

In 1992 the first publication on the use of CT pulmonary angiography (CTPA) for the diagnosis of acute pulmonary embolism (PE) appeared.[45] Since then, CTPA has become the investigation of choice in the workup of patients with suspected PE.[46] Its preference is due to the

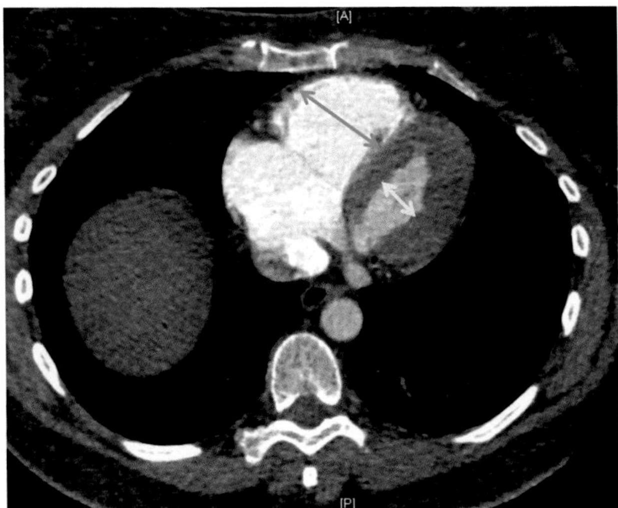

FIGURE 16-20 Significant dilatation of the right ventricle (blue arrow) and right atrium as compared to the left ventricle (yellow arrow) in a patient with massive PE.

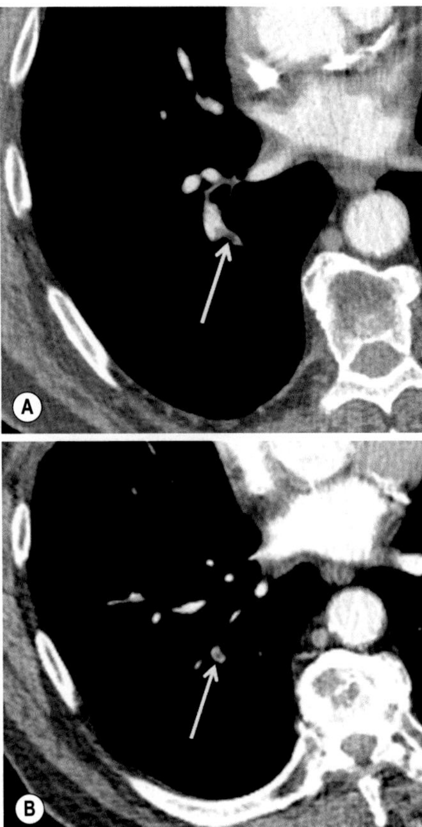

FIGURE 16-21 Small clots (arrows) in a subsegmental branch (A) and sub-subsegmental (B) branch of the right lower lobe pulmonary artery.

continuous improvement of the CT technique ensuing substantial improvement in acquisition speed, spatial resolution, image quality and, most importantly, diagnostic accuracy. Together with the broad availability, low cost and minimal invasiveness of this technique, this led to a broad acceptance in clinical practice.

With modern multi-detector CT, reported sensitivities and specificities of 83–100% and 89–97% are comparable to those of the former gold standard of PE diagnosis, invasive pulmonary angiography of 98 and 97%, respectively. This means that with a qualitatively good CT PE can be ruled out safely, at least in (out) patients without a high clinical probability of PE[47] and further testing for PE is not warranted.

The advantage of CT (and to a lesser extent MRI) over other imaging techniques is the direct visualisation of the emboli as well as the other structures of the chest, including the lung parenchyma, mediastinum and chest wall, resulting in an additional or alternative diagnosis (e.g. pneumonia, pleuritis, aortic dissection, pneumothorax and lung tumours) in a significant proportion of patients with clinical symptoms suggestive of PE.[48]

In patients with PE, CTPA can also provide parameters considered to be related to clinical outcome,[49] such as right ventricular dysfunction (RVD), the total amount of thrombus present (although contradicting results for the latter are found) and, if available, pulmonary perfusion (see below).[50] A right ventricular (RV)/left ventricular (LV) diameter ratio $\geq$ 0.9–1.5 measured on standard axial views has been shown to be directly correlated with RVD and adverse outcome.[51,52] (Fig. 16-20).

The quantitative assessment of the thrombus load for which several scoring systems such as Qanadli[53] and Mastora[54] have been proposed is very time-consuming, although this may be overcome with the use computer assisted detection (CAD) software in the future.[55]

With the improvement of the CT technique, very small PE can be detected that are at or even beyond the subsegmental level (Fig. 16-21). At the moment it is uncertain whether the risk of having solitary very small PE—reported to occur in up to 5% of patients with PE—outweighs the risk of anticoagulant treatment (minor to severe bleeding). At the moment, treatment of solitary small PE is considered indicated if patients have limited cardiopulmonary reserve, coexistent DVT, or recurrent small PE.[46] In a subgroup of patients, especially those who have a good cardiopulmonary reserve, limited timeframe of risk factors and in whom DVT is excluded, treatment for a shorter time period with anticoagulants or even withholding treatment may be considered.

CTPA Protocol. Data acquisition is performed during one breath-hold, preferably at total lung capacity. The standard CT parameters are 100–140 kV, depending on patient habitus. There is a general trend to decrease dose by lowering the kV in slim patients to 70–80 kV. The additional advantage of choosing lower kV is the increase in vascular enhancement (in HU) due to increased absorption of iodine at lower kV. Dose modulation techniques should always be used to further reduce the dose. Regardless of the number of detector rows, between 300 and 450 0.9- to 1.0-mm-thick slices using overlapping reconstruction are obtained.

The injection protocol has to provide a constant and high degree of pulmonary arterial enhancement during the complete data acquisition, which has become a challenge with the very short acquisition times. For an adequate assessment, an attenuation of at least 300–350 HU (i.e. 250–300 HU net contrast enhancement) in the pulmonary arteries is considered optimal.[56,57] Suboptimal vascular opacification is one of the major causes of nondiagnostic images, and it compounds the effect of concomitant problems such as partial volume or movement artefacts.

Combined Protocols: One-Stop-Shop Procedure. Computed tomography (CT) venography has been considered as a part of a one-stop-shop procedure in order to diagnose VTE.[58] After administering one bolus of contrast medium, first the pulmonary arteries are investigated followed by additional late-phase imaging of the deep venous system from the calves up to the inferior vena cava to detect DVT. Although this combined procedure is feasible and has the advantage of detecting DVT in pelvic veins and IVC, which is not possible with CUS, recent studies have shown that in comparison with CTPA alone, this combined technique results in only limited increase in sensitivity with a comparable specificity.[59] A major drawback of CT venography is the significant increase of radiation, which at this moment does not justify its routine use in patients with suspected PE (Fig. 16-22).

Alternatively, CTA with ECG-gating can be performed in patients presenting with acute chest pain without significant increase in radiation dose. During one data acquisition, information can be obtained on the most important vascular diseases causing acute chest pain: acute coronary syndrome, aortic dissection and acute pulmonary embolism.[60] The use of dual-source CT or systems with high numbers of detector rows may overcome the initial limitations of ECG-gated CTPA, providing faster acquisition times, better image quality in patients with abnormal cardiac rhythms, and lower radiation dose.[61] The downside of such a protocol is the increase in complexity both for the technician and the reader, with an increase in postprocessing and interpretation time.

CTPA During Pregnancy. During pregnancy and puerperium, the incidence of VTE is two- to fourfold higher and is one of the most important causes of maternal mortality. As diagnosing DVT in patients with suspected PE justifies PE treatment, leg ultrasound is considered the first diagnostic test of choice as no radiation is used,[46] at least if signs or symptoms of DVT are present.[62] Because of the concern about radiation, there is little agreement about optimal imaging during pregnancy when leg ultrasound is normal. Either CTPA or perfusion scintigraphy can be obtained, the latter being useful if the chest radiograph is normal. As an alternative, MRI has been proposed (see below).

At any time during pregnancy (including the first three months) the radiation dose to the unborn child delivered by either V/Q scintigraphy or CTA is considered negligible,[62] and the risks of a potential fatal ending due to undiagnosed PE are substantial. If CTA is performed, the CT protocol should be adapted to reduce radiation dose and to the hypercirculatory state of pregnant women to limit the number of inconclusive examinations. Furthermore, it is advised to check the thyroid function in the first week after birth, as the iodine in the CT contrast medium may decrease thyroid function.

In young women, either pregnant or not, the radiation exposure to the radiation-sensitive breast tissue (calculated to be 5.5–13.1 mSv; average 7.4 mSv) per breast has one of these must go an important issue, and to a lesser extent the exposure to the lung. Perfusion scintigraphy produces a lower breast dose. During pregnancy this would be at the expense of a slightly increased dose for the fetus as the radiopharmaceutical agent is excreted by the kidneys and may give radiation from the bladder to the neighbouring uterus. Flushing the bladder with saline via a catheter has been proposed to reduce the exposure.

CTPA Assessment. The diagnosis of PE on CTA is based on the direct visualisation of a central luminal filling defect or an eccentric partial filling defect with acute (or sharp) angle, with the vessel wall surrounded by a rim of contrast medium, or a sharp cut-off of a pulmonary artery as a result of complete obstruction by a thrombus[63] (Figs. 16-23 and 16-24). Secondary findings of acute PE may help to point attention to a certain area, such as the presence of pulmonary infarcts (Table 16-7). Signs of acute pulmonary hypertension can also be present, usually as a result of extensive obstruction of the arterial bed, such as dilatation of the pulmonary trunk and/or right heart.

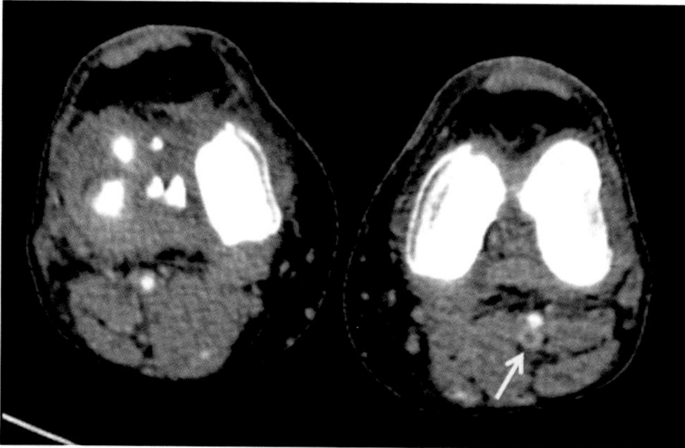

FIGURE 16-22 ■ **CT venography demonstrating thrombus in the left popliteal vein (arrows) with contrast enhancement of the vessel wall (indirect sign), not seen on the right side.**

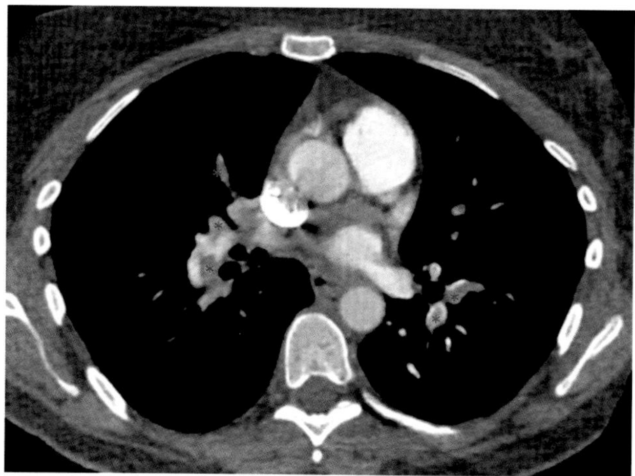

FIGURE 16-23 ■ **Patient with massive PE (asterisks).** Eccentric thrombi with acute angles to the vessel wall as well as completely occluding thrombi are present.

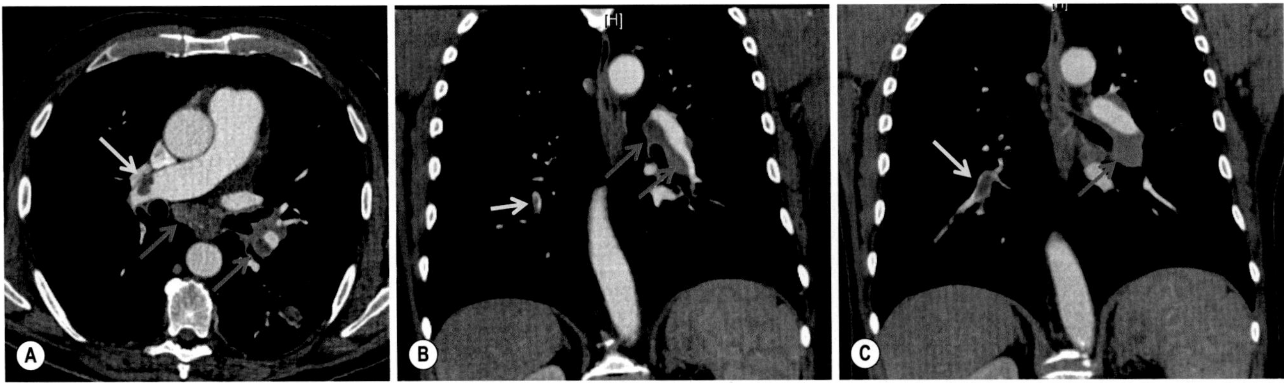

FIGURE 16-24 ■ (A) Central thrombus (yellow arrow) with smooth margins, centrally located and acute angles with the vessel wall, and lymphadenopathy (red arrows). Coronal reconstructions (B, C) may aid in the differentiation between endoluminal clots (yellow arrows) and lymphadenopathy (red arrows). Note the central position of the clot surrounded by contrast medium.

TABLE 16-7 Indirect Signs of Acute PE at CTA

- Wedge-shaped, pleural-based consolidations
- Linear densities
- Plate-like atelectasis
- Volume loss
- Focal dilatation of the pulmonary artery
- Central (proximal) or peripheral (distal) dilatation of the involved pulmonary arteries
- Pleural fluid
- Local hypoperfusion

TABLE 16-8 Causes of False-Positive and False-Negative CTA Results in the Assessment of PE

Causes of False-Positive Results

- Artefacts due to:
  - Pulsation (mainly lingula and left lower lobe)
  - Volume averaging
  - Flow artefacts (non- or only partially opacified arteries)
- Lymph nodes (esp. at the right hilum) and lymphatic tissue
- Slow flow (due to increased resistance such as in presence of atelectasis or pleural fluid)
- Tumours (e.g. pulmonary artery sarcoma)
- Complete obstruction of a vessel without visualisation of the proximal part of the thrombus (non-specific)
- Mucus-filled bronchi
- Pulmonary veins

Causes of False-Negative Results

- Artefacts due to:
  - Motion (breathing, pulsation)
  - High contrast (beam hardening)
- Suboptimal enhancement (e.g. protocol related, intracardiac shunts)
- Inadequate scan or reconstruction parameters (image noise, window settings)
- Isolated (sub)subsegmental PE

Artefacts and pitfalls frequently occur and one should be aware of them to avoid false-positive (Fig. 16-24) and false-negative results (Fig. 16-25). They are listed in Table 16-8.

CT Perfusion. Introduction of dual-source CT has led to novel image interpretation concepts[64] including the quantitative assessment of perfusion defects of the lung parenchyma,[50] which has been found to be an important determinant for patient outcome. In addition, the presence of perfusion defects may help in the detection of PE and therefore increase sensitivity, which can be beneficial, especially for less experienced readers.

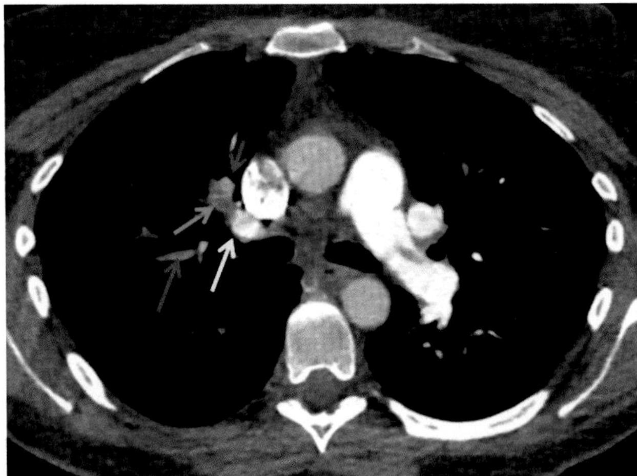

FIGURE 16-25 ■ **Beam hardening artefact in the right upper lobe pulmonary artery (yellow arrow) due to dense contrast medium in the superior caval vein.** Thrombus (blue arrow) more peripherally. Red arrows, non-opacified pulmonary veins.

Dual-source CT with dual-energy technique uses the different absorption characteristics of iodine at different kV. Fusion of the two data sets results in a 'standard' CTA. Subtraction of the lower kV data set from the higher kV data set results in colour-coded CT perfusion maps, resembling the iodine distribution in the lung (Fig. 16-26). However, this technique comes also with a number of pitfalls and artefacts, caused by underlying pulmonary disease such as emphysema, cardiac motion or diaphragm movement or beam hardening effects caused by dense contrast material in the thoracic veins. Although this technique seems promising, the potential benefit of this technique for diagnosis, prognosis and therapy monitoring still needs to be determined.

MR

Magnetic resonance imaging (MRI) is an attractive alternative to CTA as no ionising radiation is used and modern

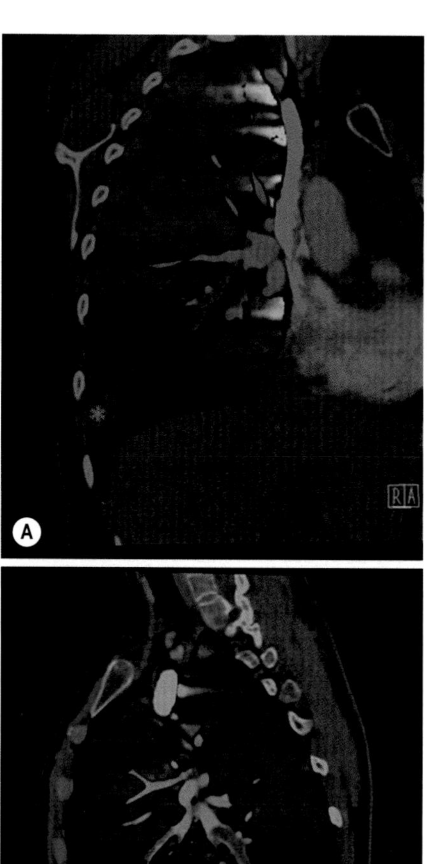

FIGURE 16-26 ■ Perfusion maps using DECT technique fused with CTA showing multiple thrombi with perfusion defects and a consolidation (asterisk) due to infarction (Hampton's hump).

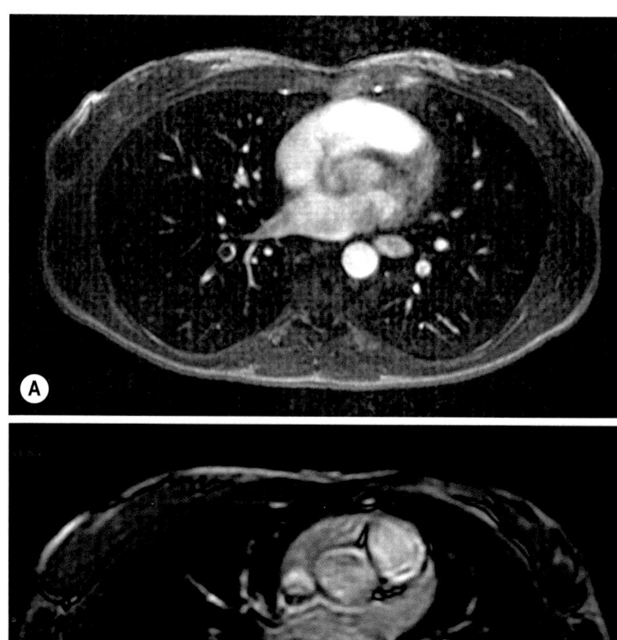

FIGURE 16-27 ■ (A) Post-gadolinium 3D TOF MR angiography image (slice thickness is 2.4 mm) demonstrates right lower lobe segmental PE. (B) Corresponding unenhanced steady-state free-precession (SSFP) sequence (FIESTA) image. (Courtesy of M. P. Revel, Georges Pompidou European University Hospital, Paris, France.)

MRI contrast media yield less risk for the development of contrast-related nephropathy and allergic reactions as compared to iodinated contrast media. Due to the long data acquisition and limited availability, especially in the acute setting, MRI is still not widely performed. On the other hand, recent improvements with respect to spatial resolution and new sequence techniques with shorter acquisition times make it a feasible technique also for the acute setting. Various MRI techniques are available (e.g. unenhanced and post-gadolinium angiography sequences, with or without MR perfusion sequences) (Figs. 16-27A, B).

According to the literature, the accuracy of MRA is comparable to CTPA for central pulmonary arteries, but still limited for PE in the peripheral pulmonary vessels. Reported overall sensitivity compared to MDCT and V/Q is 78–85% and specificity 99–100%. However, the rate of inconclusiveness ranges from 25 to 30%[65,66] and sensitivity drops down to 21–33% for subsegmental PE.[66] As with the newest CT techniques, MRI offers the option to additionally obtain functional information such as on cardiac function and lung perfusion (Fig. 16-28).

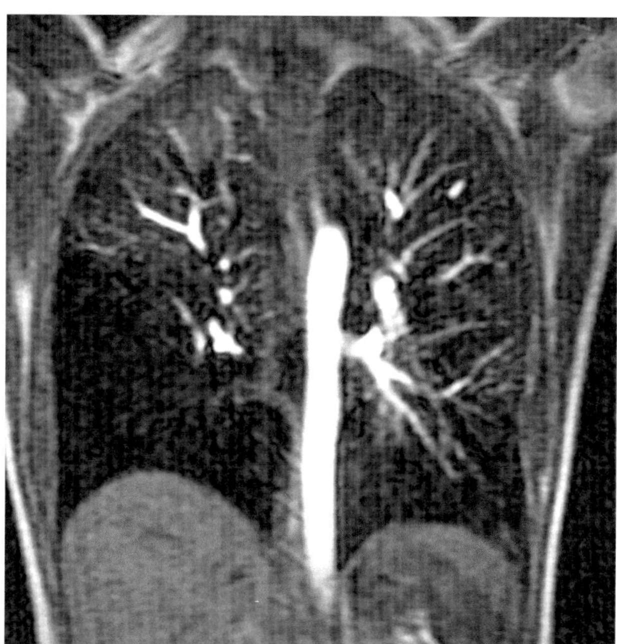

FIGURE 16-28 ■ Patient with bilateral perfusion defects due to lobar PE. (Courtesy of M. P. Revel, Georges Pompidou European University Hospital, Paris, France.)

At the moment, the technique is, however, less robust as compared to CTA and examination times remain long (up to 10–25 minutes for a combined technique protocol). However, further improvement in technique and acquisition speed is to be expected and, together with more experience, may result in better accuracies and a decrease in inconclusive results. As the specificity of MRI is high, it should be considered as a good alternative to CTPA, especially in patients with (relative) contraindications to CTA as young and/or pregnant women.

CHRONIC PULMONARY THROMBOEMBOLISM

PE becomes chronic if the clots in the pulmonary arteries do not resolve adequately. This may result in a continuously increased pulmonary arterial blood pressure, called chronic thromboembolic pulmonary hypertension (CTEPH). CTEPH is a serious and life-threatening complication, and if it occurs it is usually in the first 2 years after the thromboembolic event. The estimated incidence of CTEPH after an episode of acute PE varies, but figures as high as 4% have been described.[67] On the other hand, about half of the patients with CTEPH do not have a clinical history of acute PE. Chronic PE is one of the few causes of pulmonary hypertension that effectively can be treated by surgical resection of the thrombus (pulmonary thromboendarterectomy) if the thrombi are localised in central vessels, up to the proximal segmental arteries. Chronic PE should be evaluated in every patient with pulmonary hypertension with a known history of PE or in whom the cause is unclear. V/Q scintigraphy is the first imaging method of choice in the work-up of patients with suspected CTEPH as a normal perfusion scan confidently rules out the disease whereas multiple, bilateral segmental perfusion defects are suggestive but not specific for chronic PE. At the moment pulmonary angiograpy is still considered the gold standard for the diagnosis of chronic PE, but as with acute PE CT has gained significance in the work-up of patients with pulmonary hypertension in general and suspected chronic PE in particular. CTA may effectively diagnose or rule out other causes such as parenchymal disease, and diagnose and assess the location and extent of chronic thrombi. Although with MR important morphological and functional cardiac information can be obtained,[68] it is not performed routinely because of the known limitations: cost, availability and examination time.

As for acute PE, at CT both direct and indirect signs of chronic PE—which are related to the presence of pulmonary hypertension—have been described.[69–71] Chronic PE is described as the following:

1. A complete obstruction by a thrombus of a pulmonary artery that shows a decrease in diameter as compared to surrounding non-obstructed pulmonary arteries.
2. An eccentric partial intraluminal filling defect with an obtuse angle to the vessel wall (Fig. 16-29).
3. An abrupt tapering of a vessel which is usually the consequence of recanalisation of a previously completely obstructed pulmonary artery by thrombus.
4. A thickening, sometimes irregularly, of the pulmonary arterial wall, with narrowed lumen if recanalisation had occurred.
5. The presence of intraluminal webs or bands (Fig. 16-30).
6. An intraluminal filling defect with the morphology of an acute PE present for > 3 months.

In addition to these findings, post-stenotic dilatation or aneurysms, and calcifications of the chronic thrombi can be observed. The signs are summarised in Table 16-9. It should be noted that in patients with recurrent PE both chronic and acute PE can be present (Fig. 16-30).

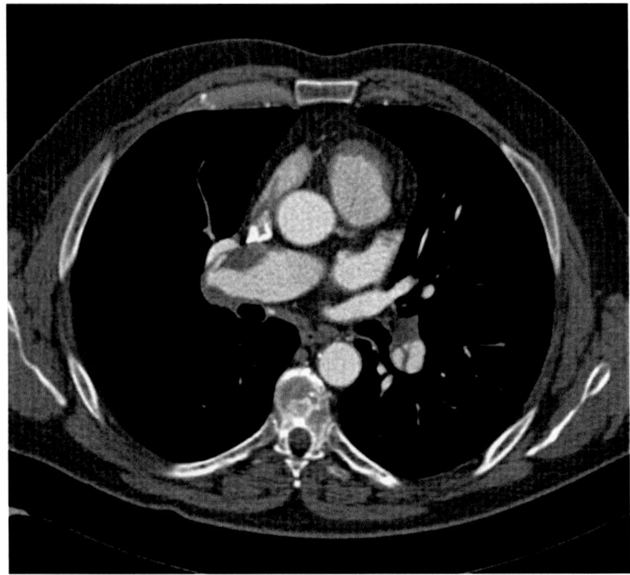

FIGURE 16-29 ■ **CTEPH.** Eccentric thrombus with obtuse angles in the right pulmonary artery and a web in the left lower lobe pulmonary artery.

TABLE 16-9 **Indirect Signs of Chronic PE at CTA**

- Dilatation of the pulmonary trunk (> 29 mm) and central pulmonary arteries
- Mosaic pattern*
- Parenchymal scars which are the sequela of pulmonary infarctions
- Dilatation of the right ventricle (often with concomitant right atrial dilatation)
- Hypertrophy of the right ventricular wall (wall thickness >4 mm)
- Tortuous pulmonary vessels
- Hypertrophy of bronchial arteries and non-bronchial systemic collateral arteries
- Retrograde flow of contrast medium into the inferior vena cava and hepatic veins due to the increased right cardiac pressure
- Cylindrical bronchial dilatation in the involved areas of vascular obstruction (less frequent)

*Mosaic perfusion is defined as sharply demarcated areas of relatively increased and decreased lung attenuation, in the case of CTEPH due to hypoperfusion of the involved parenchymal bed and redistribution of blood flow to the non-involved areas.

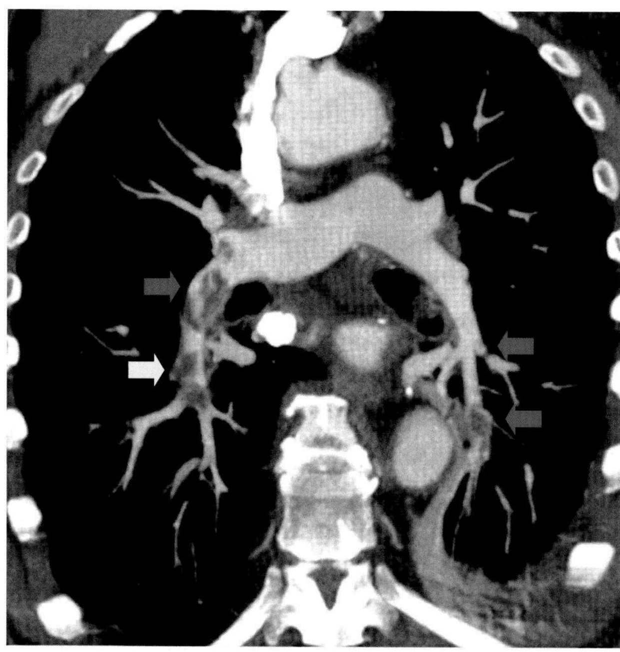

FIGURE 16-30 ■ **Patient with both acute (yellow arrow) and chronic PE (blue arrows).**

CONCLUSION

The investigation of changes in pulmonary vascular physiology has many facets. The initial clinical assessment may significantly influence further investigations. Chest radiography is still the primary method for assessing effects of pulmonary venous hypertension. CTA is the first imaging investigation in the diagnostic work-up of patients with suspected PE. In addition, CT may provide an alternative diagnosis in a significant percentage of patients in which PE is excluded. Pulmonary hypertension is a very serious disease that can be caused by a number of different diseases requiring different treatment and having varying prognosis. CT and MR play a major role in determining the different types of PH.

Acknowledgements

This chapter is based on the previous version prepared by Dr. Paras Dalal and Michael B. Rubens. Their contribution and material are gratefully acknowledged.

REFERENCES

1. Truong QA, Massaro JM, Rogers IS, et al. Reference values for normal pulmonary artery dimensions by noncontrast cardiac computed tomography: The Framingham Heart Study. Circ Cardiovasc Imaging 2012;5:147–54.
2. Edwards P, Bull R, Coulden R. CT measurement of main pulmonary artery diameter. Br J Radiol 1998;71:1018–20.
3. Nevsky G, Jacobs J, Lim R, et al. Sex-specific normalized reference values of heart and great vessel dimensions in cardiac CT angiography. Am J Roentgenol 2011;196:788–94.
4. Ng C, Wells A, Padley S. A CT sign of chronic pulmonary arterial hypertension: the ratio of main pulmonary artery to aortic diameter. J Thorac Imaging 1999;14:270–8.
5. Devaraj A, Wells AU, Meister MG, et al. The effect of diffuse pulmonary fibrosis on the reliability of CT signs of pulmonary hypertension. Radiology 2008;249:1042–9.
6. Kim S, Im J, Kim I, et al. Normal bronchial and pulmonary arterial diameters measured by thin section CT. J Comput Assist Tomogr 1995;19:365–9.
7. Remy-Jardin M, Bouaziz N, Dumont P, et al. Bronchial and nonbronchial systemic arteries at multi-detector row CT angiography: comparison with conventional angiography. Radiology 2004;233:741–9.
8. Brigham KL, Staub NC. Pulmonary edema and acute lung injury research. Am J Respir Crit Care Med 1998;157:S109–13.
9. Sommer N, Dietrich A, Schermuly RT, et al. Regulation of hypoxic pulmonary vasoconstriction: basic mechanisms. Eur Respir J 2008; 32(6):1639–51.
10. Hughes M, West JB. Last word on Point:Counterpoint: gravity is/is not the major factor determining the distribution of blood flow in the human lung. J Appl Physiol 2008;104:1539.
11. Pistolesi M. The chest roentgenogram in pulmonary edema. Clin Chest Med 1985;6:315–44.
12. Gluecker T, Capasso P, Schnyder P, et al. Clinical and radiologic features of pulmonary edema. Radiographics 1999;19:1507–31.
13. Miniati M, Pistolesi M, Paoletti P, et al. Objective radiographic criteria to differentiate cardiac, renal, and injury lung edema. Invest Radiol 1988;23:433–40.
14. Stark P, Jasmine J. CT of pulmonary edema. Crit Rev Diagn Imaging 1989;29:245–55.
15. Komiya K, Ishii H, Murakami J, et al. Comparison of chest computed tomography features in the acute phase of cardiogenic pulmonary edema and acute respiratory distress syndrome on arrival at the emergency department. J Thorac Imaging 2013;28(5):322–8.
16. McGoon M, Gutterman D, Steen V, et al. Screening, early detection, and diagnosis of pulmonary arterial hypertension: ACCP evidence-based clinical practice guidelines. Chest 2004;126:14S–34S.
17. Rubin LJ. Primary pulmonary hypertension. N Engl J Med 1997;336:111–17.
18. McLaughlin V, Presberg K, Doyle R, et al. Prognosis of pulmonary arterial hypertension: ACCP evidence-based clinical practice guidelines. Chest 2004;126:78S–92S.
19. Simonneau G, Robbins I, Beghetti M, et al. Updated clinical classification of pulmonary hypertension. J Am Coll Cardiol 2009; 54:S43–54.
20. Galiè N, Hoeper MM, Humber M, et al. Guidelines for the diagnosis and treatment of pulmonary hypertension: The Task Force for the Diagnosis and Treatment of Pulmonary Hypertension of the European Society of Cardiology (ESC) and the European Respiratory Society (ERS), endorsed by the International Society of Heart and Lung Transplantation (ISHLT). Eur Heart J 2009;30:2493–537.
21. Hachulla E, Gressin V, Guillevin L, et al. Early detection of pulmonary arterial hypertension in systemic sclerosis: A French nationwide prospective multicenter study. Arthritis Rheum 2005; 52:3792–800.
22. Junqueira FP, Lima CMAO, Coutinho AC, et al. Pulmonary arterial hypertension: an imaging review comparing MR pulmonary angiography and perfusion with multidetector CT angiography. Br J Radiol 2012;85:1446–56.
23. Marcus JT, Gan CT-J, Zwanenburg JJM, et al. Interventricular mechanical asynchrony in pulmonary arterial hypertension: left-to-right delay in peak shortening is related to right ventricular overload and left ventricular underfilling. J Am Coll Cardiol 2008;51:750–7.
24. Ley S, Grünig E, Kiely DG, et al. Computed tomography and magnetic resonance imaging of pulmonary hypertension: pulmonary vessels and right ventricle. J Magn Reson Imaging 2010;32:1313–24.
25. Devaraj A, Hansell DM. Computed tomography signs of pulmonary hypertension: old and new observations. Clin Radiol 2009; 64:751–60.
26. Devaraj A, Wells AU, Meister MG, et al. Detection of pulmonary hypertension with multidetector CT and echocardiography alone and in combination. Radiology 2010;254:609–16.

27. Grosse C, Grosse A. CT findings in diseases associated with pulmonary hypertension: a current review. Radiographics 2010;30: 1753–77.
28. Frazier AA, Franks TJ, Mohammed T-LH, et al. Pulmonary veno-occlusive disease and pulmonary capillary hemangiomatosis. Radiographics 2007;27:867–82.
29. Remy J, Remy-Jardin M, Giraud F, Wattinne L. Angioarchitecture of pulmonary arteriovenous malformations: clinical utility of three-dimensional helical CT. Radiology 1994;191:657–64.
30. Anderson FA Jr, Wheeler HB, Goldberg RJ, et al. A population-based perspective of the hospital incidence and case-fatality rates of deep vein thrombosis and pulmonary embolism. The Worcester DVT Study. Arch Intern Med 1991;151:933–8.
31. Silverstein MD, Heit JA, Mohr DN, et al. Trends in the incidence of deep vein thrombosis and pulmonary embolism: a 25-year population-based study. Arch Intern Med 1998;158:585–93.
32. Alpert JS, Smith R, Carlson J, et al. Mortality in patients treated for pulmonary embolism. JAMA 1976;236:1477–80.
33. Stein PD, Beemath A, Matta F, et al. Clinical characteristics of patients with acute pulmonary embolism: data from PIOPED II. Am J Med 2007;120:871–9.
34. Torbicki A, Perrier A, Konstantinides S, et al. Guidelines on the diagnosis and management of acute pulmonary embolism: The Task Force for the Diagnosis and Management of Acute Pulmonary Embolism of the European Society of Cardiology (ESC). Eur Heart J 2008;29(18):2276–315.
35. Moser K. Pulmonary embolism. Am Rev Respir Dis 1977;115: 829–52.
36. Ceriani E, Combescure C, Le Gal G, et al. Clinical prediction rules for pulmonary embolism: a systematic review and meta-analysis. J Thromb Haemost 2010;8:957–70.
37. Lucassen W, Geersing G-J, Erkens PM, et al. Clinical decision rules for excluding pulmonary embolism: a meta-analysis. Ann Intern Med 2011;155:448–60.
38. Goekoop R, Steeghs N, Niessen R, et al. Simple and safe exclusion of pulmonary embolism in outpatients using quantitative D-dimer and Wells' simplified decision rule. Thromb Haemost 2007;97:146–50.
39. van Beek EJ, Reekers JA, Batchelor DA, et al. Feasibility, safety and clinical utility of angiography in patients with suspected pulmonary embolism. Eur Radiol 1996;6:415–19.
40. Hudson ER, Smith TP, McDermott VG, et al. Pulmonary angiography performed with iopamidol: complications in 1,434 patients. Radiology 1996;198:61–5.
41. Goodacre S, Sampson F, Thomas S, et al. Systematic review and meta-analysis of the diagnostic accuracy of ultrasonography for deep vein thrombosis. BMC Med Imaging 2005;5:6.
42. Bajc M, Neilly JB, Miniati M, et al. EANM guidelines for ventilation/perfusion scintigraphy. Eur J Nucl Med Mol Imaging 2009;36(8):1356–70.
43. PIOPED Investigators. Value of the ventilation/perfusion scan in acute pulmonary embolism. Results of the prospective investigation of pulmonary embolism diagnosis (PIOPED). JAMA 1990;263: 2753–9.
44. Hull RD, Hirsh J, Carter CJ, et al. Diagnostic value of ventilation-perfusion lung scanning in patients with suspected pulmonary embolism. Chest 1985;88:819–28.
45. Remy-Jardin M, Remy J, Wattinne L, Giraud F. Central pulmonary thromboembolism: diagnosis with spiral volumetric CT with the single-breath-hold technique—comparison with pulmonary angiography. Radiology 1992;185:381–7.
46. Remy-Jardin M, Pistolesi M, Goodman LR, et al. Management of suspected acute pulmonary embolism in the era of CT angiography: a statement from the Fleischner Society. Radiology 2007;245:315–29.
47. Stein PD, Woodard PK, Weg JG, et al. Diagnostic pathways in acute pulmonary embolism: recommendations of the PIOPED II Investigators. Radiology 2007;242(1):15–21.
48. van Strijen M, Bloem J, de Monyé W, et al. Helical computed tomography and alternative diagnosis in patients with excluded pulmonary embolism. J Thromb Haemost 2005;3:2449–56.
49. Abrahams-van Doorn P, Hartmann I. Cardiothoracic CT: one-stop-shop procedure? Impact on the management of acute pulmonary embolism. Insights Imaging 2011;2:705–15.
50. Zhou Y, Shi H, Wang Y, et al. Assessment of correlation between CT angiographic clot load score, pulmonary perfusion defect score and global right ventricular function with dual-source CT for acute pulmonary embolism. Br J Radiol 2012;85:972–9.
51. Singanayagam A, Chalmers JD, Scally C, et al. Right ventricular dilation on CT pulmonary angiogram independently predicts mortality in pulmonary embolism. Respir Med 2010;104: 1057–62.
52. van der Meer RW, Pattynama PMT, van Strijen MJL, et al. Right ventricular dysfunction and pulmonary obstruction index at helical CT: prediction of clinical outcome during 3-month follow-up in patients with acute pulmonary embolism. Radiology 2005;235: 798–803.
53. Qanadli SD, Hajjam ME, Vieillard-Baron A, et al. New CT index to quantify arterial obstruction in pulmonary embolism: comparison with angiographic index and echocardiography. Am J Roentgenol 2001;176:1415–20.
54. Mastora I, Remy-Jardin M, Masson P, et al. Severity of acute pulmonary embolism: evaluation of a new spiral CT angiographic score in correlation with echocardiographic data. Eur Radiol 2003; 13:29–35.
55. Furlan A, Aghayev A, Chang C-CH, et al. Short-term mortality in acute pulmonary embolism: clot burden and signs of right heart dysfunction at CT pulmonary angiography. Radiology 2012;265: 283–93.
56. Bae KT. Optimization of contrast enhancement in thoracic MDCT. Radiol Clin North Am 2010;48:9–29.
57. Prokop M. Multislice CT angiography. Eur J Radiol 2000;36: 86–96.
58. Katz D, Loud P, Bruce D, et al. Combined CT venography and pulmonary angiography: a comprehensive review. Radiographics 2002;22:S3–19.
59. Stein PD, Fowler SE, Goodman LR, et al. Multidetector computed tomography for acute pulmonary embolism. N Engl J Med 2006; 354:2317–27.
60. Halpern EJ. Triple-rule-out CT angiography for evaluation of acute chest pain and possible acute coronary syndrome. Radiology 2009;252(2):332–45.
61. Becker H-C, Johnson T. Cardiac CT for the assessment of chest pain: Imaging techniques and clinical results. Eur J Radiol 2012; 81:3675–9.
62. Leung A, Bull T, Jaeschke R, et al. An official American Thoracic Society/Society of Thoracic Radiology clinical practice guideline: evaluation of suspected pulmonary embolism in pregnancy. Am J Respir Crit Care Med 2011;184:1200–8.
63. Wittram C, Maher MM, Yoo AJ, et al. CT angiography of pulmonary embolism: diagnostic criteria and causes of misdiagnosis. Radiographics 2004;24:1219–38.
64. Lu G, Zhao Y, Zhang L, Schoepf U. Dual-energy CT of the lung. Am J Roentgenol 2012;199:S40–53.
65. Stein PD, Chenevert TL, Fowler SE, et al. Gadolinium-enhanced magnetic resonance angiography for pulmonary embolism: a Multicenter Prospective Study (PIOPED III). Ann Intern Med 2010; 152:434–43.
66. Revel MP, Sanchez O, Couchon S, et al. Diagnostic accuracy of magnetic resonance imaging for an acute pulmonary embolism: results of the 'IRM-EP' study. J Thromb Haemost 2012;10: 743–50.
67. Pengo V, Lensing AWA, Prins MH, et al. Incidence of chronic thromboembolic pulmonary hypertension after pulmonary embolism. N Engl J Med 2004;350:2257–64.
68. Kreitner K-F, Kunz RP, Ley S, et al. Chronic thromboembolic pulmonary hypertension—assessment by magnetic resonance imaging. Eur Radiol 2007;17:11–21.
69. Castañer E, Gallardo X, Ballesteros E, et al. CT diagnosis of chronic pulmonary thromboembolism. Radiographics 2009;29: 31–50.
70. Wittram C, Kalra MK, Maher MM, et al. Acute and chronic pulmonary emboli: angiography-CT correlation. Am J Roentgenol 2006;186:S421–9.
71. Wittram C, Maher MM, Halpern EF, Shepard J-AO. Attenuation of acute and chronic pulmonary emboli. Radiology 2005;235: 1050–4.

CHAPTER 17

The Thoracic Aorta: Diagnostic Aspects

Rossella Fattori • Luigi Lovato

THE NORMAL AORTA

The aorta is the main artery of the body delivering oxygenated blood from the left ventricle to all parts. In common with other arteries it has three histologically distinct layers: an intima consisting of a thin endothelial layer; a media containing an elastic lamella, smooth muscle and connective tissue; and a thin outer adventitia made of connective and elastic tissues also containing nerves, lymphatics and the vasa vasorum.[1] The aortic root begins at the upper part of the left ventricle and is approximately 3 cm in diameter. A normal aorta passes superiorly and to the right for approximately 5 cm, then arches posteriorly over the root of the left lung, descending within the thorax beside the vertebral column, gradually achieving the median plane, and becoming the abdominal aorta, after it passes through the aortic hiatus in the diaphragm. The abdominal aorta is approximately 2 cm in diameter; it ends slightly to the left of the median plane at the lower border of the fourth lumbar vertebra by dividing into the right and left common iliac arteries.

The aortic root and most of the ascending aorta is contained within the pericardium. The root consists of three sinuses: the right coronary artery arising from the right coronary sinus, the left coronary artery from the left coronary sinus and a non-coronary sinus which is usually located to the right and posterior. The ascending aorta forms the right mediastinal border on a postero-anterior (PA) chest radiograph. It becomes the aortic arch at the origin of the innominate artery and also gives rise to the left common carotid and left subclavian arteries. Around three-quarters of people show this 'normal' branch pattern of the supra-aortic arteries, but in 20% the innominate and left common carotid arteries have a common origin, and in 6% the left vertebral artery arises directly from the aortic arch. The aortic arch ends and the descending thoracic aorta begins immediately beyond the origin of the left subclavian artery. At this site the ligamentum venosum (the embryological ductus arteriosus which closes within a few days of birth) joins the inferior concavity of the aortic arch to the main pulmonary artery. The aorta is fixed at this point. Occasionally the duct may persist as a short diverticulum.[2]

DIAGNOSTIC ASPECTS

The last few decades have seen an increasing recognition of thoracic aortic disease among Western people,[3] partly due to greater longevity and an increased awareness of its clinical importance.[4,5] Recent technological advances in CT and MRI have greatly contributed to the increased recognition and pathological understanding of aortic disease.

There are at least three main goals of imaging concerning thoracic aortic diseases: disease recognition, preoperative evaluation and imaging follow-up. The appropriate imaging technique depends on which of these aspects is pre-minent (Table 17-1).

Aortic disease often presents as a clinical emergency, with patients becoming rapidly haemodynamically unstable over time.[6] Accordingly, non-invasiveness, diagnostic accuracy and speed are the main properties requested in this setting, together with a comprehensive evaluation of the thoracic aorta (crucial for an accurate assessment before any intervention). *Thus the choice of the optimal imaging technique should consider these aspects and various patient-related factors (namely, acute or chronic presentation).*

Evaluation of the thoracic aorta has always been very difficult with first-line imaging techniques like chest X-ray (CXR) and transthoracic ultrasound (except for proximal aortic segments) due to its anatomical location. CXR may only identify indirect signs of aortic aneurysm or dissection such as a widening of the upper mediastinum or an abnormal aortic contour increase, but it lacks sufficient sensitivity to exclude significant aortic disease, especially in high-risk patients[7] and, almost invariably, additional imaging is required for clarification. Moreover, CXR does not give any information about

TABLE 17-1 Diagnostic Goals of Aortic Diseases and Corresponding Features Requested to an Imaging Test

Diagnostic Aspects	Appropriate Features
Disease recognition	Diagnostic accuracy Non-invasiveness Rapidity Logistic convenience Availability
Preoperative evaluation	Mutiplanarity Wide field of view High spatial resolutions 2D/3D reformatting images
Imaging follow-up	Measurement reproducibility Non-invasiveness Availability Diagnostic accuracy

anatomical details for surgical or endovascular planning. Transthoracic echocardiography (TTE) is limited by its restricted field of view, further reduced by acoustic window limitations in adult patients (e.g. due to chronic pulmonary diseases, surgical scars or obesity), and has a typical 'blind spot' at the level of the proximal aortic arch due to superposition of air in the right bronchus. Transoesophageal echocardiography (TOE) is superior to TTE for thoracic aorta evaluation[8] and it can be easily performed at the bedside. However, it is partially invasive and not well tolerated by patients. Though echocardiography is routinely used for follow-up of aortic root and proximal ascending aorta aneurysms in chronic diseases, its narrow field of view prevents a comprehensive evaluation of the thoracic aorta. Furthermore, operator dependence limits the overall accuracy. However, ultrasound still plays the main role for valvular assessment in thoracic aortic diseases (coexisting valvular disease or valvular involvement in type A aortic dissection or ascending aortic aneurysm), while intraoperative TOE is often fundamental for endovascular or surgical aortic treatment. In summary, CXR and ultrasound, although easy to perform, non-invasive and inexpensive, provide some helpful information, but alone they cannot provide comprehensive information about aortic disease.

For many decades angiography was the only available imaging technique for diagnosis and preoperative evaluation of aortic diseases. It was intrinsically invasive, relatively costly, and needed a well-organised and experienced team. It only provided limited information about the aortic wall, because angiography provides only 'luminographic' data. Thus it provided limited information about an intramural haematoma (IMH) and could be misleading in aortic dissection with a complete false lumen thrombosis. Over the past 30 years, with the advent of computed tomography (CT) and magnetic resonance imaging (MRI) and their recent technological evolutions, angiography has become progressively abandoned by physicians for diagnostic purposes.[9]

Indeed, CT and MRI combine non-invasiveness with high spatial and temporal resolution and can provide infromation about the entire length of the thoracic or thoracoabdominal aorta. Multiplanar images allow precise measurements of aortic diameters, preferably taken perpendicular to the longitudinal axis in more than one plane to avoid source of errors. In fact, the aorta has such variable geometry that it cannot usually be entirely visualised in a single plane.

MR angiography (MRA) and CT angiography (CTA) have further enhanced the non-invasive visualisation of vascular structures with a high degree of spatial and contrast resolution in all three dimensions. Different 2D and 3D processing techniques, such as multiplanar reformation (MPR), maximum intensity projection (MIP) and volume rendering (VR), play an important role for preoperative planning.[10] While thin-slice MPRs in any arbitrary plane provide high anatomical resolution, they cannot visualise the entire aorta in a single plane. MIP images of appropriate slab thickness, while demonstrating the whole aorta, only yield information of perfused lumina similar to digital subtraction angiography; as a threshold technique, MIP images may not discriminate lower-density intraluminal structures such as thrombus, plaque or intramural haematoma. MIP images also do not provide any fore- or background information, thereby limiting the perception of interstructural relationships. VR is a different 3D reconstruction technique where all tissues can be simultaneously represented. Using adequate filters, metallic stents or clips do not create artefacts and aortic wall lesions can be differentiated from the lumen. VR provides 3D anatomical information displaying the spatial relationship between aortic lesions and branching vessels. Finally, curved reformations can reconstruct even the most tortuous vascular structure in a single plane. All these processing and display options make CT and MRI measurements highly reproducible and less operator-dependent than ultrasound.

CT and MRI currently form the backbone of thoracic aortic imaging. Both techniques show comparable results in terms of diagnostic accuracy, measurement reproducibility and anatomical detail definition. MRI does not use ionising radiation and gadolinium is less nephrotoxic than iodinated contrast medium. Consideration should only be given to patient with severe renal dysfunction (creatinine clearance <30 mg/dL/min) where it is necessary to balance the clinical usefulness of gadolinium and the risk of nephrogenic renal sclerosis.[11] Recently, the development of 3D steady-state free-precession (SSFP) sequences with navigator echo seems to overcome this limitation,[12] allowing MRI to obtain angiographic images of the aorta without gadolinium administration with similar accuracy compared to traditional MRA imaging (Fig. 17-1).

The main limitation of CT imaging is the potential radiation risk,[13] especially in neonates, children and young adults. Although recent CT technologies (dual-source CT, prospective gating, etc.) are reducing radiation exposure,[14] the dose cannot be considered negligible, especially for repeated follow-up examinations of chronic aortic disease. Moreover, the use of iodinated contrast medium requires careful consideration in patients with borderline renal insufficiency or a history of previous reactions.

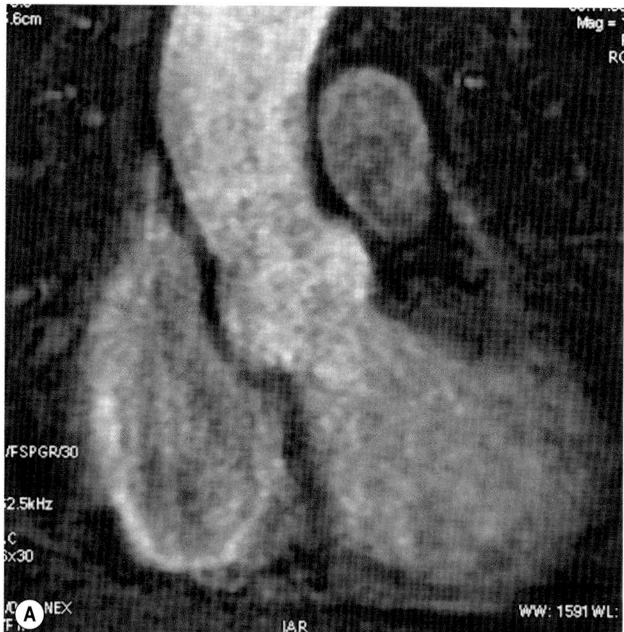

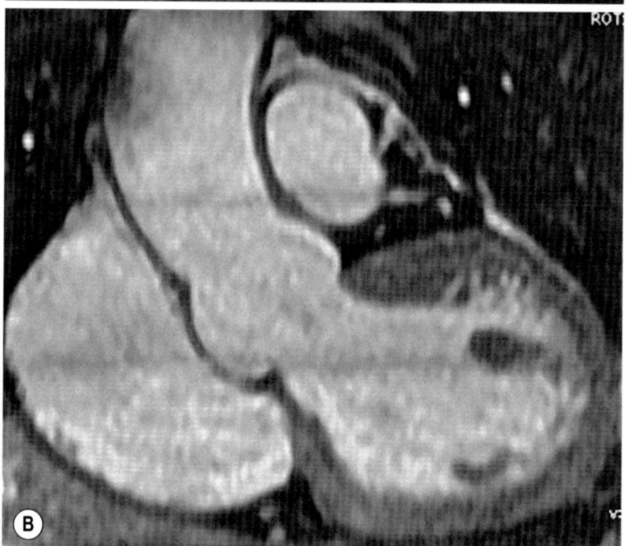

FIGURE 17-1 ■ MRA coronal oblique multiplanar reconstruction of ascending aorta. (A) Unenhanced 3D SSFP MRA with navigator echo (free breathing). (B) Contrast-enhanced MRA. Note similar or even superior image quality of 3D SSFP technique in the same patient.

Disease presentation is another aspect that influences the choice of imaging investigation. Thoracic aortic diseases frequently present acutely. MRI requires longer examination times, is less readily available and usually with less favourable logistics/locations; these factors often make it less suitable for patients with acute disease. CT is rapid and very accurate, and is particularly well-suited for the diagnosis and correct treatment planning of acute aortic problems. Modern MDCT allow for sub-millimetre, isotropic 3D data acquisition of extended anatomical ranges within comfortable (4–8 s) breath-hold duration; dedicated software provides 2D and 3D artefact-free reconstructions from virtually any angle and in any desirable plane. The introduction of the ECG gating[15] has minimised motion artefacts, increasing the sensitivity and specificity for type A aortic dissection, especially with respect to identifying intimal flaps and aortic valve morphology.

CT equipment is more widely available and often located close to the intensive care units or operating rooms. Moreover, when acute aortic dissection is suspected, MDCT is also able to exclude other potential causes of thoracic pain such as pulmonary embolism, other pulmonary diseases or coronary arteries disease[16] with high accuracy, though this requires choosing appropriate examination protocols. Thus MRI, though highly accurate for acute aortic disease evaluation, is usually confined to cases of severe renal insufficiency or absolute contraindications to iodinated contrast medium. The high diagnostic accuracy of MR in patients with acute aortic syndrome is based on its high contrast resolution between the lumen and the vessel wall provided by black-blood fast spin-echo (BBFSE) and SSFP imaging, which allows differentiation of aortic wall alterations (e.g. intramural haematoma) from atheromatous plaques or aortitis.

In patients with chronic aortic disease, follow-up and identification of findings requiring surgery are the main goals for imaging. Both CT and MRI provide highly reproducible and accurate aortic measurements, but MRI may be preferred to CT to minimise radiation exposure, especially in young adults affected by congenital aortic anomalies and genetic syndromes associated with thoracic aneurysms like Marfan's or Turner's syndrome. MRI, with cine gradient-echo sequences and phase contrast imaging, can also obtain functional informations on the thoracic aorta and quantify aortic valve regurgitation or stenosis within the same examination. CT is preferred to MRI only for aortic stent imaging follow-up. The stent material causes artefacts on MRI images, which reduce MRI's sensitivity for detection of small endoleaks or stent structure alterations.

ACQUIRED AORTIC ABNORMALITIES

Acute Aortic Syndrome

The term 'acute aortic syndrome' comprises all aortic diseases characterised by a sudden clinical presentation that require acute hospitalisation (within 15 days from symptom onset) and often need urgent surgical or endovascular repair. It includes aortic dissection, IMH, penetrating aortic ulcer, traumatic aortic rupture, suture dehiscence and ruptured aneurysm.

Aortic Dissection

Aortic dissection is the most common non-traumatic acute aortic emergency with an overall in-hospital mortality of 20–25%, which increases markedly in patients with complicated dissection.

The aetiology is frequently unknown, but is related to advancing age and hypertension. Cystic medial degeneration in connective tissue disorders such as Marfan's syndrome and Ehlers–Danlos syndrome is a predisposing factor, as are coarctation, bicuspid aortic valve, aortitis, pregnancy and blunt chest trauma.

Aortic dissection is initiated by an intimal tear, which allows blood to penetrate into the medial layer, producing a cleavage plane (false lumen) between the inner two-thirds and outer one-third of media. The true lumen is separated from the false lumen by an intimomedial flap. The blood course through the medial layer can variably extend the dissection distal or proximal to the entry tear and eventually rupture through the adventitia or back through the intima into the true lumen, creating re-entry tears. Branching vessels can be involved by the dissection process and may variably originate from the true lumen, the false lumen or both. The false lumen may thrombose completely or partially over time, while reduction in the amount of elastic tissue within the wall of the false lumen may lead to subsequent aneurysmatic dilatation.

Classification

In the literature, there are various classification systems for aortic dissection, depending on the extent of the thoracic aorta involved (Table 17-2). The most frequenly used is the Stanford classification whereby an aortic dissection is called type A if it involves the ascending aorta, regardless of the site of entry tear. Type B dissections only involve the aorta beyond the left subclavian artery. This classification is focused on prognosis and strongly influences treatment approach, because, if not surgically treated, type A dissection leads to death in the majority of cases, while type B dissection can be successfully managed with medical therapy. Even type B dissections, when unstable, may require intervention to avoid severe complications and an increasing mortality. The anatomy of the dissection indicates the type of surgery or endovascular technique and their feasibility, thus affecting the procedure success rate and the long-term results. Therefore, the goal of imaging is not only the identification of the intimal flap and the extent of dissection but also a clear definition of the presence and site of entry and re-entry tears, the relationship between true and false lumen and the aortic branches (visceral, epiaortic, iliac and femoral vessels), the presence and degree of aortic valve or coronary artery compromise.

Imaging

Aortography was traditionally the gold standard in suspected aortic dissection even though catheter manipulation and directly high-flow contrast injection in a dissected aorta increased the risk of acute complications. The advent of non-invasive imaging also demonstrated its suboptimal accuracy, especially in terms of sensitivity (77 to 90%), while specificity was 90 to 100%. CT, MRI and TOE have rapidly substituted invasive angiography.[17]

TOE can be performed at the bedside in patients too unstable for transportation and can give haemodynamic information about flow in the true and false lumen, with excellent sensitivity for the aortic dissection confirmation (85–90%). TOE also provides valuable information about the functional status of the aortic valve and can assess the degree of involvement of the coronary arteries (Fig. 17-2) in type A dissection. However, being operator-dependent, its specificity is reduced in the 'blind areas' of the distal ascending aorta and the aortic arch. Besides, TOE cannot assess abdominal aorta and its visceral branches so, in stable patients a second imaging test is advisable for a comprehensive evaluation of the thoracoabdominal aorta.

Intravascular ultrasound (IVUS) at 12.5 MHz provides intraluminal cross-sectional images of vessels and is able to demonstrate the entry tear and extent of dissection, but is particularly useful in differentiating the true and false lumen, and demonstration of dynamic obstruction. However, the transducers are single use only and expensive, most departments have limited experience of IVUS as a diagnostic tool and its role is almost exclusively confined to interventional applications.[18]

MRI is one of the most accurate tools for aortic dissection evaluation, with excellent sensitivity and specificity that approximate 100%.[19] On MRI images the excellent contrast between the lumen and the aortic wall make the detection of the intimal flap very easy. In BBFSE sequences it appears linear inside the black vessel lumen (Fig. 17-3). The false lumen can be differentiated from the true lumen by its higher signal intensity due to the slower flow (Fig. 17-4). The presence of cobwebs adjacent to the outer wall, which represent dissected media residual strands, are also useful for identifying the false lumen. A fast spin-echo sequence in the sagittal plane should be performed to define the extension of the dissection in the thoracic and abdominal aorta, including the aortic arch branches (Fig. 17-4). The accurate definition of the anatomical details of the dissection (extension, site of entry and re-entry tear, aortic branch relationships) relies on gadolinium-enhanced 3D MRA and its reformatted images, also including a complete analysis of axial MRA images to confirm and improve spin-echo information (Fig. 17-5). The SSFP technique can generate images

TABLE 17-2 **Classification Systems for Aortic Dissection**

	Classification System		
Site of Dissection	CRAWFORD	DEBAKEY	STANFORD
Both ascending and descending aorta	Proximal dissections	Type I	Type A
Ascending aorta and arch only	Proximal dissections	Type II	Type A
Descending aorta only (distal to left subclavian artery)	Distal dissections	Type IIIa—limited to thoracic aorta Type IIIb—extends to abdominal aorta	Type B

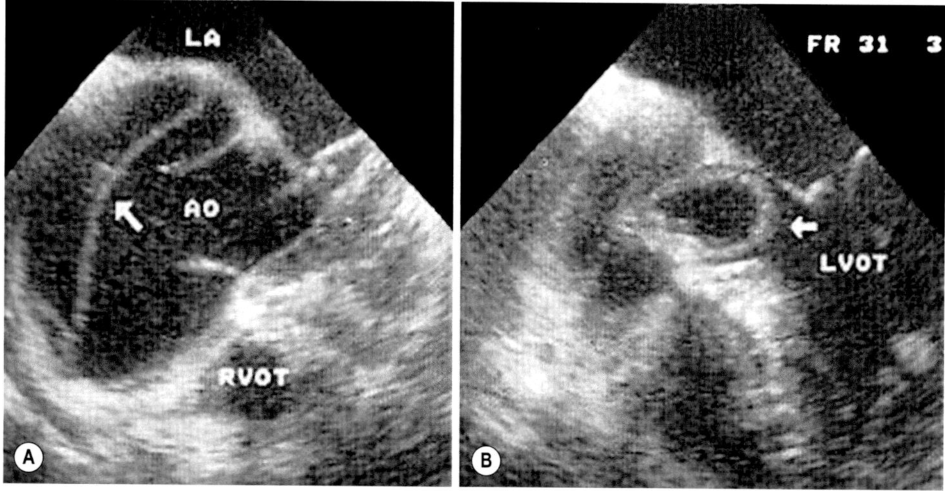

FIGURE 17-2 ■ **Transoesophageal echocardiogram of a type A dissection.** (A) The dissection distal to the aortic valve (arrow) with (B) prolapse of the dissection flap (arrow) through the aortic valve into the left ventricular outflow tract (LVOT). AO = aortic valve, LA = left atrium, RVOT = right ventricular outflow tract. (Courtesy of Dr K. E. Berkin, The Leeds Teaching Hospitals NHS Trust, UK.)

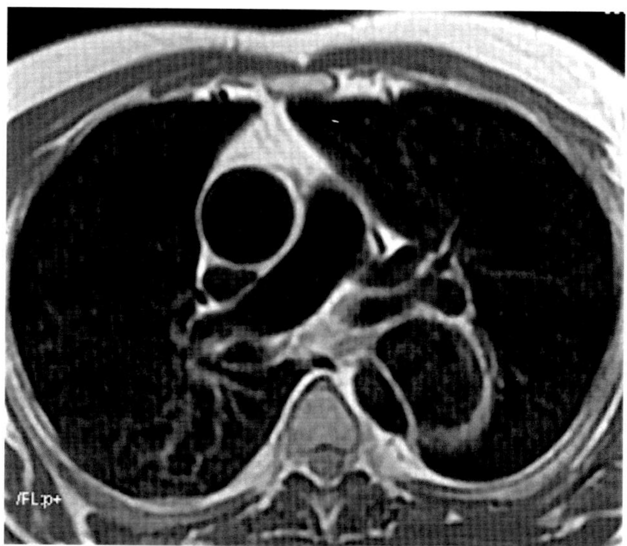

FIGURE 17-3 ■ **Axial BBFSE image of chronic type B aortic dissection.** The intimal flap is well depicted as a straight hyperintense line dividing the true and false lumen at the level of descending aorta.

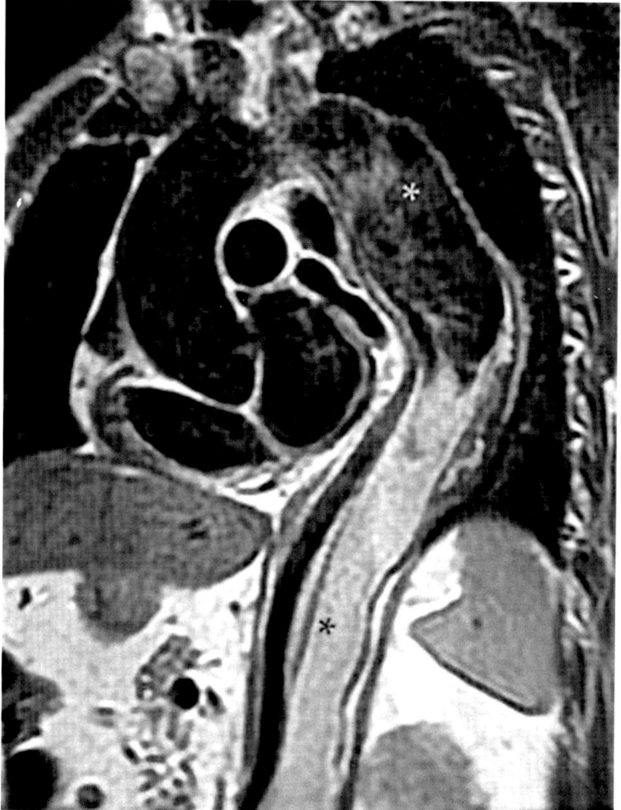

FIGURE 17-4 ■ **Sagittal oblique BBFSE image of chronic type B aortic dissection.** The intimal flap extends to the abdominal aorta. The false lumen (the posterior one) is recognised by the highest signal due to slow flow. The signal is heterogeneous in descending thoracic aorta (white asterisk) near the intimal tear, while intensity and homogeneity are increased in the abdominal aorta (black asterisk) where the false lumen flow further slows down and there are no re-entry tears or it is even thrombosed. The true lumen is small with homogeneous dark signal-like normal ascending aorta.

with a high-contrast resolution between the aortic lumen and the wall that may be used for morphological (2D or 3D images) or functional (cine sequences) analysis (Fig. 17-6). Cine sequences may be used as an additional tool to evaluate aortic valve involvement and to define the presence of an entry tear (flow turbulence). With more recent equipment 2D images can achieve a complete study of the thoracic aorta within a few minutes[20] while a patient's ECG, blood pressure and oxygen saturation can be monitored even during assisted ventilation. A 3D sequence may be an alternative to MRA in rare cases when gadolinium is contraindicated. Despite these strong capacities, which virtually make MRI an ideal imaging modality for aortic dissection, its use in acute dissection

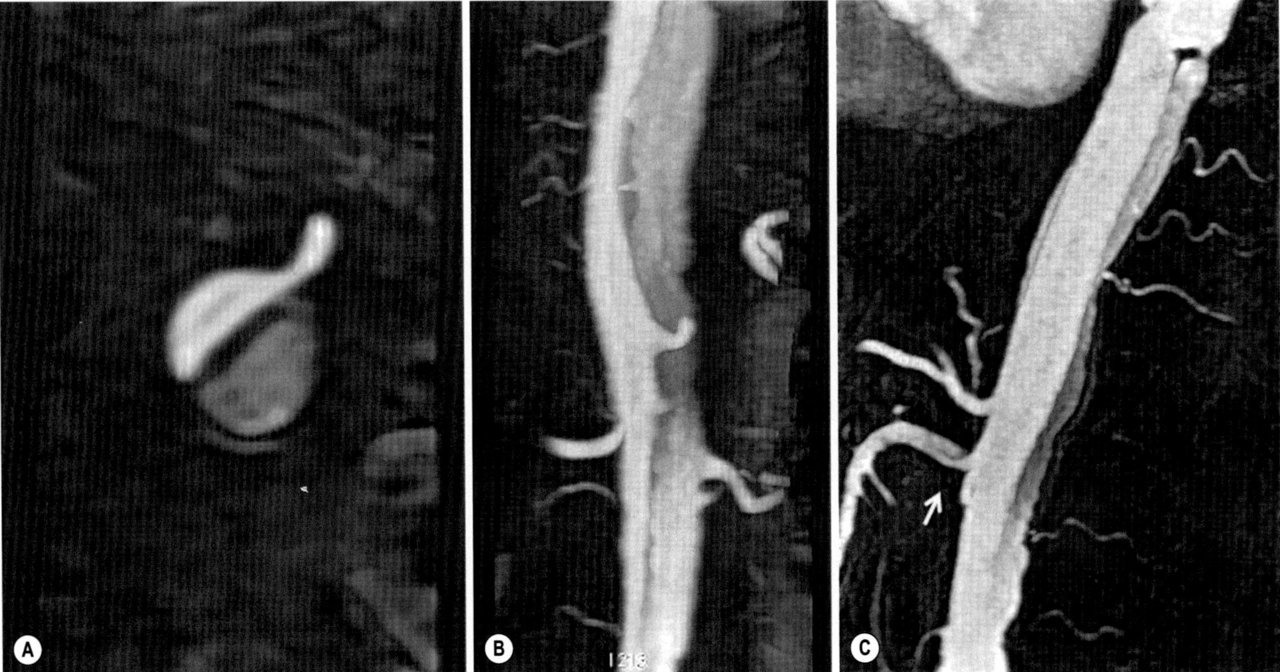

FIGURE 17-5 ■ MR angiography of type B aortic dissection. Axial image (A) displays clearly the relationships of true and false lumen with coeliac trunk, superior mesenteric artery (SMA), right and left arteries, respectively. Note that true lumen is the smaller and best enhanced one. (B, C) MIP images on coronal and sagittal oblique plane, respectively, allow a more comprehensive visualisation of these relationships. The left renal artery arises from the false lumen, while the SMA is dissected (white arrows).

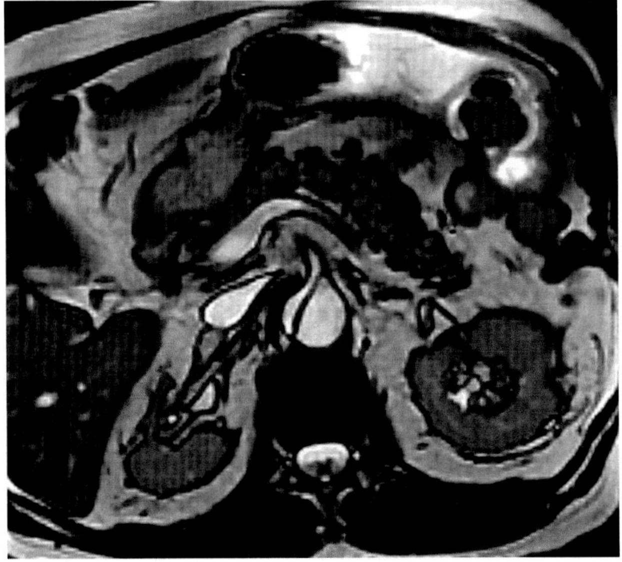

FIGURE 17-6 ■ Axial SSFP image of type B dissection at the level of the abdominal aorta. Note the optimal contrast resolution between aortic lumen and wall with an excellent depiction of the intimal flap and its relationship with the origin of SMA.

is very low,[17] because of its unfavourable logistics and restricted availability that limits its use in emergency conditions.

However, **CTA**, using modern MDCT equipment, achieves high image quality with much shorter acquisition times. In a few seconds MDCT can acquire a volume of coverage from supraortic vessels to the femoral arteries as an aortic dissection study requires, while improved temporal resolution and ECG gating acquisition minimise pulsation artefacts at the aortic root, with consequent sensitivity and specificity now approaching 100%[21] (Fig. 17-7). The wide availability, the fast acquisition and reporting times and the high accuracy make MDCT the imaging method of choice for the diagnosis of aortic dissection.

Unenhanced CT may demonstrate internal displacement of intimal calcifications (Fig. 17-8). Contrast-enhanced CT allows detection of the intimal flap as a thin linear low attenuation separating the contrast-enhanced true and false lumen.

Injection of contrast medium via the left upper limb should be avoided as the very high attenuation from contrast medium within the left brachiocephalic vein can produce streak artefact across the aortic arch, potentially causing diagnostic difficulties.

The differentiation of the false lumen from the true lumen is essential; a number of imaging findings can be helpful, like the cobweb sign, described before. In most cases the true lumen is smaller and more medially located one. On most contrast-enhanced CT images it may be identified by its continuity with the undissected portion of the aorta (Fig. 17-9). An unusual type of aortic dissection is the intimo-intimal intussusception produced by circumferential dissection of the intimal layer, which subsequently invaginates like a wind sock; CT shows one lumen wrapped around the other one, with the inner lumen invariably being the true one (Fig. 17-10). A dissection with thrombosed false lumen should not be confused with an aneurysm with calcified mural thrombus.

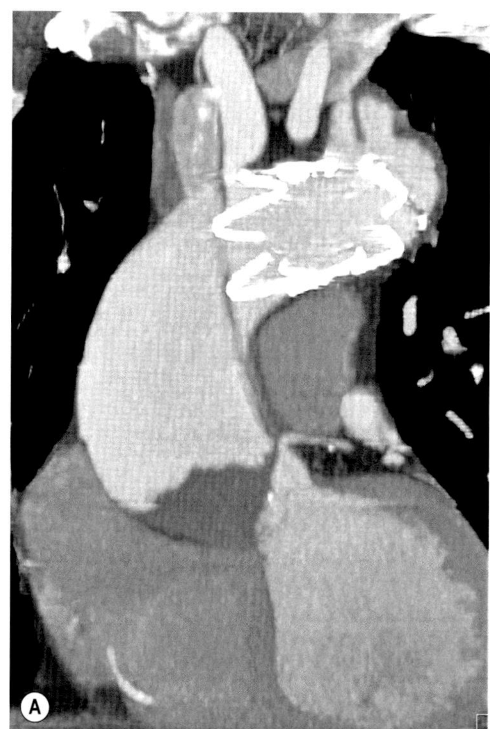

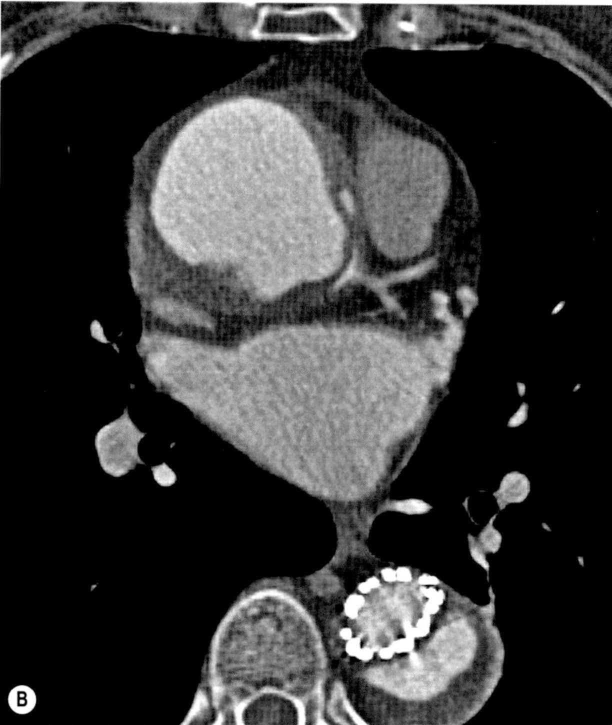

FIGURE 17-7 ■ CT images with cardiac gating acquisition of a type A retrograde aortic dissection after endovascular treatment of a type B dissection. The coronal MPR reconstruction (A) displays accurately the intimal flap extending from the innominate artery to the coronary sinus with severe true lumen compression just over the left coronary artery. The axial image (B) depicts accurately the relationships between the intimal flap and the coronary arteries without aortic pulsatility artefacts.

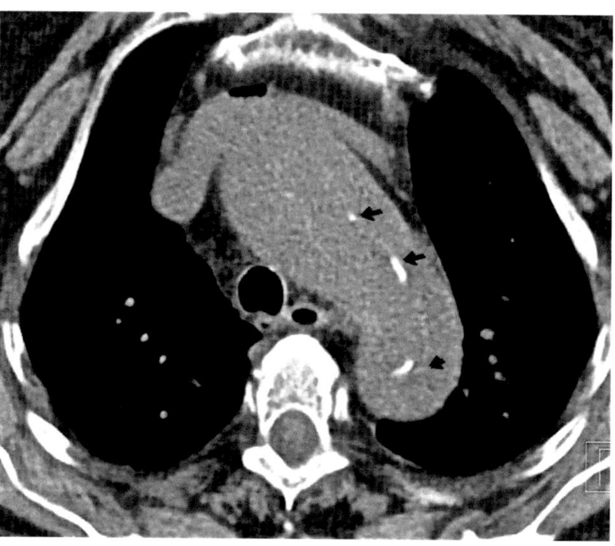

FIGURE 17-8 ■ Axial unhenhanced CT image of the aortic arch. The wall calcifications displaced inside the lumen (arrows) give the suspicion of an aortic dissection or an IMH.

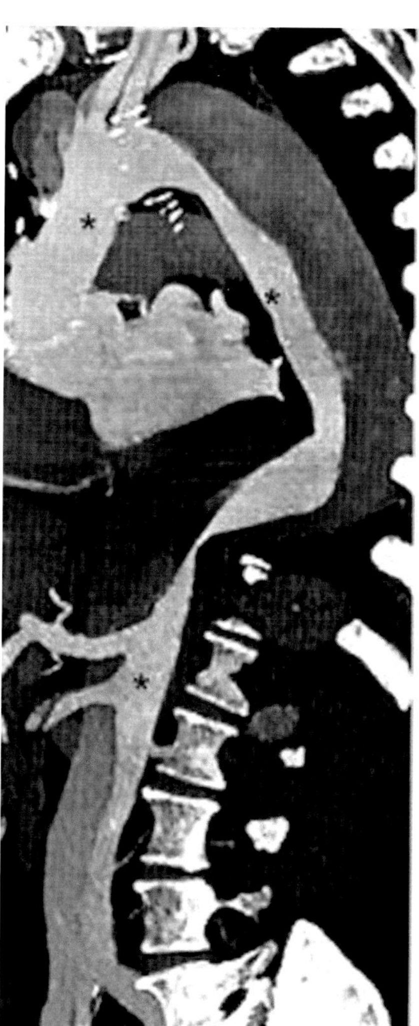

FIGURE 17-9 ■ MDCT MIP image of a chronic type B aortic dissection. The true lumen is the smallest and medial one. Note the continuity of the true lumen in descending thoraco-abdominal aorta with the non-dissected ascending aorta (asterisks).

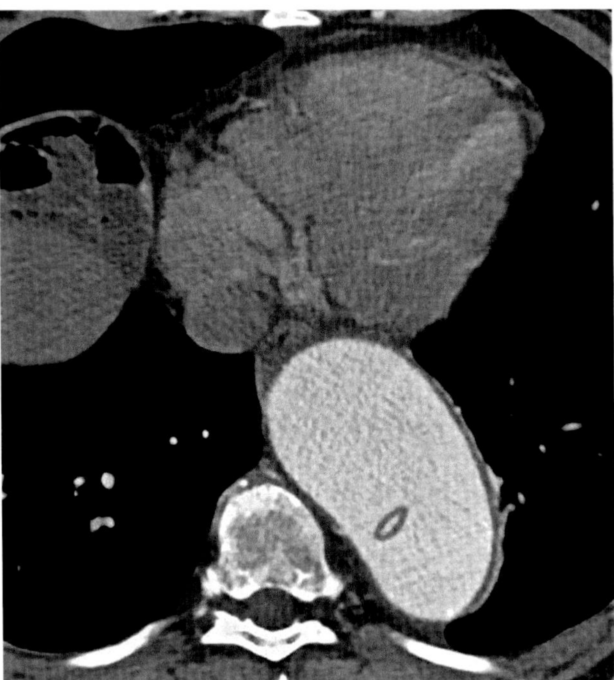

FIGURE 17-10 ■ Axial CT image of a type B aortic dissection. There is a circumferential intimal flap seen on CT as an hypodense linear image inside the aorta. The true lumen is very small and completely surrounded by the false lumen (intimal intussusception).

High attenuation within the false lumen on unenhanced images can help to identify the former. In addition, a dissection tends to spiral as it passes along the aorta, whereas a thrombus maintains a constant relationship with the aortic wall. A mural thrombus arising in an aneurysm also tends to have a more irregular internal border whilst a dissection has a smooth internal border. Finally, calcification of the intima may be identified at the periphery of the thrombus in an aneurysm (Fig. 17-11). Visceral and supra-aortic vessel involvement can account for high mortality and MDCT can reliably diagnose these aspects, also with the use of MPR reconstructions. MIP and VR images greatly contribute to surgical planning and aortic segments measurements. VR is preferred to MIP as it preserves the variable enhancement patterns of the lumina and is more sensitive for visualisation of the flap (Fig. 17-12).

Intramural Haematoma

IMH was first described in 1920 as 'dissection without intimal tear',[22] but clinical recognition of this pathological entity except for autopsy or surgical specimen was almost completely absent before CT and MRI. In fact IMH is a lesion confined to the aortic wall and invasive angiography is not able to detect it. It is considered the consequence of a hypertensive rupture of the vasa vasorum within the medial layer and eventually results in a circumferentially oriented blood collection. IMH may occur spontaneously, but may also arise from a penetrating aortic ulcer in a severely atheromatic aortic wall. It has also been described following trauma. An IMH is

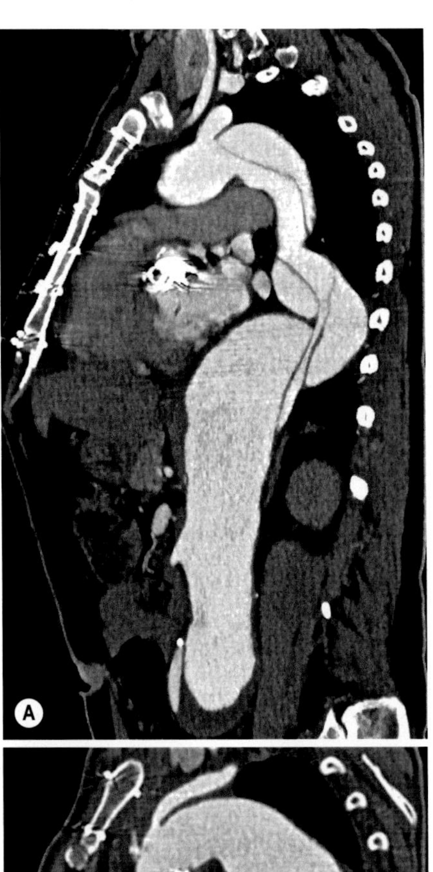

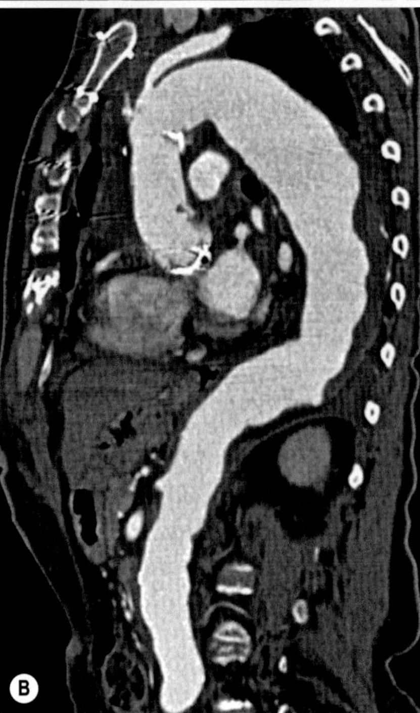

FIGURE 17-11 ■ MDCT sagittal oblique MPR images of a type B dissection (A) and an aneurysm with mural thrombus (B). Note the spiralling shape of the intimal flap and the true lumen in the descending aorta, while the thrombus maintains its relationship with the posterior aortic wall. The internal border of the thrombus is irregular, different from aortic dissection, and the calcifications are on the external border.

visualised by cross-sectional imaging as an aortic wall thickening, symmetric or asymmetric, variable in thickness from 3 mm to more than 1 cm, and it must be differentiated from mural thrombus or plaque. Intimal displacement of calcification can aid in distinguishing

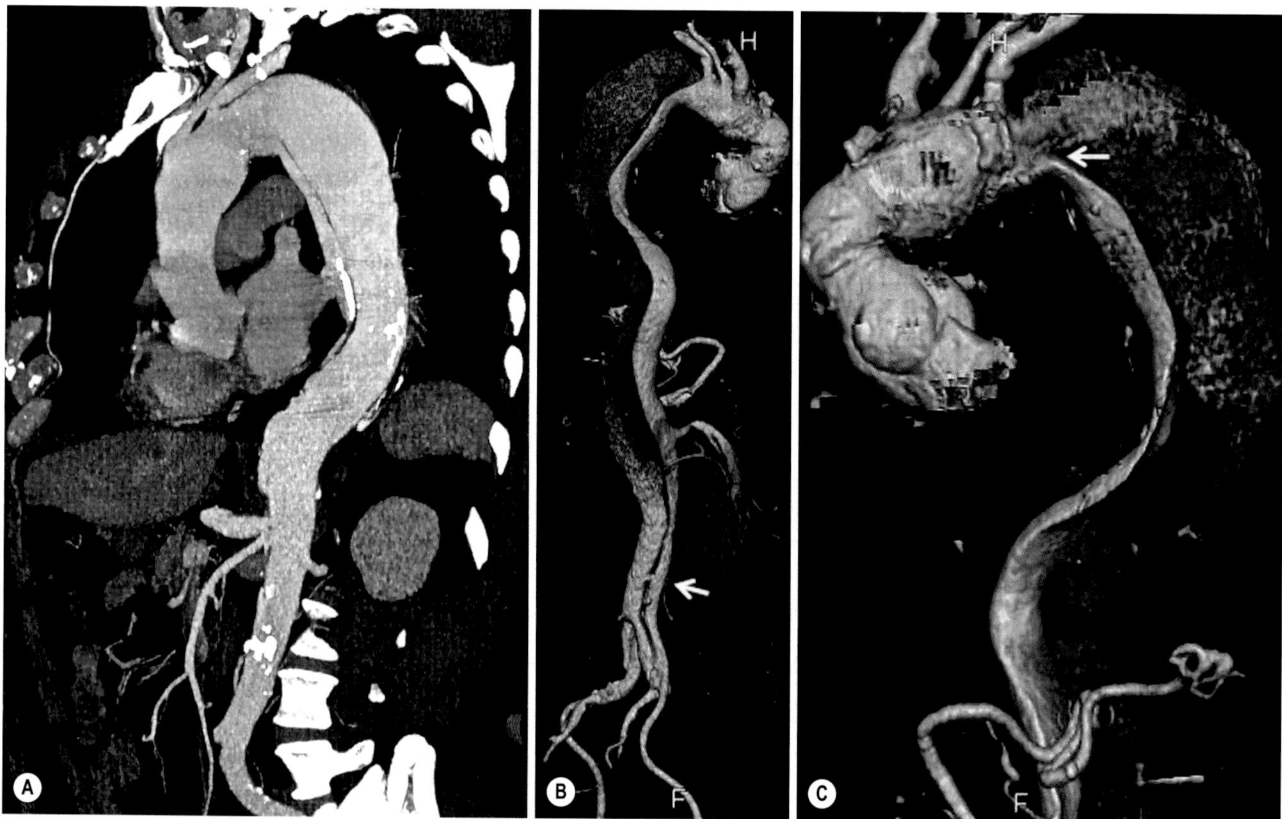

FIGURE 17-12 ■ MDCT MIP (A) and VR reconstructions (B, C) of type B aortic dissection. Both reconstruction techniques give panoramic views of the thoracoabdominal aorta and many anatomical details of the dissection. MIP images may partially obscure the intimal flap and the intimal tears (A), while VR images combine an optimal visualisation of entry and re-entry tears (arrows) as well as the intimal flap with a comprehensive evaluation of the aortic disease.

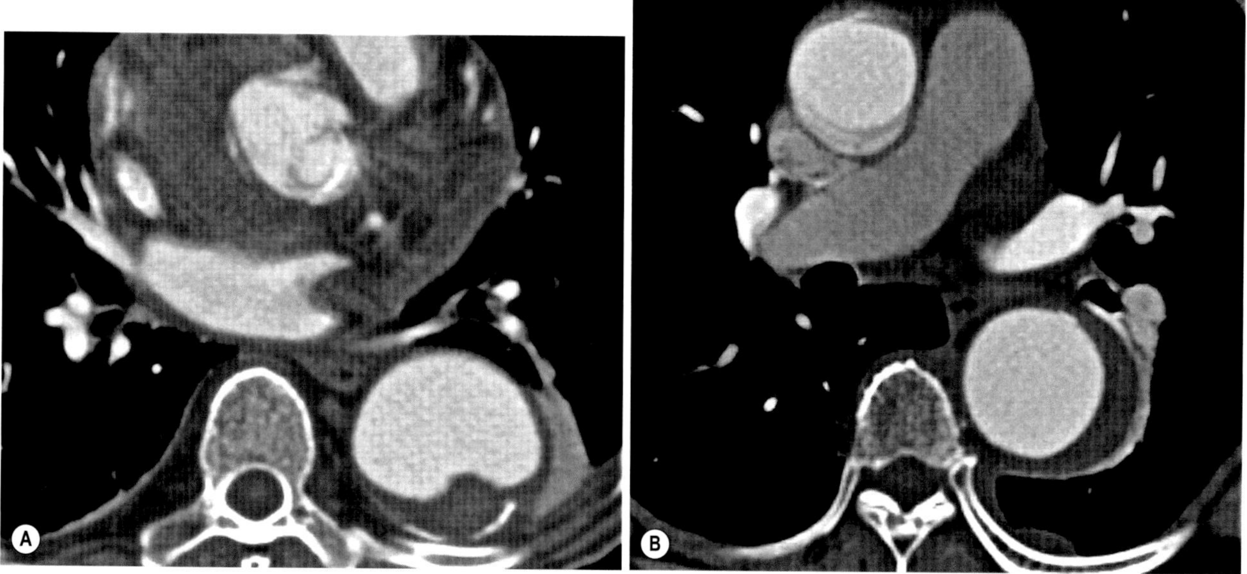

FIGURE 17-13 ■ CT cross-sectional images of a thrombosed aneurysm (A) and an IMH (B) of descending thoracic aorta. Note that IMH has a typical semilunar shape with smooth borders, while the thrombus margins are irregular.

these entities, because the IMH is a subintimal lesion, with calcifications displaced on top of the lesion facing the lumen. Acute IMH is hyperdense on unenhanced CT. Another difference is the shape of the aortic wall thickening: in IMH the borders are generally smooth, while a thrombus or a plaque are typically characterised by irregular margins (Fig. 17-13). With TOE, false-positive and false-negative diagnoses have been reported. In comparison to other imaging techniques, MRI had the best sensitivity for detecting IMH before the advent of MDCT.[23]

T1-weighted images reveal a typical crescent-shaped area of abnormal signal intensity within the aortic wall. MRI is also the only imaging modality able to assess the age of haematoma, exploiting the influence on MRI signal intensity of the different degradation product of haemoglobin: in the acute phase (0–7 days after the onset of symptoms) on T1-weighted spin-echo images, oxyhaemoglobin shows intermediate signal intensity whereas in the subacute phase (> 8 days), methaemoglobin shows high signal intensity. However, when the signal intensity is medium to low, it can be difficult to distinguish IMH from mural thrombus. T2-weighted spin-echo sequences may help in differentiating the two entities: signal intensity is high in recent haemorrhage but low in chronic thrombosis (Fig. 17-14).

MDCT, like MRI, has proven to be highly accurate in the diagnosis of IMH, with comparable sensitivity and specificity. In the suspect of IMH it is important to perform unenhanced CT: in the acute phase the haematoma appears as a crescent-like aortic wall thickening typically hyperdense on unenhanced CT with respect to the aortic lumen, while after enhancement the density of wall and lumen are reversed, with the IMH remaining unenhanced, unlike the false lumen in aortic dissection (Fig. 17-15). The differentiation between IMH and a completely thrombosed false lumen may be very difficult and the following findings are useful for differential diagnosis: IMH maintains a constant circumferential relationship to the wall (subintimal lesion), while the thrombosed false lumen tends to longitudinally spiral

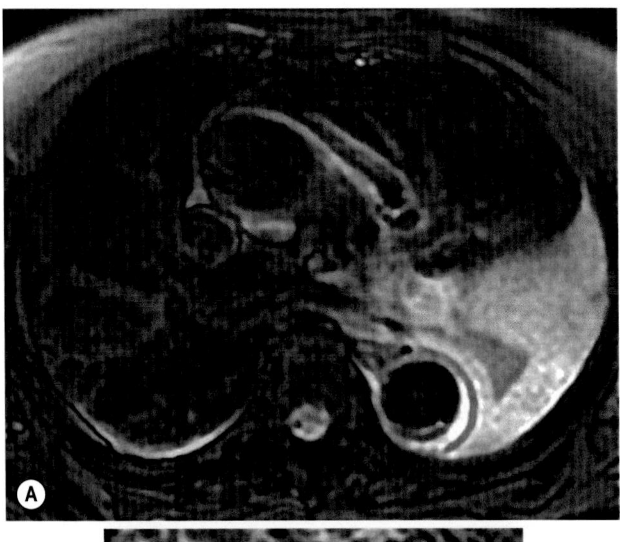

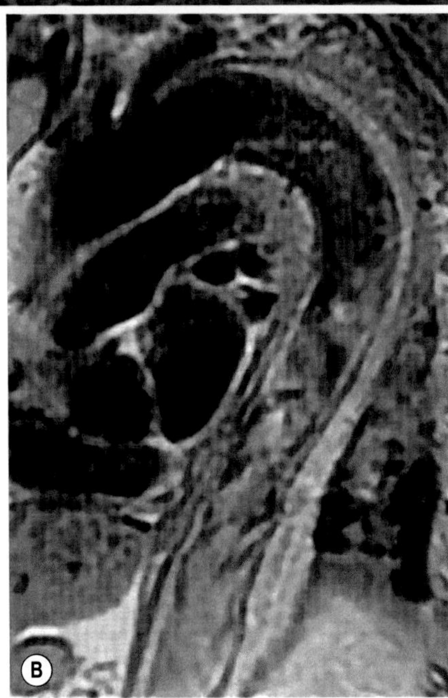

FIGURE 17-14 ■ MRI BBFSE images of an IMH 8 days after symptoms onset. In T2-weighted fat-saturated axial image (A) the signal is high, excluding a chronic disease definitely. Left serosal pleural effusion is associated. T1-weighted sagittal image (B) indicates the longitudinal extension of the IMH not involving left subclavian artery.

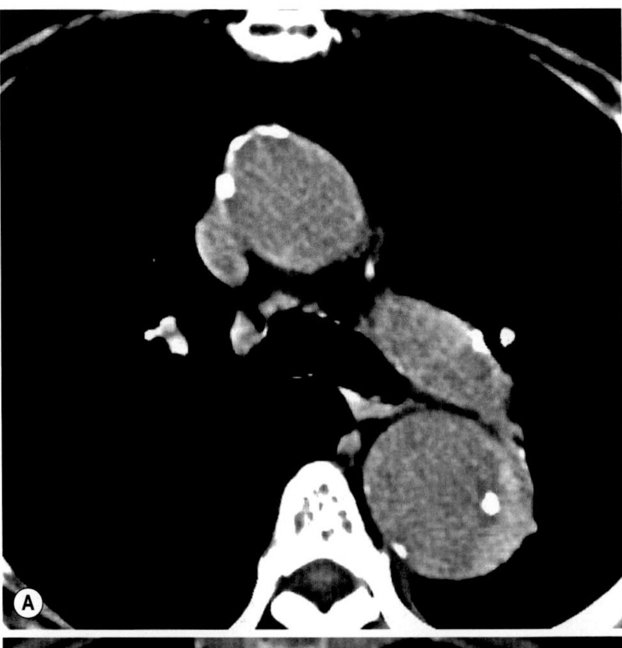

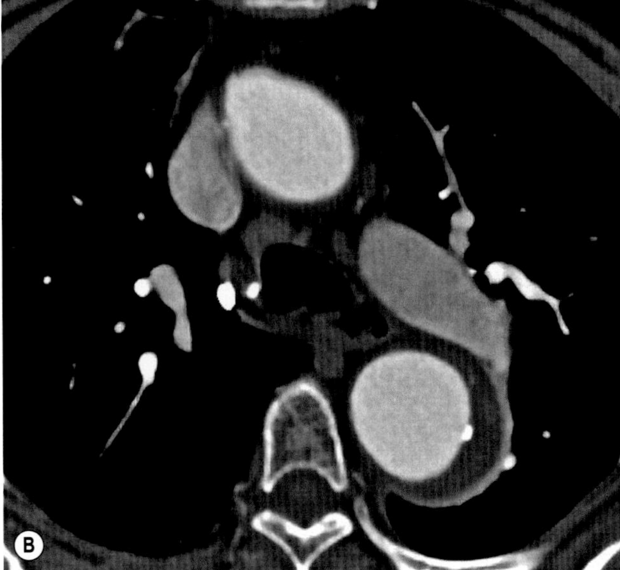

FIGURE 17-15 ■ Typical CT appearance of an acute IMH. The crescent-like wall thickening is hyperdense in relation to the lumen on unenhanced CT image (A), while the density reverses after contrast administration (B).

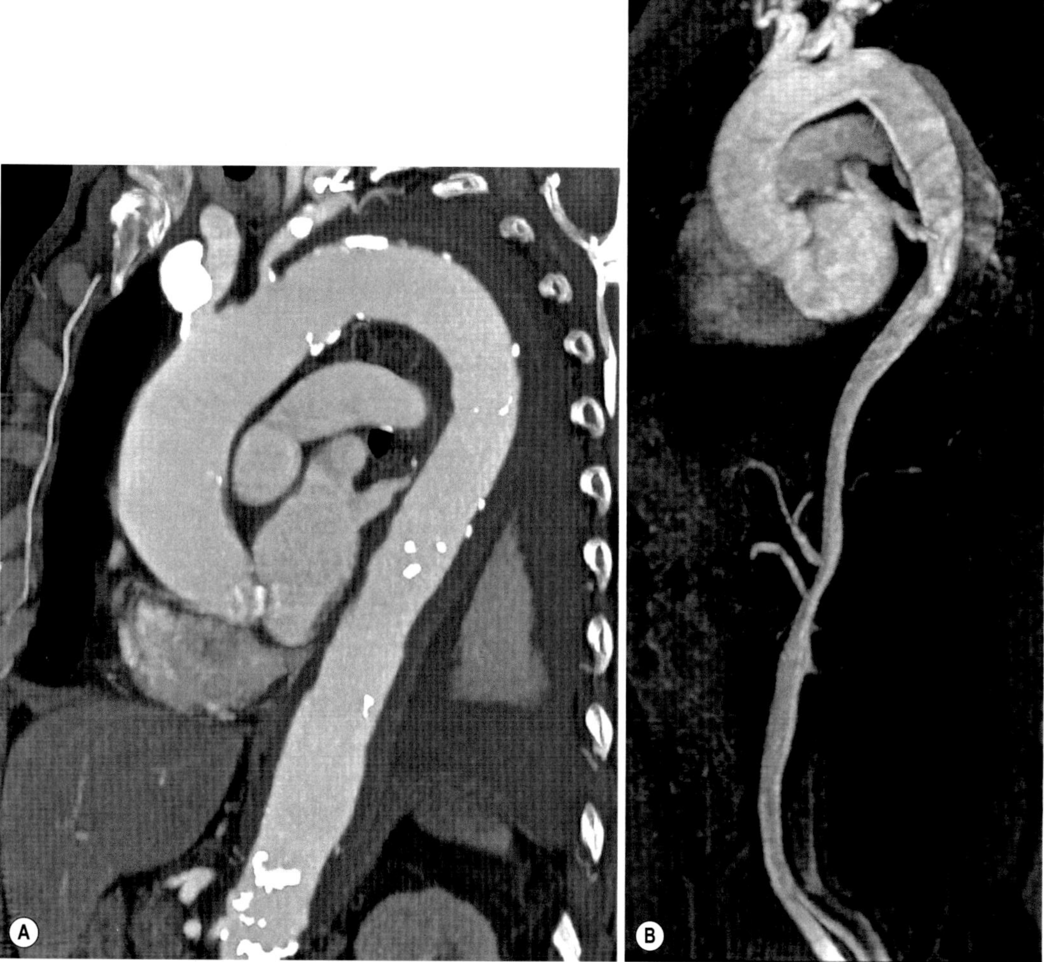

FIGURE 17-16 ■ Differentiation between false lumen thrombosis and IMH. Sagittal oblique MDCT image (A) shows no reduction of the aortic lumen along the IMH in descending aorta. MR angiography of a type B aortic dissection (B): the true lumen is reduced at the diaphragmatic level.

around the aorta. Secondly, IMH does not reduce the lumen, which maintains its regular shape, while the false lumen can variably compress the true lumen (Fig. 17-16). MDCT is highly accurate for the detection of small circumscribed intimal defects that can appear at multiple levels of the IMH; they can enlarge over time, evolving towards aneurysmatic dilation, and may eventually represent a patient subgroup with worse prognosis.[24]

The diagnosis of IMH is mainly based on axial images, but 2D reformatted images may be useful to evaluate the extent of IMH and its relationships with aortic branches. **MRA**, like conventional angiography, has poor value in IMH diagnosis because it provides only luminal information. An appropriate adaptation of the window level in reformatted images can help identify the wall haematoma.

Penetrating Atherosclerotic Ulcer (PAU)

An aortic ulcer is generated by erosion of an atheromatous plaque disrupting the internal elastic lamina, exposing the media to pulsatile arterial flow and subsequent haematoma formation. This is distinguished from an atheromatous plaque by the presence of a focal, contrast medium-filled outpouching surrounded by an IMH. An atheromatous plaque does not extend beyond the intima, is frequently calcified and lacks an IMH.

The extension of the ulceration to the medial layer can also evolve in localised dissection or even break through into the adventitia, creating an aortic pseudoaneurysm. If the adventitia ruptures, only the mediastinal tissue can contain the haematoma; otherwise, the rupture is complete. PAUs are mainly located in the descending aorta but may be also seen in the aortic arch. Ulcers can be multiple and are frequently associated with a severe atherosclerotic aortic wall. The imaging diagnosis of PAU is based on the visualisation of a crater-like, contrast-filled outpouching with jagged edges, of variable extension, which may result in a large pseudoaneurysm[25] (Fig. 17-17). Mural thickening can be associated (localised haematoma) as well as aortic dissection. Differently from IMH, conventional **angiography** has a good sensitivity for PAU, but both **CT** and **MRI** are better suited to evaluate the presence of associated lesions like

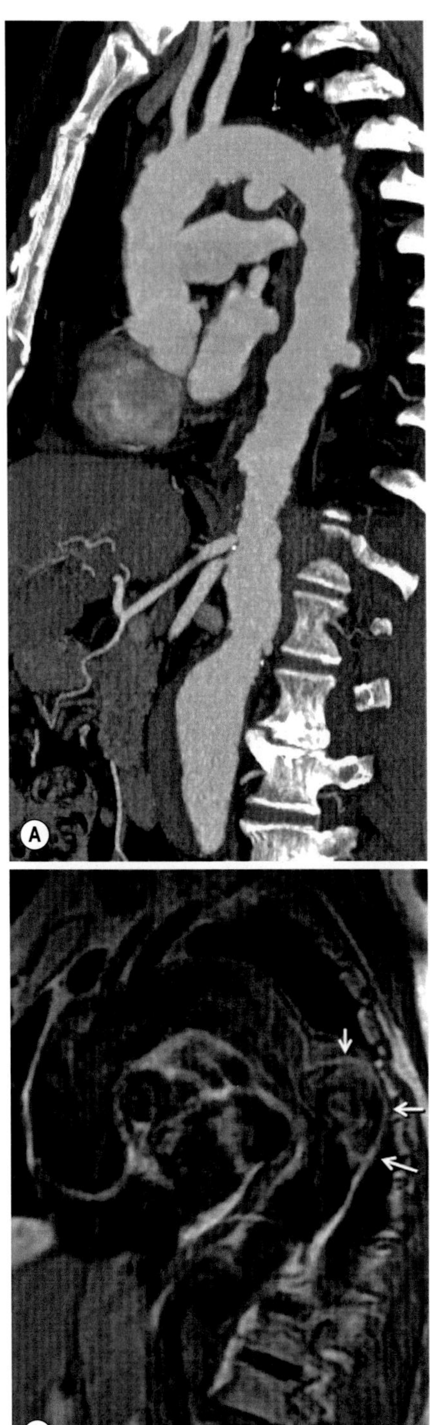

FIGURE 17-17 ■ **Penetrating atherosclerotic ulcers.** MDCT sagittal oblique MPR image (A) shows diffuse multiple finger-like ulcers of descending thoracic aorta. Severe and diffuse aortic wall atheromas are present. Sagittal oblique BBFSE image (B) demonstrates a large ulcer of descending aorta developed in a pseudoaneurysm (arrows).

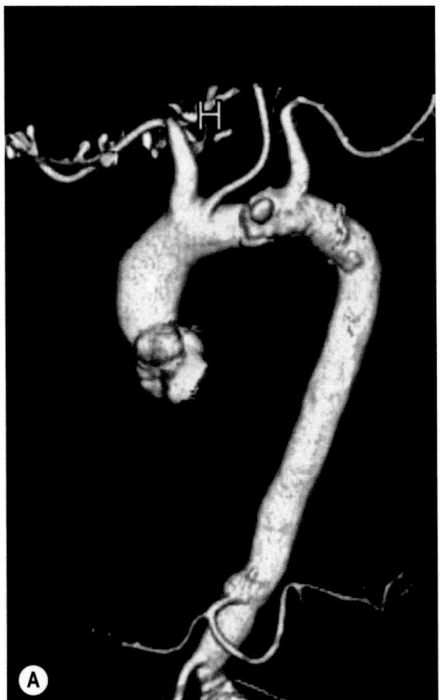

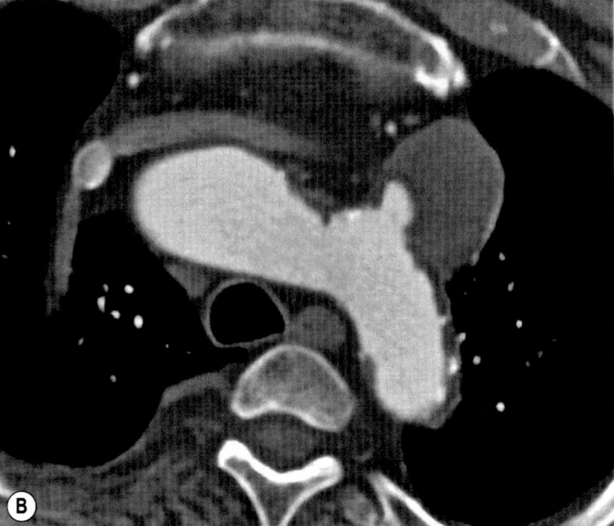

FIGURE 17-18 ■ **Penetrating ulcers of the aortic arch.** MDCT VR reconstructed image (A) clearly displays the relationships of the ulcer with the epiaortic vessels. CT axial image (B) defines the aortic wall alterations at the level and on both sides of the ulcers.

atherosclerotic disease extent, localised haematoma and dissection. Unenhanced CT has the advantage of visualising intimal calcification displacement. MRA and CTA, including 2D and 3D reformatted images, are important for analysing the often-complex spatial relationships between the ulcers and the aortic branches (Fig. 17-18).

The various aortic diseases as described so far are related to each other: PAU and IMH are both potential precursors of dissection.[25] As they are lesions that involve a more external portion of the aortic wall, they are more prone to rupture than aortic dissection and need careful monitoring in the acute phase.[26] Moreover, IMH can evolve into PAU (Fig. 17-19).

Traumatic Aortic Injury (TAI)

Traumatic aortic injury can result from both penetrating and blunt chest injuries. Motor vehicles accidents are one

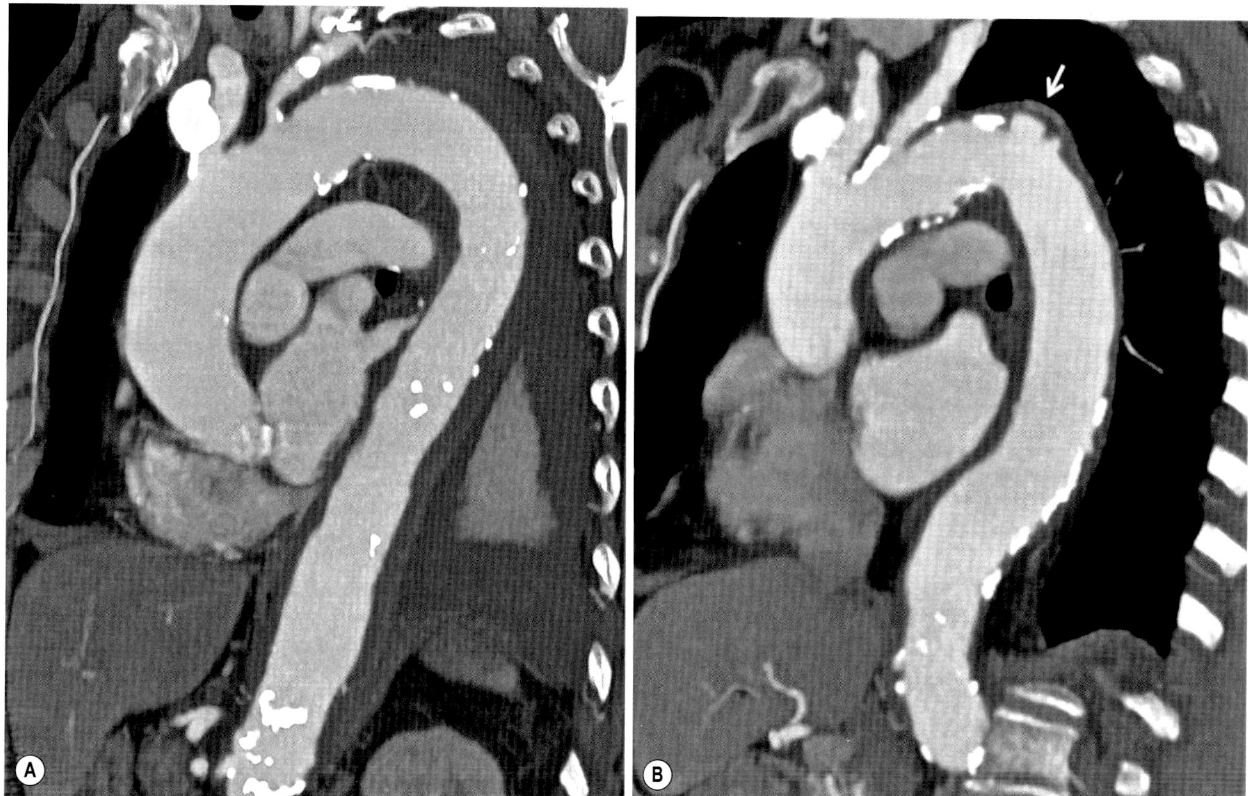

FIGURE 17-19 ■ MDCT MPR sagittal oblique image of an IMH of descending thoracic aorta (A). After 20 days from symptoms onset (B) the intramural haematoma has reabsorbed, but at the level of the isthmic aorta has evolved into a penetrating ulcer (arrow).

of the main causes of TAI. In the United States there are around 40,000 motor vehicle deaths yearly and it has been estimated that 20% of deaths are caused by aortic rupture. A number of mechanisms with an increased risk for TAI have been proposed, of which the most important is rapid and sudden deceleration during the impact. The aortic segment subjected to the greatest strain is the isthmus, where the relatively mobile thoracic aorta is fixed by the ligamentum arteriosus: 90% of aortic ruptures occur here. Another mechanism leading to TAI consists of torsion caused by displacement of the heart to the left during antero-posterior compression, which typically involves the ascending aorta close to the innominate artery or immediately superior to the aortic valve; this is seen with vertical deceleration caused by falls from large heights. Other aortic segments are less commonly involved like the distal descending (diaphragmatic) aorta or the abdominal infrarenal segment, suggesting underlying mechanisms other than the sudden deceleration strain: one process refers to the 'osseous pinch', leading to compression of the heart and aorta between the sternum and vertebral column with a trauma extended from the intima to the adventitia (Table 17-3). In the majority of patients (80–90%) there is complete rupture of the aorta, with death occurring at the scene of the accident. Those patients that reach the hospital alive have injuries that vary from a simple intimal lesion, an IMH to a false aneurysm when the laceration extends through the media into the adventitia (which may be the only layer maintaining aortic integrity). Periaortic haemorrhage is frequently seen irrespective of the type of lesion.

Imaging

The clinical diagnosis of TAI can be difficult due to the lack of specific symptoms or signs in many patients. CXR gives only indirect signs of an aortic lesion like haemomediastinum (Table 17-4), which is insufficiently specific and is more likely the consequence of venous bleeding relative to the thoracic trauma. Moreover, chest radiographs in patients with suspected TAI are taken in the supine position, so the interpretation of mediastinal widening can be problematic—especially in obese patients. Upper limits for a normal mediastinal width or the ratio of the mediastinal width to chest width at the level of the aortic arch (M/C ratio) have been proposed (8 cm and 0, 25, respectively) but have a wide range of reported sensitivities and specificities. In any case, the initial CXRs performed as part of a trauma series may suggest an aortic involvement with satisfactory sensitivity (80–90%), showing the displacement of the nasogastric tube by the haematoma (Fig. 17-20). This makes chest radiography a useful screening tool for mediastinal haemorrhage, even though a normal mediastinum does not exclude a significant aortic injury, as seen in 7.3% of patients with subsequent proven TAI.

In most of the cases, the mechanism of trauma is the crucial element that alerts the clinician to the possibility of TAI: a high degree of suspicion should be raised in case of road traffic accidents (RTAs) at speeds greater than 30 mph, falls from greater than 10 ft and severe crush injuries to the chest. Injuries to other organs are commonly associated, detracting attention from a possible TAI, strongly affecting prognosis and treatment, but overall deeply influencing the choice of the imaging approach, which often depends on the haemodynamic stability and the need of concomitant injuries diagnosis.

Thoracic aortography is no longer the preferred diagnostic test: first because it provides less information than CT and MRI about wall alterations and anatomical pre-operative evaluation and, secondly, because of its lower accuracy, with sensitivities ranging from 84 to

TABLE 17-3 **Presley Trauma Center CT Grading System: Grades and CT Findings**

Grade	Subgrade	CT Findings
Grade I Normal aorta	Ia	Normal thoracic aorta No mediastinal haematoma
	Ib	Normal thoracic aorta Mediastinal haematoma (para-aortic)
Grade II Minimal aortic injury	IIa	Small (<1 cm) pseudoaneurysm Indeterminate <1 cm intimal flap or thrombus No mediastinal haematoma
	IIb	Small (usually <1 cm) pseudoaneurysm Indeterminate (<1 cm) intimal flap or thrombus Mediastinal haematoma (para-aortic)
Grade III Confined thoracic aortic injury	IIIa	>1-cm regular, well-defined pseudoaneurysm Intimal flap or thrombus No ascending aorta, arch or great vessel involvement Mediastinal haematoma
	IIIb	>1-cm regular, well-defined pseudoaneurysm Intimal flap or thrombus Ascending aorta, arch or great vessel involvement Mediastinal haematoma
Grade IV Total aortic disruption	IV	Irregular, poorly defined pseudoaneurysm Intimal flap or thrombus Mediastinal haematoma

Modified from Gavant (1999).[56]

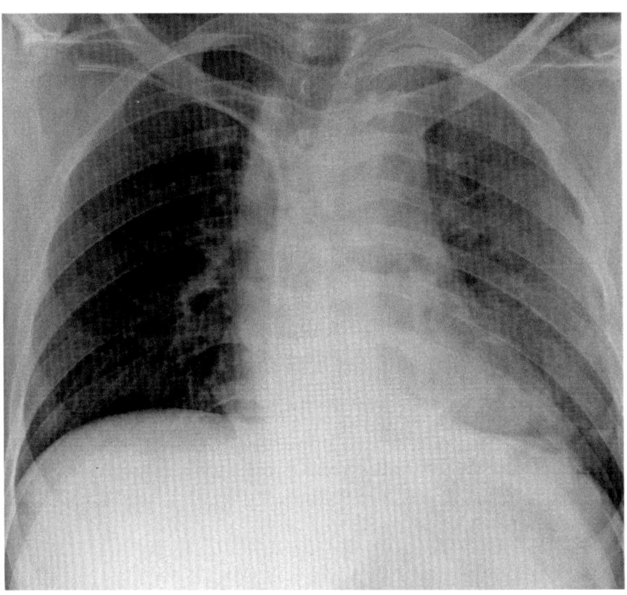

FIGURE 17-20 ■ Supine chest radiograph of a patient involved in a road traffic accident demonstrates signs of traumatic aortic injury. There is widening of the superior mediastinum (M/C ratio approximately 0.3). The right paratracheal stripe is widened and there is deviation of the trachea to the right of the midline. The contour of the aortic knuckle is enlarged and partially obscured by mediastinal haematoma.

TABLE 17-4 **Chest Radiograph Findings Associated with Traumatic Aortic Injury**

		Sensitivity (%)	Specificity (%)
Features directly related to the aortic injury	Irregularity or blurring of the aortic knuckle contour*	72	47
	Enlargement of the aortic knuckle*	35	60
Features related to the presence of mediastinal haematoma	Upper mediastinal widening*	90	19
	Aortopulmonary window opacification*	42	83
	Displacement of a nasogastric tube to the right of the midline	9	96
	Displacement of the trachea or an endotracheal tube to the right	20	92
	Anterior displacement of trachea on lateral radiograph	N/A	N/A
	Downward displacement of left mainstem bronchus	3	99
	Enlarged cardiac silhouette secondary to haemopericardium	N/A	N/A
	Right lateral displacement of superior vena cava	7	96
	Obscuration of the azygos vein	N/A	N/A
Other features	Left apical cap	5	95
	Opacification of the medial border of the left lung	12	95
	Left haemothorax	5	97
	Widened right paratracheal stripe	30	99
	Widened right or left paraspinal stripe	2	97

*Most commonly seen signs.

96%[27,28] with false positives caused by prominent ductus diverticulum, severe aortic atheroma, or double densities from overlapping adjacent vessels and false negatives due to poor opacification of the aorta or small intimal defects. Moreover, it is an expensive and invasive test, not without complications and its use in patients with multiple trauma may be hazardous.

Angiographic findings of TAI include the presence of an intimal flap, dissection, pseudoaneurysm or, less commonly, pseudocoarctation. Angiographic appearances are those of an irregularity of the aortic contour due to an intimal tear or a pseudoaneurysm (Fig. 17-21). There is usually an acute margin at the junction of the abnormal and normal aortic wall, differentiating a pseudoaneurysm from a ductus diverticulum, which classically has a smooth symmetrical contour and obtuse margins with the 'normal' aorta (Fig. 17-22). A luminal filling defect may be seen if there is thrombus formation associated with the intimal injury. Dissection results in a linear filling defect dividing the aortic lumen into two.

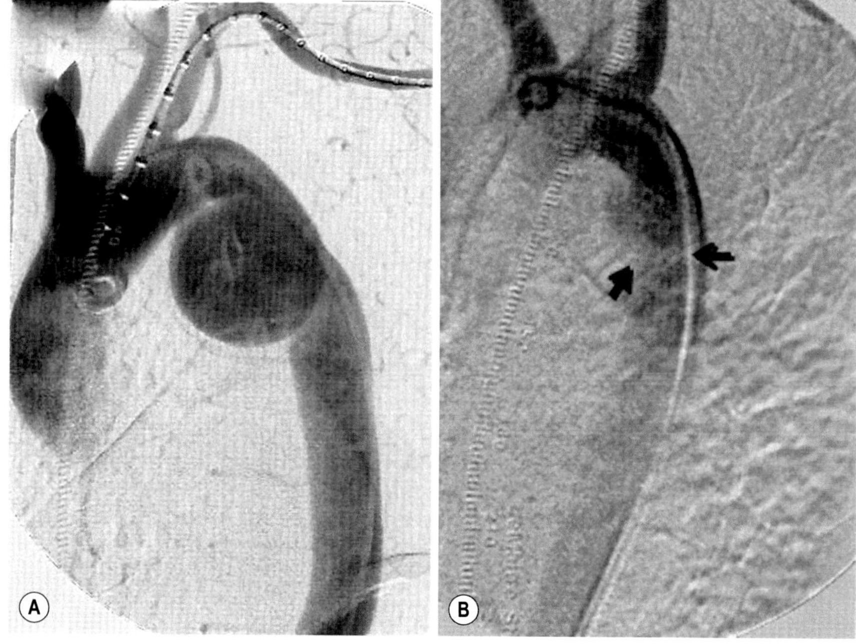

FIGURE 17-21 ■ Angiographic findings of a traumatic aortic injury. A large pseudoaneurysm (chronic traumatic lesion) is evident at the aortic concavity just distal to the arch (A). Small pseudoaneurysm of an acute TAI (B) seen as an irregularity of the aortic contour. The linear lucency (arrows) traversing the aortic lumen just below the inferior angle of the lesion represents a slight compression of the aorta by the pseudoaneurysm.

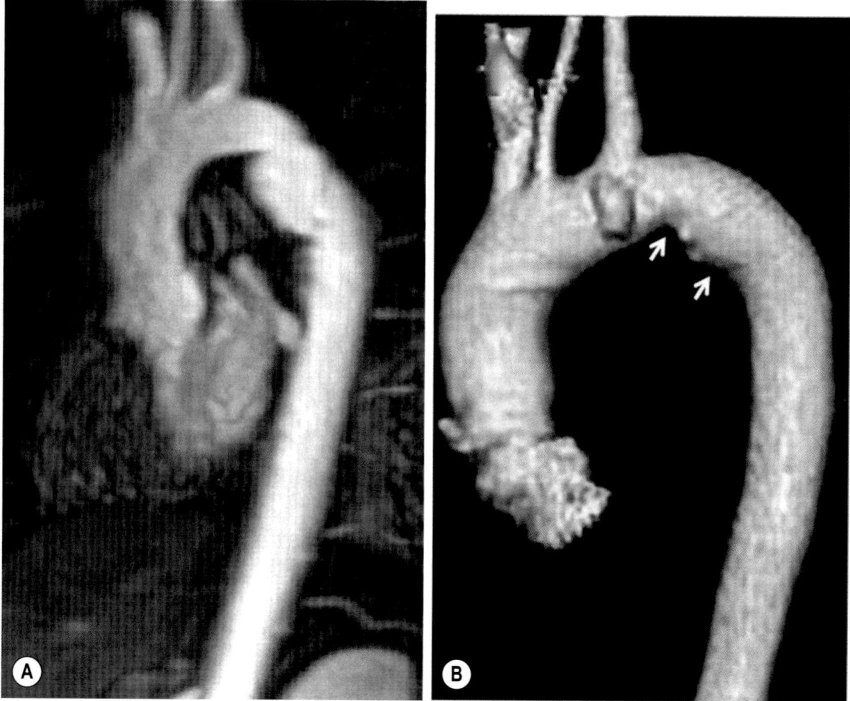

FIGURE 17-22 ■ Difference between a traumatic pseudoaneurysm and a normal ductus diverticulum. (A) The pseudoaneurysm is asymmetric and has an acute proximal margin with the normal aorta (MRA image). (B) The ductus diverticulum (MDCT VR image) has a smooth symmetrical contour with obtuse margins at its junction with the 'normal' aorta (arrows).

Transoesophageal echocardiography (TOE) has a sensitivity of 91% and specificity of 98% for demonstration of isthmic aortic injuries.[28] TOE has the advantage that can be performed at the patient's bedside in 15–20 min, even in highly unstable patients. However, it may be contraindicated in the presence of severe facial injuries or unstable cervical spine fractures. The entire aortic circumference may not be adequately visualised in approximately 30% of patients, while the aortic arch is not easily displayed, thus limiting preoperative evaluation. On the other hand, TOE is extremely useful as an intraoperative assistant tool for guiding endovascular intervention, providing excellent visualisation of the proximal aorta for accurate placement of stent grafts in relation to aortic branch vessel origins.

With the exception of extremely unstable patients, MDCT and MRI are the ideal imaging modalities for TAI, with a diagnostic accuracy approaching 100%.[28] They can demonstrate both indirect signs such as mediastinal haematoma as well as direct signs of aortic trauma, especially giving high-definition images of the aortic wall alterations like intramural haematoma, or small intimal lesions. Additionally, CT and MRI provide primary information about endovascular treatment feasibility (relationships between epiaortic or visceral vessels and the aortic trauma, vascular access) and may also evaluate other organs and structures to search for associated traumatic lesions in the same examination.

The development of fast MRI techniques has shortened the examination time to a few minutes for TAI diagnosis, even less than TOE. BBFSE images obtained in an oblique sagittal projection give a longitudinal view of the thoracic aorta, allowing for the distinction of a partial lesion (confined to the anterior or posterior aortic wall) from a lesion that encompasses the entire aorta (more than 270° of circumference). MRI may possibly achieve all this information even without contrast medium administration. A difficult access to the MRI unit, however, remains the main limitation of this imaging test. MRI may be useful for identifying and dating the IMH, when present.

CT angiography for TAI diagnosis is the most widely used imaging test, because of the extensive availability (location close to the intensive care units) and high acquisition speed, which are especially suitable in emergency conditions. Moreover, CT allows quick assessment of the entire thorax and abdomen as well as the head, which should be examined in any trauma for evaluation of head and/or abdominal injury.

Typical appearance of TAI on CT images is a frank contrast agent extravasation or a defined pseudoaneurysm (Fig. 17-23), but aortic injuries may also represent as dissection flap, a focal calibre change or a small aortic contour abnormality (representing intimal and media disruption), which may be more difficult to identify correctly. In fact, like aortography, false positives can arise from the presence of severe atheroma or a ductus diverticulum. These can be first differentiated from a small pseudoaneurysm by the absence of surrounding mediastinal haematoma. The superior intercostal vein, the bronchial artery infundibulum and movement artefacts are also sources of false-positive diagnoses. Images can also be degraded by streak artefacts from non-elevated arms and shoulders, contrast injection into a left arm vein and monitoring lines.

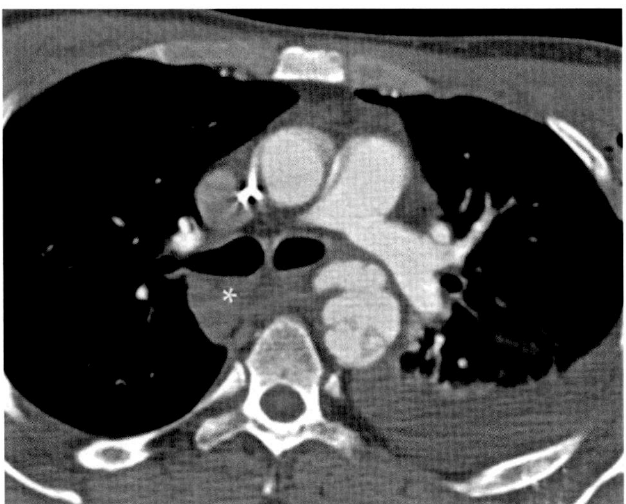

FIGURE 17-23 ■ **Axial CT image of an acute TAI.** See the large pseudoaneurysm with partial contrast medium extravasation anteriorly. Wide mediastinal haematoma (asterisk) with initial dislodgement of the left pulmonary artery.

The few cases with equivocal CT findings may eventually be resolved by intravascular ultrasound, while aortography does not add substantial elements to the diagnosis.[29]

Aortic Aneurysms

Aortic aneurysm is a localised or diffuse dilatation involving all layers of the aortic wall, exceeding the expected aortic diameter by a factor of 1.5 or more, while in a false aneurysm or pseudoaneurysm the wall is represented only by the adventitial layer. This distinction is relevant because false aneurysms result from a contained rupture and should not be considered stable.

Aneurysm development is multifactorial in nature, with both a genetic predisposition and environmental factors acting together to initiate a cascade of arterial wall degeneration.

Most aneurysms are caused by atherosclerosis, but can also be the result of a trauma, infection including tuberculosis and syphilis or genetic syndromes such as Marfan's and Ehlers–Danlos, the latter most commonly affecting the aortic root, ascending aorta and arch.[30]

Histologically, an inflammatory cell infiltrate has been demonstrated in all atherosclerotic aortic aneurysms. Matrix metalloproteinases (MMPs) play an important role in the remodelling process by degrading extracellular matrix proteins such as elastin and collagen, both of which are needed to maintain the structural integrity and mechanical properties of the aortic wall. In healthy tissue, MMP activity is tightly regulated by tissue inhibitors. Several MMPs have been identified, MMP-2 being most strongly associated with small aneurysms, while MMP-9 has been linked to medium-sized, large, or ruptured aneurysms. Furthermore, plasma concentrations of MMP-9 appear not only to be associated with

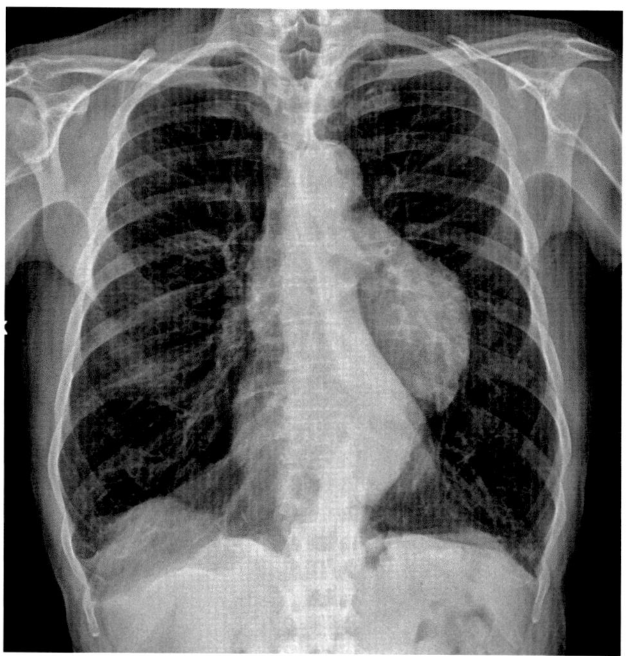

FIGURE 17-24 ■ Chest X-ray showing a large descending thoracic aortic aneurysm simulating a tumoural mediastinal mass.

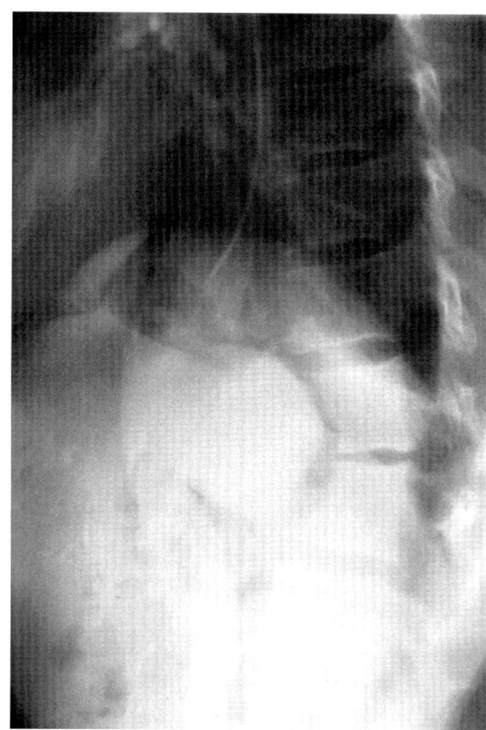

FIGURE 17-25 ■ Lateral aortogram in a patient with severe mid-back pain and lumbar spine images which demonstrated anterior erosion of the lower thoracic vertebral bodies. The angiogram demonstrates that this has been caused by a pulsatile thoracoabdominal aortic aneurysm.

aneurysmatic disease but also with the size and expansion rate of abdominal aortic aneurysms (AAAs), plasma levels falling after successful therapy of an AAA.[31]

Atherosclerotic Aortic Aneurysms

As many as 95% of atherosclerotic aneurysms affect the abdominal rather than the thoracic aorta. The natural history of aneurysms is progressive remodelling, expansion and eventual rupture. As only 14% of patients have symptoms, ruptured aneurysm is a major cause of death in Western populations. Patients usually have major co-morbidities such as coronary disease, peripheral vascular disease, obstructive pulmonary disease, diabetes and renal failure. Of patients who initially survive a ruptured aneurysm, more than 50% die during or following surgery.

The asymptomatic thoracic aortic aneurysm (TAA) is often detected as a mediastinal widening or a calcified soft-tissue mediastinal mass on a chest radiograph taken for some other reason; not infrequently, it is confused with a tumour (Fig. 17-24). Likewise, AAAs can be detected incidentally on abdominal or lumbar spine radiographs because of their mass effect and wall calcifications (Fig. 17-25).

Thoracic Aneurysms

The role of ultrasound in the evaluation of thoracic aortic aneurysms is confined to the proximal aortic segments (aortic root, sino-tubular junction and proximal ascending aorta) while CT and MRI, with their unlimited access to the thoracic structures and the superior accuracy and reproducibility of measurements, have no limitations to the diagnosis and follow-up of these diseases. **Standard BBSE MRI** sequences are useful to evaluate alterations of the aortic wall and periaortic space. Atherosclerotic lesions appear as areas of increased wall thickness, with irregular profiles and possible endoluminal projections. The high tissue characterisation of T1- and T2-weighted BBSE images allows accurate depiction of inflammatory changes or the presence of a haematoma within the aortic wall or the periaortic spaces. With a fat-suppression technique, the outer wall of the aneurysm can be easily distinguished from the periadventitial fat tissue, so that the aneurysm diameter can be accurately measured. Mural thrombus and atheromatous plaques are well visualised in the axial plane (Fig. 17-26), whereas sagittal and coronal views are used to define the longitudinal extension and location of the aneurysm and its diameters, avoiding projection effects in axial images, caused by the natural curvature and tortuosity of the aorta. Contrast-enhanced 3D MRA can provide precise topographic information about the extent of an aneurysm and its relationship to the aortic branches.

MDCT can easily detect thoracic aneurysms with 100% accuracy. It has the advantage over MRI of direct aortic wall calcifications' visualisation, which is important when planning a surgical or endovascular procedure. MPR and 3D VR applications help for the assessment of calibre, length, angle, calcification and burden of mural thrombus, as well as length, shape and angle of the aneurysm necks (Fig. 17-27).

Both imaging techniques have high reproducibility of measurements, but MRI is preferred to CT for monitoring expansion rate of chronic aortic aneurysms because it does not use ionising radiation. This is especially true

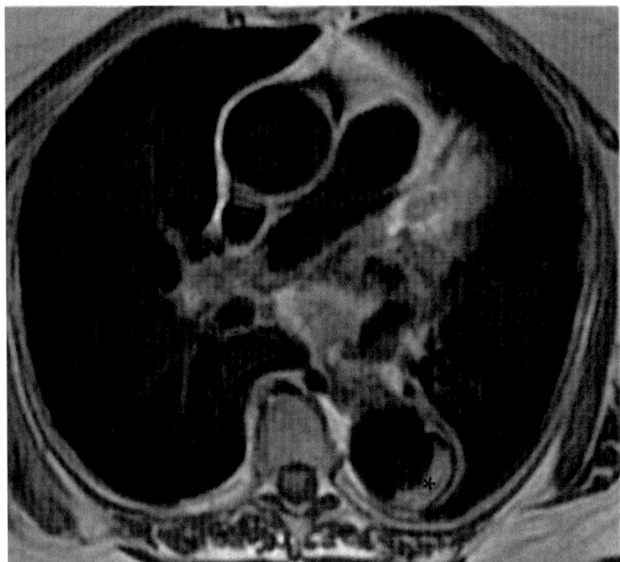

FIGURE 17-26 ■ MR BBFSE cross-sectional image of descending thoracic aorta showing an ulcerated atherosclerotic plaque. Note the thickening and the irregular internal margins of the aortic wall. The endoluminal material (asterisk) has a low signal, indicating a chronic thrombotic nature.

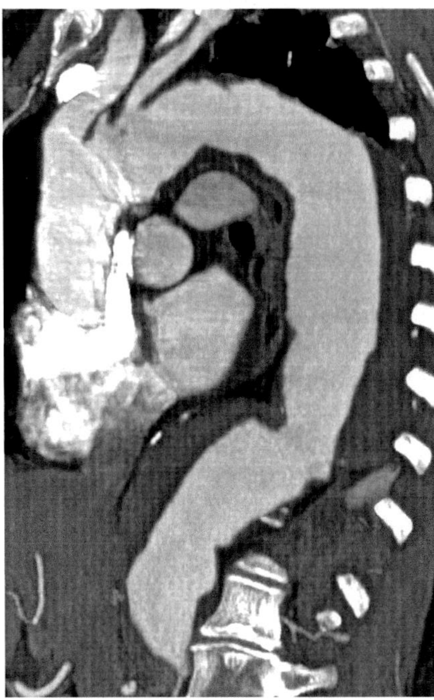

FIGURE 17-27 ■ MDCT MPR sagittal image of a descending thoracic aneurysm. The aneurysm doesn't extend up to the left subclavian artery. The proximal neck of the aneurysm is not excessively angulated.

for Valsalva sinuses and ascending aorta aneurysms, where ECG gating is mandatory in CT to avoid aortic pulsatility artefacts.

Abdominal Aneurysms

Unlike thoracic aneurysms, abdominal aneurysms are easy to access for ultrasound, which can be used for follow-up instead of CT. Recent inversion recovery BBFSE breath-hold MRI sequences with adequate suppression of the blood pool can also provide the same information as CT, except for aortic wall calcification. Fast gradient-echo SSFP sequences may cover the whole abdomen within two or three breath-holds with good contrast resolution between the aortic lumen and the wall and optimal aneurysm thrombus visualisation. Three-dimensional MRA can be helpful in planning surgical or endovascular therapy.

Abdominal aneurysms are usually monitored by ultrasound and CT. Ultrasound is the preferred imaging test for assessing abdominal aneurysm dimension; surveillance is associated with reduced mortality and no difference in long-term survival versus early endovascular or surgical treatment for aneurysm diameters <5.5 cm.[32] Thus, ultrasound is increasingly used as a screening test, with non-invasiveness and low cost.[33] CT is more accurate and widely used when dimensions are close to the cut-off values for surgical intervention. Multiplanar reconstructions provide precise definition of the size and extent of the aneurysm and its relationships with visceral and iliac vessels as well as the lumen, the wall, the extent of any inflammatory material, and the position and degree of distension of all the important adjacent structures. For these reasons CT is used to evaluate AAAs, helping with decisions about endovascular treatment or surgery (Fig. 17-28).

Inflammatory Aneurysms

Inflammatory abdominal aortic aneurysms (IAAAs) are defined as dilation of the aorta with a thickened aneurysm wall, marked perianeurysmal and retroperitoneal fibrosis, and dense adhesions to adjacent abdominal organs. IAAAs represent 3–10% of all abdominal aortic aneurysms and are more common in men. Mean age of occurrence ranges from 62 to 68 years (5–10 years younger than patients with other atherosclerotic aneurysms). Moreover, patients with IAAAs have a positive family history of aneurysms (17%) as compared to patients with non-inflammatory aneurysms (1.7%). IAAAs are more often symptomatic. In addition to abdominal or back pain, these patients also present with weight loss and elevated erythrocyte sedimentation rate (ESR).

The aetiology of IAAAs is the same as for other atherosclerotic AAAs, but the inflammatory component is more pronounced. Current aetiological thinking favours a single pathological process, with varying degrees of inflammation rather than a distinct clinical entity. The importance of the IAAA lies in its potential treatment. Its true natural history is unknown but the risk of rupture remains. Steroid therapy has been used to control the inflammatory process but no controlled studies exist. Surgery is technically difficult as the ureters can be involved in the inflammatory process and may need stenting for protection. The duodenum and left renal vein are often adherent to the aneurysm sac. IAAA repair halts the progression of retroperitoneal fibrosis but does not cure it. Complete regression of the retroperitoneal fibrosis is seen in 23–53% of cases after surgery, with partial regression or no change in the remainder. In view of the

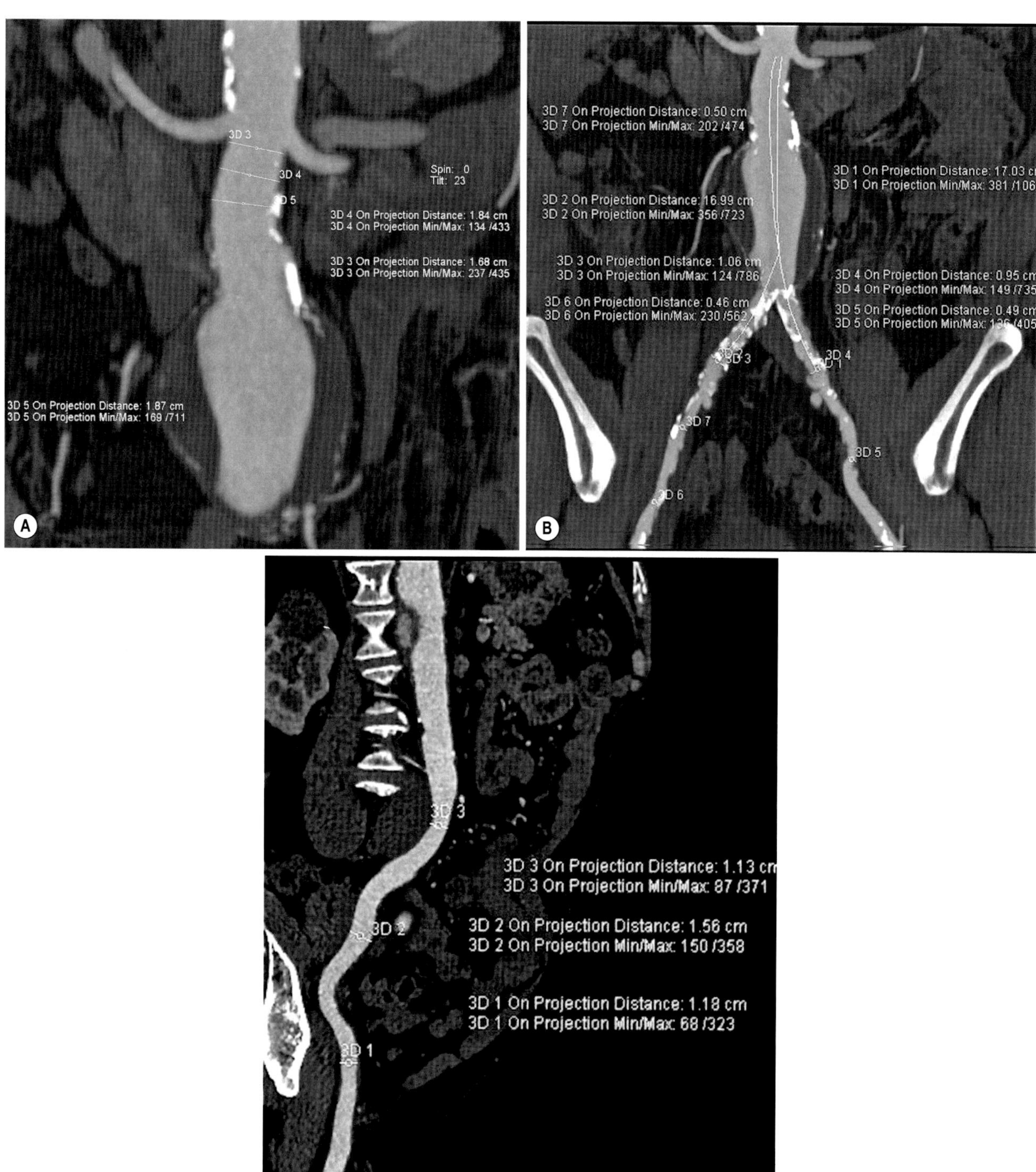

FIGURE 17-28 ■ **MDCT coronal MPR (A) and curved reformations (B, C) of the abdominal aorta in a patient affected by abdominal aneurysm.** The proximal neck, below renal arteries (A) and the distal necks (B) are measured to choose the correct prosthesis. Curved reconstructions give a comprehensive view even of the most complex structures, allowing measurements of the length of coverage required with a stent graft and the state of vascular access (B, C). Such reconstructions and measurements are vital to the successful use of stent grafts to treat abdominal aneurysms.

technical difficulty of open IAAA repair and the increased morbidity and mortality, endovascular aneurysm repair is an attractive alternative. However, the long-term regression of the perianeurysmal fibrosis seen in up to 53% after open repair is said to occur less frequently after endovascular repair, though the number of cases reported is small.

Though ultrasound is very important, CT has become the mainstay of assessing IAAAs, showing a thick cuff of enhancing soft tissue around the aorta (Fig. 17-29).

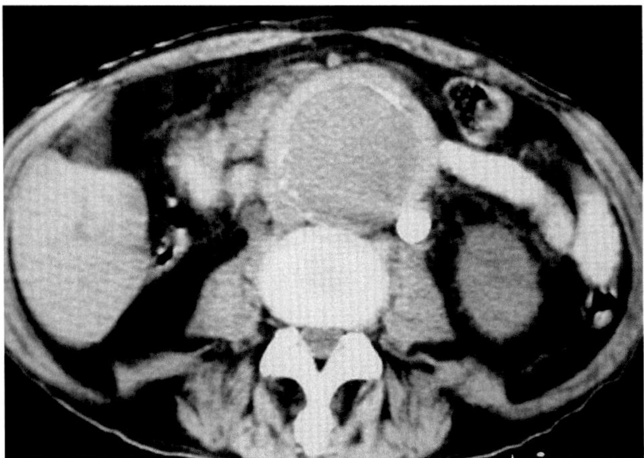

FIGURE 17-29 ■ Contrast-enhanced CT demonstrates a significantly sized abdominal aortic aneurysm with a thick well-defined outer wall. There is a hydroureter on the left and a hydroureter with a non-functioning kidney on the right. These features are typical of inflammatory abdominal aortic aneurysm.

IAAAs can usually be differentiated from other diseases such as lymphoma surrounding an aneurysm, or a tumour reaction seen in liposarcoma or bladder cancer causing a strong periaortic inflammatory fibrous reaction. Haemorrhage is another potential diagnostic pitfall. When an aneurysm has ruptured, the tissue planes within the retroperitoneum become poorly defined, which can make the identification of the inflammatory component difficult. However, fresh blood has a higher CT attenuation than muscle and usually expands into the pararenal fat further away from the aneurysm itself, except at the very point of rupture. MRI is optimal in patients with manifest or potential renal failure. SE T1- and T2-weighted sequences provide a good overall assessment of an inflammatory aneurysm. On SE images the periaortic cuff of inflammatory aneurysms has intermediate signal intensity. After intravenous administration of gadolinium, the periaortic cuff enhances significantly, so that intraluminal thrombus and aortic wall are clearly defined, along with the adjacent involved structures embedded in the inflammatory cuff.

Mycotic Aneurysms

Infection can cause thrombosis of the vasa vasorum with consequent destruction of the aortic intima and media. Commonly, such infection is due to emboli from infectious endocarditis, septicaemia, or local spread (Fig. 17-30). Imaging of mycotic aneurysms is similar to that of other aneurysms. The results of surgical treatment can be poor and often the aorta must be tied off and axillo-bifemoral grafting performed. More recently stent grafting has been tried with mixed results.

Aortic Sinus Aneurysms

These aneurysms can be congenital, particularly in Asian populations, but can also be seen secondary to infective endocarditis and in Marfan's syndrome and ankylosing spondylitis. The most common site is the right aortic sinus extending into the right ventricle or right atrium, but also the non-coronary sinus extending into the left atrium. They may rupture into the heart and present subacutely with a left-to-right shunt and a continuous murmur.

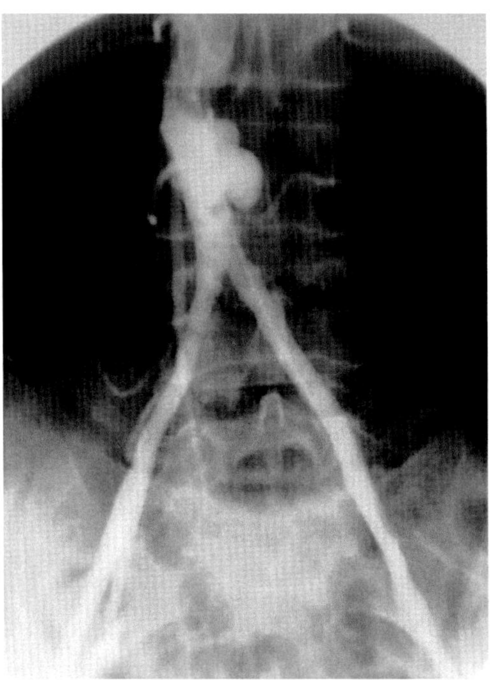

FIGURE 17-30 ■ Aortic angiogram in a patient who presented with emboli to both feet 6 weeks after an episode of acalculous cholecystitis. Aortography demonstrated an eccentric lower abdominal aortic aneurysm. This was later proved to be mycotic secondary to *Salmonella* infection. The aorta was surgically tied off and the patient underwent axillo-bifemoral grafting.

When dilatation is confined to the aortic root, it will not be seen on the PA chest radiograph, though it may be revealed on the lateral radiograph. When the ascending aorta is involved, the right mediastinal border will be prominent and, on the lateral radiograph, the aorta will obliterate the retrosternal space above the heart. Left ventricular dilatation results from aortic regurgitation. The aortic root and ascending aorta are well shown by both MRI and CTA. MRI has the advantage of adding functional information with cine gradient-echo, SSFP and phase contrast imaging that show aortic regurgitation and fistulas as flow turbulence (signal void on bright-blood images), and may quantify aortic insufficiency. In emergency conditions, TOE is also very useful and can be carried out at the bedside. Angiography is avoided in these patients, particularly in the presence of infection.

Preoperative Evaluation of Acute Aortic Syndromes

The imaging techniques must first confirm or exclude the presence of impending aortic rupture or any other signs of severe instability that deserve immediate surgical or endovascular treatment, e.g. a visceral malperfusion in aortic dissection. Secondly, the imaging test should define

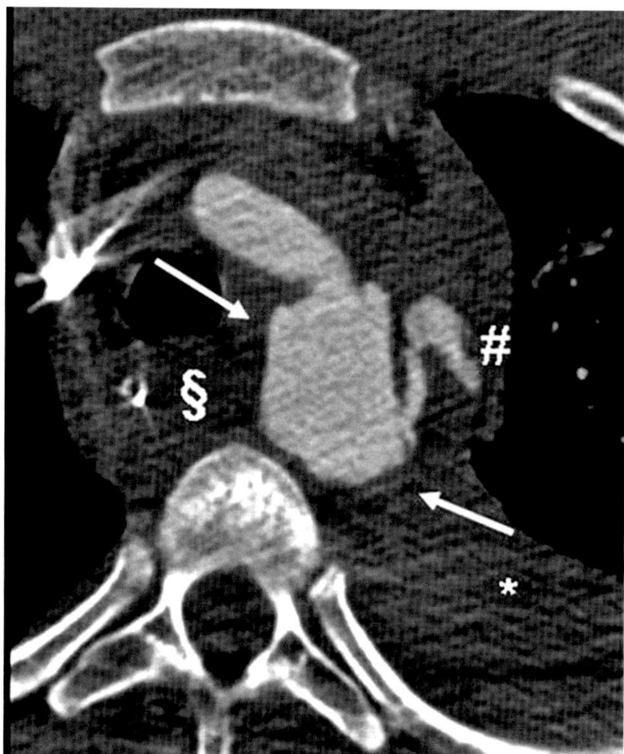

FIGURE 17-31 ■ **Axial CT image of an acute traumatic rupture of the isthmic aorta.** The extravasation of contrast medium (#) is a sign of complete rupture that needs prompt repair. See also the mediastinal haematoma (§), the serohaemorrhagic effusion (*) and the pseudoaneurysmatic sac (arrows).

whether the anatomical conditions allow an endovascular or surgical treatment of the disease.

Impending Aortic Rupture

Aortic rupture appears on CTA images as a discontinuity of the aortic wall with contrast medium extravasation and it is typically associated with a large, periaortic haematoma (Fig. 17-31). On unenhanced CT images the rupture can be suspected if there is a discontinuity of wall calcification. In the absence of evident aortic disruption, an impending rupture is indicated by various indirect signs such as haemorrhagic pleural effusion, periaortic, pericardial and/or mediastinal haematoma. A periaortic haematoma appears as a mass encompassing the aortic contour. The haemorrhagic nature of a pleural or pericardial effusion is suggested by high density values on unenhanced CT (20–40 HU). MRI is highly specific for the recognition of the haemorrhagic nature of a pleural or mediastinal effusion, exploiting the high tissue characterisation power of BBFSE T1- and T2-weighted sequences. Usually, the high signal intensity of the effusion, of periaortic tissue or the thrombus within the aneurysm as well as a periadventitial enhancement on MRA or CTA images indicate the presence of haemorrhage or acute inflammation (hyperintensity on T2-weighted images) and are signs of aneurysm instability. An emerging right pleural effusion also indicates disease evolution, as does increasing diameter of the aorta over time

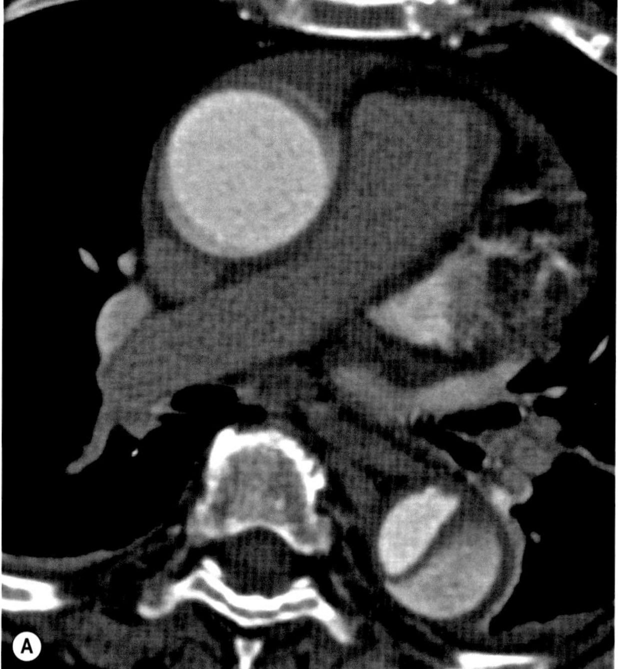

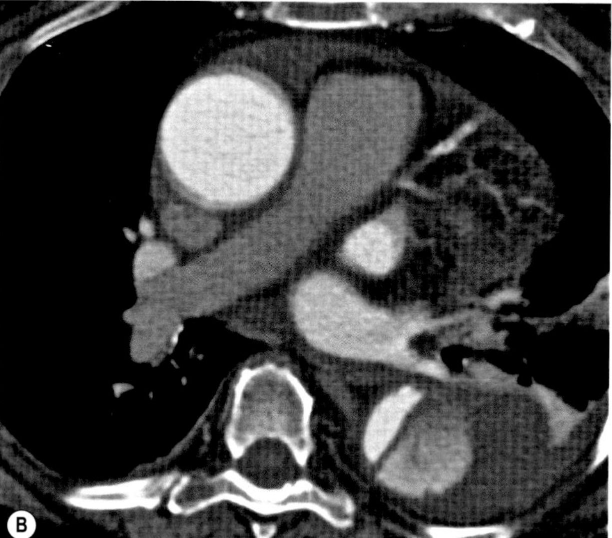

FIGURE 17-32 ■ **Axial CT images of an acute type B dissection one day (A) and 4 days (B) after symptoms onset:** note the strong increment of pleural and periaortic effusion after 4 days. The patient was submitted to urgent endovascular repair.

(Fig. 17-32). As a rule, imaging should be repeated after a few days in patients with suspected TAI to rule out or diagnose changes over time.

There are two signs in patients with acute TAI representing a 'red flag' indicative of need for urgent aortic repair:

- **The pseudocoarctation syndrome** is a partial compression of the aorta by a pseudoaneurysmatic sac just distal to the traumatic injury of the aortic wall, leading to an aortic lumen reduction as in congenital aortic coarctation. CT depicts this sign on MPR reconstructions in an oblique sagittal plane (Fig. 17-33).

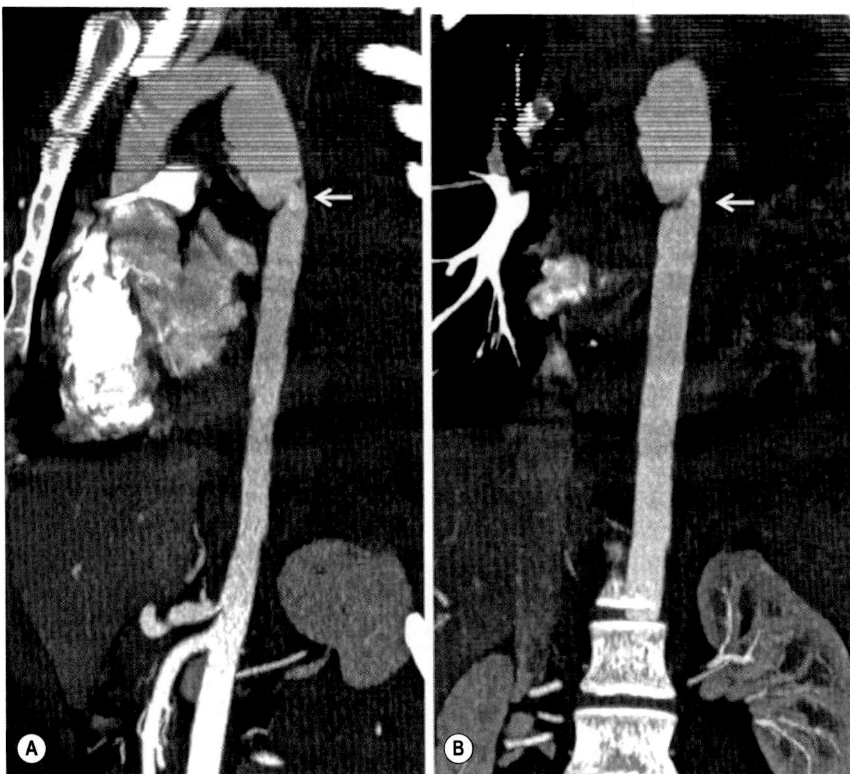

FIGURE 17-33 **CT MPR on the sagittal oblique (A) and coronal plane (B) of a TAI complicated by pseudocoarctation:** note the confined aortic lumen reduction (arrows) due to the compression excercised by the pseudoaneurysmatic sac.

- **A circumferential lesion** is a traumatic injury of the aortic wall involving more than 270° of the aortic circumference. This lesion is a strong predictor of an impending rupture. It can be diagnosed on axial images, but is best seen on 3D VR reconstructions.

Visceral Malperfusion

The instability of an acute aortic dissection is not only represented by signs of impending aortic rupture but also by the presence of partial or complete occlusion of branching vessels. The incidence of branching vessel compromise associated with aortic dissection ranges from 25 to 50%.[34] Restriction of flow into the aortic branch vessels is caused by two mechanisms leading to end-organ ischaemia (Fig. 17-34).

1. *Dynamic obstruction* affects vessels arising from the true lumen. Collapse of the true lumen is caused by bowing of the dissection flap into the true lumen, either proximal to or at the level of the ostium of the branching vessel, restricting or occluding flow.
2. *Static obstruction* is caused by extension of the dissection into the branching vessel without a re-entry point. Increased pressure or thrombus formation in the false lumen produces a focal stenosis with subsequent end-organ ischaemia.

Both dynamic and static obstruction can coexist, and identification of the mechanism of ischaemia is vital as the endovascular management of each differs (see below).

Before or in addition to clinical or laboratory signs of malperfusion, CT and MR imaging can suggest or confirm the presence of this severe pathological condition that deserves emergency treatment. The CT features of malperfusion consist of both aortic and visceral findings: a thread-like true lumen is most suggestive, but a malperfusion mechanism must be already suspected when the intimal flap shows a convexity towards the true lumen even when its dimensions are not clearly reduced (Fig. 17-35). CT may overestimate the degree of compression: in fact, an absent opacification of the true lumen does not exclude the possibility of passing the stenosis with a guidewire during an endovascular procedure.

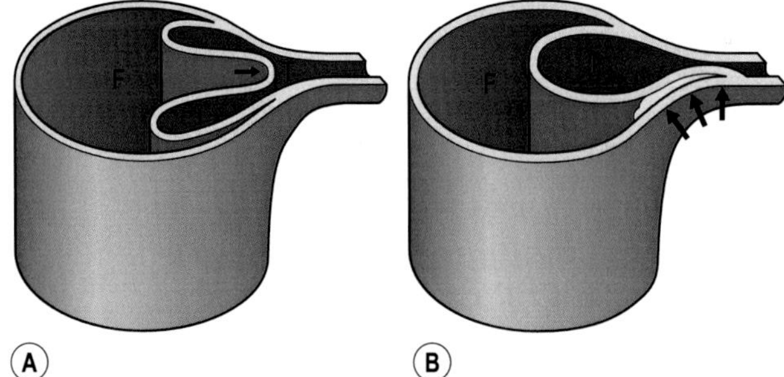

FIGURE 17-34 **Diagram of branch vessel ischaemia.** (A) Dynamic obstruction. The intimomedial flap bows across the true lumen (arrow) and obstructs flow into the branch vessel. (B) Static obstruction. The dissection extends into the branch vessel and may thrombose (arrowheads), causing stenosis of the vessel origin. F = false lumen, T = true lumen.

CT easily depicts signs of renal ischaemia such as absent or reduced opacification of one kidney. It is important to confirm the reduced opacification also in the

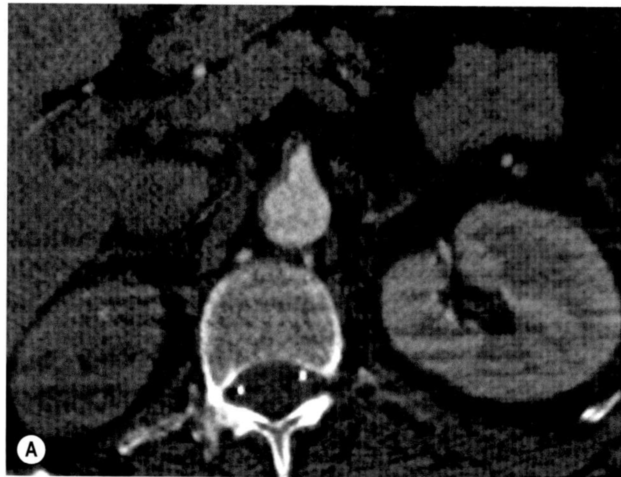

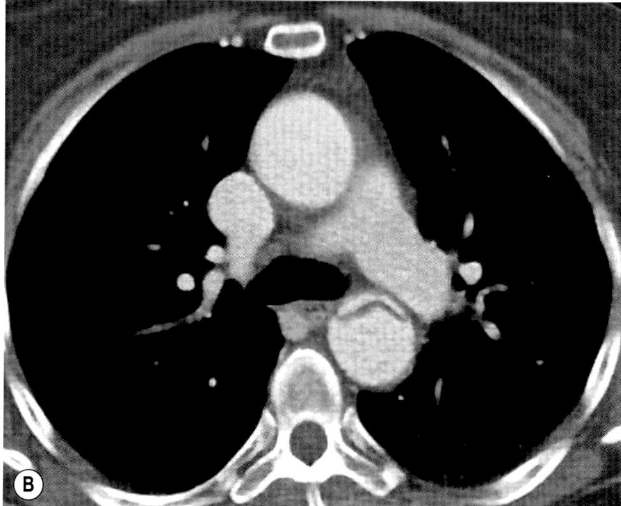

FIGURE 17-35 ■ Axial CT images of aortic type B dissection complicated by malperfusion syndrome: note the severe true lumen collapse at the level of superior mesenteric artery and the hypoperfused right kidney (A). Typical convexity of the intimal flap towards the true lumen in the absence of severe compression (B).

venous phase, because if the renal artery arises from the false lumen, the kidney may be perfused with delay due to the delayed flow as compared to the perfusion of the true lumen. A delayed acquisition after contrast administration is therefore recommended to confirm or exclude a partial or total renal ischaemia. Renal ischaemia is mostly accompanied by clinical signs such as anuria, haematuria, flank pain and uncontrolled hypertension. Hepato-mesenteric malperfusion is characterised by gastrointestinal bleeding, abdominal pain, abnormal hepatic laboratory findings and metabolic acidosis. CT shows the oedematous infiltration of the mesenterial fat during bowel distress and gastrointestinal stretching, but the venous phase is crucial to show direct signs of hypoperfusion of the bowel such as thickening and decreased enhancement in the acute phase (shock bowel). The mechanism of a static obstruction of a branching vessel is strongly indicated by an intimal flap entering the vessel with thrombus formation in the false lumen (Fig. 17-36).

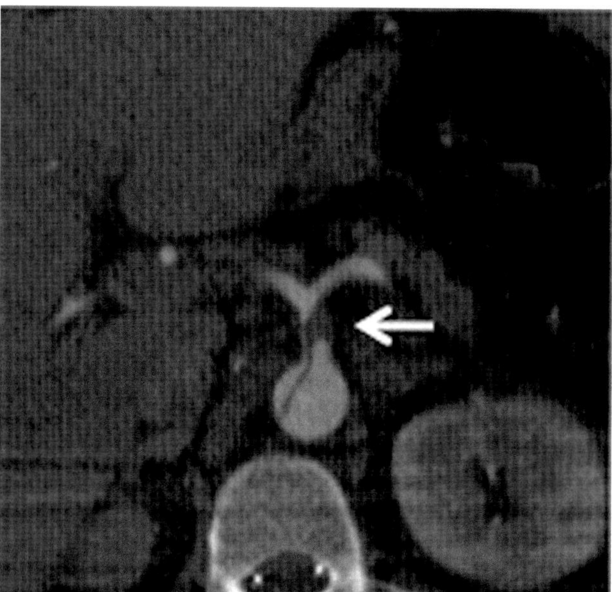

FIGURE 17-36 ■ Axial CT image showing static compression of the true lumen at the level of coeliac trunk. Note the thrombosis in the false lumen of the dissected vessel and the collapsed true lumen at the vessel origin.

Preoperative or Pre-Interventional Evaluation

Both CT and MR are equally well suited for preoperative evaluation of aortic diseases and have completely replaced conventional angiography. Especially for planning of endovascular treatment, a number of anatomical details need to be assessed to evaluate procedure feasibility and choose the correct prosthesis.[35]

For TAAs the main features that should be assessed are:

- Size and extension of the aneurysm.
- Adequate distance (>15 mm) between the proximal neck of the aneurysm and the origin of the epiaortic vessels to ensure a sufficient sealing of the stent graft, though it should be noted that, especially in emergency conditions, the left subclavian artery (LSA) can be covered, given that both vertebral arteries are patent. Overstenting of LSA may be performed in elective procedure after performance of revascularisation surgery.
- Distance of the peripheral neck of the aneurysm and its relationship to the origin of the visceral arteries (should be >15 mm) because preprocedural bypass operation or stenting are required if they have to be covered.
- Extent and type of wall alterations (e.g. amount of atheromatous material or calcium) at the proximal and distal neck that might affect the stent sealing (the oversize of the aortic diameter should be maintained by 10 to 20%).
- Diameter and condition of the abdominal aorta and vascular access (iliac and femoral arteries) and tortuosity of descending aorta which might prevent passage of the stent-graft delivery system.
- Any evidence for the presence of a large radicular artery supplying the spinal cord that could be

covered by a stent graft. The incidence of paraplegia is much lower with thoracic stent grafts than with surgery but is still around 2%. Expected length of coverage must be considered to evaluate the risk of such a complication, which can be partially prevented by CSF drainage before and after the procedure.
- Any other incidental findings in the chest, abdomen, or pelvis that should contraindicate the procedure (e.g. metastatic tumour spread)

Endovascular treatment of an AAA needs to consider other anatomical relationships of the aneurysm as most AAA stent grafts are bifurcated, though aorto uni-iliac stent grafts with surgical femoro-femoral cross-over grafting are also common, especially when the aneurysm has ruptured. Tube grafts are now the exception rather than the rule. Preprocedural CT evaluation is done to determine the following:

- Antero-posterior and transverse size of the AAA.
- Diameter of the aorta at the level of and just below the visceral arteries.
- Distance of the proximal aneurysm neck to the lowest renal artery (at least 15 mm).
- Shape of the neck (conical necks may lead to poor proximal seals or late endoleaks) and presence of excessive atheromatous wall changes potentially preventing a perfect seal.
- Angulation of the neck in the AP and lateral planes: an angle > 60° aggravates stent sealing and harbours an increased risk for stent displacement.
- The presence of accessory renal arteries that will have to be covered and makes a preproceduralassessment of split renal function necessary.
- Distance from the lowest renal artery to the aortic bifurcation determining the length of the stent-graft main body.
- Diameter, tortuosity, degree of calcification and morphology of the common iliac arteries. If they are aneurysmatic, patients need to be informed with respect to possible buttock claudication following internal iliac artery embolisation and extension of the stent graft into the external iliac artery.
- Size of the common femoral and external iliac arteries and the presence of any stenoses that might prevent the stent-graft delivery.
- Any incidental findings, especially with respect to size and function of the kidneys or the presence of a doubled inferior vena cava, especially if open surgery is planned.

The following anatomical details need to be considered for planning of endovascular treatment of aortic dissection.

- The distance between the proximal neck, the entry tear and the origin of the epiaortic vessels.
- The origin of the visceral vessels in regard to the true or false lumen must be defined. If one or more vessels arise from the false lumen, a re-entry tear ensuring vessel perfusion after stent-graft deployment has to be identified.
- Careful evaluation of ascending aorta and aortic arch dimensions and degree of atheromatous wall changes are necessary. Ascending aorta and arch aneurysms may favour a retrograde extension of the dissection if the proximal end of the stent graft (free flow extremity) is positioned in the distal arch. In patients with Marfan's syndrome or a bicuspid aortic valve, endovascular treatment of type B dissection may be contraindicated for this reason. The distal end of the stent graft is mostly localised in a part of the dissected aorta which does not represent the true aortic diameter; thus the choice of the prosthesis calibre should not exceed 80% of the sum of true and false lumen to avoid aneurysmatic degeneration of the false lumen.

CT provides optimal preoperative evaluation of stent-graft procedures under emergency conditions as well as for elective procedures due to its rapid and accurate anatomical definition; MR, though adequate for preoperative evaluation, is not able to visualise calcification and it is the less adaptable technique.

Postoperative Evaluation

Regular postoperative evaluation is mandatory after endovascular stent grafting of aortic diseases. Though stent grafting is less invasive than conventional surgery, with considerably lower perioperative morbidity and mortality rates, there are a number of short- and long-term complications, the most frequent being endoleaks (Fig. 17-37). Stent grafts may dislodge or even rupture and must therefore be monitored lifelong. Both CT and MR can be used for aortic stent-graft imaging follow-up. CT is preferred, because it provides superior visualisation of the stent-graft material. Metal artefacts on MR images limit the sensitivity for small initial endoleaks as well as for stent fractures, as the latter represent a late complication (Fig. 17-38). CXR and abdominal X-ray (AXR) may also be used to check for stent fracture in the long term.

MR provides accurate evaluation of the aorta distal and proximal to the stent graft with reproducible measurements of the excluded anurysmal sac; it is mainly reserved for the imaging follow-up of endovascular treatment of TAI, especially in young patients.

Complications may also occur after traditional surgical intervention and regular imaging follow-up should be performed, though less frequently than after stent grafting. Ultrasound is satisfactory after proximal aortic interventions (involving the aortic valve and ascending aorta), because it provides both morphological and functional information (valve prosthesis function). MR and CT are reserved for patients in which ultrasound is inconclusive or to confirm the suspected complications (e.g. suture dehiscence). MR is less affected by artefacts from surgical devices, except for old mechanical valve prostheses, and is the preferred method for repetitive post-surgical follow-up; moreover, it also provides functional evaluation of the aortic valve as opposed to CT.

Management of Aortic Diseases

Traumatic Aortic Injury (TAI)

The traditional approach of immediate repair of TAI is based on the high mortality in the first 24 h in patients

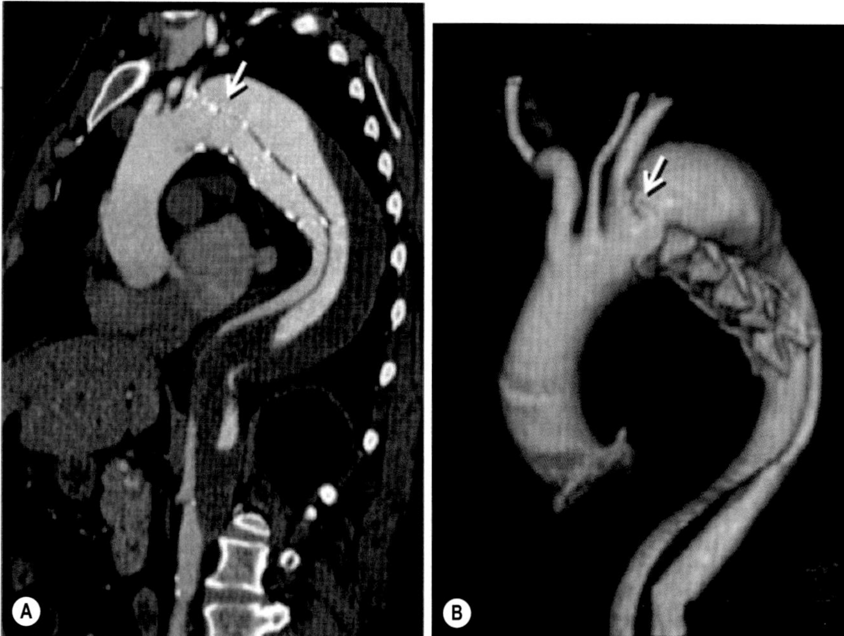

FIGURE 17-37 ■ CT MPR (A) and VR (B) images of a type I endoleak after endovascular treatment for type B aortic dissection. See the proximal flow from the aortic arch to the false lumen due to inadequate sealing of the proximal part of the stent graft (arrows). Type I is the most dangerous endoleak and requires a secondary procedure or a shift to open surgery if not solved with a moulding balloon.

who survive the initial traumatic event.[36] However, the outcome in these patients is related as much to associated injuries as it is to the TAI itself. This led to the suggestion by some investigators to delay surgical repair or even consider conservative management of TAI, allowing time to manage other serious or potentially life-threatening injuries.[37] Controlled hypotension is mandatory using beta-blockers and vasodilators to keep the mean arterial pressure below 70 mmHg. Beta-blockers reduce the rate rise of systolic ejection of the left ventricle, decreasing the shearing force on the aortic wall. This approach has been found to successfully reduce the overall morbidity and mortality in patients with other significant injuries.[38]

As surgery has a high morbidity and mortality, thoracic stent grafting (TSG) has been introduced for the management of TAI[39] as a less invasive alternative therapy (Fig. 17-39). Small cohort series have shown TSG to be a successful alternative treatment of TAI with substantially reduced morbidity and mortality compared to surgical repair and after 10 years of experience with endovascular treatment there is nowadays a definite management shift from surgery to endovascular approach.[40] Endovascular repair of TAI requires at least 15 mm long distance of aortic wall proximal to the injury to achieve an adequate seal. Given that the isthmus is the most common site of TAI and is usually very close to the origin of the LSA, the proximal distance is frequently insufficiently long. This proximal 'landing zone' may be lengthened by intentionally covering the left subclavian artery origin and extending the stent graft to the origin of the left common carotid artery. Initial concerns over acute upper limb ischaemia have not been confirmed; most patients have an adequate collateral supply via the circle of Willis and left vertebral artery and do not need carotid-to-subclavian bypass surgery. However, the risk of adverse central neurological events after endovascular overstenting of the LSA without previous revascularisation is around 10% in multiple study series.[41]

Aortic Dissection

Initial treatment in all patients presenting with aortic dissection is aimed to eliminate pain, reduce systolic blood pressure and reduce systolic pressure rise during cardiac cycle. It is achieved by a combination of intravenous beta-blockers and peripheral vasodilators. Subsequent management is based on the Stanford type and the presence of complications.

Type A Dissection. These dissections account for 75% of cases. Immediate surgical repair is indicated in all patients owing to the high mortality (>50% within 48 h) if untreated.[42] Fatal complications include aortic rupture, cardiac tamponade, acute aortic regurgitation and acute myocardial infarction. Involvement of the arch vessels harbours a high risk for neurological complications.

Type B Dissection. The current treatment of acute type B dissections is based on a complication-specific approach. In uncomplicated type B dissection (no evidence of rupture or branch vessel ischaemia) medical treatment is initiated, as both medical and emergent surgical management are associated with similar mortality rates.[43] Patients who fail under medical treatment (persistent pain and/or progression of dissection) or develop complications are referred for either surgical or endovascular intervention. Early surgery is recommended for patients with Marfan's syndrome.

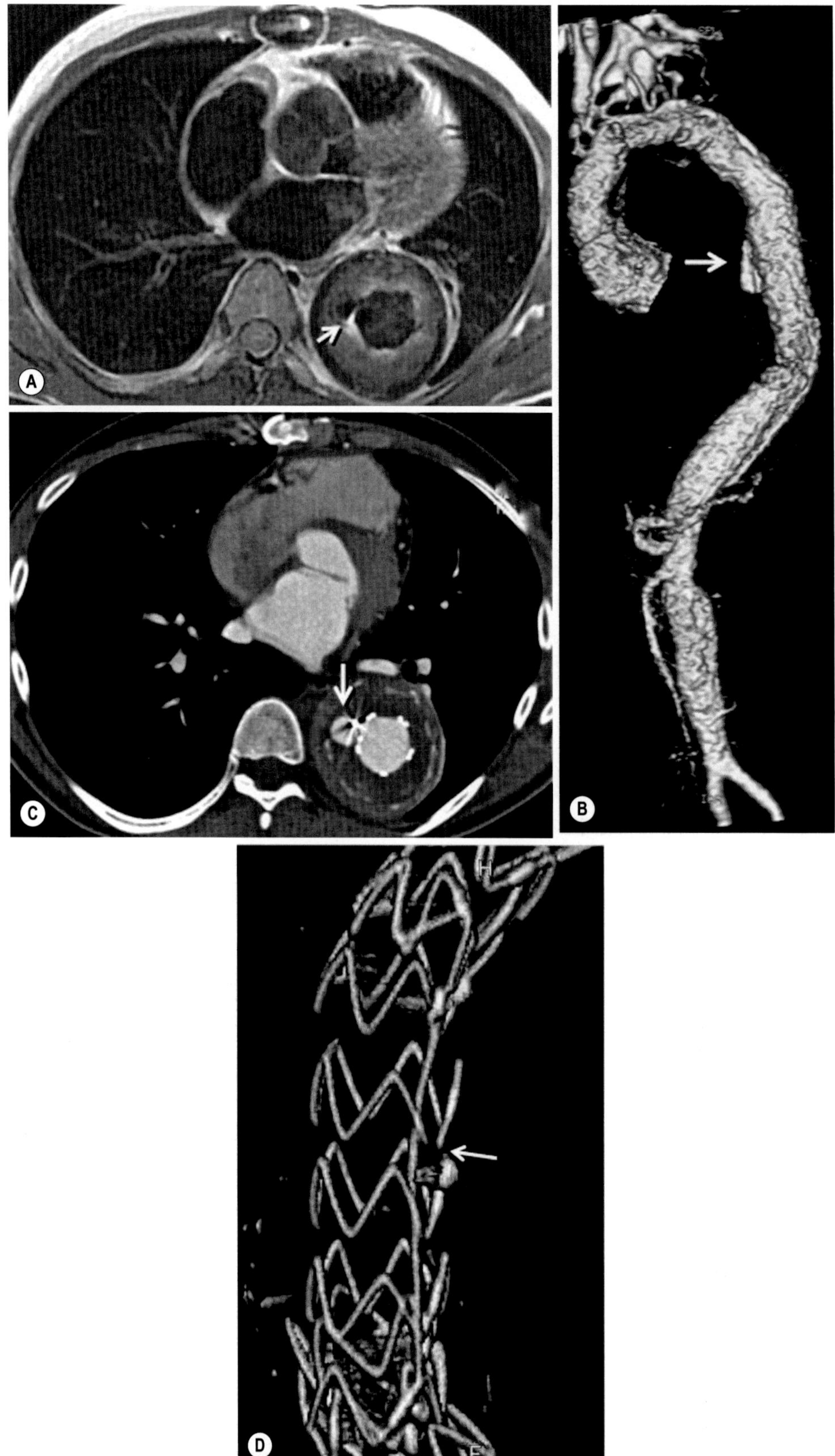

FIGURE 17-38 ■ **Imaging follow-up after endovascular treatment for type B aortic dissection.** Axial MR BBFSE image identifies a signal dysomogeneity (arrow) near the stent graft (A) and MRA VR reconstructions (B) may diagnose an endoleak (arrow), but MDCT, through the optimal visualisation of stent-graft material (C, D), may identify the nature of endoleak: a type III from a failure/fracture of the stent-graft material (arrows). This can result from a manufacturing problem or long-term wear and tear and changes in aneurysm morphology causing holes in the graft or dislocations of modular components. They can be fixed either by repeat stent grafting or open surgery.

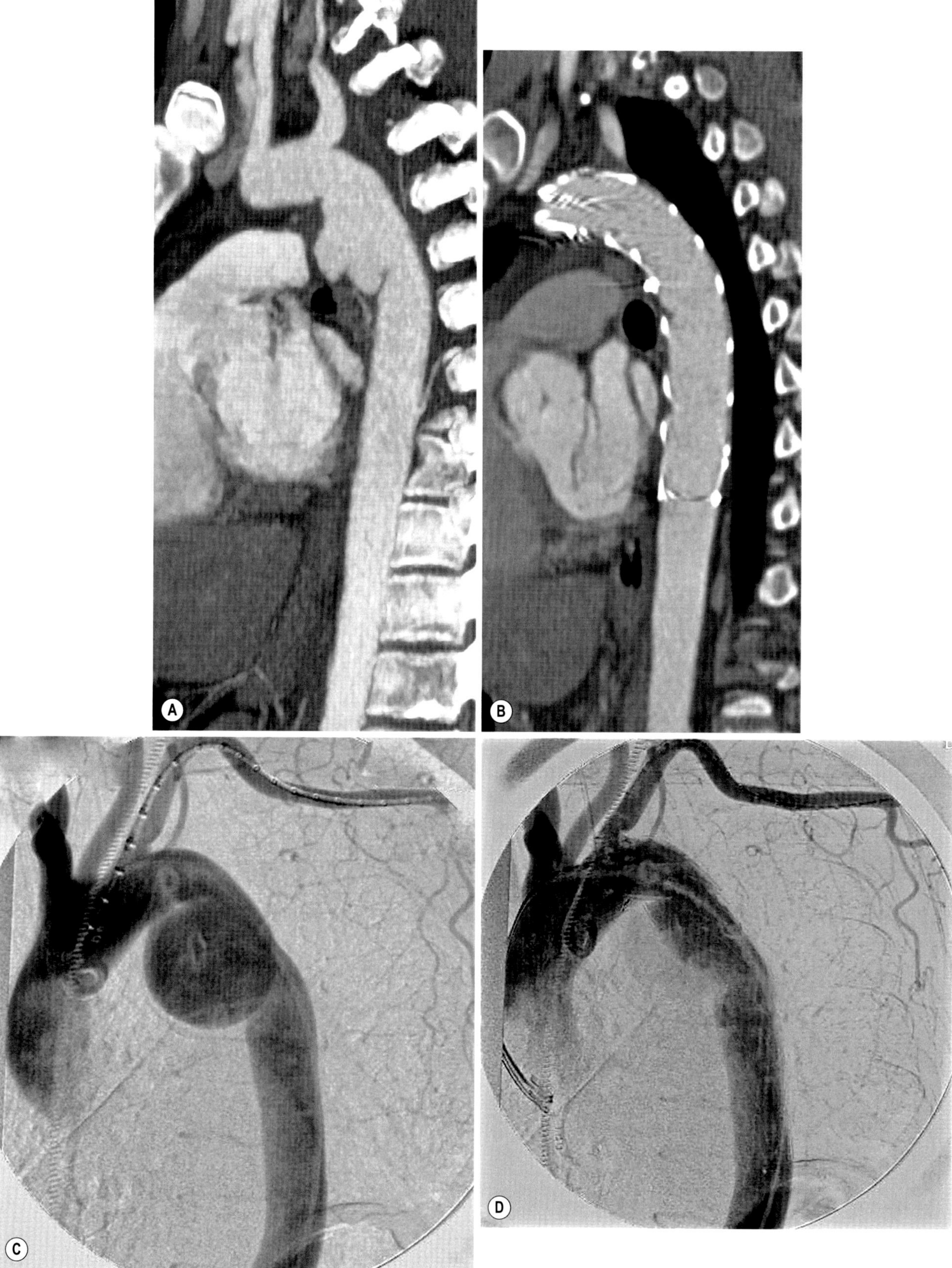

FIGURE 17-39 ■ Sagittal oblique CT MPR of a patient with acute TAI before (A) and after (B) endovascular treatment. Almost complete shrinkage of the excluded lesion on follow-up CT imaging. Intraoperative aortograms before (C) and after (D) thoracic stent-graft insertion of another patient with chronic post-traumatic aneurysm. Note the complete disappearance of the pseudoaneurysmal sac after stent-graft deployment.

Endovascular Treatment of Type B Dissection. Surgery for type B dissection is associated with mortality exceeding 50% with high risk for organ ischaemia.[44] Endovascular techniques have been successfully employed for the treatment of type B dissection with reduced morbidity and mortality.[45] The three techniques employed are stent insertion, stent-graft insertion and/or fenestration of the intimal flap.

The indications for stent or stent-graft placement in type B dissection are two-fold:

1. **Contained rupture**. Persistent flow in the false lumen is associated with aneurysmatic dilatation and increased risk of rupture of the false lumen (20–50% of patients within 1–5 years). Placement of a stent graft covering the site of the entry tear can promote thrombosis of the false lumen and stabilisation of the dissection, that way reducing the risk of rupture. Acute type B dissections are the most appropriate group to treat as the dissection flap is thin and mobile, and will readily re-appose to the aortic wall. In chronic dissections, the flap becomes thickened and rigid and, thus, endovascular stenting is less likely to result in complete false lumen exclusion.
2. **Occlusion of branching vessels**. The treatment in patients with impeding branch vessel ischaemia is dependent on the cause. Dynamic obstruction results from true lumen collapse. Sealing the entry tear with stent-graft placement directs blood flow back into the true lumen, increasing the size of the true lumen, moving the dissection flap away from the branch vessel and in that way relieving branch vessel ischaemia. Static obstruction can be successfully treated by direct stent insertion in the compromised vessel via the true lumen. In cases where the dissection extends distally to cause lower limb ischaemia, direct access to the true lumen is gained by directly accessing the involved side with weakened or absent femoral pulse.

Currently, stent grafts are mostly used in patients who have indications for surgical intervention. Given that the majority of patients undergo thrombosis of the false lumen following stent-graft placement, it is not inconceivable that, in the future, this may become the treatment of choice for all patients with acute type B dissection. However, more follow-up data are required on long-term device durability and patient outcome.[46]

Since the introduction of stent grafts, percutaneous fenestration has been less frequently employed in the management of branch vessel ischaemia due to true lumen compression. Patients who are managed conservatively require long-term follow-up with either CT or MR to monitor the false lumen for aneurysmatic dilatation and distal extension of the dissection over time. Equally, all patients that undergo endovascular treatment require long-term follow-up to assure integrity of the device.

Inflammatory Diseases of the Aorta and Mid-Aortic Syndrome

A number of conditions can lead to an inflammatory aortitis, including ergotism, radiation fibrosis, syphilis, tuberculosis, giant cell arteritis, Buerger's, Behçet's, Cogan's and Kawasaki's disease. There are also congenital inflammatory diseases that affect the aorta, such as Ehlers–Danlos and Marfan's syndrome, as well as neurofibromatosis. In the acute phase, aortitis may mimic an acute aortic syndrome, especially an intramural haematoma. Differential diagnosis can be difficult if based on clinical symptoms and laboratory tests alone. CT and MR imaging is very helpful for differentiating these two pathological entities: IMH has a typical crescent-like morphology, while in aortitis concentric wall thickening is usually observed (Fig. 17-40). Tissue characterisation with T1 and T2 BB sequences may aid to discern haemorrhagic products from mere inflammation.

Mid-Aortic Syndrome

Mid-aortic syndrome is characterised by segmental narrowing of the proximal abdominal aorta and ostial

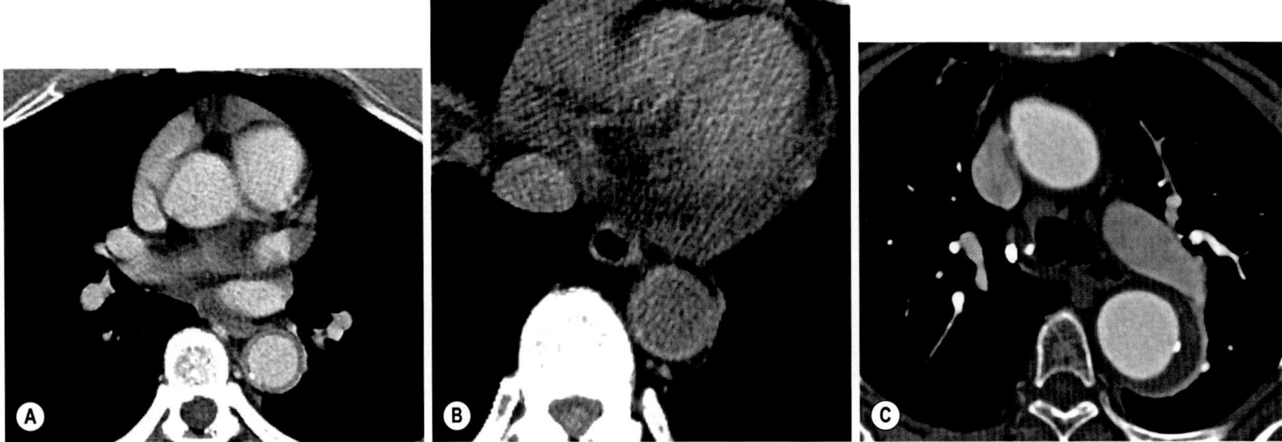

FIGURE 17-40 ■ **Axial CT images of descending thoracic aorta: imaging aspects of aortitis (A, B) and IMH (C).** Note the circumferential thickening and enhancement of aortic wall in acute aortitis (A), hyperdense on unenhanced CT (B), while IMH appears like a typical crescent-like thickening of the aortic wall (C).

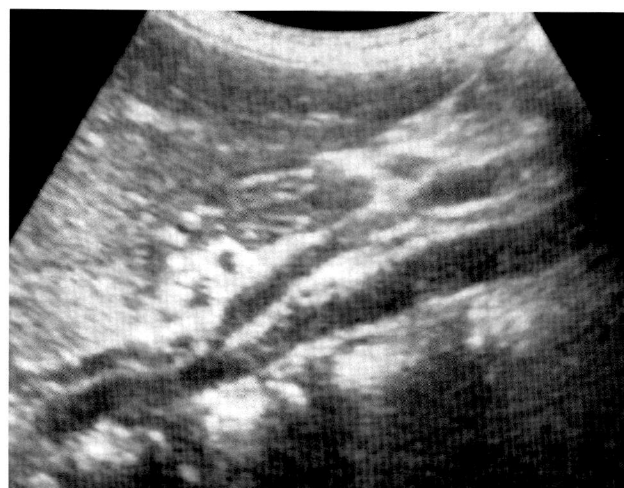

FIGURE 17-41 ■ Longitudinal abdominal ultrasound examination in a 12-year-old girl presenting with hypertension. There is clearly a stenosis at the origin of the superior mesenteric artery and narrowing and irregularity of the aorta. This is characteristic of mid-aortic syndrome. The patient had café au lait spots consistent with the diagnosis of neurofibromatosis.

stenosis of its major branches (Fig. 17-41). It is usually diagnosed in young adults, but can present in childhood. Clinical presentation and radiological findings are dependent on the underlying disease, but hypertension is a common feature in all patients.

Congenital aortic coarctation is a very uncommon cause of mid-aortic syndrome, in which the aortic narrowing occurs in the thoracic or abdominal aorta. It may be seen in fetal alcohol syndrome and then associated with intellectual disability.

Granulomatous vasculitis (Takayasu's disease) is a chronic inflammatory disease that involves the aorta, its branches and the pulmonary arteries, causing varying degree of stenosis, occlusion, or dilatation of the involved vessels; aetiology and precise pathogenesis are unknown. It is more common in parts of the world with a high incidence of tuberculosis, but also occurs more frequenly in Japan. It is predominantly a disease of young adults, but may also affect children. It is very rare in infancy. The female-to-male ratio varies from 9:1 in reports from Japan to 1.3:1 in India. The pattern of vessel involvement also varies in different parts of the world. The involvement of the aortic arch and its branches is common in Japan, whereas the thoracoabdominal aorta is mainly involved in patients from Korea and India. It is not known whether this variation reflects differing causes of the disease or differing HLA-associated genetic subtypes. Racial variation also occurs, the disease being relatively uncommon in Caucasians. The initial site of inflammation is around the vasa vasorum in the media and adventitia but later nodular fibrosis in all layers of the arterial wall is seen and the intima can obliterate the lumen. The diagnosis depends on typical angiographic morphology, a history or presence of constitutional symptoms suggestive of a systemic illness and the differential diagnosis of other, similar conditions as listed above. Atherosclerosis of the aorta is distinguished on clinical and morphological grounds, but secondary atherosclerotic changes may occur in older patients with Takayasu's arteritis.

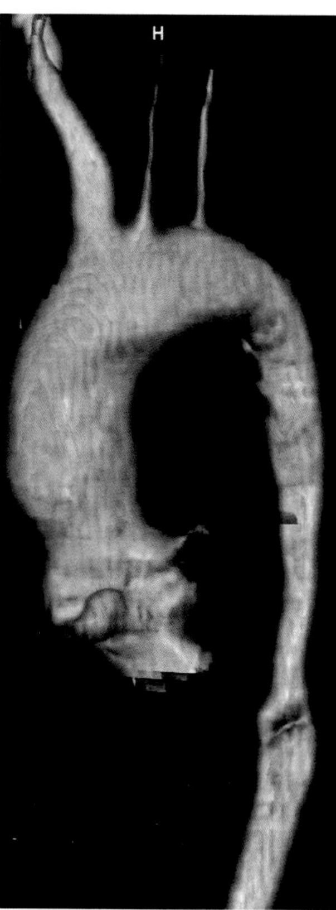

FIGURE 17-42 ■ MDCT VR reconstruction of a 20-year-old woman presenting with right arm ischaemia and hypertension with diagnosis of Takayasu's disease. Thickening of all layers of the proximal and mid descending thoracic aorta wall produced segmental lumen reduction.

The radiological features occur late in the course of the disease and include luminal irregularity, vessel stenosis, occlusion, dilatation or aneurysms in the aorta or its primary branches (Fig. 17-42). Neurofibromatosis of the abdominal aorta and some other causes of mid-aortic syndrome may produce an identical angiographic picture in children. Based on angiographic morphology, Takayasu's arteritis is divided into type I (involving the aortic arch and its branches), type II (thoracoabdominal aorta and its branches) and type III (involving lesions of both types I and II). Involvement of pulmonary arteries, in addition to any of the above types, is grouped as type IV.

The infrarenal aorta and the iliac vessels are usually not involved in Takayasu's arteritis. Similarly, the inferior mesenteric artery is rarely involved. Unlike coarctation of the aorta, intercostal collaterals rarely occur as the diffuse intimal disease in the aorta also involves the ostia of these intercostal vessels. Aortic intimal calcification may be seen.

Saccular or fusiform aneurysms of the aorta occur in 2–26% of cases and usually coexist with stenotic lesions. Aneurysms without stenosis occur in 1–2% of cases. Pseudoaneurysm or dissection of the aorta is extremely rare.

CT, ultrasound and particularly contrast-enhanced MRI and MRA provide information on mural changes of the vessels and have largely replaced angiography for

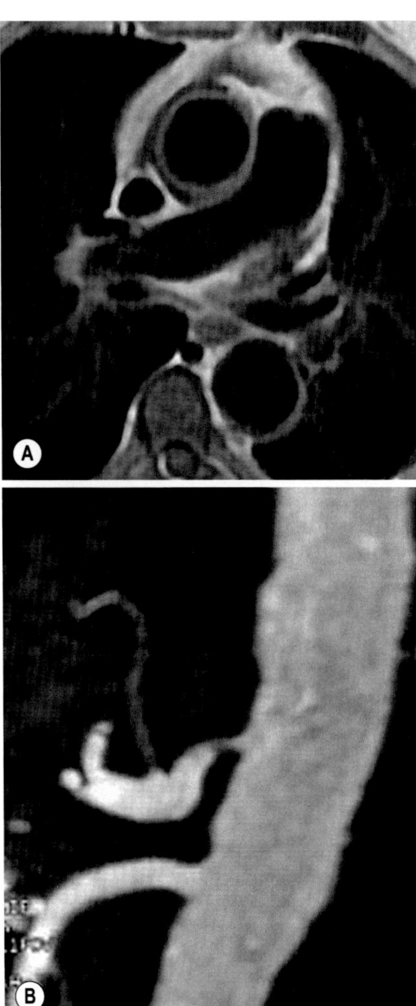

FIGURE 17-43 ■ MR imaging of aortitis. BBFSE axial image after medical therapy for aortitis (A) shows slight concentric thickening of the ascending aorta. Low signal of the aortic wall indicates absence of active inflammation. MRA of visceral vessels (B) shows a residual focal stenosis at the origin of coeliac trunk.

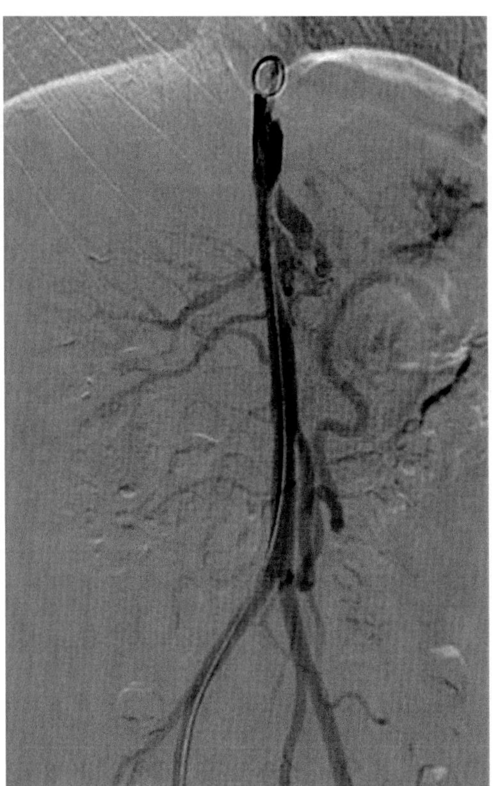

FIGURE 17-44 ■ Right oblique abdominal aortogram in a hypertensive patient with the cutaneous stigmata of neurofibromatosis. Note the mid-aortic stenosis and the coeliac axis and superior mesenteric artery stenoses with collateral supply from the inferior mesenteric artery.

diagnostic and monitoring purposes (Fig. 17-43). FDG-PET may be useful, especially in cases of fever of unknown origin,[47] by illustrating increased FDG uptake in the involved vessels.

Takayasu's arteritis in children has a mortality between 10 and 30%. The prognosis has significantly improved due to interventional procedures for the treatment of renal and aortic stenosis. Long-term follow-up data on children are not available. Five- and 10-year survival in adults is 91 and 84%, respectively. Severe hypertension, aortic regurgitation, retinopathy, aneurysms or cardiac involvement are predictors of poor outcome. In the absence of these complications, 80% of patients remain stable for years but around 20% show progression.

In the acute phase, treatment with corticosteroids leads to clinical remission in 60% of cases. Cytotoxic drugs can also be used in resistant cases. The major morbidity and mortality of Takayasu's arteritis results from stenosis and occlusion of the aorta, renal and carotid arteries. Interventional radiological techniques for stenosed segments have revolutionised the treatment of Takayasu's arteritis. Surgical treatment is not preferred for Takayasu's arteritis because of the diffuse, inflammatory, and possibly progressive nature of the disease, except for otherwise therapy-resistant, symptomatic, stenotic lesions and large aneurysms.[48]

Von Recklinghausen's disease (type 1 neurofibromatosis) can be distinguished from other causes of mid-aortic syndrome by the presence of café au lait skin lesions and neurofibromas. Approximately 2% of patients develop vascular abnormalities, including renal, aortic and mesenteric stenoses (Fig. 17-44). Vessels are surrounded by neurofibromatous or ganglioneuromatous tissue in the adventitia.

Alagille's syndrome (a multisystem autosomal dominant disorder caused by mutations in the *JAG1* gene on chromosome 20p12) and **Williams' syndrome** (a rare genetic condition estimated to occur in 1 in 20,000 births) are both associated with aortic coarctation (thoracic or abdominal).

Aortic Occlusive Disease

Atherosclerosis is the predominant cause of chronic aortic occlusive disease (over 90% of cases), with Takayasu's disease (see above) accounting for the rest; acute occlusion may result from an aortic bifurcation 'saddle' embolus or in situ aortic thrombosis.

Chronic Aortic Occlusive Disease

Atherosclerotic aortic occlusive disease affects a younger population than this generally presenting with lower limb arterial disease. Patients are typically female, heavy smokers with hyperlipidaemia, they have a small infrarenal aorta and hypoplastic iliofemoral arteries (hypoplastic aortoiliac syndrome). The infra-inguinal arteries are 'protected' by the aortic lesion and are typically disease free. Patients present with chronic lower limb ischaemia and are graded according to the severity of their disease. Aortic occlusive disease is largely associated with Fontaine grade I or II symptoms. Symptoms of critical limb ischaemia (grade III or IV) are unusual at initial presentation as these are associated with both supra-and infra-inguinal disease.

While the management of grade I and IIa patients is based solely on risk factor modification, patients with grades IIb–IV are investigated further and, in addition to risk factor modification, treated by revascularisation, if appropriate.

Investigation and Management. In the presence of significant aortic disease, the femoral pulses are diminished or absent and there is a reduction in the ABPI (grade IIb, 0.5–0.8; grades III–IV, <0.5). Duplex data acquisition plays very little role in the investigation of these patients as the aorta is often difficult to visualise and assess. Angiography is currently the investigation of choice, though MRA offers major advantages. It is non-invasive, avoiding a brachial puncture with its associated risks. It provides excellent images of not only the aortic lesion but also the run-off and negates the need for large volumes of iodinated contrast medium. It therefore allows planning of an appropriate management strategy with very little risk to the patient. A number of key points need to be addressed, irrespective of the method of investigation, as these will have impact on the surgical and endovascular options considered:

1. What is the upper limit of the lesion? Is it infrarenal or juxtarenal?
2. What is the lower limit of the lesion? Is there involvement of the aortic bifurcation?
3. Are the coeliac axis (CA) and superior mesenteric artery (SMA) normal? This is important if intervention may potentially lead to compromise of the inferior mesenteric artery (IMA).

In the past, aortic occlusive disease was treated by aortic bypass surgery or aortic endarterectomy. Though surgery is associated with excellent primary patency (75–90% and 90–95%, respectively), it is associated with considerable morbidity (9–27%) and mortality (1–7%).

Endovascular techniques have been used as an alternative since the early 1990s and are now the treatment of choice. Treatment options vary from angioplasty alone, angioplasty with selective stenting, to primary stenting. Angioplasty alone is used in short focal stenoses (<2 cm) and is associated with a primary patency of 85% and low incidence of major complications (3.6%). Stenting has been reserved for flow-limiting dissection or residual stenosis following angioplasty. Primary stenting has been advocated for the treatment of occlusions and complex lesions (eccentric, ulcerated, or calcified plaques) if there is significant concern of distal embolisation (Fig. 17-45).

Acute Aortic Occlusive Disease

Acute aortic occlusive disease is a vascular emergency resulting from either saddle embolus to the aortic bifurcation or in situ thrombosis of an aortic stenosis, aortic aneurysm or traumatic aortic dissection. Given the proximal nature of the occlusion, patients often present with neurological deficits (including paralysis) of the lower limbs, which may be initially misinterpreted and lead to investigations to rule out or diagnose spinal cord compression with consequent delay in diagnosis. If the vascular nature of the presenting symptoms is unrecognised, mortality is high (75%).[49] The key to the diagnosis is the absence of femoral pulses.

Imaging and Management. The role of imaging is dependent on the severity of ischaemia. If there is major tissue loss, absent capillary return with marbling, profound paralysis and sensory loss, or absent Doppler signals, the ischaemia is irreversible and amputation inevitable. If any of the above-mentioned findings is still missing, emergency surgery with no imaging may be appropriate. With less severe degrees of ischaemia, expedient imaging can provide useful information. As for chronic occlusion, imaging may be done by catheter angiography or MRA, with similar risks and benefits. The purpose of investigation is to determine the proximal location of occlusion, the state of the run-off vessels and to differentiate embolic from thrombotic occlusion.

If an embolic aetiology or thrombosis of an aneurysm/traumatic dissection is confirmed, surgical intervention with embolectomy or bypass grafting is the treatment of choice. In situ thrombosis of a pre-existing stenosis is suggested by the presence of collaterals. Endovascular treatment with thrombolysis can also be considered if the severity of ischaemia allows us to allocate the necessary time for this. Following successful thrombolysis, aortic angioplasty or stenting can be performed to treat the underlying lesion (Fig. 17-46). Even with appropriate intervention, overall in-hospital mortality is high (21%), being higher in those with an embolic aetiology.[48] If the occlusion is embolic, following successful revascularisation a search must be made for the underlying source. Ultrasound will exclude a cardiac source, followed by careful examination of the thoracic aorta. Emboli frequently originate from an aortic plaque or intimal flap.

CONGENITAL AORTIC ABNORMALITIES

Vascular Rings

A vascular ring is a condition in which an anomalous configuration of the arch and/or its associated vessels completely or incompletely surrounds the trachea and oesophagus and causing compression of these structures. Neonates present with respiratory distress, older children present with stridor or dysphagia. The two most common types of complete vascular rings, accounting for 85–95%

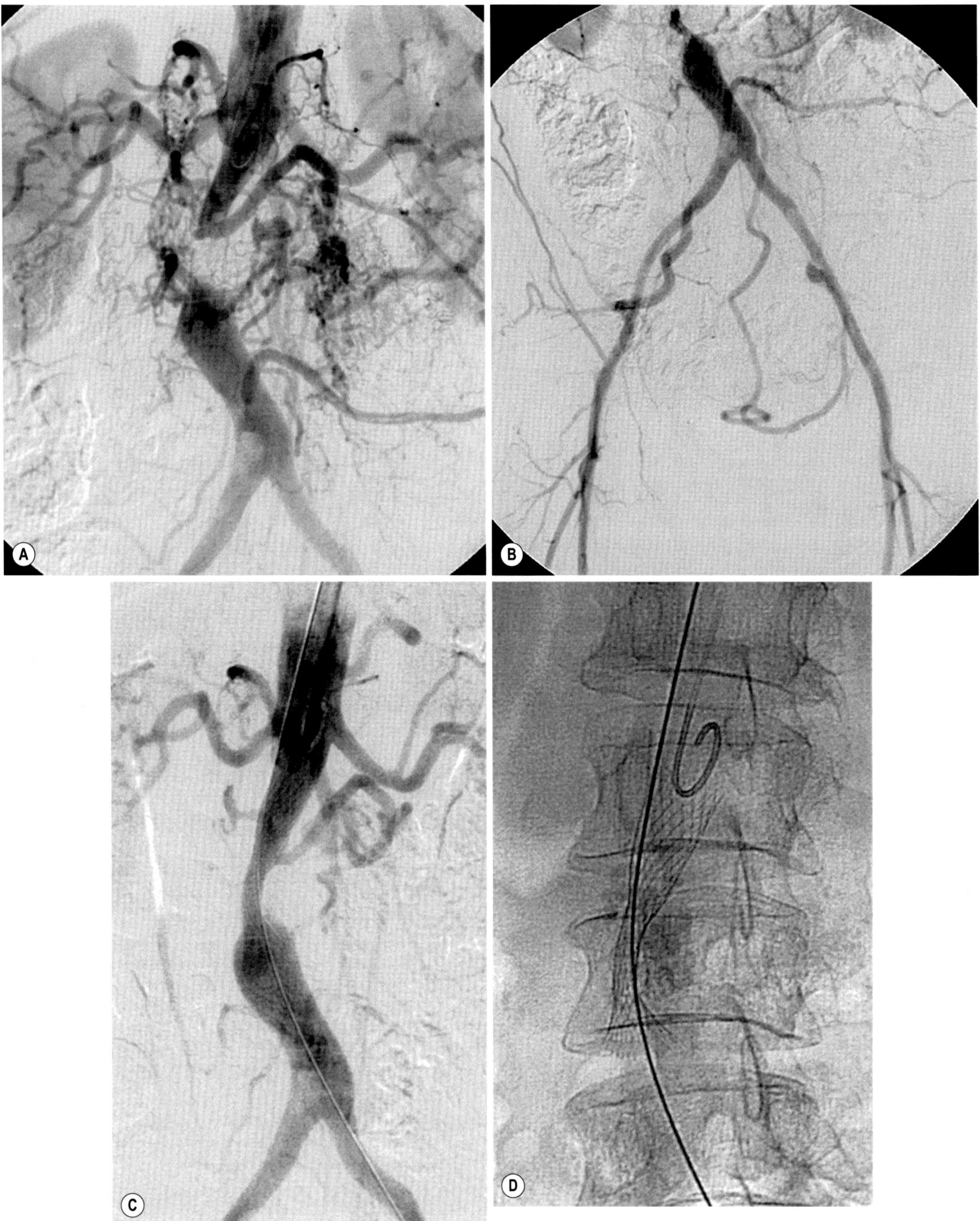

FIGURE 17-45 ■ Chronic aortic occlusion in a 56-year-old woman presenting with short-distance claudication. (A) There is a short segment occlusion of the infrarenal aorta. The aorta proximal to this is also diseased and narrowed. The lumbar arteries are markedly hypertrophied. (B) A plaque is seen at the aortic bifurcation, but the iliac arteries are relatively disease free. (C) Following primary stenting of the occlusion, the patient's symptoms subsided, despite underdilatation of the lesion. (D) The extreme calcific nature of the lesion is seen on the native image.

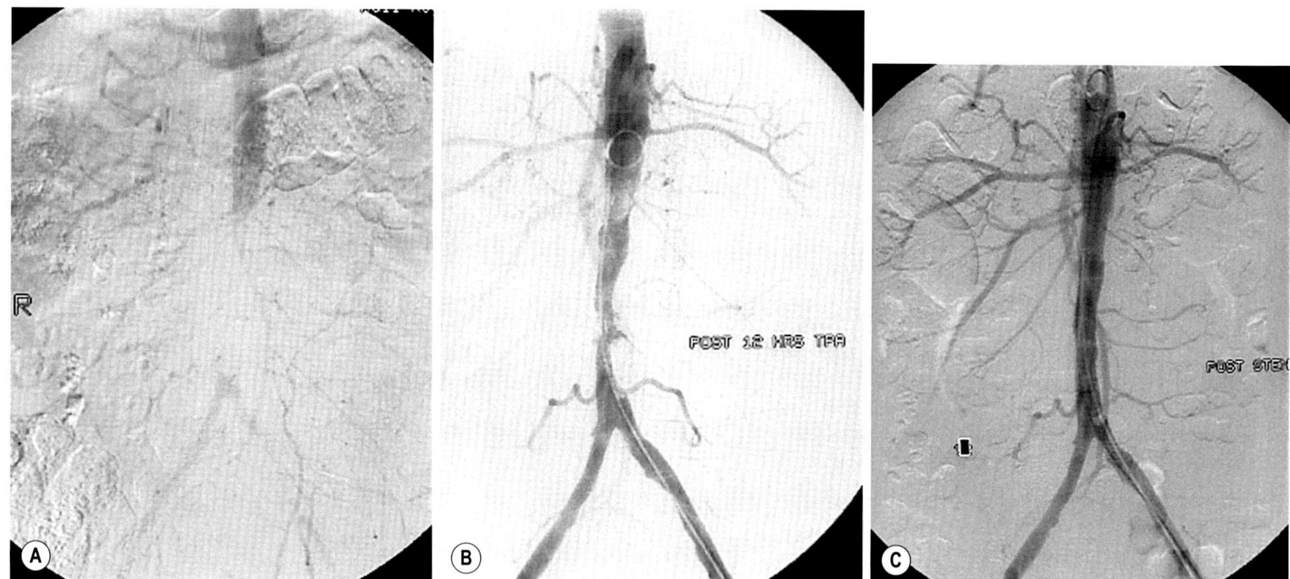

FIGURE 17-46 ■ **Acute aortic occlusion.** (A) Infrarenal aortic occlusion with meniscus sign suggests that this is an embolic occlusion. (B) However, following successful thrombolysis, an underlying stenosis is revealed which appears secondary to extrinsic compression of the aorta. (C) A good angiographic result is achieved after stent placement.

of cases, are double aortic arch and right aortic arch with left ligamentum arteriosum. Tracheomalacia may result from compression of the trachea by vascular rings.[50]

The key to understanding vascular rings lies in the development of the arch. Beyond 4 weeks' gestation there are paired ventral aortas joined to paired dorsal aortas by six pairs of arterial arches, though these are never all present simultaneously (Fig. 17-47). The fourth arch is the most important for the development of vascular rings.

Double Aortic Arch

Persistence of the right and left fourth arches lead to a double aortic arch (Fig. 17-48). In 75% the right arch is larger; in about 30% the smaller, or less dominant, the arch is atretic but remains in continuity with the descending aorta, maintaining a complete ring. This may be difficult to identify radiologically. The normally positioned left, or anterior, arch exits the pericardium and joins the left-sided descending thoracic aorta after giving off the left subclavian artery. The ligamentum arteriosum is positioned normally. The posterior, or right, arch joins the descending thoracic aorta at the same level as the anterior arch but reaches that point from an extreme posterior course behind the oesophagus. Hence the descending aorta is more commonly on the left but can be on either side.

Other Vascular Rings Associated with Aortic Arch Abnormalities

Involution of the left fourth branchial arch and persistence of the right branchial arch results in a right-sided aortic arch; it can occur in the absence of any other anomalies. Its presence is suggestive of the existence of an associated anomaly, as persistence of the right arch with involution of the left creates a situation in which the origins of the left subclavian artery and ductus arteriosus can vary with possible development of a vascular ring.

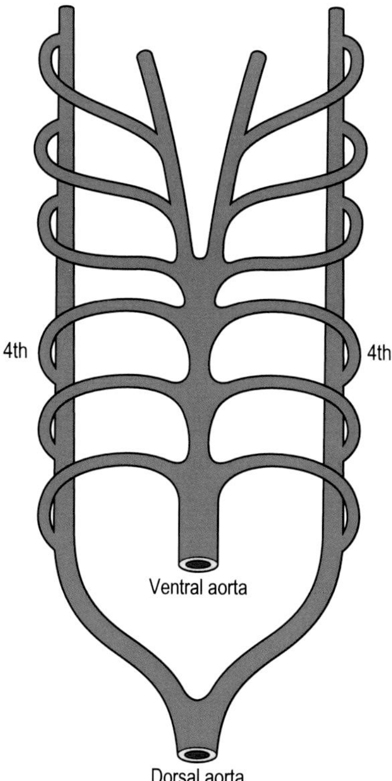

FIGURE 17-47 ■ **Embryology of the aortic arch.** Six pairs of arterial arches develop between paired ventral and dorsal aortas from approximately day 26. They are not all present at the same time and normally the left fourth arch develops into the aortic arch.

Right Aortic Arch with Aberrant Left Subclavian Artery and Left Ligamentum Arteriosum (Fig. 17-49). In these cases, the right arch first gives off the left carotid artery, which runs anteriorly to the trachea. It then gives off the right carotid, followed by the right subclavian artery, and, lastly, the left subclavian artery, which courses

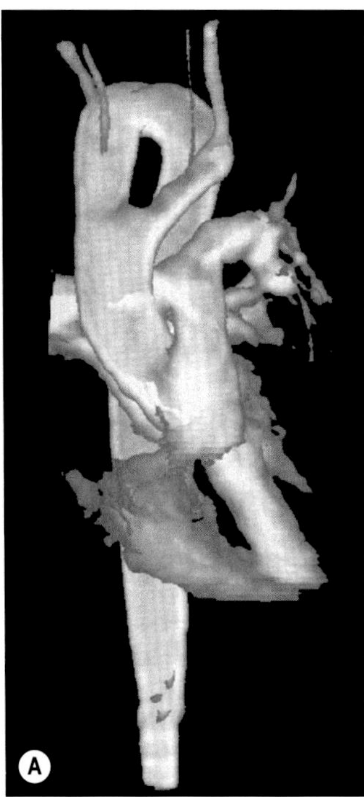

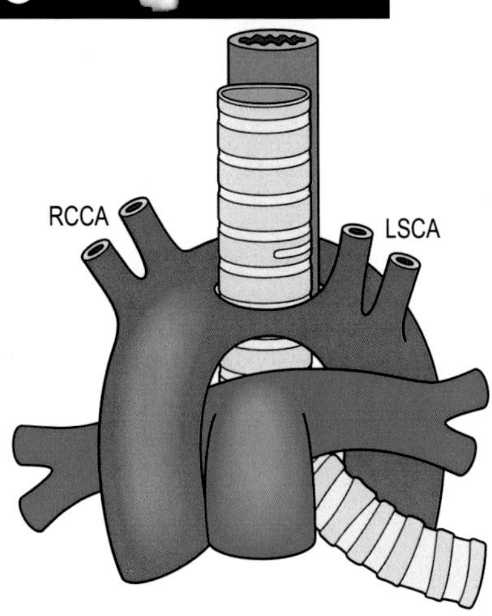

FIGURE 17-48 ■ **Double aortic arch.** (A) 3D MRA reconstruction. (Courtesy of Dr M. Shivanathan, The Leeds Teaching Hospitals NHS Trust, UK.) (B) Diagram. LSCA = left subclavian artery, RCCA = right common carotid artery

in a retro-oesophageal position and gives rise to the ligamentum arteriosum from its base, completing the ring as it attaches to the pulmonary artery.

Right Aortic Arch with Mirror-Image Branching and Retro-oesophageal Ligamentum Arteriosum. In these cases, only partial resorption of the distal left fourth arch occurs. The first vessel originating from the right arch is a left innominate artery, which, in turn, branches into the left carotid and a left subclavian artery. These course anteriorly to the trachea. The right carotid artery and a right subclavian artery subsequently arise. The ligamentum arteriosum is the final structure arising from the arch in this sequence. It originates from the Kommerell diverticulum, which represents the non-resorbed remnant of the left fourth arch and is situated at the point of merging of the right arch and the proximal descending thoracic aorta. The ligamentum passes to the left, posterior to the oesophagus and then anteriorly to join the left pulmonary artery, thereby completing the ring.

Vascular Rings Associated with Left Aortic Arch

Two extremely rare complete rings occur in the presence of a left aortic arch, and both are associated with a right-sided descending thoracic aorta:

- Left aortic arch with right descending aorta and right ligamentum arteriosum.
- Left aortic arch, right descending aorta and atretic right aortic arch.

Aortic Arch Abnormalities without an Anatomic Ring

There are also abnormalities of the aortic arch which produces compression symptoms without an anatomical ring.

Anomalous Innominate Artery. The innominate artery originates from a more distal and leftward position of the arch than normal. As it takes its course from left to right, it crosses the trachea anteriorly and in doing so compresses the trachea.

Retro-Oesophageal Right Subclavian Artery with an Otherwise Normal Left Arch. This is the most common supra-aortic vessel anomaly, occurring in about 0.5% of the population. In these cases, the right subclavian artery does not arise from an innominate trunk with the right carotid artery but originates as the last brachiocephalic branch from the descending aorta and takes a retro-oesophageal route to its destination.

Imaging

CXR is the first and most commonly performed imaging investigation. The identification of a right aortic arch on a chest radiograph in a child with airway difficulties, respiratory distress or dysphagia should alert the radiologist to the likelihood of a vascular ring (Fig. 17-50). With a double aortic arch, the arch location is often ill defined (Fig. 17-51). Findings on CXR include compression of the trachea and hyperinflation and/or atelectasis of some of the lobes of either lung.

Many authorities still consider barium oesophagography to be an important study in patients with a suspected vascular ring, and it is diagnostic in most cases (Fig. 17-52). A double aortic arch produces bilateral and posterior compressions of the oesophagus, which remain constant regardless of peristalsis. The right indentation is usually slightly higher than the left and the posterior one is usually rather wide and courses in a downward direction from right to left. If the right subclavian artery takes a retro-oesophageal course, there is a classical oblique posterior defect.

Ultrasound has been increasingly used for the diagnosis of a vascular ring using the suprasternal window but there are limitations. Structures without a lumen, such as a ligamentum arteriosum or an atretic arch, are difficult to identify, even with colour-flow echocardiography. Identification of compressed midline structures and their relationship to encircling vascular anomalies may be

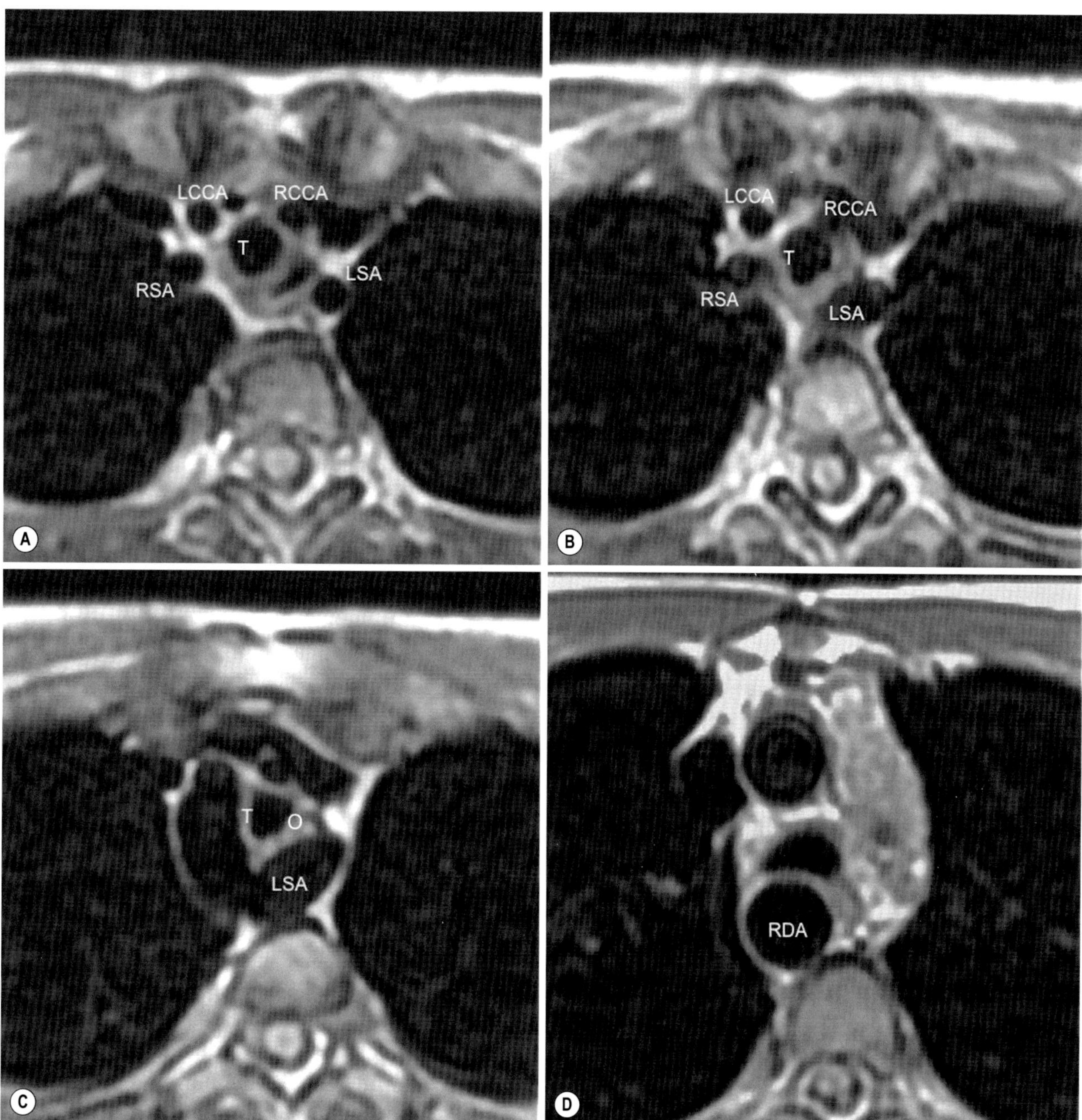

FIGURE 17-49 ■ MR BBFSE images (A–D) of a right aortic arch with aberrant left subclavian artery. LCCA = left common carotid artery, LSA = left subclavian artery, RCCA = right common carotid artery, RSA = right subclavian artery, RDA = right descending aorta, T = trachea, O = oesophagus.

difficult to detect. However, associated congenital cardiac defects can be examined.

CT, MRI and DSA are all suitable diagnostic tools because they reveal the positions of vascular, tracheobronchial and oesophageal structures, and their relationships to one another. MRA is an excellent substitute for DSA but young patients may require general anaesthesia, which might be a problem in patients with airway compromise and respiratory problems.

Coarctation of the Aorta

Aortic coarctation most commonly affects the aortic isthmus (95% of cases) and much more rarely the more distal thoracic and abdominal aorta, where it is part of a mid-aortic syndrome (see above). Presentation is characterised by hypertension and, in infants, failure to thrive. The femoral pulses are usually delayed and weakened compared to the carotid and arm pulses and there is a characteristic murmur, though this can disappear in older patients if the site of coarctation becomes occluded.[51]

Eighty per cent of patients are male. In females, coarctation is associated with Turner's syndrome. Patients can present in infancy or adulthood. The infantile type of coarctation is usually proximal to the ductus arteriosus and 50% are associated with other congenital heart defects such as bicuspid aortic valve, ventricular septal defect (VSD), or hypoplastic left heart syndrome. Cystic medial necrosis of the aorta may be also associated. At birth the ductus arteriosus closes, resulting in reduced

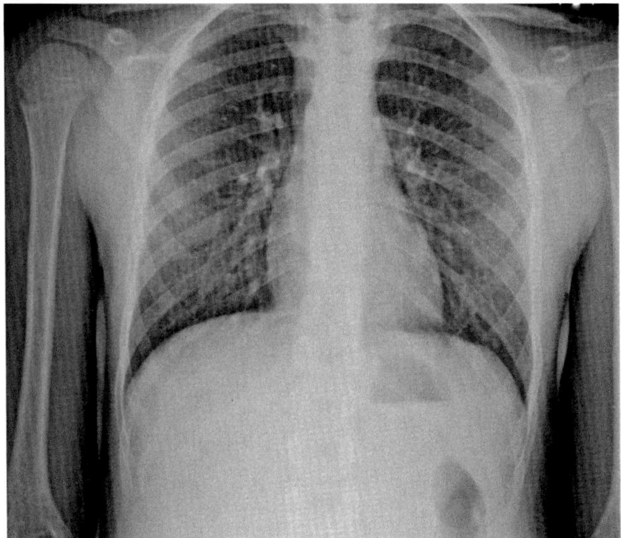

FIGURE 17-50 ■ Chest radiograph of child with right aortic arch. Stridor in this situation suggests the presence of a vascular ring.

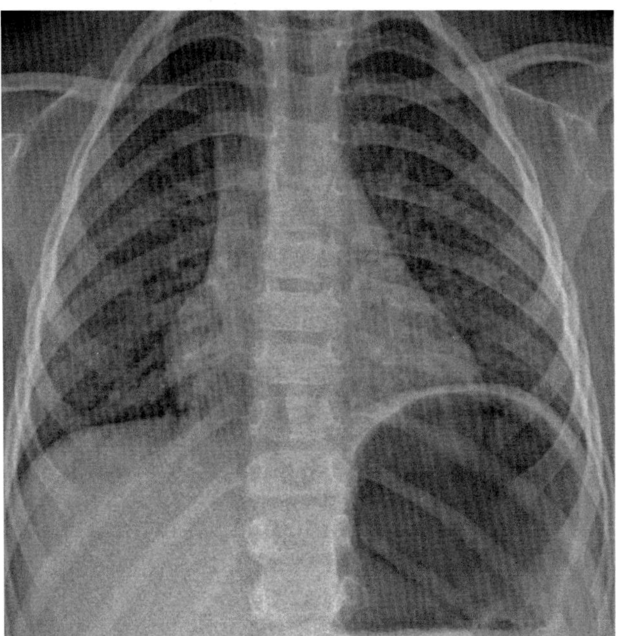

FIGURE 17-51 ■ Chest radiograph of a child presenting with stridor and swallowing difficulties. The superior mediastinum is slightly widened and the aortic knuckle is not clearly seen. The possibility of a double aortic arch should be considered.

blood supply to the distal aorta. The consequent increased strain on the heart leads to heart failure, as no collateral pathways are required in utero.

The adult type of coarctation is usually located just distal to the ductus arteriosus and the left subclavian artery and therefore collaterals develop in utero. Consequently, whereas infants present with hypertension and failure to thrive, adults present with hypertension and the classical signs of collateral vessels on the chest radiograph (Fig. 17-53). Rib notching usually takes several years to develop. It is caused by pressure erosion of the inferior aspects of the upper adjacent ribs by enlarged and tortuous intercostal arteries. It is usually bilateral but asymmetric, and

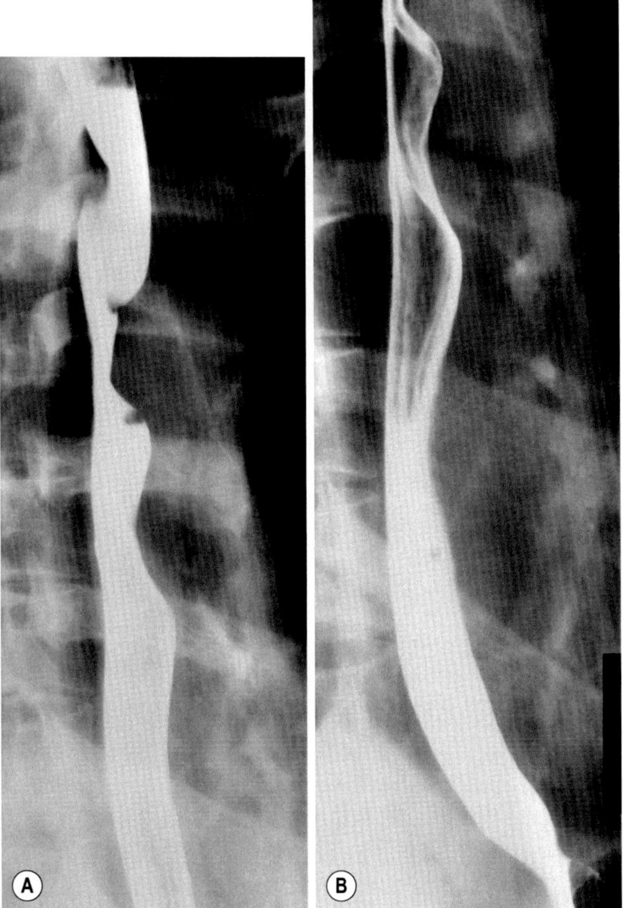

FIGURE 17-52 ■ (A, B) Barium swallow in a child with a vascular ring. Note the constant posterior impressions on the oesophagus.

most often spares the first two ribs where intercostal arteries arise from the costocervical trunk proximal to the usual site of coarctation and therefore do not form part of the collateral circulation. The rib notches may be shallow or deep and usually have a corticated margin. Unilateral absence of rib notching may also be seen according to other anomalies. Other radiographic features include cardiomegaly, particularly in older adults, a prominent ascending aorta (especially with a bicuspid aortic valve) and various aortic knuckle abnormalities. There may be a '3' sign due to enlargement of the left subclavian artery arising proximally of the coarctation, the narrowed segment itself and subsequently a localised segment with poststenotic dilatation of the aorta. Occasionally this poststenotic dilatation simulates the picture of a low aortic knuckle. The whole area of the aortic knuckle may appear small and flat. On the lateral radiograph an enlarged internal mammary artery may be seen behind the sternum.

These CXR signs may already suggest the diagnosis. Echocardiography is mostly difficult in adults and older children but in infants it might be useful for identifying the area of stenosis and associated congenital cardiac defects. Continuous wave Doppler measurements of flow velocities above and below the coarctation (and a modified Bernoulli equation) can predict the degree of stenosis.

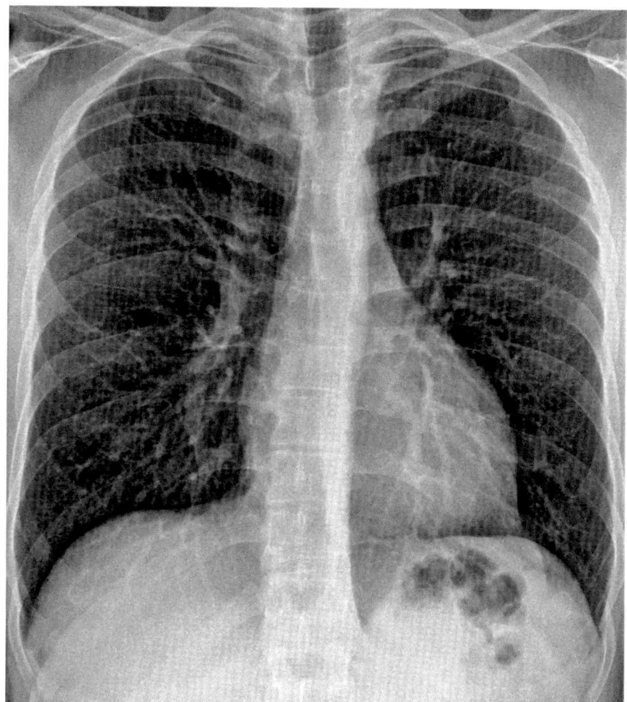

FIGURE 17-53 ■ Chest radiograph in a patient with coarctation. There is bilateral rib notching on the inferior margin of the ribs. The aortic knuckle is poorly evident.

MRI is the imaging technique of choice in both infantile and adult coarctation. It has considerable advantages as it is non-invasive, gives both morphological and functional information and is also useful for post-treatment follow-up.[52,53] T1-weighted spin-echo sequences will show the whole of the aorta, the major branches and the larger collaterals. Cine phase-contrast imaging can be used to estimate the gradient across the coarctation and quantify collateral circulation as percentage increment of flow from isthmic to diaphragmatic aorta. Gadolinium-enhanced three-dimensional (3D) MRA provides high anatomical detail (Fig. 17-54).

CT can also provide exquisite images but is used more rarely in children and young adults because of the radiation involved. CT's strongest role is the follow-up of aortic coarctation corrected by stent-graft placement, because stent metal artefacts, together with a small aortic lumen, hampers MR visualisation of complications like stent fracture or in-stent restenosis (Fig. 17-55). The prevalent role of CT versus MR is still controversial. Advocates of MR argue that MRI eventually is able to recognise all major complications like aortic dissection and identify stenosis by functional indirect signs (pressure gradient), while CT's major limitation is related to the radiation dose in the usually young population. Angiography, previously the imaging procedure of choice, is now rarely required unless cardiac catheterisation is necessary for the investigation of associated cardiac abnormalities or for interventional purposes. The coarctation can usually be crossed from the femoral arterial route, though if impossible brachial artery catheterisation is necessary. Asymmetry of the stenosis may require the acquisition of multiple views.

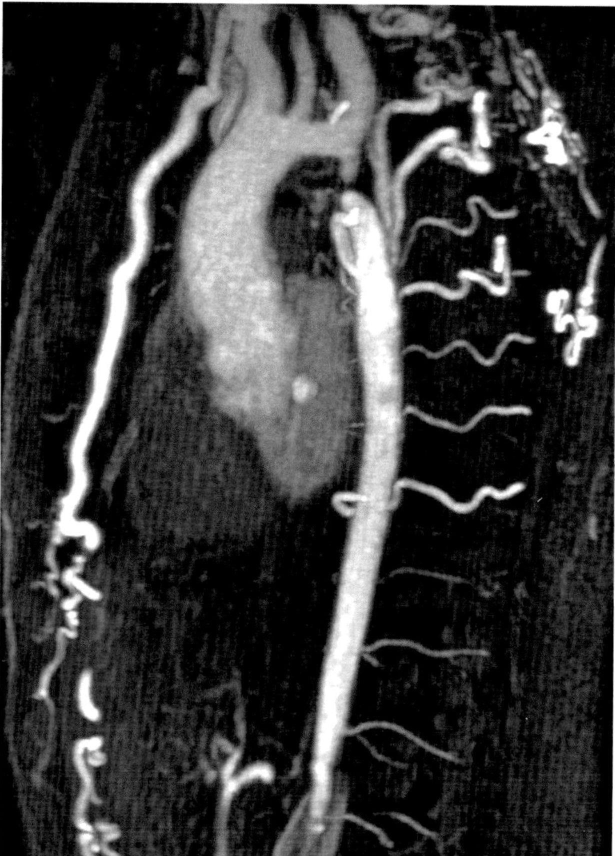

FIGURE 17-54 ■ MRA (sagittal oblique reconstruction) of a patient presenting with hypertension and femoral delay. There is a coarctation of the aorta just beyond the left subclavian artery. Huge collateral circulation is seen through intercostal and internal mammary arteries.

Management

If undetected or untreated, death from cardiac failure, aortic rupture, infective endocarditis, and intracerebral haemorrhage from associated cerebral aneurysms is inevitable, with only 50% of patients surviving into their 30s.[51]

Surgery used to be the most common treatment for significant coarctation and is still often required. If the lesion is short and the aorta can be adequately mobilised, resection and end-to-end anastomosis may be possible; this will give the best long-term result. If this is not possible, the usual procedure is repair by a subclavian patch. This involves resecting the lesion, transecting the left subclavian artery before the origin of the vertebral artery, incising longitudinally and turning it down as a patch repair. This repair will grow with the patient. Collateral supply to the left subclavian artery, which will be mainly by the vertebral artery, may cause neurological symptoms. Synthetic graft material is not suited for children because it does not stretch. There is a mortality of 2.6 to 3.1%, a 5.4% incidence of aneurysm formation and 1% risk of paraplegia.[54]

Percutaneous transluminal angioplasty (PTA) was first used in 1982 to treat a recoarctation in a critically ill patient who had undergone previous surgical repair. PTA is now considered a successful treatment option of

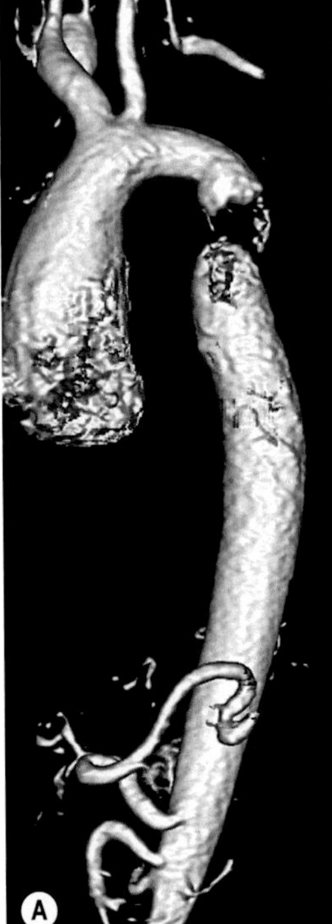

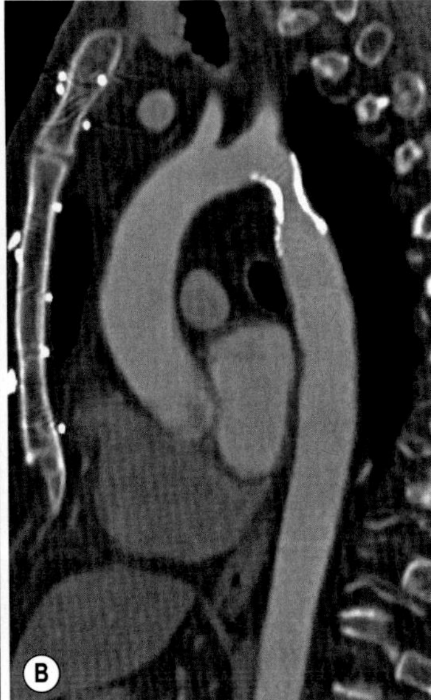

FIGURE 17-55 ■ MRA (A) and CT MIP (B) reconstructions after stent deployment for recoarctation. See large artefact on MR image (A) and insufficient expansion of the stent graft with restenosis on CT image (B).

post-surgical recoarctation, with early success rates of 90% and restenosis rates of 16–30%. The aorta is carefully measured proximal to the coarctation site and a balloon is chosen with a diameter that is 2 mm smaller than this aortic diameter. In view of the high success rate and the low complication rate compared to surgery, PTA is the primary method of treatment in adults, adolescents and children outside of infancy.[54]

Some authors state that inserting stents at the coarctation site after balloon dilatation gives better long-term results. However, there is currenly insufficient evidence for this. Stents should be reserved for initial failure of PTA due to recoil. They should not be used in infants other than as a short-term treatment in the critically ill who are not eligible for immediate surgery. Stent grafts should be available at all times in order to treat the very rare but invariably fatal complication of aortic rupture at PTA.[55]

Pseudocoarctation

An elongated aortic arch will bulge posteriorly above the point at which it is fixed by the ligament. This can produce the appearance of a '3' sign similar to true coarctation on the PA chest radiograph. There is usually no significant haemodynamic obstruction. MR or CT will demonstrate the true anatomy.

Aortic Atresia

Aortic atresia is associated with the hypoplastic left heart syndrome. The ascending aorta is variable in size but is usually very small and not larger than one of the brachiocephalic arteries. Blood flow from the heart to the aorta is through the pulmonary trunk and the persistent arterial duct, with the aortic arch filling in a retrograde direction. The brachiocephalic branches arise normally from the arch, and the coronary arteries are supplied via the diminutive ascending aorta.

Survival depends on maintaining patency of the duct by giving prostaglandin E_1.

The 'Norwood' operation converts the morphological right ventricle into the systemic ventricle, by anastomosing the pulmonary trunk to the ascending aorta. The atrial septum is excised. Blood flow to the pulmonary arteries is maintained through a modified Blalock–Taussig shunt.

An interrupted aortic arch is rare and thought to be the result of faulty development of the aortic arch system during the fifth to seventh week of fetal development. It is almost always associated with a large VSD. It can be located distally to the left subclavian artery (type A, 30–40%), distally to the left common carotid artery (type B, 53%), or distally to the innominate artery (type C, 4%). Patients with type B often have a chromosomal abnormality called the DiGeorge syndrome.

REFERENCES

1. Standring S. The anatomical basis of clinical practice. In: Gray's Anatomy. 39th ed. Edinburgh: Elsevier/Churchill Livingstone; 2005. p. 141.
2. Johnson D. The anatomical basis of clinical practice. In: Gray's Anatomy. 39th ed. Edinburgh: Elsevier/Churchill Livingstone; 2005. pp. 1021–3.
3. Olsson C, Thelin S, Ståhle E, et al. Thoracic aortic aneurysm and dissection: increasing prevalence and improved outcomes reported in a nationwide population-based study of more than 14,000 cases from 1987 to 2002. Circulation 2006;114:2611–18.
4. Tsai T, Fattori R, Trimarchi S, et al. Long-term survival in patients presenting with type B acute aortic dissection: insights from the International Registry of Acute Aortic Dissection. Circulation 2006;114:2226–31.
5. Goodney PP, Travis L, Lucas FL, et al. Survival after open versus endovascular thoracic aortic aneurysm repair in an observational study of the medicare population. Circulation 2011;124:2661–9.
6. Fann JC, Smith JA, Miller DC, et al. Surgical management of aortic dissection during a 30-year period. Circulation 1995;92:113–21.
7. von Kodolitsch Y, Nienaber CA, Dieckmann C, et al. Chest radiography for the diagnosis of acute aortic syndrome. Am J Med 2004;116:73–7.
8. Shiga T, Wajima Z, Apfel CC, et al. Diagnostic accuracy of transesophageal echocardiography, helical computed tomography, and magnetic resonance imaging for suspected thoracic aortic dissection: systematic review and meta-analysis. Arch Intern Med 2006;166:1350–6.
9. Nienaber CA, von Kodolitsch Y, Nicolas V, et al. The diagnosis of thoracic aortic dissection by noninvasive imaging procedures. N Engl J Med 1993;328:1–9.
10. Ueno J, Murase T, Yoneda K, et al. Three-dimensional imaging of thoracic diseases with multi-detector row CT. J Med Invest 2004;51:163–70.
11. Shellock FG, Spinazzi A. MRI safety update 2008: part 1, MRI contrast agents and nephrogenic systemic fibrosis. Am J Roentgenol 2008;191:1129–39.
12. Krishnam MS, Tomasian A, Malik S, et al. Image quality and diagnostic accuracy of unenhanced SSFP MR angiography compared with conventional contrast-enhanced MR angiography for

the assessment of thoracic aortic diseases. Eur Radiol 2010;20: 1311–20.

13. Brenner DJ, Hall EJ. Computed tomography: an increasing source of radiation exposure. N Engl J Med 2007;357:2277–84.
14. Ben Saad M, Rohnean A, Sigal-Cinqualbre A, et al. Evaluation of image quality and radiation dose of thoracic and coronary dual-source CT in 110 infants with congenital heart disease. Pediatr Radiol 2009;39:668–76.
15. Flohr T, Stierstorfer K, Bruder H, et al. Image reconstruction and image quality evaluation for a 16-slice CT scanner. Med Phys 2003;30:832–45.
16. Halpern EJ. Triple-rule-out CT angiography for evaluation of acute chest pain and possible acute coronary syndrome. Radiology 2009;252:332–45.
17. Moore AG, Eagle KA, Bruckman D, et al. Choice of computed tomography, transesophageal echocardiography, magnetic resonance imaging, and aortography in acute aortic dissection: International Registry of Acute Aortic Dissection (IRAD). Am J Cardiol 2002;89:1235–8.
18. Tozzi P, Marty B, Ruchat P, et al. Endovascular thoracic aortic aneurysm repair without angiography. Innovations (Phila) 2009;4: 32–5.
19. Bogaert J, Meyns B, Rademakers FE, et al. Follow-up of aortic dissection: contribution of MR angiography for evaluation of the abdominal aorta and its branches. Eur Radiol 1997;7:695–702.
20. Pereles FS, McCarthy RM, Baskaran V, et al. Thoracic aortic dissection and aneurysm: evaluation with nonenhanced true FISP MR angiography in less than 4 minutes. Radiology 2002;223:270–4.
21. Shiga T, Wajima Z, Apfel CC, et al. Diagnostic accuracy of transesophageal echocardiography, helical computed tomography, and magnetic resonance imaging for suspected thoracic aortic dissection: systematic review and meta-analysis. Arch Intern Med 2006; 166:1350–6.
22. Krukemberg E. Beiträge zur Frage des Aneurysma dissecans. Beitr Pathol Anat Allg Pathol 1920;67:329–51.
23. Moore A, Oh J, Bruckman D, et al. Transesophageal echocardiography in the diagnosis and management of aortic dissection. An analysis of data from the International Registry of Aortic Dissection (IRAD). J Am Coll Cardiol 1999;33-2(A):470A.
24. Kitai T, Kaji S, Yamamuro A, et al. Detection of intimal defect by 64-row multidetector computed tomography in patients with acute aortic intramural hematoma. Circulation 2011;124(11 Suppl): S174–8.
25. Castaner E, Andreu M, Gallardo X, et al. CT in nontraumatic acute thoracic aortic disease: typical and atypical features and complications. Radiographics 2003;23 Spec No:S93–110.
26. Coady MA, Rizzo JA, Elefteriades JA. Pathologic variants of thoracic aortic dissections. Penetrating atherosclerotic ulcers and intramural hematomas. Cardiol Clin 1999;17:637–57.
27. Wintermark M, Wicky S, Schnyder P. Imaging of acute traumatic injuries of the thoracic aorta. Eur Radiol 2002;12:431–42.
28. Fattori R, Celletti F, Bertaccini P, et al. Delayed surgery of traumatic aortic rupture. Role of magnetic resonance imaging. Circulation 1996;94:2865–70.
29. Azizzadeh A, Valdes J, Miller CC 3rd, et al. The utility of intravascular ultrasound compared to angiography in the diagnosis of blunt traumatic aortic injury. J Vasc Surg 2011;53:608–14.
30. Gillum RF. Epidemiology of aortic aneurysms in the United States. J Clin Epidemiol 1995;48:1289–98.
31. Koch AE, Haines GK, Rizzo RJ. Human abdominal aortic aneurysms. Immunophenotypic analysis suggesting an immune mediated response. Am J Pathol 1990;137:1199–213.
32. Filardo G, Powell JT, Martinez MA, et al. Surgery for small asymptomatic abdominal aortic aneurysms. Cochrane Database Syst Rev 2012;3:CD001835.
33. Cosford PA, Leng GC. Screening for abdominal aortic aneurysm. Cochrane Database Syst Rev 2007;(2):CD002945.
34. Roberts CS, Roberts WC. Aortic dissection with the entrance tear in the descending thoracic aorta. Analysis of 40 necropsy patients. Ann Surg 1991;213:356–68.
35. Mitchel RS, Dake MD, Semba CP. Endovascular stent graft repair of thoracic aortic aneurysms. J Thorac Cardiovasc Surg 1996; 111:1054–62.
36. Pate JW, Fabian TC, Walker W. Traumatic rupture of the aortic isthmus: an emergency? World J Surg 1995;19:119–26.
37. Fattori R, Russo V, Lovato L, et al. Optimal management of traumatic aortic injury. Eur J Vasc Endovasc Surg 2008;37: 8–14.
38. Demetriades D, Velmahos GC, Scalea TM, et al. Diagnosis and treatment of blunt thoracic aortic injuries: changing perspectives. J Trauma 2008;64:1415–18.
39. Dake MD, Miller DC, Semba CP, et al. Transluminal placement of endovascular stent-grafts for the treatment of descending thoracic aneurysms. N Engl J Med 1994;331:1729–34.
40. Fabian TC, Richardson JD, Croce MA, et al. Prospective study of blunt aortic injury: multicenter trial of the American Association for the Surgery of Trauma. J Trauma 1997;42:374e80.
41. Riesenman PJ, Farber MA, Mendes RR, et al. Coverage of the left subclavian artery during thoracic endovascular aortic repair. J Vasc Surg 2007;45:90–4.
42. Karmy-Jones R, Aldea G, Boyle EM. The continuing evolution in the management of thoracic aortic dissection. Chest 2000;117: 1221–3.
43. Prendergast BD, Boon NA, Buckenham T. Aortic dissection: advances in imaging and endoluminal repair. Cardiovasc Intervent Radiol 2002;25:85–97.
44. Chavan A, Lotz J, Oelert F, et al. Endoluminal treatment of aortic dissection. Eur Radiol 2003;13:2521–34.
45. Nienaber CA, Fattori R, Lund G, et al. Nonsurgical reconstruction of thoracic aortic dissection by stent-graft placement. N Engl J Med 1999;340:1539–15451.
46. Nienaber CA, Rousseau H, Eggebrecht H, et al. Randomized comparison of strategies for type B aortic dissection: the INvestigation of STEnt grafts in Aortic Dissection (INSTEAD) Trial. Circulation 2009;120:2519–28.
47. Akin E, Coen A, Momeni M. PET-CT findings in large vessel vasculitis presenting as FUO, a case report. Clin Rheumatol 2009; 28:737–8.
48. Matsunaga N, Hayashi K, Sakamoto I, et al. Takayasu arteritis: protean radiologic manifestations and diagnosis. Radiographics 1997;17:579–94.
49. Surowiec SM, Isiklar H, Sreeram S, et al. Acute occlusion of the abdominal aorta. Am J Surg 1998;176:193–7.
50. Stewart JR, Kincaid OW, Edwards JE. An atlas of vascular rings and related malformations of the aortic arch system. Charles C. Springfield, IL: Thomas; 1964.
51. Campbell M. Natural history of coarctation of the aorta. Br Heart J 1970;32:633–40.
52. Hope MD, Meadows AK, Hope TA, et al. Clinical evaluation of aortic coarctation with 4D flow MR imaging. J Magn Reson Imaging 2010;31:711–18.
53. Nielsen JC, Powell AJ, Gauvreau K, et al. Magnetic resonance imaging predictors of coarctation severity. Circulation 2005;111: 622–8.
54. Paddon AJ. Endovascular repair of thoracic and dissecting aneurysms and aortic coarctation. In: Dyet JF, Ettles DF, Nicholson AA, Wilson SE, editors. Textbook of Endovascular Procedures. Philadelphia: Churchill Livingstone; 2000.
55. Paddon AJ, Nicholson AA, Ettles DF, et al. Long-term follow-up of percutaneous balloon angioplasty in adult aortic coarctation. Cardiovasc Intervent Radiol 2000;23:364–7.
56. Gavant ML. Helical CT grading of traumatic aortic injuries. Impact of clinical guidelines for medical and surgical management. Radiol Clin North Am 1999;37:553–74.

Subject Index

Page numbers followed by 'f' indicate figures, 't' indicate tables, and 'b' indicate boxes.

Notes

To simplify the index, the main terms of imaging techniques (e.g. computed tomography, magnetic resonance imaging etc.) are concerned only with the technology and general applications. Users are advised to look for specific anatomical features and diseases/disorders for individual imaging techniques used.

vs. indicates a comparison or differential diagnosis.

To save space in the index, the following abbreviations have been used:

CHD—congenital heart disease
CMR—cardiac magnetic resonance
CT—computed tomography
CXR—chest X-ray
DECT—dual-energy computed tomography
DWI-MRI—diffusion weighted imaging-magnetic resonance imaging
ERCP—endoscopic retrograde cholangiopancreatography
EUS—endoscopic ultrasound
FDG-PET—fluorodeoxyglucose positron emission tomography
HRCT—high-resolution computed tomography
MDCT—multidetector computed tomography
MRA—magnetic resonance angiography
MRCP—magnetic resonance cholangiopancreatography
MRI—magnetic resonance imaging
MRS—magnetic resonance spectroscopy
PET—positron emission tomography
PTC—percutaneous transhepatic cholangiography
SPECT—single photon emission computed tomography
US—ultrasound

A

D

N

O

P

T

U

V

W

X

Printed in the United States
By Bookmasters